HOW WE AGE

HOW WE AGE

A DOCTOR'S JOURNEY
INTO THE HEART
OF GROWING OLD

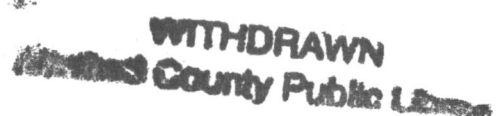

Marc E. Agronin, M.D.

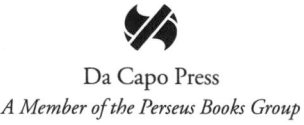

Da Capo Press
A Member of the Perseus Books Group

Designed by Pauline Brown
Set in 11.75 point AGaramond by the Perseus Books Group

Library of Congress Cataloging-in-Publication Data

Agronin, Marc E.
    How we age : a doctor's journey into the heart of growing old / Marc E. Agronin.—1st Da Capo Press ed.
        p.   cm.
    Includes bibliographical references.
    ISBN 978-0-306-81853-0 (hardcover : alk. paper)
    ISBN 978-0-7382-1415-3 (e-book)
    1. Older people. 2. Nursing home patients—Florida—Miami. 3. Geriatric psychiatry. 4. Aging. I. Title.
    HQ1061.A485   2011
    305.26—dc22

                                                                2010044261

Published by Da Capo Press
A Member of the Perseus Books Group
www.dacapopress.com

10 9 8 7 6 5 4 3 2 1

To my beloved grandparents—the elders who came before me and gave me a true appreciation for growing old—Eva, Simon, Etta, and Tany

CONTENTS

�֎֎֎

Part IV
Wisdom

Part V
A Million Sparks

A Note to the Reader

✴✴✴

It is with some trepidation that I have chosen to write about the lives of several individuals in this book. There is the risk that the retelling of a life, especially from the vantage point of a doctor, will not only fall short but will also end up trivializing certain aspects. There is the greater risk that stories of medical or psychiatric ailments end up dehumanizing the patient, portraying him or her as a disease and not as a human being.

My purpose in this book is to talk about aging by describing the lives of several individuals in a manner as humane and respectful as possible. To this end, I have retained the actual names of certain individuals with their permission only and have changed both the names and certain identifying biographical details of others so as to render them wholly anonymous. In several instances I created a composite of two similar individuals in order to retain the basic condition without allowing identification even by those who as clinicians or caregivers knew these individuals personally. Finally, there are several individuals portrayed in this book whose deaths have made it impossible to obtain permission. In those instances I have again changed names and other details to preserve anonymity. My sincere hope is that these efforts have yielded a work that respects and even extols its subjects.

Introduction

For nearly every doctor, the very first encounter in medical school with an old person is with a corpse. I discovered this fact on the first day of gross anatomy class when our instructors led us up to the dissection lab and introduced us to the rows of human cadavers that would serve as our teachers and companions for the next six months. Everyone was a little uneasy that morning, and I welcomed the nervous glances and smiles of classmates as we filtered through the room searching for what we hoped would be the perfect body. "Look for a thin woman," my labmates Steve and Jimmy each whispered to me, recalling the sage advice of an older classmate trying to steer us toward an easier dissection experience. "Who can tell?" I shot back, staring out at the dozen black slate tables in the room, topped off with human forms wrapped in heavy white gauze and covered with translucent plastic sheets. I reasoned to my labmates that it was like trying to find King Tut among a room full of mummies, and so we quickly abandoned our original plan and went for a table near the window. Even in the few short minutes we had spent in the room, the fumes of the formalin solution used to preserve the bodies were overpowering, and so I hoped that at least an open window would provide some respite from the smell.

"Please help your labmates remove the plastic coverings on your cadaver," the professor called out, "and then strip off all of the gauze to expose the entire body." A shudder went through my own body, and I cringed. The entire body? "Yes, the entire body," the instructor continued, as if she were reading my mind, "and then pick it up and flip it over—get a good look." This was surely a technique not meant to teach as much as to flood our psyches with the glory of gross anatomy, dispensing all mystery and anxiety in one fell baptism of formalin. Entering the room had been unsettling enough, but at least then the cadavers had been covered. I had honestly never seen a dead body before and was hoping to put off the experience as long as possible. But within minutes I was surrounded by teams of sweating medical students piling up strips of smelly, greasy gauze and struggling to pick up rigid and very heavy formalin-logged bodies. I remember one particularly surreal moment as I watched four classmates bearing the strangest of grins as they hoisted the cadaver off the table, grunting at its weight and struggling to grip the slippery, leathery skin.

The unmasking of the face of our cadaver unnerved me the most. I had hoped in vain to skip that altogether and heed the words of the second anatomy instructor, who was strutting through the room and cautioning against removing too much gauze so as not to dry out the body. He argued gruffly with the first instructor that her shock treatment was unnecessary, finally shouting, "If they can't stand looking at the body, they shouldn't be in medicine!" My labmates were more obedient to the initial instructions and summarily removed the plastic bag from the head and began to unravel the gauze. I stood back and envisioned seeing what archaeologists had discovered in the mummified faces of pharaohs—coal-black visages with bony physiognomy and time-scorched skin that resembled cracked china. Those ancient, royal faces looked more skeletal than human and lacked all of the machinery of expression that might have betrayed a final emotion.

When the last strip of gauze was peeled away, I looked down on the face of our cadaver, mesmerized by her silent, still expression, her upper cheek muscles and eyelids slightly scrunched as if a puff of air had been blown into her face at the moment of death. The face appeared inert, like a totem permanently carved into clay or stone and so different from the blushing, breathing face of a living person. And yet this had been a person, I realized, who once had walked the earth and lived a life like everyone else in the room—working, loving, running, eating, perhaps bearing and raising children. Although the identities of and any biographical information about the cadavers used in medical school anatomy courses are never revealed to the students, the unmasking of our cadaver revealed numerous deep facial wrinkles and a few thin strands of silver hair matted on her head that betrayed one critical fact: She had been quite *old* when she died. We later learned that she had been ninety-eight at the time of her death from a heart attack.

After we rewrapped the head and limbs of the cadaver, the dissection of the torso began in earnest, initiated by a brief instructional paragraph in the course manual: "Palpate bony landmarks on cadaver: clavicle, jugular notch, sternal angle, sternum. . . . Incise skin from jugular notch to 3 cm above the pubic symphysis in mid-line cutting around the umbilicus. . . . Then incise superficial fascia." These instructions sounded straightforward, but they underestimated the magnitude of the task. We did not merely "incise" superficial fascia (the elastic connective tissue that covers and supports the muscles), but we cut, slit, ripped, pulled, melted, and gushed it all over instruments, hands, table, and cadaver, all while we were constricted by two to three layers of gloves and heavy blue smocks.

If we were exceedingly careful and dexterous, the dissection proceeded smoothly over the ensuing months and actually taught us, as budding doctors, some human anatomy—even though a living patient is wholly unlike a cadaver in color, form, and feel. But for the average student, the time spent with the chopped and tattered remains of the cadaver cast a certain spell of nonchalance and banality over behaviors that would otherwise have been deemed inappropriate and even atrocious. One cadaver in our lab, for example, wore a pair of plastic Groucho Marx glasses throughout the course. Another cadaver in the room was decked out one morning with a party hat, balloons, and a sign that read, "Happy Birthday" for the celebrating student. And there were worse examples.

But what struck me most from the very beginning of gross anatomy was how the ninety-eight-year-old "she" lying before me was repeatedly designated an "it," a mere object to be manipulated, incised, cracked open, and explored throughout the dissection process. And this is where gross anatomy began to change from a respectful and educational part of the medical school curriculum into a dehumanizing rite of passage, what eminent cardiologist and Nobel Prize winner Dr. Bernard Lown calls a "grievous error" as a way to start off medical training. He goes on to deride the "denaturing of human values" that follows when students come to view the "repulsive formaldehyded body being dissected as an inanimate object, forgetting that it was once a fellow human being."

Lown's perspective hit me acutely one evening when I had been assigned to bring home the "bone box," a small hinged maple coffin that carried the ossified and disassembled remains of some poor soul. The bone box was meant to afford the student a more intimate educational communion with a human skeleton: a time to study the intricacies of each bone, to search for the hidden grooves where ligaments and tendons anchor themselves, and to palpate the angles and contours of the shafts and joints. Of course, the bearer of the bone box was also the subject of much, well, ribbing from other students, who warned of the midnight knocking and clacking that might emanate from the box. By that point in the course I thought I was inured to any such jibing and imaginings, but the box sat uneasily beneath my bed. I contemplated the bones and wondered whose form they had once supported. "Alas, poor Yorick!" I imagined a ghostly Hamlet cry as he cradled his jester's skull, "I knew him. . . . / Here hung those lips that I have kiss'd I know not how oft." William Shakespeare understood well the transformation from being to bone:

Imperious Caesar, dead and turn'd to clay,
Might stop a hole to keep the wind away:
O, that that earth, which kept the world in awe,
Should patch a wall to expel the winter flaw!

So too, these dry bones resting beneath the springs of my cot would remain the permanent dry relics of an unknown soul. There would be no prophetic cry from Ezekiel to God to bind them back together, to layer on muscle, sinew, and flesh and have them walk the earth again, resuming whatever holy or unholy tasks this person had once engaged in.

Over the months of gross anatomy the old woman who lay on our slate table slowly disintegrated, torn apart bit by bit until the final coup de grâce at course end: "Make a midsagittal cut completely through the entire head and neck. Leave the nasal septum attached intact to one side of the split head by cutting the septum free from the palate and skull."

From the very first day of gross anatomy, I had dreaded this lab, having already read the last page of the course manual, just as many people do with a good mystery. I was horrified then by the instructions, and yet when the time came, I found myself fearlessly and robotically sawing through the skull and neck and splitting the two halves of the head from each other. With the brain and skullcap already removed and most of the face and neck cut away, what remained looked only remotely human. This final lesson ended the course unceremoniously, and we all fled the lab, relieved to finally be free from the stink of the formalin. But a lesson on the meaning and end result of aging had been imprinted indelibly on our delicate doctor psyches.

That lesson learned in the first few months of medical training and reinforced in nearly every other experience was unmistakable: *Aging equals death*. Every course throughout the next few years, from pathology to physiology, and then to clinical work on the wards, focused on how the workings of the body could go awry. From a young doctor's vantage point, the aging process brought only decay, decline, and disease until the inevitable demise of the body. This depressing view of aging, reinforced during my years of internship and residency in medicine, neurology, and psychiatry, was then coupled with a new equation: *Aging equals dementia* (the brain disease that robs people of memory and other parts of their intelligence).

This second aging equation was represented by a common derogatory term I heard used to describe older demented patients: "gomer." I am not certain of the etymology of this word, but it was popularized by Samuel Shem's famous novel *The House of God*, a book about medical internship that has been read often by every frustrated, overworked, and cynical doctor-in-training since the book's publication in 1978. Shem's character the "Fat Man" serves as a wise but crass senior resident and mentor for neophyte hospital interns, and he introduces them to the world of gomers on day one: "'Gomer is an acronym: Get Out of My Emergency Room—it's what you want to say when one's sent in from the nursing home at 3 A.M. . . . But gomers are not just dear old people,' said Fats. 'Gomers are human beings who have lost what goes into being human beings. They want to die, and we will not let them. We're cruel to the gomers, by saving them, and they're cruel to us, by fighting tooth and nail against our trying to save them. They hurt us, we hurt them.'"

During training I discovered that these so-called gomers (or "gomes," for short) were ubiquitous figures in every medical setting. They were individuals with Alzheimer's disease or other forms of dementia who were permanently disoriented and unable to effectively communicate, care for themselves, and control their behaviors. On psychiatric wards my compatriots further nicknamed a subset of the gomes the "shriekers and smearers," inspired by episodes of blood-curdling screams or the throwing or smearing of feces that were viewed as repulsive and completely off the rails of rational human behavior. The primary care doctors and geriatricians who attended to them in nursing homes were typically referred to as "gome-docs" and dismissed as either incompetent or overly sentimental individuals who couldn't hack more illustrious or challenging medical specialties.

This perceived equating of aging with death and aging with dementia represents a pervasive societal view that stigmatizes the elderly and denigrates the individuals who tend to them. These equations are the core premises of what noted gerontologist Robert Butler first called "ageism." And they have a basis in what we all see as the undeniable truths—indeed, the defining aspects—of aging. Our bodies change irrevocably and not, it seems, for the better. We see our most beloved ones suffer from illness, frailty, and loss. Skin pales and droops. Hair becomes brittle and colorless. Voices quiver and fade. Muscles wither. And personalities who once worked a trade, soldiered in battle, or mothered a beloved child falter and fade with time. *Parents age and die.*

In response to these "grim years of debilitation and disease with which most people's lives currently end," biogerontologist

Aubrey de Grey and a small wave of researchers contend that science should be able to find a cure for aging. In this model, age is a disease that warrants treatment. And for some entrepreneurial individuals who lack both the patience and the scientific acumen of de Grey and simply want some part of the fountain of youth, aging is also an economic opportunity. Witness the rise of the multi-billion-dollar industry of antiaging products and clinics. Whether it is a costly wrinkle cream, a deluxe series of hormone shots, or a facelift, a growing number of people are willing to pay top dollar for such treatments. Many of my colleagues are less sanguine about reversing the effects of aging and focus instead on promoting a triad of physical exercise, healthy diet, and mentally stimulating activities to preserve both intellect and physical strength as long as possible.

To the extent that we think about the inevitability of aging and death, we usually have great trepidation—a sentiment captured well by Psalm 71:9: "Do not cast me off in old age; when my strength fails, do not forsake me." Face-to-face encounters with older individuals force us to look momentarily into an eternal abyss and trigger unanswerable questions about life and death that can bring wonder as easily as fear and despair. For the young doctor, the antidotes to these fears are corpse and gome—dehumanized bodies that the doctor can easily poke, cut, and crack open without a lot of emotion. When reduced to objects, the aged don't seem so bad, we reason, because *they* are not *us*. For the rest of society, there are many other ways to dehumanize the elderly and hide from what gerontologist Lars Tornstam aptly labels age-centric perceptions of the "nuisances and miseries" of old age.

✠✠✠

For many months after completing the gross anatomy course, I continued to wrestle with my experiences of working with a dead person. I would hearken back to a particularly vivid memory from class when the dissection required the corpses to be sitting upright on the slate table. Despite a somewhat human pose, everything sacred about both the body and its persona seemed stripped off the cadaver. Any small fantasies or fears of rejuvenation or zombification of the body that I still harbored by that point in the class faded away completely, and I said to myself, "There's no coming back." I now understood what the words "from dust to dust" meant. But this understanding did not bring satisfaction. I was particularly worried about how my growing lack of sensitivity toward the corpse could easily creep one step back to the extremely debilitated, aged patient. The two seemed, at times, to merge into one. I asked myself, "How does a doctor—how does anyone, for that matter—maintain a positive regard toward aging while simultaneously having to witness the loss, suffering, and utter degradation that it brings?"

I have learned since then that these dismal equations of aging with decrepitude along with the rigid and defensive attitudes that they inspire are only one side of the story. The other side is too often overlooked in our dread of aging. This realization first came to me several months after completing gross anatomy when I began volunteering at a nursing home down the street from the medical school. I was assigned to visit Esther, a one-hundred-year-old woman who, I must admit, looked uncannily like the cadaver I had just spent the previous six months with! Surprisingly, this realization was not eerie but comforting. And Esther could not have been more of a delight to be with. Her mind and wit were sharp, she smiled constantly, and she reveled in our time together. One day she described to me in detail the births of her three children, then extended their life stories over decades to the present. One moment I was hearing about her beloved young children, and the next moment I was meeting them in person—then in their seventies! There were many moments when I closed my eyes and simply listened to Esther, losing track of the nearly eighty years between us. And I began to see age in a different context: Someone living with the daily infirmities of aging and approaching death could still enjoy most of the same human experiences we find so precious in younger years. Unfortunately, we often fail to see these positive elements in the lives of our elders because we are so focused on the physical or mental decline of aging. The body will certainly reach its limits, with death beyond our ability to predict or control. But the true failure here is not old age; rather, it is the failure of our own creativity and willingness to conceive that life up until its last moments has its own ways and meanings.

In the spring of my second year in medical school, Esther died several weeks after suffering a stroke. During our last visit she struggled to talk and reach out to me despite the loss of speech wrought by a small clot in her brain. As with so many of the older patients with whom I had grown close over the years, I had put the possibility of her death out of my mind, imagining that she was actually my own age but just looked a little different. In fact, I have often employed such mental gymnastics to deal with aging and death in my own family. Shortly after my grand-parents passed away, I compressed much of my grief into an odd fantasy that in the afterlife they had moved down to Miami Beach and were experiencing eternal bliss together, with endless sunny beaches and Early Bird Specials. Florida, I imagined, was actually some form of Shangri-La where all of our deceased eld-erly could be found happily wandering around if we just looked hard enough.

As fate would have it, I currently live and work in Miami as a doctor for old people—the very profession so derided in my early years of training. In this location, I frequently encounter several unique groups of elders, including aged Holocaust sur-vivors and Cuban exiles, who have exerted a disproportionate influence on my clinical work and have inspired so much of my writing. To be more specific, I am the psychiatrist at the Miami Jewish Health Systems, the site of one of the largest nursing homes in the United States. Although people sometimes call my place of work "God's waiting room," they miss a much big-ger picture. True, the average age of my patients is about ninety years old, meaning that I see a lot of people close to one hundred. The eighty-year-olds who come to see me are like teenagers on my scale of things and the seventy-year-olds—babies! And true, my job is to tend to all of the maladies and infirmities of aging. But as I first learned from Esther and then from countless others, the true scales of aging are not one-sided; the problems of aging must be weighed against the promises. In my work as a geriatric psychiatrist I have learned that *aging equals vitality, wisdom, cre-ativity, spirit,* and, ultimately, *hope.* And for an increasing number of aged individuals, these vital forces are growing by the day.

✴✴✴

My mission in this book is to offer a more balanced perspective on aging. My intention is not to promise any cures for aging, as some books do. I am not interested in pushing certain nutritional supplements, diets, or lifestyles as fountains of youth, as other books try. I am interested solely in honestly exploring the experience of old age through the lives of my patients. I begin in Part I by defining the aging process as it is currently understood scientifically and as it is imagined and experienced psychologically. Part II is a medical rounds of sorts in which I describe the aging process of several of my most memorable patients. These cases, though quite variable in their life stories, illustrate clearly the inevitable physical, psychological, and social changes that make aging such a challenge and bring us ever closer to the end of living. Each story, in its own way, also shows the many promises of aging that transform both the ways in which our bodies and brain age and the experience of aging itself.

Part III discusses the changing role of memory in old age, telling some surprising stories of how life persists and even thrives in the face of memory loss. Part IV looks at the meaning and development of wisdom and how it is practiced by our elders— as well as by the caregivers for these elders. In both parts I highlight several sages who exemplify all that is right about aging. In Part V, I extend the discussion of aging to the very frontiers of life, exploring how certain lessons learned from the aged can serve as beacons for all of us as we head into those very same waters. These lessons promise not the end of aging, but a new beginning even as we continue to age.

Part I
What Is Old?

Age I must, but die I would rather not.

—JOHN UPDIKE, "ENDPOINT"

Heaven
Can't Wait

The old woman had drawn down the shade in her room, trying, I imagined, to stop the midday Miami sun from penetrating her grief. But the sun still hit the window full force and illuminated the shade like a Chinese lantern. She sat silently in a wheelchair, her ninety-three-year-old silhouette appearing sad and stooped in the bathing light. I entered, held her hand for a moment, and introduced myself. "Sit down, Doctor," she said politely. I asked her why she had come to the nursing home, and she described the recent passing of her husband after seventy-three years of marriage. I was overwhelmed by the thought of her loss and wanted to offer some words of comfort. I leaned in close and spoke, "I'm so sorry. What has it been like for you losing your husband after so many years of marriage?" She paused for a moment and then replied, "Heaven."

I flinched at her answer, hoping that I had misheard her. Seeing my bewilderment and understanding immediately the irony of her response, she smiled at me and proceeded to describe how she had endured decades in an unhappy marriage with a gruff, verbally abusive man. As she spoke, I realized how my instincts were so completely off. In my misguided empathy, I had committed what William James describes as the psychologist's fallacy—assuming incorrectly to know what someone else is experiencing.

With this newly widowed patient, I imagined that only a life of sadness and decrepitude remained, and I felt badly about it. But I was wrong. She had not fallen into the abyss. Rather, she was glad to have finally won a measure of freedom and was determined to make the best of it. As her life unfolded at the nursing home over the next year, she threw herself into new activities and relationships in a way that was quite unexpected to me.

All of us lapse into such mistaken impressions of old age from time to time. Our mistake stems in part from an age-centric perspective in which we view our own age as the most normal of times, regarding it as representative of how all life should be. At eighteen the fifty-year-olds may seem ancient, but at fifty we are apt to say the same about the eighty-year-olds. So what's it really like to be old? I often query my patients, who are mostly in their late eighties and nineties, and the responses are surprising. "I forgot I was so old," a one-hundred-year-old patient recently told me and then excused herself to make it to bingo on time.

This age-centrism is particularly pervasive when we gauge attitudes toward nursing homes. All too often we imagine that life stops at the doors of a facility, that the life within, if we can call it that, is loveless and lonely, with death hovering close by. We make this mistake when we refuse to see needs for intimacy even in the most debilitated elderly. Our youth-centered culture equates love with sex, but I have seen with my older patients that love can be an endlessly blossoming flower, felt and expressed in hundreds of ways. A friend's mother who suffers from Alzheimer's disease has fallen in love with another resident on her floor, and they walk around holding hands and snuggling with a newfound innocence that perhaps only their memory loss restored.

We also project our terror of death onto the aged, assuming that fear and depression must stalk the final years of life. And yet in my fifteen years of working in nursing homes, I have never heard a patient tell me that he or she was afraid of death. Sometimes there is acceptance, other times anticipation, but most often there is no great concern. Life goes on in death's shadows.

In the end there is a cost to our myopic views of aging in which only the negative images appear. We imagine the pains of late-life ailments but not the joys of new pursuits; we recoil at the losses and loneliness and fail to embrace the wisdom and meaning that only age can bring. Henry Wadsworth Longfellow captured the sentiment well:

For age is opportunity no less,
Than youth itself, though in another dress,
And as the evening twilight fades away,
The sky is filled with stars, invisible by day.

This perspective on age, filled with both curiosity and optimism, is unfortunately not the norm. In general, we understand little about aging, and what we perceive is too often a projection of our own fears. I am certain this is why I am often challenged with two specific questions when I reveal that I am a doctor for the elderly. The first question is, "What does it mean to be old?" The second question flows from the first: "Is it depressing to work with old people?" I could make it easy on myself and simply answer, "It depends," and "No," but in reality each question has a thousand different answers. "It's a gift," I might answer to the first question on some days or "a tragedy" on others. To the second question, I could confess to occasionally feeling depressed, but in truth with each patient I have a different state of mind—delight, disappointment, curiosity, consternation, *wonder*. And with both questions, I always remind myself and my questioners that I am merely an observer of age and not a member of the aged—at least not yet. Nevertheless, these questions are profound, and my answers demand some deeper explanations. Let me begin with an ending.

✹✹✹

In the spring of 1997 my beloved grandfather passed away. A week before his death, I stood vigil at his bedside while he flickered between confusion and insensibility. The once-brilliant mind of this retired doctor was soaked in a pool of morphine, and most rational thinking had already drowned. He insisted on wearing a large pair of sunglasses in the darkened room. He cursed and growled when I held his arms as he staggered into the bathroom. I am not certain that he even recognized me on that final visit, as by then his lifelong persona had largely separated from the person. Nevertheless, his voice came to me as I watched him lying in bed, breathing slowly: "Notice the abnormal rate and pitch of the breath sounds," I imagined him saying; "they are quiet at first but become increasingly labored until they stop for a moment—called *apnea*—and then the pattern repeats. This is known as Cheyne-Stokes respiration, and it is often seen just prior to death." I pictured the seriousness of my grandfather's face as he taught me to observe the ebb and flow of the respirations and then quizzed me to make certain that I had absorbed the lesson. The distinctive cadence of his voice alternated between curt instructions and impatient pauses, waiting for my answer. He had a way of repetitively flipping his outstretched hand at the wrist as he spoke, one finger extending out like Michelangelo's God, as if to say, "It can be this way, or that, but you must choose one!"

The practice of medicine was his life, and he had taught me with both an earnestness and a severity about caring for patients. My grandfather had experienced the urgency of his work while serving as a field surgeon in the U.S. Army Air Corps stationed on Okinawa during World War II. This sensibility was reinforced after the war in his fifty years as a general practitioner in the small industrial town of Kaukauna, Wisconsin. In both circumstances the survival of a patient depended on his own wit and hands; there were few colleagues or other resources to help out.

My grandfather had an instinctive sense of independence, no doubt fashioned in his childhood. He was born in 1914 and grew up in a small town in Ukraine near Kiev, alone with his mother and grandmother after his father left for America. He survived the poverty and deprivation of rural Russia during World War I and recalled hiding in haystacks or in the forest to escape from the murderous pogroms of the Cossacks. At the age of twelve he came to America in the steerage of a transatlantic steamer, landing at Ellis Island with other similarly huddled masses. My grandfather remembered seeing the gleaming torch of the Statue of Liberty as the ship glided into New York harbor. He remembered the sweet, precious taste of an orange that he ate, for the first time, while on board. His subsequent journey in America slowly took him west along the rail-lines; he lived with relatives in New York, Chicago, Madison, and, finally, Appleton, Wisconsin.

If you picture Wisconsin like the shape of a hand, Appleton is a small city located in the fleshy crook just below the thumb. It is the largest of a group of smaller towns and villages—including Kaukauna—that sit astride a shallow valley that hugs the bends and locks of the Fox River as it meanders from Lake Winnebago to Green Bay. The area is both picturesque and pastoral, surrounded by farms and woods, but with belching, steaming stacks of paper mills lying at its center. It was settled throughout the 1800s mainly by Dutch and German immigrants—farmers, dairymen, craftsmen, and small businessmen—but was no stranger to the small groups of itinerant German, Polish, and Russian Jews who found their way into its folds, including both sets of my great-grandparents.

My grandfather's father was a garrulous, backslapping businessman who ran a successful dairy and in the process befriended most of the city officials in Appleton, including a then-obscure judge named Joseph McCarthy. To his three sons, however, my great-grandfather was a firm and exacting father who fostered a competition among them better suited to the survival-of-the-fittest mentality of czarist Russia than to the open spirit of small-town America. My great-grandmother, in contrast, was a very bright and beloved woman with a good sense of humor, but she carried with her a sadness that she hadn't been able to leave behind in Russia. She was actually the first old person in my life, and I remember her as an exotic and perfumed lady with long painted fingernails, a mysterious accent, and a thick purple coat and scarf surrounding her wrinkled and wizened face. She was a babushka in purple.

Before becoming a doctor, my grandfather was, in succession, a milkman, a boxer, and a scientist. His appearance lent itself to each job, as he had the quick, thin legs of a deliveryman; the box-shaped, muscular trunk of a pugilist; and the round, balding, and bespectacled face of an intellectual. Photographs of him from youth to old age always show a dapper man, whether dressed in uniform, scrubs, or coat and tie. In 1938 he married my grandmother, and they stayed together for life. She was the consummate doctor's wife, who raised their three children, managed the books, and kept the home quiet, kosher, and revolving smoothly around his frenetic schedule.

As a doctor my grandfather worried incessantly about his patients, but he hid it behind his obsessive work habits and sometimes-gruff demeanor. He had a bad habit of throwing instruments during surgery when the wrong one was handed to him. He demanded perfection in himself, and he was relentless with his staff. By the early 1970s probably half of Kaukauna's residents were either current or former patients, a good many of them having been birthed into his hands. Neighbors, strangers, and family alike all made visits to his modest-sized, spartan clinic, where he was renowned as a diagnostician. There weren't many secrets in our large extended family living throughout Wisconsin, but whatever they were, he knew and kept them hidden as a good doctor should.

His perseverance and dedication were legendary. For example, several weeks after my grandfather's death, a former patient wrote a letter to the editor of the local newspaper to relate this story. One night during a fierce Wisconsin blizzard, the man's young daughter woke up with a high fever. He called my grandfather, who initially advised him to bundle her up and meet him at his office. Several minutes later the man's phone rang: "Stay home," my grandfather advised; "I will come to you." And as the man described, "In a time that only a man with purpose could make, there was a knock on the door and there stood a snowman." My grandfather entered, shook off the snow, and remained with the family throughout the night, tending to the man's beloved firstborn daughter. Many years later the man stood with that same daughter to watch her husband graduate from medical school. After the ceremony he pulled the new doctor aside and challenged him to repay the family's debt to my grandfather by embodying the same dedication to his craft.

Until the year before his death, aging had been a relatively benign process for my grandfather. He practiced medicine and surgery until the age of eighty and then retired not because he felt any desire to but because it just seemed logical. He played tennis, traveled, and even made a pilgrimage back to Ellis Island to see the same great hall in which he had been processed some sixty-eight years earlier. A perpetual student, he audited courses in neuroscience and German at nearby Lawrence University. I was in medical school at the time, and he would sometimes call me to discuss the role of a certain neurotransmitter or region of the brain that he was studying. He also spent his retirement tending to and doctoring my grandmother, saving her life on one occasion when her heart rate slowed precipitously.

When he became ill, however, aging caught up to him quite quickly. In the summer of 1996 he was diagnosed with an aggressive form of prostate cancer. I was called to Kaukauna immediately to offer him moral support—at a time when I was treating similarly aged and ill war veterans during my geriatric psychiatry training at the Minneapolis VA hospital. I had hoped that he would brush off the cancer like he had done with a small stroke a few years back, but within months it was clear that this would not be the case. Suddenly, he needed me for support and advice, and we spoke nearly every day about how to manage some of his physical discomfort. Of course, as a newly minted psychiatrist I was of little value to his medical management, and I left that up to my uncle, who had taken over his practice. But our conversations were not really about my grandfather's pain; they were, it seemed to me, cover for dealing with aging and death.

As the de facto family historian I also knew that I had to record his life stories, and so at Thanksgiving we sat down on the porch of my grandparents' house for a taped interview. The life review was almost too painful for him, however, and he broke down crying at several points. I had never seen him cry before, let alone show sadness, but I persisted with the camera, knowing that time was short. In my work with older individuals it is always painful to witness the crumbling of their composure in the face of loss and grief, but I can steel my own emotions because I rarely know what the person was once like. But such was not the case with my grandfather, and I vacillated between denial and despair. As I was saying my good-byes and leaving my grandparents' home at the end of the weekend, he pulled me aside and stated rather perfunctorily that this was probably the last time I would see him. His words were sterile and clinical—a doctor's way of parting with a patient. But I knew that this was his best effort at saying good-bye. A doctor myself, I brushed off his words in the same manner I might use leaving the clinic at day's end —"No, Grandpa; I'll see you soon. Call me tomorrow."

I reflected on these moments as I sat at his bedside that spring and tried to contain my emotions. He was not only my grandfather, but also my mentor, my inspiration, and, from my earliest childhood days, my own doctor. But now his life of eighty-three years was drawing to a close, and I was standing witness at the point where aging meets death. No other period of life has such a feared and mysterious ending. Childhood ends with the budding of puberty and the new challenges of adolescence. Adolescence passes away in the excitement of pulsating hormones, shedding its awkward, uncertain skin in the journey into young adulthood. The subsequent stages of adulthood bring undiscovered treasures of love, children, work, and spirit. Even in the face of failure or lost opportunities, there is always hope for something new. But aging seems to bring this process to a halt. The horizon is unknown except for the single fact that a true ending will come.

Even as my grandfather was slipping away, for me he was already changing from a presence to a memory and from a companion to a silent guide. But what I risked missing at the time was the same lesson I had learned several years earlier from my one-hundred-year-old friend, Esther—that aging is not synonymous with death. As I now contemplate the immensity of his influence on my own life, I realize that it wasn't his death but his old age that left such an imprint on me. Aging bequeathed him virtues of experience, vitality, and wisdom, but it was, in the end, simply his presence that made all the difference for me. In our last few months together I discovered what most of us instinctively know: that the primal answer to the question "What does it mean to be old?" is a beloved parent, grandparent, or other older figure.

The experiences and images of "oldness" that we absorb from aged people are immediately biased by the particulars of those people in our lives. The elders who populated my own childhood were all active, colorful, and beloved figures who conferred a delightful mystique on aging. This is why I have always felt comfortable working with the elderly. But not everyone has such vital figures in her or his life, and oldness may instead be a decrepit and mute grandfather in a wheelchair or an agitated aunt with dementia. The resultant vision of aging may be full of dread and even disgust. As I begin to answer the questions of age and refract the answers through the eyes of my many patients, I recognize that the stories capture only a piece of aging—not its entirety. But they're at least a good beginning.

Age I Must

Awareness of the difference in age between ourselves and our older caretakers is perhaps the first lesson of aging that we absorb. I am here in time and they are *there*, with there being some amorphous point farther along the timeline. At the age of four my youngest son, Sam, first made this connection, which led inevitably to some rather profound questions about age. At the time he was just beginning to count things in earnest, and what had started a year before as a show of fingers now began to flow onto objects in the environment. With each birthday came the announcement of a new age, and before long both time and space were taking on meaning as measurable dimensions. I wasn't prepared, though, for his youthful interrogation one morning.

Sam's questions began before I was fully awake and thus sufficiently attentive to his pressing curiosity. "Dad . . . do you work with old people?" he asked me. "Yes," I murmured from beneath the pillow. "Dad . . . do you *like* working with old people?" "Yes," I murmured again, still half-asleep. "Every day?" "Of course, Sam." "Even Tuesday?" "Yes, even Tuesday," I answered, again in a somnolent monotone. He paused for a minute, and I began to drift off. "Dad . . . are they just waiting to die?" This question landed like a shattered glass, and my eyes opened wide. I sat up. "Sam, why do you ask?" Even at four years old, it seemed, he had already absorbed this notion that aging somehow equaled death. He stared at me with a serene curiosity, smiling, but intent on an answer. Fortunately, his questions were coming faster than the answers I was searching for. "What is old?" he started in again, "and in how many days will I be old?"

This was a counting that I could not do for him, but the question fired my own curiosity about what being old is all about. As a doctor I measure it by years: Seventy years old has different expectations than ninety, and once you get beyond one hundred, it appears to be a whole new realm. But these distinctions, I realize, can be misleading. And they are changing by the day. At some point we see and feel changes in our minds and bodies that begin to define being old, and we ask the same questions posed by my son: What does it mean to grow old? When does old begin? And what does it entail?

For more complete answers than I could give my son, I must turn to scientists who have devoted their lives to the study of aging. One of these experts was preeminent geriatric psychiatrist Dr. Gene Cohen, who served as the head of the Center for Aging and Humanities at George Washington University. In 2009 I spent an idyllic summer morning talking to him on the large porch of his home in a quiet, wooded suburb of Washington, DC. I questioned him about aging as my own son had questioned me. In response, he began with a story from his adolescence about a fish called the longhorn sculpin.

The longhorn sculpin is not a fish you'll ever find on a plate. It's a rather ugly fish with a bulbous head, large protruding eyes, and a thin brown and olive green body that tapers to a tailfin under a phalanx of spines. For the fishermen who work the shallow coastal waters of New England, the sculpin is a nuisance because it eats up the bait intended for other fish and makes a growling noise when handled. But for Cohen, the longhorn sculpin was his entry into the study of aging. As a sixteen-year-old high school student in 1960, he developed a new technique to determine the fish's age by using a small bone in its inner ear called the otolith. When the otolith is snapped perfectly in half, its inner accretions of calcium can be read like the rings of a tree. Growing up in a small town south of Boston, Cohen was able to use a newly invented minisaw at the nearby Woods Hole Oceanographic Institute to accomplish this task for the first time ever. He used these measurements to create a database of growth norms for the sculpin and won first prize in a prestigious science fair for his project.

But it wasn't the award that inspired him so much as the way in which he imagined aging to address larger issues. Knowing the age of the fish became a way of assessing the health of the fish's habitat, which in turn allowed an exploration of even wider issues—fish stocks, overfishing, ocean currents, and pollution. For many years, however, the study of aging was like the longhorn sculpin of scientific research, both neglected and more of a nuisance compared to other, more glamorous areas of research. And yet Cohen saw how the accumulating knowledge about aging applied to many other areas. For example, discoveries about how normal cells age and die have provided a doorway into understanding why cancerous cells don't.

Over the four decades of his career, the study of aging took Cohen in many different directions. But in response to my central question, he was clear: "Aging, of course, has two paths," he told me; "there's the process and there's the people." The process tells us how and why we age and is limited by laws of physics and biology. The people, however, show us how to age, and the limits are more variable. On the one hand, the experience of aging is circumscribed by physical health, personal resources, cultural norms, and historical events that are often out of our control. On the other hand, our own efforts can bring change and meaning to the aging process that can transcend these forces in ways that biology can't.

❊❊❊

Several months after my conversation with Gene, I traveled from Miami to a large psychiatric conference in Las Vegas to deliver a talk on psychotherapy with elderly patients. As the plane crossed over the southwestern United States, I was lost in thought, pondering not the meaning of old but the breadth and beauty of the landscape below as the Grand Canyon came into view. I have discovered that it is impossible to capture the immensity of the Grand Canyon through the window of an airplane. On more than one occasion I have tried, from the confines of my seat, to snap a meaningful photograph of those sinuous cracks as they emerge and deepen in the flat desert earth below. The result is always disappointing, as the aerial vista of the canyon is just too vast and hazy amid the clouds at 37,000 feet. To really apprehend the Grand Canyon means standing right on it and then wandering down the serpentine trails carved beneath its rim. From that vantage point the profound depths of the canyon and its dazzling multilayered earthen colors emerge.

The Grand Canyon is a perfect illustration of how aging is a process of perpetual change. For the geologist, the passage of time can be seen in its ancient walls, with each epoch containing its own strata of rich colors and collections of fossils and other debris. Over millions of years the Colorado River carved away the earth and stone while the tectonic plate below lifted up an entire plateau and tilted it toward the southern rim, eventually yielding a stunning edifice. Like an old man or woman, the parched and stone-wrinkled body of the canyon stretches across the plateau, twisting and turning in the bedrock of schist and granite like an arthritic skeleton and sloughing off fossilized mollusks and corals from its sand-and-mudstone skin. The canyon was already an ancient being when the aboriginal Pueblo people first crept along its limestone spine and ribs and descended into its petrified innards. Its walls are sturdy in some places, crumbling in others, and wear an impressive timeworn face that easily distracts from the teeming wildlife on its ledges or within the impenetrable bowers of willow and brush that hug the edges of the river and gorge. The modern observer can discover a deep and meditative pleasure being around something so old, a great geological wonder that serves as a touchstone for our own origins. Such petrified nature teaches us where we've come as a species. Older people teach us where we've come as a family or a society.

For the gerontologist who studies human aging, a comparison with the Grand Canyon would seem limited. After all, people are not rocks or rivers that age without a purpose and without a genetic code to guide them. The process that continues to unfold in the earth's geography is guided only by the laws of physics, is absent of sentiment, and is still relatively young compared to the age of the universe that bore our planet. But we do have something in common with these rocks and rivers: Both people and geography are aged by two fundamental and immutable forces of nature—time and entropy.

This point was recently made to me by Dr. Leonard Hayflick, one of America's most prominent experts on aging. In 1961, Hayflick published a now-classic paper on cellular aging, informing us that contrary to prior belief, our normal cells could undergo only a limited number of divisions. The Hayflick Limit specifies the roughly forty to sixty times that fetal cells will divide before eventual death, guided in part, it is believed, by the successive shortening with each division of an end region of every chromosome known as the *telomere*. The telomere is like a built-in cellular counting mechanism, with its memory remaining intact even in cells thawed out after years in deep freeze.

At eighty-one years of age, Dr. Hayflick has spent nearly his entire career studying aging, starting in an era of scientific research in the 1950s when "it would be committing professional suicide to mention that you were working in the field" of aging.

In this time he has seen every trend and theory of aging come along, including the growth of the so-called antiaging industry. But despite the enchanted claims and pursuits of many researchers in search of a new fountain of youth, Hayflick's view of aging is quite sobering: It is not a disease to be cured, and curing all of the diseases that kill us will not extend our own life expectancy much beyond its current limits. Rather, aging is an inexorable and inescapable property of every living creature. And on one level it doesn't matter whether we're talking about a rock, a river, a cabbage, or a king; aging equals change, and change is measured by time. To reverse the aging of anything, we would have to reverse time itself.

We would also have to reverse entropy: the tendency of any organism's or system's energy to become progressively more disordered and dispersed, resulting in the weakening of its molecular structure. For example, the rushing waters of the Colorado River shake the crystalline structure of the rocks over which they run, breaking them apart piece by piece. The gearshaft of an automobile engine weathers the heat and pressure of motion until it either shatters or corrodes beyond repair. And similarly in biological systems, the molecular bonds within our cells are inherently unstable. Without constant maintenance and repair, they eventually fail. As Hayflick writes, "Consequently, the random downward spiral of molecular disorder gradually exceeds repair or turnover capability and this results in changes in the cell, tissue, and organ levels that we call aging."

All subtheories of biological aging—and there are many— stem from this basic principle. The "wear-and-tear" hypothesis, for example, describes the increasing damage to our cells wrought gradually and somewhat randomly over time by accumulating antioxidants and toxins, mutations in our DNA, and clumping of sugars and proteins that gums up the functions of cells and tissues. This process of cellular aging, called *senescence*, happens to humans (and many other species as well) once we have reached reproductive maturity. And why does aging begin in earnest then? Humans simply could not exist if we couldn't get to the point where we produced offspring. But once that's accomplished, there is no evolutionary advantage to survival.

Old age, then, is less a product *of* nature and more of a human achievement wrestled *from* nature. Biblical patriarchs aside, the life expectancy for the vast majority of our ancestors was about twenty-five years. We hit close to fifty years by 1900, and then the spectacular medical discoveries of vaccines and antibiotics in the last century enabled most of us to live into our seventies and beyond. And according to the 2000 census, the one-hundred-year-olds are the single fastest growing age group in America. And yet despite these statistics, most of the current resources being put into the science of aging are directed less toward understanding aging or extending our lives and more toward finding ways to make us *look* younger.

The ongoing obsession with finding at least some part of the fountain of youth has an honest origin in our own perceptions of aging. Starting around the age of thirty-five, the face becomes the great oracle of aging. If you look at a series of photographs of someone as he ages, you will see the slow accumulation of distinctive changes in appearance. Below the surface of the skin, a protein matrix of collagen and elastin that gives skin its elasticity begins to break down, as does a thin cushion of fat that supported the once-smooth-and-supple integument above. As a result, the skin begins to stretch, sag, and wrinkle. Small blood vessels weaken and cause the skin to become paler and more easily bruised. And years of sun exposure give the skin a leathery appearance and add dark spots, shaggy growths, moles, red spots, and scabby lesions.

Similar processes of breakdown are happening in every tissue in the body. But even though stiff, aching joints and loss of hair and posture may be both nuisances and affronts to our vanity, Hayflick points out, they are not life threatening. Loss of function in a kidney, liver, or brain due to aging, however, may be catastrophic. Is there a solution? Can we simply treat aging like we treat an infection? There are certainly no shortages of products—lotions, vitamins, supplements, and hormones—that promise to rejuvenate the body and make us physiologically younger. And some researchers have claimed that in the future we will use stem cells or gene therapy to extend life years or even centuries longer.

In response to these suggestions, Hayflick emphasizes that we have not discovered any genes that determine longevity, and so there is no possible gene therapy that could slow aging. Genes do, however, determine the relative integrity of our bodies as well as our individual vulnerabilities to certain diseases as we age. But there is a key difference here between the disease states that increase in frequency with age and the normal but inexorable breakdowns in cellular and tissue integrity that define the aging process. Unlike cancer and heart disease, which can be treated and ultimately cured, aging is not a disease, and thus it cannot be cured. "As of today," Hayflick told me, "we know of no intervention whatsoever that would interfere with the fundamental processes of aging, nor do I think that is going to come about in the future." Exercise, a well-balanced diet, and good hygiene can improve and prop up our biological dwelling places, but age will still come.

But is there any harm in wanting to do better? Hayflick likened the process to trying to extend the life of an automobile. You can repair damage and replace parts, but beyond a certain point the vehicle looks and runs like new only if you've done a complete overhaul. "But that is exactly what you can't do with biological materials," Hayflick reasoned, "and even if you could, would you want to replace your brain? And then would you be yourself?"

Changes in the brain are, in fact, the most demoralizing aspects of aging. In an 1816 letter to John Adams, Thomas Jefferson captured the sentiment well: "Bodily decay is gloomy in prospect, but of all human contemplations the most abhorrent is body without mind." Alzheimer's disease is at epidemic proportions around the world and growing by the day. We have discovered how to bring more and more people to the very frontiers of the lifespan, but at the cost of rates of dementia that exceed 50 percent by age eighty-five. Most youthful projections cast this as the dismal and inevitable reality of aging. And these fears drive an entire movement that seeks to do what Hayflick says can't be done: actually reverse aging.

One of most widely known of these "prolongevists," as they are called, is Aubrey de Grey, a brilliant British computer scientist and self-taught expert on aging who has taken as his life's mission finding a cure to aging. Many like Hayflick dismiss de Grey as a modern-day Don Quixote tilting at the immutable windmills of aging, but his unabashed confidence and omnipresent argumentativeness in the field of aging—not to mention his hippielike appearance, complete with long beard and ponytail—have made him hard to ignore. In his audaciously titled book *Ending Aging*, de Grey approaches aging solely as something that "is really bad for us, however much we would like to forget the fact." Because, in his view, aging is at the root of all undesirable bodily change and disease, it must be combated and eventually defeated. To this end, he has identified seven fundamental causes of aging that he believes can be conquered with sufficient attention and money.

For de Grey, however, the goal is not simply to live longer but to live better. For it would do no good to prolong life indefinitely if we continued to decline, much like the rare but immortal Struldbruggs in Jonathan Swift's novel *Gulliver's Travels*. "Happy Nation where every Child hath at least a Chance for being immortal!" exclaims the protagonist Lemuel Gulliver on hearing of such "excellent Struldbruggs, who born exempt from that universal Calamity of human Nature, have their Minds free and disengaged, without the Weight and Depression of Spirits caused by the continual Apprehension of Death." Such fantasy is dashed in this political satire when Gulliver learns the true fate of these poor creatures, who still live but continue to age into completely morose and decrepit societal outcasts.

Prominent gerontologists argue that de Grey's intent, while understandable, is simply not possible. Still others go even further and argue that de Grey is misguided. Such a radical extension of life would produce a dystopia in which generation after generation would coexist in unimaginable struggles for resources, status, and rank. Grandparents, great-grandparents, and great-great-grandparents ad infinitum would be indistinguishable in age from one another once each member reached a common point of designated agelessness. With a thousand-year lifespan, for example, cherished notions of family, monogamy ("'til death due us part" for nine hundred years?), family, inheritance, and government would be irreparably disrupted. Imagine an immortal Hitler or Stalin!

De Grey and others counter that any such changes in the lifespan would likely be gradual enough to allow society to adjust—just as it has over the last century as thirty years have been added (plus, there could be immortal Einsteins or Mother Teresas!). But ethicist Daniel Callahan is not convinced, arguing that "nature knew what it was doing when it arranged, through natural selection, to have all of us get old and die." Diane Schaub echoes this sentiment: "Senescence escorts us, more or less gracefully, off the stage," she asserts, "making room for fresh generations."

This entire debate reduces the questions of age to a Manichean struggle between death and immortality. Such a dichotomy is a one-way street under which everything we believe about the meaning of aging flows from inescapable biological facts. Either we accept aging as an inevitable and immutable fact, or we abhor it as a tragic and wholly unnecessary state of affairs. Either way we lose ourselves in the picture, forgetting that regardless of whether we live to be one hundred or one thousand, we still have a great deal to say about what will happen in the time of oldness, a time of potential human creativity in which, according to gerontologist Thomas Cole, "the experience and cultural representation of human aging help to constitute its reality."

This point illustrates where the *people* of aging transcend the *process*. The Hayflick Limit tells us that we are biologically finite, but there is no comparable Hayflick Limit to meaning in late life—that is the lesson from the people.

❇❇❇

An astounding discovery in 2007 by an Inuit hunting party along the northern Alaskan coast resulted in the crowning of the Bowhead whale as the oldest living mammal. Imbedded in the blubber of this leviathan the hunters found the metal tip of a harpoon dating back to the early 1880s. Not only did the young whale survive the initial wounding, but it also managed to escape and live another 120 years! This story reminded me of my former patient Eugene, a 102-year-old World War I veteran who once showed me a small bump above his eyelid that harbored a piece of shrapnel from the Battle of Vittorio Veneto in 1918. Though the Austro-Hungarian troops with whom he served lost this decisive battle, he survived to tell (and show!) the tale for another 85 years.

Both of these survivors, man and whale, illustrate important findings from research into the oldest old human beings. Through a combination of genetics and lifestyle, some individuals are able to either avoid or survive the age-associated medical problems that end most lives, shrugging them off like the whale did the ancient piece of harpoon. In fact, many nonagenarians and centenarians are often healthier and more active than their slightly younger counterparts and have mortality rates after the age of ninety-seven that are actually lower than expected. According to a hypothesis by gerontologist James Fries, disease and disability tend to be compressed into a much later and shorter period of time for those living toward the frontier of the age span, up to and beyond one hundred.

Studies of centenarians have yet to identify any genes that bring longevity (and probably never will, according to Hayflick and others), but they have elucidated several common lifestyle characteristics. Centenarians, on average, have delayed onset of most diseases, especially the main killers—heart disease, stroke, and cancer. They are rarely obese, tend not to smoke or drink alcohol to excess, and often have similarly old siblings (There are, of course, outliers like Frenchwoman Madame Jeane Calment, the oldest recorded living human being, who died in 1997 at the age of 122. She reportedly smoked and drank a glass of port twice a day up until the age of 117!). And centenarian women often had their children after the age of 35 or 40, perhaps an indication of the hardiness of their reproductive systems.

We also see that these older minds, when intact, share several common features. Compared to their younger peers, centenarians cope better with stress, tend to be more confident and independent, are generally less anxious and depressed, and have increased levels of life satisfaction, even when their functional limitations are greater. In addition, research with centenarians has found much lower than expected rates of dementia—roughly in the range of 15 to 30 percent. There may be several reasons for this, including more connections between neurons and less genetic susceptibility to Alzheimer's disease. Whatever the factors may be, they cast a ray of light along the frontier.

Despite these findings, clinicians often assign mythic status to their oldest patients and try not to intervene too much when problems arise. I remember being asked to treat a 106-year-old woman who was wheeling up and down the hallway of the nursing home and banging her cane on other residents' doors. My initial treatment plan of "do nothing and let the woman alone" lasted about one week until staff demanded that I intervene more effectively. I was squeamish, worried that my pharmacologic hand might wield the harpoon that dealt the final blow to this majestic life. I pretended she was a mere 90 years old and started her on a low-dose antipsychotic, to good effect. Her 84-year-old son appeared the next week to thank me. "She's happier, and so am I!" he exclaimed. The frontiers of aging had truly fallen, I concluded.

When it comes to the question of what old age means, I often turn to my patients for answers. As psychiatrist George Vaillant remarks, "Old age is like a minefield; if you see footprints leading to the other side, step in them." Is it possible, I wonder, for the aged to distill the lessons of extreme old age into a formula that would guide all of us into this new terrain? After all, the eighty-five-year-olds and older are the fastest-growing demographic group in the county now, and we are all headed that way. But the answers from my patients are often strikingly mundane: "I stopped counting my age years ago," teased one centenarian, whereas another insisted that she didn't feel a day over eighty. Their answers are not definitive, but that is the point. Hope is a viable response, among many, to old age.

But at the age of forty-five, I can reasonably be asked whether my thoughts are just the starry-eyed views of a young man. Am I like Aubrey de Grey but in another cloak (or beard), wanting to project a different and more hopeful view of aging based simply on my own fear of death? Even though this particular question of aging is personal to me, we all know with absolute certainly that we will age, and the vast majority of us will reach old age. And our experience of aging will be influenced by how we imagine it to be. "Just take me out and shoot me before I ever end up in a nursing home," instructs a middle-aged friend, imagining his decrepit body being cast into the bowels of a stinking nursing home before death. And yet I work in a nursing home day in and day out, and I see how life goes on and even flourishes. Under the right circumstances, the imagined grim reaper of old age can seem more like an angel.

In an unexpected encounter at a caregiver's conference, I once had the opportunity to pose this question of age to an older woman who in her day had been an icon of beauty: actress Julie Newmar. In her career, Newmar was a goddess who embodied the charms of youth: as a dancer and singer on Broadway, as a movie star in such iconic movies as *Seven Brides for Seven Brothers*, and as the sultry Catwoman in the *Batman* series of the 1960s. At one point the movie studio insured her legs for $1 million. I expected that aging would be tough for Newmar, especially because a neurological disorder has made it nearly impossible for her to walk, let alone dance. And yet at seventy-six she is an active, articulate, and deeply spiritual woman who feels as vital as ever, with her writing and countless other activities. She was direct with me on what a book on aging would look like: "The pages would be blank," she insisted, because it would be up to each one of us to fill in our own meaning. This reminded me of Cole's view of aging as a mystery that requires meaning rather than a problem that requires solution: "Human freedom and vitality lie in choosing to live well within these limits" of aging, he suggests, "even as we struggle against them."

When I interviewed Hayflick, I expected to hear about his own experience of aging, but he didn't feel that much had changed for him. Instead, he focused on the impressive effects of aging—most of them negative—on his 104-year-old mother, who at the time of our interview was living on her own in Philadelphia, still relatively cognitively intact, but unable to walk because of the severe effects of arthritis on her knee joints. I asked him whether there was the possibility for improvement. Hayflick appreciated all of the efforts to make late life more tolerable, but he was still pessimistic. "For example, I don't think anyone would operate on her knees," he lamented, "but that keeps her so confined to this one room, and her life is four walls." Hayflick also asserted that she could benefit from an attitude adjustment: "She has been led to believe that a nursing home is a terrible place to be. But she cannot be convinced [otherwise]— she insists on staying in that apartment and dying there." And Hayflick was troubled by doctors who were sometimes too negative and fatalistic to believe that anything could be done for their oldest patients.

I have worked with many patients like his mother. They have severe physical limitations and multiple ailments that sometimes evade our most intensive and compassionate efforts to help. More devastating is the loss of hope engendered by these conditions. And it is not surprising to me that Hayflick could unravel the secrets of the aging cell but struggled mightily with the secrets of an aging mother. Understanding the process of aging does not always help in understanding the people. Questions about how we grow old remain.

Long Time Dead?

No one knows what age will bring. We may plot and plan for years to ensure the best old age possible, but circumstances and fate may dictate otherwise. Pity the person who spends countless hours exercising, eating right, and engaging in any of the imagined saviors of time and age and then prematurely drops dead. And then consider the robust and happy ninety-five-year-old woman I once saw in my office who never exercised and always ate the greasiest piece of meat on the plate with all the trimmings. These anecdotes represent the extremes, of course, and certainly do not denigrate the many tried-and-true aspects of a healthy lifestyle that can increase positive outcomes for aging. But we cannot escape the uncertainly of it all.

When young, we often try to cope with this uncertainty by imagining a future in which happiness will reign only if we remain free of pain, terrible illness, severe infirmity, disfigurement, or devastating personal losses. The inverse of this image is that old age will be quite miserable if any of these factors arise. Such myopic perspectives prove depressing and lead us to put old age out of our minds or to avoid too much exposure to old people.

This avoidance can go only so far, however, and sooner or later we face our greatest fears of aging in one way or another, sometimes prematurely as a caregiver for a loved one. In that role even more uncertainty arrives as we are forced to weigh the myriad complex and confusing issues of how to deal with the underbelly of old age. Leonardo, Rosa, and Alberto taught me this well.

Leonardo's mother, Rosa, lay spread out on the bed like the Cuba of her birth. In the folds of the sheets that traced the contours of her body he imagined the mountains of the Sierra Maestra, rising then falling within the cotton-spun landscape and splaying down to the three harbors of Havana. Her rational mind, like her country, had sent its most precious memories into exile on a distant shore. Despite his deepest efforts, Leonardo couldn't find her. And yet this woman was the guardian angel who had spirited him out of Cuba as a child. When he watched her sleep, he would often conjure the indelible image of their journey to freedom together, with his mother holding his hand tightly as they emerged from a plane into the brilliant Miami sun, the warm wind lifting up the billowing folds of her shawl like wings.

Leonardo would do anything for his mother, but he could neither understand nor accept the transformation that had unfolded over the previous year. A once bright, loving mother had turned cold, confused, and compulsively agitated as she entered her seventy-eighth year. For some time he had tried to ignore or explain away her symptoms, maintaining a delusion of age, like a form of misidentification in which he still saw her as the young woman who had bravely fled Cuba with him because she feared that Castro would send her beloved son off to the Soviet Union for indoctrination. And yet anyone outside of Leonardo saw in Rosa a depressing picture of oldness, full of mental confusion, irritability, anxiety, odors of incontinence, and fits of crying and panic that quickly gave way to screaming, kicking, and flailing at any attempts to redirect or soothe her.

Leonardo's father, Alberto, had no illusions about Rosa's illness, and I witnessed many times his almost violent grief. When he spoke, his entire body seemed to convulse with each phrase, and he vacillated between expressing devastation over the loss of his partner and exaltation over his enduring love for her. His face would twist and spasm as he coughed and choked on his words of concern: "She . . . needs more . . . help . . . now!" A moment later he would calm down, and a glazed look of resignation would release the tension in the muscles around his eyes and mouth. At eighty Alberto had ceased to age well as Rosa's once mild dementia had nose-dived into a state of frenetic pacing, grabbing, and repetitive, nonsensical vocalizations. I tried to explain to both Leonardo and Alberto that such behaviors are commonplace in various forms of dementia, including its most common variant, Alzheimer's disease. But knowledge in this case brought more despair than relief, more questions than answers, and an unquenchable pleading for my expertise.

I always knew when they had arrived for appointments because I could hear Rosa's yelps grow increasingly louder as they approached the door of my office. Alberto was calling me nearly every day for a while—"Doc, I don't know what to do. I don't know what to do. You've got to help me!"—appearing to mimic both his wife's restlessness and her verbal repetition. He was trying hard to maintain some form of vital balance for them, but the days were just too unpredictable. Peaceful hours with his wife alternated with crises: She fell; she hit him; she urinated on the living room carpet. One time he lost control as she was struggling with his attempts to help her in the bathroom. In his rage he cursed at her and shook his fist in her face a bit too close, nearly knocking out a tooth and sending blood spurting from her mouth. Despite her dementia, Rosa was in remarkably good physical shape. In response to their question about how long she might live like this, I once reminded Leonardo and Alberto that the course of Alzheimer's disease, even in its severe stages, was measured in years. "That's a long time dead," Alberto lamented. Leonardo looked away in silent acknowledgment.

I worried about Leonardo's emotional state, but at least he had a supportive wife and a busy job that kept his mind distracted from Rosa much of the day. I worried more about Alberto, seeing that everything he valued in later life seemed to be teetering on a precipice. How much longer could he manage the stress? Old age for him was chaotic, dizzying, and exhausting, what English writer Ronald Blythe has described as "full of death and full of life . . . a tolerable achievement and . . . a disaster." Over time I began to see telltale signs of depression in Alberto; he was persistently sad, tearful, and dejected. He felt useless as a husband, unable to manage the household due to failing interest and concentration. His sleep was constantly interrupted by his wife's awakenings since she had lost all sense of day and night. On some days he would not eat. Eventually, she fell hard, broke her hip, and ended up in the hospital. I thought it would be a respite for Alberto, but he showed up at my office in an even blacker mood. Leonardo was in tow, now gravely concerned about both parents.

As a psychiatrist I am trained to reflexively consider a diagnosis of depression for someone like Alberto. When it's severe enough, treatment for such a depression is optimal when it involves both talk therapy and a course of antidepressant medication. Alberto's generation, however, is sometimes prejudiced against the "talk" of therapy and more interested in a pill that promises a quicker and easier resolution. And I have had many cases of late-life depression that melted away with a little pharmacology, the psychiatric equivalent of a slam dunk. It's incredibly gratifying when that occurs. The power of medications has solidified our view of depression and other forms of mental illness as mere chemical storms in the brain, prompted and whipped up by genes, stress, metabolic derangements, and a host of other factors. The older brain seems particularly vulnerable, especially when it is pockmarked by small areas of dead tissue that choke off the nerve cells that regulate mood.

At the same time, I had to consider a somewhat wider diagnostic picture for Alberto. In a controversial 1995 *Atlantic Monthly* article entitled "Overselling Depression to the Old Folks," psychotherapist Stanley Jacobson argued against the rush to judge all late-life moodiness as a disease. "Old age is reason enough to be depressed if you dwell on it," he asserted, and then broadsided his own colleagues, accusing them of reducing "the struggle of the old to an illness" and contributing "more to the prevalence of depression than to its cure." Despite his polemics, Jacobson was not actually denying the existence of depression in late life, although he did come perilously close. Instead, he was arguing for the restoration of the mind to the clinical picture, reminding us that most of us will inevitably face "the awesome incurability of oldness" and will struggle with that fact. We can't wish aging away and reduce the negative reactions to it to a dysfunctional organ in the head.

With or without a formal diagnosis of depression, however, Alberto clearly needed more from me than a pill. He needed psychotherapy, and he also needed some hope for his wife. He needed to see her somehow get better, even in small measure. Treating him meant treating her, even though she was suffering from an incurable dementia that now was erupting into furious bouts of agitation. Such agitated states are the bane of geriatric psychiatry; they are difficult to understand, notoriously difficult to treat, and the medications that work bring with them a host of new problems and risks. Not too many years ago such patients were simply medicated into oblivion as a chemical form of the chains that had once bound the mentally ill. It's an antiquated approach that I never use, but families still beg me not to turn their loved ones into zombies, preferring screaming over silence, perhaps because screaming indicates that life is still present.

In any event, I now had three patients to treat: a severely agitated wife, a depressed and exhausted husband and caregiver, and an anguished, guilt-ridden son. I spent time counseling

Leonardo individually, talking about his expectations for both parents and his fears of what may yet lie ahead. He was thoughtful and eager to get my advice, but the emotional connections with his failing parents often derailed all logic. He persisted in caring for both with an obsessive-compulsive style that overwhelmed his time and energy, sowed discord with his wife, and yet brought some relief to his crushing grief and guilt. He acted not only out of obligation as a son, but believing in a sacred emotional debt to Rosa that could never be fully repaid.

I started counseling Alberto as well and then added a low dose of an antidepressant, but despite some mild improvement in his mood, the central problem with his wife continued to be an unstoppable source of dejection for him. Rosa had been transferred to the rehabilitation floor of my nursing home and was giving the nurses hell. She refused to get out of bed, and when she was transferred to a wheelchair, she refused to get back into bed. Every effort to care for her was met with fits of panic and screaming. During the day she frequently wandered up and down the hallway in her wheelchair, intruding into other rooms and taking clothes, food, and personal effects from other residents. Even though her walking and balance were terrible following hip surgery, she would sometimes attempt to stand up and stagger out of her wheelchair, one time tumbling onto the nursing station and sending papers, charts, and an overturned vase of flowers crashing to the floor. I was forced to assign an aide to monitor her during waking hours—at the facility's expense—to prevent a catastrophe.

These behaviors went on for week after week without improvement. I took a broad approach and considered a variety of potential disorders that might have been associated with her dementia, such as depression, mania, anxiety and panic, psychosis, and post-traumatic stress. One antipsychotic medication slowed her down a bit but caused excessive drooling, whereas another made her drowsy and even more unsteady on her feet. Two alternative medications from the same class seemed to agitate her more, perhaps because they paradoxically increased the restlessness in her legs, a sure sign of a medication-induced condition called akathisia. A mood stabilizer didn't touch her fury, and several antianxiety medications caused excessive sedation alternating with periods of paradoxical agitation. Two separate antidepressant trials both caused extreme agitation and weight loss; a third one gave her a voracious appetite. I tried every psychopharmacologic trick in my bag, but to no avail. In concert with her internist and neurologist, I ran every possible diagnostic test, hoping that I was missing some hidden organic cause. Nothing revealed itself, and nothing worked. Alberto and Leonardo were initially patient with my attempts at treatment, but with time they lost faith. Eventually, I too lost faith in my ability to understand and heal her condition. This was less an illness and more an act of God, it seemed, and I was stumped.

In such moments of uncertainty, I frequently conjure an idyllic scene. The actual scene took place one evening during a bitterly cold Wisconsin winter when I was accompanying my grandfather on a call to the emergency room. I still see him leaning closely into the faces of several grieving family members, his serious yet kindly expression unwavering as he explained why he was unable to save their beloved older mother, who lay on a gurney several paces away. He held a definitive air of authority in his role as a small-town doctor, swathed as he was in a long white lab coat wrinkled by endless hours of consultations, hospital rounds, and procedures. It was a primal scene in the practice of medicine, the image of the healer at work even as his own limits are exposed. And this scene occurred in a time and place when my grandfather's role as doctor was sacrosanct. Any moments of uncertainty he faced in clinical decisions—and there were plenty—were often absolved by the respect and understanding given him by both patients and families. If he could not heal, then, his patients believed, it was simply beyond the powers of medicine to heal.

My grandfather represented an era of medicine in which doctors held unique esteem in the eyes of society: almost beyond reproach and imbued with an authority and a privilege that drove the doctor-patient relationship. This admiration for doctors has changed significantly since my medical training in the 1980s. The uncertainty of difficult clinical cases is set against a very different backdrop in which the doctor is no longer considered the ultimate authority, where patients sometimes know or think they know more than the doctor about their illnesses by virtue of in-depth Internet research, and where rigid diagnostic and treatment algorithms, managed care criteria, and public scrutiny hold doctors accountable in ways that often demoralize the profession.

Cross the complexity of aging with the plethora of age-associated illnesses and the frustration and hopes of family members, and the geriatric specialist is left with an extremely vexing situation. With Rosa, for example, it was never clear how much of her problem was due to her underlying dementia and how much to a more acute, superimposed illness. How much was due simply to the ravages of age, and how much was due to a potentially reversible illness? This is a central dilemma with all aged individuals and begs the question of how much control we ever have over the inexorable age-associated changes in both mind and body. This uncertainly is frustrating and may drive two opposing attitudes among the aged and their caregivers: a fatalism that accepts the process and is resigned to its inherent suffering and an amalgam of rejection, denial, and simple optimism that refuses to give up and accept the status (call it *stagnant*) quo.

At the same time, many physicians still hold a fantasy of absolute authority, coupled with a desire for the decisionmaking prowess described so cogently in Malcolm Gladwell's book *Blink: The Power of Thinking Without Thinking*. Gladwell holds that many expert decisions are made quickly and intuitively based on a sizing up of the gestalt of a situation. Such decisionmaking is not the realm of the novice; it requires years of training, experience, and a certain savoir-faire to accomplish. Given the inherent uncertainty of many medical situations, both patient and doctor are rallied by the confidence and *certainty* that such decisionmaking brings. Even some caregivers fall into this fantasy and imagine that they, too, by force of will, can bring about a magical transformation in an afflicted loved one with just the right decision. I have seen countless caregivers wracked with guilt when their efforts prove futile.

However, in two books with different authors but identical titles—*How Doctors Think*—physicians Karen Montgomery and Jerome Groopman both suggest that the rapid "blink" of expert decisionmaking is not always appropriate in medicine. Both authors stress that illness involves "uncertainty, loss of control, and the damage to the sense of self." In the face of this uncertainty, doctors appeal to the science of medicine and the statistical probability of healing to make decisions, but there are pitfalls here. Not every treatment can bring a 100 percent guarantee of success, and having to rely on lesser statistics (such as a 78 percent chance of success or a 5 percent chance of certain unpleasant side effects) can undermine a doctor's confidence in his or her own decisionmaking and can be anxiety provoking to patients and families. At the same time, the uncertainty of medicine allows its practitioners to hide behind numbers or theories rather than face their own inevitable vulnerabilities and even practice failures. Based strictly on the science of late-life illness, the rationale for medical care in the final days of life is tenuous at best. Not surprisingly, a term such as "death with dignity" has become more of a catchphrase in medicine than "life with dignity," as the former term may allow an easy out when there is no certain treatment or certainty of improvement. Ultimately, Montgomery is clear in stating that medicine is a practice, rather than a strict science, in which uncertainty is a normal part of the process and its engagement can bring increased choices, control, and, ultimately, hope.

Groopman, too, argues that uncertainty is an inescapable part of medicine and cannot always be resolved with scientific reasoning. This is a quite disconcerting assertion, implying that even the strictest evidence-based deductive reasoning will not always bail us out. Comparing a doctor to a sleuth, Groopman states that "human biology is not a theft or a murder where all the clues can add up neatly. Rather, in medicine, there is uncertainty that can make action against a presumed culprit misguided." As opposed, then, to the ever-popular Dr. House, like our old literary friend Sherlock Holmes (written, not surprisingly, by *Doctor* Sir Arthur Conan Doyle), who is always able to solve the mysterious illness, real-life doctors are not so easily able to wrap up medical and psychiatric conundrums with a neat bow at the end. We sometimes have no clear answers.

Rosa's case continued to stump me for some time, and so I turned back to the image of my grandfather as the consummate doctor. I realized that it wasn't his absolute knowledge or authority that made the difference in his practice but the two key virtues of persistence and courage, manifested by an unflinching involvement with both patient and family. He tolerated the uncertainty of medicine well, perhaps because he had trained in an era before CT scans, ultrasounds, and even antibiotics were available to seemingly guarantee clear diagnosis and quick healing. The practice of geriatric psychiatry often reminds me of that earlier era, because I face patients with intractable symptoms that cannot be visualized on any scan or diagnosed with any single test. With Rosa it would have been easiest to simply call in hospice and wash my hands of the case, but something in me (call it intuition) resisted. And so I sat down with Alberto and Leonardo and laid out everything we knew—and didn't know—about Rosa's condition, and we discussed all the remaining treatments that we could reasonably consider. This was not a single discussion but a dialogue that took place over many weeks.

Finally, we decided to hospitalize Rosa and try electroconvulsive therapy, or ECT, often referred to somewhat pejoratively as "shock therapy." Despite many misconceptions about ECT, it is actually one of the safest and most effective treatments for severe depression, even in older individuals. A course of ECT typically involves eight to twelve sessions spaced out over several weeks. During each session the individual is briefly anesthetized and paralyzed with medications and then administered an electric shock to the forehead to induce a seizure. We still have no clear idea of how ECT changes brain chemistry to improve depression and other mood disorders, but its effects are impressive. Nevertheless, it's usually a treatment of last resort.

ECT is used even more rarely to treat agitation associated with dementia, but with Rosa I felt we had run out of choices other than massive doses of sedating medications. I feared that the procedure would only exacerbate her underlying memory impairment, but the potential benefits still outweighed the risks. Despite how "long time dead" Rosa appeared to her family, I had to have some hope. Over the course of three weeks Rosa received eight rounds of ECT. Her memory impairment held steady, and she seemed to tolerate ECT well for the first two weeks, but without response. During the third week, however, Rosa's storm began to subside as she grew quieter and less frenetic. Her once fearsome wind became a breeze, and we saw that the treatments were working. Actually, they worked beyond our wildest expectations, and a completely different woman emerged from the hospital. She was generally calm, pleasant, and cooperative. I could actually have a conversation with her. "My wife—she's back!" Alberto exclaimed every time I saw him, and he was back, too. He stopped his antidepressant and dropped out of therapy, telling me, "I don't need it anymore!" Leonardo was equally thrilled, and now Rosa, even in her relatively severe state of cognitive impairment, seemed like a rose. It was as if an exile had returned, changed from the experience and not quite the same person, but good enough. For Leonardo and Alberto, Rosa was home.

Although in retrospect I can claim that the success of the ECT confirmed a clear diagnosis of acute mania in Rosa that was superimposed on her Alzheimer's disease, I realize that this Monday-morning quarterbacking brings no more certainty to the case. After all, every other treatment for mania failed. And so what made the difference in the end? Groopman suggests that "uncertainty sometimes is essential for success." But what does this mean?

There is a lesson here on aging, a moral to the parable of old age that begins with the question of what it means to be old and proceeds, at first, into a realm of great complexity and uncertainty. As a doctor to the aged, I have discovered that I must embrace this uncertainty and hold on tightly, often plunging in up to my elbows and hoping—sometimes against hope— that persistence and faith will prove correct. I have seen, however, that regardless of the outcome, our greatest humanity emerges in the desperate process of caring for someone old and ill. The relationship we establish with our elderly, and with their loved ones and caregivers by extension, ultimately trumps the agony of uncertainty. Over time, uncertainty buys us time, opening up doorways of possibility that reveal as much hopefulness as possible. Absolute certainty may come only with the death of the elder, but that is a fragile certainty lost in its very expression. Old age is not a long death as long as we maintain these vital connections with its inevitable practitioners. For they eventually become us.

Part II
Old Age Rounds

Listen: the sound of your going has a length of its own.

—GARY MIRANDA, "GOING"

Isaac, Erik, and Isak

Beneath the crumbling stone walls and dried-out cisterns of the ancient city of Be'er Sheva, the waters are abundant. Fed by rainfall from the nearby hills of Hebron, the massive aquifer that runs below the bedrock has allowed civilization to flourish in the desert crossroads above. It was here, the Bible tells, that the patriarch Isaac dug wells, raised his family, and sealed an oath with King Abimelech to live in peace with the nearby tribes. This is also where a primal struggle took place between two brothers over who would receive their old father's blessing to become the next head of the family.

According to Genesis 27, by around the age of one hundred Isaac "had grown old" and "the vision of his eyes had dimmed." Knowing that his life was entering its final stage, Isaac asked his son Esau to hunt some game and prepare a tasty meal for him, after which Isaac would bestow his blessing on this son.

Overhearing her husband's instructions and believing their son Jacob to be more worthy of the blessing, Rebecca devised a plan to trick the blind old man. While Esau was out in the fields, she prepared an alternative meal of goat meat for Isaac and dressed Jacob in animal skins so that he could masquerade as his hairier brother. Isaac was initially suspicious, but the ruse worked and Jacob was blessed. Later, Esau appeared with his own tasty meal, and a seemingly bewildered Isaac asked, "Who then is the one who hunted game and brought it to me . . . and I blessed him?" Discovering that he had been tricked by his brother, Esau burned with a murderous fury toward Jacob, who quickly fled Be'er Sheva. In the end it seems an old blind man was fooled and a new generation of conflict was created.

That such drama takes place in the life of a centenarian is nothing new for the Bible, as most of its early characters are wholly geriatric. After all, Noah lived for 950 years; Abraham died "at a good age, old and satisfied" at 175; and his wife, Sarah, gave birth to Isaac well after the age of 70. In the case of Isaac, there is a singular lesson on aging that I take from his story: Sometimes what we perceive only as a weakness conferred by old age may actually conceal or prompt a strength. On the surface, it is a story about a weakened and physically blind old man who could not tell the difference between a ruddy, rough, and hairy son and a smoother, more genteel one. But lying beneath this surface is a man who sees exactly what's going on and who in his deep, abiding love for both sons refuses to expose the wrongdoing of one and the deception of the other. The dimming of one attribute allowed the extension of another, and two seemingly opposite forces—vision and blindness, light and darkness, *Jacob and Esau*—were thus balanced and ultimately reconciled in the life of Isaac. Now the story could continue into the next generation.

As with the actual process of aging, we can easily miss the hidden strengths that guide and balance a person's life. Memory slows down, but knowledge and wisdom increase. The loosening of certain neural connections in the brain may enhance creativity. And the failing of physical strength may prompt the need for greater intimacy and companionship with others. Within each problem lies a solution that enables further development.

I did not learn this lesson originally from my older patients. Nor did I learn it originally from the Bible or from my studies as a psychiatrist. And though I did learn it first from a great thinker who wrote about the human life cycle, it was less the theory and more my encounters with the man behind it— the *old* man behind it, *dimmed* by age—that taught me this lesson. At the time, I was a young nineteen-year-old college student and he was my eighty-two-year-old teacher. His name was Erik Erikson. Like Isaac, Erik was a patriarch, an original force in the field of psychoanalysis and psychology. There are few textbooks in either discipline that do not mention his name and his work as fundamental to an understanding of adult development. In fact, he could accurately be called the father of all life cycle studies.

Getting to know the famous Erik Erikson was a heady experience for a college sophomore at Harvard who still had one foot in the small Wisconsin town of his upbringing. It was the fall of 1984, and during the first week of classes I ran across a flier that advertised a seminar on the human life cycle to be led by Erikson and his wife, Joan, as well as by Professor Diana Eck from the Department of Religion and Dr. Dorothy Austin from the Divinity School. Erikson was returning for a final curtain call at Harvard, where his career in America had begun some fifty years earlier and reached its zenith during the late 1960s. I immediately called the number on the flier to apply for the seminar, and within a few hours I was sitting on a brick stoop in Cambridge being interviewed by Dorothy. I did my best to tell her about myself and explain my interest in the course, but in retrospect I am not certain what I said made any difference. Something just fit, and soon I would meet the master.

❊❊❊

Erik Erikson was born in 1902 and grew up in the German city of Karlsruhe, raised by a loving mother who refused to reveal the true identity of his father—a mystery that he would never solve and that would profoundly shape his life and work. He was a Jew who looked more like a Nordic gentile, and he did not feel that he fit in either community. He was not a particularly gifted student. He gravitated toward the arts, studying how to sketch and make woodcuts. But despite his artistic interests, young Erik Homburger (as he was known at the time, taking his stepfather's last name) was moody, directionless, and depressed.

In his early twenties Erikson continued to flounder. He studied art in Munich and spent a significant amount of time traveling throughout Germany and Italy. In 1927, however, his childhood friend Peter Blos invited Erikson to help teach at a

Vienna school for the young children of visiting foreigners being analyzed by Sigmund Freud and his daughter Anna. Through his connection to the small school, Erikson was quickly inducted into the inner circle of the Vienna Psychoanalytic Society. Anna Freud provided direction, a personal analysis, and mothering for Erikson, and he bathed as well in the physical presence of Sigmund Freud himself. Erikson himself recalled the thrill of waiting for a therapy session with Anna and seeing Sigmund Freud emerge from the adjacent office and offer a bow before retrieving his next patient.

In 1930 Erikson was formally introduced to a beautiful twenty-six-year-old Canadian woman named Joan Serson, who was visiting Vienna to study dance. Joan, in contrast to Anna, was a warm and spirited woman who came to eschew the insular psychoanalytic community and its approach, which overemphasized the inner mechanics of the psyche and neglected the outer world of activity and socialization. Not only did Joan give order and stability to Erikson's life, but she also had a profound effect on the direction of his work. He had been schooled by Sigmund and Anna Freud in the strict excavation of memories that formed in childhood and attached themselves to the basic structures of the mind—id, ego, and superego. But in his own work Erikson liberated these memories from both the child and its mental template, showing how they continued to evolve and face unique challenges in the active social world of adolescence and adulthood. In many ways, this shift was all Joan.

She was also a catalyst for their move to America in 1933, where they settled in Boston. Erikson began working as one of the first child psychoanalysts in the city. Throughout the 1930s he built an impressive reputation as both an empathic and successful clinician and a serious thinker about child development. This productive time solidified his identity as a psychoanalyst and as an American, a change symbolized in 1938 by his adoption of a new family name—*Erikson*. The name hearkened back to his Scandinavian roots and proved to be a successful alliteration in his later literary fame

In 1939 Erik was invited to join the faculty of the University of California at Berkeley's Institute of Child Welfare, where he began to work in earnest on his theory of human development. Initially, he looked at how children play, at the shapes, forms, and directions of their toys and games, which are partly influenced by the effects of the developing body on the mind. But in contrast to his psychoanalytic roots, Erik saw no sense in speaking of the role of the unconscious mind forged in childhood without reckoning with the equally important roles of society, culture, and the historical moment.

When the product of his clinical work and research emerged in 1950, *Childhood and Society* had a revolutionary effect on American psychological thinking, which at the time was beginning to demand a greater equality of voices. Here was a psychoanalyst who wrote about childhood development as it took place in middle-class white households across America, on the plains of South Dakota with the Oglala Sioux, and on the Pacific West Coast with the Yurok tribe. In it he coined the term "identity crisis" to describe the process of trying to define self-identity during late adolescence and young adulthood. By the 1960s Erik's work was as apt to be found on the bookshelves of scholars as in the hands of young students protesting the war in Vietnam and trying to define a new identity for America. As his fame was spreading, Erik returned to Harvard to teach an undergraduate course entitled "The Human Life Cycle" (and aptly nicknamed "from womb to tomb" by many students). He had both an unconventional style and a relaxed charisma that resonated with students during the turmoil of the time, and his course quickly became one of the most popular on campus. He was an older man who still commanded the trust of a younger generation seeking to overthrow the establishment. In addition, many of his students were in the throes of their own identity crises and looked to Erikson as a guiding light.

Erikson's career reached its zenith between 1968 and 1973. He won both the Pulitzer Prize and the National Book Award for *Gandhi's Truth*, which traced the life of Mohandas Gandhi set against the template of the life cycle. Considered a cultural icon who graced the cover of *Newsweek*, Erikson was consulted by the academic and political elite. In 1970 he taught his famous course for the last time and retired from Harvard, but awards, honorary degrees, and prestigious lecture invitations poured in. As the 1970s drew to a close, however, Erikson was beginning to slow down considerably, beset by several physical illnesses. During this same time, his theories were subject to greater challenge as the psychopharmacologic revolution brought a paradigm shift to psychiatry and psychoanalytic approaches fell out of favor. "It's all poetry," a professor of mine once declared to me, denigrating Erikson's work as nice sounding but unscientific.

As old age loomed and Erikson faced a number of personally devastating critiques of his work, he was fortunate to have his wife and several close associates to help buffer some of the stress.

And yet ever since leaving Vienna, he had not continued with any form of personal psychotherapy, as he had previously done with Anna Freud. "There is the incredible paradox," his daughter, Sue Bloland, related to me, "in that my father is writing about psychoanalysis in such a brilliant and innovative way, and yet he was rejecting it for himself—and my mother was helping him do it." Daughter-turned-psychoanalyst Bloland believes that it was her parents' very fame that enhanced their desire to hide feelings of inadequacy that had deep roots in their childhoods.

A more profound turning point for Erik and Joan Erikson began in 1984 when they returned to Harvard from California for an encore of their seminar on the life cycle. Within a few years they moved into an intergenerational home in Cambridge with Eck and Austin, hoping that this would provide a satisfactory old age. Despite the creation of a center at Harvard to promote Erikson's work, the regard that his writings had garnered in the preceding thirty years had continued to fade, and outside of professional circles he had become much less known. In fact, other than his name none of my roommates or friends at college knew much else about the man I was about to meet. How I even knew his name was a mystery to me, as I had not read any of his works and had had little exposure to his theories. Yet something gripped my attention when the seminar was advertised, and I was drawn to it for mysterious reasons that now seem fateful.

The life cycle seminar had about twenty participants, mostly drawn from Harvard's School of Education. I was the youngest participant, and Erik was the oldest. It was held late in the day in Sever Hall, an imposing nineteenth-century red-brick-and-blood-mortared building in Harvard Yard that looks itself like a giant brick, adorned with two symmetrical round bays that extend the height of its four stories. We met in one of the ground floor bays, sitting around a long wooden table with the Eriksons at the head.

On the first day of the seminar I arrived with nervous anticipation to meet Erik and Joan. As I entered the room, Erikson stood out immediately, with a burning bush of white hair and a faint frosty mustache. His face was a melding of Semitic and Nordic physiognomies, with a beautifully carved nose and cheeks whose skin revealed the bony prominence of age. His tall frame was somewhat gaunt and slightly stooped but magisterial in its oldness. He was a cross between Moses and Thor, and I expected him to be wearing a white priestly robe and bearing in his hand a giant hammer with radiating bolts of lightning. Instead, he wore the colors of the earth: a brown tweed jacket, a stone-colored shirt, and a bolo tie fastened with a round coin of polished granite. On his feet he wore black socks and brown leather sandals. I greeted him sheepishly, and he shook my hand politely, his demeanor quiet. Joan, in contrast, wore a radiant smile, and she greeted with a burst of energy the students who were slowly ambling into the room. Her shirt, shawl, and long skirt matched the earthiness of her husband's clothes but with richer colors and thicker textures, and she was adorned with a stone-beaded necklace.

There was a celebratory mood to the seminar, a feeling of homecoming for the Eriksons. The crisp fall air outside lent a coziness to the group. Each week we explored a different concept from Erikson's work. The discussions were always led by Professor Eck and Dr. Austin, with Erikson appearing to listen intently, nodding along and occasionally offering a few words. My roommates were slightly intrigued but mostly bemused by my hero worship of him, particularly when I told them how excited I was to shake the hand of someone who had shaken hands with Freud. They called him "sandalman" and suggested that I was devoted to him like a young child skipping after the pied piper.

The fundamental theme of the seminar was Erikson's conception of the eight stages of the human life cycle. The idea of staging the life cycle goes back in history at least as far as the riddle posed by the Sphinx in Greek mythology: "What creature goes on four legs in the morning, two legs at noon, and three legs in the evening?" According to the myth, Oedipus solved the riddle because he knew that a man starts off as a crawling baby, then walks upright as an adult, and finally rests on a cane in old age. These three stages gave way to four and then seven as the notion of the rise and fall of human strength and capability across the lifespan was perpetuated by Greek, Roman, and then European writers and philosophers.

Erikson was particularly inspired by Shakespeare, whose protagonist Jaques in *As You Like It* declares,

> *All the world's a stage,*
> *And all the men and women merely players;*
> *They have their exits and their entrances;*
> *And one man in his time plays many parts,*
> *His acts being seven ages.*

Shakespeare goes on to describe each stage from infant to

Last scene of all,
That ends this strange eventful history,
Is second childishness and mere oblivion;
Sans teeth, sans eyes, sans taste, sans every thing.

Unlike Shakespeare's poetic rendering, however, Sigmund Freud was interested less in mere descriptions and more in the whys and hows of each age as it developed during childhood. He believed that successes, failures, and fixations from early childhood stages accounted primarily for the later vicissitudes of personality and that most major psychiatric symptoms had roots in this development. He proposed that symptoms could be understood and, ideally, resolved through psychoanalytic exploration of the mind. Not surprisingly, old age was a conundrum for Freud, a no-man's-land where psychoanalysis initially dared not tread, not because it lacked the means but because "old people are no longer educable." Though he himself was quite productive in his old age, the younger Freud imagined that the "mass of material" in late life would prove too much for the psychic probing of his fledgling science.

Erikson was schooled in this theory but found it insufficient to describe life after childhood and the vital interaction between the inner psychic structures of the mind and the outer influences of the social world—a process he termed the "psychosocial." The heart of Erik's theory lies in this juncture between the mind and the social environment, at once both a struggle and a merging of opposing forces. *Ego-syntonic* forces stoke the sense of self or ego and promote positive growth, whereas *ego-dystonic* forces lead in opposite directions and produce discomfort, withdrawal, or rigid defensiveness.

This theory underlies nearly everything else that Erikson wrote. In each of the eight stages from birth to old age proposed by Erikson, there is a central tension or crisis that emerges and propels development. In Erikson's lexicon, the word "crisis" "does not necessarily connote a threat of catastrophe but rather a turning point, a crucial period of increased vulnerability and registered potential."

The struggles and resolutions in each stage take place in relationships between individuals and across generations and are carried through into successive stages. The endpoint of each stage, ideally, is a tilt toward the ego-syntonic, along with the acquisition of core strengths that form the foundation of successful growth and adaptation. For example, the adolescent who is able to pick and choose among various "confirming ideologies and affirming companions" and commit to several of them as part of his or her identity can develop a strong sense of *fidelity* that will apply throughout life. In young adulthood, where intimacy versus isolation becomes the dominant theme, the acquired strength of fidelity is now applied to a partner and to work, and a new strength—love—is sought. Erikson didn't stop at the individual; he spoke of how our acquired strengths and weaknesses interact with societal values and historical trends.

At the time of the seminar, Erik fell chronologically into the eighth stage, which centers on the task of developing and maintaining a sense of *integrity* with respect to body, mind, and social network in the face of age-associated pressures and losses. In practical terms, this is a person who can examine her present circumstances and review past experiences and have a sense of completeness, understanding, and meaning. In late life "meaning" refers to both an intellectual and an emotional sense of rightness, harmony, and purpose. It may also represent a transcendent, ineffable mental sensation of connection with a larger entity, such as can be found in nature, spirituality, or love. A person may have suffered greatly in life or may still be suffering, grieving, or feeling pain, but he can still find meaning and achieve a broader sense of integrity in day-to-day existence. This is a gift of aging that can be shared across generations.

Despair—"the feeling that the time is now short, too short for the attempt to start another life and to try out alternate roads"—is the opposing ego-dystonic force in Erikson's eighth stage. Such despair may represent many dystonic forces—mistrust of caregivers, shame over a declining and dysfunctional body, an inability to be industrious, lost roles or identities, isolation from loved ones, and stagnation in daily activities—that have collapsed into one and given rise to an overall feeling of disgust with life. Although cultivating a sense of integrity seems to be the only ideal pursuit in later life, Erikson's framework is more supportive of a balance between syntonic and dystonic forces. This does not mean that a little despair is necessarily good, only that an unbridled sense of integrity without some realization of the limited horizon ahead can be problematic. The achieved balance in perspective— a recognition and tolerance of competing life forces and of the reality of death—is what Erikson aptly labeled "wisdom."

At the time of the seminar I imagined that Erikson embodied the eighth stage. His achievements were monumental, and he seemed to be a fount of wisdom and reflection. I now realize that my nineteen-year-old eyes were unable to see the reality of the situation. Erik was attentive but quiet during the seminars, occasionally adding a comment in his heavily German-accented English, along with a small gesture of his hand or a mischievous smile. Because he was revered by the participants, such responses sufficed as meaningful signs from the master. In reality, he offered little more than his presence, and Joan spoke with enough energy and expression for both of them.

One day at a small reception for the seminar, I approached Erikson to discuss the project I was working on—a replication of his 1930s study on children's play constructions. I caught his attention for about ten seconds until he waved me off, simply stating, "I am trying to eat a cookie." Still too starstruck to be angry, I felt deeply embarrassed for bothering him. My roommates howled at the scene when I recounted it later that night, suggesting that such was the fate of anyone trying to chase a guru. I laughed along with them, hoping to dissolve my own confusion and lack of self-esteem in their rather pessimistic assessment. To this day they occasionally remind me of the "cookie scene" as a hard-learned lesson in hero worship.

As I think back on the seminar from the perspective of a well-seasoned geriatric psychiatrist, however, I now realize quite clearly that Erikson was suffering from early-stage dementia—most likely Alzheimer's disease. The symptoms of this dementia accounted in part for his quiet and apathetic demeanor, his inability to make significant verbal contributions to the seminar, his distance, and even his unwillingness to engage in conversation during the cookie scene. In my clinical work I am similarly waved away multiple times a day by patients who are simply too tired, confused, or impatient to speak to me. Indeed, in a biography of Erikson entitled *Identity's Architect*, Lawrence Friedman recounts how by the early 1980s Erikson's writing projects were "erratic" and required "more energy and perseverance than he could summon."

Fittingly, then, in a revised edition of one of Erikson's last works, *The Life Cycle Completed*, a section written largely by Joan Erikson proposes a *ninth* stage to the life cycle, representing individuals in their eighties and nineties beset by the overwhelming demands and difficulties of everyday life. Much of the description of the ninth stage is quite gloomy as it depicts the unraveling of the life cycle due to bodily decline and the loss of autonomy, self-esteem, confidence, and, ultimately, hope itself, casting despair as the dominant force. She writes that "there is much sorrow to cope with plus a clear announcement that death's door is open and not so far away." This perspective depicts our greatest fears of aging, a projection of how miserable life must be without all of the capabilities we cherish in earlier stages.

The theory of the ninth stage, however, is not well developed and seems to reflect Joan Erikson's struggle with aging more than her husband's own thinking. It may also represent the loss of the attention and adulation that was critical to the Eriksons' identities. For Erikson, however, the loss of memory likely brought with it loss of insight and a loosening of his attachments to lifelong concerns, including a need for affirmation from others. Disappointments from unachieved goals that he might have felt late in his career succumbed to the creeping shadows of dementia. His aches and pains in the final years, like his joys, were those of any other individual, famous or not. It is ironic how dementia steals away personal identity just as it finally liberates the mind from traumatic memories and neurotic concerns.

For Joan Erikson, however, the clarity of her mind until her final days allowed her to care for her husband and promote the vestiges of his fame. It also brought the physical and mental burdens of caregiving and, in the words of their daughter, the "dread of being abandoned by the world should it become known that her link with greatness was no longer viable." But to the outside world, Joan Erikson was unfailingly bright and stalwart, and she seemed the embodiment of integrity.

Thus, Erikson's situation in 1984 contained a clear dilemma. On the one hand, he was an accomplished man who had achieved substantial fame and accolades in his lifetime. Though he was failing physically, he could still interact in socially meaningful ways, and he had the support of his wife and many others. On the other hand, he was suffering from cognitive impairment that made it impossible for him to participate verbally and intellectually at the high level of discourse and writing to which he had been accustomed. According to his daughter, however, no one knows if he ever received any formal medical or psychiatric work-up for these symptoms.

Joan Erikson did her best to prop up her husband and act as if he were his old self, and those who didn't know him well but were awed by his presence—as I was—didn't fully appreciate the difference. At worst, others might have chalked up his quiet demeanor to old age. "Mother did everything possible to sustain this deception," Bloland writes, describing how her mother "publicly denied Dad's intellectual decline, celebrating—and often exaggerating—every sign on his part that he understood what visitors said to him." In fact, in her preface to the revised edition of *The Life Cycle Completed*, Joan Erikson continues to project this façade years after her husband's death: "When Erik was ninety-one . . . following hip surgery, he became withdrawn, and he serenely retired. He was neither depressed nor bewildered but remained consistently observing and quietly appreciative of his caretakers. We should all be so wise, gracious, and accepting of old age when it comes our way." Although these words are poetic and comforting, such a failure to acknowledge the sad reality of dementia, in which individuals are truly bewildered and often depressed, may prompt a clash of expectations among caregivers and lead to undertreatment of legitimate illness. This unbalanced perspective limits our ability to understand the truth about aging and then educate others, particularly young people, about what is real.

Today, an individual with Erikson's symptoms would get complete physical, neurologic, and psychiatric evaluations that included a brain scan, cardiograms, blood work, and neuropsychological testing, all designed to discover the cause of the cognitive impairment and make a reasonable diagnosis. This information would guide appropriate care, which would include therapeutic activities geared for the afflicted individual's level of ability and medications to enhance cognition or improve symptoms of apathy, depression, anxiety, or agitation. Doctors did less and had less to offer in 1984, but even so, an eighty-two-year-old man with mild dementia who couldn't conduct a seminar would not, perhaps, have been put in the position to try. But in this case the man was Erik Erikson, and it was both ironic and tragic that the creator of the theory of the life cycle failed to live out his own theory. For how is integrity possible without the ability to remember, appreciate, and articulate the scope of a life?

A lesson from Isaac's old age might be informative here. If we cast Jacob and Esau as respective ego-syntonic and dystonic elements in their father's life, Isaac was able to "see" both while simultaneously elevating one over the other. And consider Isaac's blessing of Jacob: "See, the fragrance of my son is like the fragrance of a field God has blessed. And may God give you of the dew of the heavens and of the fatness of the earth. . . . Peoples will serve you, and regimes will prostrate themselves to you; be a lord to your kinsmen. . . . Cursed be those who curse you, and blessed be they who bless you." If we translate this blessing into a wish for a fruitful life cycle, we might say, "Your presence is special. May you receive what you need in life. May you grow to be your own person. May others find benefit in relations with you (or loss in rejection of you)." And in old age, we might affirm, "May your presence still be meaningful to others. May you receive the care you need. May you still retain some strengths. May you benefit from mutual interactions."

And each component of the blessing was true for Erikson regardless of his mental decline. His presence was magnificent, he received an abundance of care from his wife and others, he still retained the ability to experience life and interact in meaningful ways with others, and these relations brought great blessings to those who spent time with him. His old age showed me how to extend the promises of the eighth stage into the seeming despair of the ninth stage for the oldest, frailest, and most debilitated of our elderly, with whom I now work on a daily basis.

Integrity without the benefit of memory is lived in the moment; it is appreciated through the absence of pain and fear, through the mutuality of affection and social recognition, and through the retained strengths of sensory stimulation, laughter, and creativity. My most enduring images from the seminar are just such moments: a birthday party we had for Erikson during which he joyfully kidded with us, playfully balancing a bouquet of flowers on his head; the Eriksons walking hand in hand across Harvard Yard as they departed from each seminar. These moments, when regarded in all their glory, can serve as a powerful counterpoint to the prevailing view of despair at life's end. They represent the triumph of Jacob over Esau, a view to the heavens rather than to the hunt.

And whether we regard Isaac as an actual historical figure or a fictional character, there is no denying that this tale of a father and his sons sits at the cornerstone of three great faiths. Its lessons have shaped how Western civilization defines morality, elevating the spiritual strength of Jacob over the physical prowess of Esau. Erikson's notion of the life cycle also shows how the story of one life plays a role within the culture and history of many others. We cannot measure a life simply from the vantage point of the nursery or the schoolyard, and the shapes of our lives express more than our genetic endowment or the circumstances of our immediate family circle. The true measure of a life must take into account our place in society, in history, and among the generations.

Within the scope of our seminar, it would have been difficult to study an entire life in such depth. Instead, Erikson used Ingmar Bergman's 1957 film *Wild Strawberries* to demonstrate the life cycle, starting from old age and moving back in time. Beginning in the 1960s, Erikson frequently screened *Wild Strawberries* because "I found in this screenplay an incomparable representation of the wholeness of the human life cycle—stage by stage and generation by generation." Midway through the course, then, we joined the Eriksons for an unforgettable movie night.

The basic plot of *Wild Strawberries* revolves around a daylong journey undertaken by a distinguished seventy-six-year-old Swedish doctor named Isak Borg. He travels by car from Stockholm to Lund, where he is to receive an honorary university degree. In the opening scene, Isak is sitting at his desk the night before the trip and reflecting on his current station in life: "I have found myself rather alone in my old age. This is not a regret but a statement of fact. All I ask of life is to be left alone and to have the opportunity to devote myself to the few things which continue to interest me, however superficial they may be." This strong dystonic element of isolation thus begins the story, and we learn that it runs throughout the course of Isak's life.

The next morning Isak and his daughter-in-law Marianne set out, and the trip is laden with highly symbolic encounters, stops, recollections, and dreams that all serve to recall and reconstruct events from his life. For instance, the first stop is at a wooded summer home along the shore, where he wanders into a wild strawberry patch and daydreams about his cousin Sara, whom he loved and had once hoped to marry. He then encounters a young woman and her two male suitors who need a ride, and their presence serves as a constant reminder of his own early years. The group picks up an angry, arguing couple who are perhaps reminiscent of Isak's own failed marriage. He then visits his cold and critical old mother, in whom we see the genesis of Isak's own isolative and moralistic character. He dreams about being interrogated during a medical school examination, and he is flunked by the professor for demonstrating "indifference, selfishness, lack of consideration." It is a damning critique of Isak's life, pronounced in the dream just before he is led out into the forest, where he witnesses his wife having an affair.

As Isak and Marianne pull into Lund, we find that the events of the day and his interactions with his daughter-in-law, who reveals that she is pregnant with his grandchild, have transformed him. Even in his old age he now seems to have a deeper understanding of both the successes and failures in his life, and he is more emotionally connected to the next generation.

In the final scene of the movie, Isak falls asleep and begins dreaming, finding himself again in the wild strawberry patch with Sara. She takes his hand and leads him to the shoreline, where he sees his parents waving in the distance. He cries out but cannot make himself heard. Nevertheless, he feels at peace. Isak has now completed his journey from old age and impending death back to the first stage and his primal protectors; the cycle has come full circle.

There was an electric feeling in the room as the movie ended, the lights came on, and the group looked to Erikson—as if we were sitting with Isak Borg himself. There was a spirited discussion about the movie, but I do not remember much about Erikson's contributions other than his presence. But we did learn some interesting parallels between Erik and Isak. The movie's idyllic scenes along the Swedish shoreline were certainly a reminder of Erikson's own childhood, when he spent many happy summers at his uncle's house in Denmark only twenty miles across the Oresund waterway from Lund. As an adult, Erikson received the same honorary degree and top hat from the University of Lund as did Isak. And Erikson, like Isak, was now facing the end of his career and the ever-approaching reality of death. But how would his own journey end? Perhaps Isak's tale was an inspiration for Erikson, who had hoped that his own old age would bring similar degrees of honor and revelation. This thought hung over me as the evening drew to a close.

Throughout Isak's daylong journey, the timeline of his life jumps among memories, dreams, and encounters from various stages. One moment he is an old man sitting in an abandoned wild strawberry patch; the next he is a young man again, swooning over the beautiful Sara. Bergman's script echoed Erikson's point that the key elements of each stage of life are embedded in every other, almost like a psychosocial DNA. By the time we reach old age, all the previous lessons of the life cycle become lessons of aging. Nothing is lost from the past, and we carry with us, in one form or another, all of the people, places, and experiences we have encountered.

Perhaps this is what I have found so compelling about Erikson's work. His notion of the life cycle gives a meaningful template to life. It shows us where we've come from and where we are heading. It holds out the possibility for change at any stage, even in the last. Memories can be brought up and reconsidered within the ever-changing context of life. There is the potential for a constant resculpting of identity. We might imagine that aging, like any other stage in life, is fixed in time and form and that our declining anatomy is our destiny. But Erikson's message suggests that the trajectory of a life is more like a tributary of water cascading down the side of a hill and then curling off into the landscape below. At first the tributary follows a cohesive line predictably bent by the angle of the riverbed. But then small lines of water etch through the bedrock, twisting under the influence of unseen pores in the earth until they suddenly open like a flower into the aquifer below.

✷✷✷

More than twenty-five years have passed since the life cycle seminar, and yet I am still inspired by my encounter with Erikson. Out of nostalgia I returned to Harvard Yard in 2009 to retrace my steps. Professor Eck and Dr. Austin had aged a bit, but they were still teaching at Harvard with as much energy and enthusiasm as before, and they greeted me as if hardly a semester had passed since we last met. They both reflected on the last few years with Erikson as he struggled with his failing memory. Dr. Austin described a poignant scene in which Erikson would sometimes sit and read over and over again a page from a small notebook in which he had written the titles of his books. Even as his memory failed, he found ways to reconnect with his past. After I left her office in the basement of Memorial Church, I walked along the brick pathway to Sever Hall and stopped near the bay window of my former classroom. I lost myself in a memory about Erikson.

In 1992, I was working as a medical intern at a small hospital outside Boston when an elderly patient was admitted. It was Erikson. I stood outside his room as he lay quietly in bed, clearly in the final stages of both his physical and cognitive illnesses. There he lay, almost like an infant, unable to communicate and totally dependent on the care of the nursing staff. I had once wondered how his journey would end; now I stood witness. It was painful to be so close to a hero and yet so completely unable to make a personal connection. And yet as I reflected on that moment, I realized that a very deep bond of sorts had been established between two generations of individuals and clinicians—a bond that continues to energize my work. I am reminded of what the Eriksons wrote in their final work together: "If, then, at the end the life cycle turns back on the beginnings, there has remained something in the anatomy even of mature hope . . . without which life could not begin or meaningfully end."

And what was this hope? And for whom? One life ends and passes on, and another generation follows. Aging stands at the juncture between the two, and the enduring connection between the stages of life and all of the forces within are united in a brilliant history. Most of us *will* make it to this point, in one form or another. And we will have the chance to look on ourselves and our loved ones and bestow both a vision and a blessing for the future. This is where the trust of the child can engender the hope of the elder.

Out of blindness, Isaac blessed his son for sustenance, courage, and mutuality—what we would wish for every child. Inured to his own faults, Isak was blessed with a final vision of his life, enabling him to reset his most important family connections—an opportunity that we would wish for every elder. And Erik Erikson himself was blessed by the father of psychoanalysis, Sigmund Freud, who suggested that the role of this once young and uncertain artist would be, simply put, to allow others "to see." Erikson's life was a testament to this blessing. So many years ago he opened my own eyes—and those of countless others—to both aging and the entire life cycle that precedes it in ways that bring great meaning and a deeply felt and abundant sense of hope.

Annabe, Bartleby, and the
Doctor Who Flunks Aging

I am a rather young doctor, but the nature of my work brings me into contact with some extraordinary characters, both patients and mentors. Sometimes, no matter how many years I have practiced, I still find myself a student to the life lessons offered by these individuals. Here is one such lesson, which I will relate through the life of a patient named Annabe and through the prism of a literary figure named Bartleby, both of whom capture the essence of a condition that no diagnostic manual has yet classified.

The aged patient doesn't always listen to the doctor. In fact, some patients take pride in their resistance, seeing it as a reflection of their still-present autonomy even as they approach the end of their lives. I saw this recently with my ninety-three-year-old patient Ben. "I am trying to walk *without* my cane," he told me emphatically as he wobbled out the door of my office. The grin on his face was telling as he attempted to stride through the clinic, blissfully unconcerned that the tip of the cane held uselessly behind his back was smacking into nearly every object in its path. I grabbed his arm as he suddenly lurched toward me in the hallway and implored him; "Ben, how about walking *with* your cane, as the doctors have asked?" Ben just smiled at me, pretending not to hear, and meandered out of the clinic. There wasn't much else I could do. I did not agree with Ben, but I did admire his fortitude and positive attitude. Of course, I say this without intending to sanction or romanticize his behavior— or the broken hip that I feared would result.

Unlike Ben, there are older patients whose resistance appears to the doctor to be both negative and life threatening. Such individuals inspire a sense of obligation to help them, but their refusal to cooperate leaves both doctor and caregiver feeling quite helpless. In more extreme cases, these individuals refuse all tests, treatments, and medications, choosing instead to isolate themselves and wither away without clear reason. And herein lies the case in question, perhaps my greatest failed case as a doctor. What I hoped was a straightforward case of late-life depression ended up defying all of my diagnostic wit and pharmacologic sleight of hand.

✳✳✳

I think of a T-square when I think of Annabe, because in every clinical encounter she was lying horizontally on the bed and I was standing vertically at her side. Even when I sat down next to her, the perpendicular positioning of our meeting only reinforced the fact that we were on such different planes. If only the forty-five-year age difference between us had been the degree of an angle, we might have both had a better vantage point for talking. But that, sadly, was elusive. Her doctor had asked me—rather, *begged* me—to see Annabe because for months she had been refusing everything but food: no blood draws, no baths, no touching of her extremities, no trips out of her room, no visitors. Her soft, raspy voice was articulate, and her responses were curt: "Annabe, how about a bath today?" the nurse would ask, and Annabe would reply, "I'd rather not."

Anyone who is a fan of Herman Melville might immediately be reminded of one of his most intriguing short stories, called "Bartleby." This nineteenth-century tale concerns the struggle of a well-meaning but wholly perplexed attorney to deal with his new employee, Bartleby, who works as a scrivener (or copyist) of legal documents. Bartleby is an odd but initially industrious man who will copy documents endlessly but when asked to do anything else simply replies, "I'd prefer not to." The attorney's disbelief and then astonishment at Bartleby's audacious resistance quickly turn to frustration and then confusion over how to handle him.

For me, Annabe *was* Bartleby. Her resistance, like her very presence at our facility, seemed at first to emerge out of nowhere. She had been transferred from a hospital to our rehabilitation floor and then to a long-term unit, pushed along by an unseen force and without the benefit of any human advocate—family, friend, or otherwise. She suffered from a relatively severe post-polio syndrome and was nearly quadriplegic. She was laid out flat like a board, simply garbed in a shabby white nightgown and covered with a sheet up to her neck. Day after day she lay in bed impassively staring at the ceiling, requesting nothing and refusing everything but a few spoonfuls of broth and Jell-O and an occasional swallow of minced chicken that the nurses could coax into her. She denied feeling depressed or suicidal, but her words seemed to betray a deep hopelessness, as she stated that she would rather not have her existence prolonged any more than necessary. A review of her chart revealed several recent aggressive attempts at antidepressant treatment that had all failed. And now she refused further attempts.

Bartleby, like Annabe, eventually refuses all requests, in his case to copy documents, responding to every entreaty from his boss with the same expression: "I would prefer not to." The attorney's anger is tempered by his perplexity at such an individual as Bartleby, and at times he even feels compassion for such a pitiful figure. As the attorney begins to plot ways to rid himself of Bartleby, now an impassive figure who continues to live in the office space without agreeing to perform any work, he questions his own beliefs: "Again I sat ruminating what I should do. Mortified as I was at his behavior, and resolved as I had been to dismiss him when I entered my office, nevertheless I strangely felt something superstitious knocking at my heart, and forbidding me to carry out my purpose, and denouncing me for a villain If I dared to breathe one last bitter word against this forlornest of mankind."

Even as I felt sorry for this bewildered attorney, I fantasized that he and Melville's other literary characters could emerge from the story for a moment to discuss our mutual, parallel circumstances. In my own case, I tried repeatedly to convince

Annabe to eat more food, to accept some physical therapy, to let the nurses bathe her, and to try another antidepressant, but I was always met with the same ninety-degree sigh and terse "rather not." The nurses were growing increasingly frustrated, and the nursing supervisor fearfully envisioned the arrival one day of a long-lost relative or a crusading ombudsman who would sanction the facility and its staff for the insufficient care of this pitiful woman. During one behavioral team meeting I had a mild fit of passion and loudly questioned why we had admitted Annabe in the first place and how we could find another facility for her. Egged on by my fury, the director of nursing demanded that I immediately send Annabe to the psychiatric ward. I knew that I *could* do it—but what would that accomplish for Annabe? It would relieve us of a burden for a few days, at least, but it would have been akin to dumping Annabe on some other un-suspecting party—much like my literary counterpart attempts to do. My passion subsided as my conscience got the better of me, and I slunk away from the meeting resolved to do nothing other than continue my angular reverie at Annabe's bedside each week.

In a like manner, Bartleby's resistance is maddening to the attorney, yet he is unable to resolve any plan of action to re-move the creature from his office. Instead, he moves his entire office and staff elsewhere, leaving Bartleby alone in the empty space. Soon enough, the new tenants arrive at the attorney's doorstep, seeking his guidance on what to do with Bartleby, who now haunts the hallway outside the attorney's previous of-fice. The attorney returns briefly to confront Bartleby, pleading with him to accept some help finding a new job or a home; the attorney even offers to have Bartleby move in with him! But still the same response: "I would prefer not to."

Annabe, like Bartleby, similarly refused every entreaty. "How about a new room?" I asked, "or some fresh air? I will ask a nurse to wheel you out into the garden by the birdcage. Do you like music? We have a wonderful music therapist!" I was getting desperate, but I didn't fold. "How about a different diet? Or a friendly visitor?" I sent in one of our psychologists for a visit, followed by the geriatric psychiatry fellow when that failed, and then an eager medical student, all to no avail. In the next wave, I sent one of our most dedicated volunteers to see Annabe. When that didn't work, I ordered a new antidepressant. "I'd rather not take it," she told me. Finally, I sent in Stuart, our prized "Volunteer of the Year," known for his sense of humor. "Try jokes," I said, "or that Brooklyn routine you do that worked so well with Stanley the misanthrope upstairs." It didn't work, and Stuart was not elegant in his assessment of Annabe. "She's crazy!" he told me, "and whatever you're doing, Doc, it *ain't* working!" I was deflated. I had no good diagnosis, I had not established any doctor-patient rapport, I had achieved absolutely no progress, and I was quickly earning, I feared, the derision of all staff that had to care for Annabe.

I tried to discern some meaning in Annabe's behavior, but I knew almost nothing about her background and had no informants. On the one hand, I knew from my clinical assessment that, even though she seemed depressed, apathetic, and even suicidal at times, she was not demented. On occasion she would explain her reasoning to me, and even though I disagreed, it came from a fully oriented mind and followed a logical line of thought. Her voice was so faint at times, yet it boomed out a consistent set of wishes, and I felt obligated to respect her right to refuse treatment. On the other hand, her depressive and apathetic tone and the way it suffused her attitudes toward accepting care did seem to warp her capacity to make reasonable decisions. The case was poised on the edge of two opposing lines: Leave her alone, or send her to the hospital for electroconvulsive therapy.

I thought about the many reasons that older patients may refuse help. The most obvious explanation is that the individual is so depressed that he or she lacks the motivation, energy, or will to get better. In these cases, resistance to care is sometimes best viewed as indirect life-threatening behavior, a form of suicide. Other individuals simply deny that they have a problem that warrants treatment, perhaps due to ignorance, lack of education, or a condition called anosognosia in which brain damage, usually to the right hemisphere, has robbed them of insight into their deficits. Individuals with personality disorders are also frequent refusers, particularly those with passive-aggressive, depressive, dependent, or obsessive-compulsive traits. Annabe fit some criteria from these various categories, but none of them captured her.

As much as Melville provided some insight into my own reactions, I needed to seek higher counsel. This I found in a thick, prized volume on my bookshelf that had been inscribed to me many years prior when, as a young college student, I had spent some time in the presence of the author, who was not only a famed psychiatrist but also a great Melville scholar—Henry A. Murray. As one of the founding fathers of personality study (a distinction that had even brought him into Freud's study during a visit to Vienna in 1936), Murray saw in Melville some of the richest personality descriptions in all of American literature. In one particular essay Murray had channeled the characters from Bartleby—including Bartleby himself—into a group discussion about the meaning of their lives. I imagined that Murray's Bartleby also gave voice to Annabe as he stated, "Tired of everything, I had resigned myself to—well, a sort of death in life, and then to no life, the last resource of an insulted and unendurable existence. . . . I also derived some hidden pleasure from witnessing the disturbance I produced in the office, seeing to what extent I became the center of attention, and how, one after the other, they adopted my word 'prefer.'"

Was this it? I wondered. Annabe, like Bartleby, was no passive wisp but a lion under a sheet, displaying not the lack of adherence to treatment that we saw but a fortitude "marked by . . . adherence, despite everything, to the principle of self-sovereignty, the last stand of an oppressed ego." If I turned the angle around—now Annabe upright and me horizontal—I began to see a different configuration. This is not to deny the role of psychiatric illness here, and I take Murray's suggestions that Bartleby (and Annabe) could have suffered from a variety of maladies: anger, obsessive-compulsive disorder, regressed behaviors, and the apathy of the institutionalized. Perhaps none of these terms are adequate and a new clinical entity is required: "I will end," Murray declares, "by crediting Mr. Melville with the discovery of the Bartleby complex."

At the end of the story, Bartleby is taken away to a penal institution, where he continues to refuse all requests, even to eat. When the attorney returns for a final visit, he discovers the wasted form of Bartleby lying on the ground huddled next to a wall, his head touching the stones. "He's asleep, ain't he?" questions the cook observing the scene, to which the attorney replies, "With kings and counselors," realizing that the now-mythic Bartleby has passed on. The attorney concludes his tale by relating something he learned about Bartleby several months after his death: He had previously worked as a clerk in the Dead Letter Office. The attorney realizes the tragic journey of both Bartleby and these Dead Letters, consigned to the flames containing perhaps "a bank note sent in swiftest charity—he whom it would relieve nor eats nor hungers any more; pardon for those who died despairing; hope for those who died unhoping. . . . On errands of life, these letters speed to death."

Seized with emotion, the attorney cries out to the reader one of the most famous lines in American literature: "Ah, Bartleby! Ah, humanity!" Critics may debate the meaning of these lines, but as I hold level in my mind the visages of both Bartleby and Annabe, I understand their passionate cry, how they speak to the unfortunate but common fate of so many elderly individuals.

And thus I have tried to understand Annabe by changing the geometry of our relationship, actually upending my own expectations of her behavior. All of us caring for Annabe expected and eventually pleaded for her to act like a patient and obey two key responsibilities of the "sick role" described by sociologist Talcott Parsons: that she have a desire to get well and that she seek out medical assistance. Instead, she expressed the opposite desire and thwarted our very mission to heal her. Not surprisingly, such individuals produce a lot of unwanted conflict with doctors and come to be viewed as "bad" patients.

And so poor Annabe, like Bartleby, did not receive the sustenance intended for her, and she passed away quietly in her bed one morning, without anyone in attendance or even aware of her departure until several hours later. Sometime after her death I was finally able to review some old records on Annabe from the archives of the veterans hospital in which she had spent much time. These few details I learned: Annabe was born in rural Minnesota to a Norwegian minister and his wife, who died in childbirth. She was initially raised by a young couple in the parish, at her father's request, and then later by an aloof stepmother after Annabe's foster mother died suddenly. After high school she became a nurse in the U.S. Navy on the eve of World War II. Although she suffered from a debilitating bout of polio, Annabe recovered sufficiently to be sent to a field hospital in the South Pacific during the height of the war. Here she was traumatized sufficiently by her exposure to dead and dying soldiers and had to be discharged for psychiatric reasons, listed as alcoholism and war fatigue (and later diagnosed as post-traumatic stress disorder, or PTSD). By her early seventies Annabe's drinking had become so severe that she was unable to function and had to be placed in a veterans home with a diagnosis of dementia. Now abstinent by necessity, she slowly recovered her faculties and was discharged to an assisted living facility. Just as she was beginning to live again, she developed a severe postpolio syndrome that robbed her of her ability to walk and later her ability to coordinate her trunk and arm movements. Annabe was passed from one facility to another until she eventually reached our doorstep.

And so there it was, a life of certain emotional deprivation from the very instant of birth, never having a consistent loving parent to meet her needs. This loss was coupled with the shattering experience of tending to dying soldiers who were leaving young children waiting for fathers who would never come home, wives hoping for children who would never be born, and parents dreaming dreams that would remain forever unfulfilled. At certain moments when I think about our attempts to help Annabe, I feel a twinge of the emotional cry expressed at the end of "Bartleby." Her fate was like that of many unfortunate elders: destined to lie in bed alone, debilitated and dependent on the care of strangers, bereft of dignity, and even scorned before death!

At some point Annabe rebelled against this, refusing to accept what life had given her and declaring that perhaps it is better to be scorned than to be ignored or forgotten. Some unconscious siren called out from her stillness, luring all of us into the desired role that had proved so elusive in her life. She died alone but not forgotten and not without concerned attendants, even if that concern was not always so tender. I understand Annabe a little better now and realize the limits of my profession. Sometimes mothers and fathers or their loving surrogates must intervene where doctors cannot. Absent them, we are all in Annabe's position.

Joseph Red Hair

"I cannot compete with a holy man."

This was the solitary thought running through my mind as I sat and listened to my patient. Joseph Red Hair had many identities, some empowering, others expressing great pain and struggle—Korean War vet, PTSD sufferer, recovering alcoholic, and Lakota tribal elder. At sixty-two he was my *youngest* patient, but aged by experiences during combat that, once revealed, were beginning to unravel our work together. On this particular day he told me of his time with a *wichasha wakan*, or Lakota holy man, who had tried to cleanse him of his intense wartime guilt through a sweat lodge ritual. In my own eyes I was feeling somewhat inadequate as his therapist, wondering how I could ever understand and treat Joseph as the holy man did. What words of wisdom, comfort, or healing could I—a child of the 1970s and son of Western culture—give to this man, a child of the

1930s, son of American Indian culture, and descendent of Crazy Horse? Where was the common ground on which to meet, young doctor with older patient?

Joseph Red Hair was a member of the Lakota tribe, also known as the Oglala Sioux, and he had grown up on the Pine Ridge Indian Reservation in the Black Hills of South Dakota. The land of the Lakota was once a vast undisturbed prairie— an "ocean of grass" stretching from Wyoming to Minnesota where buffalo roamed in the tens of millions before being senselessly slaughtered by American settlers and the U.S. Cavalry. Lakota culture revolved around the buffalo, which were hunted for both physical and spiritual sustenance and from which every last piece of flesh, hide, bone, and sinew was put to use for food, shelter, clothing, utensils, and ritual items. Starting in the mid-1800s, the Lakota suffered one devastating blow after another: loss of land; slaughter of the buffalo; disease, war, and massacres brought on by settlers and soldiers; and, ultimately, an education stripped of traditional ways that was forced on Lakota children during the early twentieth century. Joseph's lineage was touched by all of these events: He was a descendent of the great Lakota warrior Crazy Horse; one of his grandfathers had fought at the Battle of the Little Bighorn in 1876, in which Lieutenant Colonel George A. Custer had been killed and the U.S. Seventh Cavalry defeated; and he had lost relatives in the 1890 massacre at Wounded Knee. Joseph was raised in a family stripped of its spiritual basis and crippled by alcoholism. He was saved, he believed, by the powerful and soothing figure of his grandmother, who plucked him from an abusive home and raised him as her own son.

In 1951, at the age of seventeen, Joseph enlisted in the U.S. Army Paratroops, and he soon found himself in ferocious combat on the frozen plains and hills of Korea. His experiences, at least the ones he shared with me, were horrific. He recalled, haltingly during one session, a battle in which an army buddy was blown up in front of him, showering him with brain tissue. He fell into a dissociative stupor afterward, and once he came to his senses, members of his platoon gave him alcohol to soothe him. Alcohol soon became the chosen medication for his intense stress, and he drank heavily. But worse things lay ahead.

In June 1952 Joseph was stationed in Japan as part of the 187th Airborne Division. He and his buddies were out drinking one night when they were recalled to base for what they thought was another drill. Joseph tucked a bottle of I. W. Harper Bourbon Whiskey under his arm and started going through the motions of preparation. Only when live ammunition was being handed out did he realize that his battalion was being sent on an actual mission. Mail call arrived just before Joseph boarded the C-46 troop transport plane, and he learned from a letter that his beloved grandmother had died. He was stung by the news, but he recalls that the pain eased after he took a shot from the whiskey bottle he had in his possession.

Flying into a thunderstorm, the plane climbed and then dropped suddenly, its fuselage shuddering back and forth and sounding like it was coming apart. Joseph was terrified. As he sobered up and grew increasingly grief-stricken over the loss of his grandmother, he became convinced that he would die on the plane, especially after hearing on the radio that another plane had gone down. "I went to a wall in that experience,"

Joseph related to me. "I kinda know when people go insane. I went to a wall where I was experiencing total fear and horror. I prayed my grandmother's prayers, and I did everything I could do in my mind and heart and spirit to take me to a place where I could accept death. I thought about my ancestors in the spirit world, and then all of a sudden I had a sense of peace."

Joseph does not recall the rest of the trip, but on arriving at Koje-do Island off the southern coast of Korea, he and his men were ordered to retake a prison camp that had been commandeered by thousands of Chinese prisoners. According to Joseph, the mission went awry when several of his men were killed during the assault on the camp, perhaps due to friendly fire in the haze of the smoke used as camouflage. Joseph described the deep rage that erupted among the troops, so that "when the Chinese dead were brought out of the compound, people drew their machetes and started cutting heads, arms, and legs off and put gasoline on them and started burning them. And if you've ever smelled burning flesh, it never leaves you." Joseph recalls incongruous feelings of fascination and rage mixed with revulsion, fear, grief, and guilt.

Decades later it was still hard for him to reconcile these actions. "I never thought I would participate in something like that. That's the thing that bothered me for a long time. I came from a peace-loving family. My grandparents were very spiritual people and very gentle, and here I was participating in something that I know now any human being would be driven to that point to act out and to commit those atrocities." It was warfare, he reasoned, and yet the trauma left an indelible mark. In his mind, he descended into a place of evil, inhabited by the Lakota spirit Iya, who is responsible for all other evil beings in the world and who brings only destruction and suffering. According to tribal legend, Iya would disguise himself as an abandoned infant who, once rescued and brought unwittingly into a tribal camp, would swallow it up in one gulp.

In the years following that mission, Joseph sensed the presence of Iya and other spirits in his dreams and visions and in the shadows of his daily life. On some nights he would be visited by a faceless buddy from his platoon who appeared out of the shadows and entreated him: "We've got to talk about this." He struggled with intense guilt and tried, for years, to drown it in alcohol. As a result, his life played out much as the Korean War had, with arduous battles advancing him forward, alternating with retreats in the face of enemy hordes, eventually culminating in a tense truce along an artificial border. For Joseph, the advances were marriage, children, an educational degree, and a stable teaching position, forced back time and time again by endless waves of beer and liquor and furious hordes of slain enemy troops who haunted his memories and visions. Most painful was the fact that when Joseph was visited by these spirits, they appeared to him like his own people, their Asian physiognomy resembling that of American Indians in general and of some of his relatives in particular. He felt unable to conduct the Lakota ceremonies once used by his ancestors to ritually honor the spirits of those they had killed in battle. He was stuck with an uneasy armistice, living both on the reservation and in a large city miles away, seeking wisdom and healing from both a wichasha wakan and a psychiatrist.

When I first began seeing Joseph, I wondered whether he was experiencing transient psychotic symptoms because his "visions" sounded like hallucinations. Yet his spiritual tradition provided a better explanation. In Lakota culture, both dreams and visions hold the key to understanding a person's life and destiny, and they are actively sought and interpreted. According to Lakota teachings, a Lakota spiritual leader once had a vision of Iktomi, a spirit of mischief and teacher of wisdom, who appeared in the form of a spider and wove for him a web in his ceremonial willow hoop. This woven dreamcatcher was Iktomi's gift to the Lakota people to help collect good ideas, dreams, and visions, while letting the bad ones flow through the open center. Many American Indians hang these circular dreamcatchers above their beds, decorated with beads, yarn, and feathers. Joseph's dreamcatcher, I imagined, had collected many good forces in his life, including warm visions of his grandmother and ancestral land, bonds with his children, and the powerful and protective image of a spirit named Standing Buffalo. At the same time, the dreamcatcher was clotted with other forces that couldn't find a way out: gruesome battle scenes, sneering faces of enemy soldiers, alcoholic binges, and infidelities. These inescapable, haunting memories drove Joseph's alcoholism for many years and remained even after he became sober for good. Sitting in my office, I saw a clear case of post-traumatic stress disorder.

PTSD, once referred to as war neurosis or combat fatigue, did not come into prominence as a psychiatric illness until the 1980s, largely driven by the experiences of Vietnam War veterans. The clinical picture of PTSD centers on the intrusive re-experiencing of traumatic memories, often in the form of flashbacks or nightmares, and accompanied by intense fear and physiological arousal. The brain of the PTSD sufferer is stuck in the trauma, unable to separate the memories from the physiological fight-or-flight response that was adaptive during combat but crippling at all other times. Persistent hyperarousal develops as a response to imagined threats and is characterized by insomnia, irritability, angry outbursts, poor concentration, an exaggerated startle response, and hypervigilance. Individuals suffering from PTSD will try to avoid thoughts, feelings, people, and places that trigger these painfully charged memories. This avoidance may evolve into loss of memory for certain aspects of the trauma, decreased interest in activities, detachment from relationships, and loss of hope for the future. PTSD is typically associated with severe depression, anxiety, and substance abuse. Ironically, in severe PTSD the very brain structure that is responsible in the first place for coding the traumatic memories— the hippocampus—is known to shrink over time and impair verbal memory function, perhaps in response to persistently elevated levels of the body's stress hormone cortisol.

When I began seeing Joseph in the mid-1990s, a number of forces were coming together at the same time to change our understanding of late-life PTSD. Veterans Affairs (VA) hospitals were, by necessity, evolving into geriatric facilities treating growing numbers of aging World War II and Korean War veterans. At the same time, veterans who had previously coped with or suppressed underlying PTSD were now appearing with old symptoms triggered by the trauma of age-associated stresses such as retirement, medical illness, or loss of spouses and other loved ones, as well as by many events of the time: the first Persian Gulf war and the growing number of fifty-year anniversaries of World War II events. Many of these veterans had always suffered from PTSD but without a formal diagnosis and thus without treatment. As word got out in the VA system, they arrived in droves, Joseph Red Hair among them.

Like many older veterans with PTSD, Joseph had been treated with both individual and group psychotherapy and was already on an antidepressant when he came to see me. His symptoms were still severe and caused a chaotic life beset by nightmares, depressed and anxious moods, and periods of suicidal thinking. He had been able to maintain a tenuous sobriety, largely due to an inpatient stay at a national treatment center and the strong support of his third wife. I was never quite sure whether he would show up for appointments, because he canceled frequently and was difficult to track down. When he missed an appointment, I could sometimes reach him by phone at his house in the city. Many times he disappeared for weeks on end, traveling either back to Pine Ridge or to some other, unknown place. Even as he began to divulge more of his life history, he resisted my treatment suggestions, asking instead that I wait until he was able to consult the wichasha wakan and revisit the sweat lodge.

As Joseph began to describe more detailed and gruesome memories, he reduced the frequency of his visits, and I started to doubt my effectiveness as a therapist. I tried to limit how much he told me, knowing that his words were triggering an overwhelming flood of emotions. There is a strong nonverbal component to memory that is easily triggered in PTSD. These experiential memories are beyond words and will persist in older individuals despite extensive talk therapy and even in the face of impairments in memory and other mental abilities. Joseph sought relief through traditional Lakota ceremony, in which the holy man sought to restructure Joseph's experiences in the sweat lodge through prayer, chanting, drumming, the burning of sage and cedar, and the interpretation of visions and dreams. The image of a braided Lakota warrior named Standing Buffalo was given to him as a form of guardian angel to guide and strengthen him in his quest.

Over time, I sensed that I was losing Joseph as a patient, and I was sure that the wichasha wakan wasn't faring any better. Joseph didn't seem ready to fully trust either one of us, because his symptoms persisted regardless of the setting, whether in the sweat lodge or on the psychiatrist's couch. His last message to the clinic spoke of his misery but did not betray the fact that I would not see him again: "The patient needs to reschedule the appointment—he's paranoid about coming in today."

Everything I knew about Joseph Red Hair was spoken to me, and yet I understood that, although healing would begin with words, resolution would be found beyond them. There was a primal emotional force sustaining his symptoms, born out of a cauldron of horrific wartime experiences and conflicting emotions that no eighteen-year-old should have to face. His ancestral world had already been shattered, and now his personal one shared the same fate. He had crawled away physically alive from the battlefield, dousing the pain with alcohol, and he had even managed to make a life, but the spirit of Iya—of evil and destruction—was his frequent companion. I suspected that as much as Joseph despised and tried to avoid this force, he also embraced it as a well-deserved punishment, a perpetual act of atonement for his self-described evil actions.

My position with Joseph was not unlike that of many colleagues in geriatric psychiatry who attempt to understand and empathize with individuals of advanced age who suffer from multiple medical problems and often come from vastly different backgrounds. Sometimes these patients are unable to even communicate verbally due to language disturbances (known as aphasia). When patients do not feel understood, or do not sense that there is a shared mission with the doctor, they often retreat—directly by not returning to the doctor or the clinic or indirectly or passively by not following treatment directives. The clinician, in turn, may lose hope in the patient's ability to get better.

The antidote, it seems, is to cultivate a sense of empathy for the patient, to be able to creatively imagine what he or she is thinking and feeling, and to mentally "oscillate from being observer to being participant to being observer." The expression of empathy requires the capacity to listen closely and the ability to respond with physical attentiveness through eye contact, physical demeanor, and voice cadence, all of which indicate some degree of emotional resonance. Empathy also extends beyond the words exchanged between doctor and patient. At the same time, a good doctor must maintain appropriate boundaries without succumbing to his or her own emotional reactions to "feeling" a patient's pain. Unbridled empathy, without boundary, purpose, or true positive regard for the patient, can become manipulative, misleading, and even destructive. It can rob the patient of autonomy.

When working with older patients, including Joseph, I cannot always empathize with experiences or emotions that are foreign to me. How can I know what it is to be ninety-eight? Or to face the death of so many beloved friends and relatives? Can I really imagine what Joseph felt in the heat of battle or after he saw the physical destruction of his buddy? Frankly, most of us do not want to even imagine such experiences and emotions. And when we do, we can wind up feeling depressed, emotionally depleted, even traumatized. Such moments are like comforting a mourner, when words fail us and the best we can do is to simply be present in his or her grief.

In these situations, there is a mutual virtue of hopefulness that is crucial to healing and that goes beyond the spoken words of the doctor-patient relationship. According to Erik Erikson, hope "is the enduring belief in the attainability of fervent wishes, in spite of the dark urges and rages which mark the beginning of existence." It is "both the earliest and the most indispensable virtue inherent in the state of being alive." Hope is a human strength shaped by the mother-infant bond prior to the formation of verbal memories, and it lays the basis for trust in others. When empathy is difficult to conjure, then, we can still share with others the hope that a better state of physical and mental health can be achieved, regardless of the situation. Even with terminally ill patients, the doctor can seek to improve health through reduction of pain, relief of depression, and restoration of personal dignity.

Thinking about Joseph, I realize that the wichasha wakan and I shared this virtue in our work with him. This hopefulness was both a nonverbal sense of communion with him and a more mature, verbally expressed hope—perhaps better termed "optimism"—that he would get better. I could not offer him the burning of sage or the beating of drums in my office, but I could offer my genuine intent to listen to him, to be present for him, and to guide him through the best that Western psychiatry could offer.

Many older individuals who successfully adapt to aging do so by returning to and reinvigorating symbolic pursuits full of meaning and hopefulness that capture the basic trust of early childhood. Others are not so successful, and lacking this hope, they become preoccupied with the immediate gratification of basic needs for food, warmth, bowel and bladder release, physical touch and affection, and relief of pain. In the first stage of life, the infant's behaviors to get needs met are appropriate and life sustaining; in the last stage of life, these strivings appear uncomfortably noisy, out of control, and undignified. Nevertheless, there is a relentless drive in later life to recapture this ineffable experience of trust that has no words and yet carries the basic promise of life.

More than fifteen years after I last saw Joseph, I became curious about what had happened to him (he was now seventy-seven). I was able to get a message to him through the alcohol treatment center where I remembered he had worked as a volunteer. Several days later I heard a familiar voice over the phone; it was Joseph. I reminded him about our work together, which he recalled fondly, and I asked him how his life had been since that time. What I discovered both relieved and amazed me: *Joseph had gotten better.* In the years since our last meeting, he became a respected tribal elder as well as a spiritual counselor for individuals with substance abuse, leading his family, his people, and many suffering addicts through ceremonies that bestowed faith and hope. Joseph returned to the reservation and reclaimed his family's ancestral land. He built a home and planted on his land, and he acquired a small herd of buffalo. He commented on his life's work by saying that the language of the spirit consists not of words but of symbols, ritual, and ceremony. True healing, he discovered, can be found only by going to this deeper level. The vision of Standing Buffalo that had sustained him for so many years was now a living reality on his own land. His life had come full circle, and age had brought him the peace and respect accorded to elders in Lakota culture.

As we finished our phone conversation, I heard Joseph calling to his wife, asking her to remind him of the name of the spirit now assigned to his own grandson, a marine on his way to Iraq. The spirit of Joseph's own grandparent carried him through Korea; now he would support and inspire his grandson in Iraq, as he would his fifty-six other grandchildren scattered around the United States. And what spirit still carried Joseph? "One of the ways we address God," he told me, "can be translated from the Lakota language as meaning *something in sacred motion*. And we know that everything is not stagnant—everything is in motion, and everything is connected." Joseph Red Hair was also Joseph the elder, the healer, and the holy man. In his old age he had discovered a timelessness to the connections among us, a spiritual force beyond the confines of words, of age, and of oldness, accessible to every generation. This was still his guide: "Just be present and open all of the doors around you. Allow the natural spiritual vibrations to come into you and heal you."

Old Pickled Brain

Every old brain has a tale to tell. Sometimes the ravages of age are apparent on simple visual inspection of the organ when it is lifted from its slotted seat in the skull and placed in the pathologist's brine. The serpentine grooves between the aged folds of the brain, once closely pressed together like the fisted fingers of a baby, are now separated by large gaps and channels and resemble the withered meat of a walnut. Remnants of previously robust elastic blood vessels appear as hardened tendrils. Many specimens contain evidence of small strokes and tumors. A slice of brain from any level or lobe, stained and prepped for the microscope, reveals numerous small plaques of toxic amyloid protein surrounded by a debris field of dead neurons.

Mr. Summerhill had such a brain, I imagined, an old brain pickled by years of heavy drinking that at one point crested at a bottle of whiskey daily. I couldn't see the actual brain, mind you, but meeting the seventy-five-year-old man himself made the point all too clearly. His wife had finally had enough of his drinking and threatened divorce one evening, triggering an episode of madness in which he ran around the house ranting and raving and threatening to kill both of them. She called the police, and they hauled him off to a nearby emergency room, where he calmed down, sobered up, and then suffered a seizure after thirty-six hours without imbibing his routine brew. It also turned out that he had been taking massive doses of an antianxiety medication, and now the receptors in his brain had revolted without their daily fix. A neurologist saw him and started an antiseizure medication. Shortly thereafter, the extremely wealthy Mr. Summerhill, now rendered homeless by his wife's restraining order against him, was spirited out of the hospital by his attorney and arrived on the doorsteps of our rehabilitation facility.

I found him ensconced in his one-bedroom suite in the VIP wing of the facility, surrounded by a retinue of personal assistants and attorneys. His secretary, Betty, was gathering and arranging papers for three suited attorneys, while his butler and driver shuttled drinks and snacks into the room. Mr. Summerhill, or Alvin as he requested I call him, was extremely cordial and even deferential when we met. "I hear you're a Harvard man, as am I," he informed me, "and I also have a medical degree from your alma mater." In fact, I noted somewhat suspiciously that most of the staff were referring to him as "Dr. Summerhill." He was dressed in baggy gray sweatpants and a neatly ironed blue tennis jacket, and his gray hairs were remarkably well coiffed for a man who had just spent several days in a hospital. His muscular build surprised me, as it resembled that of a much younger man.

The entourage was impressive, but Summerhill was having a hard time maintaining his polished demeanor. One minute he was sitting calmly, whereas the next he was snarling at his staff and threatening to fire them. Several minutes later he would turn smiling to me and his attorneys and answer questions in a seemingly logical but completely false way, what we refer to in psychiatric lingo as "confabulation." The old pickled brain was trying its best to stay on course, but ironically the absence of alcohol and prescription drugs had unleashed a growing beast. With each passing hour Summerhill grew more hyperactive, grandiose, erratic, and inappropriate.

His attorneys pressed me for a quick solution, knowing that they could never settle a multi-million-dollar divorce case with a certifiably crazy old man. "But what if he *is* crazy?" I questioned them, trying to blend in with their less-than-legal slang. Their responses ignored the growing reality of the moment: "He can't be—just fix him." I decided that the rehabilitation wing was no place for a manic and possibly demented man with a serious drug and alcohol addiction, and so I arranged for him to go to a high-class substance abuse treatment center for the elderly in Palm Beach.

As he was preparing to leave, Summerhill's mind was gyrating out of control. First, he fired—*again*—his entire staff. Second, he asked us to summon his three sons from around the country. "Money is at stake!" he roared. "We'll see who loves me best!" He then asked me if the ambulance could bring a young woman to play with his penis on the way to Palm Beach. "Alvin, I would recommend that you *not* ask that," I implored. "OK, good advice," he said, and then ten minutes later turned to the attractive female EMT, "Will you play with my penis?" She suppressed a smile, hoisted the patient onto a gurney, and answered curtly, "Time to go, Mr. Summerhill." "That's *Doctor* Summerhill!" Alvin replied with a perverse grin.

❈❈❈

Look into the brain of even the most mentally impaired young person, and, barring any recent physical trauma, you'll see a relatively normal-sized brain without anything that betrays its derailed functioning. We still know precious little about what actually is occurring in the brain to disrupt thinking, mood, and behavior, and much of what we do know is extrapolated after the fact. It was the survival of numerous head-injured soldiers during World War I that accelerated this knowledge, because we knew where they'd been hit and how they acted afterward. Damage to the frontal lobe produces changes in judgment, motivation, and language function. Damage to the occipital lobe located in the back of the brain brings changes in visual perception. But such localization of brain function tells only part of the story, because most of our abilities are spread throughout the brain, and higher-order ones, such as consciousness and compassion, lie somewhere beyond our understanding.

Seventeenth-century French philosopher René Descartes subscribed to the belief that our true God-given spirit resided in a small organ in the middle of the brain called the pineal gland and somehow exerted its ghostly vapors therein. "Ridiculous!" we scoff at such beliefs, but with what do we replace them? We speak not of "vapors" today but of "chemical imbalances" that we cannot see but can only infer from stained slices of rat brain or deduce from the fact that boosting levels of chemicals such as serotonin or dopamine in the brain has profound effects on mood, behavior, and perception. The terms and techniques have become more sophisticated since the days of Descartes, but we are still wrestling with the same question of how a human mind emerges from a gray blob of brain matter. Contemporary philosopher John Searle has tried to answer this question with a simple formula. Mind and brain, he asserts, are not two separate things but one in the same, such that "all mental phenomena, whether conscious or unconscious, visual or auditory, pains, tickles, itches, thoughts, in deed, all of our mental life, are caused by processes going on in the brain." This is true for young and old brains alike.

❀❀❀

Summerhill's brain had a rough course in Palm Beach. Though he was sober, having been off both booze and antianxiety meds for several weeks, his memory lapses and hyperactivity were worse. Increasing doses of antiseizure medication, mood stabilizers, antipsychotics, and, eventually, lithium were brought in to dowse the cerebral fire, but with limited success. When I visited him at the request of his attorneys, he was insistent on leaving and returning to his apartment. "But your wife has a restraining order against you," I reminded him. "To hell with her!" he bellowed at me. "I'll sneak in and get what I need!" These moments of willfulness worried me the most. His poor judgment and paranoia could get him into serious trouble, and he had vast financial funds to fuel such trouble. I suggested to his attorney that a legal guardianship was needed before Summerhill, left to his own devices, brought catastrophe on himself and others.

After my visit to Palm Beach, I didn't imagine seeing Summerhill again, but his absence turned out to be a brief respite from a coming storm. After being discharged from the Palm Beach facility, he bounced between one son's house in northern Florida and several five-star Miami hotels, all the time in the company of his secretary, butler, cook, and team of attorneys. I now understood how the eccentric and obsessive-compulsive billionaire Howard Hughes used to get by without ending up in a psychiatric institution. With enough money and staff, a person can call the shots, no matter how insane she or he may be. And so it went, for a while at least, with Summerhill.

One night I received a call from a hospital in Orlando where he had been admitted after having some form of either stroke or seizure. "Was he drinking?" I asked the ER physician. "No, his blood alcohol level was nil." It was becoming clear that I was the only one who really knew Summerhill's history, and even in his fog Summerhill recognized this and made it known to every doctor he saw. "Was he taking his medications?" The ER doc called up the lab results—the blood levels were all in range, except one. Summerhill had apparently taken a few doses of ibuprofen, which pushed his lithium level into a toxic range, resulting in slurred speech and muscle jerks. Lithium is perhaps the best mood-stabilizing medication available, but it is also the most toxic, having a narrow therapeutic window below which it is useless and above which it is deadly. Summerhill was the last person a doctor wanted on lithium, because his impulsivity, poor judgment, and generally uncooperative demeanor interfered with safe monitoring.

I could see where Summerhill was heading. He was sober, but years of alcohol and prescription drugs that had kept the lid on an underlying bipolar disorder were no longer in effect, resulting in mania and psychosis. He also seemed to have a mild dementia from the severe alcohol abuse, manifested in his wildly disjointed stories about his past and recent history. And finally, a survey of Summerhill's life history that I gleaned from his three sons pointed to an extremely obsessive-compulsive and narcissistic man whose very personality dysfunction had led to his financial success as a ruthless and detail-obsessed investor. At the same time, his nasty and capricious demeanor took a toll on everyone around him. I feared that without aggressive intervention he would either end up killing himself or someone else, or his slowed, clumsy, and erratic intellect would continue sputtering out until total dementia set in. I did not imagine that his old pickled brain was capable of much else.

I thus reached a point with Summerhill that I had experienced many times before with other older patients, when a doctor must make a decision in the face of supposed fate and futility. Give up and let nature take its course, or leap in and actually do what needs to be done. In practice, this is not the difference between doing nothing and doing everything, as debates on health care seem to imply. It's not the difference between pulling the plug and trying to jump-start a comatose brain. Rather, it's the difference between settling for the achievement of some physical comfort and striving to enable life *and* positive growth, comfort *and* meaning. It's about not giving up.

I conferred with Mr. Summerhill's attorneys, and we brought him back to the rehabilitation facility. They obtained a temporary guardianship, and I committed myself to going in front of a judge to support that petition. Despite the long odds, we decided to try to save Summerhill. For myself, I could honestly say that his wealth was not the issue. After all, I could charge him only the same Medicare rates I charged everyone else, and what I earned in a month of treatment was less than what his attorneys earned in one hour of billable time. For me, this was about pushing the envelope of psychiatric care and testing my own abilities to care for someone; it was about seeing if I could actually pull the brain from the brine.

From the start, however, things did not go well. Summerhill was demanding, impulsive, and just plain rude. Every other day he tried to fire staff members. He insisted on smoking cigars in prohibited areas. He called in his attorneys for endless meetings during which he would take copious, disorganized notes. As the guardianship hearing approached, we met with his three sons to discuss a long-term plan. Summerhill was paranoid about their intentions. "What do you want of my estate?" he yelled. "Who loves me most?" he demanded to know. Each son entreated him to be sensible and tried to reassure him of their intentions, but Summerhill was too far gone to understand. Amazingly, these were nice boys who had somehow survived growing up with a tyrannical, alcoholic, and manic father.

As the guardianship hearing approach, I tried my best to regulate Summerhill's medications, but they were only poor brakes on a speeding freight train. Every other day I was being called for one emergency or another. The final straw came late one Thursday afternoon when Summerhill and his sponsor from Alcoholic's Anonymous attempted to drive off campus against our explicit instructions. I was called out to the guardhouse, where Summerhill sat jumping about in the front seat of the car, wide-eyed and enraged over the guard's refusal to open the gate. "Drive though it! Knock it down!" he screamed at his AA sponsor, who sat in the driver's seat, trembling and confused at the scene. I went toe-to-toe with Summerhill. "You've got to stop this, Alvin. It's not safe for you to leave." I reminded him of the scene he had caused at a restaurant another day when he had run out without paying and then had tried to hitchhike barefoot back to his former penthouse. "It's all lies! I will sue you, sue this place, and all of you will go to jail!" Summerhill could be amazingly sharp and intimidating when he was in a fury.

It was time for the nuclear option. I wrote up a form to involuntarily send him to the county hospital for treatment and then called the Miami Police to enforce the order. After an hour of wrangling with an astonishingly patient and empathic police sergeant, Summerhill gave up and walked into the ambulance. That night he hit rock bottom. When his attorney went to check up on him in the crisis unit at the emergency room, he discovered that Summerhill had stripped himself nude and was ranting, weeping, and frenetically pacing around the quiet room in the smeared puddles of his own urine and excrement. Summerhill's madness was in full bloom. Hearing this, I thought of old King Lear's madness over the loss of his kingdom: "You see me here, you gods, a poor old man, / As full of grief as age; wretched in both."

The doctor at the county psychiatric ward was not a finesser with meds. He dropped the Daisy Cutter on Summerhill's brain using a combination of high doses of the antipsychotics Thorazine and Haldol. Within a day Summerhill was calmed, fogged, slightly rigid, and drooling. I gently suggested to his attorney-turned-guardian that we get him to a nearby geriatric psychiatry ward where I could have a colleague pursue a kinder, gentler regimen. Summerhill was three-quarters gone by now, and I wasn't certain who or what would eventually emerge.

※※※

Sometimes the brain in late life hits a tipping point where it can no longer sustain previous levels of intellect and function. At that point the effects of both medical problems and medications on the brain become exaggerated, and a normally innocuous infection of the bladder or even a toothache can cause a rip-roaring delirium. In such a state, coherent speech gives way to babbling; motor agility surrenders to aimless, uncoordinated picking and pinching; and the air fills with hallucinated images of long-lost loved ones, infestations of bug and rodents, or Lilliputian people tumbling about the room. A manic state and a psychotic state in an older brain are similar in the disorganization they produce, often likened to a mental bonfire where the roaring flames toss back and forth like the outstretched arms of a group of frenzied dancers. A doctor's instinct in the case of both delirium and mania—which can exist simultaneously—is to throw everything on the fire to put it out. But the process of smothering the fire can nearly kill what's left of the human within.

The key is to learn when to advance and when to back off, to select the medications and proper doses that help and avoid those that hurt, and to sense when it's time to act and when patience must reign. Doing so is an art as much as a science, but one best infused with an attitude of care and commitment.

Writer Jay Neugeboren, whose brother Robert suffers from chronic schizophrenia, describes the spirit of this enterprise so well. Based on his own observations over the years, Neugeboren describes the ideal approach of a mental health clinician as being a commitment to a long-term relationship, saying in effect, "I believe in your ability to recover, and I am going to stay with you until you do."

❈❈❈

In many cases with older mentally ill individuals, there is tremendous variability from day to day and from medication to medication, often too much to know with certainty which path is best. Summerhill was a particular challenge because he lit up across the entire diagnostic spectrum, from dementia to substance abuse to personality disorder to severe bipolar disorder, and he had failed most treatments. But after following Summerhill for so many months, I could recite his entire history by rote. I had produced the definitive treatise on his life and mental condition for the judge. Intellectually, I knew he was far gone, but emotionally I was still drawn to the case. Despite the long odds, I wanted badly to succeed.

At the geriatric psychiatry ward I engaged the assistance of my mentor and colleague Dr. Stone to retool the treatment plan. We stopped the medicines that were making Summerhill nonfunctional. Instead, we used a long-acting injectable medication that would guarantee both compliance and a reliable blood level of the medication. Once injected into Summerhill's gluteal muscle, the small blob of antipsychotic degraded slowly over the course of two weeks, when another injection was needed. We added on top two oral medications that would augment the first by rebalancing the chemical neurotransmitters in the brain that we believe lie at the heart of bipolar mania and psychosis without overwhelming the circuits. After several weeks Summerhill was calm, alert, and conversant. He was still somewhat stiff and slowed, but the trade-off was necessary for the time being. We had clearly pulled him back from the brink. Over the course of several months Summerhill became more mentally engaged. He behaved appropriately at the guardianship hearing, and the judge decided to hold off on a permanent guardianship. Summerhill was free, but under close supervision. He agreed to work closely with me to get better.

Over the next year something remarkable happened. Summerhill's mania, psychosis, and cognitive impairment began to evaporate. He attended AA and maintained his sobriety. He returned to my office weekly for counseling and medications, and his impulsive, inappropriate, and self-centered demeanor subsided. After his divorce was settled, he found a girlfriend and began to cultivate near-normal relationships with his sons and their families. The boozing, pill-popping, deranged Summerhill who had swaggered through the social and financial corridors of Miami for several decades was no more. One of my most impaired patients became my most compliant. Though the financial meltdown that hit the country nearly wiped out most of Summerhill's cash reserves, he endured and adapted. Out of the fog his intellect reemerged, and a man who a year prior I would not have trusted to safely walk across the street was driving, managing his finances, and seeking out new ventures.

To this day I still marvel at Summerhill. Once the bipolar disorder and substance abuse problems that had plagued his entire adult life, twisting his personality into a Frankenstein monster of a man, were resolutely treated, a normal older man emerged. With time, the old pickled brain, chemically rebalanced and freed from years of mind-numbing toxins, turned out not to be so pickled. The resilience of the Summerhill brain reminded me of a stunning discovery in 2008 when pathologists studied the donated brain of a Dutch woman, Henrikje Van Andel-Schipper. Her brain was not merely old; it was the oldest brain in existence at the time of her death that year at the age of 115. Such a brain would normally be riddled with pathological findings. But not so with this old brain; in fact, it appeared remarkably normal, with almost no evidence of any age-related changes beyond what would be found at about age 75. These findings corresponded to Van Andel-Schipper's normal performance on standardized neuropsychological tests conducted at the age of 112.

Not every old brain, of course, will be in such terrific shape. And not every older individual with the mental illness of a Mr. Summerhill can be salvaged. But there are always the promise and the possibility if we at least try to find them. My patient and friend Mr. Summerhill knows this well, and he instructed me during our last appointment to write his case down for posterity. I promised him I would try.

Lousy

It's only a guess, but something must have happened in the tank. It was December 1944, and a bitter winter had settled over the Allied forces in the Ardennes Forest in Belgium. A furious and unexpected German offensive punched a large bulge in the American and British lines, inflicting heavy casualties on both infantrymen and Sherman tankers. It may have been the threat of or even the actual explosive graze of a menacing *Panzerfaust* charge against his tank or perhaps the terrifying whine of incoming rockets from the *Nebelwerfer*s. Whatever it was, James was never the same. I was able to gather a few facts from a yellowed note in his chart at the veterans hospital dating back to 1945: He was first hospitalized in England for severe nervousness and vomiting, diagnosed with shell shock, and while in the hospital refused to take off his helmet.

Curious thing about the helmet but explainable: What was once called shell shock or war neurosis but is now called post-traumatic stress disorder involves several characteristic symptoms, including hypervigilance, intrusive flashbacks, and avoidance of any stimuli that trigger a state of panic. For James, as with every combat-related PTSD sufferer, part of his mind still lived on the battlefield. The helmet was a necessary accoutrement.

Somewhere along the line, however, James managed a truce with these memories, discarded the helmet, and moved on with his life, marrying twice, fathering two sons, and finding gainful employment as a meat-cutter. When I first met him, he was a seventy-eight-year-old widower who had retired from a large supermarket chain and was living alone in a small suburban house. Although he still had a designated service connection to the VA hospital for "neurosis" that guaranteed free treatment, he had avoided any contact with psychiatry for decades. He came to me reluctantly, then, suspicious about my intentions and insisting that he was only doing his internist a favor. His complaint was clear and about as nonpsychiatric as it could get: "I've got lice."

A year before our meeting John had appeared at the VA emergency room with a bloody nose and complaining of headache and dizziness. These symptoms were attributed to high blood pressure, and he was sent home on a higher dose of a diuretic—*and* with a prescription for a bottle of Kwell shampoo. "Shampoo?" I questioned him. "Oh, yes, I needed it *again* for the lice," he told me. He claimed to have recurrent forms of lice, or "lousiness" as he called it, using a more antiquated diagnostic term no doubt learned in the service. According to James, these lice were infesting his scalp and eyebrows and had spread to his entire body, causing terrible itching and red, oozing sores. He believed that he had acquired them from a less than sanitary barbershop and from "bedbugs" at his cabin in the woods. As proof, he pulled up his sleeves and revealed scattered red scabs in groups of three. Over the past year he had tried multiple prescriptions and over-the-counter medications, but without relief. His medical chart indicated that he had come to both the VA emergency room and the urgent care clinic on many occasions with the same complaints: itching, headache, tingling, skin lesions, and concerns about seeing lice flying around his house.

This was my first clue that something was amiss: *Lice don't fly*. And even if they did, they certainly wouldn't be biting someone's skin in groups of three. Pediculosis, as it is called, is a human parasitic infection caused by the tiny blood-sucking ectoparasite *Pediculus humanas*—or louse—a small, *wingless* crawling creature with six legs, two antennae, and retractable needlelike jaws. *Pediculosis capitis* is the most common form of infection, in which lice live and lay their eggs, or nits, in the scalp, causing intense itching and excoriation. There are also variants that infect the body and the pubic region. At the time I saw James the main form of treatment for lice was a onetime application of Kwell shampoo and ointment, which contain a neurotoxic insecticide called lindane.

It was clear to me that pediculosis was not the true diagnosis here, but rather that James had a somewhat rare and incredibly treatment-resistant form of psychosis known as a delusion of parasitosis or Ekbom's syndrome. These individuals are well known to dermatologists, presenting with diffuse complaints of itching and crawling sensations in their skin and with visible self-induced skin excoriations—sometimes secondarily infected—that they attribute to some form of parasite. Most of the time the sufferers of this particularly virulent delusion go from doctor to doctor seeking help, sometimes bringing in small vials of "bugs" that actually contain small pieces of dried, scratched-off skin. They are often smart enough to know, as James figured out quite quickly, that the antipsychotic agents given to them are *not* dermatologic medications used to treat lice.

My concern with James was not so much with his skin or even with his delusion. I was more concerned with the myriad neurological symptoms he was reporting, including headaches, tingling, dizziness, and memory lapses, and the fact that he was practically bathing himself in a neurotoxic shampoo and ointment on a frequent basis. In addition, every day he was spraying his hat, clothes, bedsheets, and furniture with an antilice spray that contained another neurotoxic insecticide. Although nowadays Kwell is considered a second-line treatment for lice due to concerns about its potential neurotoxic and carcinogenic properties, it was for James the treatment of choice given to him by half a dozen doctors over the course of a year—most of who did not realize what their colleagues were also doing.

The treatment could have been worse, I thought, knowing that previous approaches to the eradication of lice included the application of DDT powder to body and clothing or the use of other poisons containing derivatives of cyanide or mercury. The aggressive use of these obviously toxic agents had to be weighed against the fact that the common body louse was historically considered a vector for lots of nasty diseases, including typhus and trench fever. Even though I knew that James did not have to worry about such diseases, I also realized that part of him was still sitting petrified in a Sherman tank during the Battle of the Bulge, believing that the "flying lice" attacking him, like the Nazi scourge, had to be eradicated at all costs. In his mind it was "kill or be killed," and if that meant greasing up his hat, or helmet, with lindane or some other toxin, well that's what a good soldier had to do.

After a few sessions I built up enough trust with James to convince him to try an antipsychotic agent, casting it as a way to improve his sleep and lessen all of the stress he felt over his "infestation." I implored him to stop using all of the insecticidal ointments, shampoos, and sprays, telling him in stark terms that they could kill him. I referred him to a colleague in neurology, who thought it was likely that the neurotoxic insecticides were causing his various symptoms. I posted notes in James's chart, contacted all of his doctors, and even called the pharmacy he frequented, begging everyone to restrict his access to antilice products.

My notes over the ensuing year were telling. James claimed to be taking the antipsychotic agent, but he also claimed that the lice infestations were coming and going. "I still see the eggs," he told me one month. He appeared noticeably thinner over time and was slower in speech and movement. He lost his driver's license after passing out at the wheel. I called his son Bill, with whom he had intermittent contact, and expressed my concerns. Bill sighed over the phone and concurred: "I know," he said, "but my Dad will do what he wants do in order to stay safe in his own mind."

Surprisingly, James always kept his appointments with me, punctual to a fault. Other patients missed appointments now and then, but James never did, and so when he didn't show up one morning, I grew concerned. I called the VA van driver, who reported that James hadn't come out of his house at the usual time. James's phone rang repeatedly when I called, but without response. By early afternoon without word from James, I called the police. About an hour later I got a phone call back from an officer informing me that they had found James lying in bed, deceased.

What killed James? I still wonder. Was it his heart? After all, he did have both diabetes and heart disease. Or was it the antilice poisons that were probably still coursing through his skin and nervous system and permeating the fibers of the hat he kept matted to his head on most days. I don't know. But when I think of James's death, I recall the famous words of General Anthony McAuliffe during the Battle of the Bulge when he refused an order to surrender to the surrounding German troops: "Nuts!" he responded. McAuliffe and his men survived the siege of Bastogne because of the determination of Sherman tankers like James, who broke the back of the German lines several weeks later. But a part of that battle lived on, lingering in the helmet, hat, hair, and mind of James, and might have even killed him fifty years later. This, for many old soldiers, is the legacy of war.

The Strange but True
Case of Dawson da Vinci

I have learned in my practice as a geriatric psychiatrist to observe two key maxims. The first has become a cliché in every textbook: Start low, go slow, but *go*. Whether a doctor is dispensing advice, engaging in talk therapy, or prescribing medications, an older patient requires an approach that is moderate, measured, and persistent. The second is based on an old adage in medicine that instructs the doctor to treat the whole person who has the disease rather than just the disease itself. It's a reminder to the practitioner that every disease has a context that is much wider than simply a list of symptoms. Old age is certainly one key consideration, as are factors such as diet, gender, family history, daily habits, and attitude toward illness. Thus, depression in an eighty-five-year-old meat-eating, Irish Catholic, male, World War II combat veteran who loves to exercise will be different from depression in a ninety-year-old, widowed, grapefruit-juice-drinking, retired, female Asian seamstress who is a devout churchgoer. Depression—like every other form of mental illness in late life— is a coat of many colors whose expression and treatment course are fundamentally influenced by all of these unique aspects of the individual.

There is a particular category of mental illness, however, that appears to defy both maxims. In this category, the very being of an afflicted individual as expressed in daily behaviors, attitudes, and emotions is itself considered the disease. We call these mental illnesses *personality disorders*, and they are marked by a pervasive and dysfunctional weirdness, hostility, volatility, self-centeredness, or avoidance of others, to name a few symptoms. These disorders in both young and old are the scarlet letters of psychiatry, and they run roughshod over any concerted and organized attempts at treatment. And when seen through the prism of age, their appearances may be so disruptive and noxious that they appear to strip away all the individual differences that we weigh in the case. I have tried diligently, however, to understand and engage with these older patients, to liberate the person from the label.

"You are not a Michelangelo!"

I wasn't sure at first whether this declaration from my patient was a true insult or merely an observation. Mr. Dawson, the seventy-eight-year-old patient in question, continued: "You are probably in the 325 range. But I am, on the other hand, a Leonardo da Vinci." Seeing the quizzical look on my face, Mr.

Dawson dug through a jumble of papers on the tray in front of him and retrieved one particular page entitled "The Biometric Cosmos." An inverted pyramid was outlined on the page, balanced on top of another pyramid, and each was divided into subsections with various names and labels and a numbering system ranging from 0 to 800. I could see that the highest category on the top pyramid was labeled "Masters of the Cosmic Gamma," and it included da Vinci's name. I could also see that the category assigned to me by Mr. Dawson was several echelons below his, lying between "Persons incapable of true reason" and "Golddiggers." That didn't sound too complimentary. It could have been worse, though, as the levels below me went from "Unskilled workers in ultraviolet light" to "Imbeciles and Morons" and eventually to "Dust."

Mr. Dawson had been given a number of different labels from the nurses: strange, bizarre, skittish, obnoxious. He was not well liked. I realized, quite quickly, that this was nothing new for Mr. Dawson; over the years he had earned many similar labels in his encounters with staff at the VA hospital, all culminating in the more parsimonious diagnosis of a schizotypal personality disorder. The schizotypal individual is, by definition, an odd character who is uncomfortable with social relationships. Older schizotypal individuals can pose enormous challenges when they arrive, often unwillingly, in clinical settings and refuse to cooperate with standards of care. These strange patients cannot be avoided, however, and are a lot more bearable when understood.

I was asked to evaluate Mr. Dawson after his nurses reported that he was refusing his medications and threatening to sign out against medical advice. He had arrived at the hospital several days earlier with a gangrenous loop of intestine, and following emergency surgery had developed a rapid heart rate, which necessitated a transfer to the cardiac care unit. When I first went to see him, Mr. Dawson was lying in bed with the covers pulled up to his chin and a surgical cap bound tightly to his head, having obtained it after days of arguing with the nurses. I was greeted with a suspicious stare, and the reception only got chillier when I introduced myself as a psychiatrist.

"I consider myself above psychiatry," he stated, "and I don't need the heart doctor either—I have the heart of a twenty-year-old." Despite his antagonism toward psychiatry, Mr. Dawson was interested in talking about his work once I got him on the subject. "I am an evaluator," he described, "and a scientist." He claimed to be a master of evaluating the "cosmic energy" that flows as part of the life force. Handing me the diagram of the biometric pyramids along with another strange scale of "emotional tone," Mr. Dawson outlined, in grandiose terms, his ability to use both energy waves and handwriting samples to evaluate people using a special "box" at his house. And because he was at the level of da Vinci, he claimed that he could evaluate someone just by looking at the person. I asked him why he was in such a hurry to leave the hospital.

"First of all, I am not psychotic. But you have to understand the unseen forces here. The nurses send vibrations towards me but do not accept mine in return. This imbalance has caused my heart to misfire."

Mr. Dawson spoke to me coherently, even eloquently. There was no evidence of cognitive impairment or depression. He was irritable when describing his idiosyncratic demands (e.g., that he had to wear a surgical cap to keep his brain warm), but he was not particularly angry or anxious at other times. He didn't want to be around staff because he was suspicious of their motives and believed that they were causing his problems. At first listen, his thoughts sounded delusional, but as he continued to relate his work to me in such a detailed and rational way, even producing charts prepared by an actual "Biometric Society," I realized that they were—despite their grandiosity and implausibility—more odd than psychotic. After all, some individuals believe wholeheartedly in clairvoyance or astrology— why not the "biometric cosmos"?

For most of his life, Mr. Dawson had had neither the desire nor the fortitude to spend much time around others. He did not report disliking people, but he clearly did not feel comfortable in their presence. He was somewhat autistic in his approach, not being able to actually read the emotional tone of others (despite his self-described status as an "evaluator") or separate out his own emotional feelings from the reality of the environment. Though he was intelligent, he clearly demonstrated a warped interpretation of the behaviors of people around him. Over time Mr. Dawson had increasingly withdrawn from social contacts, grown suspicious of others, and developed a number of unusual interests and mannerisms. Eminent personality researcher Theodore Millon describes this process as a crucible for schizotypal personalities, in which "the more individuals turn inward, the more they lose contact with the styles of behavior and thought of those around them."

The further consequences of this isolation and the lack of social feedback from others are that schizotypal individuals "gradually begin the process of acting, thinking, and perceiving in peculiar, unreal, and somewhat 'crazy' ways." These patterns are not in essence psychotic, even though the general schizotypal personality may spin off brief psychotic episodes and share elements with a psychotic disorder such as schizophrenia. It is widely believed that schizotypal traits do not change much with aging but become more entrenched—as was the case with Mr. Dawson. By the time I saw him, he had a lifetime of odd beliefs and behaviors woven into his character.

Like many individuals with late-life personality disorders, Mr. Dawson also demonstrated other enduring and pervasive dysfunctional traits: schizotypal, obsessive-compulsive, paranoid, narcissistic, and passive-aggressive. Put together, these traits composed a man who was isolative, yet pompous, seeking to flee from the hospital, yet seemingly drawn to the presence of others who indulged his desire to talk about his work in excruciating detail. In the end, however, he was resisting and even sabotaging efforts to help him, and he was leaving everyone around him feeling angry, confused, and even frightened. Up until being hospitalized, he had retained his independence and hadn't needed to interact much with others. But now his age and medical condition demanded help and forced him into situations that he could handle only in his typically odd and hostile manner.

It is tempting to dismiss the late-life course of many older individuals labeled with chronic mental illnesses. In this scheme we focus instead on the "personality disorder" or the "schizophrenic" or the "demented" as if they were no more than a stereotyped disease. We open our treatment manual, and it spells out a clear formula of psychiatric evaluation, medication, and, oftentimes, institutionalization for each category. Being old and being mentally ill are a double whammy, bringing derision and discrimination from two different directions. Even the doctors who tend to these individuals face discrimination in terms of reduced and highly limited insurance payments and thus salaries.

In the end, Mr. Dawson signed out of the hospital against medical advice but agreed to follow up with both a cardiologist and my clinic within the week. I wasn't optimistic, because individuals with schizotypal traits can be notoriously difficult to engage in any form of psychotherapy. I wasn't surprised either when he refused to consider any medication, but I was disappointed. There is reasonable evidence suggesting that the use of low-dose antipsychotic medications in his case could improve symptoms of paranoia, thought disorder, hostility, anxiety, and even obsessive-compulsiveness that are commonly associated with the schizotypal personality.

I figured that even without medications Mr. Dawson would do best when he wasn't forced to be around people and would return to his eccentric pursuits. I remained concerned, however, about whether he was able to take care of himself, especially because he refused his cardiac medications, asserting that he knew better than the doctor. This is where clinicians often clash with schizotypal patients, becoming annoyed at their poor adherence to treatment and assuming that they are psychotic and incapable of making clear decisions. That assumption, however, is not necessarily true. In most cases decisionmaking is relatively intact though intransigent, and we have no choice but to accept their ways and their decisions, no matter how strange they may seem.

Mr. Dawson was a no-show for the appointment, and so I asked the clinic's social worker, Dan, to make a home visit. I warned Dan ahead of time that Mr. Dawson—the self-styled da Vinci—might appear and act quite strange and fill him with lots of bizarre theories of the cosmos: "Dawson da Vinci claims to actually practice with some form of a biometric box," I added, "but that is likely not true."

"Not so," Dan informed me later that day. As it turned out, there *was* an actual biometric box in Mr. Dawson's apartment, an eight foot by twelve inch square polished wooden box with a metallic meter in its center and a silken cord attached to a small woolen cap at one end. Mr. Dawson even gave a demonstration, having Dan place his hands on the box while Dawson wore the cap and appeared to enter a brief trance. He rated my colleague with a gamma score of 420, meaning that he was a "true individualist"—almost approaching the level of Galileo!

"Strange," Dan commented, giving me a wry smile, "but true!"

Part III
Memory

My history falls away, like sacks of grain from a careless farmer's wagon. I begin to forget everything.

—JOSEPH SKIBELL, *A BLESSING ON THE MOON*

If I Forget Thee

Emily was a pleasant, bespectacled woman of eighty-two years who guided herself into my office at the controls of her electric scooter. I was impressed by her careful maneuvering around the desk and assumed, prematurely, that she must be cognitively intact. But when I asked her to tell me about herself, she was befuddled. "You're not the eye doctor?" she queried, "because I need my glasses fixed." I explained my role again and asked her about her memory. "It's okay," she said, "no better, no worse than average." She recounted her history, but with many gaps. When I asked her how many times she had been married, she stated, "Two or three times." I persisted: "Was it two or three marriages?" She didn't remember and conflated two names into one. Her first husband, she thought, had died in the war. Or was that the second? I tried to imagine the missing men here, no longer even memories to Emily, just faint traces of "someone."

Alzheimer's disease was slowly engulfing her brain, and soon even Emily's notion of marriage would disappear. Place and time were fading as known entities to her, aside from the clear road directly in front of her scooter. With time, even her own name would slip away, taking with it her identity and those of all the beloved people in her life. Perhaps the only consolation would be her inability to even know whom to mourn.

Seeing Emily, I wondered about the consequences of losing such defining memories and was reminded of the oft-quoted passage from Psalm 137 in which the Hebrew exiles in Babylon cry, "If I forget thee, O Jerusalem, let my right hand forget her cunning. If I do not remember thee, let my tongue cleave to the roof of my mouth." For these ancient exiles, the imagined price of forgetting a beloved memory was a paralysis of sorts involving the loss of both physical and verbal functioning. In some respects, Emily and other aged individuals suffering from progressive dementia face a similar exile from the memories that once defined their identities. And with time they lose their very ability to act and communicate in meaningful ways.

This evolving exile is depicted quite poignantly in sequential self-portraits by artist William Utermohlen created throughout the first five years of his suffering from Alzheimer's disease. Compared to a detailed sketch of his healthy appearance from earlier years, a painting done two years after his initial diagnosis reveals distortions in both the shape and symmetry of his face along with a bewildered and anxious expression as the disease creeps in. Three years into the illness the colors of the drawn face become starker, the artist looks utterly confused, and the entire head is disembodied and trapped in a rough frame. In year four the facial expression has disappeared into a maelstrom of white and green, and the head is floating in a box with an enlarged, misshapen ear. The last portrait in year five is primitive and bereft of color, consisting of a round swirl of pencil lines with two dotted nostrils in the center. The identity is absent in this last drawing, but a trace of sensory awareness remains. By his midseventies Utermohlen had stopped painting.

The end result of dementia seems wholly tragic, a premature death in which all of the lines, shapes, colors, and memories that built a lifetime of love, purpose, and meaning have been wiped away. And this tragedy is compounded when the losses are exploited. Consider how often we discuss the conditions or behaviors of cognitively impaired individuals in their presence, assuming that they cannot understand what we are saying. I once witnessed a particularly cruel example of this exploitation when serving as a consultant at a Boston-area nursing home. A couple who had been married for more than seventy years shared a room at the facility, each suffering from severe dementia and largely unaware of the presence of the other in the adjacent bed. One morning the husband passed away, and within hours of his body being removed from the room, a new roommate was put in his bed. The widow lay silently nearby, unable, it seemed, to take notice or utter any complaints. The administrators of the facility believed that the newly widowed woman was unaware of her loss and acted without regard for her dignity. They were embarrassed and contrite when confronted, yet did nothing to prevent a future occurrence of such disrespect to a resident.

In the face of a memory disorder, then, how can we respond to the relentless loss of persona inflicted on its sufferers? We can acknowledge the tragedy and grieve the lost identities and memories, but is there anything more substantive to be done beyond maintaining the individual's physical presence? To the administrators of the nursing home, the severely demented widow was little more than a body in a bed, waiting her turn to be replaced. Most of us would not knowingly act in such an uncaring manner, but instead we may have a more passive—but equally uncaring—approach. We simply ignore, avoid, or neglect our most debilitated elderly. The problem with nursing home placement is not the placement itself or the fact of having to live in a nursing home; the problem is the abandonment and the loneliness visited on those so placed. But these are human-made problems, not products of age. The exile, then, may be twofold: exile from memory and exile from memorable, caring people. But is there anything we can do to help these exiles come home?

My patients have taught me two lessons. First, it is easy to miss sparks of the person hidden under the burden of disease. I once interviewed a ninety-five-year-old man with moderate dementia who was unable to provide much history due to his memory loss. The day was late when we finished our meeting, and I decided to take him in his wheelchair across our campus to his room. On the way we happened across a friend of his, whom he greeted warmly in Russian and with whom he carried on an animated conversation. At one point they switched to Polish, then to Yiddish, and they ended up in song together as they linked arms. For my patient, the words and cadence of a first language were like the inspiring taste of the madeleine cookie for Marcel Proust, reawakening memories and skills that flowed as naturally as in the past.

Second, we can step in to discover and even help rejuvenate the person behind the lost memories. I saw a powerful example of this role with my patient Hannah. I had first met her about ten years previously when she was a caregiver for her husband, Edwin, who suffered from Alzheimer's disease. Several years later Edwin passed away, and Hannah began to demonstrate signs of memory loss herself. I remained her doctor and referred her to a special social club for individuals with early-stage dementia. Hannah's identity revolved around several pillars: her beauty, her exile from Poland and then Cuba, and her dedication to social service. Even as she lost more and more of her independence, she struggled fiercely to maintain her dignified manner and dress. She also retained a fair amount of insight into her illness and often reported feeling depressed by her memory loss.

Then a generous neighbor stepped into Hannah's life and offered to make a scrapbook for her. With Hannah's help, the neighbor prepared a laminated book that included a narrative of Hannah's life, photos of her as a young woman in Poland and Cuba, and copies of certificates and newspaper clippings that recounted her involvement in the community. All that Hannah had difficulty remembering could be found in this amazing book, and she carried it with her everywhere as a reminder of who she was. It was astounding to see the restorative transformation in Hannah as she proudly showed the book to others. The scrapbook became, in essence, a portable identity.

I would like to think that even in the last days of dementia there are still traces of memory that allow patients to keep someone in their hearts. At the long-term care facility where I work, the music therapist, Joseph, was once working with a ninety-three-year-old severely demented woman who would sit in a wheelchair all day and make a repetitive clicking sound with her tongue. No words, utterances, or grunts—just clicks. After several hours of this noise she would become an extreme annoyance to staff and residents alike. Such repetitive vocalizations are always difficult to treat, and as her doctor I was having almost no success. More often than not, the medications that quell such vocalizations work only when they have sedated the person—a wholly unacceptable prospect.

Fortunately, Joseph had a better plan than I did, and so one day he brought the woman into a music therapy session. As Joseph played on the keyboard, each participant kept the beat in her or his own way. One older man shook a tambourine, while another tapped a small drum. Meanwhile, the old woman just clicked away. Several of the other residents were getting distracted and annoyed and began to yell at her to shut up. As Joseph listened to the woman's clicking, however, he began to sense a rhythm; "Click, click-click, click click-click." Something familiar struck him, and he began to play out the rhythm on the keyboard. As he played, a song began to fall into place, and the woman took notice. With more notes, the song became clearer, and her clicking suddenly ceased, her eyes opened wide, she took a deep breath, and she began to sing, "Let–me–call–you–sweetheart!" These were the first words anyone had ever heard her speak.

Joseph kept playing, and the woman kept singing—"I'm–in–love–with–you"—while the rest of the group sat in stunned silence, their pieces of percussion momentarily silenced.

Joseph later learned that "Let Me Call You Sweetheart" had been the song played so many years ago at the woman's wedding with her beloved husband. Ever since, it had always been "their" song. Even in the depths of dementia, one fond memory persisted, without words or tune and likely without images, only a rhythm indelibly imprinted on a clicking tongue.

I am also reminded of an elderly female patient with severe dementia who was visited daily by her husband. He doted on her, providing attention and affection even though she no longer remembered who he was. When he died unexpectedly, I witnessed this same woman wandering the floor in tears for many weeks, no doubt feeling deeply grieved over a missing presence. She had no memories of what she missed, but a part of her brain instinctively felt emotions that her caregivers were able to recognize and soothe. When her daughter and grandchildren visited with her several weeks later, there were no more tears, just embraces and laughter. They were able to help restore a small part of what had gone missing.

Fortunately, dementia is not a universal affliction of age. Being "senile" does not mean being demented; it simply means being "old"—although too often the terms are used interchangeably, and we end up equating aging with memory loss. We must realize, instead, that for many older individuals aging brings a vast repository of memories that carry with them the identity and history of the person and of the larger society. An eyewitness to history can impart memories in ways that books cannot.

The process of recalling the past, known as reminiscence, is a particularly powerful and vital activity in late life. In his autobiography, author and Holocaust survivor Aharon Appelfeld describes how "ever since my childhood, I have felt that memory is a living and effervescent reservoir that animates my being." In reminiscing about his own life, Appelfeld explains, "memory and imagination sometimes dwell together. In those long-buried years it was as if they competed. Memory was tangible, as if solid. Imagination had wings. Memory pulled toward the known, and imagination sailed toward the unknown."

This interplay between memory and imagination may explain the dreamlike quality to memories of the past, which Appelfield experiences as both "elusive and selective" in their conjuring. It is not always clear how and why we come to review certain events over others, but there is always the potential for memories to change how we look at life and for us, in turn, to overlay the memories with new meaning. Such a possibility exists in the very way our brains process memory. Sensations and events are registered and reviewed in a small snail-shaped part of the brain called the hippocampus. The most powerful memories, whether pleasant or traumatic, are imbued with strong sensations and deep emotions by a separate almond-shaped bundle of neurons called the amygdala. For example, most of my older patients can recall exactly where they were and what they were doing when they learned of the Japanese attack on Pearl Harbor on December 7, 1941, because it was such an emotional event. This type of indelible recollection is called a "flashbulb memory" because it sits almost like an exact photograph in our minds and can be easily recalled and reviewed with voluminous detail and emotion. For those and other less dramatic events, the brain prioritizes, encodes, and then spreads them like interlinking spider webs throughout its various regions.

This makes them easier to recall because there are multiple avenues of contact. The entire process, known as consolidation, forms our permanent long-term memory stores.

It is tempting to view these long-term memories as permanently shaped channels in the brain, but research indicates that they are more malleable than previously thought. When recalled, memories become like softened gels that are then reremembered or reconsolidated back to their hardened forms by neurons that reactivate the connections between them. In the softened states, however, we can change these memories by actually altering the attachment of emotions and meaning. This process may account for how individuals with post-traumatic stress disorder can be healed slowly through rote and repetitive verbalization of their traumatic memories, leaving some of the painful emotions and sensations stripped away with each retelling.

Gerontologist Robert Butler was the first person to propose a greater therapeutic role for reminiscence, or "life review," as he called it. He felt strongly that the life review process was both natural and healthy and could help aging individuals revisit and come to terms with unresolved conflicts. Tapping into remote memories and long-held beliefs as well as current thoughts and self-observations could provide an individual with a sense of continuity and strength, especially during times of rapid change or loss. Under ideal conditions, he proposed, life review held the promise of bringing increased "candor, serenity, and wisdom."

The process of life review is facilitated by several factors in late life. First, individuals may have more time for self-reflection, and second, they often face losses and stresses that trigger the need to tap into past life skills in order to cope. A number of psychologists have also proposed that the way in which we organize and think about ideas changes in adulthood in ways that support the goals of life review. Theories of cognitive development are traditionally based on the work of Swiss psychologist Jean Piaget, who proposed that a certain endpoint is reached in young adulthood with the achievement of "formal operations," a stage characterized by abstract thinking and the ability to formulate and test hypotheses. However, the concept of *post*-formal thinking posits that aging adults can develop beyond this stage, acquiring the ability to examine and balance the needs of competing relationships, systems, or perspectives. For example, postformal thinking allows an individual to balance logic and emotion in decisionmaking and to see how he or she participates in creating perspective. Life review thrives on this expanded view of reality as it allows for greater patience, acceptance, and pragmatism in complex situations, whether present or past. This is exactly the skill that Butler and others refer to as "wisdom."

Unfortunately, reminiscence can also reactivate traumatic memories and even trigger depression in other aged individuals. A life review may only highlight mistakes or losses or be rendered useless by denial, distorted or grandiose recollections, or memory loss. Other individuals may be able to acknowledge past transgressions but feel hopeless about the possibility for forgiveness. Still other individuals are too paralyzed by daily life to even engage in the process. In *The Life Cycle Completed*, Joan and Erik Erikson describe how "in one's eighties and nineties one may no longer have the luxury of such retrospective despair. Loss of capacities and disintegration may demand almost all of one's attention." As a result, life review may fail to keep despair at bay in the last, or ninth, stage of life.

Life review, then, carries with it the potential for both rejuvenation and reconsolidation of past memories, as well as the risk of retraumatization. For many of my patients, however, any talk of past events may initially seem pointless. There is often despair that no one will listen, or if they do listen, they will not care. I have learned, then, that life review is not meant to be a solo trek and that any risks can be mitigated when memories are shared, guided, or even shaped within a relationship with another caring and interested individual or even with an audience. Writing an autobiography can also serve this purpose.

This fact struck me after reading *Living in the Shadow of the Freud Family*, written and edited by Sophie Freud, a distinguished professor emerita of social work at Simmons College and granddaughter of Sigmund Freud. Sophie Freud's book is both a family history and an autobiography set within the annotated diary of her mother, Esti Drucker Freud, who was married to Sigmund and Martha Freud's second child and oldest son, Martin. It is a unique form of life review that presents memories, elaborates on them through several voices, and then tries to gain some understanding of their meaning after many decades of reflection.

Esti Drucker Freud's memoirs begin by recounting her childhood in Vienna in the early years of the twentieth century, followed by her courtship with Martin Freud while he was a soldier in the Austrian Army during World War I. After the war they married and had two children, Walter and Sophie, but their ill-fated union quickly began to break apart as economic and social pressures increased in the days leading up to World War II. Sophie Freud adds her own fascinating commentary and queries: "Do happy memories disappear in a generalized glow, while unhappy memories remain much sharper?" This question persists throughout the entire book as the story seesaws among the memories, many soaked in sadness and tragedy, of several generations of parents and children.

After the German invasion of Austria, Sigmund Freud, with international help, received seventeen exit visas enabling his immediate family to emigrate. Sigmund, his wife, his sister-in-law, daughter Anna, son Martin, and grandson Walter fled to England, separating from Esti and Sophie, who traveled to Paris. Shortly thereafter the Germans invaded France and entered Paris, and Esti and Sophie escaped in the nick of time on bicycles, heading first to Nice, then to Casablanca, and finally to the United States. Unfortunately, not everyone in the family made it to safety. Esti's mother, Ida, was caught in southwest France and sent to die at Auschwitz. Several of Sigmund Freud's own sisters were interned in Theresienstadt and then sent to the gas chambers of Treblinka.

Included in this rich life review are Sophie's recollections of her grandfather. As a young child she would visit his famous home at 9 Berggasse in Vienna most Sundays and have a brief audience with him, although these contacts were both limited and formal. "I knew him only superficially and learned about his life mostly through his numerous biographies," laments Sophie. She last saw her grandfather briefly in June 1938 in Paris, where the family had stopped en route to London. Despite physical separation, Sophie was able to have a particularly fond correspondence with him in the ensuing fourteen months before his death in September 1939.

In one letter dated October 26, 1938, Sigmund wrote to Sophie, "I don't answer you as often as you write to me, but be sure to write if you have special experiences or if you need something. I take pleasure with each of your letters." This was a kind appeal to his fourteen-year-old granddaughter, and its impact reverberates over a great expanse of time. At age eighty or so Sophie penned an updated response, which she includes in her book:

> *My Dearest and Much Loved Grandfather,*
> *Even now, in my very old age as I read your loving*
> *letters . . . I am deeply moved. Perhaps you really did care about*
> *me. . . . I was a child who craved your affection. . . . I remember*
> *you as old and sick, with your fingers in your mouth, always in*
> *pain, a grandfather of few words. Our visits in your sacred office*
> *were short—*

Sophie continues by recalling a walk in the garden with her grandfather while collecting nuts: "I knew that this was a rare and precious moment, a moment of pure joy, to be ground forever into my memory." She thanks Sigmund for the loving letters that he wrote her in the year before his death, seeing them as proof that he cared about her.

I decided after reading this extraordinary book to seek out Sophie Freud herself. I had actually met her many years back at a psychiatric conference in Boston, and so I was familiar with the great work she had done in the field of social work over the course of her long career. I made contact, and Sophie invited me to visit her at her home in the woods outside Boston. When I arrived, she greeted me warmly and expressed satisfaction that I had correctly navigated the serpentine roads to her driveway. This exciting visit felt a little bit like a pilgrimage to a holy seer by virtue of her eighty-five years and her role as a living, genetic extension of Sigmund Freud. After all, the very foundation of my life's work as a psychiatrist, including the vast majority of everything I had ever read on human nature, was shaped by her grandfather. Even so, Sophie was not Sigmund, and I had come to hear her own thoughts about aging and memory, and not those of her grandfather.

We sat together in her study, surrounded, floor to ceiling, by books, papers, paintings, and small artistic knickknacks from her life, including a miniature bronze bust of her famous grandfather. The floor of the adjacent living room was covered with a richly detailed red, orange, and blue Oriental rug reminiscent of her grandfather's iconic couch. A nearby computer was in active use, and I was impressed by her facility with both e-mailing and downloading files. Outside of the large sliding glass doors lining the wall of the room was a serene view of her wooded lot, which led down to a small pond. Over the course of several hours she spoke to me about her life, past and current, and insisted that I stay for lunch, tea, and homemade strudel.

We began by speaking about her book. Sophie acknowledged that the eight-year process of writing it had served an important function during the time she was cutting back her full-time work schedule. As she writes in the introduction: "The book project helped me with this difficult transition. It gave meaning to my suddenly senseless life; it has become my closest friend in these somewhat solitary years." The project took so long, in fact, that Sophie worried "that my age would defeat me before I could finish its conception—thus it was a race between a piece of work and my aging brain, in which my drive to work, trained through many years, did win after all." That her "aging" brain could accomplish such a task counters the view that "old people are no longer educable" espoused by Grandfather Freud. "There is often *more* change" in late life, Sophie emphasized to me, "and an enormous need for change and adaptation more than in earlier years."

Even though Sophie is extremely active for her age, she sees herself as much less involved in the world compared to previous years. On the one hand, she continues to teach and take courses at the Brandeis Lifelong Learning Institute, write poetry and short stories, exercise, spend time with her children, and keep up with correspondence. On the other hand, she no longer works full-time, travels around the world, or raises young children as in years past. She still has the sentiment of an activist but not the physical energy: "I've become more of a bystander," she told me, "but I am still sensitive to the suffering that goes on around me." These sentiments were well captured in a recently published poem by Sophie, entitled "The Old Woman and Time":

> *Was it only yesterday*
> *Or ten years ago*
> *I stood on one foot*
> *straight as a tree*

in my yoga class.
Arms over head
saluting the sun
This is so easy. I thought
I could stand here all day.
Today time's typhoon
threatens to blow me down
as I stumble along
on both feet.

During our visit, I asked Sophie about the particularly poignant and intriguing "Apologia" (best described as a defense of her philosophy) in the beginning of her book. There she speaks quite candidly with the reader about aging for her mother and for herself: "Mother, dying of cancer, complained that there was no one in her life who would make her a cup of tea. 'You should have made friends when you were younger,' I said. 'I had no time for friendships,' she responded. 'You always wanted to be left in peace . . . ,' I reproached her, 'and now you are paying the price of such a choice.'"

Her words in this Apologia are honest and harsh and signal to the reader that the book will not hesitate to examine feelings all around. Sophie continues: "In the 20 years since my first book, in this time of my own aging, I have come closer to Mother. She no longer appears so alien to me; I too want to be left in peace. . . . I live alone and now and then I feel alone. Others see me as an eccentric old lady. Many cadavers of cutoff relationships litter my life. I also might not have anyone preparing me a cup of tea when I am sick. Well, there are always electric teapots one can rely on."

I felt a degree of sadness when I read this opening passage, as it seemed to describe Sophie as someone who deliberately sought isolation. And yet the book is incredibly inviting and intimate with the reader. In person, Sophie herself could not have been more personable and hospitable. When I commented on this contrast between her words and her demeanor, Sophie responded with a smile: "I am more independent than most people I know. I need less company because I have my books, and the courses I teach. I did not have to give up my identity as a teacher . . . [and] I do not experience loneliness." Her comments reminded me of the sentiments expressed many years prior by Henry David Thoreau, in whose beloved Walden Pond Sophie swims every summer. When asked by a friend whether he was lonely out in the woods in his cabin, Thoreau responded, "This whole earth which we inhabit is but a point in space. How far apart, think you, dwell the two most distant inhabitants of yonder star? . . . Why should I feel lonely? Is not our planet in the milky way?"

In retrospect, I see how my own ageist assumptions crept in here, imaging that being alone in late life implied loneliness and sadness. But this is certainly not the case for Sophie—and for many other aged individuals. She treasures her solitude and her independence, but they do not preclude interpersonal connections. At eighty-five she is more connected to others than most of her peers. She has a timeless vitality. And my visit allowed me to understand firsthand the spirit that lies behind her written life review. As Sophie herself writes, "This book is the magic bastion Mother has bequeathed me to combat futility in my old age."

I learned an additional lesson about the powerful role of memory in late life from the title of her book—*Living in the*

Shadow of the Freud Family. Among the dozen definitions of the word "shadow" that appear in the dictionary, two in particular have seemingly opposite meanings: A shadow may represent an obstruction of light by some object, and it can serve as a place of hiding and safety. I see memories playing these same roles for so many of my patients. When painful or even traumatic, they blot out much of an individual's identity, obscuring happier memories and engendering a sense of failure, danger, and despair. Sophie herself made this observation within her mother's memoirs.

But so many other memories are like Appelfeld's imagination: They take wing and prove both soothing and elevating as they conjure people and places from the past that bring affirmation of the greatest connections and joys in life. This, of course, is the ultimate goal of reminiscence—not to restore what has been lost but to experience the gratitude that can come only with the realization that we never truly lose the gifts from the most important figures in our lives. Sophie reaches a similar conclusion in her letter to her grandfather, written when she herself had attained his final age:

> *Dearest grandfather,*
>
> *Being your grandchild has stamped my life. You were a kind and protective presence in my young life, even if emotionally distant . . . but altogether your mighty shadow has enriched my whole life, rather than curtailed it. It was my good fortune, my enormous privilege, to be born your grandchild and I thank you for all you have done for me.*
> *Your Sopherl*

Savant, of Sorts

Everyone has a photographic memory.
Some don't have film.

—Steven Wright

What does the number thirty-seven look like? Most of us visualize two black-and-white numerals side by side, but Daniel Tammet sees an image that he likens to lumpy porridge. After suffering from severe seizures at the age of four, Daniel developed a condition known as *synesthesia*, in which two or more senses are experienced together. He "sees" numbers as shapes full of light, color, and texture, allowing him to perform incredible calculations by seeing the numerical landscape in his mind. On one occasion he memorized the number pi to 22,514 digits and recited them without mistake over the course of five hours. In another jaw-dropping challenge, he studied Icelandic—one of the most difficult languages for a nonnative speaker to learn—for only one week before going on national television in Iceland and stunning the audience by being interviewed live in its native language. Daniel has what is known as the "savant syndrome," which is characterized by the innate possession of spectacular mental skills, such as being able to memorize massive lists of numbers or statistics, quickly learn new languages, or instantly perform complex mathematical calculations.

Imagine how different the world would be if we could simply look at or listen to something just one time and then remember it in its entirety. Like Daniel Tammet, the great composer Wolfgang Amadeus Mozart was believed to have this ability. One legendary story holds that at the age of fourteen Mozart went to the Sistine Chapel to hear a performance of the *Miserere*, a mass whose musical notes had been kept secret for nearly a century. Afterward, he retired to his room and transcribed the entire piece from memory! This skill has been called photographic, or eidetic, memory. Despite the numerous people who have demonstrated this ability, some memory researchers have argued that photographic memory does not really exist, that individuals who appear to have eidetic memory are actually using memory techniques. One example is retired Japanese engineer Akira Haraguchi, who on October 4, 2006, recited by memory 100,000 digits of the number pi over the course of sixteen hours. To accomplish this task, Haraguchi had spent years practicing a memory technique in which he translated a string of numbers into symbols, which he then used to create memorable stories and poems. During his sixteen-hour feat, he was actually reciting the memorized stories in his head and translating them back into numbers. But even the use of this technique begs the question, How did he remember all of those stories? That ability in itself reveals a spectacular memory.

Unlike Mozart and Tammet, neither my friend Gerald nor I have innate savant abilities. Like Haraguchi, however, we resolved to learn several memory techniques to use in our own daily lives and to teach to some of the individuals at an assisted living facility who were struggling with mild memory lapses. Gerald himself is just over eighty, and as a gerontologist he has been interested for several decades in positive approaches to aging. He had watched me grow my memory assessment clinic for some time but felt strongly that something was missing. "My friend," he instructed me one day, "it's time for action." This meant doing more than simply diagnosing memory problems; we had to engage patients in activities to pump up their mental muscles. Increasingly, research has supported the obvious point that regular cognitive exercises can improve a variety of mental skills, ranging from memory processing speed and retention to visual tracking and fine motor speed. But for countless aging adults facing a general slowdown in cognitive speed and efficiency, the benefits of mental exercise (as opposed to physical exercise) are only now being recognized.

Our first "Memory Fit" class included about a dozen individuals ranging from Susan, a seventy-two-year-old former social worker who wanted to avoid the memory problems she had witnessed in her mother, to Victor, a ninety-three-year-old snowbird and retired stockbroker from Brooklyn who spent his winters in Miami. Gerald and I cotaught the four-week course, with each session featuring a different category of items to remember: names, lists of things and topics, and numbers. We first taught and then practiced with the group a technique to remember names using stimulating mental associations. "I now remember Susan's name perfectly," exclaimed Victor after a little practice, "because her eyes remind me of my niece Susan." We then taught the Roman room technique, in which a list of items is memorized through the creation of a visual image of walking through a familiar house and seeing each item placed in a different room. This mnemonic technique was originally developed and perfected by ancient Roman orators who had long speeches to remember but lacked the teleprompters, PowerPoint slides, or even paper note cards utilized by modern-day speakers. Finally, we had a session to teach ways to break down long strings of numbers and letters into more manageable chunks and then add creative associations. "I finally remember that my license plate number is JR2845," explained Susan, "because I think of belonging to the *Jr.* Women's League from the ages of *28* to *45*."

As we were reviewing the course material during the final session, a debate over technique erupted. Victor was illustrating to the class how he always knew where he kept the TV remote: It was tethered to a bright yellow carved wooden duck that he pulled out of a bag and ceremonially placed in the middle of the table. "That's not a memory technique; that's a prop!" called out Sam, a ninety-year-old retired travel writer and World War II veteran sitting at the table. "A prop, so what?" Victor fired back. Sam sat up ramrod straight in his chair and began to deliver a short speech. "Dr. Agronin, and Gerald, with all due respect, you have tried your best to teach us these special memory techniques. But in the end, it's too much work. I have a better solution that works for me." Sam reached into his shirt pocket and pulled out a small spiral bound notepad, then continued speaking. "Whatever I need to remember, I just write it down here," he explained, holding out the notepad for all to see. A furious debate ensued, with Victor claiming that the memory techniques were necessary and Sam insisting that keeping a written list was more practical. Within minutes the debate became Talmudic. "But how many notepads do you need?" queried Victor, "and what if you lose the notepad?" Sam thrust his hand in the air, pointing toward Victor's shirt, "You will only lose the notepad if you forget to wear a shirt!" Victor was not convinced—"but my shirt has no pocket!" At this point Gerald and I jumped in. "Whatever works for each of you is best," we counseled. "Victor's duck, Sam's notepad—they both work!"

The course taught me several key lessons about memory. I started out as a teacher but finished as a student, realizing that any chronically busy multitasking individual, whether doctor, patient, student, or senior citizen, can suffer from memory lapses. Research clearly shows greater declines in memory with age, including a higher frequency of "tip-of-the-tongue" experiences, but it is equally true that training and practice can significantly improve performance, rendering some of the age-related differences meaningless. In addition, the aging brain has two advantages over younger brains: a lot more experience (and hence, a larger knowledge base) and a greater ability to see both sides of the coin, better known as wisdom. If you are comparing yourself to someone like Haraguchi, however, do not despair. Simply having an awesome memory doesn't guarantee success, as you still need "street smarts" to know how to apply it. After all, even Mr. Haraguchi once forgot his wife's birthday!

My own memory test occurred a year after completing the course. I had just finished giving a lecture on memory to a group of residents at the assisted living facility when a familiar face stood up in the back of the room. "I have a question," my former student called out. "What's my name?" I had just lectured on the importance of practicing several memory techniques, and now my snowbird friend from Brooklyn was testing me. I hesitated for an uncomfortably long pause. A few associations triggered by my former student's heavy accent tumbled from the recesses of my memory: Brooklyn, sea, fish. Fish! . . . Tuna? Cod? Haddock? And then it came to me. I smiled and reached out my arm. "Welcome back to Miami, Mr. *Herring*!" I called out. Victor smiled knowingly, a small notepad bulging in the front pocket of his shirt.

Strength in Numbers

We have all seen a flock of birds or a swarm of bees, but what about a *parliament* of owls? Or a *shrewdness* of apes? According to James Lipton's wonderful compendium, most animal groups have terms that, to a greater or lesser extent, capture the meaning of the collective. These terms might be based on certain characteristics of the animals, like a *leap* of leopards or a *knot* of toads, or on some early linguist's onomatopoetic attempt to capture the sound of the animal, as in a *gaggle* of geese. And what about human groups? Lipton suggests, to our amusement, that we might encounter a *flush* of plumbers, a *wince* of dentists, or a *void* of urologists. He even dares to propose that a group of psychoanalysts might be termed a *complex*! Whatever we call it, when people who have a common mission or plight get together, they form a stronger unit that is able to achieve on a level far above that of the individual.

So it is with memory disorders. I encountered such a group recently when I was invited to give a talk on the brain to twelve ladies who all faced a similar dilemma: Suffering from early-stage Alzheimer's disease, they were too impaired for many senior activities in the community, yet not impaired enough to benefit from the average day care program for individuals with more severe forms of dementia. To meet their needs, I worked with my staff to create a special social club designed to emphasize skills that are resistant to early-stage memory loss, such as imagination, sensory enjoyment, and camaraderie. Led by a group leader with training in memory disorders, the ladies in the club had lectures on humor and history; they read poetry, listened to music, and sang; they read a selected book and had discussions on the content; and they sat together in a leisurely luncheon to talk and laugh about whatever topics came their way.

My invitation to lecture to them on the brain was accompanied by a list of ten questions that the participants had devised the week before and inscribed on a chalkboard. My arrival was greeted enthusiastically by the group, not because they knew me as a particularly wise lecturer, but because I was their doctor, having evaluated each and every one prior to enrollment in the program. I knew their deficits well, having reluctantly conferred their very diagnoses. When they saw me in the clinic, these ladies were typically friendly and gracious but reticent, sobered by the exposure of their cognitive deficit in my presence. Individually, I rarely get many questions from them; they listened intently to my words and often turned to an accompanying husband or adult child for assistance and reassurance.

Meeting with them as a group, however, I encountered something quite different. I saw broad smiles and heard small talk that easily gave way to giggling or burst into full-bodied laughter. They did not merely ask me about the brain; they interrogated me with ten of the most sophisticated questions on brain function imaginable. How do the right and left hemispheres differ? they asked. Do male and female brains think differently? The questions flowed logically from one to another, and as I spoke, group members jumped in to discuss my responses, add in their own commentaries, and pose thoughtful follow-up questions.

Alone, each member of the group faced a growing sense of disconnection from personal memories and other aspects of her identity. Together, however, they shared not just a common ailment, but also common aspirations to feel a part of something larger than themselves, to feel loved and cared for, to care for someone else, and to laugh in the face of adversity. They interacted in ways that defied their individual limitations, with their strengths united. As I talked about the wonders of the brain, I concluded each of my responses to the ten questions with the same theme: Although short-term verbal memory may wane in the face of numerous age-related diseases, our brains have many different ways to capture life experiences, yielding a vast storehouse of persistent memories and cognitive skills. The goal of our social club was to tap into these latent skills, and as I lectured, I witnessed an extraordinary demonstration of these brain powers in tandem with others—a true strength in numbers. And what would I call this group? I recall a sketch from Lipton's book that depicts a dozen beautifully choreographed larks flying together—an *exaltation* of larks, a phrase that gives the book its very title. That is what I saw in the group that day—a joy, a dignity, a strength, and a true *exaltation* of friends.

Old Soldiers

D-Day, June 6, 1944. H-Hour + 15 minutes, 6:45 AM. Uncle Red Sector, Utah Beach. Members of the U.S. Army's 359th Infantry Regiment, including a young private named Clarence Green, hit the Normandy beaches in the third wave of attack. Several miles to the east, another young soldier named Jake Custer of the famed "Blue and Grey" 29th Infantry Division was welcomed to the hell of Omaha Beach in the early hours of the attack. Both soldiers, now in their eighties, have vivid recollections of the events of that day. It was their first time in battle, their first witness to death. Clarence recalls the intense seasickness and stench of vomit in the Higgins boat as it neared the shore. Jake remembers charging onto the beach, hearing a deafening explosion to his right, and seeing nothing but the limb of a buddy fall nearby. Several days prior, however, their spirits had been quite different. Only nineteen years old, they were full of bravado and anticipation, having no true idea of what they would face in the coming invasion. War historian Stephen Ambrose describes how young men who had never experienced the carnage of warfare had a sense of invulnerability, so much so that one young soldier, informed that likely nine out of ten soldiers would be casualties of the D-Day invasion, "looked at the man to his left, then at the man to his right, and thought to himself, You poor bastards."

In circumstances of war, such massive denial serves a function: to enable headlong, impulsive acts that, if left to older men, might never happen. This form of denial is facilitated by lack of both information and experience, coupled with poor insight into impending possibilities. And it likely has a neurological basis, sustained by not fully matured frontal lobes that allow for the excessive risk-taking, aggression, and impulsivity that are gold on the battlefield.

In the clinic, however, this denial is not so golden. For years after the war, Clarence struggled with emotional outbursts, nightmares, and panic attacks, refusing to accept the possibility of psychiatric illness. This denial was willful but not calculated and was enabled by the same ignorance and poor insight that had once sustained his warrior mind-set on the eve of D-Day. Although for a doctor such denial can be problematic, leading a patient to refuse treatments for an illness not recognized in the first place, it can itself be corrected.

There are other forms of denial that are not so amenable to correction. These are cases in which the core mechanism is not lack of understanding or anticipation but a state of forced or innate inattention. In other words, the patient cannot help it. Trauma to one side of the brain, for example, can cause an individual to ignore or even deny the existence of the paralyzed side of the body opposite the lesion. In some individuals, the loss of integrity of their basic body image turns out to be a whole-brain conspiracy, linking together visual impairments with impairments in attention, motivation, insight, and prior-itization. Neurologist Joseph Babinski originally coined the term "anosognosia" to describe this syndrome, but the word has come to mean a general state of denial of illness.

Given these linkages, patients express their difficulties in many ways: Some individuals merely ignore the paralyzed side, others actively deny its existence, and still others develop a dislike or even hatred for a paralyzed limb. The search for some mean-ing to the predicament may even lead to overly elaborate or even delusional beliefs about the limb. In "The Man Who Fell Out of Bed," neurologist Oliver Sacks describes just such a case in which he was asked to consult on a man who fell out of bed after pushing his leg out first, convinced that it was someone else's severed leg that had been attached to him in some sort of cruel New Year's Eve joke.

Despite my lack of military experience, I am always tempted to salute Mr. Custer when I visit the Veteran's nursing home and find him sitting in his wheelchair at the front door, wearing a baseball cap with the word "D-Day" scrawled across each side. What I call valor he calls duty, speaking proudly but not arro-gantly about his service. Looking back, he neither denies nor is preoccupied with the unpleasant parts of his combat experiences. He is generally satisfied with his life.

Jake Custer's contentment reminds me of a fellow soldier and veterans home resident named Ben, who is in the middle stages of dementia, most likely of the Alzheimer's type. "Do you have any memory problems?" I recently inquired of Ben, to which he resoundingly replied, "Of course not." Like the young Jake Custer predawn June 6, 1944, Ben is in complete denial of his current predicament and impending course. In the moment, he lives for lunch or for a laugh with one of his buddies. Like the current Jake Custer, Ben is generally satisfied with his life, enabled, to be sure, by his dense denial of reality. In this case, Ben's denial is both willful and pathologic, prompted by a laid-back character who never paid much attention to illness and sustained by small lesions riddling his frontal lobes and their grip on reality. He is in denial about his cognitive deficits in the same way that a stroke victim can deny a limb hanging limply. In this case, there is no point to my trying to convince him that he is ill.

Curiously, in dementia different forms of knowledge help guide a person's daily life, some in complete and blissful denial of certain facts, others acutely aware of the surrounding vista. What astounded newsmakers but generated a yawn from most geriatricians perfectly illustrated this fact: Former Supreme Court justice Sandra Day O'Connor's husband, John, suffering from Alzheimer's disease and residing in a long-term care facility, took up with a girlfriend and was acting "like a teenager in love," oblivious to his marriage of fifty-five years. Here we see complete denial of long-term biographical knowledge, yet perfect awareness of erotic emotions not experienced since his early twenties. This phenomenon takes many forms and is an everyday event in most dementia wards.

From the standpoint of the doctor, determining whether denial of illness is willful or pathologic helps guide efforts to convince the cognitively intact person of the necessity of care or, alternatively, to respect the convictions of the denier, yet work around them. After all, war may be hell, but illness does not have to be.

Memories, False and Fixed

Doctor Al, my uncle, calls it "the shrine." He was the second and now I am the third generation of doctors to sit at this old wooden desk, preserved just as it looked back in 1946 when my grandfather first opened his practice. On one side sits an old-fashioned rotary phone, next to the portable blood pressure cuff that my grandfather used to carry with him on house calls. The elegant blotter in the middle of the desk has two raised leather sides, with a yellowed piece of paper taped to the left and containing the typewritten names and phone extensions of the six other doctors who lived and worked in and near the town of Kaukauna, Wisconsin. The drawers still contain patients' note cards, old glass pathology slides, and various medical knick-knacks from a bygone era. Most interesting to me are the two medical texts I keep on top of the desk: *Stedman's Medical*

Dictionary, 10th edition, published in 1928, and James Meakins's *Practice of Medicine,* published in 1936. I look at these timepieces every once in a while, out of curiosity and out of a desire to see how far we've come in medicine today.

The references to psychiatric terms in these two worn leather tomes are particularly interesting. For example, in 1928 the terms "psychopathist" and "alienist" were two common synonyms for "psychiatrist." Attention to political correctness and risk management were not to be found in 1936, as Meakins described chronic alcoholics as "immoral" and "untruthful" and recommended a brew of toxic sedatives, including phenobarbital and sodium bromide, to treat anxiety disorders. Other terms, however, do not yield the same sense of pride and appreciation for how far psychiatry has progressed.

Take the term "psychosis" as an example. According to the 2004 version of the medical dictionary, psychosis is "a severe mental disorder, with or without organic damage, characterized by derangement of personality and loss of contact with reality and causing deterioration of normal social functioning." The 1928 version was not so specific, defining psychosis as "any mental state or condition" and "a disorder of the mind, insanity," having ten different types, ranging from "exhaustion psychosis" to "toxic psychosis." Meakins was similarly broad. I have often noted, however, that these broader, antiquated definitions of psychosis are too often applied to older individuals whose memories seem disjointed or false. When such memories or, indeed, "any mental state or condition" is painted as psychosis, the logical treatment involves relatively potent medications. Here are two illustrative cases.

Bugs

The call from the nurse on duty at the assisted living facility was brief and to the point: "Dr. Agronin, please see Mrs. Nestor and get her started on something—she's *psychotic*." Betty, the head nurse, followed up with another message: "She has bizarre complaints of bugs crawling all over her room and infesting her clothes and skin. Please see her soon."

I was surprised. Mrs. Nestor, or Francine as I called her, was a particularly friendly woman who usually came to appointments accompanied by her daughter Judy and carrying a box of family photos. I knew that her grandson was an aspiring actor and had been elected class valedictorian. One granddaughter loved ice-skating; another had just started college. Francine treated me like a long-lost cousin each time we met, discussing family and friends and recent events with a joy so refreshing in a ninety-year-old woman. But now . . . bugs?

Francine arrived without her characteristic smile or banter and was clearly preoccupied with something. Because the appointment had been scheduled at the last minute, Judy wasn't able to accompany her mother. There was no box of photos. "How *are* you?" I asked.

"Doctor, I am so upset! There are bugs everywhere!" For the next fifteen minutes Francine described to me in detail how small black bugs were coming out of her newspaper and infesting her room. I was struck by how different she appeared in both voice and demeanor as she described the pathways around the room that the bugs were traversing. She pointed out several small spots on her skin that were itching, and she attributed them to the bugs. Her concerns were overly detailed and seemed implausible, suggesting that she actually did have what we call in psychiatric parlance a "delusion of parasitosis"—meaning a false and fixed belief of being infested by insects. In addition, her visual descriptions of the actual bugs were vague and yet made them sound monstrous, suggestive of visual hallucinations. Perhaps the nurses were right—Francine was psychotic!

After my evaluation, I ordered a urinalysis, reviewed her medications, and was poised to order an antipsychotic medication. I didn't trust my own judgment, however. Francine the smiling cousin versus Francine the frightened entomophobe— I just couldn't put the two together. I put down my pen and pad and called her daughter, who was appropriately concerned by her mom's behavior. I acted on a hunch: "Judy, I need to ask you a favor. Before I do anything else, will you inspect your mom's room for me?"

Judy called me back an hour later from her mom's room. She was laughing. "It's infested! There are bugs everywhere!" Francine, I learned, kept her newspapers rolled up on the floor near the window. Ants were entering through the floorboards, crawling out of the newspapers, up along a bead of dried jelly that had spilled on her rocking chair, through her shawl and over her shoulders, and onto her end table, where she had left an open bag of candies. When seen without glasses, Francine's visual impairment made small black ants appear much larger and fuzzier. Several had irritated her skin with small bites, adding to her discomfort. Only someone sitting in her rocking chair could appreciate the extent of the infestation—but the nurses saw Francine only down in the dining hall or the activity room.

I was relieved by the discovery but not surprised. After all, this is Florida, where ants are practically the state animal, and so I should have suspected a true infestation immediately! At the same time, I realized how close I had come to mistaking Francine's recollections for a nonexistent psychotic symptom. But this was a job for an exterminator, not a geriatric psychiatrist.

Switched

I had known Ed Blum for several years because I used to take care of his wife, Shirley. She had suffered from dementia, and Ed had been her main caregiver, informant, and mode of transportation for all clinic appointments. Late into the course of her illness Shirley began to deteriorate rapidly, around the same time that Ed suffered from a bout of pneumonia with an associated delirium. Delirium is an acute form of brain impairment, often superimposed on other illnesses, and involves waxing and waning disorientation, hallucinations, and agitation. Ed was admitted to the hospital for intravenous antibiotics and then moved to the rehabilitation unit at the nursing home. It took about two months for his delirium to fully resolve.

Sadly, Shirley passed away while Ed was recuperating from the pneumonia and delirium. Ed was able to attend the funeral and appeared appropriately grieved at the time. After fully recovering from his medical problems, however, Ed was still quite weak and unable to walk, and his daughter arranged for him to move permanently into the nursing home. Several weeks later a consult request came into my office: "Please see Mr. Blum—he is *psychotic*."

When I saw Ed, he seemed at first like his old self. He was generally well oriented, in good spirits, and cracking jokes: "Doc, did you hear the one about the priest and the rabbi riding in a plane together?" I had not heard that one, and Ed had me laughing a minute later. He told me about his days as a bandleader during the heyday of Miami Beach in the 1960s, playing with Frank Sinatra and other celebrities at the time. I then turned the subject to his present condition, and Ed reassured me that he was adjusting nicely to the nursing home. There was, however, one sticking point. Ed was not convinced that his wife had really died, and he was concerned about where she was.

"But, Ed, didn't you go to the funeral?" I asked.

"Yes, I remember the funeral, but that isn't my wife in the grave. It's my *mother*—they buried her in my wife's plot. A switch was made."

I tried to reconstruct Ed's logic. He knew that Shirley was gone, but he did not remember what had happened to her, and he had no recollection of sitting at her bedside when she died. When pressed, he admitted that his mother had died years before—"I remember *her* funeral!" he told me. Then why, I asked, did he think someone would put his mother's body into a grave marked for his wife? "I don't know," he replied.

When I saw Ed a week later, I asked him again what had happened to his wife. "They tell me that she died," he related, "but I am not certain. I just don't believe it." He was still convinced that his mother had been switched into his wife's plot. When I asked where Shirley was, his thoughts were murky. "I just don't know."

On the face of it, Ed seemed delusional in his belief that his wife had not actually died, and no argument could convince him otherwise. Such a false and fixed belief might seem to be a logical flight from the reality of his wife's death—a delusional form of denial. I also wondered whether Ed had a delusion of misidentification: Was he switching the memory of his mother with that of his wife? Or was Ed merely confused?

I held off giving him an antipsychotic because he was otherwise doing well and was not overly bothered by his belief. In addition, there seemed to be a plausible explanation for this potential delusion. Because of his previous delirium, Ed had only vague memories of his wife's death and burial. He knew only that his wife was gone, and like a good husband of more than fifty years, he was appropriately concerned. It was hard for him to believe what he had been told because he could not truly remember it happening. Ed's "delusion" seemed more like a poorly reconstructed memory from a dream or, in his case, from a delirium.

✖✖✖

Francine's near-miss diagnosis of psychosis raises an important issue that many older individuals face. Lacking a blood test or a brain scan for "delusionality," the diagnosis will ultimately rest on whether the doctor or other health care professional believes in the veracity of the patient's memories or not, which in turn depends on the time and energy devoted to learning the truth. After all, the paranoid person may have a real enemy and the jealous wife may have a true romantic rival. The "Martha Mitchell effect," a term coined by my college professor Brendan Maher, describes a situation in which a mental health clinician mistakenly diagnoses a patient's description of real events as delusional. He named this effect after Martha Beall Mitchell, the wife of Richard Nixon's attorney general, John Mitchell, who was said to be mentally ill when she began reporting to the press in the early 1970s that illegal actions were happening at the White House. The Watergate investigation later proved her correct—but not before she had been vilified by friends and family for her behaviors. Older patients, in particular, are often assumed to be unreliable historians, and many end up—like Francine almost did—being treated for psychotic "symptoms" that don't actually exist.

But with Ed, his belief was patently false. It seems to qualify as a delusion on the basis of the three criteria first outlined by psychiatrist and philosopher Karl Jaspers in 1913: (1) It is a strongly held belief, (2) no argument or logic can convince the person otherwise, and (3) the belief is clearly false to other people. And yet there are many other sorts of beliefs that might meet these criteria, but we would not consider them to be delusional. Jaspers might respond to this concern by pointing out that it is the form of the delusional belief, more than the content, that elicits the diagnosis. Thus, the way in which a truly psychotic individual persists in his or her delusional thought unfazed by counterarguments, contrary evidence, or incredulous witnesses is what leads to the diagnosis. Jaspers also described primary delusions as ultimately un-understandable, meaning that they have no logical underlying context in the person's life. As before, the diagnosis of a true "delusion" in some cases comes down to the point of view of the observer and the depth of the clinical investigation.

Ed's belief might qualify as a "secondary delusion" under Jaspers's scheme, because it is understandable given his mood (he was depressed over his wife's disappearance) and recent history (he attended her funeral). In a classic work on psychopathology, British psychiatrist Andrew Sims uses the term "delusion-like idea" to describe such a belief. As Ed's grief subsides and he comes to grips with his wife's death, he may correctly believe that it is her body, not that of his mother, buried in Shirley's plot. Only time will tell.

✾✾✾

Clearly, the 1928 *Stedman's* definition of psychosis encompasses a grab bag of psychiatric disturbances and neglects to account for the extensive writings on the meaning of psychosis by Karl Jaspers and others that were well known at the time. The 2004 *Stedman's* is more specific but still allows for the diagnostic errors and ambiguities presented by the cases of Francine and Ed.

Yet this may explain why I keep the shrine in my possession, with its old instruments, weathered books and pamphlets, and aging medical knowledge inside its drawers or placed on its sturdy wooden surface. Even though my profession has journeyed across many years and successive generations of practitioners, there is still much knowledge to be gained from looking back at where we came from. And much of the wisdom of years past is still relevant today—perhaps waiting to be reawakened with a little time and effort. This shrine—my grandfather's desk—is also a tangible metaphor for the older individuals with whom I work, teaching me that studying the memories from the past is a pathway to enlivening the present and opening a doorway to the future.

Part IV
Wisdom

Days should speak,
and multitude of years should teach wisdom.

—JOB 32:7

The Elders

The summer of 1972 was a momentous one in the history of Miami Beach. In the middle of July the Democratic National Convention convened at the Miami Beach Convention Center and, after a tumultuous week of late-night sessions, selected South Dakota senator George S. McGovern as the party's presidential candidate. The political temper of the time, roiled by conflicts over Vietnam, civil rights, and women's rights, stoked the passions of the delegates and guaranteed that the final result would not come easily. McGovern's determined political team was able to prevail, but only after sufficient balloting chaos among punch-drunk delegates who selected him over twelve other candidates and his running mate, Senator Thomas Eagleton of Missouri, over seventy-six other candidates submitted for voting, including Mao Zedong and Archie Bunker. In a 3 AM televised acceptance speech, McGovern trumpeted the essence of his campaign message: "I am here as your candidate tonight in large part because during four administrations of both parties a terrible war has been charted behind closed doors. I want those doors opened, and I want that war closed."

One month later the Republicans came to the same convention center on Miami Beach to confirm President Richard Nixon as their candidate for a second term. In his acceptance speech Nixon cleverly sought to undermine McGovern's floundering attempts at party unity: "Six weeks ago our opponents at their convention rejected many of the great principles of the Democratic Party. To those millions who have been driven out of their home in the Democratic Party, we say come home. We say come home not to another party, but we say come home to the great principles we Americans believe in together."

Although the pageantry and discipline of the Republican convention far outpaced those of the Democrats that summer, all hell broke loose in the streets. Antiwar protesters flocked to Miami Beach from around the country, where they met a strong police presence and the streets filled with tear gas. Despite a wise and well-intentioned attempt to confine most protests and protesters to a safe zone, Flamingo Park, several blocks from the convention center, the days of the convention saw screaming and aggressive protests against the delegates, mass arrests, and general chaos in the streets. The outcome of the election, however, bore no relationship to the passion of the protests, as Nixon's landslide victory over McGovern was one of the largest in U.S. history.

It has been close to forty years since that hot and troubled summer. Individuals who once struggled as delegates to make the political process more inclusive are now an entrenched part of the establishment. Young protesters of various stripes are now grandparents. Many radicals of that time still push for peace or justice, but their fervor prompts no fears—real or imagined—of violence or sedition. The streets around the Miami Beach Convention Center, a mere fifteen minutes from my office, are quiet. Flamingo Park is serene, with the only strident voices being those of young people running and playing. The poor and gritty streets of South Beach have been transformed into a sheik bastion of Art Deco hotels, boutiques, and clubs. Forty years ago a cross-sectional survey of Miami Beach would have revealed, so the joke goes, that its residents were born as Hispanic males and died as Yiddish-accented Jewish ladies. The senior boom has largely passed, however, with many of them living and dying in nursing homes like the one in which I work.

As a psychiatrist for the old, I am fascinated by the remnants of such a historical time. But the details of what happened as told by its aged eyewitnesses are not the only thing I find most informative. I want to know how they think *now*. How has age changed their perspectives? It is easy to imagine that the passage of time dulls the emotions of the past, softens a person's political bent, and brings greater understanding for past opponents. I saw this reflected in some of the comments on a historical account of the Miami events of 1972 that I found on the Internet: "Looking back there is only one thing I regret in my life," commented one former protester, now nearly sixty, "and that is being conned by the Anti-American Left during my youth."

Or perhaps age brings greater entrenchment of perspective. "I am still a liberal and proud of it," stated another anonymous former protester and Internet commentator, adding that he would still "fight in the streets to end this war." At the same time, a common stereotype is that old age brings less flexibility and greater obtuseness regarding detail. Age brings more experience, that is certain, and likely greater knowledge of things, but do these elements necessarily bring wisdom? And what do we mean by wisdom in the first place?

In the spring of 2008 I brought these questions to a former history professor and Methodist minister who had a particularly keen vantage point during the events of 1972. This eighty-five-year-old retired professor had also been a pilot in the U.S. Army Air Corps during World War II, flying thirty-five missions as a B-24 Liberator bomber pilot and awarded the Distinguished Flying Cross for saving his entire crew in an emergency landing. And what was this man's role during the summer of 1972? He was the man in the middle of it all: George S. McGovern.

I met McGovern in March 2008 when he came to speak at the annual meeting of the American Association for Geriatric Psychiatry (AAGP). As the medical editor for the organization's newsletter, I decided to seek him out for an interview, to which he readily agreed. In my research prior to our meeting, I learned that McGovern had served South Dakota as a congressman from 1957 to 1961 and as a senator from 1963 to 1981. From 1961 to 1963 he worked in the White House as President John F. Kennedy's director of the Food for Peace program.

McGovern's very presence at the AAGP meeting was an exciting event for so many attendees and served as a touchstone of powerful memories for those who had been politically active during the 1972 election. One colleague excitedly told McGovern how as a high school student she had campaigned for him and had had *his* poster on the wall of her room, as opposed to a poster of, say, the Beatles. His loss had been such a blow that she had sworn off any further political involvement. Another colleague recalled working as a medical student at an emergency medical station for protesters during the street riots.

McGovern himself is tall, dapper, and unassuming. He has a quietness and a warmth that radiate compassion and thoughtfulness. He is only a moderately aged version of the middle-aged man who strode upon the Miami stage back in 1972, and he retains the intellectual acuity and formidable orator skills that have characterized his entire career. Today McGovern remains in Mitchell, South Dakota, the town of his upbringing. He lives with one of his daughters ever since the death in 2007 of his beloved wife, Eleanor, after sixty-three years of marriage. Her loss was a body blow that he has only recently begun to recover from, aided by his decision to get back on the road—often traveling alone—to reach out to people and lecture on various topics. He readily admits that the intensity of his grief after Eleanor's death disrupted both his appetite and his normal pattern of sleep. With time, both bodily functions resumed their normal rhythms, but the experience changed his views on aging. He is less concerned now with what he might achieve and more focused on the value of interpersonal experiences. "I'd give everything I own in a heartbeat to have her back for one more year or one day," he said of Eleanor.

McGovern's sentiments echoed some of the dimensions of successful aging articulated by George Vaillant. As Vaillant has discovered through decades of research in Harvard's Study of

Adult Development (which he directs), successful aging is less dependent on the maintenance of perfect memory and cognition than on the "sustained capacity for joy." The study has followed three subgroups of a total of eight hundred individuals since the 1920s and 1930s, providing one-of-a-kind longitudinal physical, psychological, and social histories for these now-octogenarian subjects. Vaillant has found that good relationships are more important than events in terms of bringing happiness and that a good marriage at age fifty predicts positive aging at age eighty.

McGovern has certainly lived these findings. He was known, and still is, for the strength of his interpersonal relationships. Ironically, this may have been his political Achilles' heel in 1972 when up against the ruthless campaign of Nixon and his minions. McGovern recounted the controversy that erupted when it was revealed that his running mate Eagleton had been hospitalized several times for depression and treated with electroconvulsive therapy. McGovern initially rallied to Eagleton's side, even declaring that he was "1000 percent" behind him, despite deafening pressure from fellow Democratic leaders and the national press to dump the vice-presidential running mate. McGovern carefully weighed the pros and cons of keeping Eagleton on the ticket, consulting with multiple insightful individuals, including "America's most famous psychiatrist," Dr. Karl Menninger, whom McGovern managed to reach in a 2 AM phone call. Within a few short weeks Eagleton withdrew as the nominee and was replaced by Sargent Shriver, but not before the entire incident and McGovern's perceived handling of it did considerable political damage and may have contributed to his landslide loss.

I was particularly curious about how McGovern viewed the events of 1972 through the lens of old age. Had it given him a different perspective? "Right now, I think I'd be a better president than I would have thirty-six years ago," he told me. "I've learned more about the importance of working across party lines. . . . As I've gotten a little older, I've found I can work with a broader range of people and be comfortable about it." I wondered aloud about what had led to these changes. McGovern pondered for a moment and then answered, "I think you just come to a practical awareness that you can't just plow straight ahead and the devil take the hindmost. It just doesn't work that way with human beings. You've got to always have some degree of openness and tolerance for opposing points of view. . . . I've even become more eager to read opposing points of view."

McGovern was quick to add that being open and tolerant "doesn't mean you become flabby about where you stand on public issues." Instead, he articulated what has become a defining characteristic of wisdom: "a capacity to see that problems are really complicated, that there are other angles that have to be considered." Such a perspective, which includes self-education about all sides of an issue, leads to different ways of approaching problems: "I don't make snap judgments as quickly as I might have in earlier times," McGovern described. "I do think one characteristic of youth is to be impetuous, to assume that they're wiser than their parents, wiser than older acquaintances. I think I've developed a growing appreciation for the insights of other people."

McGovern's thinking is in line with what both gerontologists and cognitive theorists have discovered about the capacities of the aging brain. In *The Mature Mind*, geriatric psychiatrist

Gene Cohen summarizes the growing body of research demonstrating that aging individuals develop a new ability to think, strategize, and devise solutions in ways that go beyond the abstract, or formal, reasoning that Jean Piaget described as the endpoint of cognitive development. "Postformal reasoning," Cohen writes, "helps integrate the subjective and the objective, feeling and thinking, the heart and the mind, and becomes more facile . . . [in] deal[ing] with conflicting opposites in the second half of life." Psychologist Judith Stevens-Long describes how older thinkers can "integrate logic and the irrational aspect of experience. . . . [They] see not only how truth can be a product of a particular system, but also how the thinker participates in creating the truth." According to these definitions, postformal thinking allows an older individual to look at both sides of the coin simultaneously and then reason without being hampered by the inherent ambiguity or contradiction in the situation. This ability is life sustaining and even *life saving* in the final years.

It's easy to imagine how this sort of thinking comes into play with McGovern and many of his aged peers who continue to pursue meaningful activities even after profound losses. As a younger man McGovern was a war hero who commandeered bombers and a dedicated public servant who served under President Kennedy ("like being around royalty," he told me). As a middle-aged man he stood with the great political giants of our time and counted himself among them. He was one election away from the most powerful position in the world. There were years in which he was one of the most recognized figures on the planet. Yet now he travels alone, carrying his own suitcase through airports and walking about almost anonymously in most settings. Aging has robbed him of his political stature, influence, public recognition, and life companion. His horizon of activity, even with the best of actuarial projections, is measured in a few short years. Many younger individuals project themselves and their youthful sensibility into McGovern's stage and see only futility in front of a closing doorway. And yet for McGovern, this side of the coin doesn't stop him, doesn't haunt him, and doesn't preclude his interest and ability in seeking new adventure.

Indeed, the concept of a postformal mental state embodied so well by George McGovern was envisioned centuries ago by Roman philosopher Marcus Cicero in his famous essay "On Old Age." He wrote that "the reasons why old age is regarded as unhappy are four: one, it withdraws us from active employments; another, it impairs physical vigor; the third, it deprives us of nearly all sensual pleasures; and four, it is the verge of death." Yet Cicero sought to counter these beliefs by asserting that old age should be guided by rational reflection and not by the hedonistic pursuits we value in younger years. "The arms best adapted to old age," he wrote, "are the attainment and practice of the virtues; if cultivated at every period of life these produce wonderful fruits when you reach old age."

Such an approach can help an individual to recognize and cultivate many new strengths and advantages in later life that do not depend on physical vigor or sensuality. In fact, Cicero held that the pursuit of physical pleasures was actually a burden of youth that was lifted in later life. Freed from the youthful intensity of physical passions and girded with knowledge and wisdom, the accrued influence "is the crowning glory of old age."

Like a modern-day Cicero, Cohen writes passionately that the myth of cerebral decline must be countered by the fact that the brain *can* grow new nerve connections and physically resculpt itself in later life. As a result, the aging brain has the potential for more mature and interconnected neural circuitry to regulate thinking, emotions, and creativity. A recent study in support of this hypothesis found that the brains of older individuals are less emotionally reactive when viewing negative images, and another study showed that older individuals have more positive autobiographical recall compared to younger subjects. A large-scale survey published in 2010 found that levels of self-reported well-being and happiness declined from age eighteen to age fifty and then began to improve, nearly peaking at age eighty-five. In essence, aging may enable individuals to increasingly take to heart and brain the notion "Don't worry; be happy." Even though the vicissitudes of aging are always unpredictable, both ancient and modern lines of thought encourage individuals to think and act positively in late life while suggesting that the aging brain is better able to do so.

On this basis, Cohen proposes a series of human-potential phases that "reflect evolving mental maturity, ongoing human development, and psychological growth as we age." In each phase there is a surge of energy that promotes new activities and interests. In McGovern's case, after he lost his Senate seat in 1980, he founded a liberal political action committee, went back to teaching history, and then, in 1984 at the age of sixty-two, attempted another run for the presidency. Such persistent activity represents Cohen's "liberation phase," which occurs from the fifties to the seventies and during which individuals take advantage of newfound personal freedom and creativity to explore new pursuits. At the age of seventy-two McGovern suffered the tragic loss of his daughter Terry to alcoholism. Despite his grief, he wrote a book about her struggle and started a foundation in her name. Then in 1998 he began serving as the U.S. ambassador to the UN Food and Agriculture Organization, and in 2001 he was appointed the UN global ambassador on world hunger, recapitulating his earlier work on world hunger as a young member of the Kennedy administration. These activities occurred during what Cohen describes as the "summing-up phase," which occurs from the sixties to the nineties (and overlaps to some extent Erikson's eighth stage of integrity versus despair and Vaillant's "keeper of the meaning" phase) and during which an individual searches for a larger meaning to life, energized by wisdom and a desire to contribute to the world.

The last phase in Cohen's scheme is the "encore phase," beginning in the late seventies and characterized by personal reflection and reaffirmation and celebration of the major themes in a person's life. McGovern's presence on the lecture circuit, sans entourage, brings him back to his earliest roots as a politician and even a minister, traveling around and lecturing to audiences. He has also returned to his academic roots as a historian with a 2008 book on Abraham Lincoln. In my interview with McGovern, I asked him to sum up his life wisdom: "Be intellectually honest," he advised. "Don't shade the truth. Say what you honestly think. When I ran in '72, I said that I was making one pledge above all others: to seek and speak the truth. And I really tried to do that."

Cohen has described numerous other influential individuals who provide similar evidence for his scheme of aging, such as author Alex Haley, who began in middle age a search for his family history that eventually became the best-selling book *Roots*, and iconic dancer Martha Graham, who from her retirement as a ballet dancer at the age of seventy-five to her death at ninety-six spent her time choreographing new ballets. This incredible potential for artistic creativity in late life is perhaps best exemplified by the many great folk artists producing works (and even starting careers!) in their eighties and nineties. But are these extraordinary elders the outliers? Is such potential accessible for the aging masses?

Cohen suggests the development of what he terms a "social portfolio" to enable everyone to cultivate a sense of meaning, vitality, and dignity in later life. This practical approach is analogous to management of a financial portfolio and begins with an accounting of assets, including an individual's interests, skills, resources, and relationships. The social portfolio intends a slow buildup of assets over time and includes some form of insurance for dealing with potential losses. For example, an individual categorizes personal assets according to individual and group pursuits and then segregates them according to the degree of energy and mobility that they require. A sixty-five-year-old person who loves to ski with friends (a group activity requiring high energy levels and independent mobility) will eventually need to pursue alternative group and individual activities that involve lower levels of energy and mobility. The key is to identify activities (such as hiking, nature walks, bird-watching) that can bring equal degrees of gratification and socialization but are more realistically accomplished. An individual then possesses a list of vital and meaningful pursuits, and the process of developing the portfolio, sharing it with others, and reviewing it over time can motivate and inspire those who might otherwise drift toward stagnation and despair as they age. Keeping these interests in reserve provides a form of psychological insurance, preventing the avid skier from seeing life as less meaningful when she or he can no longer safely manage the same slopes.

Cohen basically defines wisdom as a broadening of perspective that includes the cultivation of creativity and social interaction. Neuroscientist Elkhonon Goldberg looks at wisdom as a product of nerve pathways built up over a lifetime of experiences. These pathways allow decisionmaking to increasingly take the form of "pattern recognition rather than problem solving." In practice, this means that the wise elder can quickly size up a situation and render judgment, almost like the "blink" that Malcolm Gladwell describes in his best-selling book on the subject.

But most longitudinal studies on cognitive ability have shown clear declines in performance starting in the fifties and sixties and encompassing a broad range of skills, including memory processing speed, numerical ability, visual pattern recognition, and word fluency. So here's a paradox: How does the brain lose capacity at the same time it seems to grow in wisdom? This paradox emerged in a conversation I had with eighty-eight-year-old Dr. Bernard Lown, an eminent cardiologist and current professor emeritus in cardiology at the Harvard School of Public Health who invented the cardiac defibrillator. In addition to his fame as a cardiologist, Lown is equally well known for his work as an international peace activist, winning the Nobel Peace Prize in 1985 for his role as cofounder of International Physicians for the Prevention of Nuclear War.

Lown had strong feelings about aging in general. "As you grow older," he told me, "you grapple with issues of age not out of knowledge but out of ignorance because you are ill prepared for it." Lown did acknowledge the fruits of age, which bring "a

certain perspective that is not merely intellectual but is an emotional perspective on life—what time is, what sorrow is, and
what loss is." And yet as he aged, Lown took notice of declines
in the cognitive skills deemed so essential to his role as a doctor.
His short-term memory began to atrophy, and the names of
drugs or the details of patient histories that had once been at
his fingertips became more elusive. "I would engage in circuitous
conversation to not let on to somebody that I didn't know it,"
he said, adding that it became more difficult to keep up with
the latest advances in his field. At the same time, however, "I
was better in judgment, far better and far keener, and the patients
sensed that. They would say to me, 'You're a far better doctor
than you were twenty, thirty years ago.'"

As Lown expressed the paradox, he was less sharp on the details and yet somehow better in general as a doctor. But where
does this wisdom come from? In part, it derives from the use
of cognitive pathways described by Goldberg, where overall
decisionmaking has a more automatic quality. It may also represent a shift in cognitive style in which older individuals take
in more detail, which slows them down compared to younger
people but ultimately results in the retention of more information for later analysis and decisionmaking. In his own words,
Lown described acquiring "the ability to commune and perceive an emotional dimension that is pre- or post- or *extra*-
verbal. It's not words—it's gestalt. It's an ability to perceive,
but more than that, a sensibility to nuance that is so trivial
that it is overlooked."

Lown's observations suggest that wisdom may be an emotional skill as much as it is an intellectual one. I thought about

this skill when discussing the events of 1972 with Marilyn Gold-aber, who was the director of social work at the Miami Jewish Health Systems when I first began working there in 1999. Marilyn once worked closely with her husband, Irving (now deceased), a sociologist who created and pioneered the use of the "win-win" strategy in which each side in a conflict could emerge with a resolution that met its needs. In fact, it was Irving, working as a consultant to Miami Beach Chief of Police Rocky Pomerance in 1972, who suggested that Flamingo Park be designated as a safe zone for protesters during the summer political conventions. Such a venue gave the protesters a place to camp out and exercise their free speech, while at the same time it relieved the Miami Beach authorities, to some extent, of their fears of the protesters. This certainly wasn't a perfect solution, but one as close to win-win as was possible at such a fractious time.

Today, Marilyn at age eighty-two is as sharp and articulate as she was during the summer of 1972. She now has her new husband, Mac, at her side. Mac is ninety-two years old and appears as fit and trim as the dashing young World War II bomber pilot staring out of the black-and-white wartime photographs in their apartment. He still rises early to exercise and walk five miles, as he has done daily for the last few decades. When I interviewed the couple, Marilyn reported that she was taking aging in stride, but Mac was more resistant. A once compulsively organized journalist and public relations/marketing genius, Mac bemoaned the fact that he could not accomplish even half of what he did when he was younger.

He focused on the decline in his previous abilities and the potential for further calamity. In fact, his description of aging echoed his stories of the Martin B-26 Marauder bombers that he flew on 122 missions in New Guinea during World War II. The plane was a gem once aloft, with great speed, stability, and capacity to drop a devastating payload on its targets. The problem, however, lay in takeoff, when the finicky engines had a high rate of failure at critical moments, earning the plane its nickname as the "widowmaker." "If the engine coughed on takeoff," Mac described, you were a goner because it meant the plane was not achieving sufficient speed and lift to continue climbing. Mac managed a fear of crashing back then, even surviving a bailout into enemy territory in the jungle of New Guinea and a several-week trek alone back to his base, despite being given up for dead by his squadron. But aging, at one point, brought a never-before-experienced lack of reassurance for Mac, who would climb out of bed on some days already burdened by the fear and frustration of potential failure.

During my initial interview with Mac and Marilyn, however, I pushed hard on the issue of wisdom and perspective in late life because I viewed them as role models. "How do you cope with these changes?" I asked Mac. "I don't really adjust," he told me in a tense voice. "I continue to be aggravated. If I make a plan for the day, I stay with the subject, but the problem is now I find myself drifting. I forget the subjects. I lose track of things. And somewhere along the line I find that I'm off the track. I am not meeting my standards." Cognitively, Mac had begun experiencing the slowing of memory processing speed and efficiency that most ninety-year-old brains face. And it seemed to have hit him in a particularly sensitive spot, because mental efficiency had been his trademark since his days in the service.

"Is anything better with age?" I pressed. "Are there any advantages?" Mac resisted the possibility: "I see deterioration on a daily basis" he said. Marilyn, however, chimed in with a different take. "But I see positives," she said, smiling at Mac. "You are much more mellow, much less hard on yourself." Mac had to agree, but he attributed the change to his motivation to please Marilyn or at least not to aggravate her. Marilyn pointed out an increased match between his intellectual and emotional maturity. "Is this different from the relationship you had years ago when you were married to your first wife?" I asked Mac. "I am much more sophisticated now," he confessed. "I know the value of adjusting to the change in my capacities. . . . I realize that if I don't adjust my style and my behavior that I am liable to hurt myself."

Marilyn went even further, describing how Mac had developed rich, loving relationships with his sister and her children that he never had in the past. "He has the capacity he never even knew—*love*," she said. "He is concerned. His sister's as well as my own children and grandchildren adore him. It's a delight. It's a whole life he didn't have. And he has not only adjusted, he's embraced it, and I think he has grown immensely. I see real positive aging." And this positive aging has continued for Mac and Marilyn, so much so that they could barely even relate to some of Mac's original concerns when I sat down with them two years after our original interview to read them excerpts. Even in the short interval between our meetings, they had grown so much as individuals and as a couple. I thought about them later when a ninety-six-year-old patient described how his life had been turned around for the better after working with a therapist on some chronic marital issues. Even at his age and after many years of marital problems and depression, he had found new peace and happiness with his wife.

Herein lies a critical lesson of aging: Even in the context of age-related intellectual decline and other losses, the enhanced capacity to love, create, and renew relationships is a gift of growing old not to be overlooked or trivialized. Surgeon and best-selling author Sherwin Nuland elaborates on this point in *The Art of Aging*, arguing that the factors most critical to successful aging include mutual caring and connectedness, maintenance of physical capability, and creativity. Vaillant's longitudinal data support this suggestion, revealing that the key personal strengths that underlie good relationships in later life include forgiveness, gratitude, and loving-kindness.

In contrast to Mac's embrace of new relationships, previous psychological theories of aging suggested that there was a natural process of disengagement in late life. In truth, many older individuals do have an eclipsed range of personal and social involvements and relationships. This is due in part to the loss of loved ones. Bernard Lown described poignantly how his mother responded to this natural attrition. At the age of ninety-five she asked her son, "Why am I living? I am already dead. The people that defined me are gone, so who am I?" If we are indeed defined by our relationships, Lown points out, then their loss robs us of the energy and memories that keep us going.

But there is a counterpoint to this view. What some see as disengagement may actually represent a pragmatic pruning back of life's activities and relations. This form of wisdom is encapsulated in the work of Laura Carstensen, a psychologist at Stanford, who suggests that aging individuals recognize their limitations and the shrinking horizon ahead and actively place a greater emphasis on seeking more positive and meaningful emotional experiences. The work of Carstensen and others has demonstrated that even in the face of losses such as those experienced by Lown's mother, many older individuals are able to maintain a generally positive emotional state. In my own experiences at the nursing home, it is not always clear whether it is denial, resignation, or acceptance of life's vagaries that enables this mind-set, or perhaps it is something else. This something else may be a form of spiritual wisdom that proves transcendent for many individuals.

During the summer of 1972 at the height of the protests, there was, not surprisingly, a tent in Flamingo Park sporting a handwritten sign that advertised "POT." Numerous young people flocked to the tent, expecting to score some marijuana. They were surprised, even shocked, however, when a young Hasidic rabbi emerged from the tent, proffering not pot but tefillin—the little leather boxes containing Bible verses that observant Jews don during morning prayers. "Put On Tefillin—P.O.T.—that's how I got them to stop by my tent," recalled Rabbi Avrohom Korf, now the Florida regional director of the Chabad Lubavitch organization. In terms of his own spiritual wisdom forty years later, Korf points to the thinking of his own spiritual master, Rabbi Menachem Mendel Schneerson, who held that old age is to be viewed not as a failing but as an ongoing opportunity to accomplish one's purpose in life. For Jews, Christians, Muslims, and people of many other faiths, wisdom, defined as "not merely the result of accumulated information" but as "the ability to focus on the unifying element *behind* all information" represents a call to action. The commandment to "rise up before the aged" (Leviticus 19:32) is not just a call for the young to respect their elders, but for the elders themselves to "rise up before age" and continue to pursue their enhanced ability for spiritual fulfillment.

Twentieth-century theologian Abraham Heschel added an existential component to the notion of spiritual wisdom, suggesting that if late life is "an age of anguish and boredom," then the answer must be to cultivate a sense of significant being as "a thing of the spirit . . . not entertainment but celebration." He added, poetically, that "old men need a vision, not only recreation. Old men need a dream, not only a memory." In this forward-thinking view, aging is a formative time, "rich in possibilities to unlearn the follies of a lifetime, to see through inbred self deceptions, to deepen understanding and compassion, to widen the horizon of honesty, to refine the sense of fairness."

Heschel offered an antidote to the distorted equating of aging with death or dementia that I was taught as a doctor and that permeates our culture. "The effort to restore the dignity of old age will depend upon our ability to revive the equation of old age and wisdom," he wrote. "Wisdom is the substance upon which the inner security of the old will depend forever. But the attainment of wisdom is the work of a lifetime." Wisdom is thus more than an achievement of aging; it is as integral and essential to the aging process as walking is to the toddler, play is to the young child, and the pursuit of love and partnership is to the young adult.

Gerontologist Lars Torstam, influenced in part by Zen Buddhism, elevates the role of spiritual wisdom to an even greater height, suggesting that aging can bring any older indi-

vidual to a place of "gerotranscendence," where experience is
less focused on time as a horizon and more on time as a moment. For Torstam, the wisdom of gerotranscendent individuals
enables them to shed much of their fear of death as well as the
human obsession with material things and superfluous social
interactions. There is a sense of connection to a greater spirit
in the universe and to the flow of generations past and yet to
come. We could argue that this state actually represents a form
of negative disengagement, but Torstam replies that such a
view is culture-bound and ignores the positive aspects of gerotranscendence, which he equates with the supreme wisdom of
old age.

Returning to the summer of 1972, I wonder how current
politics would be transformed, for better or worse, if the surviving and now elderly players from that era returned to the
scene, armed with all their wisdoms. McGovern has many ideas
for what he would like to do, but he is content to leave it up to
younger politicians, including his grandson, who recently ran
for office in Milwaukee, Wisconsin, and lost. Perhaps there is
still some hesitation on McGovern's part; he is, after all, the
man who during the Vietnam War cried out on the Senate floor,
"I'm fed up to the ears with old men dreaming up wars for
young men to die in." If we ponder his admonition, we might
ask whether it is natural and expected for the old to step aside
and let the young assume the reins of power and decisionmaking.
But perhaps the opposite is true—the aged should have a greater
role because of their wisdom.

Any answer today is largely a thought experiment, because
most elderly retire from both the workforce and positions of

power in their mid- to late sixties—a relatively young point in the scheme of old age. But perhaps the vision of greater involvement of our elderly can at least be approximated. In 1997, for example, former South African president Nelson Mandela brought together a diverse group of prominent older world leaders for a unique forum. Could these illustrious, aged individuals serve as an influential, experienced, and independent group of peacebuilders to be called "the Elders"? Since the group's creation, several of these Elders have traveled around the globe to various sites of war and oppression, hoping to bring their collective wisdom to bear on seemingly intractable conflicts. Although their individual political bents might belie their independent labels, the existence of such a group puts to the test the questions of whether old age actually confers a unique, *wiser* perspective and whether such a perspective can be translated into action. Time may tell.

I have learned, then, that it is easy to puff up wisdom into a great force of history. But wisdom in its truest and most common form is not sitting in judgment like King Solomon or trotting the globe like the Elders to weigh the woes and conflicts of humankind. The individuals who manage such feats are few and far between. Instead, wisdom shines forth in the daily tumult of aging. And a day in the life of an elder may be like the Miami summer of 1972, where chaos and order and pageantry and protest coexisted, where hippies and politicians, radicals and Republicans, potheads and rabbis all came together in one hot, crowded, tear-gas-filled island to make a point about the future of the country. Wisdom serves to calm this maelstrom, providing a way of thinking, feeling, and experiencing that brings order, harmony, and, for many, a great measure of happiness.

Bereft

"You are no longer my son. I hate you."

The hand that penned these words is now a bony and blemished relic of a once powerful woman. I envision the actual pen as a heavyweight sterling silver Montblanc, befitting a woman of wealth and prestige who doted on her husband and his many interests. But there was neither dignity nor doting in this same woman's letter to a wayward son. Her searing words were scrawled on a piece of lined notepaper, with disjointed letters barely able to sit adjacent to each other. Whether it was true hate that motivated this woman's letter or merely the bewildered and reactive anger of a wounded mother cannot be known. It is clear, however, that the long-standing feud between this mother and her son eventually shattered the last vestiges of their relationship, and they parted ways permanently following the death of her husband. She was bereft of all family and arrived at our facility as if out of the ether, without penny or home.

In appearance Miriam was a stately woman, meticulously groomed, her white hair pulled back in a tight bun. She described the central narrative in her life in bold terms: She came from wealth and married into wealth, and her husband was a successful banker and the love of her life. But her children were "rotten thieves" who swindled her out of her personal fortune. She denied any history of abuse or neglect of the children, nor did she admit to any family trauma or other arguments. "I tried to fix things up," she argued, "but my son demanded money in order to visit me." That offense, she contended, prompted the poison pen letter. From her arrival at the nursing home to my first interview with her, Miriam had received no visitors and had had no outside contacts. She occasionally spoke of distant cousins who had lost track of her.

I have, unfortunately, seen many similarly bereft aged individuals. Some, like Miriam, are vicious in their descriptions of absent children or family, whereas others exist quietly and without protest, providing little or no explanation for their solitude. Occasionally, the person has a telltale history of substance abuse, pathological gambling, chronic mania, personality disorder, or abusive behaviors that clearly drove family members away. Other times the family members themselves suffer from mental illness or are abusive or neglectful. In most cases these older individuals appear friendly and cooperative, yet incredulous at their fate. There are almost always missing pieces to their social and clinical histories that limit attempts to understand them and prevent potential reconciliations. They arrive with so many years of broken promises, lost fortunes, and burned bridges behind them that old age seems an unlikely time to heal.

Getting involved with these individuals raises its own challenges. Sometimes I learn from probing the histories of these lonely elders that they were, in fact, abusive or uncaring individuals. One daughter told me that when she was a child, her father used to dump cold buckets of water on her head for the smallest behavioral infraction. She will call to inquire about his health, but she will not see him. Another adult child hinted that her father was a sexual predator but could not bring herself to reveal more. She never visits. Sometimes these past behaviors are repeated in small ways, such as when Miriam accused her aides of being thieves who stole several pieces of costume jewelry that later appeared hidden in her room. With other bereft individuals, their appearances are so banal that it is hard to imagine why anyone would have abandoned them.

Knowing the history, however, may require some mental juggling. For instance, how does a mental health care provider form a therapeutic bond with a known sexual predator? Or a racist? How does a clinician feel empathy for a depressed patient who used to beat his children? It may be easier for an internist or a surgeon to face these patients, because their priority and duty are to heal the physical illness or injury at hand without having to probe the social history. The Hippocratic Oath of doctors tending to wounded enemy soldiers or terrorists during wartime does not discriminate on the basis of creed, even if it is a disturbing one. And in the rush of treatment, the doctor's ignorance of the patient's past sins may provide a protective emotional barrier.

The psychotherapeutic care of these older individuals is different, however, as it requires clinicians to learn about and understand past behaviors and their underlying causes. It might also require clinicians to subscribe to treatment goals that they reject in their hearts, such as helping an abuser to feel less depressed or to sleep better. The abandoning family members may resent or even obstruct attempts to help the patient, viewing clinicians as collaborators.

I recently began working on a family tree for my paternal relatives. As I called distant cousins around the country and slowly pieced each branch together, I began to feel a profound deepening of my own connections to both my father and his kin. I also saw how easily people could lose track of one another and how branches of the tree could break off and isolate individuals or families from one another. This experience led me to imagine Miriam as a small twig pruned from a tree, falling to the ground and being blown by the wind far from its trunk of origin.

Miriam, however, was wiser and more resourceful than I gave her credit. She became an integral part of the unit by befriending many other residents and staff. She was particular about whom she associated with, but bold nonetheless, and within several months had built up a social network throughout the nursing home. She had, in essence, formed a new family consisting of members who knew nothing or cared nothing about her past. This stance, I realize, is also essential when caring for most of these bereft older individuals. Regardless of past behaviors, they have arrived and must be tended to. I rarely know the exact truth of their past, and so I have to focus on their present and future. This is not an act of absolution but one of wisdom and adaptation, and serves as a necessary act of humanity in the final stages of life.

Just Words

What a loud voice cannot convey is better carried by a whistle across the deep valleys, or barrancos, of La Gomera, a small mountainous island in the Canary Island chain off the coast of West Africa. Over centuries the shepherds of La Gomera developed a unique way to shape these whistles into an actual language, called Silbo Gomero. To untrained ears, these whistles strike the brain like any other nonsensical sounds, perceived but meaningless. To speakers of Silbo, however, these whistled communications activate the same parts of the brain involved in language comprehension and expression.

One lesson here is that a language can consist of something more than just words, be it whistles, tongue clicks, or hand gestures. This lesson is learned the hard way by older individuals with severe language disturbances, called aphasia, who struggle to find an elusive language without words that will override their jumbled linguistic circuits. In the beginning, however, this "language of one" is nonsensical because, according to the philosopher Ludwig Wittgenstein, the true meaning of a language emerges through its use among people. But with time and interaction, a new form of communication may emerge.

My older patient Rachel had once been fluent in five languages—not an uncommon skill for individuals born and raised along many European frontiers prior to World War II. At the time of our first meeting, however, the speech of this elderly polyglot had been reduced to a nonfluent cadence of chopped words that resembled some English and at least some Hungarian. As long as she didn't speak, however, she had an air of normality. I often bumped into her strolling along the brick footpaths near the assisted living facility in which she lived. She always remembered me and would greet me with a kiss on my hand and a sincere embrace.

I initially suspected that Rachel suffered from a relatively rare form of dementia afflicting the frontal and temporal lobes of her brain because her symptoms seemed to consist solely of impaired language function, including difficulty expressing words and an inability to name things. Her brain scan was unremarkable, and her medical history, physical exam, and labs were unrevealing. She refused to sit for neuropsychological testing. With time came worsening language function, behavioral outbursts, and more cognitive decline, still suggesting the rare form of dementia I initially suspected but also the more common Alzheimer's disease.

More pressing than her diagnosis, however, was the question of how best to communicate with Rachel. Once she came to the clinic in great distress, crying out unintelligibly and grimacing whenever her abdomen was touched. Her condition seemed clinically to be some form of gastrointestinal illness, and yet an extensive workup that included an abdominal X-ray, CAT scan, ultrasound, and, eventually, a colonoscopy was unrevealing. Rachel returned from the hospital calmer, but with the lingering mystery of what she had been trying to tell us.

There are many debates about the difference between words and deeds. Lofty words may invoke great power, but words not backed up by deeds may be ultimately meaningless. A student of Wittgenstein might argue, however, that because reality stems from the shared logic and meaning of our language, words *are* deeds. Anything that lies beyond the logic of our speech is otherwise meaningless, worthy only of silence. And yet I have sometimes found that the patients who speak the loudest are those in whom language has dissolved. Like the shepherds of La Gomera, they are forced by necessity to shape words into whistles.

The key question is whether these whistles—in whatever form they manifest—will hit the brains of listeners as nonsensical sounds or as meaningful expressions. I am reminded of the legend of King Solomon, who was said to have understood the language of the birds, and I ask, "Who among us has the patience and wisdom to listen closely and try to understand the whistling and warbling of our own linguistically impaired elderly?"

I came close to this ideal state one day when Rachel burst into my office, grabbed me by the arm, pulled me out of my chair, and without making a sound escorted me arm in arm down the hallway of the clinic. Several nurses watched the scene incredulously and followed behind, wondering whether Rachel had gone mad. As we rounded the corner and entered one of the bays off the hallway, Rachel pushed me up to her sister-in-law, Emma, who was sitting in a wheelchair. She gestured at Emma and let out a high-pitched whine saturated with a pained inflection. The sound made me wince, and I instinctively knew that Emma needed help. Indeed, Emma had been trying to call the doctor, and none had appeared. Rachel had felt her pain and was able to convey it to me.

Emma looked at me and raised her arms upward: "God has forgotten me," she sighed. I surveyed the scene in front of her, now surrounded by a retinue of interested and concerned staff members, with Rachel standing by, beaming proudly. In the moment, I understood Rachel perfectly. I turned to Emma. "Has God forgotten you?" I asked, and then answered, "I don't think so."

Liar, Liar

"Lies, my dear boy, are found out immediately, because they are of two sorts. There are lies that have short legs, and lies that have long noses."

—CARLO COLLODI, *PINOCCHIO*

This was a long-nosed lie, and I knew that payback was coming. Several minutes earlier Ginny had bulldozed into my office with her walker. "Why the hell am I here? What's this all about?" I stared at her for a moment in silence. "All I want from you is my scooter!" she demanded. "Give it back!" The bare truth was that Ginny was moderately demented and perpetually hostile and paranoid. I was getting calls from nursing staff telling me that she had fixated on one particular chair on her unit and was forbidding anyone else to sit in it. It had even come to blows one day when she punched poor Victor, who had unknowingly sat in "her" chair, his deaf ears not hearing her stomping and curses from behind.

Fueling her anger was the fact that for several months Ginny had been demanding the return of her electric scooter. The nursing home administrator and I had recently made a decision to restrict her from using it for safety reasons, and I was supposed to inform her that day. However, given her demeanor and her hatred of psychiatrists, I feared an explosion.

"I'm one of your doctors," I stated, intentionally leaving out my specialty. She fired back, "Can I have my scooter?" I hesitated to answer. "Well, Ginny, we haven't yet decided," I lied. Ginny's angry face seemed to scrunch up into a single point that jabbed at the fragile bubble of my lie. She could be amazingly prescient even in the fog of dementia and paranoia. "Liar! Liar!" she accused, and then stood up and shrieked at me, "Go to hell!" I quickly opened the door and let her pass. I could hear her carrying on as she traversed the long hallway of the clinic. "That doctor can go to hell!" she called out repeatedly, her words echoing back to my office several times. "He can go to hell!" In her wrath she seemed to stretch my long-nosed lie past each office bay, around the front desk, and out into the courtyard in front of the clinic. Maybe it would have been better if I had simply told the truth.

Truthfulness is the foundation of the doctor-patient relationship, both as a method of discourse and as one of the "most widely praised character traits" of a doctor. Gone are the days when doctors withheld certain diagnoses or treatment details from patients. If anything, doctors today are often forced to disclose excess and sometimes unnecessary information due to concerns about liability or to patients who have already canvassed the Internet on their own and have pressing questions. The doctor's challenge is to present what he or she knows to be true about the diagnosis and its treatment options and to do so in a manner that truly informs the patient. But there are limitations and pitfalls to this process, as illustrated in the following paraphrased conversation I recently had with a seventy-five-year-old moderately demented patient and his wife:

> PATIENT: Doctor, I know I can still drive. Just let me take a test.
> DOCTOR A: I'm sorry, Mr. K, but I can't help you with that. As we discussed, your memory impairment makes it unsafe for you to drive.
> PATIENT: Just let me take the test. I can drive just fine.
> DOCTOR A: The memory testing tells us that you would not be a safe driver.
> PATIENT: My memory is not that bad. I know I can drive.
> PATIENT'S WIFE: Honey, I told you that the car is not working now and needs to be fixed. Let's talk about it later.
> PATIENT: Okay.

Mr. K's wife did what caregivers for individuals with dementia often do—she placated his concerns for the moment and then redirected him, in essence telling a lie. Should doctors ever do the same thing?

According to a leading book on medical ethics, "Careful management of medical information—including nondisclosure,

deception, and lying—will all occasionally be justified when veracity conflicts with other obligations." Every clinician has encountered situations in which being too bluntly honest about
a diagnosis can actually be harmful to the patient, and so we
employ what is euphemistically referred to as "benevolent deception." Consider mentally fragile patients with whom full
disclosure of a devastating diagnosis may cause excessive anxiety,
abandonment of ongoing therapies, or total loss of hope. In
these circumstances, strict adherence to the clinical virtues of
truthfulness and candor risks violation of the core ethical principle to do no harm. We are left telling a series of what I term
"short-legged lies," or partial truths that take small steps toward
eventual and necessary disclosure of the complete truth.

As much as I urge eventual, complete disclosure of the truth
to every patient, there are individuals with dementia who will
not be able to appreciate the meaning of what they are told and
cannot correctly distinguish between truth and deception. Perhaps there is still an obligation to at least go through the motions. I think about how I endeavor to always formally introduce
myself to patients regardless of their mental state—even when
they seem completely insensible. There is a transcendent ethical
principle at stake here applying specifically to severely demented
individuals: the preservation of their human dignity, even when
they lack the ability to perceive its personal value. Truth-telling,
in some form, appears to be a key part of this principle.

In work with cognitively impaired patients, there is a certain
savoir faire to telling the truth, or a piece of it, without causing
unnecessary confusion or anguish. "Frank but not blunt" is how
one textbook characterizes the ideal approach, recommending

that the clinician present the reality of a medical situation without causing the patient to lose all hope. This is a difficult and sometimes impossible tightrope to walk, especially when a clinician has to convey a diagnosis in which there is no hope for cure. In those moments clergy are often more skilled than doctors at providing hope for something other than physical redemption.

I recently had to inform a relatively young couple in their late fifties of a diagnosis of Alzheimer's disease in the husband. There was no escaping a frank presentation of the data and the logical conclusion. I was girded with the knowledge of a recent study suggesting that, contrary to the fears of many doctors, patients are unlikely to demonstrate catastrophic reactions when a diagnosis of dementia is relayed. In fact, many are relieved. In this case, however, there was no visible relief. Instead, I saw the color drain out of the woman's face as the meaning of the diagnosis settled in. Her tense facial expression relaxed, no longer anticipating the verdict, but then began to absorb the tears tracing a growing look of despair. She had many questions that I knew would come in time, but I wasn't ready to lay out any more truths that day. It was not even the moment to talk of hope—of medications, therapeutic programs, and research. It was a moment instead to retreat into the practice of medicine described by the poet Virgil as *ars muta*, the "silent art." Bioethicist James F. Drane captures a more modern-day description of this form of truth-telling: "There are times for both the patient and the doctor when silence both carries deep meaning and is an appropriate expression of truth."

Rules of Four

"His head feels like a furry leaf, but softer."

This was the unintentional poetry of a six-year-old boy meeting his newborn brother for the first time. That "furry leaf" is now a wild bush of brown curls that sails through the house, jumping from couch to chair and through clutters of overturned toys, Legos, and puzzle pieces with the energy that only a four-year-old boy can expend. I am tired just watching him. I think to myself how the universe of a four-year-old has its own rules. He lives in the moment. He speaks what is on his mind. Sometimes he asks for what he wants; sometimes he screams for it. Regardless, I love every hair on his head. No matter what he does or how he looks, he is always beloved to me. And aside from the few instances in which he tells me that I'm "fired," I know that he feels the same. These guiding principles for my four-year-old son and me—or "rules of four," as I call them—are a binding force between us.

On many nights I engage in a ritual familiar to most parents and steal silently into his room just to watch him breathe. I sit next to his bed and lay my head on his pillow, my nose nestled into curls that smell of oatmeal and honey from his bath. The only sounds are his soft rhythmic breaths and the hushed blowing of the air conditioner. His expression is serene. It is in these quiet moments that I sometimes pose questions that perhaps only a geriatrician would consider: Who will attend to this precious child when he is ninety? Who will guard him as he sleeps, guide him while awake, and treasure him merely for his presence? There will come a time, I imagine, a time long in the future, when my youngest son will be an old man, bereft of his parents and siblings. Who will love him and care for him like we do?

There have been many evenings when I have walked the halls of the nursing home in which I work, attending to last-minute orders or residents' needs. I often stop to look at the photographs that family members have posted in the clear plastic shadow boxes outside many of the rooms. Black-and-white photographs of ancient childhood scenes mingle with formal wedding poses, soldiers in crisp uniforms, beloved pets, and color shots of children and grandchildren. Outside one room a twenty-five-year-old model strikes a pose in a stylish black dress with arm-length gloves, her fingers balancing an ivory cigarette holder in her lips. Inside the room, the frail body of this same woman, now eighty-five years old, lies silently in her bed. Outside another room I see an entire lifetime before me: an infant child in his mother's arms, a World War II marine, a father with children, and then a retiree sitting with his grandchildren. With one eye I regard this circle of life; with the other I peer into his room where he sits asleep in a wheelchair. And I wonder, To whom are these residents still beloved?

Rule #1: When you need something, ask. When you don't get it, scream.

Anita reminded me of this rule the other day. I sat with her in my office, thumbing through her chart and reading—*again*—that she was screaming at staff. There were a few choice words that she preferred to use to get what she needed, and they seemed to work, although at a cost. Her undergarments were clean, but she was not well liked. "Anita," I said calmly. "*Anita*," I repeated with a little more emphasis, and implored, "You cannot scream at the nurses." My face was serious, but I softened it with a half-smile, mouth closed. We had talked about this before, but I still wanted to be patient with her. "Listen, Dr. Agronin," she said, "you don't understand what *I* do, and *I* am a pro at this. If I don't scream, they won't come to help me."

Anita stared me down, and I wasn't sure what to say. I know how things work on a busy floor in a nursing home. The staff work hard, and they cannot drop everything and run instantly each time a resident rings the call bell. Sometimes screaming does work better than softness. "Remember rule number one," I thought. Anita lives in the moment. She is mildly cognitively impaired and majorly impetuous. At eighty-eight years old, confined to a wheelchair, widowed, and racked with pain from a large sore on her behind, she has lost all manner of discretion. She tells it like it is, and if a bowel movement is pressing and she needs help, you'll know it. Here is my disclaimer: I do not endorse or condone this approach in the nursing home; in fact, it is my job to treat it. But I do understand it.

Rule #2: Every hair on your head is important to me.

If you think about how precious young children are to their parents, no one is surprised when they dote over them, marveling at every word and each new hair and tooth. Then why are we so surprised when older family members do essentially the same thing? Edgar was one such son who baffled and annoyed the nursing home staff. He used to measure his ninety-five-year-old mother's temperature to the tenth of a degree, trusting neither the thermometer at the nurse's station nor the judgment of the medical staff. According to the doctors, normal body temperature is 98.6 degrees Fahrenheit, with some variation by time of day and method of measurement. According to Edgar, the normal body temperature range for his mother was between 97 and 98.2 degrees Fahrenheit; anything above was, by his empirical method, a fever that required workup. He kept a log by her bedside with his own daily measurements.

I was called one day to mediate a dispute between Edgar and his mother's doctor. For two days Edgar had recorded a temperature of 98.8 degrees, and he was panicked. He demanded a chest X-ray for his mother, along with urine, sputum, and blood cultures. The doctor refused, stating that 98.8 degrees was not a fever and that there was no evidence of infection. Edgar threatened to report the facility to the state. I pulled the doctor aside, knowing that trying to negotiate with Edgar was futile; he was worked up into such a lather that my very presence as a psychiatrist might put him over the edge. "I know that he can be unreasonable," I admitted, "and I know that he has an obsessive-compulsive personality dis—"

"Yeh think?" the doctor interrupted me. "I'm drawing a line in the sand here."

"Don't do that," I suggested, trying to reason with her without taking Edgar's side. "She has a little bit of a cough—will a chest X-ray hurt anyone? In the very least it will get him off of your back."

The X-ray was taken, and it showed, to everyone's surprise, except Edgar's, a rip-roaring pneumonia. If the doctor had waited one more day, Edgar's mother might have ended up in the hospital. Rule number two came to mind: It's not her hair but every tenth of a degree in her body temperature that is important to Edgar. He knows her and cares for her more than anyone else ever will. His observations and demands may be a burden for the doctors and staff and may challenge their clinical judgment, but they stem from a fierce sense of love and protection.

Rule #3: No matter how you look, you are adorable to me.

Jorge was in love with Marta, deeply in love. After forty years of marriage and five children, the fire might be expected to burn a little lower. The love I see in many similar couples is warm, reserved, and practical, like the glowing embers of a small fire. For Jorge, his love for Marta was like a burning torch. His request to me, then, was not surprising; "Do anything to bring her back." Marta had suffered a massive stroke several months earlier but remained in a coma. The only thing keeping her alive was the ventilator next to the bed, pumping oxygen through the ribbed blue tubing hooked into the tracheotomy site in her neck. After lingering in the hospital for several weeks, she had been transferred to our long-term vent unit.

Marta was motionless in the bed, showing an occasional flutter of her eyelids that Jorge interpreted as some form of communication. The scene in the room was intimidating to most visitors. On one side of the bed hung a bag of beige liquid nutrients being infused into Marta's stomach through a soft gray tube. Adjacent to the bed a urine bag was hanging visibly from the metal side rails. In the background was the constant, rhythmic whoosh of the ventilator. The room felt humid and had an antiseptic smell. On most days I found Jorge hovering at her side, smoothing her hair and saying, "You are beautiful, *mi amor.*" Here was a vision of rule number three: the personage of Marta, lying insensibly in bed with a full diaper and the odors of bodily fluids, surrounded by tubes and machines and pumps—but still adorable to her true love.

I had spoken to the pulmonologist about Jorge's request to try a cocktail of stimulants to bring Marta out of her vegetative state, but she was hesitant. Marta's cardiac status was fragile, and multiple brain scans and neurological exams had confirmed irreversible brain damage. We could still care for her body, but her mind had slipped too far away. Nevertheless, Jorge's torch was undimmed.

Rule #4: No matter what you do, I still love you.

I do not understand how Bonnie manages to care for her mother, Shelly, at home. Shelly is morbidly obese, confined to a wheelchair, moderately demented, and *mean.* She doesn't ask for things; she screams once, curses, and then tries to pinch or bite if she isn't tended to immediately. She wakes Bonnie up at night for no specific reason, yelling for her daughter to come to her mother's room. I have tried everything to calm Shelly, but with each new medication trial comes a new side effect: confusion, agitation, tremors, and diarrhea. Ironically, the only medication that has worked, and that she has tolerated, is Thorazine. For most of my patients, Thorazine would be the equivalent of a chemical sledgehammer, so I never use it. Even so, it merely slows Shelly down without stopping her rampages.

At our last meeting Shelly was relatively calm. She denied her behaviors, insisting that her daughter was lying to me. I contrasted the descriptions of Shelly's behavior with her beautifully dressed and manicured appearance in my office. "What did you do in the past?" I asked her. Her remote memory was still intact, and she described to me her life as a young model, actress, and singer. "It's true," Bonnie told me, gazing at her mother lovingly; "you were quite a singer, sweetie." Shelly basked in the love for a moment and then shot back, "You're my sister, aren't you?" Bonnie didn't miss a beat: "No, remember sweetie, I'm your daughter, Bonnie." Shelly was not convinced. In fact, she looked disgusted.

As I listened to a litany of problem behaviors, I looked straight at Shelly. She smiled knowingly and then confessed, "Since I don't have a mother to give me attention, I *have* to behave that way." This was a moment of lucidity and honesty, and it faded quickly. But I understood: rule number one crossed with rule number four. Shelly wanted her mother, and so did Bonnie.

✳✳✳

These rules of four represent for me the bond between parent and child, and I have learned that they do not stop at the age of four. The child may now be sixty and the parent eight-five, but the rules still apply. Some rules change with the person or context, whereas others are inviolable. I see this all the time in the nursing home, although now the roles of parent and child have been reversed. Sometimes it is an older spouse or sibling, or a niece or nephew, who fills in the dyad. As a doctor, I am sometimes surprised by how emotional or irrational these caregivers can become. But I have to catch myself at those moments, examine the relationship, and remember the rules. If I can empathize with their own rules of four or five or *eighty-five*, then I can intervene in a caring way. And my sincerest hope is that if my own precious child is the one lying in a nursing home bed someday long in the future, with my caring hand only a memory, that someone else's protective wing will be there—and let it be as emotional or irrational as is required to care for him.

Part V
A Million Sparks

Seeing, in April, hostas unfurl like arias,

and tulips, white cups inscribed with licks of flame,

gaze feverish, grown almost to my waist,

and the oak raise new leaves for benediction,

I mourn for what does not come back: the movie theater—

reels spinning out vampire bats, last trains,

the arc of Chaplin's cane, the hidden doorways—

struck down for a fast-food store; your rangy stride;

my shawl of hair; my mother's grand piano.

My mother.

> *How to make it new,*

how to find the gain in it? Ask the sea

at sunrise how a million sparks can fly

over dead bones.

—GRACE SCHULMAN, "CELEBRATION"

Final Acts

Old age is the closing act of life, as of a drama, and we ought to leave when the play grows wearisome, especially if we have had our fill.

—MARCUS CICERO, "ON OLD AGE"

Here is a scene from the final act of a man's life: A small crowd of spectators, all clad in blue and white scrubs, were gathered around the imposing figure of an eighty-five-year-old hospital patient. His outstretched arm jabbed toward the crowd while the other cradled the soiled bedsheet wrapped around his body like a toga. "Hear me! Hear me!" he bellowed at each staff member, his face wide-eyed and contorted like a crazed orator. With each shout he spun a quarter-turn from his perch on the floor, spreading out the pool of urine in which he sat. Each nurse tried, in turn, to entreat the man to calm down and return to his room. Thirty minutes into his increasing agitation, I received a phone call requesting an urgent psychiatric consultation. I entered the scene and asked that the crowd disperse, save one kindly nurse. After a few minutes without an audience, the man calmed down and was coaxed into a wheelchair.

Scene two occurred a day later and opened with this same man lying in a hospital bed. He was again agitated, begging for someone to hear him but unable to make his needs known. I prescribed a mild sedative to calm him, but with little effect. He languished for several days with spreading infection and delirium, insensible to surrounding family, and then he passed away. This short drama was all that I witnessed of the man's long life. I was one of his doctors only at the end, and I missed the last few years of kidney failure, chronic pain, and dementia. Prior to that, he had been a successful architect, an avid traveler and photographer, and the patriarch of a large family. In reflecting back on all of the pain, indignity, confusion, and agitation of his last few years, the man's son raised a logical question: "What's the point? If that is old age," he wondered, "who needs it?"

This is a common question today and has been a common question since antiquity. Indeed, the search for answers that provide some meaning to aging is an ancient pursuit, explored in depth in the Bible and in later writings by major Greek and Roman philosophers. "Rise up before the aged, and honor the face of the sage," instructs Leviticus 19:32. From the vantage point of the Bible, this is an easy task because most of the major players, from Adam to Noah and from Abraham and Sarah to Moses, remained active and influential in later life. They served as role models for aging and countered darker voices, such as are found in Job 12:1, where the reader is warned to remember days of youth, "Before the evil days come, And the years draw nigh, when thou shalt say: 'I have no pleasure in them.'"

Ancient Greek philosophy was less sanguine about aging. According to the hedonistic teachings of Aristippus of Cyrene (435–356 BC), the pursuit of pleasure was the supreme good, especially the immediate gratifications obtained by the body. The later writings of Epicurus (342–270 BC) focused less on physical pleasure and more on the measured pursuit of mental tranquility, coupled with the absence of fear and physical pain. For both schools of thought, old age presented a serious challenge because illness, pain, and infirmity often limited the pursuit of most forms of pleasure. In essence, aging was equated with death. This is not surprising given that the average life expectancy in ancient Rome was twenty-eight years.

But today the average lifespan is now close to eighty. In our deepest aspirations we hope for a *good* old age, a *golden* age where gold means a time of interpersonal richness, wisdom, and gilded reflection on the deeds of our lives. But although we can extol the sense of integrity and satisfaction that can come with a life lived long and well, we must ask what would be the meaning and value in aging for those who have failed to achieve this? In 44 BC Roman philosopher and statesman Cicero wrote in his essay "On Old Age" that "old age is respectable as long as it asserts itself, maintains it rights, is subservient to no one." If this is true, then what do we make of those aged individuals who can no longer assert themselves or who are dependent on caregivers for satisfying most of their needs? Cicero himself seemed to recognize a point of no return: "As the pursuits of the earlier periods fall away, so do those of old age, and when this happens weariness of life brings a season ripe for death."

A time for death? I call this the "enough is enough" argument, and I have heard it from countless older individuals in the throes of illness. I have also heard it from baby boomers obsessed with their independence and right to make all health care decisions as they project themselves into an imagined state of dementia and disability. Philosophers and ethicists have a version called the "fair innings argument," which postulates that those aged individuals who have already experienced many good years of life should not be endlessly preserved at the expense of younger individuals. This argument is pursued in the writings of medical ethicist Daniel Callahan, who raises concerns about the disproportionate amount of resources spent on extending the length but not necessarily the quality of the lives of older individuals. He asks whether "there is an obligation to keep the elderly alive as long as possible, regardless of the cost of doing so." Perhaps, he asserts, "there is a duty to help young people to become old people, but not to help the old become still older indefinitely." And how does Callahan define "old"? "My own answer," he states, "is that someone is old when it can be said that he or she has had a 'full life,' by which I mean enough time to do most (though not necessarily all) of the things that a life makes possible: education, family, work, and so on." Callahan imagines that between the ages of seventy-five and eighty most people have lived a full life, and he then suggests that most of us would not regard death at that time as a tragedy.

This is a well-crafted argument from a thousand feet high, but it often flounders on the ground in face-to-face interactions with older people. It may also lead to cynical and fatalistic attitudes toward both medical care and meaningful activities for the oldest and most debilitated individuals. The "what's the point?" argument engenders apathy and resignation among younger generations who could be vitally involved with their elders. It also prompts the great fear that limiting resources to the aged leads down a slippery slope toward a society like the fictional Republic of Britanura envisioned by novelist Anthony Trollope in his 1882 work *The Fixed Period*. In Britanura the "problems" of old age are solved by mandatory suicide at the age of sixty-eight. The 1967 novel *Logan's Run* is a modern version of Trollope's dystopia, as is the world in the 1973 movie *Soylent Green*, in which older individuals are gently euthanized and then turned into food.

This latter argument is exaggerated, of course, because no one would argue for such a world. But in the hinterlands of the aged, in quiet rooms where the oldest of the old dwell, there are raging arguments about what to do about aging, sometimes solved by passive or active unsanctioned neglect. And in many cases even our best intentions seem futile and they utterly fail, pushed aside by what I call the "Four Horsemen of Old Age": depression, dementia, delirium, and destitution. In nearly every tragic case of aging, one or more of these reapers are in attendance. And when they hold the mind in their grip of dissolution, any talk of potential quality of life seems comical. We pity and sometimes shake our heads at caregivers who persist in loving and attending to diseased or dying older loved ones or who rage at their attendants in hope of salvaging some last vestige of a good old age.

I have a deep and enduring fascination and affection for these aged souls. Their care is my life's work and my passion. But many of the countless older patients whom I have treated have tested me as a doctor, and I have sometimes failed. And they have forced me to admit that old age is not always what I want it to be. Thus, the sentiments behind Cicero's resignation and Mr. K's son's despair are understandable. At this point, the doctor reaches the limits of all knowledge and technique. Cicero seems to rule the day only as long as the aged mind is intact and the body is still able to secure its basic needs; after that, many elders reasonably assert, "Close the curtain. Enough is enough!"

I have seen, however, how sparks of humanity persist until the final moments, and I must state, "Perhaps we are missing something." Even without mental rationality, there are perception, emotion, and imagination. Even without the ability to walk or even move independently, there are still movement and sensation. Even for Mr. K., there were years of existence prior to his final moments that were filled with the potential for meaningful experiences. We cannot reverse death, but dementia, depression, delirium, and destitution are challenges we *can* do something about. If Cicero had the audacity to challenge both the hedonism and the ageism of Roman culture, why can't we push our own cultural envelope a bit further? Here the young can help the old to form intergenerational connections, create vital activities, relieve pain and mental suffering, and ensure a dignified existence. Cicero, too, recognized these timeless responsibilities: "When the end comes what has passed has flowed away, and all that is left is what you have achieved by virtue and good deeds." In the final act, it is not life that fails our efforts, but our lack of effort that fails the still pulsating life.

I contrast the last stage of life and its profound challenges to a vantage point one step beyond the passing of an individual. My friend Eli is a volunteer member of a *chevra kadisha*, or Jewish burial society, in which he helps to ritually prepare bodies for burial in what is known as the *tahara* ritual. This responsibility is considered one of the holiest acts in Judaism, because the deceased can never thank those who accord this final act of respect. As Eli has described to me, the ritual cleansing, washing, and enshrouding of the body are performed in a careful and dignified manner and are accompanied by the recitation of specific prayers. The four volunteers do not converse during the ceremony other than required, and they never turn their backs to the body or expose it in an undignified manner. It is a wholly anonymous task, without any thanks given or received. The holiness of the act is thanks enough.

The respect accorded to the deceased is not unique to Judaism but is enshrined and ritualized in most religious and secular burial rites. In general, both the ritual and ethics of death are well structured in our society, focusing on values of respect and dignity for the deceased and comfort and meaning for their mourners. With many older individuals, however, the final months and years of life are often folded together and considered a living death, but never given the amount of attention, ritual, or respect accorded when death finally arrives. For if we regard every second of life as precious, then the incredible degree of respect that we naturally accord to the deceased must also be extended to the living. Hospice for the dying must be preceded by a movement of meaning and vitality for the still living! Otherwise, we end up missing profound opportunities to understand our elders and, by extension, ourselves. We also miss opportunities to encourage and gather together the still present sparks of life that can transform the experience of aging into a more positive and meaningful time. My older patients have shown me what can be.

Mended

According to legend, when the Angel of Death descends to earth to take a soul from the world of the living, he stands at the head of the dying one's bed and draws the sword from his sheath, preparing for the final moment. But Aaron the peacemaker, brother of Moses, was spared this act due to his righteousness. God himself kissed Aaron's soul and brought it to heaven.

As my patient Aron lay in his hospital bed, he had a strange vision. A figure emerged from the darkness and penetrated the curtain around his bed, hovering over his face and poised to strike. Despite his physical debility, Aron gathered up his strength and swung his fist at the shadowy intruder, wrestling with it before knocking it away. He awoke the next morning and was wheeled into surgery.

✳✳✳

A month before I met Aron, the circumstances of our meeting were set in motion. As I was preparing for a trip to Boston, my assistant brought me a message from Aron's daughter-in-law begging me to see him for a second opinion. She explained that he was an eighty-four-year-old survivor of Auschwitz who had recently been diagnosed with Alzheimer's disease and was deteriorating rapidly. Although she had already learned that my clinic did not accept Aron's health insurance, she inquired whether I could still see him the following week when her husband would be in South Florida and could bring him to an appointment. Although the urgency of the consult was not clear to me, I agreed to see Aron on my return.

My trip to Boston turned out to be quite prescient of the coming events with Aron. After a nearly fourteen-year absence, I was returning to the site of my residency training in psychiatry to deliver a lecture on the topic of late-life personality development. McLean Hospital was one of America's first major asylums for the mentally ill, designed in the 1800s when a serene, park-like atmosphere was considered a mainstay of psychiatric care. Seeing the familiar panorama of rolling hills, grand oak trees, and Gothic brick buildings on campus brought back strong memories, even though I assumed that much had changed in the many years I had been away. My trip felt like a homecoming as I encountered so many of the same colleagues with whom I had worked years before—even several supervisors whom I had imagined were long retired. Appearances had changed a bit but not spirits, and I was exhilarated by the visit.

In my lecture I spoke about how, although personality seemed cast in stone early in life, there remained the great potential for positive change over time, for adaptation and even rejuvenation in the face of late-life stresses. In clinical work with the elderly, however, there is the risk of getting accustomed to the opposite: viewing constant decline as fate and restoration of the past as fantasy. As it turned out, my encounter with Aron illustrated the potentially disastrous consequences of such an attitude.

Aron arrived for his appointment late on a Friday afternoon, accompanied by his oldest son. I was immediately concerned when I saw how slowly he shuffled into my office, as if he were wearing heavy shoes magnetically stuck to the floor. He had a baffled expression on his face and could barely speak except for a few phrases in a mix of English, Hebrew, and Yiddish. His son reported that Aron lived alone in a small retirement community near Ft. Lauderdale, where he had been quite active with the large group of Holocaust survivors. Amazingly, he also reported that only four months ago Aron had been driving a car and functioning independently. The family was deeply concerned about this precipitous change in his function, and they were furious with his primary care physician, who had refused to authorize a brain scan because he reasoned that it would not change the diagnosis or management of Alzheimer's disease. Instead, he had sent Aron to a psychiatrist, who diagnosed depression and started him on an antidepressant medication.

In truth, it took only a few moments for me to realize that the clinical picture looked nothing like Alzheimer's disease but instead suggested a rapidly progressing neurological disorder that warranted immediate attention. Strokes can certainly cause the gait impairment seen with Aron, even when the actual event goes initially unrecognized. In some individuals, a variety of causes, including high blood pressure and diabetes, can cause tiny strokes in the lower regions of the brain. The silent, slow accumulation of these small areas of dead brain tissue eventually hits a tipping point where symptoms appear, often consisting of short-term memory loss, a slowing of movement and thought, and a propensity to apathy and depression. Aron's slowed gait fit this clinical picture, but his language dysfunction did not. A stroke large enough to cause his impaired speech would certainly have caused other, more devastating symptoms, which I did not detect.

Another possibility was a relatively uncommon but frequently misdiagnosed condition called normal pressure hydrocephalus, or NPH, in which the natural circulation of cerebrospinal fluid is disturbed, resulting in swelling of the inner chambers of the brain and compression of the surrounding tissue. To the doctor's eye, NPH produces a classic symptomatic triad of progressive dementia, gait disturbance, and urinary incontinence. The gait disturbance looks very much like Aron's walk, with each plodding step appearing to be strenuously resisting a strong magnetic pull to the ground. Although I certainly suspected NPH, Aron's language impairment was not consistent with its clinical picture.

Aron came to me with a diagnosis of Alzheimer's disease, but that is a slowly progressive disease of the brain where change unfolds over many years, not in just a few short months. Something else was going on with Aron that only a brain scan could show. Unfortunately, neither time nor Aron's insurance was in his favor at that moment. It was late on a Friday afternoon, and only his assigned physician could authorize the insurance company to approve a scan. I called repeatedly but did not hear back from the doctor. As Aron and his son waited, I tried repeatedly to make progress with the insurance, running a gauntlet of phone numbers and various departments, none of which took responsibility for the decision. Finally, I managed to reach a supervisor. I explained the dilemma and suggested—almost threatened—that without authorization for a brain scan I would be forced to send Aron to the emergency room at much greater cost. The supervisor relented, and within minutes I had Aron and his son out the door and on their way to our imaging facility. I went so far as to walk them out to their car and program the GPS to make certain that they made it to the facility before it closed for the day. The son called me a half hour later; they were there, but questions about whether Aron had a metal stent in his body would delay the scan for a day.

The next morning I received a phone call from the radiologist about an hour after the scan. I had never gotten such an urgent call from him before, and so I immediately suspected trouble. In fact, the news was ominous. He informed me that Aron had a huge cyst in his left frontal lobe with an associated tumor that was causing his entire brain to shift two centimeters away from its midline. The clinical symptoms now made perfect sense, because the large mass was pressing on both his brain's language center and a strip of brain tissue that controlled movement.

I reached Aron's sons to give them the news, and they were concerned but not surprised. We agreed that a neurosurgical consult was needed, and I called the primary care physician to get the ball rolling.

"Oh, yes, I know Aron," the doctor said; "he has Alzheimer's disease." "No," I countered, "he has a massive tumor in his skull." There was silence for a moment. I explained to him the findings from the brain scan and asked what the next step should be. The doctor instructed me to have Aron call his office Monday morning to schedule an appointment. Now I was angry and almost ready myself to drive Aron down to the nearest hospital. If he had been my own grandfather, I would have demanded faster action and moved heaven and earth to get it. I sought advice from a former college roommate who is now a neurosurgeon in Seattle. The news was not good, he cautioned, because such brain tumors in eighty-four-year-olds are often malignant, and without rapid treatment, Aron would soon die. Given the grim prognosis, I did not expect to see Aron again.

It took several days to get Aron to a neurosurgeon, and approximately ten days after our initial meeting he was admitted to the hospital for brain surgery that would attempt to drain the cyst and cut out as much of the adjacent tumor as possible. Although his vision of an unknown, shadowy visitor to his hospital bed the night before surgery seemed ominous, Aron interpreted it quite differently, feeling emboldened by his strength and confident that he had vanquished the intruder. As it turned out, the cyst was drained easily and the tumor was cut out completely from its perch on top of his brain. It was a completely benign growth, and Aron was cured.

Three weeks after surgery Aron himself drove to my office with his two sons as passengers in the car. "He's a little fast on the pedal," one son commented, "but that's nothing new." Aron strode into my office with a steady, *normal* gait. He threw his arms around me and hugged me, thanking me with tears in his eyes. In perfect, fluent English he told me about his desire to resume his previous independent life, despite his sons' concerns. I was so impressed that I invited him to sit and talk for an hour while I recorded his life history. Aron described his life in great detail, including his survival in Auschwitz, where he managed to fool his Nazi overseers during forced labor by rubbing charcoal on his face so that he looked as if he were working a lot harder than he actually was. And now, I thought, he had survived again by tricking fate. Recounting his experiences during the Holocaust certainly brought great sorrow to Aron, but that day he was stitched up a bit, temporarily mended by the opportunity to share an epic, defining story in his life that spoke of his bravery and faith in the face of certain doom. And in the listening, I felt a little mended myself, both amazed at his recovery and thrilled to see my elderly patient returned to a former state of function after nearly dying.

Nevertheless, I wondered deeply about Aron's presurgical vision of the shadowy intruder. Perhaps he had been hallucinating from the effects of the tumor or from the steroids prescribed to shrink the swelling in his brain. Perhaps the nurses had given him a sleeping pill that induced a mild delirium. Or perhaps the silent visitor wasn't the Angel of Death but was Raphael, the Angel of Healing, who once visited Abraham the patriarch and healed the wounds of his circumcision as a reward for his profound faith in God. I imagined that this visitor lay atop Aron like the prophet Elisha, who resurrected the dead child of the Shunammite woman who had shown him kindness and generosity: "And he went up, and lay upon the child, and put his mouth upon his mouth, and his eyes upon his eyes, and his hands upon his hands; and he stretched himself upon him; and the flesh of the child waxed warm" (2 Kings 4:34).

And what good deed on Aron's part would have merited such miraculous healing? I learned that there were many. Several years after surviving the death camps of Poland, Aron was a young father living outside of Tel Aviv. As he was riding on his motorcycle one day, he saw a large poisonous snake approaching a little girl and poised to strike. Aron gunned the engine and raced toward the girl, putting himself in the path of the snake. The girl was saved, but the snake bit Aron on the ankle. He was rushed to the hospital and saved by the timely injection of anti-venom. But even as he recovered from the snakebite, Aron was sickened from receiving too much of the life-saving antidote. He languished for weeks in the hospital in a weakened state before recovering completely. The Talmud teaches that saving a single life is like saving the world. Aron had saved a life at the risk of his own. For this alone he deserved to be healed.

Nearly a year after Aron's recovery, I received an invitation to his eighty-fifth birthday party. On the way to the party my wife wondered aloud how atypical it was for me to even consider attending the life event of a patient. In the small town where my grandfather had served as doctor, it had been common and even expected for patients to extend invitations to such occasions. But for a psychiatrist, accepting such invitations is usually considered a violation of appropriate boundaries between doctor and patient. For Aron, however, I made an exception. Never in my career had I witnessed such an amazing recovery, a return from the precipice of death. I still marvel at how Aron was not only healed but also seemed better than before, as if the hands on the clock of time had been moved a few beats backward.

Seeing Aron sitting and beaming at the head of the table, surrounded by family and friends and being feted on such a happy occasion, was a wondrous experience for me, a true moment of joy. He thanked me again and extolled what he described as my life-saving role, but I honestly felt that I was the one who needed to express gratitude. I was one small part of a transcendent chain of events, a messenger sent on a preordained mission. In every doctor's life there should be at least one such moment of satisfaction, one shining opportunity to witness the miraculous glory of healing the seemingly incurable. I witnessed the words of the Psalm 92:15 spring to life: "They will still be fruitful in old age; vigorous and fresh they will be." This was my moment, and I shall never forget it.

As my wife and I got up and prepared to leave the birthday party, a stream of Holocaust survivors in attendance approached us. Each one, in turn, rolled up his or her sleeve and pointed out the numbers tattooed on one forearm, permanent reminders of the evil that they had survived. And each survivor, in turn, expressed the same sentiment: "This person," each one said, gesturing to Aron, "this was a person to save."

Not all older individuals will have such happy endings. Many times there will be little that can be done, and the results will seem tragic. But that doesn't mean we have to give up and cast fate to the wind. Sometimes our very presence is life saving when imbued with a sense of commitment and caring. At other times, as with Aron, our desires for an individual's return to health will help us to take critical steps to actually achieve that goal. After all, we harbor these deep hopes for the health and sustenance of ourselves and our loved ones. We should want nothing less for all our elders.

Lessons from Fire

Place of fire,
place of weeping,
place of madness—

—ZELDA, "PLACE OF FIRE"

The red-hued bricks that run along Piedmont Street do not give up their secrets easily.. Dredged from shallow pits south of Boston, the alluvial clay that makes up these bricks is mixed, molded, and then fired in kilns up to 1,800 degrees Fahrenheit, where it is transformed from a soft, pliable material into its hardened final form. These bricks are then trucked to Boston and laid down in soft sandbeds, where they run like a petrified vasculature through the historical walkways and side streets of the city, pooling and clotting in courtyards and municipal plazas. Their worn, rough red faces bring a sense of history to the city.

The bricks along Piedmont Street have a sad history hidden beneath them, a lesson of fire and grief imprinted by the fleeing shoes and charred skin of victims and the steaming rubber boots of firefighters that came together at this spot on the evening of November 28, 1942. Shortly after 11 PM a great and tragic fire erupted in the basement of the Cocoanut Grove nightclub, and within minutes the flames burst furiously up the stairwell and then exploded through the shocked and panicked crowd of revelers packing the renovated speakeasy. Tens of diners dropped at their seats, instantly overcome by the toxic fumes. Hundreds of other women and men—many of them soldiers on pass—died in the stampede to the revolving door in the front of the club, which was rendered useless by the crush of bodies. The fire grew quickly to five alarms as Boston's finest tried desperately to save those individuals trapped by a building riddled with fire code violations. Hundreds of firefighters, police officers, doctors, nurses, social workers, passers-by pressed into service, and, eventually, undertakers worked throughout the night and ensuing days to attend to the survivors and then bury the 492 men and women who had lost their lives. It was the second deadliest single building fire in U.S. history. Amazingly, there is no monument on this spot today, only a parking lot and a small parting of the bricks where a bronze plaque in the sidewalk reminds pedestrians of the event.

The legacy and lessons of the fire, however, revolutionized building safety codes. They also inspired a Harvard psychiatrist by the name of Dr. Erich Lindemann to study the process of acute grief. What happens to someone who experiences such a tragedy? Lindemann asked. How does grief manifest and change over time? His observations were published in a now-classic paper in the *American Journal of Psychiatry* in September 1944. "At first glance," Lindemann began, "acute grief would not seem to be a medical or psychiatric disorder in the strict sense of the word but rather a normal reaction to a distressing situation." But such grief is of great interest to the clinician who wants to understand its vicissitudes and learn to reckon the limits of normality.

Lindemann reported several key observations about grief that we now accept as obvious but at the time had not been documented in any systematic way. He spoke of the sense of unreality that grips the mourner, accompanied by waves of somatic distress, sighing and exhaustion, and mental preoccupation with the deceased, sometimes associated with profound guilt. Morbid grief reactions may appear weeks, months, or even years later, often in distorted ways. For example, Lindemann cited one man who suddenly came down with a grief reaction twenty years after the loss of his mother, triggered, it was believed, when he reached her age at the time of her suicide. Other individuals adopt characteristics, even illnesses, of a deceased loved one or continue to function, but in a "wooden and formal way" devoid of emotion or strong interest.

For both the survivors and the rescuers of the Cocoanut Grove fire, the psychological trauma had the potential to produce its own symptomatic picture, what we commonly refer to today as a post-traumatic stress reaction. Aside from the physical trauma of burns or wounds, the subjective trauma can be equally or even more devastating. The intensely frightful, life-threatening event was a fundamental contradiction to how its witnesses viewed the world. As psychologist Jon Allen describes, such a trauma "may shatter the assumptions that the world is meaningful and benevolent, and that the self is worthy." But the trauma of a terrible fire can at least bring some answers to its victims—a revelation of highly flammable décor, faulty wiring, and locked exits. Trauma resulting from the actions of evildoers is more problematic. For survivors of war or genocide, the search for some theodicy that explains either the silent presence or the glaring absence of God may prove elusive. Worse, the work of evildoers may beg a twisted explanation, where "the most perniciously traumatic result is profound shame and guilt, a sense of oneself as evil."

Old age brings unique perspectives to loss and trauma. It is itself a trauma to many, where the inexplicable and inexorable dissolution of body and mind contradict our view of the world as "meaningful and benevolent." It is also a fundamental challenge to the sense of self, and many elders accept and even adopt ageist views of themselves as useless and decrepit. At the same time, the older mind carries within it newly recognized strengths, including the remarkable ability to adapt to enormous change and trauma, in part by filtering out negative emotions and selectively engaging in more positive activities and states of mind. In old age, survivors of great traumas from earlier in life can teach us how they sustained themselves following unimaginable losses and then went on to thrive.

I have learned from my patients that the crucial antidote is hope. And hope, defined here, goes beyond the mere desire for a better time of life. It goes beyond any rationale that explains the ways of the world, accounts for the mysteries of aging or evil, or explains the nature of God. It is a primal force woven out of both mind and heart that carries us through even the worst of conflagrations. Hope, in this sense, is formed in life's first attachment and is reactivated in all subsequent trusted attachments to others. Too often we imagine that these attachments drop one by one in old age, that they are no longer necessary or even sought. But I have seen the opposite. This is a lesson, among several others, taught by some of the most impressive survivors I have known—those now-aged individuals who survived the Holocaust.

❈❈❈

The forest still stands, but the people are gone. Only a stone memorial guards their place, surrounded by tall grasses that hide bits of ash and bone deep beneath their roots. In this spot on February 4, 1942, more than 920 Jewish men, women, and children from the town of Rakov in what is now Belarus were rounded up by Germans and herded into the town's synagogue. Several shrieking children were stabbed with bayonets and thrown over the heads of the weeping Jews just before the doors and windows were sealed and the building was doused with kerosene. An unspeakable scene of wailing ensued as the once vibrant Jewish community was annihilated in the fire. My patient, now ninety-eight, still weeps when he describes witnessing this horror from a hidden perch in a tree. He gasps audibly when he recalls watching his father being pummeled by a German soldier before he was thrust into the doomed crowd.

When this survivor first told me his story, I was speechless. He held tight to my arm, and I imagined myself as the branches of the tree that supported him during this trauma. I was now a witness. As his psychiatrist I am obliged to ease his suffering, but no medicine of mine can touch such a memory. I have tried hard to understand how he and others managed to mentally survive such traumatic experiences. These aging Holocaust survivors, in particular, have taught me what I have come to call "lessons from fire."

Lesson one is the most difficult for a doctor: *Sometimes the perpetual sadness of many older survivors is not to be healed but shared.* Over time, as memories fade and the voices of lost loved ones grow quieter, all that remains is a closely guarded sadness, persisting as a substitute for the losses. Any attempt to ease this emotion may be a threat to the painful but beloved remnants of memory. What some survivors seek is not medicine or therapy but the attentive presence of a doctor and others to serve as the next generation of witnesses.

Lesson two brings a paradox: *Surviving a grueling trauma does not inoculate a person against the stresses of aging.* A patient once told me that the small daily indignities she faced in the nursing home felt worse than her experiences in a Siberian labor camp. I realized that she could not bear feeling a victim again, even in small measure.

Lesson three gives me hope: *Survivors of great trauma can sometimes find healing when they give to others what they need themselves.* One patient, a survivor of Auschwitz, recently lost her husband of sixty years. She came to me severely depressed, with thoughts of suicide. I asked her, "How did you have any hope in the camp, knowing that each day could be your last?" She smiled briefly and told me a story: "My dear doctor, I believe in God, and He was with me in the camp. But I also had several young women from my town with me in the barracks. When we had to stand at attention for hours, we stood together, propping up one another when weak. When we dug ditches, we did it together, one holding and moving the arms and shovel for another who didn't have strength that day. We were desperate, but never alone." I referred her to a social club we had created for older people with mild memory problems, and one day I crept into the room during a discussion group and hid behind the corner to listen. One woman spoke disparagingly of her memory: "I am losing my mind," she said. "It is so painful." Then I heard my patient respond in a resolute voice, "You must have hope. We are all in the same boat here, together." As I listened, I could feel the tears welling up in my eyes, but I kept myself hidden, afraid to let the group see their doctor weeping. From my hiding place I witnessed a beloved patient begin to heal herself.

These lessons from fire are not the only points of clinical knowledge that a doctor needs to work with aging victims of trauma, but they're a good start. When facing the last generation of Holocaust survivors, I offer my presence as a doctor and I feel strengthened by their words. "Faith—I still have faith," I hear a survivor say. "Doctor, hope for me!" another commands. These are the primal gifts of life that we share.

The Seamstress

"There is nothing more you can do for me. It is time to die."

These are troubling words for a doctor. They challenge the root mission to heal disease or, in the very least, to relieve suffering. It is at these moments that I have often witnessed colleagues become less scientific and more moralistic with patients, urging them to hang in there and live or to accept some form of hospice care as they are dying. My patient Emma, who spoke these words to me, was not, however, suffering from an imminently terminal illness. Instead, she *felt* terminal in her own eyes. I frequently encounter similar older patients in my work who refuse treatment, believing that it is futile. Such attitudes risk provoking sufficient fear and confusion in both doctor and caregivers that they come to silently agree with the older, despairing individual.

Emma was my patient for nearly ten years, and she lived alone in an assisted living facility for all of that time. At the age of ninety-eight she first expressed to me her wish to die. My progress note from our meeting began the way all my notes on Emma did: "This is a 98-year-old woman with a history of recurrent depression, anxiety, and post-traumatic stress disorder. She survived the Holocaust but lost her husband and children in German concentration camps."

The not-so-subtle message was that her psychiatric illness must be considered within the context of her surviving an almost unspeakable tragedy. I hoped that all clinicians who read my note would pause before seeing Emma, notice her sorrow, and accord her a few extra minutes of time and attention. I also wondered whether other clinicians who encountered her might become consumed, as I sometimes did, in amazement at her survival and horror at her losses.

Emma was a vital young wife and mother prior to World War II. She worked as a seamstress in a small town in Czechoslovakia and lived with her husband and their three young children, ages six months to six years. When the war broke out and persecution of Jews began to accelerate, the family escaped to Antwerp, Belgium, hoping to find a safe haven for their young children, including a fourth child born shortly after they arrived. Eventually, Emma's husband was arrested, never to be seen again. She knew that her own survival was precarious, so she placed the children in a Catholic orphanage that agreed to hide them. She was later arrested by the Germans and spent the next five years in various concentration camps, eventually ending up in Auschwitz. After surviving a death march from Auschwitz and being liberated by American troops, Emma returned to Belgium on foot, only to discover that her children were no more, having been seized by the Germans and sent on a transport to certain death. She wandered around Antwerp "like a crazy woman," she told me, ill and battered physically and psychologically from the death camps and mourning the loss of her entire family. She was later arrested because she had no papers to prove her identity.

And then a small miracle happened. While in jail, she was notified that her youngest son, Chaim, had survived! Emma learned that in 1940 members of the Belgian underground had managed to pull several children out of a cattle car shortly before it left for a death camp. Chaim, then eighteen months old, was small enough to be extracted through an opening formed by several broken planks in the train's siding. Emma's older three children were not so fortunate; they were taken to Auschwitz, where they were gassed immediately on arrival.

Despite her joy over his survival, Emma recounted how it was actually quite difficult being reunited with Chaim, because the seven-year-old boy did not know who she was—he had no memory of anyone in his family—and she was in no shape to be a mother again after her experiences in Auschwitz. She described herself as an inadequate and even abusive mother during their first few years together. Even sixty years later she was consumed with guilt and anguish over her behavior. At times she expressed her own incredulity that the boy returned to her was even her son, although I have seen this grown man and he is her image. When I first met Chaim he told me, quite simply, "It is a miracle that I even stand before you."

Emma related these experiences to me during each monthly appointment, filling the minutes with a long and painful list of losses and trauma, all woven with an unbearable and seemingly unbreakable fiber of depressive and guilt-ridden memories and beliefs. She wept and beat her chest and asked me, "Why? Why?" I listened and offered support, but I had no answers for her. I initially tried to fall back on the pharmacologic moorings of my training, offering her one antidepressant or antianxiety medication after another, but none helped. Most caused dizziness and unsteadiness, which jeopardized her daily walk around campus—the one consistent activity that gave her some peace. And then, after several years of treatment, she informed me that our work had come to an end, that no efforts could overcome her agony.

Despite the great tragedy of her life, Emma at ninety-eight seemed to share a common belief with many old and frail individuals that any and all treatments for despair are futile given their advanced age and overwhelming illness. Multiple blows have taught them that modern medicine can neither slow the process of aging nor alter the inevitability of further decline and death—despite so many claims to the opposite. Even many clinicians have jumped on the bandwagon here, arguing that late-life depression is less "illness" and more a natural reaction to circumstance. As psychotherapist Stanley Jacobson writes, "The high rate of depression among nursing home residents is surely related to the mere fact of their being nursing home residents, immersed in infirmity and impending death." The end result, Jacobson believes, is that clinicians overdiagnose depression, applying a pathological label to what is actually a normal and predictable response to aging. Of course, this argument distorts the true definition of major depression, conflating it with a range of nonpathological states such as sadness and grief. However, we might conclude from this perspective that psychiatric treatment for late-life depression is often a waste of time, a fountain of youth folly no better than so many other spurious claims. I do not think that most clinicians overtly believe this, but many clinicians do hear these doubts from older patients, who in various ways express unremitting despair. In this state a patient's belief in the futility of treatment, regardless of the belief's veracity, can easily become the major barrier to all forms of therapy.

In Emma's case she did not believe that treatment could restore her will to live, because she linked her emotional state with her failing body, the failure of so many past treatments to quell her anguish, and, ultimately, the loss of her young children. And the waters run deep with her because after leaving Europe with her one recovered child, she never loved again, never married, and grew more isolated with time—even from her son and his four children.

Emma's life has been uniquely tragic, but I see bits and pieces of her in so many other older patients. Sometimes pain or immobility or unresolved grief over a dead spouse can consume the entire world of sick and debilitated older individuals, blotting out the possibility of anything other than death to rescue them. Clinicians who hear this and try and fail repeatedly to engage the patient in treatment often come to agree with the futility of treatment, out of frustration, anger, fear of failure, narcissistic injury, or their own despair.

So how does a doctor proceed? One response to an older patient's belief in the futility of treatment is to approach it as a form of suicidal thinking. There is rarely a stated intent or plan to actually commit suicide. Instead, older individuals who lack the energy, will, or physical capability to kill themselves may engage in indirect life-threatening behaviors, such as refusing to eat or drink, take life-sustaining medications, or undergo critical diagnostic tests or treatments. In these circumstances, psychiatric assessment is warranted to identify underlying causes that may yield a variety of treatments. This traditional clinical approach asserts that, even though aging itself cannot be cured, the factors distorting the patient's perspective *can* be treated. Thus, the patient refusing treatment or begging to die may be depressed and hopeless, misinformed, terrified, delirious, under the influence of a substance, or in excruciating pain. Regardless of the factor, patients may be wrong in their belief that treatment is futile because their insight and capacity to think clearly and make decisions are compromised.

This is a particularly important consideration for individuals who have limited insight due to brain damage resulting from stroke, tumor, head injury, or other forms of dementia, such as Alzheimer's disease. For example, individuals with damage to the brain's right hemisphere have impaired recognition and sometimes complete denial of specific neurological deficits or illness, and this may interfere with any sense of concern or urgency for treatment. Frontal lobe injury will also impair insight and judgment in addition to producing impaired abstract thinking, disorganization, disinhibition, or apathy. Put together, these deficits may account for an individual's refusal to consider treatment, either because he or she does not recognize the nature and severity of the disease and the potential benefits of treatment or lacks the motivation to do anything about it.

Unfortunately, when the patient expresses a sense of futility, the doctor may not be far behind. After all, the patient may be correct! A review of the scientific facts of a case may confirm that it is futile to expect improvement. The treatment of potentially reversible factors may carry unacceptable risk or may sustain life without improving its quality. Emma felt depressed and traumatized for sixty years—how could I help her now? Multiple treatments failed. I could not restore her lost children or her capacity to love again. Her lifespan had shrunk to a few more years, at best. What could be gained in that time? Was I willing to put her through treatment that would be coercive and could result in more harm than good?

A good clinician can certainly choose a number of different pathways when dealing with older patients who feel treatment is futile. The clinician can, to a reasonable point, pursue a workup to determine why the patient is refusing treatment and then consider addressing reversible factors. Once this is accomplished, the patient can again be presented with treatment options. But a clinician may agree with both patient and family that further treatment is not reasonable and pursue a less active but still caring approach. With either road, the patient's capacity to make an informed decision must be known. With Emma I was stuck between respecting her wishes, if I believed them to be sincere and rational, or shunting them aside and pushing a more aggressive approach with medications because I doubted her decisionmaking capacity. For many months I remained uncertain of the best plan.

My own bias is that we often give up too early with older ill people because of our own impatience and despair. There is a tendency for even the most caring clinician to begin to with-draw from the person who is preventing fulfillment of the root mission of any clinical practice—*healing*. But there is a counter-point to this tendency. We certainly cannot reverse aging, nor can we effectively treat many of the illnesses encountered in our older individuals. However, we can do something about the concerns that often drive them toward choosing death: loss of autonomy, loss of dignity, and loss of life-affirming activities. These are the factors—not physical pain—that have been cited year after year as the main reasons that a small number of indi-viduals have elected to end their lives under Oregon's Death with Dignity Act. It takes a good dose of hopeful imagination to consider the full potential of older individuals—even at ap-parent endpoints. We cannot give up on them even as they give up on themselves.

Emma's request arrived about the same time a poem crossed my desk by a woman from a similar time and culture as Emma: "All this misery—When will I die?" the poet asks and then con-cludes, "I scorn the hopes of the sun and the promises of blos-soms." Just as I began to anticipate Emma's fading away, another small miracle happened. Arriving suddenly on Emma's doorstep was her eighty-five-year-old sister-in-law, Rachel, who was mourning the recent death of her husband, Emma's brother. I had not known anything previously about Rachel, but here she was, suddenly living with Emma and relying on her to translate because Rachel spoke only Hungarian, Yiddish, and some bro-ken English. Emma became her caregiver, her escort to appoint-ments, and her personal translator with all staff in the clinic and at the assisted living facility. She went to meals and activities with Rachel, advised her on what doctors she needed to see, and supported her through her mourning. In turn, Rachel brought great comfort to Emma. She no longer asked for death. She started coming again to appointments, but with less weeping and less anguish.

During one appointment Rachel told me that she had something important to show me. She pulled from her purse two old, creased, black-and-white photographs. The first photo showed an extended family at a wedding. She pointed to herself in the photo, a smiling figure standing near the bride and groom, surrounded by parents, grandparents, aunts, uncles, and many children. Rachel waved her hand over the photo. "All gone," she said, "all lost." No one in the photograph except Rachel had survived the war. She then turned to the other photo, which showed three perfectly dressed and coiffed children sitting on a park bench next to a young woman. "The momma," she said, and pointed to the figure in the photo and then to Emma sitting beside her. "This is Emma and her children."

I had heard about these children for so long that I was startled to actually see their images. Emma grimaced a bit and said that the photo had been taken so long ago that she could barely recognize herself in it. "What were their names?" I asked. Emma took the photo and pointed to each child: "Yankel, the oldest, then Mendel, named after my grandfather, and then my *maidele* [little girl] Sora." I imagined that a small smile crept on her face as she stared at her lost children, but Emma's reaction was subtle and quiet and did not betray her feelings. "It's time to go, Rachel. Put them away; the doctor has other people to see." They both got up to leave, thanking me for the time, and walked away, one supporting the other. In my own eyes Emma seemed a little steadier, a little more dignified. I wasn't sure what, if anything, I had contributed to her renewal, but my own hope in Emma was certainly restored. It was, in the end, a caring relationship that seemed to offer the best antidote to futility.

❈❈❈

In 2008 Emma celebrated her one-hundredth birthday surrounded by her son, Chaim, his wife, four grandsons and their wives, eight great-grandchildren, Rachel, and a nephew. Seeing the entire family together allowed me to glimpse a small repair in the torn fabric of Emma's life. She continued to live in the assisted living facility near my office, and she witnessed the addition of four new great-grandchildren, bringing the number of her living descendents to seventeen. Rachel remained in the adjacent nursing home, because her memory and ability to speak had deteriorated significantly. Emma could no longer walk, and her failing memory had, ironically, brought her some peace as she no longer dwelled on her lost children. Nevertheless, there was no way, I was certain, for Emma to ever be reconciled with the events of her life. There were no necessary acts of retribution, forgiveness, or even forgetting that would bring sufficient understanding or justice to her losses. Old age allowed her, however, one powerful message: "I am still here." We may argue about whether there is triumph in mere survival or whether the apparent quality or meaning of a person's life must always be entered into the equation. On many days I try to take these measurements in my older patients and do what I can to improve them. When I would see Emma, however, such considerations would drop away, and I would simply marvel at her presence. In late spring 2010, Emma passed away just shy of her one hundred second birthday.

Trees

A magnificent date palm tree stands a few paces outside of my office window. Beholding its thickly ribbed and fern-bearded trunk and majestic crown of fronds, I understand why eighteenth-century Swedish doctor and botanist Carl Linnaeus labeled palm trees the "princes" of the plant kingdom. Like the tree outside my window, Jacobo was a prince of a man—a robust and bearded figure with a perpetual smile. He used to visit me often to teach me Spanish and to talk about his life both before and long after he had fled Cuba. My office was a refuge for him, a bower of books and papers that made him feel at home, as if surrounded by his own library. Over time he even planted parts of himself in my bookshelves with select volumes he brought as gifts. Several years ago he proudly presented me with a copy of his own recently completed magnum opus, *Lógica Trascendente*, the product of decades of deep thought and several years of diligent work in his study. Unlike most of the older men and women who visit me in my office, Jacobo was not a patient; he was my friend.

In my profession such a friendship is not unusual for me, even when the difference in ages spans thirty to fifty years and a generation or two. I still marvel at how both the content of our conversations and the mutual regard rarely betrayed our ages. I had first met Jacobo seemingly by chance—although he would argue that nothing is by chance—during my first year as the psychiatrist at the nursing home. While tending to several consults one afternoon, I walked by the bearded, garrulous figure of Jacobo speaking in an animated tone in Spanish to his daughter. They had arrived that day to visit a beloved family member. We exchanged greetings and sort of tumbled over each other in conversation as I tried in my halting Spanish to welcome him to the "Home," as we called it. Before I knew it, Jacobo had designated himself my personal Spanish tutor, and I suddenly had an eighty-year-old friend with whom to discuss history, religion, and the meaning of life.

Mahogany Tree

The parking lot outside the nursing home in which I work is surrounded by mahogany trees. They appear as sentries along the walkways and parking spaces, with thin, angled trunks, wizened barks, and small-leafed crowns that provide only limited, dappled shade. These trees are young, however, because the mature West Indian mahogany that once grew in abundance throughout South Florida can average up to eighteen feet in circumference and soar to more than seventy feet, earning the moniker "King of the Forest." Most captivating is the woody mahogany seedpod, which from the outside resembles a small brownish-gray potato. Once opened, however, it reveals an intricate, five-chambered array of winged seeds imbued with the rich reddish-brown color that makes mahogany such a desirable wood.

Like these trees, my patients surround and guard the passageways around the nursing home, sharing an outward appearance of frailty but containing within lustrous seeds of history and wisdom that have been spread, year after year, throughout the lives of so many others. I have grown close to these patients, even though the time I know them is short because I lose to death almost as many as I gain each year. They are patients, not friends, although sometimes the lines between can get blurry. This is one unique feature of working with the elderly that every doctor discovers with time. Even when attending to the strictest boundaries in the doctor-patient relationship, the burden of illness and the proximity of death force a special bond with patient and family. At that point small decisions, such as a medication dose or a lab test, can have far-reaching consequences.

In geriatrics, facing the death of so many patients is part of the job. Clinical decisions are often shaped by this reality, as maximal gains from therapies are necessary in minimal time frames. The emotional toll varies, but the loss of a patient who is closer to the line of friend evokes a greater level of grief. I have noticed, however, that the practice of medicine has evolved away from this line, in some ways making it easier to bear these losses. In her book *How Doctors Think*, Kathryn Montgomery describes how medicine has increasingly become a business transaction between strangers; the more objective and scientific it has become, "the more easily it can be commodified, detached from a caring physician, and judged by its 'product,' health." She does not, however, propose a "medicine of friends," despite how attractive the virtue of friendship may be to the doctor-patient relationship. For example, she notes that many physicians value the moments of deep connection with patients and their families that sometimes occur during crises as antidotes to "the alienation and detachment of medicine understood as a science." Although friendship between doctor and patient is a lofty ideal and serves a rhetorical purpose in juxtaposition to a medicine of strangers, Montgomery asserts that such friendships are fraught with risks and ethical concerns.

Instead, as a middle ground Montgomery proposes a "medicine of neighbors": "Neighborliness implies a duty, especially in time of need, but a limited duty that leaves considerable room for both self-preservation and performance above and beyond its call." This proposed metaphor for the doctor-patient relationship is valuable, especially as it stipulates "attention and respect" for patients without the emotions and obligations of friendship, which can be intrusive and burdensome for doctor and patient alike. At the same time, however, the very presence of extant or impending losses, hovering over both doctor and older patient, sometimes demands something more than just a good neighbor.

Apple Tree

During a visit with Jacobo one spring, he appeared tired and depressed. After an hour of conversation, however, he was enlivened, and I felt reassured that all was well. Several weeks passed and I didn't hear from him; I called but got no answer. I persisted, and a weakened voice finally answered the phone: "*Mi amigo, no estoy bien*. I am not well," he told me. I was alarmed and insisted, "Jacobo, I must see you soon!" The next day Jacobo came to my office, unable to walk, with an aide pushing him in a wheelchair. The color was drained from his skin, and he appeared gaunt and exhausted. We barely spoke as I beheld his image. The timelessness of our friendship had suddenly hit the reality of aging, and I knew he was dying. At that moment my friend became my patient, and I quickly made arrangements for Jacobo to go straight into the hospital. Within two weeks Jacobo was gone, drifting off to eternal sleep one morning as his liver shut down from an unknown malignancy. It was a startling departure to me, as I had previously tried to deny that, despite our close friendship, Jacobo's eighty-five years always meant that death was not far off.

And so it was with our friendship, a refuge of time we spent together that was unknowingly and perilously a little way away from the end. Jacobo knew this better than I did. He was an incredibly spiritual man who believed with certainty that God created the world and that it was logic, not just emotion or spirit, that could bring this understanding. But when he once spoke of death to me, it was not logic but pure poetry: "When I die," he offered with a mischievous smile, "perhaps I will be buried close to an apple tree, and I will reach out and pluck a fruit from the branch." I looked at him and chuckled, then reassured us both that there were no trees in the near future. But the image remained in me— this gleaming apple, the symbol of all the worldly knowledge that Jacobo so eagerly sought.

As much as I agree wholeheartedly with Montgomery, I must confess what I, and many of my colleagues, have learned: Sometimes older patients become friends and older friends become patients, either way driven by the nearness of death, which eventually comes, often stealthily, and fells another soul from our practice. We are left as the final witnesses to a life long lived, once full of dreams and memories planted lovingly in this world. This is a special honor, one that grows with time if we are able to hold fast to it:

> Beloved, gaze in thine own heart,
> The holy tree is growing there;
> From joy the holy branches start,
> And all the trembling flowers they bear.

Epilogue

In the final act of life my patient Rose taught me about the enduring passions of life. The reason for Rose's sudden decline was unexpected. It was not unusual for a ninety-eight-year-old to stop eating. I see this frequently, and the causes are legion: a broken, painful tooth; persistent, corrosive esophageal reflux; depression; a hidden cancer. The reason for Rose's decline, I learned, was love. She had been deeply in love with another man on her floor in the nursing home and had craved and reveled in the affection he provided. When a younger woman of eighty-eight moved onto the unit, Rose's boyfriend broke up with her and took up with the new resident. Rose demanded to know whether this new woman was somehow prettier or feistier, and she begged him to return—to no avail.

The following week Rose had a fit at the bingo game, screaming at her former boyfriend and calling the new woman a whore. In her fury she swept the bingo cards and chips off the table with wild, flailing movements of her arms. All that the staff and other residents could see in Rose was a woman out of control: a bitter, jealous, and belligerent woman who required, many argued, a heavy dose of sedation. Rose took to her room and stopped eating and drinking. She refused all of her medications. When I met with her, she hissed at me and insisted that I allow her to die. Her family was embarrassed and exhausted by her behavior and counseled us to respect her wishes. Several days later she slipped away, taking with her, I hoped, not a feeling of scorn but a last memory of a joyful kiss. Rose's last days might seem tragic, expressions of all the wretched indignities of old age, but I marvel not at the life lost but at the love lost. Even at ninety-eight she had been able to love so deeply that the loss of that love broke her heart.

�֎✖✖

In the final act of life my ninety-five-year-old patient Naomi taught me about the preciousness of memory. At the time of her admission to the rehabilitation unit, Naomi was suffering from short-term memory loss, mild delirium, a complete loss of her independence, and a recent hip fracture that rendered her unable to walk. I was asked to see her because every morning she insisted on attempting the same death-defying feat of trying to leave her wheelchair and walk unassisted, despite the pleadings and admonitions of her therapists.

Prior to our appointment I heard Naomi in the hallway crying out in pain and confusion: "Why am I here, Doctor?" she inquired. When we spoke, I tried to reassure her, but she struggled to understand who I was and what I could do to ease her suffering. When I asked about her past, however, she appeared soothed as she related to me many fond memories—her last and most treasured possessions. I leaned in close and smiled at Naomi. "Please tell me about your *most* precious memory, the one memory that stands above them all." "Oh, Doctor," she cooed, "that's easy. I once danced with *Fred Astaire*." My eyes widened, and the disheveled and decrepit-appearing old woman in front of me suddenly lit up like a celebrity. Many years ago, I learned, she and her husband had had a special friendship with Fred Astaire and Ginger Rogers and had spent countless enchanting evenings with the couple. "Tell me, what was it like to dance with Fred Astaire?" I sincerely wanted to know. Naomi seemed to swoon for a moment as a confident, starry-eyed expression rippled across her face. She seemed lost in the memory. "To dance with Fred Astaire, well, that was . . . *heaven*."

✖✖✖

In the final act of life my patient Benjamin taught me about hope. When I first met him, Benjamin was cradling an infant boy in his lap, his slender, bony fingers gently supporting the head and neck. Though his blind eyes could not see the form of his great-grandson below, he felt it, the pride radiating out in the rays of tears that ran down his cheeks. He appeared to me like a proud vintner holding up a prized cluster of grapes to the beaming sun. I knew Benjamin well, as I knew his daughter and granddaughter—all patients at one time. In my work with them I was able to see the lines of development across all three generations—an entire life cycle laid before me.

There is a tendency to compare youngest and oldest generations, in effect infantilizing our most aged and debilitated citizens by assigning them the same expectations for incapacity and dependence. And why not? In appearance and behavior many severely demented individuals closely resemble young children. At least they appear this way to the eyes of someone much younger. But Benjamin was no infant. He had lived for ninety-six years and was still living, despite the loss of much of what had seemed to define him in the past—his memories, his wife, his ability to walk, and his vision. But at the meeting of man and infant, I saw Benjamin in a new light.

I could see the communion of hope between Benjamin and his new great-grandson as it was developing in the infant and ripening in the elder, guiding each from moment to moment. I also saw a more mature form of trust in Benjamin, one that afforded him a sense of tranquility even as his diminishing vision and memory untied him from his past. In other ways he was very much in tune with something much larger than himself, as in the hours he spent in the arts studio running his hands over the wet clay that he would mold into countless shapes. He had an understanding of life that I could not touch—a feeling of closeness to something beyond. In this light the final act of life brings maturation, not just regression. It is a blessed height poorly imagined by the young, but one, in the words of Erik and Joan Erikson, where "the view stretches out its releasing display, and the sky and the clouds perform their slow and gracious maneuvers."

For Rose, Naomi, Ben, and the many other individuals whom I have described in this book, I am reminded that when we see only the silent darkness of old age, we miss the million sparks of life still present. As the poet Zelda writes:

> *In the morning, I thought:*
> *"Life's magic will never return,*
> *it won't return."*
> *Suddenly in my house, the sun*
> *is a living thing,*
> *and the table with its bread—*
> *gold.*
> *And the flower and the cups—*
> *gold.*
> *And the sadness?*
> *Even there—*
> *radiance.*

I began this book by telling how the place where I work as a doctor for the elderly is sometimes called a waiting room for God. It is certainly a place, for those who believe, where a sacred presence hovers close by those in the final stage of life, waiting, hoping, and carrying with it a reconnection with the force that bore us. As T. S. Eliot writes:

> *In my beginning is my end. In succession*
> *Houses rise and fall, crumble, are extended,*
> *Are removed, destroyed, restored, or in their place*
> *Is an open field, or a factory, or a by-pass.*

Old stone to new building, old timber to new fires,
Old fires to ashes, and ashes to the earth.

This house of God for the elderly is sometimes a house of pain and of loss. But it is also a house of holies, where aging has the potential to be much more than even our imaginations have conceived. For Abraham Heschel, "Just to be is a blessing. Just to live is holy." These words show me where the story of aging begins and where it ends. The final act for all of us is to listen to our elders. "Hope for me, Doctor," my older patients often ask. I turn to them and answer, "I will try my best. Hope for me, too."

Acknowledgments

I share the ancient sentiments of Socrates, who said, "I enjoy talking with very old people. They have gone before us on a road by which we, too, may have to travel, and I think we do well to learn from them what it is like." The origins of this book, then, must be traced to the myriad older relatives, friends, and patients who have been part of my life. They are too numerous to name, but I owe them my deepest gratitude. I was fortunate to grow up with four grandparents who left indelible imprints on my life and work and without whom this book would never have been possible: Simon and Eva Cherkasky and Tany and Etta Agronin. Their vital presence defied all the stereotypes of growing old that I have explored in this book.

Becoming a geriatric psychiatrist does not happen by accident, and the role in which I have encountered the patients described in this book was inspired and nurtured by numerous colleagues. Two psychiatrists, friends, and mentors from Yale Medical School who first inspired me toward psychiatry were Alan Siegal and Dan Oren. My medical school anatomy partners who joined me in the trenches and who also happen to be two of my closest friends are Jimmy Levine and Steve Ugent. During my psychiatric residency at McLean Hospital, Harvard Medical School, I learned to thrive as a young psychiatrist alongside my closest friends Stuart Anfang and Richard Herman. Gabe Maletta and William Orr were two wonderful supervisors during my geriatric psychiatry fellowship at the Minneapolis VA Medical Center. Gabe Maletta helped to secure several critical interviews for this book and continues to be a particularly important mentor in my career. Our work together as editors of our textbook *Principles and Practice of Geriatric Psychiatry* has been a true joy.

The main setting for much of the book is the Miami Jewish Health Systems (MJHS), where I have been working as the director of Mental Health and Clinical Research since 1999. Only such a unique, beautiful, and enriching setting could motivate me to make the hour-long commute each way down to Miami and back day in and day out to engage in clinical work that feels more like a calling than a job. At MJHS I have had the privilege to work with so many incredibly talented individuals who serve tirelessly to improve the lives of the elderly, and I am grateful for their presence. MJHS would not have become such an amazing place—including Florida's largest nursing home at its center—without the unparalleled leadership for more than fifty years of Irving Cypen, known to all of us at MJHS as simply the "Judge," and his wife, Hazel.

I am indebted to Daniel Carlat for reaching out to me on several occasions to do writing projects that led to many of my current endeavors, including this book. I am equally indebted to my former editor at McMahon Publishing, Donald Pizzi, who gave me my first opportunity to write regular columns for several trade publications that eventually formed the basis for this book. Kate McDuffie of the American Association for Geriatric Psychiatry has also worked closely with me as both an editor and a supporter for several writing pieces that are central to this book.

It was my agent, Rafe Sagalyn, who helped, more than anyone, to sculpt the conception for this book out of many ideas and who has been steadfast in his guidance and encouragement. He introduced me to John Radziewicz at Da Capo Press, the most superb editor and mentor I could ever imagine. I also want to thank numerous Da Capo/Perseus staff members who were instrumental in getting the book in shape and then delivered to a wide audience, including Lissa Warren, Kevin Hanover, Lindsey Triebel, Jonathan Crowe, Annie Lenth, and Josh Berman. I was extremely fortunate to have Jan Kristiansson as my copy editor. Rita Jacobs gave generously of her time to read the manuscript and offer detailed suggestions.

Having the opportunity to interview so many individuals for this book was a true honor. I gratefully acknowledge Senator George McGovern, Leonard Hayflick (who went above and beyond the call of duty in reviewing my depiction of his work and the science of aging), Gene Cohen, Sophie Freud, Bernard Lown, Sherwin Nuland, Julie Newmar, Sue Bloland, Diana Eck, Dorothy Austin, Rose and Paul Svarc, Sharon Lee, Bill and Gloria Cherkasky, Rudy and Arlene Cherkasky, James Hutson, Tom Hutson, Herta Neuman, Sandy Cohen, Susan Wohl, Joseph Goelz, Dr. Walter Richardson, Gerald Charness, Marilyn Goldaber, Alfred Friedman, and Mac Seligman.

In addition to those already cited, a good number of individuals have been extremely helpful in discussing many of the issues and cases in this book, including Stephen Scheinthal, Michael Silverman, Robert Bergman, Elliot Stein, Eli Feldman,

Mairelys Martinez, Victoria Barnett, Rita Gugel, Chrystine Kopscik, Fred and Shuli Stock, Leslee Geller, Dana Ryder, Steve Cypen, Alan Cherkasky, Lynn Cherkasky, Ben Colonomos, Jared Weinstein, Shyla Ford, Alice Sarfati, Michael Brodie, Michele Fiorot, Daniel Ghelman, Patricia Jaegerman, Niurka Colina, Jorge Riveros, Rafael Mestre, Jean Kramer, Mark Samuels, Neal Foman, Michael Druckman, Alan Bauer, Amiel Levine, Melba Canals-Hooten, Stephanie Willis, Elizabeth Andrews, Blaise Mercadante, and Leslie Cedar. Up until his premature passing in the fall of 2009, Gene Cohen was extraordinarily generous with his time and interest, and his own work stands as a pillar in the halls of my profession.

I am grateful to so many friends and family who have rallied around me as this book has moved from an idea, to a proposal, and then to its final form. My parents, Ron and Belle Agronin, and my in-laws, Fred and Marlene Lippman, continue to be my greatest inspiration for what life should be after middle age. My siblings and their families all took close interest in the book, especially in helping to come up with a title, and I thank them all: Mike, Ellen, Joni, David, and Lucy Agronin; Robin, Greg, Sarah, and Shayna Druckman,

There is only one way that this book came into fruition, and that is due to the endless love, support, suggestions, critiques, and patience of my wife, Robin, and my sons, Jacob, Max, and Sam. My three boys took acute notice of my frequent attempts over the past few years to sit in solitude in my office writing this book. Despite my best efforts, however, they would undauntedly encircle my bower of books and papers, leap on me like tigers, extort presents and favors for any mention of them in these pages, and lovingly drag me to their respective dens. May I always be blessed with their constant interruptions! In my ongoing journey into the heart of growing old, I will always observe the lesson of aging exemplified by the most successful elders among us: Hang on tightly to the people we are blessed to have in our lives! Henry Wadsworth Longfellow expresses this sentiment so well in "The Children's Hour" as he reflects on his own children's nightly raids:

> *I have you fast in my fortress,*
> *And will not let you depart,*
> *But put you down into my dungeon*
> *In the round-tower of my heart.*

> *And there will I keep you forever,*
> *Yes, forever and a day,*
> *Till the walls shall crumble to ruin,*
> *And moulder in dust away.*

I invite all readers to read my blog and post comments or send e-mails via my website: www.marcagronin.com.

NOTES

INTRODUCTION

4   **"bony landmarks"**: Taken from the Yale Medical School anatomy instruction manual, circa 1987.

5   **"repulsive formaldehyded body"**: Bernard Lown, *The Lost Art of Healing* (Boston: Houghton Mifflin, 1996), 74.

6   **"midsaggital cut"**: Yale anatomy manual.

7   **"gomers"**: Samuel Shem, *The House of God* (New York: Dell, 1978), 38.

8   **"ageism"**: Butler defined ageism as "a process of systematic stereotyping of and discrimination against people because they are old" in his Pulitzer Prize–winning book *Why Survive? Being Old in America* (Baltimore, MD: Johns Hopkins University Press, 1975), 12.

9   **a cure for aging:** Aubrey de Grey, with Michael Rae, *Ending Aging: The Rejuvenation Breakthroughs That Could Reverse Human Aging in Our Lifetime* (New York: St. Martin's Griffin, 2007), 8.

9   **age-centric perceptions:** Lars Tornstam, *Gerotranscendence: A Developmental Theory of Positive Aging* (New York: Springer, 2005), 2. Tornstam talks extensively about how societal views of aging are distorted by the age-centric views of younger individuals.

PART I   WHAT IS OLD?

epigraph John Updike, "Endpoint" in *Endpoint and Other Poems* (New York: Knopf, 2009), 4.

HEAVEN CAN'T WAIT

18   **the psychologist's fallacy:** William James, *The Principles of Psychology* (1890; repr., New York: Classics of Psychology and Behavior Sciences Library, 1988).

19   **"opportunity no less":** Henry Wadsworth Longfellow, "Morituri Salutamus: Poem for the Fiftieth Anniversary of the Class of 1825 in Bowdoin College," in *The Poems of Henry Wadsworth Longfellow*, ed. Louis Untermeyer (New York: Heritage Press, 1943), 434.

24 **the family's debt:** Tom Verkuilen, "Cherkasky Lived the Life of 'Family Doctor'" (letter to the editor), *Appleton Post-Crescent,* June 19, 1997.

AGE I MUST

31 **"two paths":** Marc Agronin, "Exploring the Mysteries of Aging: An Interview with Member Gene Cohen," *Geriatric Psychiatry News,* September–October 2009, 5.

34 **"molecular disorder":** Leonard Hayflick, "Biological Aging Is No Longer an Unsolved Problem," *Annals of the New York Academy of Science* 1100 (2007): 6.

37 **Thomas Jefferson captured:** Thomas Jefferson to John Adams, August 1, 1816, in *Familiar Medical Quotations,* ed. Maurice B Strauss (Boston: Little, Brown, 1968).

38 **"really bad for us":** Aubrey de Grey, with Michael Rae, *Ending Aging: The Rejuvenation Breakthroughs That Could Reverse Human Aging in Our Lifetime* (New York: St. Martin's Griffin, 2007), 32.

38 **fundamental causes of aging:** Aubrey de Grey, "Old People Are People Too: Why It Is Our Duty to Fight Aging to the Death," *CATO Unbound,* December 3, 2007, www.catounbound.org/2007/12/03/aubrey-de-grey/old-people-are-people-too-why-it-is-our-duty-to-fight-aging-to-the-death/.

38 **"Depression of Spirits":** Jonathan Swift, *Gulliver's Travels* (London: Penguin, 2003 [1726]), 209.

39 **nine hundred years?:** Diana Schaub, "Ageless Mortals," *CATO Unbound,* December 5, 2007, www.cato-unbound.org/2007/12/05/diana-schaub/ageless-mortals/.

39 **"through natural selection":** Daniel Callahan, "Nature Knew What It Was Doing," *CATO Unbound,* December 10, 2007, http://www.cato-unbound.org/2007/12/10/daniel-callahan/nature-knew-what-it-was-doing/.

39 **"Senescence escorts us":** Schaub, "Ageless Mortals."

40 **"representation of human aging":** Thomas R. Cole, *The Journey of Life: A Cultural History of Aging in America* (Cambridge, UK: Cambridge University Press, 1992), xxi.

41 **disease and disability:** James F. Fries, "Aging, Natural Death, and the Compression of Morbidity," *New England Journal of Medicine* 303 (1980): 10–135.

41 **hardiness of their reproductive systems:** Thomas T. Perls, "The Oldest Old," *Scientific American* 272(1) (1995): 70–75.

41   cope better with stress: Marirosa Dello Buono, Ornella Urciuoli, and
        Diego De Leo, "Quality of Life and Longevity: A Study of Centenar-
        ians," *Age and Ageing* 27(2) (March 1998): 207–216.

41–42   less genetic susceptibility: Thomas T. Perls, "Centenarians Who
        Avoid Dementia," *Trends in Neurosciences* 10 (October 27, 2004):
        633–636.

42   "like a minefield": George E. Vaillant, *Aging Well: Surprising Guideposts
        to a Happier Life from the Landmark Harvard Study of Adult Develop-
        ment* (Boston: Little, Brown, 2002).

44   "Human freedom and vitality": Cole, *The Journey of Life*, xxv.

LONG TIME DEAD?

49   "full of death": Ronald Blythe, *The View in Winter: Reflections on Old
        Age* (New York: Harcourt Brace Jovanovich, 1979), 29.

50   "Overselling Depression": Stanley Jacobson, "Overselling Depression
        to the Old Folks," *The Atlantic Monthly*, April 1995, 46.

54   doctors held unique esteem: For a cogent discussion of the changing
        societal views of doctors, see Richard Horton, "What's Wrong with
        Doctors," *New York Review of Books*, May 31, 2007, 16–20.

55   decisionmaking prowess: Malcolm Gladwell, *Blink: The Power of
        Thinking Without Thinking* (Boston: Little, Brown, 2005).

56   illness involves "uncertainty": Karen Montgomery, *How Doctors
        Think* (New York: Oxford University Press, 2006), 191; Jerome Groop-
        man, *How Doctors Think* (Boston: Houghton Mifflin, 2007).

57   "a presumed culprit": Groopman, *How Doctors Think*, 149.

59   "uncertainty sometimes is essential": Ibid., 155.

PART II   OLD AGE ROUNDS
epigraph   Gary Miranda, "Going," in *Listeners at the Breathing Place* (Princeton,
            NJ: Princeton University Press, 1978), 14.

ISAAC, ERIK, AND ISAK

70   "the incredible paradox": Sue E. Bloland, "The Power and Cost of
        a Fantasy," *The Atlantic*, November 1999, 61.

73   a no-man's-land: Sigmund Freud, "On Psychotherapy," in *The Stan-
        dard Edition of the Complete Psychological Works of Sigmund Freud*, ed.
        and trans. James Strachey (London: Hogarth, 1964 [1905]), 7: 264.

74   "period of increased vulnerability": Erik H. Erikson, "Reflections
        on Dr. Borg's Life Cycle," in Erik H. Erikson, ed., *Adulthood* (New
        York: Norton, 1978), 5.

75   **Erikson's eighth stage:** Erik H. Erikson, *Childhood and Society*, 35th anniversary ed. (New York: Norton, 1985 [1950]), 269.

77   **writing projects were "erratic":** Lawrence J. Friedman, *Identity's Architect: A Biography of Erik H. Erikson* (Cambridge, MA: Harvard University Press, 1999), 457.

77   **"death's door is open":** Erik H. Erikson, *The Life Cycle Completed*, extended ed. with new chapters by Joan M. Erikson (New York: Norton, 1997), 113.

78   **mental burdens of caregiving:** Sue E. Bloland, *In the Shadow of Fame: A Memoir by the Daughter of Erik H. Erikson* (New York: Viking Penguin, 2005), 205.

78   **"sustain this deception":** Ibid., 205.

79   **"neither depressed nor bewildered":** Erikson, *The Life Cycle Completed*, 4.

82   **"an incomparable representation":** Erikson, "Reflections on Dr. Borg's Life Cycle," 3.

82   **"not a regret":** Ibid., 2.

86   **"or meaningfully end":** Erikson, *The Life Cycle Completed*, 62.

ANNABE, BARTLEBY, AND THE DOCTOR WHO FLUNKS AGING

90   **intriguing short stories:** Herman Melville, "Bartleby," in *Billy Budd and Other Tales* (New York: New American Library, 1961), 103–140.

91   **"forlornest of mankind":** Ibid., 123.

95   **"unendurable existence":** Henry A. Murray, "Bartleby and I," in *Endeavors in Psychology: Selections from the Personology of Henry A. Murray*, ed. Edwin S. Shneidman (New York: Harper and Row, 1981), 487.

95   **"principle of self-sovereignty":** Ibid., 491.

95   **"the Bartleby complex":** Ibid., 497.

96   **"kings and counselors":** Melville, "Bartleby," 139–140.

96   **"speed to death":** Ibid., 140.

96   **"Ah, humanity!":** Ibid.

96   **the "sick role":** Talcott Parsons, *The Social System* (New York: Free Press, 1951).

JOSEPH RED HAIR

108   **a sense of empathy:** Howard E. Book, "Empathy: Misconceptions and Misuses in Psychotherapy," *American Journal of Psychiatry* 145(4) (1988): 421.

109   **"attainability of fervent wishes":** Erik H. Erikson, *Insight and Responsibility* (New York: Norton, 1964), 118.

109   **"indispensable virtue":** Ibid., 111.

OLD PICKLED BRAIN

116 **"all mental phenomena"**: John Searle, *Minds, Brain, and Science* (Cambridge, MA: Harvard University Press, 1984), 18.

118 **underlying bipolar disorder:** Bipolar disorder is a psychiatric illness characterized by recurrent episodes of depression and/or mania. Mania is characterized by a persistently and abnormally elevated or irritable mood along with three or more of the following symptoms: hyperactivity (including states of agitation), grandiosity, decreased sleep, pressured speech, racing thoughts, distractibility, and an excessive engagement in reckless or promiscuous behaviors. Common psychotic symptoms associated with episodes of severe mania include delusions (false, fixed beliefs involving jealousy, grandiosity, or paranoia), hallucinations (false perceptions, usually of an auditory or a visual nature), and grossly disorganized thinking or behaviors. More detailed descriptions of bipolar disorder can be found in the official diagnostic manual of the American Psychiatric Association, *Diagnostic and Statistical Manual of Mental Disorders, Fourth Edition, Text Revision* (Washington, DC: American Psychiatric Association, 2000), also known as the *DSM-IV-TR*.

122 **"your ability to recover":** Jay Neugeboren, "Meds Alone Couldn't Bring Robert Back," *Newsweek*, February 6, 2006, 17.

THE STRANGE BUT TRUE CASE OF DAWSON DA VINCI

135 **crucible for schizotypal personalities:** Theodore Millon, *Disorders of Personality: DSM-IV and Beyond*, 2nd ed. (New York: Wiley, 1996), 613.

136 **"somewhat 'crazy' ways":** Ibid.

136 **become more entrenched:** I have described such outcomes in two papers: Marc E. Agronin, "Personality Disorders in the Elderly: An Overview," *Journal of Geriatric Psychiatry* 27(2) (1994): 151–191; and Marc E. Agronin and William B. Orr, "Personality Disorders in a Geriatric Psychiatry Outpatient Clinic," in American Association for Geriatric Psychiatry, ed., *Abstracts, Annual Meeting, March 8–11, 1998, San Diego, California* (Bethesda, MD: American Association for Geriatric Psychiatry, 1998).

137 **even obsessive-compulsiveness:** For a more detailed discussion, see Richard A. Zweig and Marc E. Agronin, "Personality Disorders in Late Life," in Marc E. Agronin and Gabe J. Maletta, eds., *Principles and Practice of Geriatric Psychiatry* (Philadelphia: Lippincott Williams and Wilkins, 2006), 449–469.

PART III MEMORY

epigraph Joseph Skibell, *A Blessing on the Moon* (Chapel Hill, NC: Algonquin Books of Chapel Hill, 1997), 256.

IF I FORGET THEE

143 **two dotted nostrils:** See Denise Grady, "Self-Portraits Chronicle a Dissent into Alzheimer's," *New York Times*, October 24, 2006, www.ny times.com/2006/10/24/health/24alzh.html?_r=1&ex=1162616400& en=66feba45095d0e0e&ei=5070.

148 **"effervescent reservoir":** Aharon Appelfeld, *The Story of a Life* (New York: Schocken Books, 2004), v.

148 **"imagination sailed":** Ibid.

149 **held the promise:** Robert Butler, "The Life Review: An Interpretation of Reminiscence in the Aged," *Psychiatry* 26 (1963): 65.

150 **"formal operations":** Jean Piaget, The Early Growth of Logic in the Child (New York: Norton, 1969). For a succinct review of Piaget's theory, see Stanley I. Greenspan and John F. Curry, "Extending Jean Piaget's Approach to Intellectual Functioning," in Benjamin J. Sadock and Virginia I. Sadock, eds., *Kaplan & Sadock's Comprehensive Textbook of Psychiatry*, 8th ed., vol. 1 (Baltimore, MD: Lippincott Williams and Wilkins, 2005), 528–540.

150 **"wisdom":** For a particularly rich summary of postformal thinking, see Judith Stevens-Long, "Adult Development Theories Past and Future," in Robert A. Nemiroff and Calvin A. Colarusso, eds., *New Dimensions in Adult Development* (New York: Basic Books, 1990), 125–169.

150 **"such retrospective despair":** Erik H. Erikson, *The Life Cycle Completed*, extended ed. with new chapters by Joan M. Erikson (New York: Norton, 1997), 113.

151 **fact struck me:** Sophie Freud, *Living in the Shadow of the Freud Family* (Westport, CT: Praeger, 2007). All quoted excerpts are from this book.

156 **"time's typhoon":** Sophie Freud, "The Old Woman and Time," *LLI Review* 4 (Fall 2009): 77.

157 **"a point in space":** Henry David Thoreau, *Walden* (1854), www.the concordwriter.com/Thoreau Quotes.html.

SAVANT, OF SORTS

159 **"photographic memory":** www.goodreads.com/quotes/show/67855.

160 **"savant syndrome":** www.optimnem.co.uk. This is the official website of Daniel Tammet.

161 **regular cognitive exercises:** Sherry L. Willis, Sharon L. Tennstedt, Michael Marsiske et al., "Long-Term Effects of Cognitive Training on Everyday Functional Outcomes in Older Adults," *JAMA* 296 (2006):

2805–2814; Amarilis Acevedo and David A. Loewenstein, "Nonpharmacological Cognitive Interventions in Aging and Dementia," *Journal of Geriatric Psychiatry and Neurology* 20(4) (2007): 239–249.

163 **"tip-of-the-tongue" experiences:** A. S. Brown and L. A. Nix, "Age-Related Changes in the Tip-of-the-Tongue Experience," *American Journal of Psychology* 109(1) (1996): 79–91.

163 **age-related differences:** Judith A. Sugar and Joan M. McDowd, "Memory, Learning, and Attention," in James E. Birren, R. Bruce Sloane, and Gene D. Cohen, eds., *Handbook of Mental Health and Aging*, 2nd ed. (New York: Academic Press, 1992), 307–337.

STRENGTH IN NUMBERS

165 **meaning of the collective:** James Lipton, *An Exaltation of Larks*, 2nd ed. (New York: Grossman, 1977).

OLD SOLDIERS

169 **"You poor bastards":** Stephen Ambrose, *D-Day, June 6, 1944: The Climactic Battle of World War II* (New York: Simon and Schuster, 1994), 49.

170 **deny the existence:** A neglect syndrome called anosognosia is classically seen after damage to the right posterior parietal lobe.

170 **a whole-brain conspiracy:** Vision and visuospatial impairments stem from damaged occipital and parietal cortices; impairments in attention, etc., from frontal, limbic, and temporal lobe damage.

170 **"anosognosia":** M. J. Babinski, "Contributions a l'étude des troubles mentaux dans l'hémiplégie organique cérébrale (anosognosie)," *Review of Neurology* 12 (1914): 845–847.

170 **hatred for a paralyzed limb:** This syndrome is known as misoplegia.

170 **delusional beliefs:** This condition is known as somatoparaphenia. See P. W. Halligan, J. C. Marshall, and D. T. Wade, "Unilateral Somatoparaphrenia After Right Hemisphere Stroke: A Case Description," *Cortex* 31 (1995): 173–182.

170 **someone else's severed leg:** Oliver Sacks, *The Man Who Mistook His Wife for a Hat* (New York: Summit Books, 1984).

171 **cognitive deficits:** Y. Kashiwa, Y. Kitabayashi, J. Narumoto et al., "Anosognosia in Alzheimer's Disease: Association with Patient Characteristics, Psychiatric Symptoms, and Cognitive Deficits," *Psychiatry and Clinical Neurosciences* 59(6) (2005): 697–704.

MEMORIES, FALSE AND FIXED

173 **two medical texts:** Thomas L. Stedman, *Stedman's Medical Dictionary*, 10th, rev. ed. (New York: William Wood, 1928); James C. Meakins, *The Practice of Medicine* (St. Louis: C. V. Mosby, 1936).

179   **switching the memory:** Capgras syndrome is an example of this type of delusion, in which an individual believes that someone familiar has been replaced by an imposter.

179   **mistakenly diagnoses:** Brendan A. Maher, "Anomalous Experience and Delusional Thinking: The Logic of Explanations," in Thomas F. Oltmanns and Brendan A. Maher, eds., *Delusional Beliefs* (New York: Wiley Interscience, 1988), 15–33.

180   **qualify as a delusion:** Karl Jaspers, *General Psychopathology*, trans. J. Hoenig and Marian W. Hamilton (Chicago: University of Chicago Press, 1963 [1913]).

181   **"delusion-like idea":** Andrew Sims, *Symptoms in the Mind: An Introduction to Descriptive Psychopathology* (London: Baillière Tindall, 1988).

PART IV   WISDOM

THE ELDERS

189   **successful aging:** George E. Vaillant, "Aging Well," *Journal of Geriatric Psychiatry* 15(3) (2007): 181.

192   **a new ability to think:** Gene Cohen, *The Mature Mind: The Positive Power of the Aging Brain* (New York: Basic Books, 2005), 7. See also the chapter "If I Forget Thee" here for more on postformal thinking.

192   **"how the thinker participates":** Judith Stevens-Long, "Adult Development: Theories Past and Future," in Robert A. Nemiroff and Calvin A. Colarusso, eds., *New Dimensions in Adult Development* (New York: Basic Books, 1990), 133.

193   **"the verge of death":** Marcus Cicero, "On Old Age," in *The Basic Works of Cicero*, ed. Moses Hadas (New York: Random House, 1951), 140.

193   **"practice of the virtues":** Ibid., 130.

193   **girded with knowledge:** Ibid., 149.

194   **more positive autobiographical recall:** M. S. Kisley, S. Wood, and C. L. Burrows, "Looking at the Sunny Side of Life: Age-Related Change in an Event-Related Potential Measure of the Negativity Bias," *Psychological Science* 18(12) (2007): 1113–1119; Q. Kennedy, M. Mather, and L. L. Carstensen, "The Role of Motivation in the Age-Related Positivity Effect in Autobiographical Memory," *Psychological Science* 15(3) (2004): 208–214.

194   **self-reported well-being:** A. A. Stone, J. E. Schwartz, J. E. Broderick, and A. Deaton, "A Snapshot of the Age Distribution of Psychological Well-Being in the United States," *Proceedings of the National Academy of Science USA* 107(22) (June 1, 2010): 9985–9990.

194   **"evolving mental maturity":** Gene D. Cohen, "The Geriatric Patient," in Marc E. Agronin and Gabe J. Maletta, eds., *Principles and Practice of Geriatric Psychiatry* (Philadelphia: Lippincott Williams and Wilkins, 2007), 7.

197   **"pattern recognition":** Elkhonon Goldberg, *The Wisdom Paradox: How Your Mind Can Grow Stronger as Your Brain Grows Older* (New York: Gotham Books, 2005), 20.

197   **render judgment:** Malcolm Gladwell, *Blink: The Power of Thinking Without Thinking* (Boston: Little, Brown, 2005).

197   **Nobel Peace Prize:** See Bernard Lown, *Prescription for Survival: A Doctor's Journey to End Nuclear Madness* (San Francisco: Berrett-Koehler, 2008).

202   **critical to successful aging:** Sherwin B. Nuland, *The Art of Aging: A Doctor's Prescription for Well-Being* (New York: Random House, 2007).

203   **one's purpose in life:** See Menachem Mendel Schneerson, "Attaining Sagacity," trans. Eliyahu Touger (Brooklyn, NY: Sichos, 1998).

203   **"the unifying element":** Ibid., 2.

204   **notion of spiritual wisdom:** Abraham Heschel, *The Insecurity of Freedom: Essays on Human Existence* (New York: Farrar, Straus and Giroux, 1967), 77.

204   **"need a vision":** Ibid., 84.

204   **"the horizon of honesty":** Ibid., 78.

204   **"the dignity of old age":** Ibid., 84.

204   **"the attainment of wisdom":** Ibid.

205   **"gerotranscendence":** Lars Torstam, *Gerotranscendence: A Developmental Theory of Positive Aging* (New York: Springer, 2005).

JUST WORDS

211   **language comprehension:** M. Carreiras, J. Lopez, F. Rivero, and D. Corina, "Linguistic Perception: Neural Processing of a Whistled Language," *Nature* 433(7012) (January 6, 2005): 31–32.

212   **true meaning:** See Ray Monk, *How to Read Wittgenstein* (New York: Norton, 2005).

212   **rare form of dementia:** This form of dementia is called primary progressive aphasia; the inability to name things, anomia.

LIAR, LIAR

epigraph Carlo Collodi, *Pinocchio* (New York: Children's Classics, 1987 [1883]), 104.

216   **truthfulness:** Tom L. Beauchamp and James F. Childress, *Principles of Biomedical Ethics*, 5th ed. (New York: Oxford University Press, 2001), 283–284.

218 **"when veracity conflicts":** Ibid., 284.
218 **"Frank but not blunt":** Ibid.
219 **many are relieved:** B. D. Carpenter, C. Xiong, E. K. Porensky et al., "Reaction to a Dementia Diagnosis in Individuals with Alzheimer's Disease and Mild Cognitive Impairment," *JAGS* 55(3) (2008): 405–412.
219 **this form of truth-telling:** James F. Drane, *Becoming a Good Doctor: The Place of Virtue and Character in Medical Ethics*, 2nd ed. (Kansas City, MO: Sheed and Ward, 1995), 55.

PART V   A MILLION SPARKS
epigraph   Grace Schulman, "Celebration," *The Atlantic*, May 2009, 64.

FINAL ACTS
epigraph   Marcus Cicero, "On Old Age," in *The Basic Works of Cicero*, ed. Moses Hadas (New York: Random House, 1951), 158.
233 **"subservient to no one":** Ibid., 140.
234 **"a season ripe for death":** Ibid., 154.
234 **"a 'full life'":** Daniel Callahan and Kenneth Prager, "Medical Care for the Elderly: Should Limits Be Set?" *Virtual Mentor* 10(6) (June 2008): 404–410, http://virtualmentor.ama-assn.org/2008/06/oped10806.html. See also Daniel Callahan, *Setting Limits: Medical Goals in an Aging Society* (Washington, DC: Georgetown University Press, 2003).
236 **timeless responsibilities:** Cicero, "On Old Age," 152.

MENDED
242 **normal pressure hydrocephalus:** Cerebrospinal fluid (CSF) is the clear, alkaline liquid that bathes and cushions the brain within its cranial vault. Hydrocephalus—sometimes called "water on the brain"—results from an abnormally increased volume of CSF. NPH represents a chronic, insidious form of hydrocephalus.

LESSONS FROM FIRE
epigraph Zelda, "Place of Fire," in *The Spectacular Difference: Selected Poems*, trans. Marcia Falk (Cincinnati, OH: Hebrew Union College Press, 2004), 147.
250 **acute grief:** Erich Lindemann, "Symptomatology and Management of Acute Grief," reprinted in *Sesquicentennial Supplement to the American Journal of Psychiatry* 151(6) (1994): 155.
252 **"shatter the assumptions":** Jon G. Allen, *Coping with Trauma: Hope Through Understanding*, 2nd ed. (Washington, DC: American Psychiatric Publishing, 2005), 290.
252 **"profound shame":** Ibid.

253 **an unspeakable scene:** A documented account of the destruction of the Jews of Rakov during World War II can be found at these websites: www.eilatgordinlevitan.com/rakov/rakov.html; http://horwitzfam.org/histories/Rakov%20Belarus%20Report.doc; and www.eilatgordinlevitan.com/volozhin/vol_pages/vol_gb_archive_03.html. A photograph of the stone memorial to the murdered Jews of Rakov can be found at www.eilatgordinlevitan.com/rakov/rakov.html.

THE SEAMSTRESS

259 **"high rate of depression":** Stanley Jacobson, "Overselling Depression to the Old Folks," *The Atlantic*, April 1995, 47.

263 **Death with Dignity Act:** See Department of Human Services, Oregon, "Oregon's Death with Dignity Act: The First Year's Experience," February 18, 1999, http://oregon.gov/DHS/ph/pas/docs/year1.pdf; and Department of Human Services, Oregon, "Eighth Annual Report on Oregon's Death with Dignity Act," March 9, 2006, http://oregon.gov/DHS/ph/pas/docs/year8.pd.

263 **"promises of blossoms":** Zelda, "All This Misery—When Will I Die?" in *The Spectacular Difference: Selected Poems*, trans. Marcia Falk (Cincinnati, OH: Hebrew Union College Press, 2004), 61.

TREES

267 **magnum opus:** Jacobo Forma, *Lógica Transcendente* (Kearney, NE: Morris, 2006).

269 **a business transaction:** Kathryn Montgomery, *How Doctors Think* (New York: Oxford University Press, 2006), 177.

270 **moments of deep connection:** Ibid., 181.

270 **"medicine of neighbors":** Ibid., 185.

272 **"the holy branches":** William B. Yeats, "The Two Trees," in *The Rose* (1893; repr., Whitefish, MT: Kessenger, 2004), 24.

EPILOGUE

276 **a blessed height:** Erik H. Erikson, *The Life Cycle Completed*, extended ed. with new chapters by Joan M. Erikson (New York: Norton, 1977), 128.

277 **"'Life's magic'":** Zelda, "Ancient Pines," in *The Spectacular Difference: Selected Poems*, trans. Marcia Falk (Cincinnati, OH: Hebrew Union College Press, 2004), 177.

278 **"ashes to the earth":** T. S. Eliot, "Four Quartets" (1943), www.tristan.icom43.net/quartets/coker.html.

278 **"Just to be":** Abraham J. Heschel, *The Insecurity of Freedom* (New York: Farrar, Straus and Giroux, 1967), 82.

Selected Bibliography

One of the greatest joys of reading any book is that you never know where it will take you. For any such journeys into the realm of aging prompted by this book, a complete bibliography would be enormous and beyond the scope of the present effort. I therefore refer readers first to the numerous notes in the text to learn more about specific topics that I discuss. However, I would be remiss not to recommend the works of several individuals whom I have relied on to teach me both the basics and the minutiae of aging.

I am a student of the life cycle as it unfolds into later life, and I believe that the work of Harvard professor and fellow psychiatrist George Vaillant has laid the foundation for much of what we know about this process. He has built on the work of Erik Erikson, Daniel Levinson, and others to provide some of our most contemporary perspectives, and he is able to weave them into fascinating case studies. I recommend that the reader begin with the following work:

George E. Vaillant, *Aging Well: Surprising Guideposts to a Happier Life from the Landmark Harvard Study of Adult Development* (Boston: Little, Brown, 2002).

Standing shoulder to shoulder with Dr. Vaillant is Gene Cohen, one of the founding fathers of geriatric psychiatry. As

I describe throughout the book, he has taken the earlier work of Erikson and others and integrated aspects of both modern neuroscience and positive psychology. I was extremely fortunate to get to know Gene before his untimely death in late 2009. I wholeheartedly refer the reader to two of his books:

Gene D. Cohen, *The Creative Age: Awakening Human Potential in the Second Half of Life* (New York: Avon Books, 2000).
Gene D. Cohen, *The Mature Mind: The Positive Power of the Aging* Brain (New York: Basic Books, 2005).

For more detailed, historical accounts of aging, I always turn to the work of Thomas Cole:

Thomas R. Cole, *The Journey of Life: A Cultural History of Aging in America* (Cambridge, UK: Cambridge University Press, 1992).
Thomas R. Cole and Sally Gadow, eds., *What Does It Mean to Grow Old? Reflections from the Humanities* (Durham, NC: Duke University Press, 1986).

For books that provide inspiring, positive perspectives on aging, I recommend the following:

Wayne Booth, *The Art of Growing Older: Writers on Living and Aging* (Chicago: University of Chicago Press, 1992).
Barbara Myerhoff, *Number Our Days: A Triumph of Continuity and Culture Among Jewish Old People in an Urban Ghetto* (New York: Simon and Schuster, 1978).
Sherwin B. Nuland, *The Art of Aging: A Doctor's Prescription for Well-Being* (New York: Random House, 2007).
Mary Pipher, *Another Country: Navigating the Emotional Terrain of Our Elders* (New York: Riverhead Books, 1999).
Lars Tornstam, *Gerotranscendence: A Developmental Theory of Positive Aging* (New York: Springer, 2005).

There are a number of excellent books that cover not only the science of aging but also the fascinating story of the search for immortality. Without question one of the best was written by award-winning author Jonathan Weiner:

Jonathan Weiner, *Long for the World: The Strange Science of Immortality* (New York: HarperCollins, 2010).

Several other excellent books that cover the territory include the following:

Aubrey de Grey, with Michael Rae, *Ending Aging: The Rejuvenation Breakthroughs That Could Reverse Human Aging in Our Lifetime* (New York: St. Martin's Griffin, 2007).
Stephen S. Hall, *Merchants of Immortality: Chasing the Dream of Human Life Extension* (Boston: Houghton Mifflin, 2003).
S. Jay Olshansky and Bruce A. Carnes, *The Quest for Immortality: Science at the Frontiers of Aging* (New York: Norton, 2001).
Thomas T. Perls and Margery Hutter Silver, with John F. Lauerman, *Living to 100: Lessons in Living to Your Maximum Potential at Any Age* (New York: Basic Books, 1999).

A more specific (and one of the best!) book on wisdom is this one:

Elkhonon Goldberg, *The Wisdom Paradox: How Your Mind Can Grow Stronger as Your Brain Grows Older* (New York: Gotham Books, 2005).

For those interested in larger societal issues on aging, the key source is unquestionably Robert Butler, one of the founding fathers of the field of geriatrics, who, sadly, passed away in the fall of 2010:

Robert N. Butler, *The Longevity Revolution: The Benefits and Challenges of Living a Long Life* (New York: PublicAffairs, 2008).

To learn more about Erik Erikson and his theory of the life cycle, I refer the reader to Lawrence Friedman's outstanding biography as well as to the other selected works listed here:

Sue Erikson Bloland, *In the Shadow of Fame: A Memoir by the Daughter of Erik H. Erikson* (New York: Viking Penguin, 2005).

Erik H. Erikson, *Childhood and Society*, 35th anniversary ed. (New York: W.W. Norton & Company, 1985 [1950]).

Erik H. Erikson, *The Life Cycle Completed*, extended ed. with new chapters by Joan M. Erikson (New York: Norton, 1997).

Erik H. Erikson, Joan M. Erikson, and Helen Q. Kivnick, *Vital Involvement in Old Age* (New York: Norton, 1986).

Lawrence J. Friedman, *Identity's Architect: A Biography of Erik H. Erikson* (Cambridge, MA: Harvard University Press, 1999).

Finally, for readers who themselves work in the field of aging and are interested in books that provide details on the science of aging and on how to work successfully with older patients, I refer them to the following books, including several of my own:

Marc E. Agronin, *Alzheimer's Disease and Other Dementias*, 2nd ed. (Philadelphia: Lippincott Williams and Wilkins, 2008).

Marc E. Agronin, *Therapy with Older Clients: Key Strategies for Success* (New York: Norton, 2010).

Marc E. Agronin and Gabe J. Maletta, eds., *Principles and Practice of Geriatric Psychiatry* (Philadelphia: Lippincott Williams and Wilkins, 2007). A second edition is due out in 2011.

Colin A. Depp and Dilip V. Jeste, *Successful Cognitive and Emotional Aging* (Washington, DC: American Psychiatric Press, 2010).

Leonard Hayflick, "Biological Aging Is No Longer an Unsolved Problem," *Annals of the New York Academy of Science* 1100 (2007): 1–13.

Robert D. Hill, *Positive Aging: A Guide for Mental Health Professionals and Consumers* (New York: Norton, 2005).

S. Jay Olshansky, Leonard Hayflick, and Bruce A. Carnes, "No Truth to the Fountain of Youth," *Scientific American*, June 2002, 92–95.

CREDITS AND PERMISSIONS

✳✳✳

Excerpts from several of the stories in this book appeared previously in columns by Marc Agronin, M.D., in *CNS News, CNS Seniorcare, American Psychiatry News,* and *American Neurology News* and have been included with the permission of McMahon Publishing.

Excerpts from several of the stories in this book appeared previously in columns by Marc Agronin, M.D., in *Geriatric Psychiatry News,* and have been used with the permission of the American Association for Geriatric Psychiatry.

Epigraph to Part I from *Endpoint and Other Poems* by John Updike. Copyright © 2009 The Estate of John Updike. Reprinted by permission of Alfred A. Knopf, a division of Random House, Inc.

Epigraph to Part II from *Listeners at the Breathing Place* by Gary Miranda. Copyright © 1978 Princeton University Press. Reprinted by permission of Princeton University Press.

Epigraph to Part III from *A Blessing on the Moon* by Joseph Skibell. Copyright © 1997 Joseph Skibell. Reprinted by permission of Algonquin Books of Chapel Hill. All rights reserved.

From "The Old Woman and Time" by Sophie Freud. Copyright © 2009 Sophie Freud. Reprinted by permission of Sophie Freud.

Epigraph to Part V from the poem "Celebration" by Grace Schulman, which appears in *The Atlantic,* May 2009. Copyright © 2009 Grace Schulman. Reprinted by permission of Grace Schulman.

Poetry from *The Spectacular Difference: Selected Poems of Zelda.* Translated by Marcia Lee Falk. Copyright for English translations © 2004 Marcia Lee Falk. Reprinted by permission of Marcia Lee Falk.

The opening section of the chapter "Heaven" is reprinted from "Old Age, From Youth's Narrow Prism" by Marc E. Agronin, from *The New York Times* © [March 2, 2010] *The New York Times.* All rights reserved. Used by permission and protected by the Copyright Laws of the United States. The printing, copying, redistribution, or retransmission of the Material without express written permission is prohibited.

The second section of the chapter "Lessons from Fire" is reprinted from "From a Place of Fire and Weeping, Lessons on Memory, Aging and Hope"

ALISON WEIR

The Six Wives of
Henry VIII

VINTAGE BOOKS
London

Published by Vintage 2007

8 10 9 7

Copyright © Alison Weir 1991

Alison Weir has asserted her right under the Copyright, Designs and
Patents Act 1988 to be identified as the author of this work

First published by The Bodley Head Ltd 1991
First Pimlico edition 1992
Reissued in B Format 1997

Vintage
Random House, 20 Vauxhall Bridge Road,
London SW1V 2SA

www.vintage-books.co.uk

Addresses for companies within The Random House Group Limited
can be found at: www.randomhouse.co.uk/offices.htm

The Random House Group Limited Reg. No. 954009

A CIP catalogue record for this book
is available from the British Library

ISBN 9780099523628

The Random House Group Limited supports The Forest Stewardship
Council® (FSC®), the leading international forest certification organisation.
All our titles that are printed on Greenpeace approved FSC® certified paper
carry the FSC® logo. Our paper procurement policy can be found at:
www.randomhouse.co.uk/environment

Printed and bound in Great Britain by
Cox & Wyman Ltd, Reading, Berkshire

THIS BOOK IS DEDICATED TO
MY PARENTS,
DOREEN AND JAMES CULLEN,
AND MY MOTHER-IN-LAW,
MARGARET WEIR
AND IN LOVING MEMORY OF
WILLIAM BLACKWOOD WEIR

Contents

Part III How many wives will he have?

Chronology

1485	22 August	Battle of Bosworth. Henry Tudor usurps the English throne as Henry VII and founds the Tudor dynasty.
	16 December	Birth of Katherine of Aragon.
1486	19/20 September	Birth of Prince Arthur, eldest son of Henry VII.
1489	27 March	Treaty of Medina del Campo: Katherine and Arthur betrothed.
1491	28 June	Birth of Prince Henry, second son of Henry VII.
1499	19 May	Katherine and Arthur married by proxy.
c. 1500/1		Birth of Anne Boleyn.
1501	19 May	Katherine and Arthur married for a second time by proxy.
	27 September	Katherine arrives in England.
	12 November	Katherine enters London in state.
	14 November	Marriage of Katherine of Aragon and Arthur, Prince of Wales.
1502	2 April	Death of Prince Arthur.
1503	25 June	Katherine betrothed to Prince Henry.
1504	18 February	Prince Henry created Prince of Wales.
	26 November	Death of Isabella of Castile.
1505	27 June	Prince Henry secretly repudiates his betrothal.
c. 1507/8		Birth of Jane Seymour.
1509	22 April	Death of Henry VII and accession of Henry VIII.
	11 June	Marriage of Henry VIII and Katherine of Aragon.
	23 June	Henry and Katherine enter London in state.
	24 June	Coronation of Henry VIII and Katherine of Aragon.
1510	31 January	Birth of a stillborn daughter to Katherine of Aragon.
1511	1 January	Birth of Prince Henry, son of Henry VIII and Katherine of Aragon.
	22 February	Death of Prince Henry.
c. 1512		Birth of Katherine Parr.
1513	30 June–22 October	Katherine rules as regent while Henry VIII campaigns in France.

	16 August	Battle of the Spurs.
	9 September	Battle of Flodden.
	October	Birth of a son, who died soon after birth, to Katherine of Aragon.
1514	November	Birth of a son, who died soon after birth, to Katherine of Aragon.
1515	22 September	Birth of Anne of Cleves.
1516	January	Death of Ferdinand of Aragon.
	18 February	Birth of the Princess Mary, daughter of Henry VIII and Katherine of Aragon.
1518	10 November	Birth of a daughter, who died soon after birth, to Katherine of Aragon.
1519	February	Death of the Holy Roman Emperor, Maximilian, followed by the election of Charles of Castile, Katherine of Aragon's nephew, in his stead.
	June	Birth of Henry FitzRoy, bastard son of Henry VIII by Elizabeth Blount.
1520	3–23 June	The Field of Cloth of Gold, summit meeting between Henry VIII and Francis I of France.
1524		Katherine of Aragon known to be past the age for bearing children. Cessation of sexual relations between her and Henry VIII.
c. 1525		Birth of Katherine Howard.
1525	August	Princess Mary's household established at Ludlow.
1526	February	First indication that Henry VIII courting Anne Boleyn.
1527	6 May	Sack of Rome by the Emperor's troops.
	17 May	Proceedings to annul Henry VIII's marriage to Katherine of Aragon instituted in an ecclesiastical court at Westminster.
	22 June	Katherine informed by Henry of his doubts concerning the validity of their marriage.
	September	Henry VIII asks the Pope to help him gain an annulment of his marriage.
1528	29 September	Cardinal Campeggio, sent by the Pope to try the King's case, arrives in England.
1529	31 May	The legatine court opens at Black Friars, London.
	23 July	Campeggio adjourns the case indefinitely to Rome.
1530	November	Death of Cardinal Wolsey.

1531	11 February	The Reformation Parliament acknowledges Henry VIII as Supreme Head of the Church of England under Christ.
	14 July	Henry separates from Katherine and she is banished from court.
1532	1 September	Anne Boleyn created Lady Marquess of Pembroke.
1533	25 January	Secret marriage of Henry VIII and Anne Boleyn.
	12 April	Anne Boleyn first appears in public as Queen of England.
	23 May	Archbishop Cranmer declares the marriage of Henry VIII and Katherine of Aragon to be invalid and unlawful.
	28 May	Archbishop Cranmer declares the marriage of Henry VIII and Anne Boleyn to be good and valid.
	31 May	Anne Boleyn enters London in state.
	1 June	Coronation of Anne Boleyn.
	7 September	Birth of the Princess Elizabeth, daughter of Henry VIII and Anne Boleyn.
1534	23 March	Parliament passes the Act of Succession vesting the succession in Anne Boleyn's children by the King.
	23 March	Pope Clement VII pronounces the marriage of Henry VIII and Katherine of Aragon to be lawful and canonical.
	c. July	Birth of a child, sex not known, either still-born or dead soon after birth, to Henry VIII and Anne Boleyn.
1535	22 June	Execution of John Fisher, Bishop of Rochester.
	late June	Birth of a stillborn child to Anne Boleyn.
	6 July	Execution of Sir Thomas More.
	November	First mention of Henry VIII's courtship of Jane Seymour.
1536	7 January	Death of Katherine of Aragon.
	29 January	Birth of a stillborn son to Anne Boleyn.
	2 May	Anne Boleyn arrested and taken to the Tower of London.
	15 May	Trial of Anne Boleyn.
	19 May	Execution of Anne Boleyn.
	20 May	Henry VIII betrothed to Jane Seymour.
	30 May	Marriage of Henry VIII and Jane Seymour.
	7 June	Jane Seymour enters London in state.

	June	Parliament passes the Act of Succession vesting the succession in Jane Seymour's children by the King.
	13 June	Henry's daughter Mary offers him her submission.
	September 1536– March 1537	Pilgrimage of Grace.
1537	12 October	Birth of Prince Edward, son of Henry VIII and Jane Seymour.
	24 October	Death of Jane Seymour.
1539	4 September	Henry VIII betrothed to Anne of Cleves.
	27 December	Anne of Cleves arrives in England.
1540	6 January	Marriage of Henry VIII and Anne of Cleves.
	4 February	Anne of Cleves enters London in state.
	April	First mention of Henry VIII's courtship of Katherine Howard.
	9 July	Henry VIII's marriage to Anne of Cleves annulled.
	28 July	Execution of Thomas Cromwell.
		Marriage of Henry VIII and Katherine Howard.
1541	1 November	Henry VIII informed by Archbishop Cranmer of Katherine Howard's misconduct.
1542	7 February	Parliament passes the Act of Attainder condemning Katherine Howard to death.
	13 February	Execution of Katherine Howard.
1543	12 July	Marriage of Henry VIII and Katherine Parr.
1544	14 July– 30 September	Katherine Parr rules as regent while Henry VIII campaigns in France.
1547	28 January	Death of Henry VIII; accession of Edward VI.
	c. April	Marriage of Katherine Parr and Thomas Seymour.
1548	30 August	Birth of Mary, daughter of Katherine Parr and Thomas Seymour.
	7 September	Death of Katherine Parr.
1553	6 July	Death of Edward VI.
	10 July	Lady Jane Grey proclaimed Queen of England.
	19 July	Queen Jane deposed; accession of Mary I, daughter of Henry VIII and Katherine of Aragon.
1557	16 July	Death of Anne of Cleves.
1558	17 November	Death of Mary I; accession of Elizabeth I, daughter of Henry VIII and Anne Boleyn.

Introduction

The reign of Henry VIII is one of the most fascinating in English history. Not only was it a time of revolutionary political and social change, but it was also dominated by one of the most extraordinary and charismatic men to emerge in the history of the British Isles – the King's contemporaries thought him 'the greatest man in the world' and 'such a king as never before'. He ruled England in unprecedented splendour, surrounded by some of the most intriguing personalities of the age, men and women who have left behind such vivid memorials of themselves that we can almost reach out across the centuries and feel we know them personally.

Six of these people were the King's wives. It is – and was then – a remarkable fact in itself that a man should have six wives, yet what makes it especially fascinating to us is that these wives were interesting people in their own right. We are fortunate that we know so much about them – not only the major events and minutiae of their public lives, but also something of their thoughts and feelings, even the intimate details of their private lives. Henry VIII's marital affairs brought the royal marriage into public focus for the first time in our history; prior to his reign, the conjugal relationships of English sovereigns were rarely chronicled, and there remain only fragmentary details of the intimate lives of earlier kings and queens. Yet, thanks to Henry VIII, such details became a matter of public interest, and no snippet of information was thought too insignificant to be recorded and analysed, a trend that has continued unabated for 450 years, and which has burgeoned in the twentieth century with the expansion of the media.

Thanks to the wealth of written material that has survived in the form of early biographies, letters, memoirs, account books and diplomatic reports, unprecedented in any preceding reign, we know a great deal about, and are able to make sense of, the lives of these six long-dead women. That such material was for the first time available to any sizeable extent was thanks to the humanism of the Renaissance and the widening interest in learning it engendered. There was a dramatic expansion of educational facilities, with the founding of many new colleges and schools, and literacy was now seen as being of prime importance, not only for men, but – to an increasing degree as the Tudor period progressed – for women also. The development of printing gave rise to a growth industry in popular works and tracts, which coincided with a renewed interest in history, leading to a succession of books by a new generation of chroniclers. Greater care was taken, both in England and abroad, to maintain public records, and with the evolution of intelligence systems, such as that established by Thomas Cromwell, more detailed information than ever before was accumulated.

Much of the source material for the reign of Henry VIII was collated by historians and published in the late nineteenth and early twentieth centuries, giving rise to a succession of biographies, learned and otherwise, of the King, his courtiers and his wives. Yet while there have been several excellent recent individual biographies of the wives (see *Bibliography*), there has been no serious collective biography since 1905 when M.A.S. Hume's scholarly book, *The Wives of Henry VIII* was published. This present book aims to fill that gap for the general reader, with information drawn from only the most reliable of the original sources.

What were they really like, those six wives? Because of the nature of the source material for the reign, nearly all of which has a political or religious bias, a writer could come up with very different assessments of each of them, all of which might be equally valid. But this would be abdicating some of the responsibilities of an historian, whose function is to piece together the surviving evidence and arrive at a workable conclusion. What follows are the conclusions I have reached after many years of research into the subject, conclusions that, on the weight of the evidence, must be as realistic as anything can be after a lapse of 450 years.

Thus, we will see that Katherine of Aragon was a staunch but misguided woman of principle; Anne Boleyn an ambitious adventuress with a penchant for vengeance; Jane Seymour a strong-minded matriarch in the making; Anne of Cleves a good-humoured woman who jumped at the chance of independence; Katherine Howard an empty-headed wanton; and Katherine Parr a godly matron who was nevertheless all too human when it came to a handsome rogue. They were fascinating women, both because of who they were and what happened to them; yet we should not lose sight of the fact that, while they were queens and therefore, nominally at least, in a position of power, they were also bound to a great degree by the constraints that restricted the lives of all women at that time. We should therefore, before proceeding with their story, pause to consider those constraints.

'Woman in her greatest perfection was made to serve and obey man,' wrote the Scots reformer John Knox in his treatise *First Blast of the Trumpet against the Monstrous Regiment of Women*, published in 1558. In Tudor England, as in the Middle Ages, women were brought up to believe that they were vastly inferior to men. Even a queen was subordinate to the will of her husband, and – like all wives – was required to learn in silence from him 'in all subjection'. Two of Henry VIII's wives – Anne Boleyn and Katherine Parr – being highly intelligent and outspoken women, found this particularly hard, and consequently both clashed with the King on numerous occasions. Naturally, Henry won. The concept of female inferiority was older than Christianity, but centuries of Christian teaching had rigidly enforced it. Woman was an instrument of the devil, the author of original sin who would lure man away from the path to salvation – in short, the only imperfection in God's creation.

Henry VIII's wives would all have learned very early in life that, as women, they had very little personal freedom. Brought up to obey their parents without question, they found that, once married to the King, they were expected to render the same unquestioning obedience to a husband – indeed, more so than ordinary wives, for this husband also happened to be the King of England. Even widowhood brought its constraints, as Katherine of Aragon found after her first husband died and she was left to the tender mercies of her father and father-in-law until she remarried. Only during courtship might a woman briefly gain the upper hand, as both Anne Boleyn and Jane Seymour did, but woe betide her if she did not quickly learn to conform once the wedding-ring was on her finger.

The notion that women could be equal to men would have been totally foreign to the King and most of his male contemporaries. Thus women, single or married, possessed very few legal rights. A woman's body and her worldly goods both became her husband's property on marriage, and the law allowed him to do exactly as he pleased with them. Infidelity in a wife was not tolerated, but for queens Henry VIII made it a treasonable offence punishable by death, because it threatened the succession. Two of Henry's wives died on the scaffold after being found guilty of criminal intercourse, and the wife of a peer could face the same penalty if her adultery was proved and her husband petitioned the King to have her executed. A wife who murdered her husband was guilty, not of murder, but of petty treason, and the penalty for this until the eighteenth century was death by burning. Even if a wife merely displeased her husband, justifiably or not, the law allowed him to turn her out of the house with just a shift to cover her, and she had no right of redress. Wife-beating was common and, instead of provoking the horrified reaction it arouses today, 450 years ago it would have been regarded as a righteous punishment for an erring or disobedient wife, although there is no evidence that Henry VIII ever beat any of his wives.

From the cradle to the grave, the lives of Henry's queens – and of all women – were lived according to prescribed rules and conventions. Only four of the six received any formal education; Jane Seymour and Katherine Howard appear to have been barely literate. Many people in the first half of the sixteenth century still did not believe that women should be educated, holding to the medieval view that girls taught to write would only waste their skill on love-letters. But thanks to men such as the Spanish educationist Juan Luis Vives, and Sir Thomas More, whose daughters were renowned examples of womanly erudition, as well as the shining examples of both Katherine of Aragon and Katherine Parr who proved that women could be both learned and virtuous, the Renaissance concept of female education gradually became accepted and even applauded. Nevertheless, the Elizabethan bluestocking was not yet born; in Henry VIII's time, the education of girls was the privilege of the royal and the rich, and its chief aim was to produce future wives schooled in godly and moral precepts. It was not intended to promote independent thinking; indeed, it tended to the opposite.

When it came to choosing a marriage partner, high-born girls – and princesses in particular – were at the mercy of their fathers, for it was almost unheard of for them to select their own husbands. One married for political reasons, to cement alliances, to gain wealth, land and status, and to forge bonds between families; marrying for love was merely wayward and foolish. Royal marriages, of course, were largely matters of political expediency: it was not unknown for a king to see his bride's face for the first time on their wedding day, and it was still thought unusual for a king to marry one of his own subjects. Kings were expected to ally themselves with foreign powers for political and trading advantages, and had done so until 1464 when Henry's grandfather, Edward IV, had married Elizabeth Woodville, a commoner, for love alone, and caused a furore. Half a century later, a burgeoning sense of English nationalism meant that Henry VIII's marriages to four commoners passed without anyone complaining that they were not of royal blood. What did excite comment was that he had married them for love, a sensational departure from tradition. In a sense, however, these were political marriages too, since the political and religious factions at Henry's court were continually trying to manoeuvre their master in and out of wedlock.

Negotiations for marriages between royal houses could be – and often were – very protracted. It took thirteen years to arrange the marriage of Katherine of Aragon and Arthur Tudor; fortunately – as so often happened – negotiations began when both were toddlers. Royal courtship in such cases consisted of formal letters containing fulsome declarations of love, and symbolic gifts, usually rings or jewels. Unless a bride was being reared at her future husband's court, geographical barriers often prevented the couple from meeting. Kings had to rely on the accuracy of descriptions sent by ambassadors, and also on the artistry of court painters, though there were notable mishaps: Holbein painted Anne of Cleves, but in doing so unduly flattered the lady, and a distraught Henry was driven to complain that it was 'the fate of princes to take as is brought them by others, while poor men be commonly at their own choice'.

There was no legal age for marriage in the sixteenth century. Marriage between children was not unknown, but the usual age of both partners was around fourteen or fifteen, old enough for cohabitation. No one questioned whether young people were mature enough to marry and procreate at such an early age: life expectancy was short, and the average woman could not expect to live much beyond thirty. In this context, therefore, all of Henry's wives except Katherine Howard married him at quite a late age. Katherine of Aragon was twenty-four (it was her second marriage), Anne Boleyn around thirty-two, Jane Seymour twenty-eight, Anne of Cleves twenty-four, and Katherine Parr thirty-one (her third marriage). By contrast, Katherine Howard was only fifteen or thereabouts when Henry, at the age of forty-nine, took her to wife, and the bride's youth excited much comment.

A formal betrothal was called a precontract; in the case of a royal union, its terms and conditions were set out in a formal marriage treaty. A precontract could be in written form, or consist of a verbal promise to marry made before witnesses. Once it had been made, only sexual intercourse was necessary to transform it into marriage, and many couples lived together quite respectably after having conformed to this custom. Some, of course, went on to take their vows in church, but this was not a necessity except in the case of a royal or noble union, such as that between Henry VIII and Anne Boleyn, which came about in this way, but which was later regularised by a ceremony of marriage.

The dowry, or marriage portion, was always the chief issue in any betrothal contract. A dowry could consist of lands, money, jewellery, plate, even household goods, and a girl's chances of marriage depended more upon her father's financial and social status than upon her face and form, although these sometimes helped. Even the plainest girl, if she had a rich dowry, would never lack for suitors. The contract would also feature the terms of the bride's jointure, settled upon her by her husband-to-be or his father, for her maintenance after marriage and during widowhood. Yet it was never hers to control directly unless her husband permitted it, or unless she was widowed and did not remarry.

Without a precontract, sex before marriage was forbidden, although, of course, it was a frequent occurrence that was not just confined to the lower orders of society. As Katherine Howard's experiences prove, lax morality could prevail among the nobility also. Men, however, were encouraged to sow their wild oats, but a woman who did so became a social outcast and ruined her chances of making a good marriage. For this reason, Henry VIII conducted his courtships of Katherine Howard and Jane Seymour in the presence of their relatives, in order to preserve the good reputation of his future wives.

Weddings themselves were performed according to ancient Roman Catholic rites, with vows being exchanged in the church porch, followed by a nuptial mass at the high altar. Two witnesses had to be present. The old form of the service then in use required the bride to vow to be 'bonair and buxom [amiable] in bed and at board'. Henry VIII's weddings were all solemnised in private ceremonies, with only a few selected courtiers present. Only three were marked by public celebrations afterwards: those to Katherine of Aragon, Jane Seymour and Anne of Cleves. The date and place of the King's marriage to Anne Boleyn were kept so secret that even Archbishop Cranmer could not be certain about them. This is not to say, however, that the modern concept of a royal wedding, with all its attendant pageantry, was unknown. Public royal weddings had been the rule up until the reign of Henry VIII, and that of his parents, Henry VII and Elizabeth of York, in 1486 at Westminster Abbey was a very public affair, as was the wedding of Katherine of Aragon and Arthur Tudor at St Paul's Cathedral in 1501. Indeed, the ceremonies observed, the procession through the streets, and the cheering crowds, were not so very different from those that a worldwide television audience saw when the present Prince of Wales married Lady Diana Spencer on the same site 480 years later.

The English had a fondness for traditional customs, and celebrated their weddings with feasting and a good deal of bawdy revelry. Dancing would follow the nuptial banquet, and then the bride and groom would be ceremoniously put to bed by the guests, the marriage bed being blessed by a priest before the couple were left alone to consummate their marriage. There is, however, no record of Henry VIII being publicly put to bed with any of his wives, although Katherine of Aragon was with Prince Arthur, in front of many witnesses.

Once the marriage had been consummated, the couple were literally viewed as one flesh, and Sir Thomas More advised them to regard their sexual union as being similar to 'God's coupling with their souls'. Theological doctrine inclined to the view that all carnal relationships were of a base and sinful nature; only the sacrament of marriage made the 'damnable act' 'pure, clean, and without spot of sin'. However, although instances of marital sex did not have to be mentioned in the confessional, the marriage ceremony was not intended as a gateway to self-indulgent lust. The Church taught that sex was only for the procreation of children, that the Word of God might be handed down to future generations; sex was therefore a sacred duty in marriage. 'Who does not tremble when he considers how to deal with his wife?' asked Henry VIII in his treatise *A Defence of the Seven Sacraments*; 'for not only is he bound to love her, but so to live with her that he may return her to God pure and without stain, when God who gave shall demand His own again.'

Marriage brought with it further constraints for women. Matrimony was essential to the Tudor concept of the divine order of the world: the husband ruled his family, as the King ruled his realm, and as God ruled the universe, and – like subjects – wives were bound in obedience to their husbands and masters. In 1537, Sir Thomas Wyatt advised his son to 'rule his wife well' so that she would love and reverence him 'as her head'. 'I am utterly of the opinion,' wrote Thomas Lupset in *An Exhortation to Young Men* (1535), 'that the man may make, shape and form the woman as he will.' Certainly this was what Henry VIII expected to do as a husband. In his eyes, and in those of other men of his era, a loving, virtuous and obedient wife was a blessing direct from God. But for women, even queens, marriage often brought with it total subjection to and domination by a domestic tyrant.

Marriage was therefore a period of great upheaval and adjustment for young women, and even more so for those born royal, for a princess often had to face a perilous journey to a new land and a stranger she had never before set eyes on, as well as a heart-wrenching parting from parents, siblings, friends, home and native land, all of which she might never see again. If she were clever, however, a royal bride could come to enjoy considerable power and influence, as did both Katherine of Aragon and Anne Boleyn. Yet such status and power emanated solely from her husband. She enjoyed no freedoms but those he permitted her. Without him, she was nothing.

Queens of England were housewives on a grand scale, with nominal charge of vast households and far-flung estates from which they derived huge revenues. In fact, they had an army of officials to administer these for them, and only controlled their own income to the degree permitted them by the King; no major transactions would be conducted without his consent. Any decisions they made concerning finances, patronage, benefactions, estate management and household matters were subject to his approval; their privy council was an advisory body appointed by him to oversee their affairs on his behalf. There is evidence that Henry VIII was in fact happy to leave a good many domestic decisions to his wives' discretion, and was certainly generous with money when the mood took him. He could also be callous when he felt the need, and was not above reminding Anne Boleyn that he had the power to lower her more than he had raised her, leaving her in no doubt as to who held the upper hand.

What was really required of a queen was that she produce heirs for the succession and set a high moral standard for court and kingdom by being a model of wifely dignity and virtue. To depart from this role could spell disaster, as both Anne Boleyn and Katherine Howard found to their cost. Katherine was certainly promiscuous, but Anne merely lacked the necessary modesty, circumspection and humility of manner; thus it was easy for her contemporaries to believe her guilty of moral laxity.

A queen's formal dignity was reinforced by the clothes and jewels she wore, and nowhere were the constraints upon women as obvious as when it came to the rules governing their attire. The everyday dress of a married woman was preordained by convention. Hair that had been worn loose before marriage must now be hidden under a hood and veil; only queens might have their hair flowing after marriage, and then only on state occasions when it was necessary to wear a crown. Women only cut their hair to enter a cloister; most wore it long – Anne Boleyn and Katherine of Aragon both had hair so long they could sit on it. Widows were required to wear a nun-like wimple and chin-barbe, familiar on portraits of the Lady Margaret Beaufort, Henry VII's mother. This practice was dying out by the time of the Reformation, although for some time afterwards widows would wear severe white caps or hoods.

Even in summer, sleeves were required to reach the wrist, and gowns were worn long, sweeping the floor. Such were the dictates of modesty, which also required a woman to suffer agonising constriction within a corset of stiff leather or even wood. Yet it was not thought indecent to wear gowns with a square neckline low enough to expose most of the upper breasts; in an age when hand-reared babies rarely survived, the sight of a female breast was a common one and excited little censure.

The sumptuous attire of queens provided yet further limitation; the heavy velvets and damasks used, the long court trains, the elaborate head-dresses, and the cumbersome oversleeves, all had the effect of severely restricting movement. Queens walked slowly, danced slowly, and moved with regal bearing, not just because they were born to it, but because their clothes constrained them to it. Yet they did not complain – like many women in all periods of history, they were willing to suffer in the cause of fashion.

The chief function of a queen – and of the wives of lesser men, for that matter – was to bear her husband male heirs to ensure the continuity of his dynasty. Pregnancy could be, and often was, an annual event – from the male point of view, a highly satisfactory state, although not so satisfactory for those wives who were worn out with frequent childbearing, or for the high proportion of women and babies who died in childbed. Pregnancy and childbirth were extremely hazardous. As well as preparing a layette and a nursery, an expectant mother would, as a matter of routine, make provision for someone to care for her child in the event of her dying at its birth. And even if she survived the birth, she might be physically scarred for life. This is not the place to discuss the truly horrific things that could happen to a woman in childbed – suffice it to say that lack of medical knowledge (only midwives attended confinements, doctors were rarely called in unless it was to deal with severe complications) and the absence of any real understanding of hygiene were what really killed women.

A woman who bore ten children could expect to see less than half grow to full maturity if she were lucky. Katherine of Aragon and Anne Boleyn had ten pregnancies between them: two children survived. Caesarian section and forceps were unknown, and many babies died at birth. Given the problems with the feeding and management of babies that prevailed at the time, it is surprising that any survived at all. Many were given unsuitable foods, and there were no antibiotics; any chance infection could carry an infant off with hardly a warning. A mother could herself be at risk, even after the birth was successfully over, for at any time during her lying-in period, puerperal fever could strike; Jane Seymour died of this, probably because a tear in her perineum became infected. In this respect, marriage brought no real security to women; in all too many cases, they died as a result of it.

In an age of arranged marriages, a wife could not expect her husband to be faithful. Marriages were business arrangements, pleasure could be found elsewhere. Adultery in men was common, and Henry VIII is known to have strayed frequently during his first two marriages. Nor did he expect to be censured for it: he once brutally advised Anne Boleyn to shut her eyes as her betters had done when she dared to upbraid him for being unfaithful.

The medieval tradition of courtly love still flourished at the Tudor court. It was a code of behaviour by which the chivalrous knight paid court to the lady of his heart, who was usually older, married and of higher rank – and thus conveniently unattainable. A man could refer to his 'mistress' in the noblest sense, without implying that there was any sexual relationship, yet all too often the courtly ideal was merely an excuse for adultery. We shall see that Henry VIII was a great exponent of this chivalric cult, a concept inbred in him from infancy, and which inspired the courtship of all of his wives as well as the pursuit of his mistresses.

Marriage, however, was as far removed from courtly love as night from day. Once married, couples had to make the best of things, however bad, for there was rarely a way out. Divorce was very rare, and was only granted by Act of Parliament in exceptional cases, usually involving adultery among the nobility. Annulment by an ecclesiastical court, or even by the Pope, was more common, but the only grounds permissible were non-consummation of the marriage, discovery of a near degree of affinity, insanity, or the discovery of a previous precontract to someone else. Where a couple were within the forbidden degrees of affinity, the Pope was usually happy to issue a dispensation before the marriage took place. The validity of such a dispensation was accepted without question in Europe until Henry VIII brought his suit against Katherine of Aragon in 1527, claiming that the Pope had contravened Levitical law by issuing a dispensation allowing him to marry his brother's widow. Such a stand, taken at a crucial time in the history of the Church, was enough to rend Christendom asunder.

To today's liberated women and 'new men', the lives of Henry VIII's wives appear to have been shockingly narrow and hemmed by intolerable constraints. Yet, having experienced nothing else, they did not think to question these, and accepted their inferior status as part of the divine order of things. Katherine Parr even applauded it; in her book, *The Lamentations of a Sinner*, published in 1548, she exhorted wives to wear 'such apparel as becometh holiness and comely usage with soberness', and warned them against the evils of overeating and drinking wine. Young women, she said, must be 'sober minded, love their husbands and children, and be discreet, housewifely, and good'. Henry VIII was dead when these words were written, but we may certainly read in them a reflection of his own views. Jane Seymour took as her motto the legend 'Bound to obey and serve', while Katherine Howard's was 'No other will than his'. They, like the King's other wives, accepted their subjugation; it was the price of their queenship and of marriage.

Part I
Katherine
of
Aragon

I

The princess from Spain

The child, thought the ambassadors, was delightful, 'singularly beautiful'. Seated upon the lap of her mother, the Queen of Castile, she was gravely surveying the important yet deferential men who were taking such polite and fulsome interest in her. Only two years old in the spring of 1488, the Infanta Katherine of Aragon was already displaying the plump prettiness that was to enchant her two future husbands. Her wide blue eyes gazed from a round, firm-chinned face, which was framed by wavy, red-gold hair, worn loose as was the custom for princesses at that time. She sat with her mother on a dais in the midst of the court of Castile and Aragon, which had gathered for a brief respite in the wars against the Infidel to enjoy a tournament. And, during the interval, when the contesting knights had withdrawn to their tents, the English ambassadors, sent by King Henry VII, came to pay their respects.

Queen Isabella, sovereign of Castile in her own right, and her husband Ferdinand of Aragon were well aware of their purpose. They came from a king whose title to his crown was dubious, to say the least. Although three years had now elapsed since Henry Tudor had usurped the throne of England after defeating Richard III, the last Plantagenet king, at the battle of Bosworth, he was still working hard to consolidate his position. He had, in fact, no title at all to the crown by descent; therefore he professed to claim it by right of conquest and through a questionable descent from the early British kings – not for nothing did he name his eldest son, born in 1486, Arthur. Nevertheless, there were still living at least six male members of the House of Plantagenet with a better lineal claim to the throne than Henry VII, and he knew it. Ferdinand and Isabella knew it too, and they were sensible of the fact that a marriage alliance between England and one of the great European powers would imply recognition of Henry VII's title and immeasurably strengthen his position both in his own kingdom and in the eyes of the world at large.

There were, at that time, two major powers in Europe: France and Spain. English distrust of the French, engendered by nearly 200 years of war, forced Henry VII to consider a more congenial alliance for his son with Spain, then a new political entity. Until 1479, Spain had been made up of a group of minor kingdoms ruled by interrelated monarchs, and since the eighth century, much of the Spanish peninsula had been held by the Moors. Slowly, the Christian rulers had reclaimed the land. The 'Reconquest' had been going on for centuries, an internal crusade that absorbed Spanish energies and kept her to a large extent out of European politics. This long struggle against the Moors was in fact the greatest source of a sense of national identity, and the biggest single unifying factor, more so even than the marriage between Ferdinand of Aragon and Isabella of Castile that brought the Spanish kingdoms together under a single monarchy. No Spanish rulers were more zealous in eliminating the Moors than Ferdinand and Isabella, and by 1488 only the Moorish kingdom of Granada remained unconquered by the Christians. The sovereigns were rulers of the rest of the Iberian peninsula, save for the kingdom of Portugal, and it would only be a matter of time before Granada too came under their dominion. Spain was therefore taking its place as a major European power.

Ferdinand and Isabella represented everything that seemed desirable to Henry VII: they were the descendants of ancient monarchies, their position was strong, and their reputation glorious. If they could be persuaded to agree to a marriage alliance between Prince Arthur and one of their four daughters, then the Tudor dynasty would be far more secure than hitherto. Moreover, Spain and France were hereditary enemies, and therefore a joint pact between England and Spain would benefit both sides. The Spanish sovereigns were well aware of the potential advantages to themselves of such an alliance, but they were in no hurry to make a commitment. Ferdinand was as wily a politician as Henry Tudor, and was not prepared to sign any treaties until he could be sure that the English King was firmly established on his throne. Given England's susceptibility to dynastic warfare, it seemed more than likely that Henry VII might not long enjoy his regal dignity.

There was, however, something that Ferdinand desired very much, and that was military assistance against the French. In March 1488, the Spanish ambassador at the English court was Dr Roderigo de Puebla, an unscrupulous diplomat of Jewish origins. Ferdinand had instructed him to offer Henry an infanta for his son in return for an undertaking on Henry's part to declare war on France. The King of England had reacted enthusiastically to the proposal, and promptly despatched his ambassadors to Spain to view the sovereigns' youngest daughter, Katherine.

A Spanish herald, Ruy Machado, was moved to comment on the charming impression made on the envoys by both the little girl and her mother, the Queen. At the same time, in England, Henry VII was welcoming Ferdinand's representatives and enthusiastically showing off his nineteen-month-old son, first dressed in cloth of gold and then stripped naked, so they could see he had no deformity. The Spaniards saw an auburn-haired, fair-skinned child who was tall for his age, and thought him both beautiful and graceful, with 'many excellent qualities'.

Ferdinand and Isabella were impressed by their reports, but still not happy about sending their daughter to a realm whose king might be deposed at any time. As Puebla told Henry VII quite candidly in July, 'Bearing in mind what happens every day to the kings of England, it is surprising that Ferdinand and Isabella should dare think of giving their daughter at all.' But at last Ferdinand decided that assistance against France was more important to him than his daughter's future security, and instructed his ambassadors to draw up a treaty of marriage. There was some haggling between the representatives of both sides over the financial settlement to be made on the bride, but this was settled amicably and it was agreed that the Infanta should bring with her a dowry of 200,000 crowns (equivalent to about £5 million today). The alliance was ratified, and the dowry confirmed, by the Treaty of Medina del Campo, which was signed by the Spanish sovereigns on 27 March 1489. Thus Katherine's matrimonial future was decided when she was three years old, a common fate of princesses at that time.

Katherine of Aragon was named after her English great-grandmother, Katherine of Lancaster, a daughter of John of Gaunt (a younger son of Edward III), who had married Henry III of Castile in 1388 and died in 1418. Her son by Henry succeeded his father as John I, and married his cousin, Isabella of Portugal; they were the parents of Isabella of Castile. Isabella had been born into a land ravaged by war, both dynastic and holy. Her brother, Henry IV, was a spineless weakling, and her mother went insane when she was a girl. Fortunately, in 1469 a marriage was arranged for Isabella with her cousin, Ferdinand of Aragon, a vigorous youth eleven months her junior. In 1474, Henry IV died childless, and Isabella became Queen of Castile in her own right.

The new Queen was of middle height with a good figure that would soon be ruined by ten pregnancies in quick succession. She had skin so fair it looked white, and her eyes were a greeny blue. She was graceful, beautiful, modest and pious, but was also blessed with a sense of humour and boundless energy. She was both clever and sensible, and turned a blind eye to her husband's many infidelities, although she loved him dearly. Her only fault, as noted by her contemporaries, was her love of ostentation in dress, for, like her daughter Katherine in later years, she was 'a ceremonious woman in her attire', favouring the rich velvets and cloth of gold so typical of the period.

In 1479, the King of Aragon died and Ferdinand succeeded him. Thus, for the first time in her history, Spain became united under centralised rule, with only the Moorish Kingdom of Granada refusing allegiance to the sovereigns. The reconquest of this Infidel bastion was to be the great enterprise of their reign, to which they would devote most of their time and resources. Campaign followed campaign, with the ever growing family of the King and Queen being trailed after them in the wake of their army, from city to city, through inhospitable and hostile territory, the monarchs themselves sometimes suffering gruelling privation in their quest for a holy victory.

This left the Queen with little time to devote to her children. Her first child, Isabella, was born in 1470, and was followed in rapid succession over the next fifteen years by nine others. Sadly, all the campaigning took its toll: five babies died young. However, the rest grew to maturity. An heir to the throne, the Infante John, was born in 1478; then there was Juana, born in 1479, Maria in 1482, and Katherine (who was called Catalina in her native land), born on the night of 15–16 December 1485 in the palace of the Bishop of Toledo at Alcala de Henares, in the midst of war. The Queen had been in the saddle all day, and rose from her bed the day after the birth to go back on the march, consigning her youngest daughter to the care of nurses. Nevertheless, she cared deeply for all her children, and personally supervised their education. They, in turn, all loved and respected her, especially Katherine, who grew up to be the most like her in looks and character.

While Isabella lived, Katherine had a champion who would consider her welfare and security before all else. Yet Katherine was Ferdinand's daughter as well, and he was very different from her mother. In appearance he was of medium height with a well-proportioned body, and had long dark hair and a good complexion. He was genial, charismatic and a good conversationalist. Like his wife, he possessed great energy which he put to good use on military campaigns but also expended on women. His contemporaries thought him compassionate, yet this did not always extend to his own family; he later abandoned one daughter to penury and had another declared insane in order to seize her kingdom. He was notorious as a great dissimulator, and for being fond of political intrigue. Yet for all his failings, he loved his wife, and theirs was a dynamic and successful partnership.

The only glimpse we have of Katherine of Aragon during her childhood is at the tournament where she was presented to the English ambassadors. Yet she was an innocent witness to most of the great landmarks of her parents' reign: the fall of Granada in 1492, the discovery of America by Christopher Columbus, and the establishment of the notorious Spanish Inquisition. All of these things served to enhance the reputation of Ferdinand and Isabella as champions of the Catholic Church; Spain's prestige in the world had never been higher.

After the conquest of Granada, the four infantas were sent there to live in the Moorish palace of the Alhambra. There they grew to maturity and were educated among the arched courtyards and splashing fountains where once the caliphs had kept their harem. The Christian princesses rarely left their sunny home, except for the great occasions of state at which their presence was required. Katherine's tutor, appointed by her mother, was a clerk in holy orders, Alessandro Geraldini, who would later accompany her to England as her chaplain. Her education was very much in the medieval tradition, although Erasmus, the celebrated Dutch humanist, who met Katherine in England, tells us that she was 'imbued with learning, by the care of her illustrious mother'. She learned to write with a graceful hand, and improved her mind with devotional reading, but she was also taught the traditional feminine skills of needlework and dancing, lacemaking, and embroidery in the Spanish 'black-work' style, which she would later popularise in England. Before her eyes was the image of her pious mother as the supreme example of Christian queenship, an example that Katherine would try to emulate all her life.

Ferdinand and Isabella arranged advantageous marriages for all their children, although none turned out as successfully as they had hoped. Isabella was married in 1490 to the Infante Alfonso of Portugal. Although it was an arranged marriage, the young couple quickly fell in love, but their happiness was shattered when, only seven months later, Alfonso was killed after a fall from his horse. His widow returned to Spain declaring it was her intention to enter a nunnery, but Ferdinand was having none of this, and after protracted negotiations sent her back to Portugal in 1497 to marry Alfonso's cousin, King Manuel I. In 1498, Isabella died giving birth to a son, the Infante Miguel, who only lived two years. Manuel would later remarry, and his bride would be Isabella's younger sister Maria.

Juana, the second daughter of the sovereigns, was volatile and highly unstable, yet her parents arranged for her an even more glorious marriage. Their fame had led many princes to seek alliance with them, one such being the Holy Roman Emperor, Maximilian I, Hapsburg ruler of vast territories, including Austria, parts of Germany, Burgundy and the Low Countries. He had two gifted children, Philip and Margaret, and Ferdinand and Isabella were happy to ally themselves with Maximilian by marriages between

Philip and Juana and Margaret of Austria and the Infante John, the heir to Spain.

Juana and Philip were married in 1496. Philip was not for nothing nicknamed 'the Handsome', and Juana fell violently and possessively in love with him, with the predictable result that he soon tired of her and took mistresses. This provoked his wife to terrible rages, and her behaviour became a public scandal both in Flanders and Spain. Reports of it reached Queen Isabella, who was deeply troubled by them, yet powerless to do very much to alter the situation. However, Juana's mental instability did not affect her fertility, and she produced six children, her eldest son Charles being born in 1500 at Ghent.

Her brother John fared rather better in his marriage, which took place in 1497. He was a pleasant youth who excelled in all the knightly virtues and who had captured the hearts of his future subjects. His constitution, however, was delicate, and Ferdinand and Isabella were concerned that his spirited and robust bride would wear him out. Their fears were well founded, too, for the Infante died only six months after his marriage, leaving Margaret of Austria pregnant with a child that was later stillborn. This meant that the Infanta Isabella was now the heiress to the Spanish throne, and when she bore her son Miguel in 1498, there were great celebrations, in spite of her death in childbirth, for Spain once more had a male heir. Yet when Miguel succumbed to a childish illness in 1500, the unstable Juana became heiress to the sovereigns, which was naturally a matter of concern to them, though at least she had a healthy son of her own.

Queen Isabella grieved deeply for the loss of her children and grandchildren, which made her remaining unmarried daughter, Katherine, seem all the more precious to her. Throughout these years of marriages and tragedy, negotiations had dragged on for Katherine's wedding to Prince Arthur, and Isabella was now determined to ensure that her daughter's future would be as secure and happy as she could make it. In 1493, when Katherine was seven years old, it had been decided that she would go to England in 1498, when she was twelve. In 1497, Henry VII sent her 'a blessed ring' as a token of his fatherly affection. She could not remember a time when she had not been referred to as the Princess of Wales, and from the age of two she had been schooled for her destiny as Queen of England. She had been brought up in the knowledge that one day she must leave Spain and her parents for ever, being told that such was the fate of all princesses like her. As she had been reared to absolute obedience to the will of her parents, she did not question this.

In August 1497, Katherine and Arthur were formally betrothed at the ancient palace of Woodstock in Oxfordshire, Dr de Puebla standing proxy for the bride. Katherine did not go to England in 1498; the date of her arrival was postponed until September 1500, when Prince Arthur would be fourteen and capable of consummating the marriage. There was concern at the English court that the bride would find it difficult to make herself understood when she arrived there, and both Queen Elizabeth and the Lady Margaret Beaufort, the King's mother, requested the sovereigns of Spain to ensure that Katherine always spoke French – the diplomatic language of Europe – with her sister-in-law Margaret of Austria, as they themselves did not understand Latin or Spanish. They also suggested that Katherine accustom herself to drink wine, as the water of England was not drinkable. In December 1497, Queen Elizabeth wrote to Queen Isabella asking to be kept informed of the health and safety of her future daughter-in-law 'whom we think of and esteem as our own daughter'.

The Spanish marriage alliance was popular in England, and Henry VII and his subjects were impatient to see the girl who would one day be Queen Consort of England. Spain's second ambassador at the English court, Don Pedro de Ayala, boldly suggested to the sovereigns that it would be a good thing if Katherine came to England soon in order to accustom herself to the way of life and learn the language. He thought she could only lead a happy life by 'not remembering those things which would make her less enjoy what she would find here'. However, considering the manners and way of life of the English, he thought it best if she did not come until she was of marriageable age. Ferdinand was in no hurry: the recent appearance of a new pretender to the English throne, Perkin Warbeck – an imposter – and the continued existence of the Earl of Warwick, who had a very good claim to it, had made him cautious, and if another, better match had presented itself for his daughter at that time he would have accepted it. However, he did agree to a proxy wedding taking place on 19 May 1499 at Prince Arthur's manor house at Bewdley near Worcester. Again Dr de Puebla acted as proxy for the bride, and the Prince declared to him in a loud clear voice that he much rejoiced to contract the marriage because of his deep and sincere love for the Princess his wife, whom of course he had never seen. Such courtesies were the order of the day, however superficial.

Prince Arthur wrote several letters to his bride, of which only one survives, dated October 1499 and written in Latin to 'my dearest spouse'. In it he acknowledges the 'sweet letters' sent to him by her (none of which are extant), which so delighted him that he fancied he conversed with and embraced her. 'I cannot tell you what an earnest desire I feel to see your Highness, and how vexatious to me is this procrastination about your coming. Let [it] be hastened, [that] the love conceived between us and the wished-for joys may reap their proper fruit.' Such florid and adult sentiments from the pen of a thirteen-year-old boy hint at the assistance of a tutor, yet nevertheless it must have been a comfort to Katherine to receive encouragement from her future husband.

There remained only one obstacle to Katherine's departure for England, and that was the young Earl of Warwick, the nephew of Edward IV and Richard III, who was then a prisoner in the Tower. Ferdinand now made it very clear to Henry VII that unless Warwick were eliminated Katherine would never set foot in England, and Henry, anxious to preserve at all costs his friendship with Spain and the benefits the marriage alliance would bring, acted at once. Warwick was arraigned on a charge of conspiring with the pretender Perkin Warbeck; the simple-minded youth, beguiled by an *agent provocateur*, pleaded guilty, but was sentenced to death for his co-operation and beheaded on Tower Hill in November 1499. There was now nothing to stand in the way of Katherine's wedding to Arthur. Yet not for nothing would she one day say that her marriage had been made in blood, nor would she ever cease to feel an irrational sense of responsibility for the young Earl's death.

In 1500, assured by Dr de Puebla that 'not a doubtful drop of royal blood remains in England', the sovereigns began to prepare for their daughter's departure from Spain. Henry VII, in turn, was commanding the Mayor and aldermen of the City of London to arrange a lavish reception for his son's bride. He also requested that only beautiful women be sent in the Princess's train, stipulating that 'at least, none of them should be ugly.' We do not know if Queen Isabella took this into account when appointing the ladies of her daughter's household; for her, the main criterion was that they should come from the noblest and most ancient families of Spain. There was also a trousseau to be assembled. Katherine was to take with her many fine gowns of velvet and cloth of gold and silver, cut in the Spanish fashion, as well as undergarments edged with fine black-work lace, and hoods of velvet braided with gold, silver or pearls. The latter she would need after her marriage, when convention required a wife to cover her hair; only on state occasions would she wear it loose. Then there were night robes edged with lace for summer and fur for winter, cloth stockings and wooden stays, as well as the stiff Spanish farthingales that belled out the skirts of her gowns. Also in the trousseau was the gold and silver plate which was part of Katherine's dowry, and her jewellery, some of which was very fine and included heavy collar chains and crucifixes, and large brooches to be pinned to the centre of Katherine's bodices beneath the square necklines that would stay fashionable, and plunge ever lower, for the next sixty years. Lastly, a reminder to the Princess of where her duty lay, the Queen packed a beautifully embroidered christening robe.

When Isabella heard of Henry VII's extravagant plans for Katherine's reception, she was quick to write and tell him that she and Ferdinand would prefer it if 'expenses were moderate', as they did not want their daughter to be the cause of any loss to England; 'on the contrary, we desire that she will be the source of all kinds of happiness.' Isabella hoped, she said, that 'the substantial part of the festival should be his love'. But Henry was determined that this, the first major state occasion since his coronation, should be celebrated on a lavish scale in order to underline the splendour of the Tudor dynasty. In March 1501, he paid £14,000 for jewels alone for the wedding, and the City of London was sparing no expense in its plans for a magnificent reception for the Infanta. Already, workmen were building a great platform outside St Paul's Cathedral so that the crowds might witness the young couple taking their vows, and as this was a popular marriage there was mounting excitement in London.

In April 1501, Queen Isabella announced that her daughter was ready. Accordingly, on 19 May, another proxy wedding ceremony took place at Bewdley, just to make sure that nothing could be found lacking in the first. Two days later, Katherine left the Alhambra for ever, and began the first stage of her journey to the port of Corunna, whence she was to take ship for England. She took her final leave of her parents in Granada, knowing full well that she might never see them again. Isabella had carefully chosen a duenna for her, Doña Elvira Manuel, a noblewoman of mature years, who would act as chief lady-in-waiting, governess, chaperon, and general mother substitute. Doña Elvira was stern and proud, yet she was zealous in protecting her charge and concerned for her welfare. Only in later years, when Katherine began to resent the strict etiquette she imposed, did a rift develop between them.

The Infanta's household was headed by the Count and Countess de Cabra. It included the Commander Mayor Cardenas, Don Pedro Manuel (the duenna's husband), a chamberlain, Juan de Diero, Katherine's chaplain Alessandro Geraldini, three bishops and a host of ladies, gentlemen and servants. Travel in those days was by litter or on horseback; the strict conventions of the Spanish court demanded that Katherine's face be veiled in public, and that she travel behind the closed curtains of a litter, even during the hot summer months.

Katherine and her suite arrived at Corunna on 20 July, but could not embark for England until 17 August because of unfavourable winds. The sea crossing was terrible: a violent storm blew up in the Bay of Biscay, and the ship was tossed for four days in rough seas. Katherine was very sea-sick and later wrote to her mother to say 'it was impossible not to be terrified by the storm'. The captain was forced to return to Spain, and docked at Laredo on the Castilian coast for a month while the tempests raged. At last, on 27 September, the winds died down, and Katherine once more stepped on board the ship that would take her to England. Five days later, it arrived at Plymouth in Devon.

2
A true and loving husband

As Katherine walked down the gangway, followed by her retinue, the first thing she saw through her veil was the Mayor of Plymouth and his aldermen, come to welcome her to England. The townsfolk were there too, cheering and waving, and there were banners in the streets. Señor Alcares, a gentleman in the Infanta's train, wrote to Queen Isabella that Katherine 'could not have been received with greater joy if she had been the saviour of the world'. After being served a great feast by the citizens of Plymouth, Katherine heard mass and gave thanks for her safe arrival in her adoptive land. Meanwhile, a royal messenger was speeding away to the King, to tell him that the Princess whose arrival he had awaited for thirteen years was actually in his kingdom.

From Plymouth, Katherine travelled eastwards on the road to London. Along the way, people who had heard of her coming lined the roads to see the mysterious veiled lady who would one day be their queen. When Henry VII received news of her arrival, it was already November, and he set off at once from the royal manor at Easthampstead, Berkshire, with Prince Arthur. In Hampshire, word reached the King that Katherine was lodged at the bishop's palace at Dogmersfield; Henry, Arthur and the lords of the Privy Council arrived there on the evening of 4 November, eager to see her.

The Count de Cabra and Doña Elvira met Henry at the door and politely informed him that Katherine had retired for the night and could see no one. Henry was first astonished and then, typically, suspicious. Why would they not let him see his daughter-in-law? What was wrong with her? Was she deformed or ugly? His temper rose; he insisted he would see her, even if she were in bed. After some argument, the Spaniards had to agree to his demand and admit him to the Princess's rooms. Here, a mute and outraged Doña Elvira presented the Infanta, heavily veiled, to King Henry, who, with a marked lack of patience, lifted the veil. His relief was evident, for the ambassador had not lied: Katherine was a very pretty girl, with no sign of any blemish or deformity.

There are still in existence several portraits of Katherine of Aragon, painted at different stages of her life. Two early ones, said with good reason to portray her, were painted by the Spanish artist, Miguel Sittow. The earlier, thought to be Katherine posing as Mary Magdalene, is in the Berg Collection, and shows a plump, heavy-featured girl with loose wavy golden hair, aged perhaps around fifteen years. The other portrait, now in the Kunsthistorisches Museum, Vienna, was executed around 1505, and shows what must be the same young woman, with round face and golden hair, eyes demurely lowered, wearing a brown velvet dress and a black velvet hood called a béguine. The sitter wears a heavy gold collar decorated with Ks and pomegranates; this fruit, symbol of fertility, was Katherine's personal badge. On this, and the strong resemblance to Isabella of Castile, rests the identification of the sitter with Katherine of Aragon.

These two portraits give us a good idea of what Henry VII saw when he lifted Katherine's veil on that November evening in 1501, a girl with a fair complexion, rich reddish-gold hair that fell below hip level, and blue eyes. It would be interesting to know Katherine's first impression of her father-in-law, that unknown Welshman who had usurped the Plantagenet throne sixteen years earlier.

Henry Tudor came from bastard stock. His mother, Margaret Beaufort, was his only link by blood to the Plantagenets, and she herself was descended from the bastards born to John of Gaunt, Duke of Lancaster, fourth son of Edward III, and his mistress Katherine Swynford. These children, all surnamed Beaufort, were legitimised by statute of Richard II in 1397, after Gaunt married their mother; however, ten years later, Henry IV, confirming this, added a rider to the statute which barred the Beauforts and their heirs from ever inheriting the crown. Thus Henry Tudor could claim only a disputed title to it through his mother. His father, Edmund Tudor, who died before he was born, was one of the offspring of Henry V's widow, Katherine of Valois, by her liaison with the Welsh groom of her wardrobe, Owen Tudor; there is no proof that they ever married. Henry VII therefore had an extremely dubious claim to his throne, and was well aware of the fact that every single surviving member of the Plantagenet House of York had more right to occupy it than he. Nevertheless, after half a century of civil war, what England needed was firm, stable government, and this Henry VII had provided. He had also eliminated his most dangerous rivals for the crown. His marriage to the Plantagenet heiress, Elizabeth of York, had in the eyes of many gone a long way towards cloaking his usurpation with the mantle of legitimacy, although Henry himself insisted he occupied his throne by right of conquest, and not as Elizabeth's husband. Now, after sixteen years, he had obtained recognition by one of the greatest monarchies in the known world, and this in itself did much to consolidate his position.

According to the description of the King given by the Tudor chronicler, Edward Hall, Henry VII was tall and lean, his seeming fragility concealing a sinewy strength. He had gaunt, aquiline features, with thinning, greying hair and grey eyes. He presented to the world a genial, smiling countenance, yet beneath it he was suspicious, devious and parsimonious. He had grown to manhood in an environment of treachery and intrigue, and as a result never knew security. For all this, he ruled wisely and well, overcame plots to depose him, and put an end to the dynastic warfare that had blighted England during the second half of the fifteenth century.

Henry was miserly by nature, but he was also highly sensitive about the dubious validity of his claim to the throne, and therefore took much care to emphasise his majesty on as grand a scale as possible, thus setting a precedent for his Tudor successors. He was prepared to spend huge sums to impress the world with the splendour of his welcome to his daughter-in-law.

When, through an interpreter, pleasantries had been exchanged between the King and the Infanta, Katherine was presented to her future husband, the Prince of Wales, who later informed his parents that he 'had never felt so much joy in his life as when he beheld the sweet face of his bride'. The only portrait to survive of Prince Arthur is in the Royal Collection at Windsor, and shows a marked resemblance to youthful likenesses of Henry VIII. Arthur had reddish hair, small eyes and a high-bridged nose. In November 1501, he was fifteen years and two months old, while his bride was a month short of sixteen. He was well educated, thanks to his tutors, Dr Thomas Linacre and the poet Bernard André, and much beloved by the English because he so resembled his maternal grandfather, the popular Edward IV. Much of his childhood had been spent at Tickenhill, his manor house at Bewdley, which still survives camouflaged by a Georgian façade; the King favoured this thirteenth-century, oak-beamed house because it was near the Welsh marches, a suitable place for a Prince of Wales to live, particularly this one, who had more Welsh blood in him than any of his predecessors since the native line of Welsh princes died out.

Katherine and Arthur conversed together in Latin; later that evening, Katherine entertained the King and his son in her chamber with music and dancing. She and her ladies danced the slow, stately pavan that permitted two beats to a step; when Arthur joined in, Katherine and one of her ladies taught him a dignified Spanish dance, after which he danced with Lady Guildford in the English style 'right pleasantly and honourably'. In the morning, Henry and Arthur took their leave of Katherine and returned to London to prepare for the wedding, due to take place in ten days' time. The Infanta and her household followed at a more leisurely pace, arriving on 9 November by river at Deptford, where they were received by the Lord Mayor, aldermen and guildsmen of the City, who saluted her from their barges before escorting her to the landing stage at Lambeth. Here, Katherine was welcomed by Edward Stafford, third Duke of Buckingham, one of the few remaining members of the older nobility and a descendant of Edward III, and by the King's younger son, Henry Tudor, Duke of York, a big robust boy of ten with red-gold hair and glowing skin, who was there as his father's representative. These two conducted Katherine to her lodging in Lambeth Palace, where there awaited a letter from the King, expressing his great 'pleasure, joy and consolation' at her coming, and telling her that he and the Queen intended to treat her 'like our own daughter'. These were doubtless heartening words to a girl who had weathered a long and terrible journey to a strange land, with the prospect ahead of marriage to a virtual stranger. It says much for Katherine's strength of character that she was coping so well; beneath her docile, demure manner, there was an inner toughness and a strong will to succeed that sustained her.

Katherine made her state entry into London on 12 November, two days before her wedding. The streets were lined with expectant citizens jostling for a good view of the procession. The Infanta entered London from Southwark, passing over London Bridge with its huddle of shops and houses and its chapel dedicated to St Thomas à Becket, with her Spanish retinue following her. One person who saw her that day was the young Thomas More, future Lord Chancellor of England, who was then a lawyer at the London Charterhouse. He later wrote of the 'tremendous ovation' Katherine had received from the people: 'She thrilled the hearts of everyone; there is nothing wanting in her that the most beautiful girl should have. Everyone is singing her praises.' About her household, however, he was less than complimentary: 'Good heavens! What a sight! You would have burst out laughing if you had seen them, for they looked so ridiculous: tattered, barefoot, pygmy Ethiopians, like devils out of hell!' The chronicler Edward Hall, relying on the accounts of other eyewitnesses, later described the costly garments of the Princess and her ladies as 'strange fashions adorned with goldsmiths' work and embroidery'.

Katherine had on a wide gown with a gathered skirt over a farthingale with bell-shaped sleeves. The English had never before seen a lady thus attired, and, since she was small in stature, thought the hooped skirt made her look as broad as she was high. She also wore a little hat with a flat crown and wide brim, like a cardinal's, held in place with a gold lace under her chin. Beneath it she wore a Venetian coif covering her ears. Gone was the veil, gone also the litter; instead the Princess showed her face to the world and rode a gaily caparisoned horse. She was accompanied by a retinue of prelates, dignitaries, nobles and knights, all richly dressed in her honour.

The procession wound its way over the bridge, along Fenchurch Street to Cornhill, and then to Cheapside where Katherine was formally welcomed to London by the Lord Mayor. At six places on her route she stopped to watch elaborate pageants that had been prepared for her entertainment, and on which vast sums of money had been spent, tableaux depicting heraldic, Christian or mythical figures whose purpose it was to laud and praise the future Queen with music and verse. There was even a prefabricated castle surmounted by a fierce Welsh dragon representing the King. In another pageant, the 'Archangel Gabriel' reminded Katherine that her chief duty was 'the procreation of childer', and that this was why the deity had given mankind the capacity for 'sensual lust and appetite'. Later, 'God' himself appeared to her, saying 'Blessed be the fruit of your belly; your substance and fruits I shall increase and multiply.'

When the Lord Mayor and civic dignitaries had presented their loyal address beneath the Eleanor Cross at Cheapside, Katherine and her train passed on to St Paul's Cathedral, where a magnificent service of thanksgiving was the climax to the day's celebrations. Katherine had been the centre of it all, for the King, the Queen and Prince Arthur had watched the procession from the window of Master William Geffrey the haberdasher's house in Cheapside. When the service was over, Katherine rode back to Lambeth through the crowds who shouted acclaim from every street corner.

Two days later those same crowds were back in force for the royal wedding itself. The King and Queen, wearing their crowns and velvet robes trimmed with ermine, sat enthroned on the temporary platform erected outside St Paul's. Elizabeth of York was then thirty-five, and still retained something of her former beauty. Polydore Vergil, Henry VII's official historian, described her as a woman of great character whose chief qualities were wisdom and moderation, and the Venetian ambassador spoke of her great beauty and ability. Yet for all that, she had no political influence, and very little authority in her own household even, which was ordered by the King's mother, the learned and pious Margaret Beaufort.

Elizabeth had borne her husband seven children; three had died young, one, the Princess Mary, was still in the nursery, and the rest now sat with their parents, waiting for the marriage ceremony to begin: Prince Arthur, clad in white satin for the occasion, twelve-year-old Margaret, a headstrong girl who was shortly to marry James IV of Scotland, and Prince Henry, whose duty it was to give the bride away. Katherine also wore white satin, in the Spanish style, with bell sleeves and a full pleated skirt over a farthingale. On her head she had a huge white-silk coif edged with a border of gold, pearls and precious stones 1½" wide; the coif overshadowed her face, and its lappets hung to her waist. Her ladies, following behind, were similarly attired.

The marriage ceremony was conducted by Henry Deane, Archbishop of Canterbury, assisted by William Warham, Bishop of London. Prince Arthur and his bride made their vows in full view of the crowds before proceeding into the Cathedral for the nuptial mass, which the whole court attended. Then the Prince and Princess of Wales emerged into the November daylight, man and wife at last after thirteen years of hard bargaining; they nodded and bowed to the cheering throng, then rode off in procession to the riverside mansion known as Baynard's Castle, where the wedding banquet was to take place in the great hall. Here, where Richard Plantagenet, Duke of York, Edward IV and Richard III had once held court, the couple were entertained by 'the best voiced children of the King's chapel, who sang right sweetly with quaint harmony'. Later, after the feast, doves and rabbits were let loose into the hall, giving much 'mirth and disport' to the company.

Marriage feasts at that time were occasions for hilarity and bawdiness, and this one was no exception. In the evening there was dancing. Whilst Katherine danced in very stately manner, clicking castanets, the young Duke of York threw off his gown and whirled his sister Margaret around the floor, leaping and twirling to the music. The King and Queen were much amused, and watched their son with evident pleasure. Katherine, too, delighted them, dancing gracefully with her new husband; she looked, said an onlooker, 'delectable'.

It was now time for the bride and groom publicly to be put to bed. Arthur, we hear, was feeling 'lusty and amorous', and was anxious to be alone with his pretty wife. The young couple were undressed by their attendants, then brought to the nuptial chamber where they sat side by side in the great tester bed whilst the Archbishop of Canterbury and the Bishop of London blessed the bed and prayed that their union might be fruitful. The guests departed amidst much mirth and ribaldry, leaving Arthur and Katherine alone behind the closed curtains. Thus began one of the most controversial wedding nights in history.

What happened? According to Katherine, testifying on oath twenty-seven years later, nothing. To the end of her life, she maintained that her marriage to Prince Arthur was never consummated. The Prince was fifteen at the time of his marriage, and afflicted with a weak constitution. It is doubtful that he was capable of achieving full intercourse. Certainly, according to later reports by eyewitnesses, he bragged about feeling 'lusty', and on the morning after the wedding he boasted that he 'had been in Spain', saying that marriage was 'thirsty work', but these were probably the self-conscious boasts of a boy who had failed in his duty and wanted no one to guess it. It was automatically assumed at the time that the union had been consummated, although when Katherine was widowed she immediately declared that she was still a virgin and that she had only shared a bed with her husband for six or seven nights. At her coronation in 1509, when she was newly married to Henry VIII, she dressed herself in virginal white, and in 1529, she publicly affirmed that, when she married for the second time, 'I was a true maid, without touch of man.' She also swore as much on her deathbed, believing that she was about to meet her Maker. Although she had her own interests to protect, she was a religious woman of sound principles; it is far less likely therefore that she was guilty of deception than that she was telling the truth.

As Princess of Wales, Katherine ranked second lady at court after the Queen, taking precedence even over the King's mother, the formidable Lady Margaret Beaufort, whose word was law on domestic matters until her death in June 1509. For her personal motto, Katherine adopted the device 'Not for my crown', and her badge was the pomegranate. For many days after her wedding there were banquets and revels at court, interspersed with pageants and a tournament.

Outwardly, all was well with the marriage. Arthur wrote to Ferdinand and Isabella, telling them how happy he was and assuring them he would be 'a true and loving husband all of his days'. At the end of November, the Spaniards delivered to King Henry the sum of 100,000 crowns, the first instalment of the Princess's dowry, whereupon he immediately sent a letter to the sovereigns in which he praised the 'beauty and dignified manners' of their daughter. In himself, he declared, 'you may be sure that she has found a second father who will ever watch over her happiness.'

That night, the wedding celebrations ended with another pageant, acrobats, and singing by the children of the King's chapel. On the following day, those Spaniards who were not to remain in England with Katherine departed for Spain, laden with costly gifts from King Henry. This breaking of yet another link with her homeland was upsetting for the Princess, but the King diverted her by showing her his library and allowing her to choose a ring from a selection presented by his jeweller. Yet this untypical generosity was only one side of the picture. In reality, Henry had his eye on the remaining portion of Katherine's dowry, which was not yet due, and he was well aware that part of it comprised the plate and jewels she had brought with her from Spain, which were not for her personal use but to be given to the King when Ferdinand so directed. Henry, however, preferred hard cash so, with the assistance of the unscrupulous Dr de Puebla, he conceived a plan whereby Katherine would be forced to use the plate and jewels; then, when the time came, he could refuse to accept them, and could ask for their value in money. Puebla had already tried to involve Katherine in this duplicity, but Henry VII told her that, although such an arrangement would be of advantage to them both, he would not consent to it. He would be content with what the treaties stipulated, he told her, and advised her to warn her parents of Dr de Puebla's treachery. Thus, when matters came to a head, they would blame the doctor and not Henry for what had happened.

The King had the ideal opportunity in December to put his plan into action. It had been arranged that after their marriage the Prince and Princess would go to live at Ludlow Castle on the Welsh marches, so that Arthur could learn how to govern his principality and so prepare himself for eventual kingship. But there was concern about the Prince's delicate health. He seems to have been consumptive, and had grown weaker since his wedding. The King believed, as did most other people, that Arthur had been over-exerting himself in the marriage bed. Fate was playing into Henry's hands in this, because it gave him the ideal opportunity to pretend that he did not want Katherine to accompany her husband to Ludlow. However, he did not wish to risk offending her parents, so he consulted the Spanish envoy, Ayala, who advised that Katherine remain with the court. The King, making a great pretence of deliberation, then asked Katherine herself if she thought it wise to go with Arthur to Ludlow whilst he was in such poor health; Katherine would only say that she would be 'content with what he decided'. Prince Arthur, on the King's instruction, tried to persuade her to go with him, but she was frightened of going against the King's wishes, and in the end Henry, with a great show of reluctance, commanded her to accompany her husband.

Because of all this procrastination, nothing was ready for the Princess's departure, nor had any provision been made for her at Ludlow. All that had been decided was the number of Spanish servants who would accompany her. Prince Arthur, the King had decreed, would pay their salaries out of his own privy purse. Ferdinand was informed by Pedro de Ayala, who had by this time realised what the King planned to do, that Henry had given nothing to Arthur with which to furnish his house, nor any 'table service'; this was a significant omission, for it meant that Katherine would be obliged to use her plate.

Seemingly, Henry VII cared more for money than for the welfare of his son and heir. However, if Henry had shut his eyes to the possible consequences of allowing the Prince and Princess to live together, Ayala and Doña Elvira had not. Both pleaded with the King to let Katherine stay at court, saying the sovereigns would prefer it. Henry replied that Dr Puebla had told him, on the contrary, that Ferdinand and Isabella did not wish the young couple to be separated on any account, and this view had already been endorsed by Alessandro Geraldini, the Princess's chaplain. Defeated, Ayala wrote again to Ferdinand, urging him to command that the plate and jewels be given to Henry at once, to avoid further trouble.

On Tuesday, 21 December 1501, the Prince and Princess left Baynard's Castle for the Welsh marches and Ludlow. It was the middle of winter, and the landscape bare and unforgiving, with skeletal trees blowing in the bitter winds. Katherine travelled by litter, wrapped in furs and accompanied by her duenna; everyone else was on horseback, the Prince included, which cannot have done much to improve his state of health.

Ludlow Castle was an eleventh-century fortress that had been transformed into a palatial residence of imposing grandeur during the thirteenth and fourteenth centuries. It had once been the seat of the powerful Mortimer family and their descendants, the Yorkist Plantagenets. Edward IV had sent his young son, the future Edward V, to be educated here in the 1470s, and it was from Ludlow that the boy king Edward V had set out in 1483 on the road that was to take him to London, the Tower and death. No royal person had lived in Ludlow Castle since then, but a staff had been maintained, and the royal apartments kept in good repair. When the Prince and Princess arrived in January 1502, their servants quickly transformed these rooms with tapestries, roaring fires, personal belongings and the controversial plate. With Prince Arthur was his council, whose members were there to help him learn the art of government; not a hard task, as the Welsh border was quiet now after many centuries of warfare. A Welsh-born king occupied the throne, and his son enjoyed great popularity locally.

Henry VII told Ferdinand and Isabella that Alessandro Geraldini, Katherine's chaplain, 'a venerable man for whom we have the greatest regard', would be keeping him informed of her welfare and Arthur's. It is unfortunate that none of Geraldini's letters survive, as they would have provided us with much valuable information about Katherine's early married life. We can only surmise that hers was the conventional routine of a lady of rank: taking responsibility for the smooth running of her household, entertaining local worthies, and attending to religious and charitable duties. Doubtless she did embroidery and occasionally went hunting. What is certain from her own testimony, is that she did not share a bed with her husband.

In late March, both Katherine and Arthur were struck down with a virus, 'a malign vapour which proceeded from the air'. People died frequently from such illnesses then, but Katherine was lucky, for she was basically healthy and made a quick recovery, although she would suffer unpleasant after-effects. Not so Arthur, who succumbed to the virus on 2 April, leaving his bride of six months a widow in what was still to her a strange land.

At once, a messenger was despatched to the King, who was then at Richmond Palace in Surrey. He had to be roused from sleep by his confessor, who said in Latin: 'If we receive good things at the hands of God, why may we not endure evil things?' The King was puzzled, wondering why his confessor should be quoting Job to him at this time of night. Then the friar said gently, 'Your dearest son hath departed to God.' Henry burst into harsh sobbing, whereupon the Queen, laying her own grief aside, came to comfort him, reminding him that God had left him three other children, 'and God is still where he was, and we are both young enough'. Then she too broke down, and it was Henry's turn to comfort her.

The Prince's body was embalmed, and conveyed on a chariot to the Abbey of St Wulfstan in Worcester, now the cathedral, where it was interred in its own chantry chapel, later to be adorned with the statues of saints and of the wife with whom Arthur had shared such a brief time. Katherine, conforming to royal tradition, did not attend the funeral. Much sympathy was felt for her; barely out of her sick bed, she was a wan figure in her widow's black and mourning barbe, which swathed her chin and face like a nun's wimple. There was also great grief in the country for the popular Prince who had been cut down in his youth. The new heir to the throne, Henry, Duke of York, was not well known, having been kept out of the public eye for most of his life.

A question mark hovered now over Katherine's future. As soon as she was well enough, she travelled back to London, shrouded in black and hidden from public view by the curtains of a closed litter. When she reached Richmond, she was conducted at once to the Queen, with whom she shared a mutual sorrow. Elizabeth of York would play a mother's part until such time as Katherine's future was decided.

3
*Our daughter remains
as she was here*

O n 10 May 1502, Ayala having been recalled, King Ferdinand instructed his new ambassador in England, Hernan Duque de Estrada, to demand the immediate return to Spain of the Princess Katherine and repayment of the first instalment of her dowry. This was intended to frighten Henry VII into agreeing to a new proposition Ferdinand was about to make, that a marriage be arranged between Katherine and the new heir to the English throne, Prince Henry. Ferdinand could foresee only two objections to such a union: first, Katherine, at sixteen, was five and a half years older than the Prince; and second, the Bible forbade a man to marry his brother's widow. Age was deemed to be of little account: in that period, the marriage of children was not unknown, and it was not that long since an octogenarian Duchess of Norfolk had married a man sixty years her junior. Nor would the age gap seem too great when young Henry was of an age to be married.

That left the delicate matter of the couple being within the forbidden degrees of affinity. Ferdinand was certain that the Pope would be only too happy to provide a dispensation if it could be shown that Katherine's marriage to Arthur had not been consummated – and immediately the intimate details of their short-lived union became a matter of international importance. 'Be careful to get the truth as regards whether the Prince and Princess of Wales consummated the marriage,' Queen Isabella instructed Estrada, who, prevented by decorum from asking Katherine outright, was driven to making discreet enquiries of the ladies of her household and even of her laundresses.

Henry VII was not so delicate, and bluntly asked Katherine if she were still a virgin. He, too, had seen the advantages of her marrying Prince Henry, but he was also hopeful that she might be pregnant with Arthur's child. She replied, quite candidly, that although she had slept with Arthur for six nights, she remained a virgin, and had confided as much to her duenna. Henry told her he was thinking of suggesting that she be betrothed to Prince Henry, but that he would prefer it if the matter was first broached by her parents. Whatever happened, he wanted to preserve the Anglo-Spanish alliance intact.

Gossip travelled fast in the court, and it was not long before the proposed betrothal was common knowledge. Reaction was swift, especially among some churchmen. William Warham, Bishop of London, who had officiated at Katherine's wedding, thought the idea 'not only inconsistent with propriety, but the will of God Himself is against it. It is declared in His law that if a man shall take his brother's wife, it is an unclean thing. It is not lawful.' This was one of the finer points of canon law, and a heated debate ensued which resulted in the King being assured by learned divines that the Pope would almost certainly grant a dispensation, since the Princess was still a virgin. Even if she were not, the Pope, were he so inclined (and persuaded with financial incentives), still had the power to dispense in such a case: there were precedents. Nevertheless, although their voices were muted, Warham and several other churchmen still maintained their stand.

Henry VII and Ferdinand and Isabella were now agreed on the match; Henry had written to Isabella, recounting his conversation with Katherine, and the Queen pronounced herself satisfied that 'our daughter remains as she was here' – that is, a virgin. The sovereigns made the signing of the new marriage treaty a priority, as there were rumours of a proposed French marriage for Prince Henry; Louis XII of France was said to be trying to block the betrothal to Katherine. Estrada was given full powers to draw up the treaty; Henry VII would be allowed to keep the first instalment of Katherine's dowry, and the final payment would be handed over when the Princess's marriage to Prince Henry was consummated. Isabella instructed Estrada to ensure that King Henry provided Katherine in the interim with whatever was necessary for her maintenance; in return, he should have the final say in how her household should be constituted, provided Doña Elvira remained as duenna. If Henry proved difficult, the ambassador was to make immediate arrangements for Katherine's return to Spain with her dowry intact. 'The one object of this business is to bring the betrothal to a conclusion as soon as you are able,' wrote the Queen.

Several weeks passed in negotiation. Naturally, no one saw fit to consult the two people most closely concerned: Henry was a boy of eleven, Katherine not yet seventeen, and both were drilled in strict obedience to their elders. The prospect of betrothal to a mere child cannot have been welcome to the Princess, deferring as it did her prospects of motherhood, yet she had been told that her destiny was to be Queen of England, and that she very much wished to be. At present, her life was humdrum, filled with religious observances, needlework, and quiet sociability in the Queen's apartments. As a widow, it was not thought fitting for her to dance in public or take part in court entertainments. A betrothal to Prince Henry would end all that, however, and thus Katherine may well have come to view it as a desirable escape from her present situation.

But there was to be further delay. Just as Estrada proceeded to draw up the marriage contract, Queen Elizabeth, who had conceived her eighth child soon after Prince Arthur's death, bore a daughter in the royal apartments in the Tower of London, and died soon afterwards on her thirty-seventh birthday, 11 February 1503. 'Her departing was as heavy and dolorous to the King as ever was seen or heard of,' and the court was plunged into mourning. Katherine, keeping vigil by the Queen's body with the other ladies of her court in the Norman chapel of St John the Evangelist within the Tower, sincerely mourned her gentle mother-in-law, and no doubt felt lonelier than ever. Prince Henry, too, felt the loss of his mother deeply. It has been suggested that his future matrimonial career reflected his subconscious efforts to replace her; it cannot be doubted that Elizabeth's memory always held a special place in his heart, and in time to come he would name one of his daughters after her.

No sooner had the Queen been buried in Westminster Abbey than the matter of the King's own remarriage was broached. Only the life of Prince Henry stood between stable Tudor government and bloody civil war, and it was thought imperative that the King remarry and provide his realm with more male heirs, especially as he was 'but a weak man and sickly'. It was at this juncture that the odious Dr de Puebla stepped in and suggested to the King that, rather than marry Katherine to his son, he marry her himself. The idea appealed to Henry, but it left Isabella and Ferdinand shocked and furious. The Queen wrote to Puebla, severely censuring him for his meddling, but her anger was provoked not so much by sensitivity about a middle-aged widower of eight weeks proposing himself as a groom for a young girl, as by her fears for Katherine's status. Henry VII was known to be ailing, and was probably in the first stages of the consumption that was eventually to kill him; the best Katherine could hope for from such a marriage was a brief reign as queen consort, then a long widowhood, commencing perhaps in her twenties, with no political influence. Marriage to Prince Henry would assure her of a far more stable and glorious future.

The practical Isabella suggested an alternative bride for the King, the widowed Joan of Naples, a relative of King Ferdinand, who was young and beautiful, as her portrait by Raphael shows. At the same time, Isabella commanded Estrada to tell Henry VII that a marriage between him and Katherine was 'a thing not to be endured'. Estrada played his part well: Henry, not wishing to offend Spain, and realising that he stood to lose not only Katherine but her dowry if he did so, immediately abandoned any notion of marrying her himself, and proceeded at once to conclude the treaty of betrothal between the Princess and his son. There was further haggling over the dowry, but eventually it was agreed that the remaining 100,000 crowns would be paid as soon as the marriage was consummated, and would be made up of 65,000 crowns in gold, 15,000 crowns in plate of gold and silver, and 20,000 crowns in jewellery, the plate and jewellery already being in the possession of the Princess.

The marriage itself was to take place in 1505, when Prince Henry reached his fourteenth birthday. In the meantime, Ferdinand and Isabella and Henry VII would request the Pope for a dispensation that would resolve all canonical difficulties. The treaty was signed by Henry VII on 23 June 1503, and two days later the Duke of York and Katherine of Aragon were formally betrothed in the Bishop of Salisbury's house in London's Fleet Street. Mourning weeds discarded,

Katherine appeared once more garbed in virginal white, her golden hair unbound and falling loose as a token of purity, with her future assured and her status at court preserved.

Prince Henry, who was not quite twelve, had conceived for her from the first both affection and respect. She aroused the chivalrous instincts of a boy who had been bred on knightly precepts, and who was already manifesting the charm and charisma that would in time attract people of both sexes to him. Katherine, for all her five and a half years' seniority, was beginning to fall under the spell. There was in her a strong maternal streak, and this boy had just lost his mother. She would be the one to comfort and console him, perhaps even guide him. Thus was set, early on, a pattern for the future.

The future Henry VIII had been born on 28 June 1491 at the Palace of Greenwich, which remained a favourite residence to the end of his life. In 1492, when he was less than nine months old, his father appointed him Lord Warden of the Cinque Ports and Constable of Dover Castle, and in that same year a sister, Elizabeth, joined him in the nursery; unfortunately, she died at the age of three. Later, there were other siblings, Mary, Edmund, Edward and Katherine (the baby born in the Tower), but only Mary survived infancy. Henry was particularly fond of Mary, much more so than of his elder sister Margaret, who married the King of Scots in 1503.

The young Prince was made Lord Lieutenant of Ireland at the age of three, as well as being admitted to the Order of the Bath. He was then created Duke of York, following the precedent set by Edward IV, and continued to this day, whereby the second son of the monarch is always given this title. To celebrate the event, the King held a joust and set his son on a table so that he could see properly. A portrait sketch of Henry at two shows him to have been a chubby, solidly made toddler with wide, intelligent eyes and a straight fringe of Tudor red hair; he wears a gown with a square neck and a wide-brimmed bonnet with a coif beneath, tied under the chin; altogether a child to be proud of.

The young Duke was made a Knight of the Garter in 1495, just before his fourth birthday. Shortly afterwards, he commenced his formal education, with the poet laureate John Skelton as his first tutor, who taught him reading, writing and spelling. Later, a more classical curriculum was introduced, and Henry would study the works of Homer, Virgil, Plautus, Ovid, Thucydides, Livy, Julius Caesar, Pliny, and other Greek and Roman authors. He was taught to write a sprawling Italic script, and received instruction in mathematics, French and music, a subject at which he would excel. The growing Prince found an outlet for his energy in the coaching that was given him daily in horsemanship, archery, fencing, jousting, wrestling, swordsmanship and royal (real) tennis. Erasmus, who saw Henry in 1499, when he was eight, called him a 'prodigy of precocious scholarship'. At only seven years old, he had performed his first public duty, attending a meeting of the City of London trade guilds to be presented by the Lord Mayor with a pair of gilt goblets. The Prince thanked them in a clear high voice for their 'great and kind remembrance', and told them he would not forget their kindness. Nor did he, for to the end of his life Henry VIII enjoyed a relationship of mutual liking with the City of London.

He was maturing fast. At eight, according to Erasmus, he already had 'something of royalty in his demeanour, in which there was a certain dignity combined with singular courtesy'. The death of Prince Arthur in 1502 brought about a cataclysmic change in Henry's life, since it made him the heir to his father's kingdom and immeasurably increased his importance. Yet for all that he enjoyed no greater freedom. His father, who had already lost three sons, insisted that the Prince lead an almost cloistered life with his tutors, avoiding the public eye, and Henry's bedchamber was only accessible from a door in his father's room. His contact with his future wife was to be strictly limited for the present.

In August 1503, Ferdinand instructed his ambassador in Rome to procure the necessary dispensation from the Pope, saying that while it was 'well known in England that the Princess is still a virgin', he thought it 'more prudent to provide for the case as though the marriage had been consummated'. A watertight dispensation was vital because 'the right of succession depends on the undoubted legitimacy of the marriage'. The Pope, Julius II, was disposed to prevaricate, saying he did not know if he was competent to grant it. Moreover, there were conflicting texts in the Bible: Leviticus forbade a man to marry his brother's wife and warned that such unions would be cursed with childlessness, while Deuteronomy positively encouraged them. There had, however, been precedents, which proved that other Popes had had fewer qualms. In the end, ambassadorial pressure persuaded Julius to relent, and on 26 December 1503, he issued the desired Bull of Dispensation permitting Henry and Katherine to marry, notwithstanding the fact that she had 'perhaps' consummated her first marriage 'by carnal knowledge'. The young couple were now free to marry when Henry was fourteen in June 1505. On 18 February 1504, he was formally created Prince of Wales.

During 1504 Katherine suffered a period of poor health, with intermittent attacks of a mysterious sickness that has been attributed to her inability to adapt to the English climate and food. The illness seems to have been gastric, producing symptoms of shivering and fever, and it was at its worst during the summer, when the Princess was unable to eat very much. She grew alarmingly pale, and there were fears that she would die. For weeks she lay ill at Greenwich, until she was well enough to travel to Fulham Palace, a country house owned by the Bishop of London which had been placed at her disposal. The move did her little good, for in August she was reported to be 'rather worse' and in a serious condition. The King sent every day to ask after her health, offering many times to visit her, though she was too ill to receive him. Perturbed, Henry wrote to inform her parents of her illness. The news could not have reached them at a worse time, for Queen Isabella herself was mortally sick. Katherine, of course, had no knowledge of this, yet as her condition improved, so her mother's deteriorated, and by November Isabella herself realised she was about to die. On her deathbed, she voiced her inner doubts about the validity of the dispensation issued by the Pope, but these were unresolved and largely ignored when she died on 26 November 1504.

There was great mourning in Spain for the death of a queen who had been a legend in her lifetime, but it was not only because of her passing. The kingdom would once more be divided, if only for the lifetime of King Ferdinand. He, not being Isabella's heir, could no longer hold sovereignty over Castile: that kingdom would pass to the Queen's eldest daughter, Juana, and Ferdinand – who had for thirty years ruled a united Spain – now found his authority confined solely to the minor kingdom of Aragon. It would not be long before this situation had repercussions for Katherine.

Katherine wrote to her father on the very day Isabella died, chiding him for not having written to her for some time. Weakened by her illness, she may well have been suffering from depression, for she felt there was something ominous about Ferdinand's silence. 'I cannot be comforted or cheerful until I see a letter from you,' she wrote; 'I have no other hope or comfort in this world than that which comes from knowing my mother and father are well.'

Any depression Katherine felt was not just the result of her illness, however. Since arriving in England, she had come to know a freedom she had never dreamed of in Spain, where women were kept in seclusion and observed an almost conventual style of life. They wore clothes that camouflaged their bodies and veiled their faces in public. Etiquette at the Spanish court was rigid, and even smiling was frowned upon. But in England, women enjoyed much more freedom: their gowns were designed to attract, and when they were introduced to gentlemen they kissed them full upon the lips in greeting. They sang and danced when they pleased, went out in public as the fancy took them, and laughed when they felt merry. Of course, there were rules of behaviour governing their conduct at court, which was expected to be decorous and formal, but this bore favourable comparison with the conventions then existing in Katherine's native land. To the maturing Princess, exposure to these unfamiliar freedoms brought with it a desire for some measure of independence and liberation from the restrictions hitherto imposed upon her. Several courtiers had told her that she 'ought to enjoy greater freedom', and, indeed, since her betrothal to Prince Henry, she had by degrees entered into the wider life of the court whenever her illness permitted. She had danced and sung, gone riding, taken part in the chase, and generally begun to enjoy herself.

Doña Elvira had been scandalised by such behaviour on the part of her charge, and was concerned that Katherine might cheapen herself in the eyes of the English. So concerned was the duenna that she complained both to King Henry and King Ferdinand. Ferdinand replied that Katherine must behave 'as was fitting for her honour and dignity', and commanded his daughter to observe the same rules at court as Doña Elvira insisted upon in her own house, and Henry VII endorsed this, saying the Princess must obey her father's orders. Katherine therefore had no choice but to do so, but from that time on relations between her and Doña Elvira were merely civil at best.

Katherine's spirits, therefore, were at a low ebb: she was debilitated by a lengthy illness, depressed by the lack of news from Spain, and chafing at the unwelcome restrictions imposed upon her, feeling very much that she was kept apart from the normal mainstream of life. And then came the news that her mother was dead.

There is no record of how Isabella's death affected Katherine on a personal level. We do know that politically it affected her a great deal, because, when news of it reached England in December 1504, and Henry VII had had time to think about its implications, he realised that he had concluded a marriage alliance, not with a strong, united Spain, but with the kingdom of Aragon, to which far less prestige was attached. This fact devalued Katherine's importance overnight and diminished her status in the world. Henry VII was the first to perceive that she was no longer the personification of a great Spanish alliance. Other, more advantageous marriages might be considered more appropriate for his son and, with this in mind, Henry VII now acted: he stopped Katherine's allowance.

By February 1505, Katherine was beginning to feel the pinch. Although she was living with the court at Richmond and did not lack for daily comforts and food, she had no money with which to pay her servants, and this was very embarrassing for her. She had also noticed a certain coolness in the King's attitude towards her, which troubled her, for she did not understand how she had offended him. She asked Dr de Puebla to remind Henry 'of the misery in which she lives, and to tell him, in plain language, that it will reflect dishonour upon his character if he should entirely abandon his daughter,' but Puebla did nothing except write to King Ferdinand asking him to clarify the position concerning financial provision for Katherine. In the meantime, Katherine's circumstances worsened. The clothes she had brought from Spain were now growing shabby, and she could not afford to replace them. Her attendants made no complaints, but she could sense their concern over the non-payment of their salaries. Then there was Doña Elvira clucking about decorum and propriety and the correct behaviour to be observed by a princess of Spain.

Katherine, still grieving for her mother, was nearly at breaking-point.

Ferdinand did not reply to Puebla until the end of June, and when he did it was to say, quite correctly, that it was King Henry's responsibility to 'provide abundantly for the Princess and her household'. This was little help to Katherine: etiquette prevented her from asking the King of England outright for money, and Puebla would not do it for her, so she was obliged literally to tighten her belt and endure what could not be remedied. Nor was there any end to her plight in view. On 28 June 1505, Prince Henry reached his fourteenth birthday, and by the terms of the marriage treaty should have been married to Katherine soon afterwards. However, it was becoming increasingly obvious that no immediate plans for a wedding were being laid. Henry VII had decided that, if a better match presented itself for the Prince, he would take it, but at the same time he was reluctant to forgo Katherine's dowry. Hence his policy was to delay the marriage for as long as possible to see what transpired.

Katherine, of course, did not know this, and could only guess at the reason for her marriage being postponed. Fortunately for her peace of mind, she was unaware that on the day before the Prince's birthday, the King had marched him before the Bishop of Winchester and made the boy solemnly revoke the promises made at his betrothal, on the grounds that they were made when he was a minor and incapable under the law of deciding such things for himself. The purpose of this little drama, which took place in secret, was to ensure that, if a better match presented itself, there would be no difficulty in breaking his precontract to Katherine.

4
Pain and annoyance

In October 1505, Henry VII entered into secret negotiations with the new King and Queen of Castile for the marriage of the newly created Prince of Wales to Philip's and Juana's six-year-old daughter Eleanor. Philip, antagonistic towards his father-in-law because of Ferdinand's interference in Castilian affairs, saw this marriage as a means of exacting revenge. At the same time, it was widely believed in diplomatic circles that King Henry was having doubts as to the validity of a union between his son and Katherine of Aragon, despite the Pope's dispensation: it was said to weigh 'much on his conscience'. However, the main reason for his change of direction was that Eleanor was a far greater matrimonial prize than Katherine: not only was her mother Queen Regnant of Castile and heir to Aragon, but her father was heir to all the Hapsburg territories and might one day be Holy Roman Emperor as well.

It is clear that Katherine herself had not yet understood how her mother's death had led to her own devaluation in the marriage market; it was some time before she thought she knew why Henry VII was treating her so shabbily, and why the Prince, whom she saw sometimes about the court, was dutifully ignoring her. Eventually, it occurred to her that perhaps her father's failure to hand over the second instalment of her dowry might be the cause of the problem, and in December she asked Ferdinand to substitute a payment of gold for the jewels and plate in her possession, as she felt certain that the King of England would refuse to receive them as part of the instalment. Ferdinand promised to do as she asked, but failed to keep his word. By April 1506, Henry VII – who had been led by Katherine to expect prompt payment of the second instalment – complained bitterly about the delay, and began to cast doubt upon Ferdinand's good intentions.

By the terms of the marriage treaty, Ferdinand was well within his rights to withhold the remainder of the dowry until the union between the Prince and Princess was consummated, but he did not stand on this and chose instead to prevaricate, make excuses, and offer promises he did not keep, primarily because he needed to retain the friendship of Henry VII. According to Katherine, this provoked rage and fury in Henry VII, and she bore the brunt of it. In March 1507, he granted Ferdinand a further six months' grace in which to hand over payment, although he sanctimoniously reminded him at the time that 'punctual payment' was a 'sacred duty', and warned him that 'many other princesses have been offered in marriage to the Prince of Wales with greater marriage portions'. For Katherine, it was vital that her father complied with King Henry's wishes in order to 'prevent these people from telling me that they have reduced me to nothingness'. Yet when October arrived, Henry magnanimously extended the term of grace until March 1508. Katherine, rightly, saw this as ominous, for while the dowry remained unpaid, 'he regards me as bound and his son as free.'

In December, Ferdinand was in Castile, doing his best to raise the enormous sum required to complete the dowry, and promising Henry VII to deliver it before March. But when March came, and Ferdinand had still not paid up, Henry VII lost patience and reopened negotiations for a marriage between the Prince and Eleanor of Austria.

During the summer of 1508, Ferdinand, fearing for Katherine's future, insisted Henry VII keep faith with the terms of the treaty. But Henry, whose health was failing, was determined to have the dowry before committing his son to the marriage. 'Your King has many crowns,' he sneered to the Spanish ambassador, 'but he hasn't 100,000 to pay his daughter's dowry!' The ambassador, a tactless man named Fuensalida, retorted that his master did not 'lock away his gold in chests' – a direct reference to Henry VII's legendary miserliness – 'but pays it to the brave soldiers at whose head he has always been victorious'. The obvious insult stung Henry to fury, and he marched the ambassador along to Katherine's apartments, saying, 'The Princess shall see how you handle her affairs!' In front of an astonished and distressed Katherine, he accused Fuensalida of jeopardising her marriage by his failure to press her father for the dowry, and warned her that he was not obliged in the circumstances to honour his part of the treaty.

In April 1509, at last, the final instalment of the dowry, 100,000 crowns in gold – Ferdinand had graciously consented to make good the value of the used plate and jewels – was ready to be delivered. Furthermore, a new ambassador, Don Luis Caroz, was to be sent to England empowered to inform Henry VII that it would be paid as soon as the King agreed to proceed with the marriage. However, when Caroz arrived in England, he found the King too ill to see him: Henry VII was dying, and the political situation was about to change dramatically.

During those four years of tortuous negotiations over Katherine's dowry, she herself suffered untold misery and humiliation. Her marriage to Prince Henry was never a certainty, and this placed her in a highly invidious position at the English court. At best, she was regarded there as a possible but ill-advised bride for the Prince, at worst as an unwanted dependant. Throughout this time she was very much the pawn of ambitious men, her happiness subject to the shifting vicissitudes of European politics.

Katherine's domestic life during her widowhood was anything but tranquil. In 1505, Durham House on London's Strand was placed at her disposal by the Bishop of Ely, whose town residence it was. Hitherto, she had lived either at court or at Fulham Palace, a house belonging to the Bishop of London. Durham House was sited to the east of Charing Cross, just beyond the City boundary and in an area populated mainly by the nobility and gentry, whose houses lined the Strand. Here, in peaceful and attractive surroundings, Katherine's household was briefly established. The house was built around a courtyard, and had two towers, one at each extremity. There were lawns and gardens leading down to the River Thames, where there was a jetty and landing stage. In those days persons of rank rarely travelled through London's noisome and congested streets, preferring to go by barge along the river.

In November 1505, Katherine was deprived of this peaceful refuge. Her duenna had to go abroad for a time, and Henry VII summoned Katherine to live at court, in order to save the cost of maintaining a separate establishment for her. Reluctantly, and with a depleted household, she obeyed the King's command, but she was extremely unhappy about doing so, knowing that there was little privacy to be had at court and that she would doubtless be the object of much speculation and gossip. Nevertheless, she was obliged to remain there for the next year.

Her lack of money brought further problems, especially concerning her household. In 1505 she employed mostly Spaniards on her staff, the majority of whom had come from Spain with her. Many were girls from noble families who had come to England in the hope of attracting aristocratic husbands, and Katherine knew she was obliged to provide dowries for them, when the time came, out of the income due to her from the King, which of course had ceased in the summer of 1505.

A case in point was that of Doña Maria de Salinas, who had once been a maid of honour to Queen Isabella. Her family had arranged her marriage to a noble Fleming, whom she was anxious to marry. Katherine, having no money at all, begged her father to provide a dowry, 'as Maria has served me well', but Ferdinand ignored her request. As a result, plans for the marriage had to be abandoned, to Katherine's great embarrassment and sorrow. Yet such was her ability to inspire devotion in others that Maria de Salinas remained close to her for three more decades until death severed the friendship.

Lack of money affected Katherine personally too. By December 1505, nearly a year after Henry VII had stopped her allowance, her financial situation was grave. Her father had failed to send her any money, despite repeated requests, and all King Henry had given her was a small pittance for food – she was often reduced to eating yesterday's fish from the market. She was also in debt to some London merchants for household necessities, and the gowns she had brought from Spain four years before were so shabby that she felt, as she told her father, 'nearly naked'. At Christmas, she had a humiliating interview with King Henry, who refused to pay her even a small allowance. An argument ensued, which resulted in Katherine bursting into tears, something her rigid training had schooled her not to do in public. But even this did not move Henry.

Katherine wrote again and again to her father, but Ferdinand was adamant that Henry VII should honour his undertaking to defray Katherine's living expenses, and would not help her. In Spain, her suffering aroused indignation and sympathy. It was generally felt that it was Henry VII's duty to support her and that, in failing to do this, he was guilty of a serious breach of his sacred oaths of knighthood and kingship, by which he was bound to protect defenceless maidens such as his daughter-in-law.

By the end of 1505, Katherine had come to realise that the King no longer desired her marriage to his son, and warned her father that she would 'be lost if I am not assisted from Spain'. Alas for Katherine, Ferdinand had no knowledge of Henry VII's secret negotiations with Philip of Castile, and consequently had no reason to believe that the English King wanted to break the alliance; nor did he himself wish to prejudice it, for he now needed Henry more than Henry needed him. As a result, he chose to ignore his daughter's complaints.

It was unfortunate that Katherine was ill-served throughout her widowhood by the men who should have championed her: her father's ambassador, Dr de Puebla, was more interested in ingratiating himself with Henry VII and serving his own ends than in carrying out his master's wishes. In December 1505, Katherine decided that all her troubles were 'on account of the Doctor', and begged Ferdinand to consider 'how I am your daughter' and help by sending another ambassador, 'who would be a true servant of your Highness', since Dr de Puebla had caused her so much 'pain and annoyance that I have lost my health in a great measure', and might 'soon die'.

There was, at that time, another Spanish envoy in England, Hernan Duque de Estrada, who was sympathetic towards Katherine and tried to offer her some comfort. For a time she confided in him, and he, highly indignant on her behalf, wrote to King Ferdinand endorsing her requests, but to no avail. Later, however, Katherine was to say that he had not done as much as he could have done to assist her when she most needed it. Certainly his pleas, like hers, fell on deaf ears. Ferdinand was in no hurry to replace Puebla, and instructed Katherine to make use of him before another ambassador could be selected, which would not happen for more than a year.

All of these problems had indeed, as Katherine complained, taken a severe toll on her health. She had been unwell since shortly after her arrival in England, when she suffered a viral infection at Ludlow in 1502. Since then, she had continued to be susceptible to fevers and stomach upsets, which may be attributed in part to the changes in climate and diet to which she had had to accustom herself. She does not seem to have suffered one long illness, but a succession of ailments following one upon the other, and from April 1502 until early in 1507 was constantly unwell.

The likelihood is that much of her ill health was the result of stress. She herself attributed the 'severe tertian fevers' she suffered during the autumn of 1505 to all the aggravation to which she was being subjected. She wrote to tell her father that she had been 'at death's door for months', but this may have been an exaggeration born of depression, for she was 'in the deepest anguish'. Again, in March 1506 she informed Ferdinand she had been 'near death' for six months, although she was then 'somewhat better, but not entirely well'.

Her partial recovery may have been due in some measure to a brief reunion with her sister Juana. In January 1506, Juana and Philip were sailing from the Low Countries to Spain when they were shipwrecked off the English coast and welcomed at Windsor Castle as guests of the King. Although Juana was Queen Regnant of Castile, she was mentally unstable, and real power lay in the hands of her husband, King Philip. Because of the hostility between Philip and Ferdinand, Philip was anxious to conclude the betrothal of his daughter Eleanor to the Prince of Wales, thereby driving a wedge between Henry VII and his own father-in-law, and he welcomed this opportunity of a meeting with the English King.

Katherine, who knew nothing of these negotiations, was at Windsor for the visit, and was naturally elated at the prospect of seeing her sister, being hopeful also that Juana would use her influence with their father to improve her own situation. Henry VII made sure that Katherine had a prominent role in the festivities. Wearing Spanish dress, she danced for her good-looking brother-in-law, or sat with the King's daughter Mary Tudor at table or around the fire while the Kings talked. She may have wondered whether her inclusion really signified her return to favour or whether the King merely intended that Philip should return to Spain with the impression that she was being well treated and was accorded all the dignities and privileges appropriate to her status. Nevertheless, it would not have escaped Philip's shrewd eyes that all his meetings with Katherine took place under Henry VII's watchful supervision, thus preventing her from airing her grievances to her brother-in-law. Nor was Katherine allowed more than half an hour alone with her sister.

Katherine's expectations of Juana proved greatly overestimated; the sisters had not met for ten years and had very little in common. Juana was sunk in depression, obsessed with jealousy of her wayward husband, and not in the slightest interested in the problems of her younger sister. Katherine did not even attempt to ask for her help.

The two Kings spent several hours closeted together discussing the possible betrothal between their children, but nothing was finally concluded. Philip and Juana left England in April 1506, with Katherine in no doubt that they were completely unaware of her suffering. She never saw her sister again, even though Juana was to outlive her by nearly twenty years.

Philip and Juana returned to Spain, where only six months later Philip fell ill and died at the early age of twenty-eight. Queen Juana's mind, never very stable, became unhinged, and she suffered a complete nervous collapse. This gave her father the chance he had been hoping for to take over the reins of government in Castile on his daughter's behalf, and since it was obvious to everyone there that Juana was incapable of ruling for herself, there was little dissent. The widowed Queen seemed to be under the impression that her husband was not dead, and would not surrender his corpse for burial. Her attendants were horrified when she insisted upon opening the coffin and embracing and kissing what lay within, even though the body was rapidly decomposing; only with difficulty could she be parted from it and persuaded to allow it to be laid to rest.

Ferdinand had had long years of experience of governing Castile, and once he regained power there he was determined never again to relinquish it. After two years, he declared his daughter mad and unfit to reign, and had her shut up in the grim castle of Tordesillas, where she remained until her death fifty years later. She was deemed to have abdicated in favour of her son, now Charles I of Castile, but as the boy was only eight real power remained in the hands of his grandfather, who would govern both Castile and Aragon until his death.

Katherine's health might have been slightly improved when her sister left England, but her financial situation was worse than ever. In April 1506 she was deeply in debt, 'and this not for extravagant things', but for food. She had no decent clothes to wear, and not even enough money to buy a new chemise. Since arriving in England she had had only two new gowns, and the only serviceable ones left from her trousseau were two made of damask. It would be seventeen months, however, before she was able to afford to buy herself some decent clothes, and in that time she would appear ever shabbier. Mindful that she should maintain the standards suitable to her rank in an age when appearances counted for a lot, she felt she 'dared not neglect my own person', and consequently had to sell or pawn other items from her dower plate and jewels just for necessities. By the summer of 1506, she could no longer pay her servants their salaries, and told King Ferdinand that her people were 'ready to ask for alms', which caused her more anguish than Maria de Salinas's dowry. Predictably, she fell ill again at this time, suffering recurrent bouts of fever, doubtless exacerbated by anxiety over her situation.

In the autumn, however, she was somewhat better, thanks to the King allowing her to spend more time with the Prince of Wales. Young Henry, ever obedient to his father, had never hinted of his secret repudiation of his betrothal to Katherine, and in 1506 was still referring to her as 'my most dear and well-beloved consort, the Princess my wife'. When they were together during the late summer and autumn, a bond of affection began to develop between them, and the gap between their ages to seem narrower. The King, realising what was happening, deemed it prudent to separate them, as it now seemed unlikely that their marriage would ever take place. Saying he was concerned for her health, he sent Katherine to live at Fulham Palace once more; it was still unoccupied, having been put at the disposal of the Castilian ambassadors, who had not used it. The King told Katherine that 'if she preferred any other house, she had only to say so, and it would be kept for her'. She told him she was content to go to Fulham, but she does not appear to have lived there long, and was soon reinstalled in apartments at court, where she remained for the rest of her widowhood. Henry VII took care to keep her apart from the Prince, and from January to April 1507 she did not see him. This distressed her, and she thought it ominous. She told Ferdinand that the hardest thing she had to bear was to see her betrothed 'so seldom. As we all live in the same house, it seems to me a great cruelty.'

In 1507, Henry VII negotiated with the Emperor Maximilian a betrothal between the Princess Mary Tudor and Maximilian's grandson, Charles of Castile, an alliance that would be highly advantageous to England with her trade links through the wool-cloth trade with the Low Countries, of which Charles – as Archduke of Austria – was heir; it would also counterbalance a recent political alliance between Ferdinand and Louis XII of France. Henry VII had decided he no longer needed Ferdinand, and Katherine was made aware of this by what she described as his 'want of love'; she told her father it was 'impossible for me any longer to endure what I have gone through and am still suffering'.

By April 1507, Katherine's servants were walking about 'in rags' and existing 'in such misery it is shameful to think on it'. She begged her father to succour them, as there were 'no persons to whom your Highness is more indebted'. They had served her with unfailing goodwill through prosperity and increasing adversity. Now, however, their patience was, like their clothes, becoming rather frayed at the edges.

During the sixteenth century, servants were treated far more familiarly than, for example, they were in Victorian times. Friendships could flourish between royal personages and those who served them, since 'condescension' was expected and not resented. Servants often performed the most intimate tasks: ladies of rank were always given assistance with dressing, coiffure and even bathing. Ladies-in-waiting and maids of honour would keep their mistress company for hours, sewing, reading aloud, chatting or making music in the intimate panelled rooms of the period. They would take it in turns to sleep on a pallet at the foot of her bed when she was alone at night. Indeed, there would be no time of the day when she was unattended, no bodily function that did not have its rituals, and no private emotion that went unwitnessed.

In return, a lady of rank was responsible for her servants' physical, moral and spiritual welfare, for housing, clothing and feeding them, and in some cases for arranging marriages for them and providing dowries. The strong bonds that developed between Katherine of Aragon and many of those who served her were no doubt forged not only from her innate kindness but also the shared experience of being foreigners together in a strange and hostile land, almost the only people there who spoke their native Spanish. There were in her household, however, some who took advantage of her kindness, or let self-interest stand in the way of their duty. Certainly intrigue was rife among the Princess's servants.

Katherine's patience and forbearance were by now little short of saintly. Trained from the cradle to be submissive to the men of her family, she did not venture to criticise, but contented herself with pitiful pleas for assistance, which were calculated to flatter the powerful men with whom she had to treat. Honest and sincere to a fault, and perhaps lacking humour, her humility and self-effacement were at odds with her staunch pride in her royal blood and lineage. Yet it was her pride that helped her to cope with the many tribulations laid upon her, not the least of which was being besieged daily by creditors demanding payment.

Yet some relief was at hand. In April 1507, Ferdinand wrote to ask Katherine for her views as to the kind of ambassador who should be sent to replace Dr de Puebla. She replied that he should be someone 'who dared to speak an honest word at the right time'. Ferdinand had suggested Don Guitier Gomez de Fuensalida, Knight Commander of the Order of Membrilla, a high-minded Spanish aristocrat who had already spent some time in England, and although he was not Katherine's first choice – she preferred Pedro de Ayala, who had visited England with Philip and Juana in 1506 – she made no objections to Fuensalida, as she believed him to be 'a man of great experience, knowledge and high status'. Meanwhile, she told her father that, when the new ambassador came to England and made his first report, Ferdinand would be 'frightened at that which I have passed through'. If Puebla were any kind of man, he would not have consented to her being treated as 'never knight's daughter was in the kingdoms of your Highness'. This alarmed Ferdinand, who, prompted by 'royal and paternal solicitude', and impressed by the way in which Katherine was handling a very difficult situation, took the unprecedented step, on 19 May 1507, of appointing his daughter to act as his ambassador in England until a replacement could be found. Never before in Europe had a woman acted in such a capacity, and the appointment naturally enhanced Katherine's status at the court of Henry VII. It was also a timely appointment, as Puebla was ill and having to be carried from his house to the palace in a litter. Henry VII, hearing the news, 'rejoiced', although it is obvious that he and his advisers believed Katherine to be a lightweight who could easily be manipulated. To some extent she would confound them.

In her role as ambassador, Katherine grew more confident in her dealings with the King, disputing with him, flattering him, even telling him she was 'very well treated and very well contented'. She never used the Doctor as an intermediary, for she feared the 'injurious consequences'; Puebla was still playing a double game, and she viewed him with jaundiced eye as 'the adviser to the King' whose chief interest was to make his own life in England as comfortable as possible. Staunchly moral herself, she was finally beginning to appreciate the lack of scruple in the men with whom she was dealing, and slowly, painfully, she was learning to play the game of power politics their way. Nevertheless, she realised that she now was getting nowhere with Henry VII on the main issues, and continued to press her father for a new ambassador.

Acting as her father's ambassador certainly had a beneficial effect on Katherine's health, however. In May 1507, her physician, Dr Johannes, reported to Ferdinand that she was entirely recovered 'from the long malady which she has suffered ever since her arrival in England', and had regained 'her natural healthy colour. The only pains she now suffers are moral afflictions beyond the reach of the physician.' Money was still a problem, yet worry over it did not affect Katherine as badly as previously, and her health remained stable for the next eighteen months. Being allowed once more to see the Prince doubtless helped.

During May and June, Katherine was present at the tournaments held to celebrate young Henry's sixteenth birthday, and delighting to watch him showing off his prowess in the lists. Already he was a skilful horseman and jouster, being very tall and of strong build, 'most comely of his personage', and so amiable that he was perfectly happy discussing warfare with 'gentlemen of low degree', something his contemporaries marvelled at. Prince Henry was popular with his future subjects for his common touch, something his father had never had. He dreamed of war and glory and chivalry, and since he was openly pro-Spanish and anti-French the prospect of marriage to the Princess Katherine was very attractive to him. For the present, however, he was bound to obey his father, and could only exchange pleasantries with his betrothed. The King had seen to it that his life was sheltered and secluded during his formative years, and Henry had learned to keep his own counsel.

The age gap between Henry and Katherine seemed to be narrowing as Henry grew to manhood. The time was now ripe for their marriage, and yet, in July 1507, it still seemed to be a long way off. 'Nothing has changed,' Katherine told Ferdinand then. She herself was now twenty-one, old by Tudor standards for marriage, and to her the delay was extremely distressing. An indication of her true feelings was given in September, when she overheard speculation that her marriage would never take place and told Henry VII 'she could not bear to have such a thing said'. Prince Henry was the husband she wanted. 'There is no finer youth in the world,' wrote Dr de Puebla at this time; 'he is already taller than his father and his limbs are of gigantic size. He is as prudent as is to be expected for a son of Henry VII.'

By the autumn of 1507, Ferdinand had firmly established himself as ruler of Castile and Henry VII began to look upon Katherine in a more favourable light, something that substantially increased the esteem in which she was generally held at court. Katherine herself believed that her marriage to Prince Henry might now go ahead as planned if only her father would comply with Henry VII's demands for payment of her dowry. Yet while Ferdinand prevaricated, he instructed her to 'always speak of your marriage as a thing beyond all doubt', as though 'God alone could undo what has been undone'.

But it was not just Ferdinand's extended power that provoked Henry VII to a change of heart; since January 1507, the English King had cherished a desire to marry Queen Juana and thereby rule Castile himself, and to do so now he needed Ferdinand's goodwill and his permission. It was this that precluded him from breaking off his son's betrothal to Katherine, and this that influenced his dealings with Ferdinand throughout the year.

It was to Katherine that Henry had first disclosed his intentions, telling her he did not care about Juana's mental derangement; he had seen for himself her sultry, almost oriental beauty, and knew she was capable of producing healthy children. From the first, Katherine favoured an alliance between the King and her sister. Family feeling apart, she saw it as a surety for her own marriage taking place. She did not perceive that Ferdinand would never allow Henry VII to marry Juana, and that he meant to continue ruling Castile himself without foreign interference. Yet at the same time, he did not wish to alienate his ally, and therefore, when the King's proposal was put to him by Katherine, he instructed her to tell Henry that it was 'not yet known whether Queen Juana be inclined to marry again', although it was certain that if she became so inclined, 'it shall be with no other person than the King of England'. Ferdinand continued to dangle the carrot of Juana, believing that this was the best way to induce Henry VII to proceed with the marriage of his son to Katherine, but by September 1507 Henry was chafing at the delay and looking elsewhere for a wife, telling Katherine that the whole business had 'occasioned him great perplexity', and begging her to urge her father to think again. She did her best to bring negotiations for the marriage to a successful conclusion, which resulted in Ferdinand promising, in October, to persuade Juana 'by degrees' to it.

Katherine took advantage of this situation, and her authority as ambassador, by asking both her father and King Henry to redress the wrong done to her servants, who were still 'in absolute misery'. At long last, Ferdinand's conscience pricked him, and in September he sent her 2,000 ducats, not a large sum but enough to clear some of her debts, although she was somewhat perplexed as to which should have priority. Her creditors must be satisfied, her servants paid, her depleted plate needed replacing, and she herself needed new clothes. Then Henry VII, eager to ingratiate himself with her father, stepped in, telling her he loved her so much he could not bear the idea of her being in poverty, and would give her, without delay, 'as much money as you want for your person and servants'.

For the present, it seemed that Katherine's troubles would soon be over. She had also achieved tranquillity in her spiritual life with the advent of a new confessor. Early in 1507, she had been forced to apply to the General of the Order of the Franciscan Friars Observant in Spain for a new confessor, as Alessandro Geraldini had gone home a year earlier, leaving her virtually without spiritual comfort. She still could not speak English, and her father had failed to send a replacement, despite repeated requests. The confessor sent by the Order, who arrived later in the year, was in Katherine's opinion 'very good': he was a young Spanish friar called Fray Diego Fernandez, a man of magnetic charm and forceful personality, who rapidly gained a powerful influence over the Princess, to whom he offered the kind of devoted friendship and support she had so often found lacking in England. Moreover, he was a learned young man, and had about him an air of authority that commanded respect.

Before long, Katherine was showing herself reluctant to take any step without the friar's advice and blessing. She was a deeply pious person, but also a woman of twenty-one who had for long lacked a male figure – father, lover or husband – in her restricted life. It is perhaps no coincidence that she recovered her health shortly after Fray Diego's arrival. The friar certainly knew his power over her, and soon capitalised on it. He told her there was no need to suffer any more humiliating delay in waiting for her marriage to take place; the marriage treaty had been concluded conditionally, Henry VII had defaulted on its terms, and she was free to renounce it. But King Ferdinand was unimpressed by this view, and ignored the letter in which Katherine set it forth.

Katherine's marriage prospects received a major setback early in 1508 when Henry VII finally lost patience with Ferdinand over the delay in arranging his marriage to Juana. When he was informed that she was completely deranged, he retorted that he did not believe it. In fact, though, he now realised only too well that Juana was not in the marriage market, and the matter of their betrothal was quietly dropped without further recriminations. But the damage had already been done. By March 1508 relations between Henry and Ferdinand had deteriorated badly, and that month saw the King re-entering into negotiations with the Emperor Maximilian for the marriage of the Prince to Eleanor of Austria. Young Henry himself was behaving as if he was 'hardly much inclined' towards marrying Katherine; it was what his father expected of him, especially as Henry VII was becoming convinced that their union would be of questionable validity anyway.

In the spring of 1508, Ferdinand finally granted Katherine's request for another ambassador and sent Fuensalida to England. Unfortunately, the new ambassador proved to be as proud, pompous and dogmatic as only a Spanish grandee could be; the first thing he did was ruffle King Henry's feathers over the sensitive matter of Juana, thus setting a pattern for diplomatic relations over the next year. Katherine took an instant dislike to Fuensalida, and accused him of behaving with 'too great rigour towards the King'. She did not trust him, and she resented the fact that the respect formerly shown to her as her father's official ambassador had diminished with the Knight Commander's arrival in England. Fuensalida, for his part, immediately assessed how matters stood between Katherine and Fray Diego, and decided that the friar was a bad influence and should be removed at the earliest opportunity. In this he had Katherine's best interests at heart, since he could foresee a scandal brewing; Katherine, however, resented his animosity towards the friar, and preferred to heed the vitriol poured in her ears by Fray Diego about Fuensalida than Fuensalida's warnings about the integrity of Fray Diego.

Negotiations for the betrothal of Prince Henry to Eleanor of Austria broke down early in the summer of 1508, and before long Henry VII was scouring the courts of Europe for another possible bride for his son. At seventeen, the Prince was approaching manhood and should be fathering heirs to safeguard the dynasty and the peace of the realm. Unfortunately, Ferdinand's spies told him what was afoot, and he wrote heatedly to Fuensalida, saying, 'The King of England must keep faith in this matter!' He also threatened war if Henry VII broke the treaty. Fuensalida was further instructed to ingratiate himself with the Prince of Wales, and 'use all the means in his power for bringing the marriage to a speedy conclusion'. Fortunately, many of the English nobility were eager for it to take place. In January 1509, when the King was trying to negotiate a French match for his son, a deputation of them confronted him and pressed him to marry the Prince to Katherine, as they had heard that her dowry was ready for payment and, more important, they had noted the sickness of their sovereign and feared for the succession. The King, who was indeed ill with consumption, agreed to consider their request, but Katherine was not hopeful of his agreeing to it, and there was even talk of her returning to Spain to await another acceptable marriage.

During the early months of 1509 she was 'in deep despair', feeling herself unable to endure much more. She told Ferdinand that her sufferings continued to increase, and that she felt so depressed that life seemed not worth living. She feared, she said, that she 'might do something which neither the King of England nor your Highness would be able to prevent'. In Lent, she was physically unwell again, which commonly happened to her at that season, perhaps because she was confined to a diet of mainly fish, which may not always have been fresh or agreed with her. She was not seen about the court, and was probably still unwell in April, when an event occurred that would dramatically change her life. It is significant that, when her circumstances improved, as they did within two months, her illnesses disappeared for good.

Money had again become a problem during the early months of 1509, and had been since September 1508, for Henry VII, piqued by Ferdinand's duplicity, had once again ceased paying Katherine's allowance. In March she told her father that 'my necessities have risen so high that I do not know how to maintain myself'. She had sold all her household goods and most of her dower plate – 'it was impossible to avoid it' – and had since spent the money thus raised. Once again, she was driven to begging King Henry for help, though he told her he was not bound to give it; nevertheless, he added that the love he bore her would not allow him to do otherwise, and grudgingly gave her enough to defray the expenses of her table. She found this humiliating, and wrote to Ferdinand: 'From this your Highness will see to what a state I am reduced, when I am warned that even my food is given me almost as alms.'

To add to Katherine's woes, there was a good deal of tension within her household, due not only to the uncertainty overshadowing her future, but also to petty disputes and jealousies. Early in the year, Katherine quarrelled with Doña Elvira over the latter's constant intrigues and dismissed her, leaving no suitable person to supervise her servants and protect her reputation. Katherine was now twenty-three and mature enough to order her own affairs, and circumstances would shortly dictate that the duenna would never be replaced. Her desperate lack of money meant that her servants were once more facing destitution, for again they had not been paid, 'which hurts me and weighs on my conscience'. This time, they were not so forbearing. The Princess's chamberlain, Juan de Diero, responded by treating her with great 'audaciousness' and failing to order her household properly, and because she could not pay him the arrears of salary due to him, she could neither reprimand nor dismiss him.

Much of the tension in Katherine's household was generated by Fray Diego. The friar had already acquired a reputation as a womaniser, and most of the ladies in the Princess's household, not to mention some about the court, were a little in love with him. His hold over Katherine was stronger than ever, and the relationship between them intense. Fuensalida had watched the Princess and marked her complete dependence on Fray Diego, and by March 1509 was so alarmed about it that he confided his fears to his master, alleging that the friar was 'unworthy' to hold his office. Katherine was 'full of goodness' and 'conscientious', but her confessor was making her 'commit many faults'. The ambassador did not elaborate, but sent his servant to Spain to inform Ferdinand in person 'of the things which for two months past have happened'.

Fuensalida called Fray Diego 'light, haughty, and scandalous in an extreme manner'. Even Henry VII had heard of his promiscuity and had spoken to Katherine 'in very strong words' about her confessor's behaviour. But the friar, perceiving that Fuensalida was hostile to him, 'put me out of favour with the Princess, so that if I had committed some treason she could not have treated me worse'. Fuensalida accordingly begged Ferdinand to recall the friar and replace him with 'an old and honest confessor'.

The implication was clear: Katherine was placing herself in moral danger and risked ruining her reputation by associating with Fray Diego, a confessor who was stressing the avoidance of sin on one hand and fornicating with women on the other. Fuensalida feared that Katherine too would succumb, for if this had not been the issue at stake, then the nature of the complaints against the friar would have been stated more specifically by the ambassador.

Today, it is hard to assess the precise nature of the relationship between Katherine and Fray Diego. In view of Katherine's character, and her repeated later assertions that she had come to Henry VIII 'a true maid, without touch of man', it was certainly not a sexual one – Henry VIII's retention of the friar in his office after his marriage to Katherine is sufficient proof of this. Katherine's respect for the friar's vows and for her own rank and person were enough to deter her from overstepping the bounds of accepted morality, but the men around her were hardened realists, and saw life in basic terms; they well knew what could develop from such a potentially explosive situation. To them, the removal of Fray Diego was therefore imperative for the sake of Katherine's as yet unblemished reputation and her future marriage prospects.

Katherine, meanwhile, could see no wrong in her confessor; in her view, he was 'the best that ever woman in my position had'. She reacted with passionate anger to Fuensalida's criticism, not perhaps fully comprehending why he should be so concerned, and wrote to inform Ferdinand 'how badly the ambassador has behaved' towards the friar. By March 1509, she would have nothing to do with him, and was demanding that her father replace him with someone else. 'Things here become daily worse,' she wrote, 'and my life more and more insupportable. I can no longer bear this.' Fuensalida, she went on, had 'crippled your service'; Henry VII did not want him, and would undoubtedly welcome a replacement. Whatever Fuensalida wrote in his reports, she warned, 'might not be true'. Because of this, Ferdinand immediately ordered the recall of Fuensalida: Luis Caroz could take his place. Later on, after the accession of Henry VIII, Fuensalida did make his peace with Katherine, thanks to the intercession of the new King, before leaving England in May 1509. At the same time, Katherine also bade farewell to Dr de Puebla, who was likewise returning to Spain, where he died a few months later.

By defending her confessor to her father, Katherine had provided a credible reason for her rift with Fuensalida, but at the same time she had exposed her emotional and spiritual dependence on the friar. By now, she would do nothing without the friar's consent. When the court moved to Richmond and he told her to remain behind, for no apparent reason, she obeyed him without protest, even though no provision had been made for her to stay. When the King heard, he was 'very much vexed', and when Katherine did arrive at Richmond the next day, after a comfortless night, she met with a very chilly reception. The King did not speak to her for three weeks after the incident.

The friar had also managed to alienate most of the senior members of Katherine's household, including the chamberlain, Juan de Diero, and when Katherine wished to sell her remaining plate 'to satisfy the follies of the friar', Diero spoke out against it, with the result that the Princess behaved towards him as though he had 'committed the greatest treason in the world'. Fuensalida, seeing this, continued to press Ferdinand for the removal of the friar, whom he referred to as 'this pestiferous person'. He was writing, he said, 'not so openly as I would desire'; instead, he was sending one of Katherine's devoted servants who would disclose more sensitive information. Katherine, learning of her servant's departure and guessing what was afoot, warned Ferdinand not to credit anything that was written or said to him about 'my confessor, who serves me well and loyally'. She herself refused to believe the rumours then circulating about the friar, nor could she see the damage he was causing. In fact, he had brought about a rift between Katherine and Henry VII, and when it became obvious in April 1509 that Henry was dying, Katherine's fortunes were at a low ebb. She was ill and depressed, even suicidal, and once more in grave financial difficulty.

Nevertheless, an end to her troubles was in sight. That month, Luis Caroz arrived to replace Fuensalida as ambassador, and brought with him the reassuring news that her dowry was ready for payment. This was comfort indeed, but Katherine was anxious about what would become of her once the King was dead. Already the courtiers were behaving towards her with a new respect, believing she might shortly be Queen of England, but she had as yet heard no word from Prince Henry, who was so distraught at the prospect of losing his father that all other matters had temporarily been banished from his mind.

Henry VII died a hard, difficult death from tuberculosis on 22 April 1509. On his deathbed, he admitted to his son that his conscience was troubling him over his poor treatment of the Princess Katherine, and commanded young Henry to do the honourable thing and marry her, something that was much in accord with the Prince's own inclinations.

When Henry VII died, England's reputation in Europe was so impressive that it was said that all Christian nations were eager to forge alliances with her. Much of Henry's power lay in the wealth he had accumulated over the years; there was well over £1 million in the treasury at his death, a fantastic sum in those days. In this wealth lay England's strength and security. Yet when Henry VII was buried in the chapel named after him in Westminster Abbey early in May, few mourned his passing. The English had always underestimated his greatness, seeing him as a parsimonious schemer who was not to be trusted, rather than the wise founder of a strong dynasty and the guardian of a precarious peace.

There was little doubt in anyone's mind that the new King, Henry VIII, had already chosen the lady who would share his life and his throne. The Princess had always been on close and affectionate terms with the young Henry before his father's death, even though the old King had kept them apart for much of their five-year engagement. Although the Prince had secretly renounced his vows on his father's orders in 1505, few knew of it, and in the eyes of the world Henry and Katherine were still betrothed. As a result, Katherine found herself treated with a new and gratifying deference by courtiers. It was, of course, a matter of absolute necessity that the King marry and get himself an heir as soon as possible: there were still living some members of the House of York who thought they had a better claim to the throne than he, and the spectre of civil war still loomed large.

After the funeral of Henry VII, the court moved to Greenwich, the red-brick hilltop palace on the Thames where Henry had been born. Here, where the windows afforded magnificent, panoramic views of London, the new King made it clear that he intended to pursue traditional foreign policy and revive Edward III's ancient claim to the throne of France and have himself crowned at Rheims. The possibility of war with France, England's hereditary enemy, made an alliance with Spain all the more desirable. King Ferdinand was urging him to marry Katherine without delay, and was promising him 'all the advantages which were denied to his father, on the sole condition that the marriage is immediately consummated'. The dowry, he promised, would be 'punctually paid'.

But, briefly, Henry VIII hesitated: his councillors told Fuensalida that, unexpectedly, he was suffering 'certain scruples of conscience' and wondering whether he would 'commit a sin by marrying the widow of his deceased brother', as such unions were forbidden in the Bible. It seemed that certain churchmen had been whispering in Henry's ear, Warham amongst them; and the King's conscience was a rather tender organ, as many would later find to their cost. Informed of Henry's doubts by Fuensalida, Ferdinand hastened to reassure the young King that 'such a marriage is perfectly lawful, as the Pope has given a dispensation for it, while the consequence of it will be peace between England and Spain'. He drew Henry's attention to the King of Portugal, who had married two of Katherine's sisters in succession and was 'blessed with numerous offspring, and lives very cheerfully and happily'. Ferdinand felt certain that 'the same happiness is reserved for the King of England, who will enjoy the greatest felicity in his union with the Princess of Wales, and leave numerous children behind him'. Fuensalida told Katherine that Ferdinand loved her 'the most of his children and looks on the King of England like a son'. It was Ferdinand's intention to give advice about everything to Henry VIII, 'like a true father'; Katherine's duty would be to foster an understanding between the two men and ensure that her future husband would heed Ferdinand's guidance in all matters of state.

Early in June 1509, the Privy Council urged the King to marry Katherine and fulfil the terms of the betrothal treaty. They did not have to spell out why the matter was urgent, as Henry was more than cognizant of the insecurity of his dynasty. Instead, they extolled Katherine's virtues, saying she was 'the image of her mother, (and) like her possesses that wisdom and greatness of mind which win the respect of nations'. As for Henry's scruples about the canonical legality of the marriage, 'we have the Pope's dispensation,' they said; 'will you be more scrupulous than he is?'

The King could only agree that there were many good reasons for the marriage; above all, he told them, 'he desired her above all women; he loved her and longed to wed her.' Most of the Councillors knew this: since the age of ten, Henry had looked up to and admired his pretty sister-in-law; and, as he had grown to manhood, and had seen how well Katherine had coped with the adversity and humiliations she had suffered, his admiration had deepened, not to passion – it would never be that – but to love in its most chivalrous form, blended with deep respect. This apart, honour demanded that Henry should marry her, as by so doing he would rescue her from penury and dishonour, like a knight errant of old, and win her unending gratitude. It was a plan that appealed vastly to the King's youthful conceit. Indeed, there was even a certain smugness in his approach to his marriage, for he was later to inform King Ferdinand that he had 'rejected all the other ladies in the world that have been offered to us', which, in his view, proved beyond doubt the depth of the 'singular love' he bore to his 'very beloved' Katherine. Undoubtedly he found her attractive, with her long golden hair and fair skin; he was impressed by her maturity, her dignity, her lineage and her graciousness. Everything about her proclaimed her a fit mate for the King of England, and Henry, who was no fool, realised this.

Yet in some ways she was an unwise choice. Doubts that the marriage might be uncanonical were well founded in the opinion of some churchmen of the time, though they, knowing the King's will in the matter, kept silent for the most part. Then there was the matter of the five-and-a-half-year age gap, and the fact that Katherine, at twenty-three, was well past her first youth by the standards of her day, and rather old to be contemplating motherhood for the first time. Many girls married at fourteen and bore a child the following year, while the average age at death for women in Tudor times was around thirty. Henry VIII could have had his pick of the young princesses of Europe, but he needed the alliance with Spain, he wanted Katherine's dowry to add to his already rich inheritance, and, above all, he wanted Katherine herself.

And what Henry VIII wanted, he usually got.

5
Sir Loyal Heart
and the Tudor court

One day in early June 1509 Henry, in a buoyant mood, made his way from the Council Chamber at Greenwich to Katherine's apartments. He came alone, and dismissed her attendants. Then he raised the Princess from her curtsy with a courtly gesture, declared his love for her, and asked her to be his wife. Without any hesitation, she joyfully agreed, relief and happiness evident in her face and voice.

This was the culmination of all Katherine's hopes during the last six years: God had now seen fit to answer her prayers, and she was filled with thankfulness. She would be Queen of England, raised by this magnificent young man to be the bride of his heart and the mother of his heirs. Those courtiers who had scorned her and tried to humiliate her would now have to defer to her, and she would not have been human if she did not relish the prospect. The days of want were gone for good, for very shortly she would be the wife of the richest monarch ever to reign in England.

Fray Diego was all but forgotten now, as Katherine gave her heart unreservedly to her future husband. That she fell quickly in love with him we may easily believe as she had long ago responded to his charm and good looks, and he, now that the matter had been decided, saw no need to wait much longer before they could legally share a bed. His coronation was planned for midsummer, and he wanted Katherine to share it with him as queen.

Henry VIII and Katherine of Aragon were married privately on

11 June 1509, the feast day of St Barnabas, in her closet at Greenwich, by William Warham, who was now Archbishop of Canterbury, and had once spoken out against their union. Katherine wore virginal white with her long hair flowing free under a gold circlet, and vowed to be 'bonair and buxom in bed and at board' as was laid down in the more robust form of the marriage service then in use.

The Archbishop pronounced the young pair man and wife, then the small wedding party proceeded to the Chapel of the Observant Friars within the palace precincts to hear mass.

There is no record of the King and his new Queen being publicly put to bed together; their wedding was private, therefore it is likely that they were accorded some privacy afterwards. However, there was never any doubt that Katherine's second marriage was ardently consummated that night.

To his contemporaries, Katherine's bridegroom was the true heir in blood to both Lancaster and York, and the reincarnation of his magnificent maternal grandfather, Edward IV. He was a man of great physical beauty, above the usual height, being around 6'3" tall (his skeleton, discovered at Windsor in the early nineteenth century, measured 6'2" in length, whilst his armour, preserved in the Tower of London, would fit a man of nearly 6'4"). He was magnificent to look at, being lean and muscular, with an extremely fine calf to his leg of which he was inordinately proud, and had skin so fair that it was almost translucent; we are told that it glowed, flushing a rosy pink after the King had exercised. All were agreed that he was extremely handsome, and the ambassadors who visited Henry VIII's court during the early years of his reign were united in their praise of his personal endowments: 'His Majesty is the handsomest potentate I ever set eyes on,' wrote the Venetian Sebastian Giustinian in 1514, adding that Henry had 'a round face so beautiful that it would become a pretty woman'. Five years later, that same ambassador was still singing the King's praises: 'Nature could not have done more for him. He is very fair, his whole frame admirably proportioned.' He had strong features, with piercing blue eyes, a high-bridged nose, and a small but sensual mouth. His voice was slightly high-pitched. He had 'auburn hair combed straight and short in the French fashion', and until 1518 he was clean-shaven. He then grew a beard, saying he would not shave it off until he had met with and embraced his ally, the King of France. Queen Katherine protested, for she did not like this new bearded Henry, but the beard remained until 1519. Many thought it attractive – 'it is reddish and looks like gold' – but Katherine continued to complain about it, and by November that year the King had given in to her entreaties and shaved it off. An international catastrophe was only narrowly averted by Henry's ambassador to France, who told King Francis the truth, whereupon the French courtiers, far from being indignant, were amused to learn that the mighty sovereign of England had capitulated to his usually complacent and meek wife. Thus, peace was preserved, and the Queen was kept happy.

Henry VIII had boundless energy and a strong constitution. When, in 1514, he contracted smallpox, his doctors were afraid for his life, yet within days he was up, having 'risen from his bed to plan a military campaign'. However, throughout his life he had a pathological hatred of anything to do with illness and death, and he was as terrified as a child of the plague that troubled his kingdom during hot summers.

Giustinian thought Henry 'the best dressed sovereign in the world; his robes are the richest and most superb that can be imagined, and he puts on new clothes every holy day.' As the calendar was full of saints' days and religious festivals, that meant a lot of new clothes. There were outfits of cloth of gold, Florentine velvet, silver tissue, damask and satin, mantles lined with ermine, heavy gold collars with diamonds the size of walnuts suspended from them, ceremonial robes with trains four yards long, and jewelled rings worn on fingers and thumbs. Some clothes were cut in 'Hungarian' or 'Turkish' fashion, and many had raised embroidery in gold or silver thread. It was an age in which men strutted like peacocks in their finery, although none was finer than the King, who looked upon costume as a visual art.

Henry's contemporaries thought he was 'the most gentle and affable prince in the world'. He was quick to laugh and 'intelligent, with a merry look'. He had great charisma and a strong personality that won golden opinions. In 1509, Katherine's future chamberlain, Lord Mountjoy, told the Dutch humanist scholar Erasmus that the

King, 'our Octavius', had an 'extraordinary and almost divine character. What a hero he now shows himself, how wisely he behaves, what a lover he is of goodness and justice! Our King does not desire gold or gems, but virtue, glory, immortality!' As Henry himself declared in one of his songs, idleness was the chief mistress of all vice, and he meant to follow the path of virtue, something by which he set great store throughout his life. That his expectations often related to others rather than himself he did not regard as inconsistent, for in his opinion his own deeds and behaviour were always morally justified. He was bursting with confidence, 'prudent, sage, and free from every vice'.

On the debit side, he was quick-tempered, headstrong, immature and vain. In 1515, he asked the Venetian ambassador if the King of France was as tall as he: 'Is he as stout? What sort of legs has he?' 'Spare,' he was told. 'Look here!' crowed Henry, 'I also have a good calf to show!' And he opened his doublet to display his shapely, muscular legs. He 'could not abide to have any man stare in his face' when in conversation, yet he himself would often turn a steely gaze on people, and Sir Thomas More was not the only one to stammer under the 'quick and penetrable eyes' of his sovereign.

As the years passed, Henry continued to attract praise and acclaim. He was well aware of his glorious reputation, and on occasions boasted about it. Yet as early as 1514 there were indications of the kind of ruler he would one day become, and the Spanish ambassador was moved to warn his master, King Ferdinand, that if a bridle was not put on 'this colt, it will afterwards be found impossible to control him'. His words were echoed seven years later by Sir Thomas More, who advised Thomas Cromwell, then newly admitted to the King's service, that he should handle Henry with caution: 'For, if the lion knew his strength, hard were it to rule him.'

Henry was gifted with acute powers of reasoning and observation, as well as the ability to evaluate a person or situation almost immediately. He had a vast store of general knowledge that he used to good effect. Above all, he was an intellectual with 'most piercing talents'. According to Sir Thomas More, he had 'cultivated all the liberal arts' and possessed 'greater erudition and judgement than any previous monarch'. From infancy, he had been imbued with a passion for learning, thanks to the good offices of his grandmother, the austere Lady Margaret Beaufort and was the most learned king yet to have ascended the throne of England. He was 'so gifted and adorned with mental accomplishments of every sort' that the Venetian ambassadors 'believed him to have few equals in the world'. 'What affection he bears to the learned!' wrote Lord Mountjoy in 1509, informing Erasmus of Henry's intention to establish a haven for scholars at his court. Europe was then on the brink of a period of cultural flux, when men were beginning in earnest to question and rationalise in matters of religion or philosophy. During Henry's own lifetime, two great movements would affect his realm: the Renaissance, which would have a profound effect upon England's cultural life; and the Reformation, which was to overthrow the traditional conception of a Christian Republic of Europe for ever.

Henry's education had been extremely thorough. He could speak and write fluent French and Latin, understood Italian well and spoke it a little, and by 1520 was conversant with Spanish. He loved reading, and his favourite books during his younger years were the works of St Thomas Aquinas and Duns Scotus. However, in 1519, he began to suffer from recurring headaches and migraines, which made reading and writing 'somewhat tedious and painful'. The headaches continued to plague him for the rest of his life, and may well account to some extent for his later irascibility.

The King wrote several treatises during his life, and his letters to the Vatican were said to have been the most eloquent received there, for which reason they were exhibited in the consistory. His literary talents extended to passionate love letters, as well as poetry. His chief interest was theology; he was a master of doctrinal debate, of which he was 'very fond', and would hear others out with 'remarkable courtesy and unruffled temper'. He was good at mathematics, and also keenly interested in astronomy, a passion he shared with Sir Thomas More, who would often join him on the leads above Greenwich Palace to look at the night sky.

Henry VIII professed all his life a deep and sincere faith in God, and for many years regarded himself as a true son of the Church of Rome. He was known to attend as many as six masses in a single day, and at least three on days when he hunted. Every evening, at 6.0 p.m. and 9.0 p.m., he went to the Queen's chamber to hear the offices of vespers and compline. At Easter, he 'crept to the Cross' on his knees, with all due humility. He also held himself up as an authority on doctrine, and was acknowledged as such by his contemporaries because 'he is very religious'.

In 1521, while convalescing after a fever, the King added the finishing pages to a Latin treatise he had been working on for some time with assistance from others, notably Sir Thomas More. It was entitled *A Defence of the Seven Sacraments against Martin Luther*, and was an attack upon the heresies propagated since 1517 by a former monk of Wittenburg in Germany, who would – thirty years later – be hailed in England as the founder of the Protestant religion. Henry was well aware that information about Luther's controversial teachings was already filtering through to England, and had gained hold in Germany. Yet although he himself enjoyed disputing points of doctrine, heresy was another matter entirely, and he was appalled that any credence should be given to the corrupt teachings of 'this weed, this dilapidated, sick and evil-minded sheep'.

Henry VIII, like most of his contemporaries, was well aware that there were certain abuses within the established Church that needed reforming, but he was a religious conservative at heart, and would not countenance heresy as a means of achieving this. To Henry, and men like him, heresy was a poison that threatened the very foundations of the superstructure of Church and State as one body politic. It encouraged disaffection among the lower classes, challenged the divinely appointed order of things, and – worst of all – meant eternal damnation for those who succumbed to its lure. In sum, it represented every evil that could be manifested in a well-ordered world, and must therefore be eradicated.

In his book, the King's central argument was for the retention of the seven sacraments – Luther had rejected all but two. Marriage, in particular, was upheld by Henry, for it turned 'the water of concupiscence' into 'wine of the finest flavour. Whom God hath joined together, let no man put asunder.' Luther had also rejected the authority of the Pope, but the King exhorted all faithful souls to 'honour and acknowledge the sacred Roman See for their supreme mother'. When Thomas More suggested that this was a little extravagant, Henry protested that he was so 'bounden' to the See of Rome that he could not do enough to honour it: 'We will set forth the Pope's authority to the uttermost,' he declared – words he was later to regret.

Although Luther himself accused Henry VIII of raving 'like a strumpet in a tantrum' in the book, and spoke of 'stuffing such impudent falsehoods down his throat', the Pope received the treatise with rapturous praise, and in the autumn of 1521 rewarded Henry with the title *Fidei Defensor* (Defender of the Faith) in gratitude. Elizabeth II still bears this title today, though Britain has been an independent Protestant state for more than four centuries.

Apart from religion, Henry loved gambling, good food, and dancing, in which he did 'marvellous things, both in dancing and jumping, proving himself indefatigable'. He was obsessive about hunting, which he preferred above all else. The 'grease season' was traditionally in the autumn, but Henry also hunted at other times of the year, both for pleasure and to provide for his table. In the autumn, however, he would take a rest from state duties and go on a progress through parts of his kingdom, chiefly for the purpose of discovering the delights of different chases. 'He never takes his diversion without tiring eight or ten horses,' wrote the Venetian ambassador in 1519; 'when he gets home, they are all exhausted.' In fact, he exhausted most of his male companions too by 'converting the sport of hunting into a martyrdom'. And, after a successful day, it was not unknown for him to boast about his success for three or four hours at a time. Queen Katherine enjoyed hunting too, and sometimes accompanied her husband.

Being an excellent horseman and an expert in the martial arts, Henry was also passionately fond of that other great medieval sport, the jousting tournament, which was almost a weekly event during the early years of his reign. He was a fine jouster who was conspicuous in the combats, both on horseback and on foot, excelling everyone else 'as much in agility at breaking spears as in nobleness of stature'. At one tournament in 1518, Henry performed 'supernatural feats', causing his magnificent charger to 'jump and execute other acts of horsemanship'. Then, changing mounts, he made his fresh steed 'fly rather than leap, to the delight and ecstasy of everybody'. The Queen would never miss a joust if she could help it, and watched with her ladies from specially erected pavilions at the side of the lists.

Another sport at which he excelled was tennis, not the game played at Wimbledon today, but 'royal' (real) tennis played on a hard, enclosed court – Henry's court is preserved at Hampton Court – an altogether tougher and more dangerous game. The Household Accounts for the year 1519 record a payment for 3¼ yards of black velvet for a 'tennis coat for his Grace'. 'It is the prettiest thing in the world to see him play, his fair skin glowing through a shirt of the finest texture,' reported the Venetian ambassador.

Henry enjoyed hawking, 'running the ring', 'casting the bar', wrestling, and archery. He practised daily at the archery butts and passed a law requiring every man in England to spend an hour doing the same on Saturday afternoons, such was his faith in the reputation of the longbow as the traditional instrument of English military success; he himself could 'draw the bow with greater strength than any man in England'. He also wished to ensure that the young men of his court were expert in the martial skills, and on one occasion in 1510 arranged for a fight with battle axes to take place in the presence of the Queen and her ladies in Greenwich Park, thus mixing military exercise with pleasure.

Henry had a lifelong love of the sea and all things maritime. He ordered the building of several great ships – including the *Henry-Grace-à-Dieu* and the *Mary Rose* – and has been rightly acclaimed as the founder of Britain's modern navy. In 1515, he went with the Queen to review his fleet at Southampton, wearing a 'sailor's coat and trousers of frieze cloth of gold' and carrying 'a large whistle with which he whistled almost as loud as a trumpet'. He was in his element that day, on board his flagship, where for a couple of hours he enjoyed himself immensely, acting as pilot.

His pleasures were not always so boisterous. He inherited from his Welsh forbears an abiding love of music, and could play a number of instruments, sing and compose. He was particularly accomplished on the lute, harpsichord, recorder, flute and virginals, and would often entertain the court by singing and playing his own compositions. He could 'sing from the book at sight', often set his own verses to music, and composed anthems and hymns. One, 'O Lord, the maker of all things', is still sung in churches today. Yet Henry preferred writing secular songs, mostly in the courtly tradition, with English or French lyrics. The most famous were 'Green groweth the holly' (probably written for Katherine of Aragon), '*Adieu Madame et ma maîstresse*' (written much later for Anne Boleyn), and 'Pastime with good company', which vividly portrays his mood at the commencement of his reign.

In these early years, Henry VIII's pleasures took precedence. His attitude to kingship and the duties of state he was required to perform was a different matter entirely. He had had a cloistered upbringing before suddenly finding himself in a position of power, honour and wealth, a heady experience for a youth of eighteen. Perhaps it was not surprising that he spent his days in pursuit of amusement rather than learning statecraft. Matters of state, he felt, could safely be left in the hands of his Privy Council; in fact, 'he did not care to occupy himself with anything but the pleasures of his age'.

The mature men appointed to advise him were so slow that they caused him 'much disgust': Henry preferred the company of the young men of the court with whom he had shared his boyhood. His councillors were alarmed to see him squandering his father's carefully amassed wealth on expensive and frivolous pastimes when he should have been learning about the government of his kingdom, and they were at pains to persuade him – not without difficulty – to sit in on meetings of the Privy Council, 'with which at first he could not endure to be troubled'. As the French ambassador observed, 'Henry is a youngling, cares for nothing but girls and hunting, and wastes his father's patrimony.'

His councillors hoped that, given time to mature, he would settle down and fulfil their expectations. Yet it was a slow process. In 1514, the Milanese ambassador complained that the King had put off their discussion about politics to another time, 'as he was then in a hurry to go and dine and dance afterwards'. Affairs of state, even after five years on the throne, were still ranking fairly low on Henry's scale of priorities. Even as late as 1519, the Papal nuncio reported that he was 'devoting himself to accomplishments and amusements day and night, being intent on nothing else'. All business was left to Cardinal Wolsey, 'who rules everything'. This was the situation that endured until the late 1520s, when Henry began to take the reins of government into his own hands.

It was the outward trappings of kingship that were important to Henry VIII during these early years: the pageantry, the ceremonial, the gorgeous robes, the priceless jewels, and the glittering court, and he passionately believed that they all served to enhance the image of royalty. It was Henry who was the first English King to express a preference to be styled 'Your Majesty' rather than the customary 'Your Grace'. He saw himself, indeed, as a hallowed being set apart from the ordinary species of men, and it was a persona he consciously cultivated, so confident did he become of his own divinity. No King of England before him enjoyed such power, nor ever would after him.

A man of contrasts, he personified for the average Englishman all the strengths and virtues of his race, and it was this that lay at the root of his vast popularity. As Prince of Wales his charm had won the hearts of his people, and now, exalted to kingship, he was fêted as the herald of a new age, a golden epoch that would witness a return to England's former glory, the revival of the days of chivalry, and the ultimate conquest of France – the new King's ambitions were well-publicised. The English loved Henry for his youth, his beauty, his high courage, his accomplishments, and above all for having identified their interests as his own. He was very knowledgeable about most of the issues that touched their lives, having been born with a talent for absorbing information, and there was 'no necessary kind of knowledge, from King's degree to carter's, but he had an honest sight of it'. He was fond, in his younger years, of mingling incognito among his subjects, in order to learn their views on the issues of the day.

In 1509, it was said that the whole world was 'rejoicing in the possession of such a King'. The passing of years did not dampen this enthusiasm, for in 1513 we are told that 'love for the King is universal with all who see him, as his Highness does not seem a person of this world but one descended from Heaven'. Erasmus, later still, described Henry as 'more of a companion than a King', a view that would have earned the hearty agreement of those courtiers with whom the King hunted, tilted, and otherwise amused himself. This common touch came naturally to him, and would serve to hold the love and loyalty of his subjects until he died.

In an era of arranged marriages, men were not censured for taking their pleasure when they found it. In his youth, the King was commendably discreet about such matters, so much so that we know absolutely nothing about his sexual activities, if any, before his accession. As Prince of Wales, he had led a cloistered life and had cultivated a chivalrous attitude towards the opposite sex, seeing himself as the knight errant whose role it was to flirt, offer elegant compliments, and profess undying love. When he came to the throne, women were waiting for him in droves, and freed from the confines of his princely existence, he made the most of his position and took what they offered. In this respect, though he was far from virtuous by modern standards of morality, by the standards of his time, and compared to other princes of the age, he was quite circumspect. Thanks to his discretion, Queen Katherine never knew of these early infidelities, which were fleeting anyway, and as far as Henry was concerned, they had nothing to do with her. His love for her was on a different plane completely.

Having sex was one thing, talking about it quite another. The King was very prudish, and was known to blush at bawdy remarks. He abhorred lightness in married women, even though he was not above pursuing them himself. And from his wife, he expected total fidelity and absolute obedience.

Katherine of Aragon first appeared at court as Queen of England on the day her marriage to the King was proclaimed, 15 June 1509. Henceforth, she would be at Henry's side at all state and court functions. She had already adopted the pomegranate, symbol of fertility, as her personal badge, and now she took the motto 'Humble and Loyal' for her personal device. In the royal palaces of England, an army of carpenters, stonemasons and embroiderers were already carving, chiselling and stitching her initials and Henry's, 'H' and 'K', on every available surface, and her throne was set beside the King's under the rich canopy of estate.

In 1509, Fray Diego described Katherine as 'the most beautiful creature in the world'. Marriage certainly made her seem so. She was twenty-three, and had kept her looks thus far. She was plump, pretty, and still had beautiful red-gold hair that hung below her hips when loose. Yet, within six years, she had lost her youthful bloom and her figure, and in 1515 was described by the Venetian ambassador as 'rather ugly than otherwise'. Sadly, he spoke the truth. By 1515, Katherine had suffered several bitter disappointments and five pregnancies, and these had aged her considerably. A miniature of her painted by Lucas Hornebolte (now in the National Portrait Gallery) survives from this time, and shows with cruel clarity that the pretty girl depicted in Miguel Sittow's portrait of 1505 had in fact aged almost beyond recognition in ten years. Hornebolte's portrait is of a stout, mature woman with a face overshadowed by anxiety and sadness. The red–gold hair seems to have darkened (although this may be due to pigment in the paint), and is gathered into a bun or plait on the nape of the neck, being surmounted by a Juliet cap, a rare fashion in England at that time.

This miniature should be compared with a portrait painted about five years later, which has been attributed to Johannes Corvus. Several versions exist, the most famous being in the National Portrait Gallery in London. Katherine is here shown wearing the gable hood traditionally associated with her, with long frontlets that would shortly become unfashionable. She is in a rich brown velvet gown with a low square neckline and furred sleeves, and is portly in build, with no pretensions to beauty, having a pale face in which the mouth has a slightly disdainful look and the firm chin juts out. A similar portrait, probably painted from a lost original during the reign of Mary I and until recently in the possession of the Royal Academy of Arts, is kinder, and shows the Queen smiling graciously. Yet the face is the same, that of a woman no longer young, obviously well–bred, with the marks of sadness etched upon it. And the figure, camouflaged in dark velvet furred with ermine with ropes of gold chains slung across the bodice, has likewise gone to ruin, spoiled by frequent childbearing. Perhaps the best existing likeness of Katherine in her later years is the fine miniature in the collection of the Duke of Buccleuch, which shows a stout woman, with large attractive blue eyes, holding a monkey.

Katherine's gradually fading looks were brought increasingly into contrast by the maturing beauty of her younger husband. She selected her ladies for their looks as well as their background, which showed up even more her own ageing face. To compensate for this, she took care to dress herself as magnificently as she could, being, like her mother, 'a ceremonious woman in her attire'. On marrying the King, she had been provided with a sumptuous new wardrobe, most of it in the English fashion. After her marriage, she rarely wore the farthingale, although she did very occasionally appear in Spanish dress. Her new gowns would have had court trains several yards in length, and were of rich materials such as satin, velvet – often with raised gold embroidery – or cloth of gold. If one had wealth, it was not considered vulgar to display it.

Katherine did not dictate fashion, like Anne Boleyn who came after her, but she had a lifelong love of rich clothes and jewellery. In fact, her jewellery was magnificent, and comprised two sets: the crown jewels, pieces that had been worn by former queens of England, and which were not her own but public property; and those items that the King had given her personally, which alone were worth a fortune. She favoured ropes of pearls from which hung suspended pendants made of diamonds in the form of a cross or a St George medal or religious symbols such as the IHS, representing Christ. Like many people at that time, the Queen wore several rings at once, and her corsage was rarely without a jewelled brooch pinned in the centre. On her head, she would usually wear the English gable hood and black veil made popular twenty years before by Elizabeth of York, although on occasion she would wear a different head-dress such as the Flemish hood which 'gave her additional grace', or the Juliet cap already mentioned. Her crown, which was melted down in the time of the Commonwealth, was worn only occasionally, for the great occasions of state; then she would wear her hair loose.

Katherine had all the personal qualities needed for a Queen of England. She had adapted to the customs of her new land, although she would continue actively to further Spanish interests for several years to come. She had strong principles, and set a high moral tone for her household. Beneath her outward air of meekness and submissiveness to her husband, she concealed a tough and tenacious character that would help her to bear the blows later dealt her with calm dignity. Those who served her invariably became devoted to her, for she was both kind and unfailingly courteous. In 1514, she was described by a Flemish diplomat as 'a lady of a lively, kind and gracious disposition, and of quite different complexion and manner from the Queen her sister.' Unlike Juana, Katherine was neither given to tantrums, hysteria or bouts of melancholia, nor was her love for her husband as obsessive as Juana's had been. Yet it was a deep love and would survive until death; in this, as in everything else, the Queen displayed singlemindedness and a trusting naïvety.

Katherine had received a good education, comparable to or better than that given to most girls of her rank. Erasmus called her 'a miracle of learning', and while this was probably an exaggeration in the best courtly tradition, there is every indication that there was some truth in it. The Queen was literate, well read and thoroughly conversant with the Scriptures, although her intelligence and her powers of perception were somewhat limited. Nevertheless she was far more erudite than most women at the court, and her qualities were justly recognised by the scholars who gathered there at the King's invitation. Katherine herself thrived in this cultural atmosphere, for she was interested in humanism and matters of religious doctrine and, as she grew older, she turned to intellectual pleasures more and more, finding little to stimulate her mind in the daily round of courtly revels. In 1526, she was very impressed by Erasmus's new book, *The Institution of Christian Marriage*, which was shown to her by Sir Thomas More. More himself warmly praised the work, and remarked that 'her Majesty the Queen correctly regards it as being of supreme importance'.

Katherine also took an interest in the universities. When she visited Merton College, Oxford, in 1518, she was welcomed by the students with 'as many demonstrations of joy and love as if she had been Juno or Minerva'. She also lent her support to Wolsey's foundation at Oxford, Cardinal College (now Christ Church), and when, in 1523, the King brought his confessor, Dr Longland, to show her the plans for it, she showed herself 'joyous and glad' to learn that she herself was 'particularly prayed for' in the chapel of the new establishment.

Since her arrival in England, when she spoke only Spanish, Katherine had laboured to learn English. It was a long process, for languages were not a strong point with her, but by the time of her marriage to the King she was able to speak English passably well, and her command of it would increase considerably over the following years. Yet she still spoke with a Spanish accent which never left her; this is evident from the phonetic spelling in her letters, in which, for example, Hampton Court becomes 'Antoncurt.'

According to Erasmus, Katherine was 'more pious than learned', and 'as religious and virtuous as words can express'. The great humanist praised her warmly to Henry VIII, saying: 'Your wife spends that time in reading the sacred volume which other princesses occupy in cards and dice.' From her youth, Katherine spent a considerable part of each day at her devotions, hearing mass, kneeling privately at prayer at the prie-dieu in her chamber, reading the Bible (then in Latin, which she understood to a degree) and other religious works, and hearing the Divine Offices of the day, which her chaplains performed in her private apartments. As she grew older, her faith deepened and, since her philosophy was a passive one, she faced up to and accepted what she understood to be the will of God without question or complaint.

By 1519–20, the Queen was leading an almost conventual existence. She withheld herself to some extent from the mainstream of court life, preferring to devote her time to her religious observances, and there are frequent references in the sources for the period to her being in her chapel, or 'just come from hearing mass', or on pilgrimage, our Lady of Walsingham being a favourite shrine of hers. From now on, religion would be the mainstay of her life and her chief consolation.

Her life was nevertheless lived under the public gaze. Nearly everything she did was attended by ceremony and performed according to strict rules of courtly etiquette. She was never alone. As Queen of England, she was given a household of 160 servants, and several of these – usually ladies-in-waiting, maids of honour and pages – were always in attendance upon her. Her meals were frequently taken in public, in full view of the court (and, on occasion, the common people, when they were admitted to watch their betters at meat); sometimes they were served in her apartments, where she was waited on by pages, her ladies standing in attendance behind her.

There were many demands on the Queen's time: charitable enterprises, religious observances, ambassadors come to pay their respects, domestic matters to be discussed and acted upon, and meetings with her own council. Such leisure time as she had she spent mainly at needlework, embroidering tapestries, altar-cloths, vestments, rich gowns and head-dresses for herself, shirts for her husband worked with the Spanish black-work lace that she herself had popularised, linen shifts to wear beneath her gowns, infant layettes on occasion, and clothing for the poor. Sometimes she and her ladies would entertain themselves with music – although there is no record of Katherine herself being able to play any instrument, she certainly enjoyed hearing others – with dancing – she herself would sometimes partner her ladies in the privacy of her chamber – in discussion, or even gambling with cards, dice, backgammon or other table games.

Even her sex life was surrounded by ritual. Traditionally, kings and queens had separate apartments in the royal palaces. If the King wished to sleep with his wife at night – a matter of public interest, since the succession must be assured – he went in procession, escorted to her chamber door by members of his guard and gentlemen of his privy chamber. Katherine, in turn, having been undressed by her ladies, would be sitting up in the great tester bed waiting for him. On the nights the King did not honour her with his company, a maid would occupy a truckle bed at the foot of her bed, but she was banished whenever the King arrived unannounced, as he often did. Then his guards would be posted outside the doors to the Queen's apartments. Henry VIII was very sensitive about security, and any bed he slept in was always made up by his servants according to an elaborate ritual which involved a sword being thrust between the mattress and the feather bed, just in case an intruder had secreted himself there.

As queen, Katherine was more often than not an observer, rather than a participant, in the pageants and entertainments performed at court, even though she had in her teens been a good dancer. But dignity and gravity now sat heavily upon her in public, and probably in private also, and as she grew older, pageants and court balls lost their appeal. Nevertheless, she was always at Henry's side on state occasions or whenever foreign dignitaries visited the court. Indeed, we know very little else of her activities during the middle years of her marriage to the King; in the foreign dispatches and the chronicles of the period, she is very much a background figure, gracing these state occasions but doing little else of note.

Katherine was always an extremely popular queen, partly because her marriage had strengthened the vital commercial links between England and the Low Countries. This, however, was only one reason for the affection in which she was held. The main reason for it lay in her personal qualities, her unfailing graciousness and dignity, and her kindness. Not for nothing was it said of her that she was 'more beloved than any queen who ever reigned'. The English had taken her to their hearts; they rejoiced on her marriage, grieved with her in her sorrows, and – much later – were ready to champion her cause in the face of the King's displeasure.

Henry VIII established the first Renaissance court in England, using a large portion of his father's fortune to finance it and to refurbish the palaces in which it would be housed. The court in those days was a nomadic institution, moving between Greenwich, Richmond, Windsor, Westminster (until the royal apartments were destroyed in the fire of 1512), the Tower of London in the early years of the reign, Eltham Palace, Hampton Court after 1514 and a host of smaller palaces and manor houses. It comprised noblemen, churchmen of every degree, privy councillors, officers of the King's household, gentlemen of the Privy Chamber, the Queen's household, ladies, servants and menials, and could on occasions number several thousand people, especially when most of the aristocracy were in residence with their attendants.

It was a very splendid court; the King was extremely liberal, and enjoyed displaying the riches at his disposal. Following in his father's footsteps, he insisted on the observance of elaborate ceremonial on state occasions, though at other times he preferred to be more relaxed. Venetian envoys visiting the English court in 1515 were astonished at the lack of formality, and delighted when the King himself, while walking in the gardens, actually stopped under their windows and called up to them, then stayed there some time chatting and laughing with them, 'to our very great honour'. These same ambassadors reported to the Venetian Senate that the whole of Henry's court 'glittered with jewels and gold and silver, the pomp being unprecedented'. It was noticed that the Queen's ladies in particular were of 'sumptuous appearance', being very handsome.

Scholars, notably those from Italy, then the hub of European culture, were particularly welcome at the English court. The King wished to surround himself with learned men and bask in their reflected glory, preferring them – according to Erasmus – to the 'young men lost in luxury, or women, or gold-chained nobles'. Sir Thomas More applauded Henry VIII for cultivating all the 'liberal arts', and Erasmus thought that 'under such a King, it may not seem a court, but a temple of the Muses'. When Henry dined, he was attended by writers, divines, humanists, poets and artists, with whom he eagerly conversed and exchanged ideas.

One of the scholars who ranked highest in the King's estimation was Thomas More, a friend of Erasmus and a fellow humanist. A man of upright character with a gentle, dry wit, More was also a brilliant lawyer and well read in theology. In 1516, he published a book entitled *Utopia*, which described the ideal political state and earned him a generous measure of fame. He was also renowned for his exemplary family life and for his learned daughters, the products of his advanced views on female education. His eldest daughter, Margaret, the future wife of the Protestant writer William Roper, could speak both Latin and Greek. Henry and Katherine admired More, and the King invited him to court, though he only accepted with great reluctance, being unhappy about leaving the peace of his Chelsea home for public life; in later years, Henry would often throw up More's lack of enthusiasm for the court 'in a joke in my face'.

As he had feared, he hated it. 'I am as uncomfortable there as a bad rider is in the saddle,' he wrote. However, the King was 'so courteous and kindly' and did all in his power to make More welcome, singling him out for special friendship and showing he realised what a sacrifice More had made to humour him. 'I should not like to think that my presence had in any way interfered with your domestic pleasures,' he told him, intrigued by this rare, unworldly man who seemed content with his family, his books and his animals.

More's integrity, and his conservatism in matters of religion – he advocated the burning of heretics – appealed to Queen Katherine, and theirs was a friendship that would remain untarnished by events. 'He is an upright and learned man,' the Spanish ambassador would one day say of More, 'and a good servant of the Queen.' When the King and Queen dined privately, they would often send for Thomas More to be 'merry with them', and so much did they enjoy his company that, according to his son-in-law, William Roper, 'he could not once in a month get leave to go home to his wife and children'. The King would frequently summon More to his private study, where the two men would sit for hours discussing astronomy, geometry and divinity.

All of this brought its rewards, of course. In 1518, More was admitted to the Privy Council; three years later he was knighted. Yet he himself had few illusions about his standing at court. When William Roper congratulated his father-in-law on his advancement, More replied: 'Son Roper, I may tell you I have no cause to be proud thereof, for if my head would win the King a castle in France, it should not fail to go off!'

By 1517, Henry VIII's court had a magnificent reputation. 'The wealth and civilisation of the world are here,' enthused the Venetian ambassador; 'I here perceive very elegant manners, extreme decorum and great politeness.' Yet it all had to be paid for, and by 1518, Henry had dug so deep into the fortune left by his father to finance his pleasures and his court that his treasury was emptying at an alarming rate. This meant that for a time there would have to be fewer pageants, fewer tournaments, fewer entertainments than in earlier years. It is even possible that the King had grown a little bored with these things. He seems also to have got into bad company at this time, and whereas previously he had won praise for 'putting a silence on all brawlers', in 1519 he was attracting criticism for preferring the company of 'youths of evil counsel, intent on their own benefit, to the detriment, hurt and discredit of his Majesty' rather than seeking the society of 'demure, sober and sad' persons. In the eyes of many, these young bloods were bringing scandal on the throne by encouraging their young master to go amongst his people in disguise and behave in 'a foolish manner'. Their habits were scathingly described as 'French', and they were said to indulge in 'French vices'. They poked fun at 'all the estates of England, even the ladies and gentlemen of the court'. The King was for a time coming increasingly under their influence, and his Council was resolved to put an end to his associating with them. Fortunately, the Council prevailed, and Henry agreed to banish the offenders from court, having been convinced that his hitherto glorious reputation was at stake.

The court itself was an extravagant, wasteful institution. It moved from palace to palace so that each royal residence it had occupied could be cleansed. There were carpets on the floors of the royal apartments only; elsewhere there were rushes, which were anything but sweet-smelling when the court had been in residence for a few weeks. Gentlemen did not always bother to use the privies, which were primitive anyway; they sometimes urinated on the rushes, as did the many pets owned by the courtiers. The food waste from the kitchens mounted up; in the summer, it stank, and the stench from the privies on hot days was terrible indeed. Thus the court had to move on, so that the palace might be cleansed. This arrangement meant that a skeleton staff had to be maintained in all the palaces.

Cardinal Wolsey, the King's chief minister, was concerned about the way in which the royal household was run, and anxious to make economies, especially after the crippling of the Exchequer by the Field of Cloth of Gold in 1520, when the courts of England and France met amid scenes of unprecedented splendour. Thus, in 1526, after much research, the Cardinal drew up the Eltham Ordinances. The Ordinances, which were strictly enforced, rid the court of hangers-on and laid down rules of etiquette and practice, streamlining finances and cutting back on expenditure. Restrictions were placed on the number of retainers allowed those visiting the court, and also on the number of pets permitted (not only dogs but birds and monkeys were favoured by the courtiers); scullions were forbidden to go about the kitchens naked, and were given new clothes. The King's servants were to wear the Tudor livery of green and white at all times. Even the food was rationed, although fairly generously: from this time on, the Queen's maids would each breakfast on two small loaves and a gallon of ale. The result was a far more efficiently run household and a saving of both money and resources.

During the early years of the reign, when the young King and Queen passed their time in 'disports', there were hunts, tournaments, banquets, balls, sporting events, and 'disguisings'. The latter were elaborate masquerades in which the King and his gentlemen would dress up and disguise themselves – sometimes in the strange costumes of other lands – and then come upon the Queen and her ladies unawares, dance for her, or perform other scintillating feats, and then disclose their identity, 'whereat the Queen and her ladies were greatly amazed'. It afforded Henry great amusement to come thus attired upon Katherine and see her astonishment. It was a game of which, in his youth, he never tired; and she, for her part, never spoilt his pleasure by disclosing that she knew who it was, even when these 'disguisings' had been going on for several years.

But perhaps the most popular and spectacular of the entertainments staged for the pleasure of the Tudor court was the pageant, an early dramatic form. Pageants followed a set pattern: the male participants would enter the hall clad in matching costumes with a certain significance; then the ladies, in complementary attire, would emerge from a kind of stage on wheels, which could be made to resemble a castle, a forest, a mountain, the sea, or anything else that the King's Master of the Revels could devise. Pageants usually followed allegorical or classical themes, such as 'The Garden of Hope', or they could be based on English legends such as Robin Hood. When the ladies had appeared, the gentlemen would invariably show off their prowess in a mock fight, then the ladies would descend and dance with them as a reward. Often the participants were disguised. The King frequently took part in these pageants, partnering his sister Mary since the Queen preferred to watch rather than join in.

The pageants give us some idea of the opulence of the Tudor court: the materials used for the costumes were all of the richest quality, and purpose-made; the gold and jewels were all genuine. The King's intent was not entirely frivolous. Visiting princes, ambassadors, and other foreigners watching them would quickly gain the impression that the King of England was extremely wealthy and that his court was the most splendid in Christendom. Wealth and its trappings were evidence of political and military strength, and Henry used pageantry to build up the reputation of the Tudor monarchy in Europe.

The first pageant to be staged in Henry VIII's reign took place at Christmas 1509, when twelve men, dressed as Robin Hood and his Merry Men danced with the Queen's ladies in Katherine's chamber to the music of a consort of minstrels – Robin Hood later turned out to be the King in disguise. From then on, pageants were held whenever there was something to celebrate at court, and often when there was not. Sometimes the male dancers wore masks, which would be removed after the dancing by the ladies to the accompaniment of much laughter and flirtation.

The pageants to celebrate the birth of a son to Henry and

Katherine in 1511 were particularly elaborate: one took the form of 'a mountain glistening at night' with a golden tree adorned with Tudor roses and pomegranates. The celebrations for the birth of the prince continued for well over a month, culminating in the day when the palace doors were thrown open to the common people, so that they could watch the pageants. Unfortunately, matters got rather out of hand when they rushed into the hall and 'rent, tore and spoiled' the stage and its props. Pandemonium reigned as the courtiers ran for the shelter of the thrones on the dais, but the King was enjoying himself enormously, playing the role of a benevolent prince indulging his subjects. Laughing, he stood unresisting as they stripped him down to his hose and doublet, carrying off his clothes as souvenirs. The other courtiers had no choice but to follow their monarch's example, and they too were forced to suffer the indignity of losing their clothes and jewels; the unfortunate Sir Thomas Knyvet was stripped stark naked, and had to climb a pillar for safety! But when the mob began to despoil the ladies' costumes, the King called a halt. Fortunately, the people obeyed him, and the day ended in 'mirth and gladness', with Henry's popularity greater than ever.

Pageants were staged frequently during the early years of the King's reign. Perhaps the most original was that which took place on May Day 1515, for the benefit of the Venetian ambassadors, when Henry and Katherine, who was richly robed in the Spanish fashion, entertained their guests to a woodland picnic in Greenwich park, which had been made to resemble Robin Hood's hideout in Sherwood Forest. Henry and his nobles appeared dressed in Lincoln green as Robin and his men, and carried bows. Yet this was not a simple rustic idyll, for no detail had been left to chance: singing birds in cages had been hidden in the trees, and 'carolled most sweetly'; the court musicians sat in a bower, and the tables set beneath the trees groaned with a feast of gastronomic splendour; an archery contest took place for the visitors' entertainment. Afterwards, a procession formed and the May Queen and the court were brought back to the palace in triumphal cars adorned with figures of giants, escorted by the King's guard. Music played, courtiers sang, and the King and Queen brought up the rear with an estimated crowd of '25,000 persons' (a slight exaggeration, perhaps).

After 1518, there were fewer pageants, due to the depleted state of the King's finances and also to his growing preference for Italian masques. The last opulent court pageant of these years took place in May 1527, to celebrate a new treaty between England and France. On this occasion, a banqueting house was set up in the tiltyard at Greenwich, where the King and Queen sat under canopies of estate. A masque was performed first, after which a pageant in the form of an artificial mountain was performed in the great hall of the palace. One of the participants was the King's daughter, the Princess Mary, who, like her ladies, was dressed in Roman fashion with robes of 'cloth of gold, and so many precious stones that the splendour and radiance dazzled the sight'.

Masques differed from pageants in that there was more plot to them; whereas a pageant was merely a tableau with music and dancing, a masque incorporated a story, and was the forerunner of the modern musical. The first masque ever seen in England was performed at court in January 1512, and greatly impressed the King: in it, the participants were disguised by visors and caps of gold and told their tale with singing and dancing. In 1517, he and Katherine watched a masque entitled 'Troilus and Cryseide', based on an old tale made popular by Geoffrey Chaucer, at Eltham Palace as part of the Christmas festivities. After that masques were staged more frequently at court, and eventually replaced pageants as its chief form of dramatic entertainment.

Pageants and masques were often used to entertain foreign guests. Henry VIII always extended a magnificent welcome to visiting princes, ambassadors and churchmen, and was anxious to impress them with the splendour of his court. The Queen was always present, unless she was in an advanced state of pregnancy, and played her part as hostess, being particularly skilled at the courteous conversation required in diplomatic circles. In 1515, when she received the Venetian ambassadors, who had come to present to her the Doge's compliments, they spoke to her, they reported home, 'in good Spanish, which pleased her more than I can tell you'. Katherine spent some time discussing Spanish affairs with them, and was happy to share her memories of her mother, Queen Isabella.

Central to this lavish entertaining was the court banquet, the first of which took place in February 1510, when Henry and Katherine entertained all the foreign ambassadors then in England at the Palace of Westminster. The King led the Queen in procession into the great hall, followed by her ladies, the ambassadors, and all the nobility. Henry himself showed the ambassadors to their seats, then sat down beside Katherine at the high table on the dais, beneath the canopy of estate. However, he would not remain seated for long, for he was soon walking around the tables, chatting to his wife and guests. He then disappeared and came back wearing Turkish robes with a troupe of mummers in tow, who proceeded to perform for the assembled company.

The food at such banquets would have consisted of several courses, each with several dishes. Meat was served throughout the year, except in Lent, when fish was the main entrée. The meat or fish would be spiced and served in a sauce, and accompanied by bread soaked in gravy. There were few vegetables; however, Queen Katherine would sometimes have a salad in season, which she had introduced into England from Spain; her salad, however, would have been served hot, as raw vegetables were considered dangerous. Desserts were elaborate: fruit pies with decorated crusts, 'subtleties' of sugar resembling castles or coats of arms, and marchpane comfits. Wine flowed freely throughout the meal, as well as ale or mead for the lower tables. After the banquet had ended, the guests chatted as the tables were cleared for the pageant which usually followed. When the entertainment had ended, there was dancing for up to two hours, to the music of a consort of flute, harp, fife and violette, then spiced wine or hippocras was served, after which the King and Queen would retire to bed. Sometimes, the King himself would serve the food at a banquet, and at other times, when the Queen was heavily pregnant, he would bring the guests into her private apartments after dinner, to be entertained with music, conversation, 'disguisings' and dancing. Katherine never forgot to praise Henry's munificence on such occasions.

No effort was spared to make guests feel welcome. When Henry's sister, Queen Margaret of Scotland, visited London in 1515, Katherine sent a white palfrey to her for her state entry into the capital. The Queen of Scots had her own London residence at Scotland Yard near Westminster, but it was not ready for her, so Baynard's Castle was placed at her disposal. The King organised jousts in her honour, and a lavish banquet in the Queen's chamber at Greenwich.

In 1518 the French ambassadors were entertained to a banquet consisting of 260 dishes, followed by a 'very sumptuous' pageant. In 1519, Katherine herself hosted a banquet for the Duke of Longueville at her manor house at Havering-atte-Bower in Essex, a house once owned by several medieval queens. The King was present at this 'sumptuous' feast, which the Queen had arranged in 'the liberallest manner'. When it ended, Henry thanked her 'heartily', and the French guests were full of praise. Six weeks later Henry himself hosted a banquet at Newhall in Essex for these same envoys; afterwards, the Queen unmasked eight dancers, who all turned out to be 'somewhat aged; the youngest was at least fifty!' On the following day, Katherine again acted as hostess at yet another banquet.

Tournaments, too, were often staged in honour of specific events, and they could go on for some considerable time. One joust in November 1510 lasted for several days, during which 'the King broke more staves than any other'. In 1511, the Queen watched the jousts, held at Westminster to celebrate the birth of her son, from a pavilion hung with cloth of gold and purple velvet and embroidered with the letters 'H' and 'K' in fine gold. Her young husband appeared in the lists as 'Coeur Loyal' (Sir Loyal Heart), being her champion, and this device was emblazoned for all the world to see on his armour and his horse's accoutrements.

Thereafter, the King held tournaments frequently, being an active participant at every one. Usually they were staged in the spring, to celebrate May Day, but they also took place in winter and at other times of the year. Jousts were usually held 'in honour of the ladies', who often followed medieval tradition and gave their favours to their chosen knights. At one joust, Queen Katherine and her ladies received the men's jousting apparel as 'largesse'. In December 1524, the Queen took part in a pageant that heralded the commencement of a tournament at Greenwich, sitting in a prefabricated castle in the tiltyard. Two elderly knights then appeared and craved her leave 'to break spears'; however, when Katherine 'praised their courage' and gave her consent, they threw off their robes to reveal a laughing Henry and his friend and brother-in-law, the Duke of Suffolk.

Tournaments took place mainly in the spring, Easter was spent at Windsor, followed by the feast of St George with its attendant Garter ceremonies, then there were more jousts on May Day. In the autumn came the King's customary progress, which combined a break from court routine with the opportunity to see his realm and meet his subjects, as well as to avail himself of the hunting to be had in other parts. In 1511, the King and Queen made the first of these progresses, visiting the West Midlands, where they saw 'a goodly stage play', a mystery play performed by guildsmen at Coventry.

The annual routine of the court culminated in the twelve days of merrymaking that constituted a Tudor Christmas. Henry VIII usually kept the festival at Greenwich Palace. Christmas Day itself was then a holy day, devoted to acts of worship, but the days after it were given over to feasting and 'disports', the King celebrating Christ's birth with 'much nobleness and open court'. The festivities reached their climax on Twelfth Night, the Feast of the Epiphany, when they were usually brought to an end with a sumptuous banquet.

Gifts were exchangd on New Year's Day, not on Christmas Day. On New Year's Day 1510, Katherine's first Yuletide gift from Henry was a beautifully illuminated missal inscribed in his own hand: 'If your remembrance be according to my affection, I shall not be forgotten in your daily prayers, for I am yours, Henry R., forever.' Touched by this, Katherine immediately added a further inscription of her own beneath: 'By daily proof you shall me find to be to you both loving and kind.'

At Christmas, the court was usually thrown open to the public, who were allowed in to watch the 'goodly and gorgeous mummeries'; festive fare was distributed, boar's head and roast peacock served in its feathers being the chief meats at this season. There were pageants, disguisings and feasts, and carols danced and sung in the great hall while the Yule log crackled on the hearth, 'to the great rejoicing of the Queen and the nobles'.

Unusually at Christmas 1517, the court was closed, but there was a very good reason for it. Plague was a notorious killer, and during an epidemic drastic measures had to be taken to avoid the spread of infection, for it was no respecter of persons. And plague struck often, particularly in sixteenth-century summers. The plague that had hit London in the July of 1517 was of a type known to be extremely deadly – the sweating sickness, a scourge prevalent only in Tudor times, having first appeared in England in 1485; some saw it as a judgement of God upon the usurping dynasty.

Illness in any form horrified and disgusted Henry VIII, but the sweating sickness reduced him to a state of abject fear. It was a loathsome disease: the victim would suddenly feel unwell, break out into a profuse sweat, and continue to sweat until a crisis was reached, at which point death usually occurred. This could happen with frightening speed, taking only three to four hours from first symptoms to last breath. Recovery was rare, and those that did recover were often weakened for life. Above all, the sweating sickness was highly infectious, and spread with terrifying rapidity.

At the first sign of plague in July, the King had given orders for the court to leave the capital and move into the country, which he much preferred anyway, leaving behind him strict instructions that those people who had been in contact with the disease were under no circumstances to approach him. There were fears for a time that Queen Katherine had contracted the dreaded plague, as she complained of feeling unwell for a few days, though she soon recovered. By September, the plague was spreading further still, and the death toll was rising. Henry, fearful for the succession, as he still had no son to succeed him, and petrified of catching the disease, took himself and the Queen, with only a few attendants, off to a 'remote and unusual habitation' that has not been identified, and there he remained, whilst the sweating sickness continued to ravage his kingdom. By December, however, it was on the wane, although it was deemed prudent of the King to keep 'no solemn Christmas' that year because there was still some risk of infection.

As well as presiding over a glittering, cultivated court, Katherine of Aragon also administered her own household. This numbered some 160 persons, many of them Spaniards who had come to England with her in 1501. There were also some English officers and servants in her entourage, because the King preferred her to be served by English people, and on her marriage several members of her former household had returned to Spain, including the chamberlain, Juan de Diero. This was not so much the King's doing as the Queen's, for many of those dismissed her service at that point had in the days of her widowhood grown insolent, not treating her with the respect she should have been shown. Nevertheless, at Katherine's command they were all paid the arrears of salary due to them, though she did ask her father to administer a mild rebuke in certain cases.

After her marriage to the King, the chief officer in the Queen's household was Lord Mountjoy, the celebrated humanist, who became her chamberlain. The King was indulgent enough to allow her to retain most of her Spanish ladies, although they were now supplemented by the wives of some of the great English nobles. Katherine had grown very attached to a number of her Spanish attendants, several of whom would remain with her until she died, but the one she favoured the most, 'whom she loves more than any other mortal', was Maria de Salinas, who had once been a maid of honour to Queen Isabella. Maria was the daughter of a Castilian grandee, Don Martin de Salinas, by Doña Josepha Gonzalez de Salas. She had come to England with Katherine in 1501, and the two girls had quickly struck up a lasting friendship, which was cemented by sharing the enforced privations of Katherine's long widowhood. In 1509 Katherine told her new husband that she wished to keep Maria as 'the girl desires of all things to remain with me'. Henry VIII agreed to Maria staying on, and never resented the influence she had upon his wife, who treated her as her chief confidante.

In 1516, Maria de Salinas became a naturalised subject of the King of England as a preliminary to her marriage in June that year to William, Lord Willoughby d'Eresby, who had been courting her for some time. After her wedding, she left the court, but it was gratifying for the Queen to know that her friend, whose earlier betrothal had been broken because she could not give the girl a dowry, had at last made a good marriage. The Queen may have attended the christening of Maria's son Henry in 1517, and it is probable that she was godmother to the daughter born two years later and named Katherine in her honour. Sadly, Lord Willoughby died in 1526, leaving his widow with two young children to rear. She was still close to the Queen, and probably visited Katherine at court during her widowhood. Later still, she would brave the King's wrath for the sake of her friendship with the Queen.

When Maria de Salinas left court upon her marriage, Katherine turned to another lady with whom she had formed a close friendship, Margaret Pole, the niece of Edward IV and Richard III, and, some said, the rightful heiress of the Plantagenets. In 1513 the King had restored to Margaret Pole part of the inheritance forfeited under the Act of Attainder passed on her father the Duke of Clarence in 1478, prior to his death in the Tower – by drowning in a butt of malmsey, it was said. Henry obviously had no reservations about Margaret Pole's loyalty to the Crown at that point, for he created her Countess of Salisbury, a title she should have inherited in 1499 on the execution of her brother, the Earl of Warwick. Katherine had always felt a sense of guilt because Warwick's death had paved the way for her coming to England, and she had singled out his sister for special friendship. This was warmly reciprocated, and in later years the two women would cherish a shared hope that their children would marry and thus further cement the bond between Tudor and Plantagenet.

In 1513, Margaret Pole was forty, and had been a widow since 1505. She had several children, of whom the most gifted was Reginald Pole, who also benefitted from the King's generosity when Henry arranged for, and funded out of his own privy purse, the boy's education at Oxford, where Reginald justified the faith of his royal patron by obtaining an honours degree after only two years of study. His mother was a learned woman, whose erudition was much respected by the Queen, and, in later years, Katherine would choose Lady Salisbury as her daughter Mary's state governess, knowing that her many qualities made her eminently suitable for such a post.

In 1513, Katherine had to enlist the aid of the King's chief minister Thomas Wolsey when she wished to rid herself of a former lady-in-waiting, Francesca de Caceres, who had been in her entourage prior to her marriage to the King, and was now asking to be readmitted to her service. Francesca had once intrigued with Fuensalida to get rid of Fray Diego, and had been privy to most of Fuensalida's information about the time when Katherine had foolishly succumbed, to whatever degree, to the charms of the friar. Much of what Francesca knew was mere supposition, but the Queen felt that nevertheless it would be 'perilous and dangerous' to employ her, or even to send her abroad with a reference recommending her to a foreign princess. She dared not risk having her former maid of honour gossiping about that unhappy episode with Fray Diego at foreign courts. Happily, Wolsey, who was probably unaware of the real reason for the Queen's concern, arranged for Francesca to return to Spain, where she could do least harm.

Fray Diego himself remained in the Queen's service for five years after her marriage to the King. 'I hope to keep him all the time I shall be able,' she told her father. However, it was not long before he began to cause trouble once more. He did not trust Ferdinand's ambassador, Luis Caroz, believing that Caroz had come to England with the prime objective of having him removed from the court. As a result, though he behaved towards the ambassador with elaborate courtesy, he did not deceive Caroz, who rightly deduced that the friar was 'very suspicious and fearful of me'. Undoubtedly, he concluded, 'his mind is not quite right.'

Fray Diego still retained considerable influence over the Queen, but this was nowadays confined mainly to spiritual matters. However, he kept her 'engaged' to such an extent that it was difficult for Caroz and others to obtain an audience with her and, so the friar believed, criticise him to her face. Lesser members of her new household went in fear of Fray Diego, and dared not cross him, as they knew he could have them dismissed if he so pleased. Caroz saw what was going on, and informed Ferdinand's secretary of state that he had 'never seen a more wicked person in my life'. He had tried to warn the Queen about him, he said, but Katherine would not listen.

This state of affairs continued until 1514, when several members of the Queen's household went to the King with complaints about Fray Diego, accusing him of fornicating with women of the court. Henry at once confronted the friar, and warned him that such behaviour would not be tolerated in one so close to the Queen. Fray Diego was highly indignant: 'If I am badly used, the Queen is still more badly used!' he retorted, pointedly referring to Henry's latest mistress. At this, the King's anger erupted, and it was not long before the friar was summarily dismissed from the Queen's service and ordered to return to Spain. Shocked and angry, he left in November, but not before he had written a letter to the King, reminding him how he had served Katherine faithfully for seven years, 'enduring evil for her sake, even lack of meat and drink, of clothes and fire'. He swore he was no fornicator: 'Never, within your kingdom, have I had to do with women.' He had been 'condemned unheard', and those who had accused him were 'disreputable rogues'. But Henry was implacable, and the friar's protestations only served to confirm his belief that Fray Diego was a liar as well as a womaniser.

As for the Queen, she lifted no finger to save her confessor. She too must have been shocked by what she had heard about him, and her submission to the King's will was absolute; from henceforth she would suffer no man but her husband to rule her.

6

A chaste and concordant wedlock

On Friday, 22 June 1509, the King and Queen went by royal barge from Greenwich to the Tower of London, where custom decreed the King must spend the night before his coronation. Henry had ordered the refurbishment of the old royal apartments in the Norman keep, and here, that same afternoon, he created twenty-four Knights of the Bath. On the following morning, the grand procession formed within the Tower precincts. Henry rode on horseback, Katherine in a litter through cheering crowds via Cheapside, Temple Bar and the Strand to the Palace of Westminster, through streets hung with rich tapestries, where on every corner stood priests swinging censers.

Crowds had turned out to see them, Henry in a robe of crimson velvet trimmed with ermine over a coat of 'raised gold', which was embroidered with diamonds, rubies, emeralds, great pearls and other rich stones, and Katherine in virginal white satin. At Westminster, there was a lavish banquet, after which the King and Queen retired to the chapel of St Stephen to pray.

The 24th of June was midsummer day. A long scarlet runner had been laid from the Palace doors to the great west door of the Abbey of Westminster and, at the appointed time, the King and Queen went in procession along it, Henry walking beneath a canopy of estate borne by the five barons of the Cinque Ports, and Katherine riding in a litter of rich cloth drawn by two white palfreys. She was dressed like a bride, in an embroidered gown of white satin, with her hair – 'of a very great length, beautiful and goodly to behold' – falling loose down her back beneath a coronet set 'with many rich Orient stones'. Her officers and ladies followed her, in chariots and on palfreys. 'There were few women who could compete with the Queen in her prime,' wrote Sir Thomas More, many years later. Katherine might have been past her first youth by Tudor standards, yet marriage, and the knowledge that the King loved her, had enhanced her buxom charm and her still-pretty face.

The coronation ritual followed the form laid down by St Dunstan in AD 973, which in turn had been modelled on the ceremony devised for Charlemagne in AD 800. Now it was the turn of Henry VIII to sit in Edward I's coronation chair and receive the Crown of St Edward the Confessor, whose shrine lay only a few feet away in the Abbey; and when he had been accepted and acclaimed as England's King by the assembled lords spiritual and temporal, and due homage had been paid by all who owed him fealty, Queen Katherine received from the Archbishop of Canterbury the smaller crown of the Queen Consorts of England. For her, this was a sacred moment in which she would dedicate her life to God and to the service of her husband's realm.

Outside the Abbey, however, behaviour was anything but sacred, for the crowds had descended like vultures upon the scarlet runner along which the King had walked and ripped it to shreds, each person carrying off a piece as a souvenir of the day. So elated were the King and Queen when they at last emerged from the Abbey that they did not notice its removal, and proceeded to Westminster Hall to the acclaim of the crowds. There, in the vaulted edifice built by William Rufus and beautified by Richard II, Henry and Katherine sat down to their coronation banquet, where 'sumptuous, fine and delicate' food was served in abundance. Half-way through the proceedings, the King's champion entered and dared anyone to challenge his master's right to the throne. There was, of course, no response, and the champion was presented with a golden cup before he withdrew. This little ceremony had been performed at coronation banquets since the early Middle Ages, and always provided excitement at what was usually a very long and ceremonious occasion.

Several days of celebrations followed the coronation, with

tournaments in the gardens of the old Palace of Westminster, where a timber pavilion had been erected so that the King and Queen could watch the proceedings in comfort. There were pageants and banquets, all paid for out of the vast wealth that Henry VIII had inherited from his father. Queen Katherine was present at every festivity, and presided over the jousts with her ladies in true courtly fashion. To some extent she shared Henry's love of hunting, and was not squeamish about it. When the bloody bodies of deer killed in a hunting pageant were laid at her feet as trophies, the Queen did not flinch at the sight, but thanked the hunters and commanded that the venison be served at yet another court banquet. Blood sports were a pleasurable way of providing entertainment as well as meat for the table.

Henry VIII spoke openly of the 'joy and felicity' he had found with Katherine. According to Fray Diego, he adored her, and she him. Yet his love for her was no grand passion; it epitomised rather all his ideals about women and chivalry. Throughout their marriage, he would treat Katherine with the respect due to his wife and queen, and with genuine affection, long after love and desire had died. Her gratitude for his rescue of her from penury and humiliation was flattering to his highly inflated ego, which was further gratified by her submissiveness. She happily conceded that Henry was intellectually her superior, and deferred to him accordingly, as a wife was expected to. This, to Henry, was a most satisfactory state of affairs, and he congratulated himself on having chosen such an amiable bride. Because he was young and inexperienced, he did not perceive the steel beneath the meek exterior, and he certainly underestimated Katherine's tenacity. It is possible that he regarded Katherine almost as a mother figure. The loss of his own mother when he was eleven had affected him deeply, and Katherine, to a degree, was a substitute. She was older than he, more mature, and was always ready with advice when he needed it, and sometimes when he did not.

Katherine herself had always been solemn, with a gravity beyond her years, but for a time now her Spanish training was forgotten and she was able to laugh with the pure happiness of being in love with her young husband and free at last from care. She was, according to her confessor, Fray Diego, 'in high health, with the greatest gaiety and contentment that ever there was'. Gone were her traumatic ailments, gone her depression. She was rational enough in love to realise that Henry was in many ways immature, and sensible enough not to let him know it. She seems to have had a good insight into the youthful mind of the King, and common sense cautioned her to treat him with due respect. This came naturally from years of long training, and it was not difficult, for she was in love.

Henry wrote to Ferdinand that summer: 'My wife and I be in good and perfect love as any two creatures can be,' and Katherine also wrote to her father, thanking him for seeing her 'so well married' to a husband she loved 'so much more than myself'. Ferdinand answered that he 'rejoiced to find you love each other so supremely, and hope you may be happy to the end of your life; a good marriage being not only for the blessing of the man and woman who take each other, but also to the world outside.' It must have seemed to Katherine that her marriage was built upon a sure foundation of love, respect, desire and good political sense. How could it fail to succeed?

Within a year, however, matters were to deteriorate significantly.

In August 1509, Katherine informed the King with delight that she was to bear a child in the spring. In November, the baby stirred for the first time, and a proud Henry informed King Ferdinand of the fact, to signify to him 'the great joy thereat that we take, and the exultation of our whole realm'. The public announcement of the Queen's pregnancy had given rise to great rejoicing in England, for the birth of an heir to the throne would stabilise the dynasty and remove the ever present threat of civil war.

The court was in residence in Henry VIII's great gothic palace at Westminster when, on 31 January 1510, the Queen went into labour prematurely. Her infant, a daughter, was stillborn, which, although considered a calamity, was not an uncommon misfortune with first babies at that time. But Katherine suffered a strong sense of failure, compounded by guilt, because 'she had desired to gladden the King and the people with a Prince'. Henry, however, was philosophical, but even his reassurances and attempts to comfort his wife were to little avail, for she was profoundly shaken by her loss and remained depressed for several weeks, tormented by irrational feelings of guilt. When she wrote to break the news to her father, she begged him: 'Do not storm against me. It is not my fault, it is the will of God. The King, my lord, took it cheerfully, and I thank God that you have given me such a husband.' Again, she repeated, as if to reassure herself, 'It is the will of God.'

The King wasted no time in fathering another child, believing that it was the only thing that would cure Katherine of her depression, and in May 1510, Fray Diego was able to inform King Ferdinand that 'it has pleased our Lord to be her physician, and by His infinite mercy He has again permitted her to be with child'. She was already 'very large', which indicates that the baby was almost certainly conceived during February and that Katherine was one of those women who 'shows' early. The friar hoped this would be 'the beginning of a hundred grandsons' for King Ferdinand.

There are hints in diplomatic records that the young King had been pursuing other women at the time of his accession; whether these adventures continued after his marriage is not recorded, but in 1510, when Katherine was pregnant with her second child, Henry strayed. He had become a complacent husband, secure in his wife's devotion, and Katherine had changed from a young woman 'who cannot be without novelties' into a grave, sedate matron, who had to adjust to a second pregnancy coming hard on the heels of the first. Henry felt he had done his duty by the Queen, and now he was going to enjoy himself. By the standards of his day, his attitude was not unusual.

Henry's first known mistress was his second cousin Lady Elizabeth FitzWalter, sister of the Duke of Buckingham. In her late twenties, she had recently arrived at court with her sister, Lady Anne Herbert. The King immediately pursued her, while his friend, Sir William Compton (who had been close to Henry since being appointed a royal page in 1493) provided a front for his master by pretending to carry on an intrigue with Lady Elizabeth himself. Thus, for a time, Henry was able to make love to his mistress in secrecy.

It was not long, however, before Lady Anne noticed the attention Compton was paying to her sister, who was after all a married woman; in some agitation Lady Anne called a family conference, at which she confided her suspicions to her brother the Duke and to Sir Robert FitzWalter, Elizabeth's husband. As a result, a furious row broke out between the Duke and Compton when the Duke shortly afterwards found Compton in his sister's rooms at court. Buckingham used 'many hard words' and 'severely reproached' Compton, who slunk off to the King and warned him what was happening. Henry, in a simmering rage at the prospect of being deprived of his pleasures, summoned Buckingham and reprimanded the Duke angrily, whereupon Buckingham left the court in a fury. Meanwhile, Lady Elizabeth had confessed to her incensed husband the truth of the matter, and had been forcibly removed by him from the court and immured in a convent sixty miles away. By then, the real identity of her lover was known to the whole Stafford family, Lady Anne included.

Deprived of his mistress, Henry VIII cast his eye about to see where blame could be laid, and guessed that the prime mover in the matter had been Lady Anne Herbert, whom he knew to be one of the Queen's closest friends. Exacting revenge, he banished Lady Anne and her husband from the court, and had a mind to turn out a lot of other ladies also, believing that they had been set by Lady Anne to spy on him. However, he could not quite face the scandal such drastic action would give rise to and, moreover, the worst had already happened: someone, probably Lady Anne, had told the Queen. This resulted in a stormy confrontation between husband and wife, in which Katherine reproached Henry for his infidelity, and he upbraided her for daring to censure him for it. They both ended up 'very vexed' with each other, and the whole court knew it.

Luis Caroz, the Spanish ambassador, feared that Katherine might prejudice her considerable influence with the King by being so openly hostile about what was, after all, a common failing amongst men of rank whose marriages were arranged for them. Yet, to Caroz's dismay, she continued to berate Henry for betraying her, and made matters worse by her evident ill will towards Compton. She was now suffering as countless other queens before her had suffered, having found themselves neglected for the less dignified charms of the ladies of the court, and although she was behaving badly, she could not help herself. The honeymoon was undoubtedly over, and Katherine was shattered by the realisation.

Henry himself could not see what all the fuss was about. In fact, he saw himself as the injured party, Katherine having dared to challenge his right to do as he pleased. He had been discreet, had not intended publicly to humiliate her, and he felt he was being unfairly treated. Of course, in the end, Katherine capitulated, and faced the fact that it was a wife's duty to turn a blind eye to her husband's extra-marital affairs. The onus was on her to adapt to circumstances. It was a hard lesson to learn, but she learnt it well. Never again would she publicly call Henry to account for his behaviour, even under the most extreme provocation. She had emerged from this affair without dignity or pride – even her friend Caroz had criticised her behaviour. Now she resolved to accept what could not be altered with as much grace as she could muster, and on the surface the relationship between the royal couple reverted to its former happy state. It would never, however, be quite the same.

Late in 1510, the Queen 'took to her chamber' at Richmond in readiness for the birth of her baby. Strict regulations, laid down by the Lady Margaret Beaufort in the preceding reign, governed the correct procedures to be observed when a queen was confined. The appointed chamber must be hung with tapestries which covered the walls, ceiling, windows and doors, and these tapestries must depict scenes of light romance only, so that neither the Queen nor the newborn infant should be 'affrighted by figures which gloomily stare'. Fresh air was not considered necessary, indeed it was thought to be dangerous, but one window was left uncovered to admit light to the chamber.

The rich tester bed in which the royal infant was to be born was truly magnificent. It was made up with sheets of fine lawn, a counterpane of scarlet velvet edged with ermine and a border of cloth of gold, with curtains and hangings of crimson satin embroidered with crowns of gold and the Queen's coat of arms. Four silver damask cushions were provided for the royal head to rest upon. When her labour was over, the Queen would put on a circular mantle of crimson velvet trimmed with ermine, in which she would receive visitors while still in bed.

Men were not admitted to the Queen's presence during the last weeks of her pregnancy; even the King stayed away. Her chamberlain, Lord Mountjoy, arranged for the duties of all male officers within her household to be taken over by her ladies and gentlewomen, who became, for a few weeks, 'butlers, servers and pages', receiving all 'needful things' at the door to the Queen's apartments. When the Queen 'took to her chamber', she bade her chamberlain and other male retainers a formal farewell, and Mountjoy in return desired all her people, in her name, to pray 'that God would send her a good hour'.

Katherine's labour began on 31 December 1510, and on New Year's Day 1511, she was at last 'delivered of a Prince, to the great gladness of the realm'. In honour of the occasion, a jubilant Henry ordered beacons to be lit in London and the distribution of free wine to the citizens. Churchmen went in procession through the streets, and in the churches the *Te Deum* was sung. The child was given his father's name, Henry.

The little Prince was christened at Richmond before he was a week old, his godparents being the Archbishop of Canterbury, the Earl of Surrey, and the Countess of Devon, who was the daughter of Edward IV and the King's aunt. Katherine's happiness was now complete, for she had done her duty by providing England with an heir, and the King could not do enough to honour or praise her. Messages of congratulation were arriving hourly at the palace, and in the streets, people were chanting, 'Long live Katherine and the noble Henry! Long live the Prince!' After the birth, Henry went to the shrine of our Lady of Walsingham, the special patron of mothers and babies, to give thanks for his boy, and, on his return, the court moved to Westminster. Katherine had now been churched and had resumed public life; her child had been left at Richmond in the care of nurses, and if this caused her any qualms she did not show it, but immersed herself wholeheartedly in the celebrations arranged by the King in honour of his son's birth.

Then tragedy struck, and the festivities were brought to an abrupt halt when the King and Queen were informed that the little prince had died on 22 February at Richmond. The chronicler Edward Hall says that Henry, 'like a wise Prince', was deeply grieved yet still philosophical; his concern was mainly for Katherine, who, 'like a natural woman', was devastated by the news and 'made much lamentation'. However, her husband comforted her 'wondrous wisely', and in time she came to accept the death of her baby as the will of God. The King 'made no great mourning outwardly', but spent a lavish sum on a funeral for Prince Henry, who was buried in Westminster Abbey, and the daily routine of the court was very quiet for the next two months, during which time Katherine remained mostly in seclusion, regretting no doubt that she had spent so little time with her child during his short life, and also facing up to the fact that England still needed an heir. In September that year she was rumoured to be pregnant again, but nothing more is heard of it, and it may have been a false hope.

By 1511, there was a new power in the ascendant at court. Thomas Wolsey was then thirty-six, and had been born the son of an Ipswich butcher. He had had the good fortune to be educated at Oxford, and after that had taken holy orders, becoming chaplain to Henry VII in 1507, and Dean of Lincoln in 1509. When Henry VII died, Wolsey, ever industrious in his own interests, had quickly ingratiated himself with Henry VIII, proving his abilities by sheer hard work and well-timed, sound advice. The young King liked this affable cleric, and by 1511 Wolsey was already enjoying considerable influence, besides being honoured with the friendship of the King, who was coming increasingly to rely upon him. Wolsey would shoulder the matters of state that Henry hated, and never let the King guess that it was Wolsey, and not Henry Tudor, who was, in effect, taking over the government of England. Yet this was what happened, with Wolsey becoming the real power behind the throne to a greater degree as the years passed, while his young master rode in the lists, planned glorious but impractical campaigns, and wrote love songs.

Wolsey was resented at court by the older nobility, who were jealous of his power which they felt should be theirs by right; nor did his increasingly lavish lifestyle endear him to his colleagues. The King's favour had brought with it a string of lucrative honours: Wolsey was made Bishop of Lincoln, and then Archbishop of York, in 1514, and in 1515 the Pope made him a cardinal. He was then supporting a household that rivalled that of his master for luxury, and he had his own palace, Hampton Court, built in 1514 on the site of an old priory by the Thames. When completed, it far exceeded any of the King's palaces for luxury and grandeur. Wolsey's private rooms were lined with linenfold panelling and wall paintings by Italian masters, and his ceilings were carved, moulded and painted in gold leaf. There was space for thousands of retainers. Wolsey could well afford such extravagance, for the King had been generous to him on a grand scale. By 1515 he was virtually running the country; the King was content to leave everything to the capable

Cardinal, who was the most powerful man in England after himself. At Christmas 1515, Wolsey was appointed Lord Chancellor of England, an office he would hold for the next fourteen years, and in 1518, the Pope made him Papal Legate in England.

Katherine of Aragon did not like or trust Wolsey for several reasons. She felt that he was ousting her from her rightful place in the King's counsels, and she thought him insincere and lacking in the humility desirable in a prince of the Church. She also deplored his pro-French foreign policies, and the fact that he was working against the interests of Spain. In fact, after 1521, the Cardinal became ever more antagonistic towards Spain, because the Emperor had lifted not a finger to help Wolsey achieve his greatest ambition, that of being Pope; there had been two papal elections in 1521, and Wolsey – a candidate at both – had been overlooked, which he blamed upon Charles V's influence.

As the years went by, Wolsey's arrogance grew as, simultaneously, did his unpopularity. There was criticism from both nobility and commons, some of it calculated to make the King jealous. For a time, Henry resisted: Wolsey was an able and efficient statesman, whose grasp of European affairs was second to none. But, by 1526, heavy hints about the Cardinal's excessive power and riches were beginning to have an effect, and the King started to make meaningful comments about how much richer than his sovereign he was. Wolsey, seeing that some sacrifice was expedient, took the hint, and promptly surrendered to the King the deeds of Hampton Court. It was a magnificent gesture that had the desired effect and, through it, the Cardinal hoped to reap greater benefits in the future. Besides, he did have another residence, York Place by Westminster, the London house of the Archbishops of York, which had been refurbished by him to almost the same degree of luxury as Hampton Court.

From the first, Katherine of Aragon was mindful of the fact that she was in England to represent her father's interests, and in the early days of their marriage her influence over the young Henry VIII was very strong indeed. Henry would do nothing without her approval; even when it came to matters of state, he would say to his councillors, or to visiting ambassadors, 'The Queen must hear this,' or 'This will please the Queen.' And his advisers, dismayed though they were at their master's reliance on his foreign wife's judgement, were powerless to do anything about it. Nevertheless, there was a good deal of head shaking and muttering that, at this rate, England would shortly be ruled at one remove by Spain.

This, of course, was what Ferdinand of Aragon intended should happen, and he was duly gratified when Katherine spoke of her husband as being 'the true son of your Highness, with desire of greater obedience and love to serve you than ever son had to his father'. She would have done well at this stage to have studied the example of certain queen consorts in the past, who had put the interests of their own families before those of the kingdom into which they had married. Such queens had at best courted vilification, and at worst been suspected of treason. Already the King's councillors were complaining about the extent of the Queen's influence, and they had cause, for Katherine, reared to obey her father in every respect, and not really understanding the attitude of the English towards foreign interference in their politics, saw nothing amiss with manipulating Henry. 'These kingdoms of your Highness,' she wrote to Ferdinand, forgetting that her husband owed no allegiance whatsoever to his father-in-law, 'are in great peace, and entertain much love towards the King my lord and me. His Highness and I are very hearty towards the service of your Highness.'

It was easy to foresee, as Henry's councillors did, that the Queen would soon be prevailing upon the King to favour Spain's interests above those of England; already she viewed her husband's realm as an extension of her father's, and never ceased reminding the King of the virtues of King Ferdinand, whom he was coming to regard as the fount of all wisdom. Henry would take no step without first discussing it with Katherine, Katherine would not approve anything without her father's sanction, and unfortunately Henry was too inexperienced to realise what was happening.

With her father's warm approval, Katherine set about turning Henry's mind against France, the traditional enemy of England and Spain. This was not difficult; Henry detested the French anyway, and was intent on making war on France in the not too distant future, the conquest of that realm and the fulfilment of England's ancient claims to its throne being his ultimate goal. In November

1511, Ferdinand's scheming, and Katherine's, reached a successful conclusion with the signing of the Treaty of Westminster, whereby Henry and Ferdinand pledged to help each other against France, their mutual enemy. Katherine had done her work well, and Ferdinand was proud of her.

Henry VIII sent an army under Lord Dorset into France in 1512, but the campaign ended in inglorious failure. It was therefore relatively easy for Katherine to persuade the King to mount a second campaign in 1513, which he would lead himself. By doing this, the Queen was rendering a signal service to her father, who was also planning to take the offensive against the French. Henry was excited and enthusiastic about the coming campaign, even though his councillors tried to talk him out of it. As the Venetian ambassador put it, 'the King is bent on war, the Council is averse to it; the Queen will have it, and the wisest councillors in England cannot stand against the Queen.' Katherine had assured Henry of the full co-operation of his allies, King Ferdinand and the Emperor Maximilian, and Henry seems to have persuaded himself that those two wily old self-seekers would support him in his bid to take the French throne. For the young King the glorious adventure was about to begin, and he saw himself returning victorious from his righteous war, crowned with laurel wreaths and the ultimate prize, the crown of France.

By June 1513, all was ready for the King's departure. Katherine was to be Regent in his absence, and due precautions had been taken to guard the northern border against an attack by the unpredictable Scots, France's traditional allies. At last, on 30 June, Henry rode from London to Dover at the head of 11,000 men, with Katherine by his side. In Dover Castle, he formally invested his wife with the regency, and commanded the Archbishop of Canterbury and the seventy-year-old veteran Thomas Howard, Earl of Surrey, to act as her advisers. The Earl was to escort the Queen back to London and then travel north to be at hand in the event of trouble with the Scots. Katherine cried when the King bade her farewell, being fearful for his safety, but Surrey gallantly comforted her on the ride back to London, and she rose to the occasion with courage, remembering that, if only for a short while, she was now the effective custodian of her husband's kingdom.

Henry and his magnificent fighting force created a sensation when they arrived in France – 'you will never have seen anything so gorgeous!', reported an imperial envoy. Yet, in reality, his presence was anything but welcome to Ferdinand and Maximilian when they discovered that his ultimate purpose was to depose Louis XII and have himself crowned King of France. Alarmed, they resolved to pack him off home as soon as possible, and wasted no time in drawing up a secret treaty with Louis XII whereby the young King of England would be permitted one or two inconsequential victories, which would hopefully satisfy his craving for military glory before the advent of winter forced him to return to England. On 24 July, Henry and Maximilian laid siege to the town of Thérouanne, and on 16 August an Anglo-Imperial army routed the French at what became known as the Battle of the Spurs, so called because the French army took one look at the superior forces of England and the Empire and fled. It was not a decisive victory, but it sufficed for the present.

Wolsey, who had gone with the King to France, had arranged to keep the Queen regularly informed of Henry's progress, but letters were sometimes held up, and then her fears grew. 'I shall be never in rest until I see letters from you,' she wrote to Henry. Accounts of the risks he was taking filled her with alarm, especially when she learned that he insisted on being present in the ranks before Thérouanne, well within range of enemy cannon, and she begged Wolsey to remind the King 'to avoid all manner of dangers'. As for herself, she was 'encumbered' with matters arising from the war. 'My heart is very good to it,' declared the daughter of Ferdinand and Isabella, 'and I am horribly busy with making standards, banners and badges.'

Not all of these were destined for France, for in the midst of this activity, news reached Katherine at Richmond that the Scots were planning an invasion of England, and were mobilising their forces. Not for nothing was Katherine her mother's daughter, and she threw herself with courage and zeal into preparations for defence, informing Wolsey that the King's subjects were 'very glad, I thank God, to be busy with the Scots'. On 22 August, the 80,000-strong army of Henry VIII's brother-in-law, the 'false and perjured' James IV, invaded England, advancing into Northumberland. At the same time, an English force led by the Earl of Surrey was moving north to meet them.

Three days later, the Queen received news of the fall of Thérouanne to Henry VIII and the King's triumphant entry into the town; immediately, she dashed off a letter of congratulation, opining that 'the victory hath been so great that I think none such hath been seen before. All England hath cause to thank God for it, and I specially.' In early September the Queen travelled north to Buckingham, where she would await news from Surrey. Here she made a speech to the reserve forces camped outside the town, urging them to victory in a just cause. But there was to be no need for their services, for on Friday, 9 September 1513, the Earl of Surrey scored a resounding victory over the Scots at the Battle of Flodden, one of the bloodiest combats ever seen in Britain, and at the end of the day, ten thousand Scotsmen lay dead on the moor, among them their King and the flower of his nobility. Scotland would now be ruled by a council of regency, for the new King, James V, was only a baby; the war with England would of necessity have to be shelved.

The impact of Flodden and its consequences was immediately felt in England. Surrey wrote at once to the Queen, informing her of the victory, and sent her James's banner and the bloody coat he had died in as trophies; Katherine duly sent them on to Henry by a herald. Then she gave devout thanks to God for Surrey's success, and returned in triumph to Richmond. On the way, she stayed the night at Woburn Abbey, and it was here that she took time to write to her husband, referring, perhaps rather tactlessly, to 'the great victory that our Lord hath sent to your subjects in your absence. To my thinking, this battle hath been more than should you win all the crown of France.' Not that Katherine intended any offence; indeed, she was praying that God would 'send you home shortly, for without no joy can here be accomplished'.

If Henry felt somewhat disgruntled by the implication of Katherine's words, he was soon to forget it, for on 21 September he captured another town, Tournai. He had thoroughly enjoyed his first taste of warfare, and was disappointed that it was now autumn and time to return to England, for no commander ever campaigned through the winter months by choice. It was agreed between the allies that they should launch a combined invasion of France before June 1514, and also that the marriage of Henry's sister Mary to Charles of Castile should take place in the spring. After a short sojourn in Lille, the court of Maximilian's daughter and Katherine's former sister-in-law, the Archduchess Margaret, Henry returned to England, landing at Dover on 22 October after an absence of four months. With only a small company, he rode at full speed to Richmond to see his wife, and when he arrived, 'there was such a loving meeting that everyone rejoiced who witnessed it'.

Katherine had been pregnant for the third time during the Flodden campaign, and after the victory celebrations were over, she went to Our Lady of Walsingham to pray for the safe delivery of a son. The war had drained her energies, and there were fears that she might miscarry: 'If the Queen be with child, we owe very much to God,' wrote Sir Brian Tuke, Henry's secretary, to Wolsey. Yet in October, just prior to the King's homecoming, Katherine was delivered of a premature son, who died shortly after his birth. It was a bitter disappointment, but mitigated to some extent by her joyful reunion with her husband later that month. Both Henry and Katherine were becoming increasingly anxious about the succession and the King's lack of a male heir. Nevertheless, time was still on their side, and in June 1514, the Queen was visibly pregnant once more.

This was not, however, to be a happy pregnancy, for by that time, the King had been forced to the realisation that he had been duped by his so-called allies, Ferdinand and Maximilian, who had made it very clear that they had not the slightest intention now of pursuing the war with France. Nor would the Council of Flanders accept Mary Tudor as a bride for the Archduke Charles. This was an insult, which, together with his humiliation over Ferdinand's betrayal, inspired Henry to an outburst of righteous anger against his father-in-law and the Emperor, calling down the wrath of Heaven upon them for having deceived him. The person who suffered most was Katherine, who had for years urged Henry to heed the advice of her father. This would now cease, he warned her icily, 'upbraiding the innocent Queen for her father's desertion', and informing her that 'the Kings of England had never taken place to anyone but God', according to the chronicler Peter Martyr. In future, he would govern his kingdom by himself, with the aid of Wolsey, and without any outside interference. One after the other, 'he spat out his complaints against her'. Katherine was distressed at the realisation that her husband and her father were now enemies, and that her own role as

Henry's confidential adviser would in consequence be much diminished, and all at a time when Wolsey's influence was growing ever more powerful. It was doubtful if the King would ever listen to her again to the same extent, or trust her advice.

Katherine's friends, notably Fray Diego before his dismissal and Maria de Salinas, now urged her to forget the interests of Spain and render her loyalty wholly to her adopted land, for only by doing this could she hope to avoid further censure by the King. Katherine accepted that this was the wisest option, for she dared not antagonise her husband further. Luis Caroz, however, felt that it would be catastrophic for Spain if her remaining link with England was severed. 'The Queen has the best of intentions,' he reported, 'but there is no one to show her how she may become serviceable to her father.' Maria de Salinas realised that Katherine's services on her father's behalf had brought her to this impasse, and she effectively blocked all Caroz's attempts to persuade Katherine to place Ferdinand's interests before those of her husband. As for the King, he behaved 'in a most discourteous manner' whenever King Ferdinand's name was mentioned.

What Katherine, Caroz and Ferdinand had failed to take into account was the growing effect of regal responsibility upon Henry VIII, and his developing egocentricity; nor did they allow for the ever increasing influence of Thomas Wolsey, who was even now urging the King towards a French alliance. In October 1514, Henry married his sister Mary to the King of France, who now became his friend and ally, peace between the two kingdoms having been proclaimed with the signing of a new treaty in August. This was all Wolsey's doing, and naturally it was unwelcome to Queen Katherine, not only because of her inbred distrust of the French, but also because it meant that Wolsey's influence was unlikely to be dislodged, which could only be detrimental to her own interests and Spain's.

It was essential that she regain the King's confidence, yet Henry never came to her now for advice on political matters, and she was obliged to retire into the background and settle for a purely domestic and decorative role. For someone who had, for several years, been at the centre of events, this was hard to take, yet take it she did, with patience and humility, never betraying her sense of isolation or her distaste for her husband's new allies. If she could bring him an heir, she might yet win him back, but in November 1514 her latest pregnancy ended with the birth of yet another prince who died within hours of his birth. In Spain, it was the general opinion that this tragedy had occurred 'on account of the discord between the two kings, her husband and father; because of her excessive grief, she ejected an immature foetus.' It was a bitter blow, and Katherine herself commented that the Almighty must love her to confer upon her 'the privilege of so much sorrow'.

She was destined, however, to bear a living child. A fifth pregnancy was confirmed in the summer of 1515, and at four o'clock in the morning of 18 February 1516, Katherine gave birth to a healthy daughter. Although the baby was the wrong sex, the King was delighted with her, for she was 'a right lusty princess', and he named her Mary. Katherine's emotions when she beheld her 'beauteous babe' may well be imagined – even the news of the death of her father, King Ferdinand, which had been kept from her until after her confinement, could not dampen her joy. God, it seemed, had spoken at last, and – as Henry confidently said – 'if it is a daughter this time, by the grace of God, boys will follow. We are both still young.' The Princess Mary was christened with 'great solemnity' three days after her birth in the chapel of the Observant Friars at Greenwich. In accordance with tradition, neither parent attended the ceremony, and the infant was borne to the font by her sponsors, or godparents, under a canopy of estate.

In August 1517, Queen Katherine was again supposed to be pregnant, but it was either a rumour or a false hope. Her sixth and last child was conceived in February 1518, when she was thirty-two, well past her youth by contemporary standards, and possibly aware that this might be her last chance to present Henry with an heir. 'I pray God heartily that it may be a prince, to the universal comfort and security of the realm,' wrote Richard Pace, the King's secretary, to Wolsey; sentiments echoed by the Venetian ambassador, who hoped God would grant the Queen a son, 'in order that his Highness, having a male heir to follow him, may not be hindered, as at present, from engaging in affairs of the moment'. This was a veiled reference to Henry's reluctance to lead an army against the Turks, who were encroaching upon Eastern Europe.

The forthcoming birth was announced in June as 'an event most earnestly desired by the whole kingdom', and in churches throughout the land prayers were said for Katherine's safe delivery. She herself was then at the old palace of Woodstock, and could there take the air in gardens where Henry II had once courted his mistress, 'Fair Rosamund' Clifford, and perhaps see traces of the maze built for that lady. Here, too, in 1330, another beloved queen, Philippa of Hainault, had borne a son, the Black Prince. All seemed well when, in July, the King visited Woodstock; Katherine greeted him at the door of her chamber, proud to show him 'for his welcome home her belly something great'. Then before all the courtiers, she told him that the child had stirred in her womb; Henry was so delighted that he gave a great banquet to celebrate, and fussed around his wife to ensure that she took good care of herself, for – as he wrote to Wolsey – he knew by now that a happy outcome to her pregnancies was 'not an ensured thing, but a thing wherein I have great hope and likelihood'.

Tragically, his hopes were to come to nothing yet again, for on 10 November Katherine had a daughter, 'to the vexation of as many as knew it. Never had the kingdom desired anything so anxiously as it did a prince.' The baby was very weak, and died before she could be christened. The Queen found this latest disappointment almost too much to bear, and openly wondered if the loss of her children was a judgement of God 'for that her former marriage was made in blood'.

The Queen had conceived six, possibly eight, times, yet all she had to show for it was one daughter. She had borne her losses with amiability, resignation and good humour, yet the burden of failure was great. In the patriarchal society of Tudor England, blame for stillbirths and neonatal deaths was always apportioned to the woman, and some were of the opinion that Henry had made a grave mistake in marrying a wife older than himself. 'My good brother of England has no son because, although young and handsome, he keeps an old and deformed wife,' was the King of France's cruel comment at this time. It was true that Katherine had begun to show her age, and that her figure had been ruined by her pregnancies. Her youthful prettiness had gone for ever, while Henry, at twenty-seven, was approaching his physical peak. Yet, to his credit, he did not once reproach Katherine for his lack of a male heir, although he was himself desperate for a son, and beginning to wonder why this one crucial gift should be denied him.

By 1519, with no sign of another child on the way, the succession had become the King's most critical problem. Although his throne was based on firmer foundations than his father's had been, he still had to contend with a legacy of stray Plantagenets, and, though at present these descendants of the House of York appeared to be behaving themselves, one could never anticipate what they would do if the King died suddenly, leaving a three-year-old girl on the throne. There would, without doubt, be factions formed and a return to civil war; Mary's very life might well be threatened. Of course, the Queen might yet conceive, but that was a possibility which seemed more remote with each passing year. Henry later hinted that she suffered from some gynaecological trouble, possibly as a result of her last confinement, and that this made intercourse with her distasteful to him. At any rate, he ceased to have sexual relations with her in 1524, by his own admission, made seven years later, and by the spring of 1525, it was well known that Katherine was 'past that age in which women most commonly are wont to be fruitful'. There would be no more children.

For the King, this was a bitter pill to swallow; it was galling in the extreme for a robust and virile man of thirty-four to face the fact that he would have no more legitimate issue of his body. It was almost a slur on his manhood. Sex with Katherine had long become just a means to an end, and when the Queen's menopause came upon her, it became glaringly apparent that Henry's desire for her had long since died; nevertheless, he would still visit her bed for some years to come, if only for appearances' sake.

In August 1514, a curious rumour had been reported in Rome, to the effect that 'the King of England means to repudiate his present wife because he is unable to have children by her, and intends to marry a daughter of the French Duke of Bourbon.' Then in England, in September, it was being said that 'the King wishes to dissolve his marriage.'

Did Henry, as early as 1514, seriously consider divorce? The main argument against these reports having any basis in fact is that Katherine was pregnant when they were written, and it is unthinkable that the King would have contemplated putting her away when he was hopeful of her bearing him an heir. Rome, however, was a long way from England, and a report of something Henry had said in June, when he was furious with Katherine because of her father's treachery, would not have reached Italy for several weeks, and may well have been embroidered in the process, as nowhere else do we hear this tale of a French marriage for the King. It is therefore, on balance, highly improbable that he seriously thought of divorce at this stage.

He was, however, at that time enjoying a flirtation with fourteen-year-old Elizabeth (Bessie) Blount, a distant relative of the Queen's chamberlain, Lord Mountjoy. Her name was first mentioned in connection with the King's in October 1514, in a letter written to Henry by Charles Brandon, Duke of Suffolk, which implies that the King and Brandon were partners in flirtations with Elizabeth and another girl, Elizabeth Carew. The King was discreet about his love affairs, so we know very little about this one, except that it was what Fray Diego was referring to when he accused Henry of having 'badly used' the Queen in the autumn of 1514. Katherine, however, was by then growing used to her husband's infidelities, writing resignedly in one letter that 'young men be wrapped in sensual love'. Hence she kept her peace. The King's affair with Bessie Blount would last for the next five years at least, but it was conducted well out of sight of his wife. Thus, in 1519, Erasmus would still feel moved to extol Henry's virtues as a husband: 'What house among all your subjects presents such an example of a chaste and concordant wedlock as your own? There, you find a wife emulous to resemble the best of husbands!'

Of course, unknown to Erasmus, Henry had been anything but chaste. He was rumoured to be still in love with Elizabeth Blount, who shared with him a passion for singing, dancing and 'goodly pastimes'. In 1519 Elizabeth disappeared from court for several months; Henry had arranged for her to go to 'Jericho', a house he leased from St Lawrence's Priory at Blackmore in Essex; it was a house with a poor reputation, where the King maintained a private suite. When he visited, he took with him only a few attendants. No one was allowed to approach him during his stay, and pages and grooms of the privy chamber were warned 'not to hearken and enquire where the King is or goeth, be it early or late', and to refrain from 'talking of the King's pastime' or 'his late or early going to bed'. Obviously Jericho was a trysting place where Henry could pursue his affair with Elizabeth Blount, and perhaps other women whose names are lost to history. Elizabeth certainly lived there for a time, for in 1519 she gave birth to the King's bastard son in the house. Henry was delighted to have a boy at last: here was proof indeed that he himself was not responsible for the lack of a male heir, though it must have seemed to him ironical that his only son should be born out of wedlock. He named the child Henry, and bestowed upon him the old Norman-French surname FitzRoy, which means 'son of the King'. News of the birth soon leaked out at court, and in due course the Queen learned of it, to her sorrow and humiliation.

Henry's affair with Elizabeth Blount seems to have ended with the birth of her child, and he arranged through Wolsey to have her honourably bestowed in marriage as a reward for services rendered. Late in 1519 she married Lord Tailboys, although Wolsey was savagely criticised for his part in this, and accused of encouraging young women to indulge in fornication as a means of finding a husband above their station. Yet Elizabeth Blount would go on to make an even more impressive second marriage after her husband's death, to Lord Clinton, later Earl of Lincoln. She died in 1539. Her son by the King, Henry FitzRoy, was sent at a young age to live with a tutor, Richard Croke, at King's College, Cambridge, where he would receive part of his education.

Although she could not approve of the Princess Mary's marriage to King Louis of France, Katherine – wearing a gown and Venetian cap of ash-coloured satin – attended the banquet given after the proxy wedding ceremony at Greenwich in August 1514, and shortly afterwards rode with the court to Dover to say goodbye to her sister-in-law, of whom she seems to have been fond.

The 'amorous marriage' of Louis XII and Mary Tudor lasted less than three months; worn out with making love to his beautiful, giddy bride, the middle-aged Louis died of exhaustion at the beginning of January 1515, to Mary's great relief, and was succeeded by his distant cousin, Francis, Count of Angoulême. Francis I was just three years younger than Henry VIII, and already had a dire reputation where women were concerned. Henry was immediately distrustful of him, and not a little jealous. In fact, the strong sense of rivalry between the two monarchs would endure until their deaths, which occurred within weeks of each other. Henry's jealousy was rooted in the awareness that, until Francis's accession, he had been the youngest, most charismatic and most good-looking sovereign in Europe – all were agreed on that. But this new King of France might now be about to send Henry's star into eclipse, and Henry was determined that should not happen.

Francis, who played a significant role in the history of Henry VIII's marital adventures, was far from handsome, being dark and saturnine with an over-long pointed nose, which gave him the look of a satyr and earned him the nickname 'Foxnose'. Living up to this epithet, he could be as devious as any of his predecessors when it came to politics. Yet he was also a true prince of the Renaissance, a lover of the arts, and the patron of Leonardo da Vinci. His court was at once a school of culture and elegance and a cesspit of vice and debauchery, his palaces without peer in northern Europe.

Francis made ineffectual attempts to seduce Queen Mary during her brief widowhood, but he was pre-empted by Charles Brandon, newly created Duke of Suffolk, whom Henry had sent to convey her back to England. Unknown to the King, Mary had long cherished a secret love for Brandon, and the effect of his arrival in Paris was cataclysmic. She wanted no more arranged marriages, she told him, and begged him to marry her himself. Such was the pressure she brought to bear upon him that Brandon capitulated, and secretly made her his wife.

Charles Brandon had since childhood been very close to the King. Born in 1485, he was the son of Henry VII's standard bearer, Sir William Brandon, who had been killed at the Battle of Bosworth. Young Charles had then been taken into the royal household to be brought up with Prince Henry, whom he much resembled in looks, build and colouring. A great favourite with the ladies, Brandon had already disentangled himself from two disadvantageous marriages. Now, realising the enormity of what he had done, he wrote at once to Wolsey, confessing that he had married Mary 'heartily, and lain with her'. When he heard, the King was furious – so furious he wanted Brandon's head. But thanks to Wolsey's intervention and his suggestion that the Suffolks make reparation by payment of a crippling fine, Henry forgave them, and allowed them to return to England, where he arranged a splendid public wedding for them at Greenwich. Afterwards, the couple retired to live somewhat frugally for a time in the country, where Mary bore three children, one of whom, Frances, would later become the mother of Lady Jane Grey.

By the autumn of 1515, Henry VIII's anger against Ferdinand of Aragon had burnt itself out, and there was a renewal of friendship between them before Ferdinand's death in January 1516. He was succeeded in Aragon by his grandson, Charles of Castile, who was from now on effective ruler of a reunited Spain. Henry and Katherine welcomed Charles's ambassadors to England in March 1516, and entertained them with a banquet lasting seven hours, and a joust in which the King gave a practised display of horsemanship, 'making a thousand jumps in the air'.

Peace now existed between the great European powers. By 1517, many foreigners had come to London to set up businesses or to see the sights; many were Spaniards. This created a certain amount of tension, for the English disliked the 'strangers', as they called them, and on May Day 1517, this resentment bubbled into hatred and boiled over, as fighting broke out between mobs of London apprentices and any foreigners who were unlucky enough to cross their paths. What made these riots so ugly was the fact that they were almost certainly premeditated.

The King was picnicking with Katherine at Greenwich when news reached him of the disturbances in his capital, and he left for the City at once, sending his guards ahead, who swiftly brought the rioters under control. The youths who had caused the violence were all arrested and brought to Westminster Hall, where the King, determined to avenge the outrage committed against the foreigners under his protection, wasted no time in condemning them all to the gallows. At this, the wives and mothers of the apprentices, who had gathered at the back of the hall, burst out into pitiful weeping and wailing. Queen Katherine, seated on her throne behind the King, heard them, and her heart was touched. Without hesitation, she rose from her place and knelt before her husband, begging him with tears in her eyes: 'Spare the apprentices!' Wolsey added his pleas to hers, rightly judging that such an act of mercy would greatly enhance his own and the King's popularity with the people. Henry could resist neither his wife, nor his minister, nor could he turn down this opportunity of winning golden opinions. He therefore pardoned the prisoners and gave them back their liberty, thus turning this 'Evil May Day' into a day of rejoicing, as the apprentices threw their halters into the air and hastened to be reunited with their families. Some of the mothers went up to the Queen and thanked her for her intervention, praising her for championing Englishmen above the Spaniards who had suffered injury and loss in the riots. Katherine answered them 'gently' and then departed, more beloved than ever.

The French alliance held good for six years. In 1518, it was agreed that Henry's daughter, the two-year-old Princess Mary, should one day marry the Dauphin, Francis I's heir. Henry, still hopeful of a son to succeed him, was enthusiastic about the match, as it would guarantee Mary a glorious future as Queen of France. Katherine, however, was not happy at all at the prospect of her only child being given to France, though she did not venture to criticise.

In February 1519, the Emperor Maximilian died. His death was to have far-reaching consequences for the whole of Europe. His grandson Charles was elected Holy Roman Emperor in his place, at the age of nineteen. The new Emperor Charles V now ruled Germany, Austria, the Low Countries, parts of Italy and, from 1526, Hungary also, as well as Spain: half of Europe, in fact. Such unity had not featured in the Holy Roman Empire since the days of Charlemagne. However, Charles's title was based on tradition rather than fact: the Empire was no longer based in Rome, neither was it particularly holy. Not only were the Emperors often at loggerheads with the Popes, but the Empire itself was shortly to be divided by schism as Luther's doctrines gained currency. The 'Christian republic' of the European Middle Ages was about to become a thing of the past, although in due course Charles V would follow in the steps of Charlemagne to Rome, there to be crowned by the Pope.

The election of Charles V had the immediate effect of improving Katherine of Aragon's status in England. She was his aunt, and could command greater respect as such than as Henry VIII's barren consort. In England, she now represented the combined might, and reflected glory, of Spain and the Empire, a formidable heritage. Yet, for all this, her life continued as quietly as before. The gulf between her and the King was widening all the time; her influence was still minimal, and her function now merely ceremonial. She had failed in every way that mattered, and beside this her considerable personal qualities paled into insignificance.

Katherine's two consolations were her religion and the emotional fulfilment she found in her daughter Mary. The Queen was a very maternal woman, and fiercely protective of her child, who was a pretty little girl. 'This child never cries!' the King proudly told the French ambassador when Mary was two. She had inherited her father's colouring and her mother's air of gravity, and was 'decorous in manners', having been schooled rigidly to good behaviour from the cradle. In time, she would display a profound piety that would even exceed Katherine's, and her first recorded words – 'Priest! Priest!' – were strangely prophetic.

The Princess was brought up in an atmosphere of domestic harmony. A lady governess, Lady Margaret Bryan, looked after her daily needs from an early age. Any tension between her parents was concealed by the fact that they both doted upon her. Henry was fond of showing her off to visiting dignitaries, and when Katherine had led her by the hand into his presence, he would sweep her up in his arms and carry her round, bursting with pride. She, in turn, adored him. 'See how she jumps forward in her nurse's lap when she catches sight of her father!' exclaimed the Bishop of Durham, an entranced observer. As she grew older, she was allowed to take part in court festivities and pageants, and at four she was receiving foreign envoys and entertaining them with music played rather shakily on the virginals. At seven, she was an expert dancer, and – according to a Spanish envoy – twirled 'so prettily that no woman could do better'.

Mary's formal education began in 1523. The King and Queen wished it to be a classic grounding in all the subjects appropriate to a Renaissance princess, with sound religious teaching at its core. They had taken advice from Juan Luis Vives, a Spanish educationist with a reputation for advanced views on female education, and with his approval the King appointed Richard Fetherston, who had been chaplain to Queen Katherine and was a gentle, devout man, to be Mary's first tutor. Vives himself drew up a plan for her formal curriculum, which would later be the basis for his treatise *The*

Institution of a Christian Woman, which was dedicated to Queen Katherine. He also taught Mary Latin, while Katherine herself helped the child with her translations.

Vives's curriculum was, by modern standards, severe for a child of seven, and involved much learning of the Scriptures, the works of the early Fathers of the Church, as well as the study of ancient classics and history. Light reading was forbidden, in case it encouraged light behaviour.

In August 1525, the King sent Mary with her own household to live at Ludlow Castle. Although she was her father's heiress, she had never been formally invested with the principality of Wales, but Henry now decided to follow tradition and send her with 'an honourable, sad, discreet and expert council' to the castle on the Welsh marches where Katherine had spent most of her brief married life with Prince Arthur nearly a quarter of a century before. Here, Mary would learn something of the art of government. Lady Salisbury, her mother's close friend, was appointed state governess, and the Queen and Wolsey worked together on a plan for the regime to be followed by the Princess at Ludlow, giving 'most tender regard' to her age, education and moral training. She was to enjoy plenty of fresh air walking in the gardens, to practise her music, and continue learning Latin and French. Her lessons were not to fatigue her, and her diet was to be 'pure, well-dressed, and served with merry communication'. Her private apartments and her clothes must be kept 'pure, sweet, clean and wholesome', and those in attendance on her must treat her with 'humility and reverence'. It is not difficult to read into this remarkable document a mother's anxiety that her child should suffer no diminishment of care while they were apart.

Katherine bore the separation with stoicism, although she wrote to Mary that it troubled her. Mary's own letters were the chief joy in her life during the long months apart, as was the finished written work that the Princess sent her; 'it was a great comfort to me to see you keep your Latin and fair writing and all,' replied her mother. Katherine did not see Mary again until the Princess came to Greenwich for the Christmas festivities of 1526, when Henry led her out with him to dance before the court. After Twelfth Night, she returned to Ludlow, but was back at court in April 1527, when it was noted that, at eleven, she was 'the most accomplished person for her age'. Thereafter, Mary remained at court, where she completed her education – as she had begun it – under her mother's supervision.

In February 1520, preparations for the long-awaited summit meeting between Henry VIII and Francis I began. After discussion between Wolsey and the French ambassador, it was agreed that the English court should cross to France in May, and stay at Henry's own castle at Guisnes in the Pale of Calais, then in English hands. The French visit was Wolsey's brainchild, and he was in charge of all the arrangements, drawing up a code of etiquette which cleverly solved all questions of precedence and courtesy that might vex 'the King of England and the Queen his bedfellow'. The Cardinal then set about planning what was to be one of the most expensive charades ever staged in history, the Field of Cloth of Gold, so called because no expense would be spared in displaying the wealth of England and France to each other.

Katherine had been against the French visit from the first, and spoke out against it to her council, who were surprised she had dared be so bold. However, Henry VIII himself was having second thoughts about his alliance with Francis I, and was beginning to find the prospect of friendship with the new Emperor more appealing. He therefore paid some heed to his wife's protests, for once, and thus Katherine found herself 'held in greater esteem by the King and his Council than ever'. Nevertheless, Wolsey was so far forward with plans for the visit that it was too late to cancel it, and Henry never could resist an opportunity to show off. Katherine recognised that it was expedient to go to France with as much grace as she could muster.

Charles V himself was eager to form a tie of friendship with England, and in May 1520 he paid Henry and Katherine a visit. The King spent lavishly on new clothes for himself and his wife in honour of his 'well beloved nephew', while Katherine was elated at the prospect of coming face to face with Juana's son, whom she had never seen and of whom she had such high hopes. 'I thank God I shall see his face,' she said; 'it will be the greatest good that I can have on earth.' The meeting took place at Canterbury at Whitsun, with Emperor and King embracing 'right lovingly'. Charles greeted his aunt in his customary distant and correct manner, with little outward warmth, but she did not seem to mind, and 'most joyfully received and welcomed him'. He was not the most prepossessing figure, being graced with a pronounced version of the heavy Hapsburg jaw, which made it impossible for him to close his mouth, and gave him a somewhat vacuous look. For all this, and his inbred reticence, Charles was a hard-headed realist, already evincing something of the strength and single-mindedness with which he would rule his vast dominions for the next third of a century.

Charles's purpose in coming to England was to persuade Henry not to attend the proposed meeting with Francis I. However, Henry explained why the meeting must go ahead, and arranged to meet with Charles afterwards in Flanders. After attending mass together in the Cathedral on Whitsunday, the two monarchs presided over a banquet; Katherine was there, resplendent in a gown of cloth of gold and violet velvet embroidered with Tudor roses. Four days of feasting followed, then Charles left England, on the same day that Henry and Katherine, with a huge retinue – Katherine's train alone numbered 3,000 persons – travelled to Dover and there took ship for Calais, where they would stay briefly at the Palace of the Exchequer before moving to Guisnes on 3 June. Here, in a temporary palace erected to Wolsey's specifications, the Queen found herself occupying rooms of unsurpassed magnificence. Her closet was hung with cloth of gold and jewels; it had an altar adorned with pearls and precious stones, with twelve golden statuettes; even the ceiling was lined with cloth of gold and precious stones.

The Field of Cloth of Gold would for ever after be remembered for the riches and splendour witnessed there. On 7 June, the two kings met in the Vale of Ardres, in what is now a turnip field, but was then dotted with silken pavilions and thronged with the members of the English and French courts. It was a most satisfactory encounter; after saluting and embracing each other, Henry and Francis exchanged gifts and signed a new treaty of friendship; Henry then spoke to Francis about his hopes for a reconciliation between France and the Empire. However, as the Venetian ambassador observed, 'these sovereigns are not at peace. They hate each other cordially.' Nevertheless, this did not prevent them from indulging in three weeks of festivities to celebrate their meeting, an empty charade that would cost a fortune and achieve virtually nothing, except to cement the rivalry between them, and drive Henry directly into the arms of the Emperor. Thus what should have been a politically advantageous meeting quickly degenerated into a mere masque for the prodigal entertainment of two extravagant courts, whose sovereigns postured in new outfits of increasing splendour every day and ended up barely able to conceal their jealousy of each other.

Both their queens did what they could to calm the troubled waters. Katherine and Claude liked each other immediately; at mass, after arguing in the friendliest manner over who should kiss the Bible first, each indicating the other, they compromised by kissing each other instead. And both intervened at a wrestling match between their lords, when Francis threw Henry and Henry, red with fury, was about to retaliate.

On 11 June, the two kings tilted in their wives' honour; Katherine arrived in a crimson satin litter embroidered with gold, and sat to watch the jousts under a canopy of estate lined entirely with pearls. She wore a Spanish head-dress, with her long hair loose beneath it, and a gown of cloth of gold. Three days later, she entertained King Francis at Guisnes 'with all honour', while Henry went to Ardres as the guest of Queen Claude. Katherine sat beside Francis at a 'right honourably served' banquet, and afterwards her ladies danced for his pleasure. Later, she would call him 'the greatest Turk that ever was', for she had seen with her own eyes the effect he had on the opposite sex.

And still the extravagant festivities continued, to the ruin of both the English and French treasuries. Jousts, sporting events, banquets, balls all followed in quick succession, and at every event Queen Katherine appeared superbly dressed and displayed exquisite courtesy. At last, on 23 June, the great charade came to an end when Wolsey celebrated mass before the assembled courts; then there was a farewell banquet, and fireworks to end the day. On 25 June 1520, the English court returned to Calais, where it remained at the Exchequer. Two weeks later, Henry rode to Gravelines to meet the Emperor, and conducted him back to Calais where he and the Queen hosted an impressive banquet for their nephew before bidding him farewell and returning to England. When news of this meeting reached King Francis, he was not best pleased, and the already tense relationship between France and England was dealt a death blow on 14 July when Henry concluded a new treaty with Charles in which each agreed not to make any new alliance with France during the next two years.

Wolsey quietly arranged the breaking of Mary's betrothal to the Dauphin, to the great relief and joy of the Queen, and in the spring of 1521 Katherine's happiness was further compounded when Charles asked for Mary's hand in marriage; she had always hoped for a Spanish match for her child. Charles was undoubtedly the greatest matrimonial prize in Europe, and Mary would be assured of a brilliant future. The marriage treaty was signed in August, and Katherine found herself feeling unusually cordial towards Wolsey, who had helped arrange it. In May 1522, Charles returned to England for the betrothal ceremony, and three days after his arrival England declared war on France. Katherine had dreamed of and prayed for a Spanish alliance for the past eight years: it was now a fact.

The Emperor was met by King Henry, who brought him in the royal barge to Greenwich, where they were met at the doorway of the great hall by the Queen and her daughter. Charles knelt for his aunt's blessing and expressed great joy at seeing her, then greeted his future bride, who was still small for her age, but promised to be 'a handsome lady'. During the visit there were the usual banquets and jousts, as well as a masque, then the whole court rode to Windsor for the formal ceremony of betrothal on 19 June. Mary was due to go to Spain when she was twelve, but Charles asked if she might come earlier, to be educated as befitted a future Empress and Queen of Spain. Henry told him that if he should search all Christendom for 'a mistress to bring her up after the manner of Spain, then he could not find one more meet than the Queen's Grace, her mother, who, for the affection she beareth to the Emperor, will nurture her and bring her up to his satisfaction'. Katherine felt that Mary was not strong enough for 'the pains of the sea' or 'the air of another country', remembering her own voyage to England and how ill she had been for six years after her arrival.

Nevertheless, although Charles left England without his bride, relations between England and the Empire were never better than at this time. Charles declared war on France, and in February 1525 scored a resounding victory at Pavia in Italy, where King Francis was taken prisoner; later, he was sent to Madrid. Henry VIII was jubilant when he heard the news, and told the messenger he was 'like the Angel Gabriel announcing the birth of Jesus Christ'. In April, he sent Charles an emerald ring on Mary's behalf, with a loving message; Charles replied he would wear it for her sake. He continued to press for her to be sent to Spain, but Henry was adamant that she should not go until the appointed time, and would not budge on this point. Charles then demanded payment of her dowry as an act of good faith, but again Henry refused: it was not due for another three years. This wrangling went on until August 1525, when Charles suddenly announced that, as he had received neither his bride nor her dowry, he considered his betrothal null and void. He had, in fact, found a richer bride, Isabella of Portugal, another of Katherine's nieces, who had a dowry of one million crowns, was very beautiful, and also of an age to bear children.

Even before Henry had learned of Charles's perfidy, Wolsey had begun to edge him back into the open arms of the French, who needed a strong ally. This new alliance was Wolsey's project from start to finish: he had not forgiven or forgotten being ousted from the contest for the papacy. Of course, these events caused Queen Katherine great distress, and when, in September, Henry formally released Charles from his promise and ratified the treaty with France, her dream of a united England and Spain was finally shattered. Politically she would once more be a nonentity in her husband's realm, and for this she blamed Wolsey.

Nor was her domestic life particularly congenial. She could not have failed to guess the reason for the promotion of Sir Thomas Boleyn to the peerage as Viscount Rochford in 1525, just the latest in a string of honours accorded to a man who had been one of Henry's favourite courtiers since 1511. Yet this latest honour had undoubtedly been bestowed as a reward for services rendered to the King by Boleyn's elder daughter Mary, who had for some time been Henry's mistress. As usual, the affair was conducted discreetly, and for this reason it is impossible to pinpoint when it began or ended. Mary Boleyn had married William Carey, a gentleman of the King's household, in February 1520; the King attended their wedding, offering 6s. 8d. in the chapel. Mary accompanied Queen Katherine to the Field of Cloth of Gold later that year. Henry had just discarded

Elizabeth Blount, and it would not be fanciful to conclude that Mary Boleyn was the reason why he did so. In 1533, Mary's son, Henry Carey, who had been born around 1524, would claim he was 'our sovereign lord the King's son', but Henry never acknowledged him as such, which should be taken as conclusive evidence that the boy was William Carey's, for the King had been eager enough to acknowledge Henry FitzRoy as his own.

Mary Boleyn had spent some time at the French court, which was far more licentious than Henry's, in the train of Henry's sister the Duchess of Suffolk and had succumbed early on to the temptations there, becoming so easy with her favours that the papal nuncio called her 'a very great and infamous whore'. King Francis himself boasted of having 'ridden her', and fondly referred to her as 'my hackney'. This may have been the reason why her father removed her from the French court and brought her back to England. It seems likely that her affair with Henry VIII began around 1519–20, and that it was still continuing in 1523, when Henry named one of his ships the *Mary Boleyn*. The relationship seems to have ended in 1525, or thereabouts.

By then, the Queen was known to be incapable of having any more children and, while Henry still displayed affection for her and there was no obvious breach between them, he had reached the stage where he was prepared to go to any lengths to have an heir. Of course, he already had a son, Henry FitzRoy, who was now six years old and much resembled his father in looks. It was therefore in Henry's mind to have the boy declared legitimate by Act of Parliament and name him his heir; he even contemplated marrying him to his half-sister Mary. There was, of course, no precedent in English history for the succession devolving upon a bastard son, and no way of knowing if the King's subjects would accept FitzRoy as the lawful successor to his father, but Henry was desperate. It is highly significant that, as soon as it was confirmed that the Queen was 'past the ways of women', FitzRoy was brought to court to receive a host of honours, having the royal dukedoms of Richmond and Somerset conferred upon him in 1525, being admitted to the Order of the Garter and appointed Lord High Admiral. From then on, he was 'well brought up like a prince's child' and 'furnished to keep the state of a great prince', and it was quickly understood that he might 'easily, and by the King's means, be exalted to higher things'.

Queen Katherine was deeply offended by FitzRoy's ennoblement, which amounted, in her view, to a public snub on Henry's part. For once, she could not hide her disapproval, and the Venetian ambassador clearly perceived she was resentful and 'dissatisfied'. However, she was in no position to complain, and was 'obliged to submit and have patience', a virtue of which she was to need vast reserves in the years to come.

In the summer of 1526, Francis I, released from captivity, offered himself as a husband for the Princess Mary, Queen Claude having died in 1524. Henry was enthusiastic, as was Wolsey, who expected some hostility from the Queen but discounted it as unimportant, not rating her influence very highly. Yet from December 1526, Katherine was not to be entirely isolated in England, for in that month there arrived at court the new Spanish ambassador, Don Diego Hurtado de Mendoza, a man of very astute judgement and deep integrity, who was to prove a loyal and gallant friend to Queen Katherine. He quickly summed up the situation in England, and guessed that the Queen was very unhappy. In his opinion, 'the principal cause of her misfortune is that she identifies herself entirely with the Emperor's interests.' After the arrival of Mendoza, Katherine's life is better documented, and from this date the Calendar of State Papers relating to Spain is full of information about her life.

What was immediately apparent to Mendoza was that Katherine was kept in isolation on purpose, and that Wolsey was taking care to be present whenever the new ambassador had an audience with the Queen, having no desire to let her unburden her troubles into the ear of a Spaniard. Hence Katherine found it very difficult to pass any messages or information to Charles V, although one letter did reach him, in which she bewailed the fact that she had not heard from him in two years; 'such are my affection and readiness for your service that I deserve better treatment.' Yet Wolsey's spies were everywhere, and letters were intercepted; Charles might not after all have been at fault.

In the spring of 1527, Francis sent an embassy to England headed by Gabriel de Grammont, Bishop of Tarbes, to discuss the forthcoming betrothal of the Princess Mary to Francis himself or one of his sons. There were the usual jousts and banquets in honour of the visitors, then the two parties settled down to business. It came as something of a bombshell when the Bishop of Tarbes suddenly began questioning the legitimacy of the Princess and 'whether the marriage between the King and her mother, being his brother's wife, were good or no'. As a result of the Bishop's queries, negotiations were suspended for a short while, during which time Wolsey apparently managed to reassure him that Mary had indeed been born in lawful wedlock. Then talks resumed without further complications.

The envoys also saw the Queen, who made some pointed and rather hostile remarks about King Francis, and they left with the correct impression that there was only one alliance that would satisfy Katherine, and that would not be with France. She would, they felt, have done 'anything in her power to preserve the old alliance between Spain and England', but however strong her desire to do so, 'her means for carrying it out are small'.

The new marriage treaty, which provided for the marriage of Mary Tudor to Francis I or his second son the Duke of Orléans, was ratified by Henry VIII in May 1527 – Francis shortly afterwards became betrothed to the Emperor's sister Eleanor, and Henry of Orléans was substituted as the bridegroom. At the banquet and ball which followed, Queen Katherine put on a brave face, watching her husband and daughter dancing together. At one point, Henry, anxious to display Mary's charms to the Frenchmen, pulled off the jewelled garland she wore on her head and let fall 'a profusion of fair tresses, as beautiful as ever seen on human head'.

The festivities were brought to an abrupt end, however, by news of the sacking of Rome on 6 May by the unfed and unpaid mercenary troops of the Emperor, who was then campaigning in Italy. Lacking a commander, they surged into the eternal city and unleashed an orgy of violence and murder that went on for several days; details of the atrocities they committed shocked even that brutal age. The Pope was forced to take refuge in the Castel St Angelo, where he soon afterwards found himself a virtual prisoner of the Emperor. Charles had not been personally responsible for the sack of Rome, and was as appalled as anyone else by it, but he was not averse to having the Pope in his power.

The sack of Rome was to have far-reaching consequences for Henry and Katherine. Their marriage had failed, for many reasons. On a personal level, the age gap seemed wider than ever, and there had long ago been a divergence of interests. With the French alliance newly signed, it no longer seemed desirable for the King to have a Spanish queen. More importantly, Katherine had failed in her crucial duty, that of bearing an heir. But, above all, the King, for some years past – or so he later claimed – had, when reading the Bible, turned again and again to the passage in chapter 20 of the Book of Leviticus, which warned of the severe penalty inflicted by God on a man who married his brother's widow: 'And if a man shall take his brother's wife, it is an unclean thing: he hath uncovered his brother's nakedness; they shall be childless.' To Henry's mind he was as good as childless, lacking a male heir, and years of worrying whether the prohibition in Leviticus applied to his own marriage had by now crystallised into the conviction that indeed it did. He and Katherine had offended against the law of God by their incestuous marriage and, because of this, God, in His wrath, had denied them sons. By the spring of 1527, the King was 'troubled in his conscience' about this; the more he studied the matter, the more clearly it appeared to him that he had broken a divine law, and that something must be done to rectify the situation.

Just how long the King's conscience had been troubling him we do not know. In 1527, he declared he had had doubts about his marriage 'for some years past', though there is no mention of the matter in contemporary records before May of that year. It is likely that these doubts first became serious around 1524, when Katherine went through the menopause and Henry ceased to have sexual relations with her; but they could have been in the King's mind as far back as 1521, for in that year he quoted the critical verses from Leviticus in his treatise against Luther, an indication that he was already aware of a possible impediment to his marriage. At the same time, Dr John Longland, Bishop of Lincoln, became the King's lord almoner (or confessor), and it was to him that Henry first confided his doubts; Wolsey's secretary, George Cavendish, confirms this in his biography of his master, quoting Henry as saying he himself 'moved first in the matter, in confession to my lord of Lincoln, my ghostly father'. Longland later bore this out, revealing that for a time he and Henry had waged a spiritual battle over the issue. 'The King never left urging me until he had won me to give my consent,' declared the Bishop in later years.

By 1524, Henry's conscience had become tender as far as his marriage was concerned; although he no longer desired his wife, and may have found sex distasteful because of the mysterious female ailment she suffered, these were not the only reasons why he decided to cease having intercourse with her. He had persuaded himself that their marriage was incestuous, and that any sexual congress would be a sin. Nevertheless, it was not until three years later that he resolved to act upon his doubts and seek an annulment of his marriage.

Two separate factors combined in the spring of 1527 to provoke the King to action. One was the questioning by the Bishop of Tarbes of the Princess Mary's legitimacy, which only served to compound Henry's own doubts. Nor was this the first time that the validity of his union with Katherine had been questioned. Others, among them his own father and the conservative William Warham, now Archbishop of Canterbury, had spoken out about it as far back as 1502. Henry VII, however, had inclined to the view that the law as laid down in Leviticus only applied where the first marriage had been consummated, and he had been satisfied that Arthur had left Katherine a virgin. However, as a precaution, Ferdinand and Isabella had insisted that the Bull of Dispensation issued by Pope Julius II in 1503 provided for the marriage of Katherine and Henry, even in the event of her first marriage having been consummated.

For Henry VIII, Katherine's virgin state when she came to his bed was not the issue to be disputed, although he did his best to cast doubts upon it. Katherine, on the other hand, would come to see it as the crux of the matter, for, to her understanding, Leviticus only applied when the first marriage had been consummated, and hers had not. Henry, of course, must have known this, and realised that for his case to succeed he had to take his stand on the Levitical law applying whether the marriage had been consummated or not. Here he was treading on dangerous ground, for of course the dispensation of 1503 permitting his marriage to Katherine had had precedents, notably in the case of Katherine's own sisters, Isabella and Maria, who were married in turn to the same King of Portugal. What Henry VIII was really questioning, therefore, was the power of the Pope to dispense at all in such a case as his. This was not immediately apparent as the central issue in the affair, but it would soon become so, and then the shock waves would reverberate around Europe, for to question the Pope's authority, which all good Catholics believed was invested in him by Christ, was tantamount to heresy. Yet the European climate was ripe for it: for two centuries the papacy had been recognised as corrupt, and was held in disrepute by those who argued the need for reform of a church riddled with abuses, not all of them followers of Luther. Given this, it is not perhaps surprising to find a devout Catholic, as Henry undoubtedly then was, calling the Pope's authority into question over a matter of canon law.

The other factor spurring the King into action in the spring of 1527 was that he was, by a fortuitious coincidence, passionately in love for the first time in his life, and wished to remarry. This has often – and erroneously – been understood to have been the real basis for the King's doubts of conscience, which has tended to trivialise the whole issue. In fact, Henry VIII did, desperately, need a male heir; his wife of eighteen years was now barren. His concern for the succession and the future of his kingdom was sincere and genuine. He had been questioning the validity of his marriage for several years, long before he had fallen in love with this latest mistress. Moreover, he and the Queen had had little in common for years. It was a sensible decision, therefore, to consider applying for the annulment of his marriage and taking another wife who could bear him children. Falling in love was merely the final spur to action.

Like all the others, this latest affair was conducted in the strictest secrecy, yet Henry was hinting at it in courtly fashion from the beginning of 1526, when, on Shrove Tuesday, at a joust held at Greenwich, he appeared in the lists decked in a splendid outfit of cloth of gold and silver, on which was embroidered in gold the device *Declare je nos* ('Declare I dare not'), which was surmounted by a man's heart engulfed in flames, typical of the symbolism so beloved by the Tudor court. The King's affair with Mary Boleyn had ended, probably in the previous year, so this pretty conceit could only mean that he had found someone else. The Queen was by now used to his infidelities, and probably attached little significance to this evidence of a new one.

In May 1527, the affair was still going on, although the identity of the chosen lady was still a well-kept secret. Yet Henry could not resist dropping hints, for he was now completely enslaved by her, and wanted the world to know it. One evening, he entertained the court with a poignant song he had written that told of the heart's torment when spurned by the beloved:

> The eagle's force subdues each bird that flies;
> What metal can resist the flaming fire?
> Doth not the sun dazzle the clearest eyes,
> And melt the ice, and make the frost retire?
> The hardest stones are pierced through with tools,
> The wisest are with princes made but fools.

Few present were aware to whom the song was addressed, nor guessed that she was probably present at the banquet in her official capacity as one of the Queen's maids of honour. Nor did anyone realise that this love affair, which had now been gathering momentum for more than fifteen months, was to be the most significant of them all. For the King was passionately, abjectly in love, a novel experience for him. Even more novel was the fact that the object of his desire was holding herself tantalisingly aloof, and would not even agree to being named his mistress in the courtly sense. This was surprising indeed in an age when it was considered almost honourable, and was at least lucrative, to become the mistress – in the sexual sense even – of a king. Yet this lady was keeping him firmly at arm's length and loudly proclaiming her virtue, which of course only served further to inflame the King's passion. She would have marriage, and the crown of England, or nothing.

Her name was Anne Boleyn.

Part II
The
'great matter'

7
Mistress Anne

The story of Henry VIII and Anne Boleyn began with passion and ended with a bloody death. At its outset, Henry VIII was still a youthful ruler much praised by his contemporaries; by the time it ended he had degenerated into a ruthless tyrant, feared by his subjects, vilified throughout most of Europe, and capable of sending the woman he had so passionately loved to her execution.

Throughout those years, Henry's motives remained clear, even though he was fast gaining a reputation for keeping his own counsel and being excessively secretive. Anne Boleyn, conversely, is an enigma. Her biographers, both before and after her death, were never impartial. On the one hand, we have the Jezebel portrayed by hostile Catholic writers, the 'Concubine' who would use any means at her disposal to ensnare a king and be rid of his wife and child, and who would not stop at adultery or incest to provide her husband with a son and so save her own skin. This violent hostility towards Anne Boleyn began in her own lifetime, and when she was beheaded in 1536 there were few who did not believe her to be guilty of at least some of the crimes attributed to her. The Spanish ambassador, who detested her, referred to her at this time as 'the English Messalina or Agrippina', and Reginald Pole, the son of the Princess Mary's former governess, openly called Anne 'a Jezebel and a sorceress'. In many ways, Anne was her own worst enemy: she attracted the enmity of Catholics because she openly espoused the cause of church reform, and was widely, but erroneously, reputed to be a Lutheran. She was also indiscreet, arrogant, vindictive in her treatment of her enemies, and given to abrupt mood swings. Although there is very little evidence that she was ever promiscuous, she was regarded as immoral from the first simply because she was the 'other woman' in the King's life. Her enemies, and they were many, thought her a she-devil, a tigress, and – according to a later Catholic source – the 'author of all the mischief that was befalling the realm'.

On the other hand, we have the saintly queen of the Protestant writers, who did so much to further true religion in England, gave her protection to the followers of Luther, and produced the great Queen Elizabeth. These writers saw Anne as a veritable saint. 'Was not Queen Anne, the mother of the blessed woman, the chief, first and only cause of banishing the beast of Rome with all his beggarly baggage?' asked John Aylmer, the renowned Protestant scholar, in the reign of Anne's daughter. Likewise George Wyatt, grandson of the poet Thomas Wyatt and Anne's first biographer, who compiled his work at the end of the sixteenth century from the reminiscences of his family and those who had known her, such as her former maid of honour, Anne Gainsford; he concluded that 'this princely lady was elect of God'.

Both these conflicting portraits of Anne Boleyn have in them some degree of truth; and both are partially inaccurate. Anne was no saint, but neither was she an adulteress nor guilty of incest. She was however, ruthless and insensitive, and if she was not as black as the Catholics tried to paint her, it is likely they were nearer the truth. Nevertheless, she was a remarkable woman of considerable courage and audacity, who knew exactly what she wanted, and made sure she got it. Once she had achieved her goal, and was expected to conform to conventional ideals of queenship, disaster overtook her, for she was demonstrably unsuited to her role, and incapable of playing the part of a docile, submissive wife.

Much is known about Anne, but there are also vital gaps. Her date of birth was not recorded, and even the date and place of her marriage to the King were kept secret. The best-documented period of her life is the last seventeen days of it, which were spent in the Tower of London, when her courageous bearing at her trial and execution were in stark contrast to her hysterical fits on her arrest, and a world away from the days when she held sway over the court with such hauteur as the King's mistress.

Anne Boleyn was only the second commoner to be elevated to the consort's throne in England – the first had been Elizabeth Woodville, wife of Edward IV. Anne's origins were uninspiring, although, like all Henry VIII's wives, she could trace her descent from Edward I. She was well-connected on her mother's side, but her father's origins were in trade. The Boleyn family came from Norfolk, where there are no records of them before 1402. Anne's forbears lived at Salle, near Aylsham, which was then a thriving community grown prosperous as a result of the profitable wool trade with the Low Countries. Salle is now a deserted hamlet, and the only trace remaining of its former prosperity is its incongruously large church where several early Boleyns are buried.

Geoffrey Boleyn, who died in 1471, was the first member of the family to make a name for himself. A mercer by trade, he became an alderman of the City of London in 1452, and Lord Mayor in 1457. By then he was a wealthy man, having purchased the manor of Blickling in Norfolk from Sir John Fastolf in 1452, and a 200-year-old castle at Hever in Kent in 1462. His wife, Anne, was the daughter of Lord Hoo and Hastings, and his marriage to her was of great social value; he now mixed with the local gentry – such as the Paston family – and the lesser nobility, and even with the much more exalted Howard family. It was probably through their influence that Geoffrey was knighted by Henry VI.

Sir Geoffrey's son, Sir William Boleyn, made an even more impressive marriage, to Margaret Butler, daughter of the Irish Earl of Ormonde. Lady Margaret bore four sons: Thomas, James, William and Edward. Thomas was the eldest, being born around 1477, when his mother was only twelve years old. When he was twenty, he fought with his father for the King, Henry VII, against the men of Cornwall, who had risen in protest against high taxation. The Boleyn family was loyal to the Crown, and came early on to the favourable notice of the Tudor kings, who preferred 'new men' of merchant stock to members of the old nobility.

At around the turn of the century, Thomas Boleyn was married to Elizabeth, the daughter of Thomas Howard, Earl of Surrey. It was fortunate for Thomas that the Howard fortunes had suffered a reversal after the Battle of Bosworth, when Surrey's father had fought on the losing side, otherwise Elizabeth might have been considered too grand for him. Yet it was still in every way a brilliant match: Elizabeth's brother, Lord Thomas Howard, was then married to the Queen's sister, Anne Plantagenet, and as the Howard family was gradually received back into favour, Thomas Boleyn's status increased accordingly.

Elizabeth Howard proved a fertile bride. 'She brought me every year a child,' Thomas recorded later, remembering what a struggle it had been to provide for them all on an income of only £50.00 per annum. But only three of the children grew to maturity: Mary, Anne and George. Of those who died in infancy, Thomas was buried in Penshurst Church in Kent, and Henry in Hever Church. There has been some dispute as to which of the surviving Boleyn children was the eldest, but it seems clear that Mary was. In 1597, her grandson, George Carey, Lord Hunsdon, referred to her in a letter to Lord Burleigh as 'the eldest daughter' of Sir Thomas Boleyn. This is supported by the wording of the Letters Patent creating Anne Boleyn Marquess of Pembroke in 1532, which refers to Anne as 'one of the daughters' of Sir Thomas Boleyn. Had Anne been the elder, the Patent would surely have said so.

Even more controversy surrounds the dates of birth of Anne and her siblings. Their parents married around the turn of the century, and thus the earliest date for Mary's birth would have been around 1499–1500. George was the youngest of the three: he was not more than twenty-seven when he was preferred to the Privy Council in 1529, and therefore cannot have been born before 1502. It is likely also that his dead brother Thomas was the eldest son, and that George was actually born after 1502, probably in 1503–4.

Until recently, it was accepted that Anne Boleyn was born in 1507; this was the date noted by William Camden in the margin of his manuscript copy of his biography of Elizabeth I, printed in 1615; another late source, Henry Clifford's *Life of Jane Dormer, Duchess of Feria*, based on the reminiscences of one of Mary Tudor's maids of honour as told to her secretary in old age, published in 1645, also gives Anne's date of birth as 1507, stating that she was 'not 29 years of age when she was executed'. However, if Anne was born in 1507, she could not have been more than six years old when she entered the service of Margaret of Austria in 1513, an impossibly early age. For a more realistic date we must turn to Lord Herbert of Cherbury's biography of Henry VIII, written during the early seventeenth century and based on many contemporary sources now lost to us. Herbert states that Anne was twenty when she returned from France in 1522; this would place her date of birth in 1501–2, and make her around eleven or twelve when she entered the Archduchess's household. Two other late sources support an even earlier date of birth: Gregorio Leti's suppressed life of Elizabeth I, which suggests 1499–1500, and William Rastell's biography of Sir Thomas More, both written in the late sixteenth century.

If Anne Boleyn was born in 1500–1501, she would have been around thirty-five when she died, middle-aged by Tudor standards. Life had not been kind to her, and stress had aged her prematurely. In 1536, the Spanish ambassador referred to her as 'that thin old woman', and there is other evidence that Anne was ageing visibly: the portrait of her (in a private collection) painted at this time is in striking contrast to earlier portraits, which show her as youthful and vivacious. None of this evidence is conclusive, but it all points to an earlier date of birth than 1507, probably 1501.

Finally, there is conflicting archaeological evidence. In 1876, during restoration work in the Chapel of St Peter ad Vincula within the Tower of London, workmen found Anne Boleyn's bones beneath the altar pavement. Victorian archaeologists described the bones as those of a woman of delicate frame; the neck vertebrae, which had been severed, were very small. They estimated that Anne had been aged between twenty-five and thirty at her death. It is a fact, however, that the science of pathology was then in its infancy, and this estimate may easily have been inaccurate.

If we date Anne's birth to around 1501, we are able to establish exactly where she was born, for – prior to Sir William's death in 1505 – Thomas Boleyn and his family lived at the manor house at Blickling in Norfolk. Anne's chaplain, Matthew Parker, confirmed her birth here in later years when he referred to himself as her 'countryman', in the sense that he came from the same part of the country that she did; he, too, was born in Norfolk. It has sometimes been claimed that Anne was born at Hever Castle, but her father did not move his family there until after Sir William Boleyn's death. As the eldest son, Thomas inherited both properties, but made over Blickling to his brother James, preferring to settle at Hever which was more convenient for the court.

Here, in the moated castle amid the Kentish countryside, Anne Boleyn spent most of her childhood. If we are to believe Lord Herbert, Thomas noticed early on that Anne was an exceptionally bright and 'toward' girl, and 'took all possible care for her good education'. As well as receiving the usual 'virtuous instruction', Anne was taught to play on various musical instruments, to sing and to dance. She quickly became accomplished in all these things, excelling on the lute and virginals, and soon learned to carry herself with grace and dignity. Her academic education was limited to the teaching of literary skills, including a fine Italianate hand and – achieved after some struggle – French. Under her mother's guidance, she became expert at embroidery, and also learned to enjoy poetry, perhaps as a result of associating with the young poet Thomas Wyatt, who lived nearby at Allington Castle. Anne, too, had a talent for composing verse. In sum, her education was similar to that enjoyed by many girls of her class, its purpose being to perfect those feminine accomplishments that were so prized, both in the marriage market and at court. With this behind her, and her undoubted charm and vivacity, she would not fail to attract the right kind of husband.

During Anne's childhood, her father's career traced an upward curve. After the accession of Henry VIII in 1509, he was often at court, and by 1511 already figured prominently in the King's circle of intimates. He was an affable man and highly cultivated, if at times somewhat brusque, and he was a natural diplomat, sent by the King on a succession of embassies to foreign courts. Henry's favour also brought a string of honours his way, and with them came increasing wealth and status. Some attributed this to sexual favours bestowed upon the King by Lady Boleyn, but this was categorically denied by Thomas Cromwell, in Henry's presence, in 1537. Thomas Boleyn was nothing if not ambitious; when sent on an embassy to the court of Margaret of Austria, Regent of the Netherlands, at Mechelen in Brabant, he quickly ingratiated himself with his hostess and wasted no time in extolling to her the virtues and accomplishments of his daughter Anne, the brightest of his children. Margaret responded by offering to take Anne into her household as one of her eighteen maids of honour, and when Thomas returned to England in the spring of 1513, Anne was despatched immediately to the Low Countries in the care of a knight surnamed Broughton.

The Regent was delighted with her new maid of honour, and wrote to thank Sir Thomas for sending her, for Anne was

> a present more than welcome in my sight. I hope to treat her in such a way that you shall be quite satisfied with me. I find in her so fine a spirit, and so perfect an address for a lady of her years, that I am more beholden to you for sending her than you can be to me for receiving her.

To improve Anne's command of the French language, Margaret appointed a governess called Simonette to tutor her, and insisted that Anne's letters to her father be written in French, so that Sir Thomas, who spoke that language fluently, would be suitably impressed. Anne herself later wrote and confessed to him that these early letters were dictated by Simonette but 'the work of my hands alone'. By then, however, she would be as proficient in French as if it were her native tongue.

Anne stayed at the court of Brabant for about eighteen months, until her father found a better position for her as maid of honour to Mary Tudor, who was betrothed to Louis XII of France in August 1514. There was the usual rush to obtain places in the future Queen of France's household, and Sir Thomas was influential enough to secure two, for both his daughters. Yet only one 'Mistress Boleyn' was listed amongst her attendants when she sailed to France in October 1514; this was probably Mary, for it appears that Anne travelled to France direct from Mechelen. Anne's position in Brabant had latterly become slightly uncomfortable due to the deteriorating relationship between England and the Empire, though the Regent recorded in a letter that she was sad to lose her. Anne herself was delighted at the prospect of serving Mary Tudor, and wrote to her father:

> Sir, I find by your letter that you wish me to appear at court in a manner becoming a respectable female, and likewise that the Queen will condescend to enter into conversation with me. At this

I rejoice, as I do think that conversing with so sensible and eloquent a princess will make me even more desirous of continuing to speak and to write good French.

The transition to Mary Tudor's service could only be to her advantage, she reasoned. She and her father were kindred spirits in their desire for advancement, their ambition, and their self-interest. Even at this age Anne had a shrewd eye to the future.

Once in France, Anne was reunited with her sister Mary, and they were among the six young girls permitted to remain at the French court by King Louis XII after he had dismissed all Mary's other English attendants. When Louis died in 1515, Anne and Mary remained in the service of his young widow until she married Suffolk and returned to England. They were then invited to serve Queen Claude, the long-suffering wife of the new King, Francis I – perhaps because both of them by this time spoke French so well.

Claude of Valois was a virtuous woman, crippled from birth by lameness; her household resembled nothing so much as a nunnery. Places in it were much sought after, and the Boleyn girls were honoured to be accorded them. They would now be expected to follow the Queen's example and conduct themselves with modesty and decorum by observing an almost conventual routine based upon prayers, good works and chastity. Claude's marriage had brought her little happiness; she was constantly pregnant, while her philandering husband entertained scores of mistresses and set the tone for one of the most licentious courts of the period. Because Claude was ill at ease in such an environment, she lived mainly at the châteaux of Amboise and Blois in the lush countryside of the Loire valley. On the occasions when her presence was required at court, the Queen was extremely watchful over her female attendants, knowing full well that they were morally at risk from Francis and his courtiers.

In such contrasting worlds did Mary and Anne Boleyn grow to maturity. The experience would shape their characters in strikingly different ways. Mary succumbed early on to the temptations so feared by Queen Claude, briefly shared her favours with Francis I, and then went on to become Henry VIII's mistress. Anne, however, was more discreet, and learned from the example set by her sister. She benefited from the regime observed in Claude's household in that she learned dignity and poise. 'She became so graceful that you would never have taken her for an Englishwoman, but for a Frenchwoman born,' wrote the French poet, Lancelot de Carles. She adopted becoming French fashions, and the French courtier Brantôme tells us in his memoirs that she dressed with marvellous taste and devised new modes which were copied by all the fashionable ladies at court; Anne wore them all with a 'gracefulness that rivalled Venus'. Later, she would be responsible for introducing the French hood into England, a fashion that would last for sixty years. Even the Jesuit historian, Nicholas Sanders – who was responsible for some of the wilder inaccuracies that later gained currency about Anne Boleyn, such as the tale that she was raped by one of her father's household officials at the age of seven – felt moved to praise her inventiveness, saying she was regarded in France as 'the glass of fashion'.

Brantôme remembered Anne Boleyn in his later years as 'the fairest and most bewitching of all the lovely dames of the French court'. According to Lancelot de Carles, her most attractive feature was 'her eyes, which she well knew how to use. In truth, such was their power that many a man paid his allegiance.' She used her eyes, he tells us, to invite conversation, and to convey the promise of hidden passion. It was a trick that enslaved several men. Even King Francis was smitten by the fascinating Anne, and wrote:

> *Venus était blonde, on m'a dit:*
> *L'on voit bien, qu'elle est brunette.*

Anne's charm lay not so much in her physical appearance as in her vivacious personality, her gracefulness, her quick wit and other accomplishments. She was petite in stature, and had an appealing fragility about her. Her eyes were black and her hair dark brown and of great length; often, she would wear it interlaced with jewels, loose down her back. But she was not pretty, nor did her looks conform to the fashionable ideals of her time. She had small breasts when it was fashionable to have a voluptuous figure, and in a period when pale complexions were much admired, she was sallow, even swarthy, with small moles on her body. George Wyatt says she had a large Adam's apple, 'like a man's'. This was described by the hostile

Nicholas Sanders as 'a large wen under her chin', which Anne always concealed by wearing 'a high dress under her throat'. Nowhere is this borne out by other contemporary writers, or by portraits. Anne did, however, have a small deformity, which her enemies sometimes delighted in describing as a devil's teat. Wyatt tells us she had a second nail 'upon the side of her nail upon one of her fingers', about which she was rather self-conscious, for she took pains to hide it with long hanging oversleeves, another of her fashionable innovations. Sanders described it as a sixth finger, as did Margaret Roper, the daughter of Sir Thomas More.

Even Sanders, however, conceded that Anne was 'handsome to look at, amusing in her way, and a good dancer', while John Barlow, a divine who was later in Anne's service, thought her 'very eloquent and gracious', but less beautiful than Elizabeth Blount, Henry VIII's former mistress. Anne Boleyn undoubtedly had charm and personality in great measure, as well as that indefinable quality, sex appeal. It was this that made her appealing to so many men. Though not beautiful in the conventional sense, she had the gift of making men think she was.

Her portraits – and there are several extant – show in nearly every case a dark-haired woman with a thin face, high cheekbones and a pointed chin – facial characteristics all inherited by her daughter, Elizabeth I, who resembled her in everything but colouring. Portraits claiming to be of Anne Boleyn as a young woman at the French court are all spurious. The most famous portrait of her is that in the National Portrait Gallery, a copy of a lost original, painted between 1533 and 1536. The Gallery portrait, as well as other versions (notably at Windsor Castle, Hever Castle, and the Deanery at Ripon), once formed part of a long gallery set of royal portraits, popular in Elizabethan and Jacobean times. This portrait type still has something of the charm and vivacity that made Anne so attractive. She wears a black velvet gown with furred sleeves, a French hood edged with pearls, and a rope of pearls with a 'B' pendant. Anne was fond of initial pendants, and had at least two others – an 'A' and an 'AB', both of which were inherited and worn by her daughter. Some versions of the portrait show Anne wearing a golden filet and carrying a red rose in her hands. The miniaturist John Hoskins made a fine copy of the lost original of the National

Portrait Gallery picture in the seventeenth century; now in the collection of the Duke of Buccleuch, its quality is striking, reflecting the artist's great skill in this medium.

Other authentic representations of Anne Boleyn are little known. Her features were faithfully depicted on a medal struck in 1534 bearing the legend 'A.R. The Moost Happi'; Henry may have intended to issue it when Anne presented him with a son, for she was pregnant with her second child that year. Now it is defaced, but, in spite of this, the image is clear, in essence the same as the portraits already discussed, and the face depicted on an enamelled ring now at Chequers, the Prime Minister's country house. This was made in 1575 for Elizabeth I by an artist who had perhaps seen Anne Boleyn, or copied a lost portrait.

Some portraits said to be of Anne are of doubtful authenticity, such as the Holbein sketch at Weston Park. The sitter wears an English gable hood of the 1530s, and has dark hair, large eyes, a long nose and full, sensual lips; her face is fuller than shown in authentic portraits, and her chin not so pointed. Copies in oils exist; one is at Hever Castle, and one was at Warwick Castle until recently. (At Hever, there is a companion portrait of Mary Boleyn, of doubtful authenticity.) Yet is this Anne? Because the sitter is shown from a different angle, it is hard to tell. Holbein was a far better artist than any of the workshop limners who produced copies of authentic portraits, and his portraits are stunningly realistic when compared with the flat portrait panels produced in the studios of the age. Moreover, the portrait was first identified as Anne Boleyn in 1649, not too late to be accepted as proof of a reliable tradition of authenticity.

Anne Boleyn was highly accomplished, intelligent and witty, and in her younger years, according to George Wyatt, 'passing sweet and cheerful'. She loved gambling, played both cards and dice, had a taste for wine, and enjoyed a joke. She was also fond of hunting and the occasional game of bowls. At the glittering French court, she shone at singing, making music, dancing and conversation, and became friendly with the King's sister, the blue-stocking Margaret of Alençon, a lady of great talent and humour, who encouraged Anne's interest in poetry and literature.

Not surprisingly, the young men of the court swarmed round her.

Francis I was impressed by the way she handled them, and told her father in a letter that she was discreet and modest. He had heard a rumour that she desired to be a nun; 'This I should regret,' he wrote. It is highly unlikely that Anne Boleyn had any inclination whatsoever towards the religious life; perhaps she used it as a weapon with which to ward off unwelcome suitors, or whet the appetites of those men she found attractive. There is some later evidence that she was perhaps not so virtuous during her years in France as has hitherto been supposed. Brantôme tells us that 'rarely, or never, did any maid or wife leave that court chaste', and in 1533, Francis I confided to the Duke of Norfolk, Anne's uncle, that she 'had not always lived virtuously'. More tellingly, Henry VIII told the Spanish ambassador in 1536 that Anne had been 'corrupted' in France, and that he had discovered this when sexually experimenting with her. Whatever the extent of Anne's sexual experience in France, however, she was certainly much more discreet than her sister Mary, for no breath of scandal attached itself to her at the time. Nor would this have been in her interests, for she was eager to make a good marriage. One slip, and that ambition would be finished.

Anne's prospects of marriage came under discussion while she was still in France. In 1515, her great-grandfather, James Butler, Earl of Ormonde, died without any male heir of his body to succeed him. The earldom was claimed both by his cousin, Sir Piers Butler, and by Sir Thomas Boleyn, his grandson. It was a contest that would drag on for fourteen years before a solution was reached, although in 1520 Sir Thomas saw a way of resolving the dispute. He proposed a marriage between his daughter Anne and James Butler, the son of Sir Piers. James was described by Cardinal Wolsey as 'right active, discreet and wise', and Thomas was agreeable to the earldom devolving upon him if he married Anne. Boleyn's brother-in-law, the Earl of Surrey, agreed to lay the proposal before the King, whose consent was necessary in such matters. Anne, of course, was not consulted, and no one thought to question whether she would be happy to exchange the sophistication of the French court for a primitive castle in Ireland.

Henry VIII told Surrey he would consult Wolsey on the matter, and Surrey immediately wrote to the Cardinal, hoping to enlist his support, for James Butler was at that time a member of Wolsey's household, one of many young artistocrats who were sent to him to complete their education and gain experience of the court.

Wolsey took his time. It was not until November 1521 that he informed the King that he intended to 'devise with your Grace how the marriage betwixt [James Butler] and Sir Thomas Boleyn's daughter may be brought to pass'. However, although negotiations dragged on, they were mysteriously abandoned in the autumn of 1522. It may be that Sir Thomas Boleyn had had second thoughts, and decided to pursue his own claim to the earldom of Ormonde after all. Whatever the reason, at the end of 1522 Anne Boleyn was no nearer to being betrothed than she had ever been.

Anne had left France early that year. The recent pact between Henry VIII and Charles V had brought England and France to the brink of war, and English subjects living in France were advised to return home. Anne left Paris around January 1522, when English scholars were curtailing their studies at the Sorbonne. Queen Claude regretted losing a valued attendant, and King Francis, in a letter to Wolsey, expressed himself saddened by the 'strange' departure of the fascinating Boleyn.

The Anne Boleyn who returned home to Hever was a very different person from the girl who had left it more than eight years before. Everything about her was now very French: her mode of dress, her manners, her speech, her behaviour. Having lived at the most civilised court in the world, she stood out by reason of her wit, her grace and her accomplishments. It was no time at all before Sir Thomas had secured her a place in the household of Katherine of Aragon, which she entered around February.

At the English court, Anne's social skills brought her instant admiration from all quarters, and she was immediately chosen by the Master of the Revels to take part in one of the pageants planned for Lent. On 4 March Cardinal Wolsey gave a great banquet for the King and Queen at York Place, his London palace near Westminster. After dinner, the hall was cleared and a model of a castle called the *Château Vert* was wheeled in; from it issued five ladies and five gentlemen, who danced together before the court, the King, as Ardent Desire, being one of the dancers. However, he had eyes for no one but his partner, Mary Boleyn, who was then his mistress. The other ladies were the King's sister, Mary Tudor, his aunt the

Countess of Devon, Jane Parker, daughter of Lord Morley, who was betrothed to Anne's brother George, and Anne. All wore gowns of white satin embroidered with gold thread.

In April 1522, Sir Thomas was appointed Treasurer of the royal household. Rather than deploring his daughter Mary's immorality, he was in fact capitalising on it, and hoping for greater rewards to come. Nor did he have to wait long, for in 1525 he was elevated to the peerage as Viscount Rochford. But by that time, Henry's interest in Mary Boleyn had waned: if Wolsey's secretary and biographer, George Cavendish, is to be believed, he was casting amorous eyes in her sister Anne's direction, and had in fact been doing so since 1523. However, he had refrained from actively pursuing her, and had not disclosed his secret inclinations to anyone, least of all to the lady herself. Cavendish's information was probably correct; he was an eyewitness of the events of the period who was often taken into Wolsey's confidence, and Wolsey, of course, knew nearly all his master's secrets and made it his business to learn about the private intrigues of the court.

In 1523, Anne Boleyn's life revolved around her duties within the Queen's household. Katherine liked to surround herself with attractive young women, often to her own detriment, and was a benevolent mistress to those who served her, never failing in courtesy towards them, and taking an almost maternal interest in their lives. Young men were made welcome in the Queen's apartments, and there were plenty of opportunities for flirtation. Anne had attracted a number of suitors, and one young man who was smitten with her charms was Henry Percy, the 21-year-old heir to the earldom of Northumberland. Percy had served on the Council of the North in 1522 before joining the household of Cardinal Wolsey, hoping like many other young men of similar rank to find preferment. Percy was the Cardinal's servitor at table; whenever Wolsey went to court, Percy would go with him, but as soon as he had been excused from his duties, he would resort to the Queen's apartments, there to chat and flirt with the maids of honour. Thus he had met Anne Boleyn, and before very long he had eyes for no one else.

Anne Boleyn was not for nothing her father's daughter; she saw in Henry Percy not only an ardent suitor to whom she was attracted, but also the heir to one of the greatest and most ancient earldoms in England. The prospect of becoming Countess of Northumberland and chatelaine of Alnwick Castle, was a glorious one, and falling in love with Henry Percy was consequently very easy. He was quick to declare his feelings for her, and that summer he proposed marriage and secretly contracted himself to marry Anne before witnesses. But although their betrothal was to be kept a secret for the time being, the lovers could not conceal their feelings, and there was talk. It reached the ears of Cardinal Wolsey and alarmed him, for he was aware that Percy had been betrothed since 1516 to Lady Mary Talbot, daughter of the Earl of Shrewsbury. Percy had been very rash to involve himself with Anne Boleyn, a precontract being then as legally binding as a marriage. Anyway, in Wolsey's opinion, Anne Boleyn was no fit bride for a Percy, and it was unlikely that the Earl of Northumberland would ever have agreed to such a match.

Wolsey wasted no time in laying the matter before the King, without whose permission no aristocratic marriage could be contracted and who was angry at not being consulted. According to Cavendish, who relates the whole episode as one with inside knowledge of it, the thought of Anne Boleyn betrothed to another man disturbed him, so much so that he reluctantly confessed to the Cardinal the 'secret affection' he had been nurturing for her, and ordered Wolsey to break the engagement. This Wolsey agreed was the best course, and when he arrived back at York Place, he summoned Percy and proceeded to lecture him sternly over his folly in involving himself with 'that foolish girl yonder in the court, Anne Boleyn'. In front of Cavendish and other onlookers, the Cardinal accused the young man of having offended his father and his sovereign; Anne was 'one such as neither of them will be agreeable with the matter', and anyway, 'His Highness intended to have preferred Anne Boleyn unto another person, although she knoweth it not'. Henry, of course, had done no such thing: he was reserving Anne for himself.

Percy was dismayed at his master's words, but he outfaced the Cardinal and argued that he was 'old enough to choose a wife as my fancy served me best', emphasising Anne's 'right noble parentage, whose descent is equivalent with mine'. But Wolsey was not to be swayed, and called Percy a 'wilful boy'. Percy retorted that he had 'gone so far, before so many worthy witnesses', that he knew no way of extricating himself from his engagement without offending his conscience. Too late, he realised his error, for the Cardinal, well-versed in canon law, swooped. 'Think ye that the King and I know not what we have to do in as weighty a matter as this?' he interrupted smoothly. Percy was beaten, and he knew it. His father was sent for, and he was commanded in the King's name not to resort to Anne's company again. When the Earl of Northumberland arrived, he soundly berated his son, threatening to disinherit him if he did not do his duty. Then he had a long talk with the King and Wolsey, which resulted in a decision that Percy should marry Lady Mary Talbot as soon as it could be arranged. After that, Wolsey put in hand the legal process whereby Percy's contract with Anne Boleyn was 'clearly undone'.

Forbidden to see Anne, Percy was frantic with worry about her, having no means of knowing what she had heard. In desperation, he sent her a message via his friend, James Melton, begging that she would never allow herself to be married to another man: 'Bid her remember her promise, which none can loose but God only.' But Percy's hopes were futile. In September 1523, he married Lady Mary Talbot, and went home to Northumberland. His marriage would prove a very unhappy one, blighted not only by incompatibility but by his own advancing ill health.

Anne's first reaction, upon hearing that her betrothal to Percy had been broken, was not sorrow but anger. The Cardinal had ruined her life, the upstart butcher's son had dared to dismiss her as a 'hasty folly', and had had the effrontery to refer to her as 'a foolish girl'. Worst of all, he had proclaimed her unfit to mate with a Percy. Of the King's involvement in the affair, she suspected nothing; it was Wolsey with whom she was 'greatly offended'. If ever it lay in her power, she openly declared, 'she would work the Cardinal as much displeasure as he had done her.' However, it seemed she would have little opportunity to do so, for an order arrived almost immediately for her to return to her father's castle at Hever for a time. This made her so angry, says Cavendish, that 'she smoked'!

Anne was left to simmer and sorrow at Hever for a year or more. As for the King's interest in her, this would seem to have been a case of out of sight out of mind; he was still preoccupied with her sister anyway, although his interest in Mary dwindled as the months went by. Anne's life during her exile is not documented. She may have attended the wedding of her brother George to Jane Parker in 1524; as a wedding present, the King granted George the manor of Grimston in Norfolk, which proves that any displeasure he may have felt towards the Boleyns on account of the Percy affair was transitory.

Anne returned to court some time in 1524 or 1525, and resumed her duties in the Queen's household. In the months of her absence she had learned the hard way to be wary of men, although she still attracted them and once more established herself as one of the brightest young women at court.

In 1525, the King's interest in Anne reawakened. He was intrigued by her grace and her sharp wit, while her sophistication and sexual allure were in delightful contrast to Queen Katherine's piety and grave dignity. Anne was twenty-four, Katherine approaching forty: in every way Anne was in direct contrast to his ageing wife. He himself was still magnificent, larger than life, in his middle thirties, and ripe for an affair. When he looked at Anne, he found himself drawn to her as he had been to no woman before her; and in view of the ease with which he had made his past conquests, he did not doubt that he would succeed in seducing her.

He was destined to be quickly disillusioned, for no sooner was the object of his desire firmly established back at court than she seemed to be encouraging the advances of the poet Thomas Wyatt, a married man whose wife's adulteries were notorious. In reality, Anne's participation in this affair was at best half-hearted, for she knew there was no brilliant future in it. She did not see any more in Wyatt's attentions than the polite conventions of the courtly affair, nor did she have any intention of granting sexual favours to the poet, for all his fervent protestations of love. For her it was an enjoyable flirtation, but the King, of course, did not know this and, suspecting the worst, grew tense with jealousy.

Wyatt's grandson, George Wyatt, later recounted how the poet had been taken with Anne's beauty and her witty and graceful speech, and tells us that Wyatt was supposed to have expressed his feelings for her in some of his verses. In fact, his poems tell us very little about the affair, as few of them can be proved to relate to it, while one or two of those once accepted as referring to Anne Boleyn are now thought not to have been composed by Wyatt at all. One verse, which is in the form of a riddle about a disdainful lover, has as its answer the name 'Anna'; but which Anna cannot be proved. What is clear, though, is that Wyatt was far more interested in Anne Boleyn than she was in him, and before his courtship went too far she 'rejected all his speech of love' as kindly as she could, encouraging friendship rather than amorous advances. Wyatt went on hoping and dreaming, writing of 'the lively sparks that issue from those eyes, sunbeams to daze men's sight', and seeking her company. What he failed to realise was that it had dawned at last upon Anne Boleyn that other, more august eyes were upon her.

In February 1526, Henry VIII appeared in the tiltyard wearing the jousting dress embroidered with the words 'Declare I dare not'. This was the first indication that he had begun paying court to Anne Boleyn in secret, and doubtless his courtiers assumed that once more their sovereign had taken a new mistress. They would have been wrong: Henry had asked Anne to become his mistress, but – to his astonishment – she had refused. She would not be his mistress in the courtly sense nor in the physical sense. She had seen what had happened to her sister, who had been cast off without so much as a pension, and she told the King (according to George Wyatt):

> I think your Majesty speaks these words in mirth to prove me, but without any intent of degrading your princely self. To ease you of the labour of asking me any such question hereafter, I beseech your Highness most earnestly to desist, and to take this my answer in good part. I would rather lose my life than my honesty, which will be the greatest and best part of the dowry I shall have to bring my husband.

Henry, who was used to women surrendering the instant he beckoned, was intrigued. It was new for him to be placed in the position of having to beg for sexual favours; far from being angry or irritated, he was captivated, and Anne at once became infinitely more desirable. 'Well, Madam,' he told her, 'I shall live in hope.' But then it was Anne's turn to express astonishment: 'I understand not, most mighty King, how you should retain such hope! Your wife I cannot be, both in respect of mine own unworthiness, and also because you have a queen already. Your mistress I will not be.' Besides, she added, referring to the Queen, 'how could I injure a princess of such great virtue?'

Whether these were Anne's actual words is really immaterial; she must have said something of the sort, for she made it very clear to Henry VIII that she would only surrender her virginity after marriage. The only way that Henry would ever enjoy her would be by making her his wife, and that, as she pointed out, was impossible. It may be that he had told her already of his doubts about the validity of his marriage; if not, he would soon do so. Nor was it long for the seed once sown to take root in Henry's mind. Wyatt says the King told Wolsey he had spoken with a young lady with the soul of an angel and a spirit worthy of a crown who would not sleep with him. Wolsey, who failed to see the significance of what the King was really saying, observed in his worldly-wise way that if Henry considered Anne worthy of such an honour, then she should do as he wished. 'She is not of ordinary clay,' sighed the royal lover, 'and I fear she will never condescend in that way.' 'Great princes,' Wolsey insisted, 'if they choose to play the lover, have means of softening hearts of steel.'

Henry chose to play the lover. He sent Anne expensive gifts as tokens of his affection; these she accepted, which led him to hope that she might come to relent, given time. Yet already Anne was playing for the highest prize of all. As soon as she learned from the King of his doubts about his marriage, she saw her advantage. If he obtained an annulment, which might not be very difficult in the circumstances, then he would be free to marry again and father the heirs he so desperately needed. A Percy had considered her worthy, and a strain of Plantagenet blood ran in her veins. Why should she not become Queen of England?

Anne was setting out on a dangerous path, which she would have to tread with the utmost care. Whatever happened, she must not surrender to the King: his interest cooled too quickly. For the moment, she contented herself with dropping subtle hints, intimating that in the right circumstances she was ready to give heart, body and soul to him, and Henry, like any man kept at bay, grew daily more intent upon having her. Her studied aloofness only added to his torment lest she was harbouring some secret passion for Wyatt.

Anne was on friendly terms with the poet, who, blithely unaware of his sovereign's interest, was still paying court to her. One day, he playfully snatched a small jewel hanging by a lace out of her pocket, and thrust it into his doublet. Anne begged for its return, but Wyatt kept it, and wore it round his neck under his shirt. Presently, Anne forgot all about it, the jewel being of little value. However, not long afterwards, Wyatt was the King's opponent at a game of bowls; Henry thought the winning cast was his, and pointing to it with a finger on which a ring Wyatt recognised as Anne's was displayed, said, 'Wyatt, I tell thee, it is mine!' Thomas, not to be outdone, rashly produced Anne's trinket from about his neck, and taking the chain, said, 'If Your Majesty will give me leave to measure it, I hope it will be mine!' The winning cast was indeed his own, but he had not been referring to that, and the King, to whom his meaning had been clear, lost his temper. 'It may be so, but then I am deceived!' he snapped, and broke up the game.

Henry was not only jealous, he was hurt, because the ring he wore had been given to him by Anne, under some pressure, as a token of her affection. It was not, as has sometimes been supposed, a betrothal ring, because Anne had not received one in return. Nevertheless, it was not long before Henry did make up his mind to 'win her by treaty of marriage'; in his mind, he was a free man, having convinced himself that his marriage was uncanonical, and that for the Pope to declare it so would be a mere formality. He now wanted Anne more than anything else in the world, except, perhaps, a son, and he could see no reason why he should not enjoy lawfully what she would not permit him illicitly. His proposal to her was made in the latter part of 1526 or early in 1527, yet there was a delay of some months before he sought Wolsey's advice about obtaining an annulment. This delay was caused by Anne's reluctance to commit herself, a ploy calculated to banish any regrets the King might have had after asking her to become his wife. She had cleverly manoeuvred him into proposing marriage; now she would make him play a guessing game, while she affected to consider whether she would accept him.

Anne had assured the King that Wyatt meant nothing to her, and that the poet had taken her trinket without her permission. She had also made it clear to Wyatt that his courtship of her must end. Henry was taking no chances, however, and sent Wyatt off on a diplomatic mission to Italy, from which he would not return until May 1527, when it was becoming obvious to everyone just how serious the affair between the King and Anne Boleyn was. Wyatt accepted defeat with good grace, and drowned his sorrows in some very apt verse:

> Who list her hunt, I put him out of doubt;
> As well as I may spend his time in vain.
> And graven with diamonds, in letters plain,
> There is written her fair neck round about:
> *Noli me tangere*, for Caesar's I am,
> And wild for to hold, though I seem tame.

Wyatt soon recovered from his loss and shortly afterwards found a new love, Elizabeth Darrell, who remained his mistress until his death in 1542. Soon, he was celebrating her in a new poem:

> Then do I love again;
> If thou ask whom, sure since I did refrain
> Her, that did set our country in a roar;
> The unfeigned cheer of Phyllis hath the place
> That Brunette had.

Later, Thomas amended the third line of this verse to 'Brunette, that set my wealth in such a roar,' deeming it wiser to delete all references to his affair with Anne Boleyn, which is perhaps why very few of his poems about it survive today.

Having eliminated his rival, the King may now have hoped that his way was clear to ecstasy with his sweetheart. Anne found his ardour hard to deal with, and retaliated by withdrawing from the court to Hever Castle. This only inflamed the King more, and he began sending her passionate love-letters, of which this is one of the first:

My mistress and my friend,

I and my heart commit ourselves into your hands, beseeching you to hold us recommended to your good favour, and that your affection to us may not be by absence diminished. For great pity it were to increase our pain, seeing that absence makes enough of it, and indeed more than I could ever have thought; remembering us of a point in astronomy, that the longer the days are, the farther off is the sun, and yet, notwithstanding, the hotter; so it is with our love, for we by absence are far sundered, yet it nevertheless keeps its fervency, at the least on my part, holding in hope the like on yours. Ensuring you that for myself the annoy of absence doth already too much vex me; it is almost intolerable to me, were it not for the firm hope that I have of your ever during affection towards me. And sometimes, to put you in mind of this, and seeing that in person I cannot be in your presence, I send you my picture set in a bracelet. Wishing myself in their place, when it should please you. This by the hand of your loyal servant and friend,

     H.R.

Anne was better able to cope with separation than Henry, for she was not so deeply involved emotionally. Seven years in France had taught her skill in the game of courtship, and she sent the King the gift of a jewel fashioned as a solitary damsel in a boat tossed by a tempest. The allusion was clear. At the same time, she wrote her lover a warm letter, hinting at her inner turmoil, but implying that she might, with some reassurance from him, see her way to accepting him as her future husband. Sadly, this letter, and all the others written to the King by Anne, have not survived. His to her, however, she kept, but they were stolen by a papal servant in 1529, and today rest in the Vatican archives.

Anne's letter and love-token provoked a passionate reaction from Henry, who wrote:

For so beautiful a gift, I thank you right cordially, chiefly for the good intent and too-humble submission vouchsafed by your kindness. To merit it would not a little perplex me, if I were not aided therein by your great benevolence and goodwill. The proofs of your affection are such that they constrain me ever truly to love, honour and serve you, praying that you will continue in this same firm and constant purpose, ensuring you, for my part, that I will the rather go beyond than make reciprocal, if loyalty of heart, the desire to do you pleasure, even with my whole heart root, may serve to advance it. Henceforth, my heart shall be dedicate to you alone, greatly desirous that my body could be as well, as God can bring it to pass if it pleaseth Him, Whom I entreat once each day for the accomplishment thereof, trusting that at length my prayer will be heard, wishing the time brief, and thinking it but long until we shall see each other again.

Written with the hand of the secretary who in heart, body and will is your loyal and most ensured servant.

H. autre 　AB　 ne cherche R.

'Henry the King seeks no other than Anne Boleyn.' And around Anne's initials the King drew a heart, as lovers have done from time immemorial. Anne may have been flattered, yet her resolve remained firm, and she stayed tantalisingly out of reach. When Henry, driven to desperation, made a brief visit to see her at Hever, she told him she was returning to court. Then, when he had gone, she changed her mind, and sent a message to say she could not come after all, even in her mother's company, which Henry had suggested as a means of preserving her good name. Frantic in case her feelings had cooled, he complained bitterly in his next letter that she had not written often enough and that she was being unduly hard on him:

To my mistress,

Because the time seems to me very long since I have heard of your good health and of you, the great affection that I bear you has prevailed with me to send to you, to be the better ascertained of your health and pleasure, because since I parted with you I have been advised that the opinion in which I left you has now altogether changed, and that you will not come to court, neither with my lady your mother, nor yet any other way. I cannot enough marvel, seeing I am well assured I have never since that time committed fault; methinks it is but small recompense for the great love I bear you to keep me thus distanced from the person of that she which of all the world I most do esteem. And if you love me with such settled affection as I trust, I assure me that this sundering of our two persons should be to you some small vexation. Bethink you well, my mistress, that your absence doth not a little grieve me, trusting that by your will it should not be so;

but if I knew in truth that of your will you desired it, I could do none other than lament me of my ill-fortune, abating by little and little my so great folly.

Unknown to Anne, the King had already made the decision to test the validity of his marriage in the ecclesiastical courts; this was a matter too sensitive to be written of in his letter, so he entrusted the bearer with a message for Anne, 'praying you to give credence to that which he will tell you from me'. The news had the desired effect, and elicited a prompt reply, in which Anne, as his humble subject, professed her love and devotion to a gracious sovereign. This was not quite what Henry had hoped for, but it was enough to provoke him into a fervent declaration of his intentions towards her in his next letter, written in the spring of 1527. He was in great distress, he said, because he did not know how to interpret her last letter, and he prayed her,

> with all my heart, you will expressly certify me of your whole mind concerning the love between us two. . . . If it shall please you to do me the office of a true loyal mistress and friend, and to give yourself up, heart, body and soul to me, who will be and have been your very loyal servant, I promise you that not only shall the name be given you, but that also I will take you for my only mistress, rejecting from thought and affection all others save yourself, to serve you only.

He ended by beseeching her for an answer, if not in writing, then in person.

It is clear from this letter that the King was using the word 'mistress' in its honourable, courtly context, yet equally clear that he meant Anne to interpret it in its fullest sense. But there is more to the letter than that. She was to be placed above all others, including, presumably, the Queen herself. Henry was not yet free to marry her, and saw no reason why they could not be lovers while he was waiting for his freedom: he wanted Anne to commit herself publicly to the relationship. For her, this was a prospect fraught with danger and insecurity, and therefore not to be considered. If she became the King's mistress now, she might never become Queen of England.

Nevertheless, she could not go on absenting herself from Henry for ever, and it was at this stage that she consented to return to court. It was the right psychological moment, for Henry was ready to do whatever she asked, and was adamant that their futures lay together. Almost immediately, Anne found herself in a position of unparalleled influence: even Queen Katherine had never held such sway over the King. But Anne had an old score to settle, and she was now in a position to exact vengeance. Since 1523 she had blamed Cardinal Wolsey for publicly humiliating her, and her burning desire since then had been to teach him that one did not mishandle members of the Boleyn family with impunity. She had never guessed that it had been the King, and not Wolsey, who was the prime mover in the affair, and Henry had not seen fit to enlighten her.

When Anne returned to court, the King made no secret of his love for her, nor that she was from henceforth to play a prominent role in affairs. He began showering her with fine jewellery and clothes, and saw that she was lodged in splendid apartments. The courtiers made much of her, using her as an intermediary between themselves and the King, and she was soon revelling in her growing influence and power. According to George Wyatt, she began to look 'very haughty and proud'.

The Queen had both heard by report and seen with her own eyes what was going on between her husband and her maid of honour, yet she showed neither of them any grudge or displeasure, but accepted the affair with good grace and commendable patience, openly declaring herself to be a 'Patient Grizelda', and telling her ladies, according to George Cavendish, that she held Anne Boleyn 'in more estimation for the King's sake than she had before'. Had she known just what her husband's intentions were towards Anne, she might not have accepted the situation with such equanimity, but as far as she was concerned, Anne was merely the latest in a line of royal mistresses and would be discarded in due course.

Others at court were more perceptive, and correctly assessed the intensity of the King's passion for Anne Boleyn. One was Anne's maternal uncle, Thomas Howard, third Duke of Norfolk, son of the victor of Flodden, who had died in 1524. In 1527, Norfolk was a hardened soldier and statesman of fifty-four, who would retain his position as premier duke of the realm and one of the most prominent members of the Privy Council until his disgrace in 1546. After the death of his first wife, Anne Plantagenet, Henry VIII's aunt, Howard had married Elizabeth Stafford, daughter of the Duke of Buckingham who had been executed for treason in 1521, and by her had three children, the eldest being Henry, Earl of Surrey, who would become one of the greatest poets of the Tudor age. The Duke and Duchess were not happily married; he had taken for his mistress the low-born Elizabeth Holland, whom his wife described as 'a churl's daughter, who was but a washer in my nursery eight years'. Norfolk's involvement with his laundress lasted more than twenty years and in 1539 the Duchess was still complaining about him keeping 'that harlot' and other whores also, vindictive women who had bound and restrained the Duchess while one sat on her breast 'till I spat blood'. By that time, the ducal couple had long since gone their separate ways, and the Duchess reckoned that 'if I come home, I shall be poisoned'.

Thomas Howard might have been brutal and callous in his domestic life, but his male contemporaries considered him to be a man of the utmost wisdom, solid worth and loyalty. His portrait by Holbein shows a granite-faced martinet, and it is difficult to imagine him being the prudent, liberal, astute and affable man he was reputed to be. Nevertheless he had the common touch, and associated with everybody regardless of rank. What made Norfolk valuable to Henry VIII was his astute judgement and his ruthless expediency. He had great experience in the administration of the kingdom, and could discuss affairs of state in depth. Like all his clan, he was ambitious.

Norfolk, like most of the older nobility, hated Wolsey. Because he and several other lords believed the Cardinal was preventing them from enjoying the power that should rightly be theirs, they meant to use Anne Boleyn as 'a sufficient and apt instrument' to bring what Cavendish calls 'their malicious purpose' to fruition. To this end, they very often consulted with her as to what was to be done, and she, 'having a very good wit, and also an inward desire to be revenged upon the Cardinal, was as agreeable to their requests as they were themselves'. Thus Anne began her long campaign to discredit Wolsey in the King's eyes, and then bring about his ruin, not only for the sake of her pride but also in the interests of her family.

Wolsey was at first unaware of her enmity. He had virtually forgotten the Percy affair and the furious girl he had dismissed so lightly four years earlier. Now, to please his master and ingratiate himself with the new favourite, the Cardinal entertained them both to sumptuous banquets at York Place. Then, wrote Cavendish, 'the world began to be full of wonderful rumours' because 'the love between the King and this gorgeous lady grew to such a perfection that divers imaginations were imagined'. Nor were the rumours without foundation, for in the late spring of 1527, Anne finally accepted the King's proposal of marriage and agreed to become his wife as soon as he was free.

She was well aware of the domestic politics of the court and the struggle between factions for power, but she was not afraid. With the King at her side, an ardent lover, she had no cause to be. Her hardest task, as she viewed it, was to keep his love and maintain his desire at its present pitch without giving way to it. It was this that would test her resolve to the utmost during the years to come, and this that lay at the root of the chronic insecurity she later manifested.

As soon as he had Anne's consent, the King took her father, now Viscount Rochford, into his confidence, 'to whom we may be sure that the news was not a little joyful', observed George Wyatt with exquisite understatement. Rochford was no less ambitious than his daughter, yet the prospect of being the father of the next Queen of England, and possibly grandfather to a future monarch, was more than he had ever dreamed of. Such a position automatically brought with it not only wealth, power, fame and honour such as he had always craved and worked so hard to obtain, but also a considerable amount of influence in public affairs. From the first, he would be his daughter's greatest supporter. Like her he was also an enemy of the Cardinal. Rochford was bitter because when, in 1525, he had been created a Viscount, he had been forced to resign his post as Treasurer without any financial compensation. For this, he blamed Wolsey.

It did not take long for the Cardinal to realise what was happening: a faction was forming around Anne Boleyn, and he knew it to be hostile towards himself. For the present he could afford to be sanguine about this, for the King had not acquainted him with his true intentions towards Anne. Like the Queen, Wolsey saw her as just another mistress, who could go the way of the others. Yet to keep the King happy he paid court to the lady, sending her gifts – she had in particular expressed a desire for carps, shrimps and other delicacies from his famous ponds – and putting on entertainments for her. On the surface, cordial relations existed between Anne and Wolsey, and no doubt he was privately of the opinion that she was as light-minded and foolish as he had thought her four years earlier, having no great opinion of the intelligence of women. This particular young woman, however, did have brains, and was determined to use them to good effect when it came to manipulating Wolsey's downfall. First, however, she would make use of the Cardinal, for Henry had made it clear that he was the one man who could effectively negotiate the annulment of his marriage. Then she would do her best to discredit him in the King's eyes, and take her revenge.

Anne was now constantly in the King's company. She ate with him, prayed with him, hunted with him, and danced with him, but she did not sleep with him. Henry had no leisure to ponder his thraldom, however, for he was about to embark on the greatest enterprise of his life: the annulment of his marriage to Katherine of Aragon, which would come to be known as the King's 'great matter'. When Henry set out to obtain what has often, but erroneously, been called his 'divorce', he little dreamed it would take him six years, nor envisaged the far-reaching effects it would have on himself, the woman he loved, or his kingdom and people.

8
A thousand Wolseys for one Anne Boleyn

In the spring of 1527, Henry VIII finally set in motion the ecclesiastical machinery that he hoped would bring about the dissolution of his marriage to Katherine of Aragon; what he desired was a declaration that their union had been invalid and unlawful from the first. When news of his intentions leaked out, several people believed that Anne Boleyn had been the cause of his doubts about his marriage. In fact, she was merely a catalyst, and the indications are that Henry would have pursued an annulment at some stage anyway, for overriding all other considerations was his desperate need for a male heir.

Throughout the course of the 'great matter', Henry behaved like a man possessed, on two counts. One was his conviction that he was right, the other was his passion for Anne Boleyn: the French ambassador thought him 'so much in love that God alone can abate his madness'. Under Anne's influence, he was beginning to display the character traits that would govern his later behaviour, and this period of his life saw the beginning of the transition from knight errant to tyrant. It was a slow metamorphosis, however, and would only be accomplished once the King had thrown off first the tutelage of Wolsey, and afterwards the influence of Anne Boleyn. Then he would at last be his own master.

Once the King had made his decision to take proceedings, and because she was the butt of so much speculation at court, Anne Boleyn resolved to return to Hever again. Hever Castle has changed immeasurably since Anne's day. By the eighteenth century it was a ruin, and it was gutted and refurbished at the beginning of the twentieth century, when the present gardens were laid out and the lake dug. Apart from the stone fabric of the building and the moat very little remains from the sixteenth century; yet the restoration has been so harmonious that it is easy to picture Henry and Anne there, in formal gardens very like the present ones.

Anne was rarely at court between May 1527 and the summer of 1529. She joined the King at his manor of Beaulieu in Essex in August 1527, and spent the greater part of a month hunting with him and supping each evening in his privy chamber. From Beaulieu, Anne returned to Hever. She paid a brief visit to court at the end of September, but spent most of the winter at Hever. In March 1528, she and her mother, who acted as chaperon, were the King's guests at Windsor, whither Henry had gone with only a handful of attendants. It was a brief idyll: when the weather was fair, Henry and Anne would ride out hunting or hawking every afternoon, not returning until late in the evening, or would go walking in Windsor Great Park. At other times they occupied themselves with the pastimes they both enjoyed: cards and dice, music, poetry, and dancing. Anne and her mother were again at court during July and August 1528, but by September the political situation was such that Henry sent them back to Hever.

Throughout these long absences, the King found himself once more playing the role of scribe, and his letters to Anne, whom he referred to as 'mine own sweetheart' or 'darling', were written with increasing intensity. He would often abase himself as a courtly suitor should, thanking her 'right heartily for that it pleaseth you still to hold me in some remembrance'. Occasionally, he would end his letters in a code that has never been deciphered, or sign himself 'by the hand which fain would be yours, and so is the heart', or 'by the hand of him which desires as much to be yours as you do to have him'. He needed to see her

more than any earthly thing; for what joy in the world can be greater than to have the company of her who is the most dearly loved, knowing likewise that she, by her choice, holds the same, which greatly delights me.

He spoke often of his 'fervency of love', and told Anne that their frequent separations 'had so grieved my heart that neither tongue nor pen can express the hurt'; she could not begin to imagine 'the sufferings that I, by your absence, have sustained', nor 'the great loneliness that I find since your departing'.

There is a strong sexual tone to these letters. The King spoke often of his need to be 'private' with Anne, and wished he was, 'specially an evening, in my sweetheart's arms, whose pretty dugs [breasts] I trust shortly to kiss'. 'Mine own darling,' he wrote on another occasion, 'I would you were in mine arms, and I in yours, for I think it long since I kissed you.' It would not be long, he assured her, before 'you and I shall have our desired end, which shall be more to my heart's ease than any other thing in this world'. There is no evidence, however – despite rumours to the contrary – that Anne Boleyn surrendered to the King before the autumn of 1532. Even the imperial ambassador, who would become her sworn enemy, had to admit that there was no positive proof of adultery. Some intimacies she may have permitted, but never full intercourse. This is substantiated, not only by the King's repeated denials that she was his mistress in the sexual sense, but also by the fact that, once the affair was consummated, Anne became pregnant immediately and conceived regularly thereafter. Of course, there were rumours that she had borne children in secret before then, but they were without foundation, for it is certain that if Anne had conceived during these early years, the King would have moved heaven and earth to have the child born in wedlock, and many people would have known about it. Above all, Anne's surrender was her trump card, and she would have been a fool to play it with the future so uncertain and with the memory of her sister ever before her.

Anne's biographer, George Wyatt, asserted that she was not in love with the King and had hoped for a future husband who was 'more agreeable to her'. He also says she resented the loss of freedom she had suffered as a result of the King's courtship. There was probably an element of truth in these statements. Certainly her feelings for Henry were less intense than his for her; she handled him with such calculated cleverness that there is no doubt that the crown of England meant more to her than the man through whom she would wear it. Nor was she a good correspondent. She often failed to reply to the King's letters, probably deliberately, for everything she did, or omitted to do, in relation to Henry was calculated to increase his ardour. In this respect she never failed. He always wrote again, chiding her for her 'tardiness', begging her 'to advertise me of your well-being', and sending gifts of venison or jewels to please her. If she detected a hint of irritation in his letters, she dealt with it by quickly reverting from the unattainable to the affectionate, and sending a loving reply.

It was Wolsey to whom the King had turned for help and advice about his doubts concerning his marriage. When the Cardinal learned that his master was seeking an annulment, he was horrified, and fell to his knees, begging Henry to proceed no further since the matter would be fraught with difficulties. The King ignored this, insisting the Cardinal take steps to instigate proceedings and, with grave misgivings, Wolsey, as papal legate, convened in secret an ecclesiastical court, which opened on 17 May 1527 at Westminster, its purpose being to consider the King's collusive suit. William Warham, Archbishop of Canterbury, presided, assisted by Wolsey and a host of bishops and canon lawyers. The King was summoned, and asked to account 'to the tranquillity of his conscience and the health of his soul, for having knowingly taken to wife his brother's widow'. He admitted the charge, confessed his doubt, and asked for judgement to be given upon his case. Thereafter, the court reconvened for two further sessions and debated the matter, yet on 31 May the commissioners announced that the case was so obscure and doubtful that they were not competent to judge it. The King then consulted his Privy Council, who agreed there was good cause for scruple, and advised him to apply to the Holy See in Rome for an annulment, the Pope being the only authority qualified to pronounce on the matter.

Elaborate precautions had been taken to keep what was going on a secret, especially from the Queen, but these were not proof against the perception of the Spanish ambassador, who, only the day after proceedings started, was writing to inform Charles V that 'the Cardinal, to crown his iniquities, is working to separate the King and Queen'. That same day, Mendoza sent a secret message to Katherine, informing her of the convening of the Westminster court, and requesting an urgent audience. She sent word that she 'was so afraid she has not dared to speak with me'. The Cardinal's spies were watching.

Mendoza's note shattered the Queen's peace of mind, though she very quickly convinced herself that the proceedings were all Wolsey's doing since they could not be her husband's. Mendoza, fearful that the court and, subsequently, the Pope would be provided with false statements purportedly from the Queen, wanted Katherine to be on her guard. She was grateful for the warning, and acted quickly, asking Vives to represent her at Warham's court. However, not wishing to offend the King, he refused, and the Queen, whose moral courage was never in doubt, withdrew his pension. Nevertheless, events were in her favour. At the beginning of June, news reached England of the sack of Rome, and not only was the King shocked and outraged at reports of the atrocities, but also sensible of the fact that, with the Pope now a prisoner of the Emperor, Katherine's nephew, a favourable decision on his nullity suit was unlikely to be forthcoming for the time being. Wolsey now suggested that he himself should go to France to enlist the support of King Francis, who might prevail upon the Pope to extend Wolsey's legatine powers and thereby enable him to adjudicate on the King's case. Henry agreed that this might be the best solution, and Wolsey began to prepare for his journey.

By late June, events were moving at such a pace, and rumours proliferating so alarmingly, that it was impossible to keep the 'great matter' from the Queen any longer. Henry, of course, was unaware that she had already found out about it from Mendoza, and thus, when he went to her apartments on 22 June 1527, he was feeling distinctly uncomfortable. As soon as Katherine had risen from her curtsey, he blurted out that he was much troubled in his conscience about their marriage, and had resolved to separate himself from her at bed and at board. All he asked was her co-operation, and that she choose a house to retire to, at least until the matter was settled.

As Mendoza reported later, Katherine was 'in great grief' when she heard this. Her usual self-control deserted her, and she wept uncontrollably. The King hastened to pacify her, saying he hoped he might be allowed to return to her, and that he only wished to find out the truth about their marriage. All would be done for the best, he assured her, begging her at the same time not to speak of the matter to anyone – he feared that news of his collusive suit would provoke a hostile reaction from Charles V. But Katherine was beyond comprehension, and continued to sob her heart out. Unable to do anything with her, Henry fled.

After she had pulled herself together, Katherine was able to assess her situation. She was alone and without counsel, far from her friends in Spain, with spies watching her every move. Yet she was not for nothing the daughter of Isabella of Castile: her principles were firm, her moral courage undoubted, and she believed her marriage was good and valid. Pope Julius had permitted it, and that was enough for her. She was the King's true wife, and the Princess Mary his legitimate heir, and on these premises she would take her stand. She was convinced that both Wolsey and Anne Boleyn had led the King astray and planted doubts in his mind, and she saw it as her sacred duty to rectify the situation and persuade her husband that he was in error.

To Katherine, what Henry was contemplating was morally reprehensible: the casting off of a blameless and devoted wife after eighteen years of honourable wedlock, and the setting aside of an innocent child. She was at a loss to understand how he could countenance such a thing, though this was a somewhat blinkered view, which did not take into account England's desperate need for a male heir. Henry himself came to feel that Katherine was allowing her earthly pride in her rank to stand in the way of his moral scruples, but it was not so much this as the fact that her pride would never allow her for a minute to acknowledge that she had been, not his wife, but his harlot for eighteen years. That pride, the abiding love she bore him, and the deep conviction that right was on her side would enable her to stand firm in her resolution until the day she died.

In every respect other than that which touched her conscience, Katherine was ready to obey her husband, but in the event her conscience was to prove every bit as formidable as Henry's. Both were strong-willed people, and beneath the Queen's apparent meekness there was a layer of steely determination. The battle once engaged, neither would give any quarter. As Katherine told the Pope's legate in 1528:

Neither the whole kingdom on one hand, nor any great punishment on the other, although she might be torn limb from limb, could compel her to alter her opinion; and if, after death, she should return to life, rather than change her opinion, she would prefer to die over again.

She failed to appreciate that by taking her stand upon the power of the papacy to dispense in a case such as hers, she was in fact doing as much as the King to place its position in jeopardy.

Throughout the course of the 'great matter', Katherine rarely reproached Henry. She could not accept, and never would accept, that his love for her was dead. Affection and respect remained, he observed all the courtesies when they were together, and this led her to believe that all was not lost. If Anne Boleyn's influence were to be removed, she was certain he would return to her and abandon all ideas of annulment. She therefore ignored his initial suggestion that she retire from court, and continued with her daily routine as if nothing amiss had occurred. He wanted no more scenes, and was happy for the present to maintain the pretence that all was well; above all, he wanted to be judged in a favourable light by the Pope when the time came, and Wolsey had warned him to handle Katherine 'both gently and docilely'. He therefore kept her at his side for state functions and visits to their daughter, who had been sent to live at Hunsdon where she owned a manor house. Henry and Katherine were together to welcome the French ambassadors to court in September 1527, and three days later sat side by side to watch a tragic masque in Latin, played by children. In public, the Queen would appear smiling and cheerful. Even the Duke of Norfolk, a man of little feeling and the uncle of Katherine's rival, was able to find words to praise her fortitude in showing such a brave face to the world: 'It was wonderful to see her courage,' he said; 'nothing seems to frighten her.'

Sexual relations between Henry and Katherine had ceased in 1524; since then, they had occasionally shared a bed for form's sake. Now, Henry's confessor advised him not to do even this until a decision had been given on his case. However, Henry chose to ignore this advice, and as late as 2 December 1528, the Spanish ambassador was reporting that the King and Queen were sleeping together at

Greenwich, though on that very day Henry declared himself 'utterly resolved and determined never to use the Queen's body again', and thereafter left her to sleep alone.

Towards Anne Boleyn Katherine never betrayed any sign of jealousy, even though she believed – and continued to believe even after Henry's outright denial of the fact in November 1529 – that he and Anne were lovers. As for Anne, George Wyatt says she had been reluctant to accept the King's advances because of the great love she bore the Queen. This may have been so at the beginning of the affair, but her love for her mistress quickly turned into antipathy and then into hatred as she realised that Katherine meant to fight back.

The Queen sought guidance in prayer before making up her mind to ask her nephew, the Emperor, to intercede with the Pope for her. She realised this would not be easy, because of Wolsey's spies about her, but had thought of a plan to outwit the Cardinal. She announced that one of her servants, Francisco Felipez, was to visit his widowed mother in Spain, and obtained for him a safe conduct from the King. In fact Felipez was to carry a message from the Queen to Charles V, and knowing how suspicious Henry could be, Katherine pretended that she did not want him to go. Unfortunately, this did not deceive the King, and Felipez was arrested at Calais and sent back to England. The episode proved to Henry that his wife was not going to submit meekly to having her marriage annulled.

Later in 1527, Katherine did succeed in sending Felipez to the Emperor, and her physician Vittorio also slipped unnoticed out of England to acquaint Charles with further details of her plight. The Emperor had already heard from Mendoza of her situation; in May, the ambassador had told him that 'all her hope rests, after God, upon your Imperial Highness,' and advised him to put pressure on the Pope to tie the hands of the papal legate, Wolsey, and have the case referred to Rome for a decision. Charles V knew perfectly well that Clement VII, a weak and vacillating man, would not dare to give a decision in Henry's favour while he was the Emperor's prisoner, and was perfectly willing to let Henry apply for an annulment if he wished. The Queen, had she known it, was in a very strong position indeed. Nevertheless, in July 1527, Charles expressed to Mendoza his indignation at 'so strange a determination. We do not believe it possible. For the honour and service of God, put an end to this scandalous affair.' And in August, he wrote to Katherine:

> You may well imagine the pain this intelligence caused me, and how much I felt for you . . . I have immediately set about taking the necessary steps for a remedy, and you may be certain that nothing shall be omitted on my part to help you.

Mendoza, Charles's ambassador, was a true friend to Queen Katherine during this period, and did his best in a difficult situation. It was almost impossible to communicate directly with the Queen, but he too had his spies, and with their help he tirelessly gathered together every scrap of information he could discover, and kept his master extraordinarily well-informed. It was Mendoza who predicted, correctly, in May 1527, that 'there will be many more voices in her favour than against her, both because she is beloved here, as because the Cardinal, who is suspected to be at the bottom of all this, is universally hated.'

The King's 'great matter' first became public knowledge beyond the confines of the court in the early summer of 1527; by July, it was as notorious as if it had been proclaimed by the public crier. Rumour had it that the King was planning to marry the French King's sister, Margaret of Alençon. Henry was irritated by the rumours, and commanded the Lord Mayor of London to ensure that the people ceased such communications upon pain of his high displeasure. This achieved absolutely nothing, and the rumours became, if anything, more widespread. In June 1527, Wolsey informed all the English ambassadors abroad of the situation, and by the spring of 1528 the 'great matter' was common knowledge throughout the courts of Europe, thanks to the diplomatic network. Outside the dominions of the Emperor, there was a good deal of support for Henry VIII, it being generally felt that his marriage was of doubtful validity.

As Mendoza had reported, Katherine was indeed very popular, both at court and in the kingdom at large, so much so that the King feared demonstrations within her household, once her staff learned what was afoot. Mendoza too had contemplated the possibility of 'some great popular disturbance', but observed that the English 'will probably content themselves with grumbling only'. Nevertheless, from the beginning, Henry believed that Katherine was quite capable of inciting a war with the Emperor or a rebellion of his subjects against him, and had her watched closely.

When Katherine appeared in public, crowds would gather and cry: 'Victory over your enemies!' Women, in particular, spoke out in her favour, believing that the King only sought to be rid of her for his own pleasure, and the French ambassador drily commented that 'if the matter were decided by women, the King would lose the battle'. Nevertheless, those at court and those who looked for preferment tended to support the King, though there were honourable exceptions. In the summer of 1527, Sir Thomas More told the King he believed his marriage to be good and valid. Though disappointed, Henry accepted this in good part, for he respected More. John Fisher, Bishop of Rochester, a man with a reputation for wisdom and sanctity, told Wolsey in June 1527 that it could by no means be proved to be prohibited by any divine law that a brother may marry his wife of his deceased brother, and said he had been powerfully moved to declare himself in favour of the validity of the royal marriage.

Another staunch supporter of the Queen was Reginald Pole, the son of the Princess Mary's governess, Lady Salisbury; he had been studying in Italy at the King's expense and planned to enter the Church. Pole later expressed the belief that Anne Boleyn was responsible for 'the whole lying affair', and became quite outspoken in his views. Later still, when his opposition to the King had made his position in England too uncomfortable and unsafe, Pole fled abroad, remaining a continual thorn in the King's side. Nor did the King enjoy the full support of Archbishop Warham. Warham had been one of those who had advised Henry VII against marrying Katherine to Prince Henry, though the Pope's dispensation had at the time set his mind at rest. He was King's man enough to support his master's pursuit of the truth concerning the validity of his marriage, and told Wolsey in 1527 that 'however displeasantly the Queen might take it, yet the truth and judgement of the law must be followed'. Yet when it came down to basics, Warham was a traditional churchman who would not countenance any attack on the authority of the Holy See. As for Vives, he was reconciled to the Queen in 1528, when she confided to him her profound distress, saying her grief was the greater because she loved Henry so much. Later, Vives wrote: 'Can anyone blame me for consoling her? Who will not praise her moderation?' Even the King's sister Mary supported the Queen, of whom she was very fond, and she hated Anne Boleyn so much that she refused to come to court while she was there.

Some of Katherine's supporters she could have done without. Symbolic of widespread public feeling was the appearance in Kent of a nun, Dame Elizabeth Barton, who suffered from epileptic fits but was reputed to have the gift of prophecy and to have had holy visions. In the summer of 1528, the Nun would prophesy that if the King put away his lawful wife, God would ensure that he should no longer be King in England, and he would die a villain's death. Although it was not yet treason to foretell the King's death, Elizabeth Barton would be fortunate in that for the time being the authorities were prepared to dismiss her as a harmless lunatic; nor did they molest her when she persisted in repeating her prophecies and threats. However, Queen Katherine wisely refused to have anything to do with her.

Wolsey left for France in July 1527. Apart from enlisting the support of King Francis, he hoped also to discuss the possibility of a French marriage for the King, being still unaware that Henry had already decided to marry Anne Boleyn as soon as he was free. However, by August 1527, rumours were circulating in England to the effect that, when Henry had set aside his lawful queen, he would marry his mistress. Such rumours gathered momentum with alarming speed, and provoked a highly undesirable reaction, for if the Londoners as a body had looked unfavourably upon the news that the King intended to put away Queen Katherine, they were scandalised at the reports that he intended to replace her with Anne Boleyn, who was considered an upstart who was no better than she should be. From the first Anne was openly called a whore and a sorceress; nor was there anything the King could do to stop this. Anne might pretend it did not bother her, but her flippancy concealed anger and disappointment.

Before very long, the rumours spread across the Channel to France and beyond. Mendoza told the Emperor that Henry was 'so swayed by his passions, that if he can obtain a divorce, he will end by marrying a daughter of Master [sic] Boleyn'. Some foreign governments recognised that Henry was acting in the interests of his kingdom, but most were scandalised. In France, Wolsey heard the rumours with mounting dismay, and a letter from the King forbidding him to mention to Francis I the question of remarriage only served to confirm his worst fears. He knew Anne to be his enemy now, and he realised that he would in future be working to bring about a marriage that would almost certainly be his own downfall. He had no choice: his loyalty to his master as well as his sense of self-preservation were such that he would continue to spare no efforts to have Henry's marriage annulled, whatever the consequences. He told the King that he was occupied with solving his problems as if it were his only means of obtaining Heaven, and Henry, in turn, made it clear that 'we trust, by your diligence, shortly to be eased out of that trouble'.

Anne Boleyn and her supporters took advantage of Wolsey's absence by doing their best to poison the King's mind against him. Word soon reached him of what was going on, and he was dismayed to learn that Anne, Rochford, Norfolk and Suffolk had all spent the greater part of August at Beaulieu with the King, doubtless undermining his influence and criticising him to his master. He was right to be concerned. The Boleyn faction repeatedly warned Henry that, far from working to secure an annulment, Wolsey was actually doing his best to prevent the Pope from ever granting one. And once this doubt was planted in Henry's mind, the first breach in his friendship with the Cardinal had been successfully made.

To make matters worse, Wolsey had failed to elicit King Francis's support. His mission a failure, he returned home on 17 September; Anne and her supporters were waiting for him. If he thought he was going to be joyfully received by the King, he was very much mistaken.

It was customary for the Cardinal to send a messenger to Henry upon his return from trips overseas; this was the signal for the King to join him in his closet for a briefing. This time, the King was relaxing after dinner with Anne and his courtiers when the messenger arrived and informed him that the Cardinal waited outside and wished to know where he should speak with him. Before Henry could answer, Anne exclaimed, 'Where else should the Cardinal come? Tell him he may come here, where the King is!'

Henry, somewhat taken aback, merely nodded at the messenger. Thus the Cardinal was received like any other courtier, with Mistress Anne looking on triumphantly.

It now occurred belatedly to the King that his former relationship with Mary Boleyn placed him in exactly the same degree of affinity to Anne as he insisted that Katherine was to him. Yet while he saw this as an impediment to his union with Katherine, when it came to the prospect of marrying Anne, he still believed a papal dispensation – like the one he was doing his best to have declared invalid – would put matters to rights as far as Mary was concerned. In September 1527, Henry sent his secretary, Dr William Knight, on a secret mission to Rome with instructions to obtain such a dispensation and apply to the Pope for a general commission which would give Wolsey, as papal legate, the authority to examine the King's marriage. His findings could then be submitted to Clement, who would hopefully act upon them, and Katherine would have no right of appeal. What Henry did not know was that, soon after Knight left England, Charles V told the Pope that he was 'determined to preserve the Queen's rights', and commanded Clement not to take any steps preparatory to annulling her marriage, and not to allow the case to be tried in England.

Knight was joined in Italy by Gregory Casale, an English diplomat who had been sent by Wolsey formally to request Clement for a dispensation annulling Henry VIII's marriage to Katherine of Aragon on the grounds that the dispensation of Pope Julius was founded on 'certain false suggestions'. Wolsey was hoping that, out of consideration for the King's services to the Church, the Pope would find a way to ease his conscience and, to this end, Casale was to stress 'the vehement desire of the whole nation and nobility that the King should have an heir'. He was also to assure Clement that, if he granted what the King was asking for, Henry was ready to declare war on the Emperor to procure the freedom of the Holy Father.

Knight and Casale saw Pope Clement in December 1527, and implored his 'prompt kindness', but were told it was not at present possible for him to grant a dispensation annulling the King's marriage. However, he was willing to grant one enabling Henry to remarry within certain prohibited degrees should his first marriage ever be declared unlawful – this was issued on 1 January 1528 – and he also granted Cardinal Wolsey a general commission to try the King's case, though not to pass judgement.

Clement was aware of the constraints placed upon him and terrified of the Emperor. Secretly, he urged Casale to advise Henry to take matters into his own hands and remarry without involving the Holy See, something that would not appeal to the King, who had the future stability of the succession to consider.

Wolsey, meanwhile, had written to Rome to request the appointment of a fellow legate with power to pronounce judgement on the King's case. He suggested Cardinal Lorenzo Campeggio, who had begun his career as a lawyer and, after the death of his wife, had entered the Church and quickly risen to the rank of cardinal. He had visited England and been ordained Bishop of Salisbury on the King's recommendation. Clement said he could not spare Campeggio, and hinted that Wolsey should 'pronounce the divorce' himself and afterwards seek the confirmation of the papal consistory, another course too fraught with uncertainty to meet with Henry's approval.

By December 1527, Wolsey was aware that Anne Boleyn and her faction had undermined his influence with the King to such an extent that Henry was now growing resentful of his power and wealth. He had already handed Hampton Court over to the King in 1526, but now Anne was constantly urging Henry to assert his own authority. Yet he still needed Wolsey, whom he knew to be the most able of his ministers and the only man capable of securing an annulment. Wolsey was bombarding the envoys in Rome with instructions, promises, threats and inducements. Of his own anxiety, he made no secret: 'If the Pope is not compliant,' he wrote, 'my own life will be shortened, and I dread to anticipate the consequences.' At the same time, he was spending large sums on banquets for the entertainment of the King and Anne Boleyn, and doing his best to counteract the slanders heard by the Pope about Anne by praising her for her

excellent virtues, the purity of her life, her constant virginity, her maidenly and womanly pudacity, her soberness, chasteness, meekness, humility, wisdom, descent of right noble regal blood, education in all good and laudable manners, and apparent aptness to procreation of children.

On 22 January 1528, England and France together declared war on the Emperor, an unpopular move in England, since it threatened trade links with the Low Countries. A month after this, a committee of canon lawyers assembled by Wolsey at Hampton Court reached the conclusion that the King should press the Pope to grant a decretal commission, which would empower Wolsey to pronounce a definitive sentence on Henry's case. In February, the King sent to Rome Edward Fox, a doctor of divinity who was well versed in canon law, and Stephen Gardiner, a doctor of both civil and canon law and a religious conservative with a ruthless streak whose loyalty to the King was unswerving. Both he and Fox were advocates of an annulment, and could be relied upon to present Henry's case with conviction.

Gardiner and Fox saw the Pope in March 1528, when Clement told them that he had heard that the King wanted an annulment for private reasons only, being driven by 'vain affection and undue love' for a lady far from worthy of him. Gardiner sprang to Henry's defence, pointing out his dire need of a male heir and declaring that Anne Boleyn was 'animated by the noblest sentiments; the Cardinal of York and all England do homage to her virtues'. He also pointed out that the Queen suffered from 'certain diseases' which meant that Henry would never again live with her as his wife. Then he presented the Pope with a treatise that Henry had written on the case, which Clement later pronounced to be 'excellent'. Gardiner and Fox wheedled, begged and bullied over a period of several weeks, but Clement only dithered and procrastinated. In the end, he agreed to send Campeggio to England to try the case with Wolsey, but refused to grant either of them a decretal commission. This was not quite what the King wanted, but it was a start, and the envoys felt reasonably optimistic when they left Rome in April 1528. Fox wrote to Gardiner that Henry heard the news with 'marvellous demonstrations of joy', and Anne Boleyn was so elated that she confused Fox with Gardiner and kept calling him 'Master Stephen'! Yet Wolsey was sceptical about the Pope's intentions. 'I would obtain the decretal bull with my own blood if I could,' he told Casale privately. However, on 4 May, he told the King he was satisfied with the general commission granted to him and Campeggio. It was as well to let Henry believe there was cause for optimism.

In June 1528, the sweating sickness returned to plague London and, later on, the rest of the country. This was a particularly virulent outbreak, and the King, learning with horror that some members of his household had succumbed to the disease, fled with the Queen and Anne and a small retinue to another house, and then another after that, until he was sleeping in a different place each night. Finally, he arrived at Tittenhanger, the Hertfordshire residence of the Abbot of St Albans, where he decided he was far enough from the contagion to stay put for a time. Fearfully, he wondered whether this plague was a visitation from an angry God who was displeased with him for having remained married incestuously to Katherine for so long, or whether the Almighty was wrathful because he was thinking of putting her away. For a time, he believed it might be the latter, and spent the months of May and June almost exclusively in the Queen's company, though as his fear of the sweating sickness abated, so did his doubts.

In the middle of June, one of the ladies assigned to wait on Anne Boleyn caught the plague. A petrified Henry uprooted his decimated court and hastened to an unidentified house twelve miles from Tittenhanger, while Anne was ordered home to her father at Hever. Henry would not have her near him in case she had contracted the deadly virus – his fear of illness and death was stronger than his love for any woman. His anxiety for her was nevertheless acute; 'I implore you, my entirely beloved, to have no fear at all,' he wrote. 'Wheresoever I may be, I am yours.' Wolsey, fearful of a wrathful God, wrote to Henry at this time and begged him to abandon his nullity suit. The French ambassador was present when the King opened the letter, and saw him explode with rage. 'The King used terrible words, saying he would have given a thousand Wolseys for one Anne Boleyn. . . . No other than God shall take her from me,' he had cried.

No sooner had these words been spoken, it seemed, than news reached the King in the night that Anne had fallen ill of the sweating sickness. She had taken to her bed on 22 June, the same day that her sister Mary's husband William Carey, died of the disease. The King was thrown into a frenzy of agitation. He sent for his chief physician, Dr John Chambers, only to be told that he was away from the house attending the sick. However, Dr William Butts, Chambers's second-in-command, was at hand, and Henry dispatched him immediately to Hever, bearing a hastily scribbled letter for Anne. He told her he would willingly bear half her malady to have her well again, and lamented the fact that her illness would lengthen the time they would have to be apart. Dr Butts would 'soon restore your health', he told her, and he himself would then 'obtain one of my chief joys in this world, which is to have my mistress healed'. Anne was to 'be governed by Butts's advice in all things concerning your malady'.

As it happened, when Butts arrived at Hever, he found his patient already recovering, having been visited with only a mild attack of the plague. In fact, she was showing much of her old spirit, declaring that she would have died content if she could die a queen. The King, when he heard the news, was enormously relieved, and sent letters and gifts to aid his sweetheart's recovery, while Wolsey did likewise, knowing it would please Henry. And knowing that Anne was concerned about her sister, who had been left destitute with one child of three and another on the way, the King commanded that Lord Rochford make necessary provision for her, Rochford having hitherto shown himself impervious to his elder daughter's appeals for succour. He then wrote to Anne, telling her what he had done, and, 'seeing my darling is absent', sending her a haunch of venison, 'which is hart flesh for Henry, prognosticating that hereafter, God willing, you must enjoy some of mine . . . I would we were together an evening.'

By the end of July, the plague had died out in London, and both Henry and Anne returned to court. The Queen knew very well that Anne was hoping to supplant her, yet she still maintained her attitude of placid forbearance, although she did make one gentle thrust during a game of cards – Henry saw nothing unusual in including both wife and sweetheart in such pastimes – when Anne won by drawing a king. Katherine, with a dry smile, observed, 'My Lady Anne, you have the good hap ever to stop at a king, but you are like the others: you will have all or none.' History does not record the reactions of Anne or the King to this remark.

Cardinal Campeggio left Rome at the end of July 1528. It took him two months to travel to England because he was prone to agonising attacks of gout, something Clement may well have taken into account when appointing him legate, for Clement was playing for time, hoping that the Emperor might set him at liberty, or that Henry would tire of Anne Boleyn and forget about an annulment. In his luggage, Campeggio carried a decretal bull which had been secretly issued on 18 June; the legate had strict instructions not to divulge its existence to Wolsey unless authorised by the Pope, something which would only happen if Charles V relaxed his grip on affairs.

The King and Anne Boleyn were much elated at the prospect of the legate's arrival; 'I trust within a while after [Campeggio's arrival] to enjoy that which I have so longed for, mine own darling,' wrote Henry. They would not have been pleased to learn that Campeggio had in fact been instructed to do his best 'to restore mutual affection between the King and Queen', and, if this was not feasible, 'to protract the matter for as long as possible'. Suffolk, in France to welcome the legate, warned Wolsey that Campeggio's mission to England 'will be mere mockery', but the King did not believe him.

Meanwhile, Anne and her faction had continued their efforts to bring about the destruction of the Cardinal, Anne's malice all the more deadly because it was concealed under a cloak of friendship. When, in 1528, Wolsey brought the long-standing dispute over the earldom of Ormonde to an end by pronouncing in favour of Anne's father, she wrote him a letter couched in the warmest of terms, and promised that, when she was raised to queenship, if there was 'any thing in this world I can imagine to do you pleasure, you shall find me the gladdest woman in the world to do it'. She also assured him of her 'hearty love unfeignedly through my life'. In another letter, she acknowledged that Wolsey was doing everything possible 'to bring to pass honourably the greatest wealth that it is possible to come to any creature living'. And in June 1528, she wrote: 'I do know the great pains and troubles you take for me are never likely to be recompensed, but only in loving you next unto the King's Grace, above all creatures living.'

In April 1528, Anne challenged Wolsey on a new front. The abbess of the ancient and rich foundation at Wilton had just died, and there was fierce competition for the vacant position. Anne's candidate was Dame Eleanor Carey, sister of Mary Boleyn's husband William, and Anne recommended her warmly to the King, knowing that Wolsey favoured the election of the prioress, Dame Isabel Jordan. But Wolsey had heard unsavoury rumours about Eleanor Carey – who had not only had two children by different fathers, both priests, but had also left her convent and lived for a time as the mistress of a servant of Lord Willoughby de Broke – and when Anne was absent from court, he seized his advantage and appointed Isabel Jordan abbess. This earned him a public reproof from the King, who had concluded that Wolsey had gone out of his way to offend Anne, and prompted an abject apology from the Cardinal. Later, when Henry learned the reasons why Eleanor Carey had been passed over, he arranged that neither she nor Dame Isabel should be abbess, writing to Anne to explain the situation and telling her he would not 'for all the gold in the world, clog your conscience nor mine to make her ruler of a house which is of so ungodly demeanour', and that 'the house shall be better reformed, and God the much better served' if someone else were appointed. To mollify Anne, Wolsey sent her an expensive gift, for which she thanked him in a letter in which she begged him never to doubt that she would vary from her loyalty to him. On the surface all was well again.

In the autumn of 1528, though, the Boleyn faction was busy spreading rumours that the Cardinal was working in secret in the Queen's favour. Even the Spanish ambassador believed this, as did many other people, and although Wolsey was in reality as anxious as the King to have the royal marriage annulled, he was powerless to stop this damaging gossip. At present, Henry was disposed to treat it as malicious talk, but if the Pope's sentence ultimately went against him, he might take a very different view, which, observed the Boleyns and their adherents with satisfaction, would mean the end of the Cardinal.

Campeggio arrived at Dover on 29 September 1528. The King had offered him a state welcome to London, but he refused it, remembering that the Pope desired him to execute his commission with as little publicity as possible. Nor did he wish to provoke any public demonstrations, so he travelled quietly by barge to Bath Place, the London house of the bishops of Salisbury by Temple Bar – and took straight to his bed.

The next day, 9 October, he spent three or four hours discussing the 'great matter' with Wolsey, and told him that the best solution would be a reconciliation between the King and Queen. However, as he told the Pope later, he had 'no more success in persuading the Cardinal than if I had spoken to a rock'. Wolsey urged the expediting of the business with 'all possible despatch', alleging that 'the affairs of the kingdom are at a standstill'. If he had not known it before, Campeggio realised then that his sojourn in England would be fraught with difficulties.

The legate first saw the King on 22 October at Bridewell Palace by the Thames, near the monastery of the Black Friars. The interview did not begin well, for Henry was angered by Campeggio's suggestion that he return to the Queen. To pacify the King, and because the Pope had just authorised him to do so, Campeggio produced the decretal bull, saying the Pope had granted it 'not to be used, but kept secret; he desired to show the King the good feeling by which he was animated.' Henry visibly relaxed. The discussion then continued more amicably, although it was clear to the legate that the King wanted nothing less than a declaration that his marriage was invalid. Campeggio realised that, 'if an angel was to descend from Heaven, he would not be able to persuade him to the contrary.'

The legate put forward a suggestion made by the Pope, that Katherine be persuaded to enter a nunnery. If she could be assured that her daughter's rights would not be prejudiced, it might be in her best interests to make a graceful exit and so save everyone a lot of trouble. There were precedents, and her piety was renowned. The Pope could issue a dispensation allowing the King to remarry, and the Emperor could not possibly object. Henry could then make Anne his wife, and England, God willing, would in due course get its heir. Most important of all, the peace of Europe and the stability of the Holy See would no longer be threatened. This sensible idea met with the King's wholehearted approval; he hastened to assure Campeggio that Katherine would only lose 'the use of his person' by entering religion; as matters stood in the convents of the age, she could still enjoy any other worldly comforts she desired.

The two legates waited upon the Queen two days later in her apartments at Bridewell Palace. She was on her guard and very tense, and when Campeggio suggested that entering a nunnery was the ideal solution to her troubles, she refused out of hand on the grounds that she was the King's wife. 'Although she is very religious and extremely patient, she will not accede in the least,' the legate told the Pope. Katherine then swore on her conscience that Prince Arthur had never consummated their marriage, and declared that 'she intended to live and die in the estate of matrimony to which God had called her.' None of Campeggio's arguments could persuade her to change her mind, and when Wolsey warned her it might be better to yield to the King's displeasure, she turned on him, retorting that

> Of this trouble, I thank only you, my lord of York! Of malice you have kindled this fire, especially for the great grudge you bear to my nephew the Emperor, because he would not gratify your ambition by making you Pope by force!

Wolsey excused himself, saying it had been 'sore against his will that ever the marriage should come in question', and promised, as legate, to be impartial; Katherine, knowing him to be first and foremost the King's servant, did not believe him. Afterwards, Campeggio wrote to Clement to say he had 'always thought her to be a prudent lady, and now more than ever'.

On 26 October, the legate heard Katherine's confession, at her request, in which she affirmed, upon the salvation of her soul, that she had never been carnally known by Prince Arthur. Campeggio did not doubt she was telling the truth, but he still did his best to persuade her to take the veil, begging, cajoling and bullying in turn. None of it had the slightest effect. She declared she would abide by no sentence save that of the Pope himself, and that she did not recognise the authority of the legatine commission to try the case since she believed it to be biased in Henry's favour.

With Katherine proving obdurate, Henry pressed Wolsey to wrest the decretal bull from Campeggio, but the legate stood firm, and refused to hand it over, saying he could only do what the Pope instructed. It seemed that matters were still weighted strongly in the Queen's favour.

Outwardly, relations between the King and Queen were still cordial, although there was a good deal of tension below the surface. Henry resented the fact that Katherine was able to ignore what was staring her in the face; he also was irritated by the way in which she seemed able to rise above her misery, and in October 1528 he complained to the Privy Council about her behaviour. She was too merry, too richly dressed; she should be praying for a good end to her case rather than gracing courtly entertainments with her presence. Worst of all, by riding out and acknowledging the cheers of the crowds, she was inciting the King's subjects to rebellion. It seemed to Henry that she did not care for him, and he felt she might at least show some sorrow at the prospect of losing him. He even inferred that she was involved in a mysterious plot to kill himself and Wolsey, which can only have been the product of his imagination. Nevertheless, the Council wrote to the Queen, warning her that 'if it could be proved she had any hand in it, she must not expect to be spared.' She was also informed of the King's other complaints about her, and advised that the Privy Council, who thought 'in their consciences that his life was in danger', had urged him to separate from her entirely and take the Princess Mary from her. She was told bluntly that she was 'a fool to resist the King's will'.

The letter was devastating indeed to Katherine, realising as she did that the Council's censure proceeded directly from the King himself. Yet even this did not make her less conscientious regarding her duty to obey him, and she obeyed him now, by taking care to dress more soberly, spending more time at her devotions, adopting a more solemn and grave demeanour, and not venturing out of the palace so often, nor going where she might excite public interest. For all this, she was well aware that she was still under constant observation by the Cardinal's spies, who were usually women in her service who had been bribed with money, gifts and – according to the reformer William Tynedale – sex, in order to get them to betray anything of interest their mistress might have said or done. At least one of these ladies left court because she could no longer injure the Queen in such a way. All of this placed Katherine under an intolerable strain, and when Campeggio saw the Queen in October 1528, he thought she was fifty, when in fact she was just forty-three.

Henry rarely visited her now. When he did, he never stayed long, fearing Anne Boleyn's jealousy, though in public he was anxious to appear as the afflicted husband pining for a wife barred from him by canon law. Few were deceived by this charade – Anne Boleyn being too much in evidence – but Henry persisted with his role-playing, and made sure he was seen in public with Katherine as often as possible. When he saw her in private, they often quarrelled. In November 1528, he told her it would be better for her if she went of her own volition to a nunnery, but she cried out that it was against her soul, her conscience and her honour. 'There will be no judge unjust enough to condemn me!' she said hotly, whereupon Henry, in a very bad temper, left without answering her.

From the autumn of 1528 courtiers left Katherine to herself while they flocked in droves to pay court to Anne Boleyn. Anne was not easily carried away by the great events that had overtaken her, but she was now beginning to enjoy the trappings of power and the adulation that went with them. In July 1528, the King had placed an apartment off the tiltyard at Greenwich at her disposal; at around the same time, she had left the Queen's service. However, her anomalous position, both as an unmarried woman with a reputation to protect and as the future Queen of England, presented a problem. Wolsey thought it more in keeping with propriety for her to have an establishment of her own, and ordered the refurbishment of a London house for her. This was either Durham House on the Strand, where Katherine had once briefly stayed years before, or Suffolk House near Westminster; she would have preferred a house near Greenwich, but one could not be found.

Anne's new residence was made ready for her by her father in his capacity as comptroller of the King's household, and he ensured that it was renovated to a standard fit for a royal bride-to-be. When work was completed, an army of servants and ladies-in-waiting were engaged to serve Anne, and she moved into her new home, where she would keep as much state as if she were queen already. 'Greater court is now paid to Mistress Anne than has been to the Queen for a long time,' observed the French ambassador in November 1528. 'I see they mean to accustom the people by degrees to endure her.'

In December 1528, Mendoza noticed that Wolsey 'was no longer received at court as graciously as before', and reported that 'the King had uttered angry words respecting him'. Nevertheless, when Christmas that year was held at Greenwich, Wolsey and Campeggio were the guests of honour. The King arranged jousts, banquets, masques and disguisings for their entertainment, but the Queen, who was present, took no pleasure in them and hardly smiled. Anne Boleyn was also at Greenwich, lodged separately, attended by a host of servants, and being treated as if she were queen. She kept open house throughout the season, and people flocked to visit her, but she held aloof from the main festivities because, as the French ambassador correctly surmised, 'she does not like to meet the Queen'.

During the first months of 1529, Henry was showering Anne with jewels. His account with his goldsmith, Cornelius Hayes, settled at the end of March, records gifts of diamonds, rubies, bracelets, borders of gold set with gems, pearls for edging sleeves, heart-shaped head ornaments and diamond brooches. In April, Anne took it upon herself to perform a duty normally reserved for anointed queens, that of blessing rings for distribution amongst those afflicted with severe cramps.

By May 1529, she was making headway. With the help of Norfolk, Rochford, Suffolk and their supporters, she had begun to convince Henry that Wolsey had not advanced his nullity suit as energetically as he might have done. When Wolsey denied this, Henry would not listen, and the Cardinal was driven to pleading with the French ambassador to urge Francis I to use his influence in Rome to 'forward the divorce'.

Campeggio, seeing Anne with the King, thought Henry's passion 'an extraordinary thing', and told the Pope: 'He sees nothing, he thinks of nothing but Anne. He cannot do without her for an hour, and it moves me to see how the King's life, the stability and downfall of the whole country, may hang on this.' The King was constantly 'kissing her, and treating her as if she were his wife'. In spite of this, Campeggio was nevertheless almost certain that the lovers 'had not proceeded to any ultimate conjunction'.

Future queen she might be, yet Anne remained exceedingly unpopular with the King's subjects. The notoriety of his 'great matter' and the public enmity displayed towards Anne Boleyn had for some time been a matter of concern to the King. He was horrified to learn that the main topic of discussion among all classes of society was his private life. 'Lack of discreet handling must needs be the cause of it,' he told Anne. Katherine's supporters also felt that such public exposure could only be injurious to her cause. In November

1528, the King had invited his subjects to Bridewell Palace, and, standing before the throne, resplendent in his robes of estate, he had done his best to justify his need for an annulment of his marriage, reminding his audience how peace had prevailed during his reign, and confiding to them his fear of dying without a male heir to succeed him, when, 'for want of a legitimate King, England should again be plunged into the horrors of civil war'. This, he had assured them, was his only motive, and, as touching the Queen, if it was judged that she was his lawful wife,

> nothing will be more pleasant or acceptable to me, for I assure you she is a woman of most gentleness, humility and buxomness – she is without comparison. So that if I were to marry again, I would choose her above all women.

When he had gone, many Londoners expressed compassion for him, some said nothing, and others were of the opinion that he should never have raised the matter in public. Nevertheless it had been a shrewd move: it had enlisted the sympathy of a section of the public who had hitherto been hostile, and who would now be more aware of the wider issues involved in the 'great matter' and perhaps not be so eager to listen to wild gossip.

Henry's speech had failed in one respect: it had made no impact on the hatred felt by the public for Anne Boleyn. Not only did they see her as a whore and an adulteress, but also, latterly, as a heretic who had succumbed to the lure of Martin Luther's teachings. Anne herself was to some degree responsible for this, although she was not, and never would be, guilty of heresy. She had been brought up in the traditional Catholic faith, and would continue to observe its rites faithfully until her death. Not until the final week of her life would she display the kind of religious devotion exhibited by Katherine of Aragon, yet she was sincere in her beliefs, and became more interested in religious matters as she grew older.

Anne was never a Lutheran – a term not invented until 1529. She was, however, like her father and brother, a fervent champion of the movement for reform within the Church, and she took an enlightened view of so-called heretical literature. She was so interested in it, and presumed upon her influence with the King to such an extent, that she openly read books that he had banned in

England, and even asked Henry for his opinions on them. One such book, *The Supplication of Beggars* by Simon Fish, argued the case for translating the Scriptures into English so that all could read them. Anne was sent this from abroad in 1528 and showed it to Henry, telling him that Fish had fled from England for fear of persecution by Wolsey. The King read the book, which also argued an early form of communism, and decided it should remain on the banned list, but he did not censure Anne, and allowed her to continue reading works like it unchecked.

In 1529, Anne's copy of another forbidden book, William Tynedale's *The Obedience of a Christian Man, and how Christian Kings ought to Govern*, found its way into Wolsey's hands. Discovering this, Anne went straight to the King, begging him on her knees to help her retrieve it. At Henry's command, the Cardinal returned it personally to Anne, knowing he could not touch her in spite of the heresy laws. Anne then lent Henry the book, which challenged the authority of the Pope and his cardinals; he expressed approval, being impressed by some of the arguments it contained, and declared it 'a book for me and all kings to read'.

Thanks to Anne's influence over him, Henry, increasingly disillusioned with the Church of Rome, was becoming more interested in the subject of reform and more liberal in his views, although his observance of his faith was as conventional as ever. It was apparent that if Anne became queen, there might be radical changes in the Church, and while this prospect elated some people, others trembled at it.

In January 1529, Queen Katherine lodged an appeal in Rome against the authority of the legatine court. During the previous months, she had not been idle, but had marshalled her defences to the best of her ability. In October, she had announced that she had in her possession a copy of a brief of dispensation purportedly issued by Julius II in 1503 at the request of Queen Isabella, which provided for Katherine's marriage to Prince Henry while assuming that her first marriage with his brother had been consummated. If genuine, the existence of this document would demolish the King's argument that his marriage was uncanonical because Katherine had been his brother's wife in the fullest sense. The brief differed from the original bull of dispensation in that it omitted the word 'perhaps' when referring to whether or not the first marriage had been consummated. Yet as no one until now had ever heard of the brief's existence, the King and his councillors concluded that it must be a forgery given to the Queen by Mendoza. Mendoza had indeed given Katherine the copy, but he insisted that the original, in the possession of the Emperor, was genuine. The Council therefore decided that it must be removed, by fair means or foul, from the imperial archives and destroyed. Katherine was duly instructed to send to Spain for it, and had no alternative but to comply, although she guessed that once it was in England the brief, genuine or not, would conveniently disappear.

The original brief was filed among the papers of the late Dr de Puebla, but the Emperor, no fool, would not part with it. Wolsey insisted that a search be made for the copy that should be in the Vatican archives, and sent a five-man embassy to Rome for the purpose. As well as finding the brief and checking its authenticity, they were also to ask the Pope if the King could follow Old Testament precedents and have two wives, the issue of both being legitimate!

Meanwhile, the Emperor sent yet another copy of the brief to London with a subscription attesting it to be genuine, signed by the most eminent Spanish bishops in his presence. Nevertheless, both Wolsey and Henry suspected trickery, and Wolsey asked the Pope to declare the brief a forgery, knowing that, if Clement agreed to do so, the Queen's case would founder. Clement, however, refused. The English envoys could find no record of the brief at the Vatican, and two English divines sent to Spain to see the Emperor's copy wrote to Wolsey in April 1529 to say that it was undoubtedly a forgery. After that, Katherine realised that it would be useless to produce her copy as evidence at the legatine court; her case would have to stand on its own merits.

That April, Henry ordered her to choose the lawyers who would act as her counsel; she could pick from the best in the realm, he said. She chose Archbishop Warham, the Bishops of Ely and St Asaph, and her staunch supporter, John Fisher, Bishop of Rochester. In naming them, she had shown herself to be an obedient wife, though she still refused to acknowledge the authority of the court. Staunch as her counsellors were, they remained her husband's subjects, and if the verdict should go in her favour, the King's anger, and Anne Boleyn's, might be visited upon them. She did not therefore expect them to give her totally disinterested advice. If the case was heard in Rome, however, she would have more chance of receiving an impartial judgement, and on 16 June, she made yet another formal protest against the legatine court at Baynard's Castle and again appealed to the Pope to hear the case in Rome.

Very little was accomplished with regard to the 'great matter' during the early months of 1529, mainly due to the illness of the Pope, but by March Clement had recovered, and the judicial machinery began to grind slowly into action. Henry was warned by his ambassador in Rome that 'the Pope will do nothing for your Grace'; Clement's hands were well and truly tied by the Emperor, and he told Stephen Gardiner that it would be better 'for the wealth of Christendom if the Queen were in her grave'. Henry, hearing rumours that the Pope was about to revoke the legatine commission, tackled Campeggio, but was assured that Clement was, in fact, 'extremely well disposed' towards him, and that the Emperor 'had not moved him by a hair's breadth from whatever he could rightly do in your Grace's favour'. Charles, however, recalled his ambassador, Mendoza, to Spain in May 1529, and did not replace him until August, wishing to demonstrate his disapproval of the King's case by not being represented in England while it was being heard.

As the date for the hearing approached, Anne Boleyn grew pessimistic and even panicky. The French ambassador reported her as being so agitated about the outcome of the case that she could not conceal her anxiety. She was now twenty-eight, almost middle-aged by the standards of her time, and the likelihood of her producing a healthy child grew less with each passing year. She distrusted Wolsey, believing he was secretly conspiring with the Pope to get rid of her, and she was well aware of how poor her reputation was both in England and abroad. Such power and influence as she had had no basis in law. She knew that, once the King's case came before the legates, she would have to leave London, but where once she would have welcomed a separation, she now dreaded it, and remained in the capital until the last possible moment. Then in June she went to Hever, there to await the outcome of the hearing.

At last, on 30 May 1529, Henry VIII formally authorised the legates to convene their court and hear his case. The court was to sit in the great hall of the monastery of the Black Friars in London, where Parliament sometimes met. Bridewell Palace, where the King and Queen would stay for the duration of the case, was adjacent.

Great care was taken in preparing the courtroom: two chairs upholstered in cloth of gold were placed ready for the legates behind railings on a dais at the end of the hall opposite the door; before them was a table covered with a Turkey carpet for their papers. To the right, in the body of the court, stood the King's throne beneath a cloth of estate, and to the left was a similar seat for the Queen. The court was officially opened on 31 May, but because the workmen were still busy preparing the hall, the actual proceedings did not commence until 18 June, when crowds gathered to see the King and Queen arrive.

It was unheard of for an English sovereign to be summoned to appear in a court of law, still less to await the judgement of a subject, and in the courtroom, where nobility, lawyers, theologians and prelates had gathered, the atmosphere was tense. The day's business opened with the legatine commission being read, followed by a brief summary of the case. To the great disappointment of the crowds waiting outside, the King did not appear but sent two proctors instead. Queen Katherine made a brief appearance, with the four bishops appointed as her counsellors and a great train of attendants. She walked up to the legates, curtsied to them, and reiterated her formal appeal against them as judges not competent to try the case, asking that it be referred to Rome. Then she left. Her appeal was ignored, and a further citation to attend the court three days hence was issued to her. This made her very angry – 'I be no Englishwoman but a Spaniard born!' she cried. If she was not the King's wife, then she was not his subject. Nevertheless, when the three days were up, she was in her place, opposite her husband, before a packed court.

At the appointed time, the crier demanded silence, then called: 'King Harry of England, come into the court!' The King answered in a loud firm voice: 'Here, my lords!' The crier than called: 'Katherine, Queen of England, come into the court!' The Queen did not answer. There was an uncomfortable pause, and then the King turned to the legates and told them he wished to have his doubts resolved for the discharge of his conscience. All he asked was that they determine whether or not his marriage was lawful; he had had doubts about that, he said, from the beginning. Katherine interrupted at this point, saying that this was not the time to say so after so long a silence, but Henry excused himself by reason of the great love he had had, and still had, for her, avowing that he desired, above everything else, that their marriage should be declared valid. Katherine's request to have the case referred to Rome he dismissed as unreasonable, due to the Emperor having the Pope in his power. 'This country is perfectly secure for her, and she has the choice of prelates and lawyers,' he told the court.

Katherine was again called when the King had finished speaking, and all eyes turned to the small stout figure attired in a gown of crimson velvet edged with sable, its skirt open at the front to display a petticoat of yellow brocade. The Queen made no answer to the crier; instead, she rose and walked over to where the King sat on his throne, weaving around the crowded benches and tables. Then she fell on her knees before him, and made a dramatic plea for justice. Several versions of what she said survive, but what follows is extracted from the account given by Wolsey's secretary, George Cavendish, an eyewitness. Speaking in broken English, with a heavy Spanish accent, the Queen's voice echoed in the hushed courtroom:

Sir, I beseech you, for all the loves that hath been between us, and for the love of God, let me have justice and right. Take of me some pity and compassion, for I am a poor woman and a stranger born out of your dominion. I have here no assured friend, and much less indifferent counsel. I flee to you as the head of justice within this realm.

Alas, Sir, where have I offended you? Or what occasion have you of displeasure, that you intend to put me from you? I take God and all the world to witness that I have been to you a true, humble and obedient wife, ever conformable to your will and pleasure. I have been pleased and contented with all things wherein you had delight and dalliance. I never grudged a word or countenance, or showed a spark of discontent. I loved all those whom ye loved only for your sake, whether I had cause or no, and whether they were my friends or enemies. This twenty years and more I have been your true wife, and by me ye have had divers children, though it hath pleased God to call them out of this world, which hath been no fault in me. And when ye had me at the first, I take God to be my judge, I was a true maid, without touch of man; and whether it be true or no, I put it to your conscience.

[A pause. Then:] If there be any just cause by the law that you can allege against me, either of dishonesty or any other impediment, to put me from you, I am well content to depart, to my shame and dishonour. If there be none, I must lowly beseech you, let me remain in my former estate and receive justice at your princely hands.

The King your father was accounted in his day as a second Solomon for wisdom, and my father Ferdinand was esteemed one of the wisest kings that had ever reigned in Spain. It is not therefore to be doubted but that they gathered such wise counsel about them as was thought fit by their high discretions. Also, there were in those days as wise, as learned men, as there are at this present time in both realms, who thought then the marriage between you and me good and lawful.

It is a wonder to hear what new inventions are invented against me, who never intended but honesty, that cause me to stand to the order and judgement of this new court, wherein you may do me much wrong, if you intend any cruelty. For ye may condemn me for lack of sufficient answer, having no indifferent counsel. Ye must understand that they cannot be indifferent counsellors which be your subjects, and taken out of your Council beforehand, and dare not, for your displeasure, disobey your will and intent.

Therefore, most humbly do I require you, in the way of charity and for the love of God, to spare me the extremity of this court, until I may be advertised what way and order my friends in Spain will advise me to take. And if ye will not extend to me so much favour, your pleasure then be fulfilled, and to God I commit my cause.

Throughout Katherine's speech, Henry said nothing, but sat staring past his wife. Nor did he make any comment when she had finished. After a few moments, the Queen rose, curtsied, and made her way out of the hall on the arm of her receiver-general, Griffin

Richards. The King commanded the crier to call her back, but she paid no heed, commenting to Richards: 'It is no indifferent court to me, therefore I will not tarry.' Outside the monastery she was greeted by crowds of Londoners, many of them women, who shouted words of encouragement. She acknowledged their support with nods and smiles, and briefly addressed them, requesting their prayers, before returning to Bridewell Palace.

Back in the courtroom, Henry was declaring that Katherine had been to him 'as true, as obedient, and as conformable a wife as I could in my fantasy wish or desire'. He had been fortunate to be blessed with such a queen. 'As God is my witness, no fault in Katherine moved me!' he cried. Then, as his listeners were trying to equate what he was saying about his love for the Queen with what they knew of his passionate pursuit of Anne Boleyn, he reminded them how all his legitimate sons had 'died incontinent after they were born'. That, he believed, had been a punishment from God. His concern was chiefly for the succession; he had not brought these proceedings 'for any carnal concupiscence or mislike of the Queen's person or age, with whom I could be well content to continue during my life if our marriage might stand within God's laws'.

The King then produced a parchment on which was set forth the case his bishops had agreed he had to answer, saying that every bishop in England had set his hand and seal to it. He was interrupted, however, by John Fisher, Bishop of Rochester, one of the Queen's counsellors, who denied he had ever signed or sealed such a document. 'Is this not your hand and seal?' asked the King. 'No, Sire,' answered the Bishop, in a rage. 'Well, well, it shall make no matter,' said Henry testily, 'you are but one man.' Fisher reluctantly sat down, but he had in effect scored a minor victory for the Queen, since he had exposed what was obviously a forged signature and seal and had thereby cast doubts in the mind of Campeggio at least upon the integrity of the King's advisers.

The court sat again on many successive days. Katherine did not appear, despite several citations, and Henry was absent from most of the sessions. Both, however, were represented by their counsel, who spent much of the time arguing about whether the Queen's first marriage had been consummated. They even quarrelled among themselves – Warham and Fisher had a heated dispute over the validity of the royal marriage, and Nicholas Ridley, acting for the Queen, expressed disgust that her private life had ever come under scrutiny in open court.

Meanwhile, Wolsey was doing his best to gain possession of Campeggio's decretal bull, but on 24 June the legate told him that the Pope had written expressly to forbid its use. Wolsey paled. 'That will be my ruin!' he lamented. The King would not be pleased when he found out.

The hearings continued, as did the arguments. At the end of June, the legates were no nearer a conclusion than when the court first sat, notwithstanding a visitation from the King, who begged them to reach a 'final end' as he was so troubled and could not attend to 'anything which should be profitable for my realm and people'. Thereafter, the court met daily without the principal parties. The general consensus of opinion was that the King and Queen's marriage could only be lawful if Katherine had been left virgo intacta by Prince Arthur. Katherine had sworn on the Blessed Sacrament, and in open court, that she had, but the King – who was the only other person who knew the truth of the matter – alleged otherwise, and had gone to great lengths to seek out witnesses to that first wedding night. Nineteen of them gave evidence at the end of June, much of it deeply embarrassing to the Queen, and all of it inconclusive. Prince Arthur's boastful remarks on the day after his wedding were recalled, and several elderly peers were happy to attest that they had been sexually active at Arthur's age and even younger. A few of the witnesses, such as Rochford and Norfolk, belonged to the Boleyn faction.

The King's 'inconceivable anxiety' about the case prompted him, at the beginning of July, to send Wolsey to the Queen in an attempt to persuade her to be reasonable and accept the authority of the court. But she asked the Cardinal to stop and think: 'Will any Englishman counsel or be friendly unto me against the King's pleasure? Nay, my lord. I am a poor woman, lacking in wit and understanding.'

Henry, whose patience was almost at breaking-point, now heard that Campeggio had said he meant to prorogue the court until October, as the papal curia enjoyed a holiday during the summer months, and since the legatine court was an extension of the court of

Rome, the same rules must apply to it. This meant that judgement was unlikely to be given this side of the summer recess. On 13 July, Campeggio informed the Pope that some people were expecting a sentence within ten days, but assured him: 'I will not fail in my duty. When giving sentence I will have only God before my eyes, and the Holy See.' Four days later, Clement gave way to imperial pressure and revoked the general commission granted to Campeggio and Wolsey, thus invalidating any further proceedings at the Black Friars court, which was still going ponderously about its business.

In England, rumour had it that Campeggio would pass sentence on 23 July. On that day, the King himself attended the court, sitting with the Duke of Suffolk in a gallery above the door, facing the legates. But it was only to hear Campeggio announce that he would give no hasty judgement in the case until he had discussed the proceedings with the Pope. So saying, he adjourned the court indefinitely.

The effect of his words was tumultuous. The King rose and walked out, his face thunderous, whereupon uproar broke out in the court. The Duke of Suffolk shouted from the gallery: 'By the mass, it was never merry in England whilst we had cardinals amongst us!' Wolsey retorted loudly that 'If I, a simple cardinal, had not been, you should have had at this present time no head upon your shoulders wherein you should have a tongue to make any such report in despite of us!' Suffolk did not answer, and stalked off in search of the King. The legates were left sitting looking at each other.

It might well be a matter of years, and not months, now before the Pope reached a decision. Worse still, the waiting might be in vain: Wolsey knew with bitter certainty that, if the case were heard in Rome, judgement would go in the Queen's favour. If the King went to Rome, he warned the English ambassadors at the Vatican, it would be at the head of a formidable army, and not as a supplicant for justice. And the King, when letters citing him to appear before the papal curia arrived in August, was speechless with rage: 'I, the King of England, summoned before an Italian tribunal?' he cried. But that same month, Charles V and Francis I made peace, which left Henry isolated in Europe. Even now, it was being rumoured at court that the King would take matters into his own hands and force

Parliament to grant him an annulment, and although this was not his immediate intention, his anger with the Holy See was mounting, and he was already casting about for another solution.

The referral of the case to Rome had been a consolation to Queen Katherine: the Pope had listened to her, and she was still confident that her husband would eventually return to her. But the King, as if to underline his determination to have his way, left her behind when he went on progress that August, and took Anne Boleyn instead. When he returned, matters were very strained between the royal couple, and at the beginning of October a heated exchange took place, when Katherine told Henry that she knew she had right on her side, and that as she had never been a true wife to his brother, their marriage must be legal.

Katherine now had a new champion in England. In the autumn of 1529 the new Spanish ambassador arrived. Eustache Chapuys was a cultured attorney from Savoy, a man of great ability and astuteness. Never afraid of speaking his mind, he was devoted to the service of the Emperor and those connected with him. He had been well briefed about the treatment meted out to Queen Katherine by her husband, and when he arrived in London he was already committed to her cause. Nor would it be long before, having come to know her, he conceived the deepest admiration and respect, and a very sincere affection, for the Queen.

From the first, Chapuys carried out his duties with more zeal than any of his predecessors, even Mendoza. His initial brief was to bring about a reconciliation between the King and Queen by using 'gentleness and friendship'. But it would only be a matter of time before Chapuys had far exceeded these instructions and became a continual thorn in the side of Henry VIII. He was distrusted by the King's courtiers and advisers, and hated by the Boleyn faction, who feared his influence. The enmity was mutual. Chapuys would never refer to Anne Boleyn as anything other than 'the Concubine' or 'the Lady'. Sir William Paget, one of the King's secretaries, did not consider Chapuys to be a wise man, but a liar, a tale-teller and a flatterer, who had no regard for honesty or truth. Paget, it must be said, was biased, but his comments should be borne in mind, for the dispatches of Chapuys form a major proportion of the source material for this period.

By October 1529, Chapuys had met the King, the Queen, Cardinal Wolsey, and the Privy Council, and had assessed the situation in England. 'The Lady is all powerful here, and the Queen will have no peace until her case is tried and decided at Rome,' he told Charles V. He was right. Henry could not do enough to make up for the disappointment Anne had suffered at the prorogation of the legatine court. In October 1529, the ambassador reported: 'The King's affection for La Boleyn increases daily. It is so great just now that it can hardly be greater, such is the intimacy and familiarity in which they live at present.' In October 1529, Lord Rochford boasted to the French ambassador that the peers of the realm had no influence except what it pleased his daughter to allow them.

It now pleased her to urge them to seek revenge on the man whom she considered to be responsible for her present position, Cardinal Wolsey. After the legatine court had been formally closed on 31 July, this was brought home to Wolsey himself by a letter Anne sent him, in which she accused him of abandoning her interests in favour of those of the Queen. In future, she said, she would rely 'on nothing but the protection of Heaven and the love of my dear King, which alone will be able to set right again those plans which you have broken and spoiled'. There would be no more need for hypocrisy.

For the moment Henry was still reluctant to proceed judicially against Wolsey. Nevertheless, it was soon obvious to the court that the Cardinal had fallen from favour. In August, Henry and Anne went on progress, visiting Waltham Abbey, Barnet, Tittenhanger, Holborn, Windsor, Reading, Woodstock, Langley, Buckingham and Grafton before returning to Greenwich in October. When they were at Grafton in the old royal hunting lodge deep in the Northamptonshire countryside, Campeggio, accompanied by Wolsey, arrived to take formal leave of the King before returning to Rome. No accommodation had been prepared for Wolsey, and he was left standing at a loss in the courtyard until Sir Henry Norris, the King's Groom of the Stole, came and offered him his own room. Norris also advised the King of his arrival, and later brought a summons from Henry, requiring the Cardinal to attend him in his presence chamber with Campeggio.

Wolsey approached the packed room with trepidation, fearing

public humiliation, and seeing Norfolk, Suffolk, Rochford and their supporters waiting like birds of prey for the kill. But when the King entered, he greeted Wolsey warmly and helped him up from his knees, gripping him on both arms. Then he led him to a window embrasure where he chatted affectionately to him until dinner was announced. Meanwhile, Norfolk and Rochford had gone straight to Anne Boleyn and warned her what was going on. Consequently, when Henry dined with her that evening, she was in a dangerous mood, showing herself – according to George Cavendish – 'much offended' with him, and reminding him that 'there is never a nobleman within this realm that if he had done but half so much as the Cardinal had done, he were well worthy to lose his head.' 'Why then, I perceive that you are not the Cardinal's friend,' said Henry, with devastating naïvety. 'Forsooth, Sir,' cried Anne, 'I have no cause, nor any other that loves your Grace, if ye consider well his doings.'

She was still sulking when, later in the evening, Henry resumed his talk with Wolsey, but the next morning, knowing that the King had planned to sit in council with the Cardinal, she seized her opportunity and persuaded Henry to go hunting with her instead. Thus, when the Cardinal appeared, he found the King, dressed for riding, already mounted in the courtyard. Henry ordered him to return south with Campeggio, and bade him a fond farewell with the whole court looking on. They would never meet again.

Campeggio left England on 5 October. He took with him Henry's love letters to Anne Boleyn, which had been stolen from Anne's London house by one of his agents. Nor were they ever returned, for they are still in Rome today in the Vatican archives. The King's officials searched Campeggio's luggage at Dover, in the hope of securing the decretal bull. They never found it, or the letters.

Anne and her faction did their work thoroughly. In October 1529, the King stripped Wolsey of his office of Lord Chancellor of England and demanded that he surrender the Great Seal. He also commanded his attorney general to prepare a bill of indictment against the Cardinal. In a desperate attempt to placate the King, Wolsey surrendered to him York Place and most of his other property, before retiring to his more modest house at Esher in Surrey. The

King was elated at the acquisition of York Place, and in October 1529 he announced it was to be renamed Whitehall and renovated as a palace for Anne Boleyn. That same month, he took Anne and her mother to inspect it, and notwithstanding the presence of a great army of workmen, all engaged upon refurbishment, Anne moved in at once. Whitehall boasted no lodging suitable for Queen Katherine, and Anne was tired of giving precedence to her rival. Now she had her own court and was queen in all but name.

In November, Wolsey, in an agony of anxiety over his future, sent the King a message begging for mercy, and Henry, whose anger had to a great extent been dispelled by the acquisition of his property, placed the Cardinal under his own protection, graciously permitting him to retain the archbishopric of York. And when, thanks to Anne's adherents, Parliament presented the King on 1 December with a list of forty-four articles or charges against Wolsey, Henry declined to punish him further. Anne must perforce wait.

Henry VIII met the man who would present him with a solution to his marital problems in the autumn of 1529. When Stephen Gardiner and Edward Fox were returning from Rome in September, they lodged in a house belonging to Waltham Abbey in Essex. There they met a cleric called Thomas Cranmer, who had sought hospitality in the same house because there was plague in Cambridge, where he was resident in the university.

Cranmer was then forty. Cambridge educated, he had gained a degree in divinity, but soon ruined his career by marrying a barmaid called Black Joan. Marriage was then an impediment to any career in the Church; however, when Joan died in childbirth, the university readmitted Cranmer, who shortly afterwards took holy orders and devoted himself to a lifetime of study. Fox and Gardiner had been fellow students of Cranmer's in their youth, so their meeting turned out to be a friendly reunion, the envoys treating Cranmer to a good dinner. Over the meal, they asked him his opinion on the King's nullity suit. He had not really studied the matter, he said, but he ventured the opinion that the King's case should be judged by doctors of divinity within the universities, and not by the papal courts. 'There is one truth in it,' said Cranmer, and the Scriptures would soon declare it if they were correctly interpreted by learned men trained for such a task; 'and that may be as well done in the universities here as at Rome. You might this way have made an end of the matter long since.' The case, so his argument ran, should be decided according to divine law, not canon law, therefore the Pope's intervention was unnecessary. If the divines in the universities gave it as their opinion that the King's marriage was invalid, then invalid it must be, and all that was required was an official pronouncement by the Archbishop of Canterbury to that effect, leaving the King free to remarry.

This was a radical solution, but to Gardiner and Fox it made sense, and when the King returned to Greenwich in October after his progress they told him about Dr Cranmer's suggestion. 'Marry!' exclaimed Henry, 'This man hath the sow by the right ear!' Cranmer was duly sent for, and came to Greenwich, where Henry was impressed with the sober, quietly spoken, rather timid cleric. He ordered Cranmer to set all other business aside, and 'take pains to see my cause furthered according to your device'. He could begin by writing a treatise expounding his views.

Lord Rochford, Anne's father, was asked to prepare accommodation for Dr Cranmer at his London house, so that he could write in comfort. Rochford gladly complied, and seeing the admiration Dr Cranmer conceived from the first for Anne, he made much of his guest. Not only was Cranmer learned and reassuring, but he was also interested in the new learning and in the arguments for Church reform that were so often aired in the Boleyn household. In no time at all Rochford made Cranmer his family chaplain, and he stayed in that capacity for some time, being allowed frequent access to the King.

Henry VIII's acceptance of Cranmer's suggestion to sound out the universities marks the beginning of a new phase in the 'great matter'. Hitherto, the King's main concern had been to have his marriage declared invalid by the Pope, but now he began to take cognizance of the wider issues involved. He was politically isolated in Europe, and, disillusioned with the Holy See, he perceived himself also as an outcast from a corrupt Church of Rome. Even before the advent of Cranmer, Henry had contemplated severing the Church of England from that of Rome. Now, this seemed a very real possibility for the future if the King wanted his marriage dissolved, for it was almost certain that the Pope would not help him. In this way what began as a matrimonial suit became transformed, very gradually, into a political, theological and ultimately a social revolution. The period of Wolsey's tutelage was over; the lion was at last discovering the full extent of his strength and power. The King was now intent on becoming absolute ruler in his own realm, and More's prophecy, made eight years earlier, would soon be fulfilled.

9
It is my affair!

In November 1529, Henry VIII was as much in love with Anne Boleyn as ever, and still showering her with gifts; although these were now more in the way of peace offerings, for the relationship between them was by then often a stormy one. Anne felt that time was passing her by. She accused the King of having kept her waiting; she might, in the meantime, have contracted some advantageous marriage, she said, and had children – a pointed barb, this. Peace was bought with a length of purple velvet for a gown, linen cloth for under-clothes, a French saddle of black velvet fringed with silk and gold with a matching footstool, and a black velvet pillion saddle and harness so that Anne could ride in intimate proximity to her royal lover.

Often, she would threaten to leave Henry, as in January 1531, when they quarrelled violently. At the prospect of losing her, Henry went hotfoot to Norfolk and Anne's father, and begged them with tears in his eyes to act as mediators. When the quarrel was made up, he placated Anne with yet more gifts: furs and rich embroideries. This charade was repeated on several occasions, with Anne lamenting her lost time and honour, and Henry weeping, begging her to desist and speak no more of leaving him. And, always, there were the peace offerings.

As the months, and then the years, went by, Anne became increasingly difficult to deal with. The long delays and the resultant stress, coupled with the constant strain of holding Henry at arm's length, tested her endurance to the limit. Her position was insecure, and she knew it. Yet she seemed unable to avoid friction with her royal lover. She was furious to discover that the Queen was still mending Henry's shirts. She herself was an expert needlewoman, and the King's admission that the shirts had been sent to Katherine on his orders did little to sweeten her temper. After such quarrels, however, Anne would soon be fervently assuring Henry how much she loved him. 'Even if I were to suffer a thousand deaths,' she told him – referring to an old prophecy that a queen would be burned at this time – 'my love for you will not abate one jot!' Chapuys drily observed that, 'As usual in these cases, their mutual love will be greater than before.'

Once installed at Whitehall Palace, Anne was attended like a queen and courted like one. In December 1529, her father was formally created Earl of Wiltshire which meant that she herself would from henceforth be styled the Lady Anne Boleyn, and her brother be known as Viscount Rochford. To celebrate Wiltshire's elevation, the King gave a banquet at Whitehall, at which Anne took precedence over all the ladies of the court and sat by the King's side on the Queen's throne. Chapuys was present and, after seeing the lavish feast, the dancing and the 'carousing', came away with the impression he had just witnessed a marriage feast: 'It seemed as if nothing were wanting but the priest to give away the nuptial ring and pronounce the blessing.' Anne also presided over a magnificent ball hosted by the King on 12 January in honour of the departing French ambassador, who was sympathetic to her cause.

For all Anne's prominence in the life of the court, the King was at pains to convince everyone that he and the Queen were still on good terms, and kept Katherine constantly with him. She even followed the hunt each day. The Venetian ambassador observed that 'so much reciprocal courtesy is being displayed in public that any one acquainted with the controversy cannot but consider their conduct more than human'. Both were good at concealing the tensions that lay below the surface.

In private, however, it was a different story. On 30 November 1529, when Henry paid a rare visit to her after dinner, Katherine blurted out that she had been suffering the pangs of purgatory on earth, and that she was very badly treated by his refusing to dine with her and visit her in her apartments. He told her she had no cause to complain, for she was mistress in her own household, where she could do as she pleased. He had not dined with her as he was so much engaged with business of all kinds, the Cardinal having left the affairs of government in great confusion. As to his visiting her in her apartments, and sharing her bed, she ought to know that he was not her legitimate husband. He had been assured of this by many learned doctors.

'Doctors!' retorted Katherine, in a passion. 'You know yourself, without the help of any doctors, that you are my husband and that your case has no foundation! I care not a straw for your doctors!' For every doctor or lawyer who upheld Henry's case, she went on, she could find a thousand to hold their marriage good and valid.

But she was getting nowhere. Henry was immovable on that issue, and the quarrel ended with him leaving to seek comfort from Anne Boleyn. Yet she, knowing he had been with Katherine, was decidedly unsympathetic. 'Did I not tell you that whenever you argue with the Queen she is sure to have the upper hand?' she scolded. 'I see that some fine morning you will succumb to her reasoning, and cast me off!' With this, Henry had had enough, and fled back to his own apartments in search of peace.

Gradually the concept of radical change had become firmly rooted in Henry Tudor's mind, and on Christmas Eve he told the Queen that if the Pope pronounced sentence against him, he would not heed it, adding that 'he prized and valued the Church of Canterbury as much as the people across the sea did the Roman'. Severing the Church of England from the main body of Christendom was an idea entirely repugnant to Katherine, and she had difficulty in believing that this was what the King really intended. But, as far as his own case was concerned, Henry was being realistic. The long silence from the Vatican was proof that his suit was being deliberately shelved, and it seemed inevitable that he would soon have to take matters into his own hands.

In February 1530, Charles V went to Bologna to be crowned by the Pope, and Henry, resolving to turn the situation to his own advantage, sent an embassy headed by Cranmer and Wiltshire – newly appointed Lord Privy Seal – to stress to the Emperor that the King had pressed for an annulment only 'for the discharge of his conscience and for the quietness of his realm'. The embassy was not a success, due partly to the aggressive and provocative attitude of Wiltshire, an ardent reformist, and although Charles told the ambassadors that he would abide by whatever decision the Pope reached, he added that he thought Julius II's dispensation was 'as strong as God's law'. It was painfully obvious that Clement would not dare gainsay him, and in April Henry told the French ambassador that he intended to settle the matter within his own kingdom by the advice of his Council and Parliament, so as not to have recourse to the Pope, 'whom he regards as ignorant and no good father'. Katherine, conversely, was relying entirely on the Pope. In April, she wrote to Dr Pedro Ortiz, whom the Emperor had sent to represent her interests in Rome, and begged him to put pressure on Clement to give a ruling in her case. 'I fear that God's vicar on earth does not wish to remedy these evils,' she wrote. 'I do not know what to think of his Holiness.' Throughout the summer months, she sent letter after letter to Clement, beseeching him to take pity on her and pass sentence, but he ignored them, fearing that a decision in the Queen's favour might provoke Henry into creating a schism within the Church.

Henry's subjects were as supportive as ever of Katherine, and in the spring of 1530 a rumour was circulating widely that the King had separated the Queen from her daughter out of spite. This was not true, and to prove it Henry summoned the Princess to Windsor to be with her mother, and left them there together when the court moved on elsewhere. Mary was now fourteen, old enough to realise what the presence of Anne Boleyn at court betokened. Hitherto, she had been studiously sheltered from her parents' troubles, thanks to the diligence of her mother and her governess, Lady Salisbury. When Katherine left Windsor to rejoin the court, Mary went back to Hunsdon, where her father visited her on 7 July. He had seen very little of her in recent years, and one purpose of his visit was to reassure himself that she had not been infected by what he was pleased to call Katherine's obstinacy. Yet when he left Hunsdon, he almost certainly carried with him the realisation that both Mary and her governess were already staunch supporters of the Queen.

In July 1530, a petition was sent to the Pope from all the lords spiritual and temporal of England – including Wolsey – beseeching

His Holiness to decide the case in Henry's favour. Clement peevishly accused them of having troubled him for little cause, and warned them that he had to consider all the interested parties. Nor could he deny the Queen's right of appeal to Rome.

Meanwhile, Henry's agents had canvassed most of the European universities on the issue of the validity of the King's marriage, and where it was felt necessary, bribes were issued to the learned divines in order to obtain the opinions the King hoped to hear. In July 1530, Henry tested his Council's reaction to the prospect of him declaring himself a free man and marrying Anne Boleyn without the Pope's sanction. One councillor threw himself on his knees, and begged his master to wait at least until winter to see what transpired, and Henry, seeing the others to be of like mind, reluctantly agreed. Even the Emperor, however, was certain that the King would marry Anne with or without the Pope's permission. After three years of tortuous negotiations to end his marriage, Henry was still obsessed with her, and more than ever convinced that God was guiding his actions. He described his flexible conscience as 'the highest and most supreme court for judgement and justice', and – according to Chapuys – told the Queen he 'kept her [Anne] in his company only to learn her character, as he had made up his mind to marry her. And marry her he would, whatever the Pope might say.' He was, in truth, no longer the same man who had lodged a plea in Archbishop Warham's ecclesiastical court in 1527. The despot was emerging, determined to have his own way, and even if necessary to alter the process of law to get it.

Throughout 1530, the Emperor pressed Clement VII to pronounce in 'the sainted Queen's' favour, and he urged him to order Henry to separate from Anne Boleyn until judgement was given. In August, Charles granted Chapuys special powers to act on the Queen's behalf, and this gave the tireless ambassador the freedom he desired and needed; from that time on, he would be more zealous than ever in the Queen's cause. Katherine herself liked and trusted him implicitly, and her warm feelings were reciprocated. Years later, after his retirement in 1545, Chapuys would remember her as 'the most virtuous woman I have ever known, and the highest hearted, but too quick to trust that others were like herself, and too slow to do a little ill that much good might come of it'. Here, Chapuys was referring to Katherine's continual refusal during the 1530s to agree to an imperial invasion of England on her behalf. Chapuys would try again and again to convince her that this alone would put an end to her troubles, but such was her loyalty to the man she considered to be her husband that she consistently refused to have anything to do with the plan. Her attitude exasperated Chapuys, but it also increased his admiration for her.

In spite of the pressure from Charles V, Dr Ortiz and Chapuys, the Pope avoided giving a definitive sentence on the King's case. In March 1530, he issued a brief forbidding Henry to contract a new marriage before sentence was given; in May, another brief was issued forbidding anyone to express an opinion on the case if prompted by bribes or unworthy motives – even Clement had heard how Henry had bought off some of the universities. Then, in August, a papal encyclical forbade all persons to write anything against their consciences concerning the 'great matter'; this was a threat to the unity of the English government itself, as the new Lord Chancellor, Sir Thomas More, was known to be against annulment on moral grounds. Then, to add insult to injury, in September the Pope suggested that Henry 'might be allowed two wives', as he could permit this with less scandal than granting an annulment. The King's anger was further fuelled in December, when he was cited to appear in Rome to defend his case. He ignored this, and also a brief issued by Clement in January 1531, ordering him to 'put away one Anne whom he kept about him', and forbidding his subjects to meddle with his case.

Thanks to Clement's conduct, Henry was losing all respect for the Holy See, and paying greater heed to the clamour of Anne Boleyn's faction for reform of the Church in England. This prompted him to consider that the English Church might be better off with himself as its head than owing allegiance to a weak and vacillating Pope. It was a notion that appealed vastly to the King, and once it had taken root in his mind, a break with Rome was inevitable. Both he and Anne were anticipating that much would be accomplished in the new session of Parliament that was due to commence in January 1531, and that their marriage could not be far off. 'The Lady feels assured on it,' commented Chapuys.

By late 1530, Henry was beginning to feel a certain amount of resentment towards Anne Boleyn, and was not above reminding her on one occasion how much she owed to him and how many enemies he had made for her sake. She remained unimpressed. 'It matters not,' she shrugged, refusing to be baited. Nevertheless, according to the Venetian ambassador, her will was still law to him. This had been demonstrated clearly in what had happened to Wolsey.

Just after Christmas 1529, the Cardinal had fallen ill and was thought to be dying. The King sent Dr Butts to him with a message saying he 'would not lose him for £20,000', and bade Anne 'send the Cardinal a token with comfortable words'. Anne knew when not to oppose the King, and meekly detached a gold tablet from her girdle, which she handed to the physician. As a result of these signs of goodwill, Wolsey's health improved daily, though the longed-for summons back to court never arrived.

But while Anne was sending comforting messages to the sick man, she was still plotting his downfall. In February, she remarked in Chapuys's hearing that it would cost her a good 20,000 crowns in bribes 'before I have done with him'. She also made Henry promise not to see Wolsey, for, as she told him, 'I know you could not help but pity him.' Chapuys was convinced that 'to reinstate him in the King's favour would not be difficult, were it not for the Lady'. Because Henry would not order Wolsey's arrest, Anne sulked for several weeks, and was enraged when, on 12 February 1530, the King formally pardoned the Cardinal and confirmed him in his See, which meant he ranked second only to the Archbishop of Canterbury within the Church hierarchy. After that, Anne was 'incessantly crying after the King' for Wolsey's blood. Wolsey himself realised that 'there was this continual serpentine enemy about the King, the night crow, that possessed the royal ear against him.' She was, he told Cavendish, the enemy that never slept, 'but studied and continually imagined his utter destruction'.

At heart, Wolsey was a conventional churchman, and had never supported an annulment of the royal marriage. During the summer of 1530, he began taking an interest in the progress of the Queen's case, and in a letter to Chapuys urged strong and immediate action as the key to its success. In July, he supported Charles V's call for Clement to order Henry's separation from Anne Boleyn, and in August, he wrote to the Pope to urge a speedy conclusion to the

King's case, and to ask why the Queen's cause was 'not more energetically pushed'. In Chapuys's opinion, Wolsey was hoping for a return to power once the 'great matter' was settled, but this would only be possible if it were settled in Katherine's favour. With Anne Boleyn out of the way, and a grateful Queen Katherine exerting her influence upon a contrite husband, the path would be clear for him. But Wolsey, like many other people, underestimated the strength of the King's feelings for Anne Boleyn, and this time the miscalculation would be fatal.

Rumours of Wolsey's activities provoked Anne to fresh efforts. Her uncle, Norfolk, was a willing ally, and was not above bribing the Cardinal's physician into falsely accusing his master of having urged the Pope to excommunicate Henry VIII and lay England under an interdict in the hope of provoking an uprising on the Queen's behalf, perhaps dethroning the King and seizing power for himself. When this information was laid before him, Henry, who had recently been informing his councillors that Wolsey 'was a better man than any of you', was shocked and suspicious. For a while, images of the two Wolseys warred in his mind: the mentor of his youth who had devoted his energies to running the kingdom, the kindly avuncular man whom he had chosen as godfather to the Princess Mary; and the arch-traitor of Anne Boleyn's imagination and the evidence put forward by her party.

Anne won. On 1 November, a warrant was drawn up for the Cardinal's arrest and – in a form of poetic justice – was sent to Henry Percy, Earl of Northumberland, Anne's former suitor. Percy waited on Wolsey at his episcopal palace at Cawood in Yorkshire, and apprehended him on a charge of high treason. Then began the slow journey back to London, the Tower, and inevitable death. But Wolsey was a sick man, and on the way he succumbed to the ill health that had plagued him in recent months, dying at Leicester Abbey, where his escort had been obliged to find him shelter. 'If I had served God as diligently as I have done the King,' he said on his deathbed, 'he would not have given me over in my grey hairs.' He was buried next to Richard III in what Chapuys was pleased to call 'the tyrants' sepulchre'.

The King was saddened by news of his death: 'I wish he had lived,' he remarked. Anne Boleyn, however, was jubilant, and staged a masque for the edification of the court entitled 'The going to hell of Cardinal Wolsey'. Though Henry found this distasteful, Anne's temper was such these days that he dared not cross her. Early in 1531, Chapuys reported:

> She is becoming more arrogant every day, using words in authority towards the King of which he has several times complained to the Duke of Norfolk, saying that she was not like the Queen who never in her life used ill wòrds to him.

Henry did not have the courage to say these things to Anne's face, for he was afraid of losing her, although she had no such qualms. Her thwarted ambition and repressed sexuality had turned her into a virago with a sharp tongue, with which she managed to alienate many of her former supporters. For all this, her power over the King remained, based as it was on sexual blackmail and shared aims.

With Cranmer's plan now being put into effect, Anne was preparing for queenship. In December 1530, she commissioned the College of Arms to draw up a family pedigree that invented a descent from a Norman lord who had supposedly settled in England in the twelfth century. 'The King is displeased with it, but he has to be patient,' Chapuys wryly commented. On the same day she ordered new liveries for her servants embroidered with the device: *Ainsi sera, groigne qui groigne* (Thus it will be, grudge who grudge). When the court rocked with suppressed mirth, Anne was at a loss to know why, until the King bade her get rid of the device, explaining that the motto was meant to read: *Groigne qui groigne, Vive Bourgogne!* (Grudge who grudge, long live Burgundy!), a device used by the Emperor.

Anne's attitude towards the Queen had by January 1531 deteriorated into outright hatred. Chapuys wrote:

> The Lady Anne is braver than a lion. . . . She said to one of the Queen's ladies that she wished all Spaniards were in the sea. The lady told her such language was disrespectful to her mistress. She said she cared nothing for the Queen, and would rather see her hang than acknowledge her as her mistress.

Because of Anne's attitude, and the King's resentment of the Queen's stand, Katherine's supporters were finding that their lives were becoming increasingly uncomfortable. There were also signs that the King was no longer prepared to tolerate any defiance on his wife's behalf. Late in 1530, the Duchess of Norfolk was smuggling letters received from Italy to the Queen concealed in oranges. Katherine passed them to Chapuys, who sent them on to the Emperor. The Duchess's actions were noticed, and she was warned not to help the Queen, Anne using 'high words' to her aunt in front of the courtiers. Katherine was of the opinion that the duchess had sent the letters 'out of the love she bears her' and because she loathed Anne Boleyn, but Chapuys suspected that she might have sent them at the behest of the Duke, who perhaps hoped to implicate the Queen in a conspiracy. His fears were without foundation, for, in 1531, the Duchess again acted as go-between for the Queen and the Spanish ambassador, and when the King found out, he banished her from court.

Then there was Thomas Abell, one of Katherine's chaplains. In 1530, he published a book in her defence, entitled *Invicta Veritas*, which argued that 'by no manner of law may it be lawful for King Henry the Eight [*sic*] to be divorced'. It was a very brave thing to do, for Abell incurred the King's severe displeasure, and the book went immediately on to the banned list, although not before some copies had been circulated. It would soon be apparent that one supported the Queen at one's peril.

On 21 January 1531, the Convocations of the clergy of Canterbury and York met at Westminster, and anyone with any grasp of English affairs would have reckoned this significant, for it was only with the assent of Convocation that important ecclesiastical reforms could be implemented. Something momentous was indeed at hand: the meeting marked the beginning of the English Reformation.

It was Thomas Cromwell who had finally convinced the King of the advantages of severing the Church of England from Rome. Cromwell's promotion to the King's service from Wolsey's had been arranged in 1521 by the Cardinal, when Cromwell was thirty-five. The son of a blacksmith, a thick-set bull of a man with black hair and small, porcine eyes, Cromwell had led a somewhat disreputable early life, and had soldiered as a mercenary in Italy, where he may have learned to admire the Machiavellian ideal of political expediency. Upon his return to England in 1513 he had taken up law, and in this capacity had attracted the attention of the Cardinal, to whose service he had been recruited the following year. To great intelligence and ability Cromwell added a complete lack of scruple, although he always professed to be a devout Christian. It was this facet of his unattractive personality that would in time make him essential to the King. Unscrupulous and efficient, his spy network, instituted after his rise to favour following the disgrace of Wolsey, was to become a model for future governments.

Henry was aware that England's relations with the papacy had often lacked harmony over the centuries: several medieval kings had come into conflict with the pontiffs, and the English had always resented paying the burdensome levy to Rome known as 'Peter's Pence'. In the late fourteenth century, John Wycliffe and his Lollards had spoken out against the wealth and corruption of churchmen, and now, in the more enlightened world of Renaissance Europe, there was even more cause for criticism. Henry was no heretic, but he was determined to govern his kingdom 'in concert with his lords and commons only', and even some supporters of the Queen were disillusioned with the Holy See, which had become an institution increasingly at odds with the burgeoning nationalism of the English people. It was in this climate that the English Reformation was planned.

On 7 February 1531, the King stood in Parliament and demanded that the Church of England recognise and acknowledge him from now on to be its 'sole protector and supreme head'. Neither Parliament nor Convocation dared defy the King, and on 11 February, Archbishop Warham announced that the clergy were prepared to acknowledge the King as supreme head of the Church of England 'as far as the law of Christ allows' – a qualification conceded by Henry after some heated negotiations. From henceforth the English Church would not recognise the Pope, who would be referred to as the Bishop of Rome, and he would not receive allegiance from the English bishops or enjoy any canonical jurisdiction in England.

Henry VIII's Church of England remained Catholic in its precepts. The only immediate change was in its leadership, which since that day has remained vested in the sovereign. Parliament at once passed an Act confirming the King's new title, and the news was conveyed to the people of England by proclamation. They learned that Henry VIII was now effectively King and Pope in his own realm, with complete jurisdiction over his subjects' material and spiritual welfare. There was little resistance. Anne Boleyn was ecstatic, and Chapuys wrote: 'The woman of the King made such demonstrations of joy as if she had actually gained Paradise.' Her father, sharing her enthusiasm, offered to prove from scripture that 'when God left this world He left no successor or vicar.' Like Wiltshire, most of the nobility supported the King, and the clergy had no choice. Even Chapuys conceded that the Pope's 'timidity and dissimulation' had been the cause of Henry's break with Rome, and had done much harm to the Catholic Church.

Yet one or two brave voices were raised against the King. John Fisher, Bishop of Rochester, made no secret of his opinion that it was against God's law for the King to be Head of the Church of England. Henry was becoming increasingly irritated by Fisher's resistance, and Anne Boleyn and her faction were so furious that they made plans to remove the Bishop from the scene. On 20 February 1531, Fisher's cook, Richard Rouse, added a white powder to the soup which was served to Fisher and his household. Several men died at table, others fell seriously ill, but Fisher himself ate only a little soup and, although he suffered terrible stomach pains, he escaped what was obviously an attempt on his life. Rouse was arrested, even though it was widely believed he had been acting on the instructions of Wiltshire who was said to have given him the poison, and that Anne herself was privy to the plot. However, the King refused to credit the rumours, and pressed Parliament into passing a new law providing for harsh treatment of poisoners: in future, they would be publicly boiled to death, a punishment meted out to the unfortunate Richard Rouse. Chapuys thought the King had been wise to deal so severely in this case; 'nevertheless, he cannot wholly avoid some suspicion, at least against the Lady and her father.' Anne's involvement was confirmed in October 1531, when she sent a message to Fisher warning him not to attend the next session of Parliament in case he should suffer again the sickness he had almost died of in February. If she had not actively intrigued for Fisher's death, she had at the very least condoned the attempt to murder him.

Thomas More was appalled by the break with Rome, the more so because, as Lord Chancellor, he could not do other than condone it. His reluctance to become involved in the 'great matter' was widely known, and he had made enemies because of it. His old friendship with the King had been strained to the limit, and Cromwell, recently appointed to the Privy Council, had taken his place as Henry's chief adviser. How long he could continue in his office was anybody's guess, but he feared it would not be long before he and the King came into open conflict, something he would have given much to avoid.

In July 1531, Chapuys was writing: 'The Lady allows only three or four months for the nuptials. She is preparing her royal state by degrees, and has just taken an almoner (Edward Fox) and other officers.' Visiting ambassadors were warned to 'appease the most illustrious and beloved Anne with presents'; she went about decked like a queen and dispensed favours as one. Save for the crown and the title, her reign had in effect begun.

Although Anne was not, as Chapuys alleged, 'more Lutheran that Luther himself', she certainly supported the idea of radical reform in the Church, while at the same time observing all the conventions of traditional Catholicism. One of the staunchest advocates of the royal supremacy, she was now openly flaunting her controversial views, and was still reading forbidden literature with the King's knowledge. She also had in her possession more conventional works: a volume of the letters of St Paul, as well as a beautifully bound edition of Lord Morley's translation of *The Epistles and Gospels for the LII Sundays in the Year*, presented to her at Christmas 1532, and several devotional and other works in the French language, among them the *Ecclesiaste* and a letter-writing treatise by Louis le Brun, the first book ever dedicated to her, as 'Madame Anne de Rochefort'.

One reason for Anne's strong anti-clericalism was because she felt there were too many priests supporting the Queen. When Henry put in a good word for an erring priest brought before his justices, Anne said loudly to her father that the King 'did wrong to speak for a priest, as there were too many of them already'. She had no love at all for the Church of Rome, and because she supported the newly established Church of England with such conviction it was widely believed that she would urge the King to do away with traditional forms of worship as well. At the end of 1532, Queen Katherine would warn the Emperor that, thanks to Anne Boleyn, Henry had already seized a great deal of Church property. Like Chapuys, Katherine believed Anne to be a heretic, and Anne's own behaviour tended to confirm this: in 1532, she obtained a reprieve from the stake for a noted Protestant, John Lambert, who had been examined and found guilty of heresy by Warham. Her patronage of such people suggested she was one of them, though in truth she was merely putting into effect her own views on religious enlightenment, which were revolutionary enough in her time.

Parliament had, as yet, done nothing about the King's nullity suit, but every day leave of absence was being granted to those Members who supported the Queen, which Chapuys thought ominous. From the pronouncements made by the universities – all of which had now been received – it was easy to see which way the wind was blowing. So confident was Henry of receiving favourable opinions, and of the effect of his bribes, that there was no room in his mind for the possibility of the body of learned opinion being against him. Nor was it. Of the sixteen European universities canvassed, only four supported the Queen. The majority of the finest and most learned minds in Europe – not all of them susceptible to bribes – pronounced the King's marriage to be incestuous and against the law of God; it was therefore null and void, and the papacy had had no business in the first place to dispense with it.

The verdicts of the universities were read out in Parliament at the end of March, and were later published. Most of the King's subjects accepted them, but women, who were, according to Hall, 'more wilful than wise or learned', spoke out and accused the King of having corrupted the learned doctors. A similar reaction was met with by Henry's own treatise on the 'great matter', entitled *A Glass of the Truth*, which was published that year.

In the spring of 1531, Henry tried again to force Katherine to withdraw her appeal to Rome. Again, she refused, and wrote to the Emperor, begging him to press Clement to give a ruling before October, when Parliament was due to reconvene. In April, a papal nuncio arrived in England, and told the King his case could only be tried in Rome and nowhere else. Henry told him he would never consent to such a thing, even if the Pope were to excommunicate him. 'I care not a fig for his excommunications!' he stormed.

It was Archbishop Warham who now stood in Henry's way. Warham was old and ailing, a staunch religious conservative who had already gone against his principles to acknowledge the King's supremacy, but without him there could be no annulment. Henry, knowing Warham to be near death, did not press the point. He could afford to wait a little longer, and when Warham was dead, Cranmer, who had already shown Henry the way out of his dilemma, could take his place.

Henry was now seeing as little of Katherine as possible, and when they did meet he only pestered her to retire to a convent or withdraw her appeal to Rome. She had been ill in November 1530, and he left her to recover at Richmond while he went to London with Anne. 'He has never been so long without visiting her now,' wrote Chapuys a few weeks later. However, the Queen was well enough to travel to Greenwich for the Christmas season, sitting enthroned with the King in the great hall on Twelfth Night to watch a masque and some dancing. Henry made a point of dining with her every night, and showed her every respect.

After Christmas, Katherine confided to the Pope that her complaint was

> not against the King, my lord, but against the instigators and abettors of this suit. I trust so much in my lord the King's natural virtues and goodness that if I could only have him with me two months, as he used to be, I alone would be powerful enough to make him forget the past. They know this is true, so they try to prevent his being with me.

This was a viewpoint from which Katherine never wavered, whatever the King might do to prove she was wrong: she could never accept that Anne Boleyn's influence was more powerful than hers could be, given the chance.

In March 1531, Henry was still playing the part of a man who had been forced to set aside a beloved wife against his will, and was visiting the Queen regularly, even though it was a charade he had grown heartily sick of. 'The Queen is now firmer than ever,' wrote

Chapuys in April, 'and believes the King will not dare to make the other marriage.' In fact Henry was doing his best to provoke Katherine into giving him grounds for a divorce by deserting him. When the Princess Mary fell seriously ill with a digestive disorder in March, Katherine, learning that her daughter had not kept any food down for eight days, wanted to go to her. Henry, seeing his advantage, replied meaningfully that 'she might go and see the Princess if she wanted, and also stop there.' The implication was ominous, but Katherine guessed his purpose and refused to leave his side, even though she was desperate to see her child. Throughout the course of her marital problems, her chief aim had been to protect her daughter's interests. According to canon law, a child conceived of a marriage made in good faith could not be declared illegitimate if that marriage were found to be invalid. Mary therefore had a lawful right to a place in the succession, either as Henry's heiress or after any legitimate sons born to the King. Yet Katherine feared that any issue of a marriage between Henry and Anne would oust Mary from her place in the succession. For this reason, she was determined to preserve Mary's rights, with her own life-blood if need be.

Mary's illness marks the beginning of the bouts of ill health that were to ruin her constitution and her life. At fifteen, she was fully aware of the rift between her parents and her ailments were almost certainly the products of anxiety. Her problems were further complicated by a difficult adolescence and the onset of painful and irregular periods and debilitating headaches. Mary loved her father, but, from the first, her sympathies had lain with her mother. She rarely saw either of them, and in her loneliness and grief she turned to her religion for solace: it would very soon become the dominant influence in her life.

Ten days after their confrontation, Henry and Katherine dined together in public. Chapuys was present, and heard the Queen, 'with supernatural courage', ask Henry once again to dismiss 'that shameless creature', Anne Boleyn. He angrily refused. Undeterred, Katherine again asked if she might visit the Princess Mary, who was still very poorly. 'Go if you wish and stop there!' he snapped, to which she replied quietly: 'I would not leave you for my daughter or for anyone else in the world.'

Henry now, belatedly, began to feel concerned about his child's health, and guilty for having deprived her of the comfort of her mother's presence. On 24 March, he arranged for Mary to be brought by litter to Richmond Palace, and for Katherine to join her there. By April, Mary was much better, well enough for Katherine to return to court and leave her in the care of Lady Salisbury. On 4 May, Katherine suggested that Mary visit the court, but Henry was in a cantankerous mood and refused, although a month later he arranged for the Princess to join her mother when the court moved to Windsor.

Henry was still trying to make Katherine withdraw her appeal to Rome. On 31 May 1531, he sent a deputation from the Privy Council to wait on her at Greenwich, its purpose being to ask her to 'be sensible'. She refused to do as the King asked. She denied his supremacy, declaring that the Pope was 'the only true sovereign and vicar of God who has power to judge in spiritual matters'. Then she said:

> I love and have loved my lord the King as much as any woman can love a man, but I would not have borne him company as his wife for one moment against the voice of my conscience. I *am* his true wife. Go to Rome and argue with others than a lone woman!

Then, when the bishops attempted to prolong the dispute, she cut them short, saying, 'God grant my husband a quiet conscience, but I mean to abide by no decision save that of Rome'. Afterwards, Chapuys told Charles V that the deputation had been 'confounded by a single woman', and the Duke of Suffolk told Henry VIII that Katherine was ready to obey him in everything save for the obedience she owed to two higher powers. 'Which two?' Henry fumed. 'The Pope and the Emperor?' 'No, Sire,' replied Suffolk, 'God and her conscience.'

This incident provoked Henry's decision to separate from Katherine for good. The court was then at Windsor, but was due to move to Woodstock on 14 July. On that day, Henry left Windsor Castle early, without informing the Queen of his departure, and she, left behind with only her daughter and her attendants for company in the deserted royal apartments, was not immediately aware of the momentous step he had taken, nor that she would never see him again. Then she was informed by a messenger that it was the King's pleasure that she vacate the castle within a month, and in that moment everything fell into place. He had gone, had left her, without saying goodbye. Even in her distress, she remained calm. 'Go where I may, I remain his wife, and for him I will pray,' she told the messenger, and bade him convey a message of farewell, saying how sad she was that Henry had not said goodbye to her, and enquiring after his health as a good wife should. The King, hearing her message, fell into a violent rage, crying,

> Tell the Queen I do not want any of her goodbyes, and have no wish to afford her consolation! I do not care whether she asks after my health or not. Let her stop it and mind her own business. I want no more of her messages!

Nor did his spite end there. He wrote to Katherine warning her it would be better for her if she spent her time in seeking witnesses to prove her 'pretended virginity' at the time of their marriage than in talking about her cause to whoever would listen to her; she must cease complaining to the world about her imagined wrongs. To be fair to Henry, it is likely that, had she agreed to the annulment of their marriage, he would have treated Katherine generously and remained on good terms with her – his later treatment of Anne of Cleves argues this. Yet time and again she had opposed him, seemingly blind to the very real dilemma he was in with regard to the succession, and when thwarted Henry could, and frequently did, become cruel.

Katherine remained at Windsor until early August 1531, when she received a message from the King commanding her to leave court. Having seen Mary off to Richmond, she moved with her household to Easthampstead, where, on 13 October, she was visited by another deputation of the Council, come to explain to her what the determinations of the universities meant and to inform her that Julius II's dispensation was 'clearly void and of none effect'. Katherine remained unmoved, declaring on her knees that she was the King's true wife; he had succumbed, she said, to 'mere passion'. And when the lords warned her of what the King might do to her if she persisted in her defiance, she answered, 'I will go even to the fire if the King commands me'. A few days later, Henry sent her to The More in Hertfordshire, a manor house formerly owned by Wolsey, very well appointed and set in excellent parklands. Here, for a time, Katherine kept great state, being attended by 250 maids of honour. At the end of October, thirty Venetians were her guests and were impressed by her vast household and the splendour of their surroundings. On that day, they noticed, thirty maids of honour stood round the Queen while she dined, and a further fifty waited at table. As for Katherine herself, they found her of short stature, 'inclined to corpulence, of modest countenance; a handsome woman of good repute. She is neither disheartened nor depressed,' but 'virtuous, just, replete with goodness and religion, constant, resolute, prudent, good, and always smiling.' But while foreigners were happy to visit The More, Henry's courtiers stayed away.

When winter came, Katherine's mask slipped, and in November, she told the Emperor that

> what I suffer is enough to kill ten men, much more a shattered woman who has done no harm. I am the King's lawful wife, and while I live I will say no other. At The More, separated from my husband without having offended him in any way, Katherine the unhappy Queen.

In another letter written that month, she begged Charles, 'for the love of God, procure a final sentence from His Holiness as soon as possible. May God forgive him for the many delays!' The Emperor, touched to the heart by her pleas, summoned the papal nuncio and told him he thought it 'a very strange and abominable thing, that the lust of a foolish man and a foolish woman should hold up a law suit and inflict an outrageous burden upon such a good and blameless Queen'. Then he ordered the nuncio to press for Henry VIII's excommunication, in the hope that that would bring the King to his senses. The Pope, as usual, refused to do anything that might provoke Henry to further excesses against the Church: 'His conduct cuts me to the soul,' wrote Katherine of Clement.

On 10 November 1531, Henry and Katherine hosted two separate banquets for dignitaries of the City of London at Ely Place in Holborn, Henry in one hall and Katherine in another. They did not meet, and this was to be the last state occasion that Katherine would attend. On her way home to The More afterwards, crowds gathered to see her and to shout words of encouragement, which greatly displeased the King. He did not invite the Queen to court that Christmas, and the absence of mirth from the festivities at Greenwich was put down to her absence. Mary, too, was absent, being at Beaulieu in Essex. Nevertheless, Katherine sent Henry a gift of a gold cup, with a humble message, for they had always exchanged presents at Yuletide. Henry sent it back with a curt message commanding her not to send him such gifts in future, for he was not her husband, as she should know. 'He has not been so discourteous to the Lady,' observed Chapuys; Anne had given him 'darts of Biscayan fashion, richly ornamented', and in return he had given her a room hung with cloth of gold and silver and crimson satin heavily embroidered. And he even remembered Mary Boleyn, who received a shirt with a collar of black-work lace.

Anne was still as unpopular as ever. Her reputation throughout most of Christendom was dire, and she was openly called a whore, an adulteress, and sometimes even a heretic in the courts of Europe. At home public feeling made itself felt in an incident that occurred on 24 November 1531. On that day, Anne went with only a few attendants to dine with one of her friends at a house by the Thames. Word spread quickly through the City of London that she was there, and before very long a mob of seven or eight thousand women, or men dressed as women, were marching upon the house with intent to seize her, even lynch her. Fortunately for Anne, she received warning of their coming, and escaped by barge along the river. She was, however, badly shaken by this evidence of just how unpopular she was with her future subjects. Since Henry could not arrest every woman in London, he was powerless to do anything about it; all he could do was hush up the affair, so that word of it should not incite further incidents, though the Venetian ambassador learned what had happened, and recorded it for posterity.

News that Anne Boleyn had usurped the Queen's place at court during the Christmas season provoked an outcry in London, and in March 1532, the Abbot of Whitby made history by being the first man brought to justice for calling her a 'common stewed whore'. The Nun of Kent had continued to prophesy against the King, accusing him of wishing to remarry for his 'voluptuous and carnal appetite', and by the winter of 1531, the government had begun to view her as a threat to national security since she was inciting disaffection among the King's subjects, and was secretly believed by Cromwell to be in league with the Bishop of Rochester. From this time on, she would be watched by Cromwell's agents.

On Easter Sunday 1532, Friar William Peto preached before Henry and Anne at Greenwich, and warned the King that if he made 'an unlawful marriage' with the woman sitting next to him, he would be punished as God had punished Ahab, and the' dogs would lick his blood. Henry, hearing this, went purple with rage and walked out, with Anne hard on his heels. A month later, one of his own priests, Dr Richard Curwen, delivered a sermon denouncing Peto as a 'dog, slanderer, base and beggarly rebel and [a] traitor. No subject should speak so audaciously to his prince!' Peto was then banished; he went to Antwerp, and later to Rome, where he was eventually made a Cardinal, dying in 1578.

Anne had not only made enemies of the people and Katherine's supporters, but she had also alienated some of her own supporters by her behaviour. By the summer of 1531, she was on increasingly bad terms with Norfolk, although he would for some time to come continue to promote her cause, seeing in her advancement future benefits for himself. Yet he could not approve of the way she treated the King. It was to Norfolk that Henry came running, often in tears, when Anne had been unkind to him, and the Duke's estranged wife told Chapuys that her husband had confided in her that Anne would be 'the ruin of all her family'. Anne had also managed to offend the Duke of Suffolk in the spring of 1530, and he had gone straight to Henry with lurid tales of her supposed affair with the poet Wyatt. Henry refused to listen, lost his temper, and temporarily banished Suffolk from court, but the rift upset him. Suffolk was a close friend and a staunch supporter, even in the face of opposition from his wife, Mary Tudor. Lastly, there was Sir Henry Guildford, the comptroller of the King's household, who in 1531 said complimentary things about Queen Katherine in Anne's hearing. Furious, she threatened him with the loss of his highly remunerative and prestigious office. 'You need not wait so long!' he retorted in anger, and immediately offered the King his resignation. Henry tried to talk him out of it, saying he should take no notice of women's talk, but Sir Henry was adamant: he would go.

On New Year's Day 1532, Anne returned to court after visiting her family at Hever, and was lodged by the King in the Queen's old apartments with almost as many female attendants as Katherine had had. Two weeks later, the King reconvened Parliament 'principally for the divorce [sic]'. In May, as a penalty for their past loyalty to the Pope, he exacted a heavy fine from Convocation. This open defiance of the Holy See was not without repercussions, for the next day Sir Thomas More resigned from his office of Lord Chancellor and surrendered the Great Seal of England to the King. He could no longer reconcile his conscience to Henry's reforms, and he wanted nothing to do with the King's plans to marry Anne Boleyn. The King was upset, disappointed, and rather angry, but he let More go, and Sir Thomas was grateful to retire to his house at Chelsea, his family, and his books. Sir Thomas Audley, a staunch King's man, was shortly afterwards appointed Lord Chancellor in his place.

In May 1532, Henry was busy spending a small fortune on providing Anne Boleyn with a wardrobe fit for a queen. One gown was made entirely of gold-embroidered velvet, and cost over £74. Then there was the glamorous nightgown, supplied in June, made of black satin lined with black velvet, which was not to be worn in bed, but to keep warm and to receive guests out of it. That same month, Henry granted Anne the manor of Hanworth, which boasted a fine house in which she frequently stayed.

Meanwhile, in Rome, the King's case still dragged on. A hearing had been set for November 1531, but then it was adjourned again until January 1532, when 'that devil of a Pope' (as the French ambassador described him to Chapuys) once more postponed it. It would not take place until after Christmas, even though Francis I had told Clement, at Henry's behest, that if he agreed to an annulment then Henry might forget all about his new-found supremacy and once more become a dutiful son of the Church. Clement was waiting for Henry to appear in Rome and answer for himself, which Henry dismissed as a foolish 'fantasy'. He would never go, he said. Then the Pope sent a solemn injunction to the King, ordering him to restore Queen Katherine to her rightful place at court and remove 'that diabolic woman' from his bed forthwith; whereupon Henry, who had waited so long and with such impatience to manoeuvre Anne into that bed, reacted with hot fury. 'It is my affair!' he cried. How dared the Pope interfere! But interfere Clement did, threatening excommunication, a threat that Henry ignored. And in May, he issued a brief ordering Henry to treat Katherine with more kindness. In July, in secret consistory, he decreed that if the King did not appear in Rome by 1 November, he would be declared contumacious, and the hearing would go ahead without him.

The Queen also received support from other quarters. In January, Reginald Pole, then studying in Paris, spoke out against the King, after having once used his influence to cause a division of opinion in Henry's favour in the Faculty of Theology at the Sorbonne over the question of the validity of the royal marriage. Henry ordered Pole to explain himself, which he wisely refused to do; later the King tried to gain Pole's support for his reforms, but again, Pole proved uncooperative. In June 1532, John Fisher, Bishop of Rochester, preached a sermon in favour of the rights of the Queen, thereby incurring the King's grave displeasure. And in February that year, Archbishop Warham, fearing an earthly king less than a celestial one, formally protested in Parliament against all legislation passed since November 1529 that was derogatory to the Pope's authority, thereby effectively denying the royal supremacy. This was a setback for the King, but he let it pass, for Warham could not live much longer. But he could not silence his own sister, the Duchess of Suffolk, who, in April 1532, used what Chapuys called 'opprobrious language' about Anne Boleyn, and who still stayed away from court on her account. Nevertheless, finally, Mary Tudor would be reconciled to the King before her tragic early death in June 1533, and would tell him in her last letter that 'the sight of your Grace is the greatest comfort to me that may be possible.' Lastly there was Chapuys, who was still as zealous as ever in the Queen's cause. He had even obtained an assurance from the Earl of Shrewsbury, Keeper of the Queen's Crown, that he would not allow it to be placed on any other head than Katherine's.

There were signs in 1532 that the government meant to deal harshly with those who persisted in supporting the Queen. In August, Maria de Salinas, Lady Willoughby, Katherine's closest friend, was ordered to leave her household and not communicate with her royal mistress. And in that same month, Thomas Abell was sent to the Tower of London for publicly upholding Katherine's cause. However, he was released at Christmas, with a stern warning not to meddle in the King's matrimonial affairs. Most ominous of all was Katherine's separation from her daughter. In January, Mary had made a much publicised visit to her mother at Enfield, Henry being anxious to placate his subjects. When the visit ended neither mother nor daughter realised that they would never be allowed to meet again. It suited the King to keep them apart; now that Mary was growing older, he feared they might well intrigue with the Emperor against him. Besides, keeping Katherine from seeing Mary was a good way of punishing her for her obstinacy.

And there were other ways, too. In May 1532, the King ordered Katherine to leave The More and move to the palace at Bishop's Hatfield in Hertfordshire, a red-brick edifice built in the late-medieval style by Henry VII's chief minister, Cardinal Morton, in 1497. Built around a courtyard – all that remains nowadays is one wing containing the great hall – it was a royal enough residence that would later be used as a nursery palace for the King's children. Katherine was installed there by the end of June, but she did not stay long, for on 13 September, Henry sent her to Enfield, where she would be less comfortably housed. She went meekly enough, still holding firmly to her conviction that she was right.

In June 1532, England and France signed a mutual treaty of alliance. Henry now expected to be able to count on Francis I's support when it came to dissolving his marriage and marrying Anne Boleyn, and the two Kings agreed to meet at Calais in the autumn to discuss those matters and to formulate their policy towards the Emperor. In the summer, Henry told Chapuys that he meant to marry Anne as soon as possible, and would celebrate their nuptials in 'the most solemn manner'. Yet for a while it seemed there might be an impediment to their union. The Countess of Northumberland was petitioning Parliament for a divorce from her husband, Anne's former suitor Henry Percy, on the grounds that there had been a precontract between him and Anne Boleyn. Henry had Percy closely questioned by the Archbishops of Canterbury and York, who made him swear solemnly on the Blessed Sacrament that there had never been such a precontract. Parliament, accordingly, threw out his wife's petition, and the unhappy marriage of the Percys had perforce to continue.

In August, Henry took Anne on a progress with him through the southern counties, but was forced to cut it short as a result of the hostility shown by the crowds who lined the roadsides and hurled abuse at her. Some cried out that he should take back the Queen, others that Anne was a whore and a heretic. 'The Lady is hated by all the world,' observed Chapuys with satisfaction. It was around this time that Anne found a book of prophecies in her apartments at Whitehall, obviously left by one of her enemies for her to find for one crude picture showed her with her head cut off. Anne was unperturbed, and told her maid of honour, Anne Saville, that she thought it 'a bauble', adding that she was resolved to marry the King 'that my issue may be royal, whatever will become of me'.

On 22 August 1532, Archbishop Warham died, and the King wasted no time in appointing Thomas Cranmer to the vacant See of Canterbury. Chapuys wondered if the Pope knew of 'the reputation Cranmer has here of being devoted heart and soul to the Lutheran sect', a reputation that was not undeserved, although the new Archbishop had to keep his heretical views a strict secret from Henry. 'He is a servant of the Lady's,' the ambassador informed his master, 'and should be required to take a special oath not to meddle with the divorce [*sic*]. It is suspected that the new Archbishop may authorise the marriage in this Parliament.'

Of course, Cranmer had every intention of meddling with the annulment, not only because he believed in it, but because his appointment was enthusiastically supported by the Boleyns, whose chaplain he had been; the new primate had a sincere affection for Anne Boleyn, and saw her as a means whereby he might push through the ecclesiastical reforms that were so dear to him. The Queen, like Chapuys, regarded his promotion as ominous, and was also concerned about her daughter, having heard that Anne Boleyn's enmity towards the Princess was as great as it was towards herself. It was said that the King dared not praise Mary in Anne's presence for fear of provoking her vicious temper, and that she had made spiteful remarks about the girl. By September 1532, Henry was having to keep his visits to Mary as brief as possible because Anne was so jealous, and not long afterwards she was boasting that she would have Mary in her own train and might one day 'give her too much dinner, or marry her to some varlet'. Chapuys, hearing her, was concerned, remembering the attempt on Bishop Fisher's life; he had no doubt that Anne was perfectly capable of putting her threats into effect.

Henry VIII took the first step towards making Anne Boleyn his queen on Sunday, 1 September 1532. On that day, at Windsor Castle, he bestowed upon her a peerage in her own right, something that had never before been granted in England to a woman. He created Anne Marquess – using the male style – of Pembroke, Pembroke being a title borne in the fifteenth century by Henry's great-uncle, Jasper Tudor. The ceremony of ennoblement was performed with great pomp, with the King enthroned in his vast presence chamber attended by the Dukes of Norfolk and Suffolk and the lords of his Council, while Anne was conducted into his presence by a great train of courtiers and ladies. She had on a surcoat of crimson velvet beneath a short-sleeved overgown trimmed with ermine – traditional robes of nobility of a style dating from the fourteenth century – and her hair hung loose down her back. She curtsied three times as she approached the King, then knelt, as the Letters Patent conferring her new title were read out. As the herald spoke, the King placed a crimson velvet mantle of estate about her shoulders and a golden coronet on her head. She then gave him humble thanks, and retired to the sound of trumpets. Afterwards, she and Henry heard mass in St George's Chapel, where a *Te Deum* was sung in honour of the occasion.

The wording of the patent of creation left some room for speculation, however, as the phrase 'lawfully begotten' had been omitted when referring to the male issue to whom the title might one day descend. Some thought this an indication that Henry had tired of Anne and was pensioning her off and providing for any bastard she might bear him, but this was not the case. Henry was enhancing Anne's status for the coming French visit, and the unusual wording of the patent was devised to ensure that any child conceived out of wedlock would be provided for in the event of the King dying before his marriage to Anne took place. This was highly significant: it could only mean that Anne had at last surrendered to the King.

Henry's and Anne's sexual relationship had begun only a short time before, probably during the previous week. The death of Archbishop Warham on 22 August had broken Anne's resolve to remain chaste, for she knew that it would now only be a matter of time before the King was free to marry her. Thus she took a final gamble, and it was this, not her imminent dismissal, as some courtiers speculated, that prompted her ennoblement. The ceremony on 1 September was arranged at very short notice, so that Anne would have rank and financial security if the King died suddenly.

Those who had predicted Anne's fall were soon to be speedily disappointed. The consummation had only enhanced Henry's passion, and the Venetian ambassador was amazed at his 'great appetite' for Anne. 'The King cannot leave her for an hour,' wrote Chapuys, and it was true: Henry was more infatuated than ever, if that were possible. Thereafter, he and Anne would live together quite openly; in December, the Venetian envoy reported that 'the King accompanies her to mass – and everywhere'.

Undoubtedly, the sexual relationship between Anne and Henry was to begin with a very satisfactory one. Henry was an attractive man. In the despatches of the Venetian ambassadors we find that 'in this eighth Henry, God has combined such corporeal and intellectual beauty as to astound all men! His face is angelic rather than handsome, his head imperial and bald, and he wears a beard, contrary to English custom.' He had a 'bold address', and still excelled with ease at

> manly exercise: he sits his horse well, jousts, wields the spear, throws the quoit, and draws the bow admirably. He plays at tennis most dextrously. He has an air of royal majesty such has not been witnessed in any other sovereign for many years.

Anne was certainly not immune to Henry's charm, and he found in her a bedmate at once loving and adventurous – perhaps too adventurous, in fact, for he would later declare with disgust that she had been 'corrupted' in France in her youth. The discovery that she had had some sexual experience after all, though it may be that she was still technically a virgin, was doubtless a disconcerting one for Henry, especially after Anne's constant protestations that she meant to preserve her virtue until she married. However, at this stage of their relationship he was too much in love to let it concern him overmuch; though in time to come this would undoubtedly be one of the grounds for his disillusionment with her.

With her marriage reported to be imminent, Anne had gathered her own court about her, and in its inner circle were young people with wit, charm and intelligence who could be guaranteed to ensure that life was never dull. Among them were Anne's brother, Lord Rochford, of whom she was very fond, his wife, the former Jane Parker – with whom he was not happily matched – Sir Francis Bryan – known, with good reason, as 'the Vicar of Hell' – Sir Francis Weston, William Brereton, Sir Thomas Wyatt, and various relations of the Boleyns and their supporters. The older nobility, who as a rule represented the more conservative element at court, were not welcome and resented their exclusion.

There were now only a few weeks to go before the French visit. Henry had expressed a desire for Anne to accompany him as his future queen, and she threw herself happily into preparations for the trip to Calais, confident that Francis I, once her admirer and now Henry's friend and ally, would surely support her forthcoming marriage. There was just one formality to be disposed of, and that was the vexing question of which royal lady would receive Anne in France. Queen Eleanor was the Emperor's sister, and refused to do so; besides, Henry was adamant that 'he would as soon see the devil as a lady in Spanish dress'. Nor would Francis's sister, now Queen of Navarre – whom Anne had known well and admired when she lived at the French court – agree to go to Calais; in fact she delivered a humiliating snub by refusing to have anything to do with one whose behaviour was the scandal of Christendom.

The bickering went on for weeks. Without any lady of rank to receive her, Anne could not go officially to France. King Francis was at pains to find a solution that pleased everybody and would soothe the ill feeling among all the ladies involved, and, at the last minute, suggested that his *maîtresse en titre*, the Duchess of Vendôme, do the honours. It never occurred to Henry that most people regarded Anne as his *maîtresse en titre*, and he angrily protested that this would be an insult to Anne and her ladies. At last, it was decided – with reluctance on both sides – that Anne would remain in Calais while Henry went to meet King Francis in French territory. There was no question of her being left behind in England – Henry wanted her with him, and many people thought they would secretly marry while in France, for which reason the trip was not popular at court. But Anne Boleyn, hearing the rumours, made it very clear that she would not consent to being married abroad; she wanted to enjoy the moment of her triumph in England.

She and Henry spent the weeks before their departure at Hanwell, where they hunted daily, and here Anne conceived the idea of further humiliating the Queen. She told Henry that she wished to take to France those jewels that were the official property of the queens of England which were still in Katherine's possession; some of them were centuries old, and of great historical importance. Henry dutifully sent a messenger to Katherine demanding that she deliver them to him. These jewels were of particular significance to Katherine; although they were Crown property, and not her own, she considered it her right, and hers alone, to wear them. She therefore refused to surrender them without the King's express command in writing, saying that to do so would 'weigh upon my conscience'. Nevertheless, she had no choice but to do so when the King's written order came.

Katherine was well aware that Anne Boleyn was behind Henry's harsh treatment of herself, and knew she would try to humiliate her at every turn. Proof of this was forthcoming that same month, when Anne appropriated the Queen's barge with Henry's knowledge and consent. Afterwards, without consulting him, Anne had Katherine's coat of arms deliberately defaced as belonging to a usurper before it was burnt off. When he learned of this, the King was 'very much grieved', and Chapuys commented: 'God grant that she may content herself with the said barge, the jewels, and the husband of the Queen!'

On 7 October, Henry and Anne, with a vast train, left Greenwich and began their journey to Dover. At Canterbury, the Nun of Kent was waiting for them. Anne had seen her two months earlier, when the Countess of Wiltshire had suggested she neutralise the Nun by making her one of her waiting women, but Elizabeth Barton made no secret of her distaste and turned down the position. In Canterbury she repeated her prophecies, though the King ignored her, and went on his way, but after he had gone to France, she continued to speak out publicly in favour of the Queen, and large crowds came to hear her. Cromwell, whom Anne Boleyn called 'her man', now had her under surveillance, and was waiting to pounce.

Henry and Anne sailed to France in the *Swallow* on 10 October; the voyage took seven hours. They were welcomed in Calais by a deputation of civic dignitaries led by the Governor, and conducted in procession to the Church of St Nicholas, where they heard mass. They then took up residence in the Exchequer Palace, where they had interconnecting bedchambers. There followed a week of merry-making before, on 21 October, Henry rode out of Calais to meet Francis I and discuss with him his nullity suit. Francis showed himself sympathetic, and at Henry's invitation, he came to Calais on Friday, 25 October, as the King's guest. For two days, Anne Boleyn kept out of sight, but on the Sunday evening, when the supper table had been cleared, she made her entrance, accompanied by seven ladies in gorgeous gowns and masks; her own outfit was of cloth of gold slashed with crimson satin, puffed with cloth of silver and laced with gold cords. She advanced boldly to King Francis and led him out to dance, the other ladies following suit with King Henry and the other gentlemen present. Henry took great pleasure in removing the ladies' masks, and after the dancing Francis spent some time in conversation with Anne. Two days later, he left Calais. The English court stayed on at the Exchequer for another fortnight, while Henry and Anne enjoyed what was effectively their honeymoon. The Milanese ambassador to the French court, seeing them together, thought they had already married in secret, and referred to Anne as 'the King's beloved wife' in dispatches. The idyll came to an end at midnight on Tuesday, 11 November, when a convenient wind made departure for England imperative. The lovers took ship for Dover, and then made their way to Eltham Palace.

Now that she was the King's mistress, Anne realised that becoming pregnant would both consolidate her position and expedite her marriage. Her hopes of this were awakened during the Christmas festivities at Whitehall, and with the coming of the new year of 1533, hope turned to certainty: she was, indeed, pregnant. When the King learned of it, he made up his mind that they should be married at once. As far as he was concerned, he had never been lawfully married to Katherine, and was therefore a free man. The best scholars in Europe had said so.

Just before dawn, on the morning of 25 January 1533, a small group of people gathered in the King's private chapel in Whitehall Palace for the secret wedding of the King to Anne Boleyn. The officiating priest was either Dr Rowland Lee, one of the royal chaplains, or – according to Chapuys – Dr George Brown, Prior of the Austin Friars in London and later Archbishop of Dublin. As Lee was preferred to the bishopric of Coventry and Lichfield in 1534, he seems to have been the likelier choice. There were four, possibly five, witnesses, all sworn to secrecy: Henry Norris and Thomas Heneage of the King's privy chamber, and Anne Savage and Lady Berkeley, who attended Anne. William Brereton, a groom of the chamber, may also have been present. Thus, in a hushed ceremony quite unlike the one she had hoped for, Anne Boleyn become Henry VIII's second wife.

Although their marriage and Anne's pregnancy remained strictly guarded secrets for some time, neither Henry nor Anne could resist dropping hints about what had happened, and Chapuys took them so seriously that he was thoroughly alarmed. Anne Boleyn was going about in a mood of high elation and, in February, Chapuys heard her say to Thomas Wyatt, before a large crowd of courtiers, that she had

an inestimable wild desire to eat apples, such as she has never had in her life before, and the King had told her it was a sign she was with child, but she had said it was nothing of the sort. Then she burst out laughing loudly.

Wyatt, whose desire for Anne was long since 'sprung and spent', told Chapuys afterwards that he was ashamed of her. A few days later, Anne told Norfolk that if she did not find herself pregnant by Easter, she would go on a pilgrimage to Our Lady of Walsingham. On 24 February, she and the King held a great banquet at Whitehall. Henry behaved like a bridegroom; Chapuys watched him fawning upon Anne and showing every sign of uxoriousness. By the end of the evening he was very drunk and roaring with laughter; much of what he said was incoherent, yet the Duchess of Norfolk heard him refer to Anne Boleyn's 'great dowry and a rich marriage' – waving his hand to indicate their sumptuous surroundings.

During that month, the Privy Council once again examined the facts of the King's case, and recommended that he proceed at once 'to his purpose by the authority of the Archbishop of Canterbury' and the Queen was officially informed of Henry's intentions.

Katherine had spent a wretched Christmas in isolation at Enfield, and the news filled her with dread. Little information reached her nowadays. She was forbidden to communicate with Chapuys, but both defied this order whenever possible, although it was difficult for Katherine, as she knew Cromwell's spies were watching her. In January, she had got a message through to the ambassador, begging him to press for a papal sentence on her case, and saying she took full responsibility for the consequences. Even if the King refused to return to her, she would 'die happy' if their marriage was decreed good and valid, knowing that the Princess Mary would not lose her place in the succession. Furthermore, she believed the people of England would support a papal decision in her favour.

In February, when the King had decided to proceed to the annulment of their marriage, Katherine was ordered to move to Ampthill. As this new abode was some way from London, the move amounted to virtual banishment, which Henry hoped would break the Queen's resistance. Built in the early-fifteenth century, Ampthill had hitherto been a favoured residence of the court while on progress. Nothing remains of it today, for it was demolished in 1616, and by the eighteenth century only traces of the gardens could be seen. Katherine had been there several times, and tried with good grace to make herself feel at home. Yet she would not be left untroubled in her new home for long, for in early March Henry sent a deputation to Ampthill in another vain attempt to make her withdraw her appeal to Rome.

The Pope had several times threatened Henry with excommunication, yet even the threat of this, the most dire sentence that could be meted out to a devout Christian, did not move the King. Nor did appeals to take back Katherine and dismiss Anne. When the papal nuncio ordered Henry, in the Pope's name, in January 1533, to recall Katherine to court, Henry refused 'for good reasons', notably 'her disobedience and her severity towards me'. In February, the Pope and the Emperor concluded a new alliance, and Clement promised Charles that the Queen's case would be heard in Rome and nowhere else. Yet no date was set.

Charles V was then fully occupied with driving back the Turks from the eastern borders of his Empire; he had for the present neither the leisure nor the resources to invade England on his aunt's behalf. This, and the knowledge of Anne Boleyn's advancing pregnancy, prompted Henry VIII to the decision that now was an opportune moment to resolve his marital problems. Moreover, it was essential that the succession of Anne's child be lawfully assured, for the infant's rights must be undisputed from the first. What Henry was planning was for a time kept entirely confidential. Anne's brother Rochford was sent to France on 13 March with a secret message for Francis I, but no one knew what it was. After his return on 7 April, the King summoned his Council and informed them that he had married Anne Boleyn two months ago, and that she was carrying in her womb the heir to England. On hearing this staggering news, the Council advised the King to inform Queen Katherine at once. Henry chose Norfolk and Suffolk to perform the unpleasant duty, and on 9 April they saw Katherine at Ampthill and warned her she must not attempt to return to the King, seeing that he was married. From henceforth, she was told, she was to abstain from the title of Queen and be referred to as the Princess Dowager of Wales. The King, in his generosity, would allow her to keep her property, although he would not pay her servants' wages or her household expenses after Easter. Katherine took the news quite calmly, although her inner turmoil must have been considerable. Afterwards, she told her chamberlain, Lord Mountjoy, that as long as she lived she would call herself Queen of England. Failing food for herself and her servants, she would go out and beg 'for the love of God'.

When Chapuys heard that Katherine had refused to allow her servants to address her as anything but Queen, he resolved never to refer to Anne Boleyn by that title, and he urged Charles V to declare war on Henry VIII, reminding him of

the great injury done to Madam your aunt. Forgive my boldness, but your Majesty ought not to hesitate. Your Majesty must root out the Lady and her adherents. When this accursed Anne has her foot in the stirrup, she will do the Queen and the Princess all the hurt she can, which is what the Queen fears most.

Charles was in no position to act; he had enough to do in fending off the Turks. However, the English government had no means of knowing where his priorities lay, and even the King anticipated trouble with the Emperor, fearing that he might have brought England to the brink of war by marrying Anne. He knew also that public opinion was not with him.

None of these things deterred him. One by one he had removed all the obstacles in his way, and he would remove any others that presented themselves. When, on 11 April 1533, Archbishop Cranmer requested permission to proceed to the 'examination, final determination and judgement in the said great cause touching your Highness', Henry VIII wasted no time in granting his request.

10

Happiest of Women

The eve of Easter Sunday fell on the 12th of April in 1533. On that Saturday morning, Anne, dressed in robes of estate and laden with diamonds and other precious stones, proceeded as Queen of England to her closet to hear mass; sixty maids of honour followed her. At last she had achieved her chief ambition, and she had adopted for her motto the legend 'Happiest of Women'. Her success now seemed assured, and she was confident that the child she carried would be the son for which the King had always craved.

The court looked on with ill-concealed dismay. According to Chapuys, even some of Anne's own supporters felt that the King should have waited for his marriage to Katherine to be formally dissolved before taking another wife. The King, sensing that his nobility were less than enthusiastic about their new queen, commanded them to pay court to her, announcing that he would have her crowned on Whitsunday, 1 June. Within days, the Lord Mayor of London would have been ordered to prepare a lavish civic welcome, with pageants, for the occasion. Henry had taken an irrevocable step; he might have gained his heart's desire, but he now had to face the consequences to himself and his kingdom and the censure of most of Europe.

On the evening of 12 April, the King authorised Cranmer to pass judgment on his union with Katherine, believing, rather naïvely, that his marriage to Anne would put an end to any opposition from the former Queen. He also set about appointing the officers of the new Queen's household: Lord Burgh was to be chamberlain, Edward Baynton vice-chamberlain, Anne's uncle Sir James Boleyn of Blickling would be chancellor, and John Uvedale secretary. Another Boleyn relative, William Cosyn, was master of her horse. Her ladies included Anne Saville, Anne Gainsford (now Lady Zouche), Lady Berkeley, Jane Seymour (who had served Katherine of Aragon), Anne's cousin Madge Shelton, and Norfolk's mistress Elizabeth Holland. As soon as all these had sworn their oaths of allegiance, Queen Anne summoned them to attend the first meeting of her council, and exhorted them to be virtuous and discreet. Male servants were forbidden to frequent brothels, on pain of instant dismissal.

On 15 April, Chapuys saw the King and tackled him on the subject of his marriage to Anne. 'I cannot believe that a prince of your Majesty's great wisdom and virtue will consent to the putting away of the Queen,' he said. 'Since your Majesty has no regard for men, you should have some respect for God.' 'God and my conscience are on good terms!' retorted Henry. Chapuys tried further remonstration, but to no avail. 'You sting me!' cried the King, at which the ambassador apologised, knowing he would never be able to help Katherine if he fell foul of Henry. But he had already overstepped the mark, for in May he was summoned before the Privy Council and warned not to meddle further in the Queen's affairs, an order Chapuys chose to ignore.

News of the King's new marriage spread quickly; it was anything but well received. Courtiers and subjects alike resented Anne. Her elevation to queenship spelled disaster for Anglo-Flemish trade, and might well plunge the country into a war with the Emperor. Moreover, by her behaviour she had alienated many people who might have supported her.

In April, there was a spate of public protests against the marriage: a priest, Ralph Wendon, was hauled before the justices for saying that Anne was 'the scandal of Christendom, a whore and a harlot'; another priest in Salisbury, commending the King's new wife to his flock, suffered greatly at the hands of his female parishioners. When, at the end of the month, the order went out that Queen Anne was to be prayed for in churches, one London congregation walked out in disgust: the Lord Mayor later suffered a reprimand when the King learned of it. The Dean of Bristol lost his office for forbidding his priests to pray for Henry and Anne. Some people even suffered imprisonment for slandering the new Queen, such as Margaret Chancellor, who had not only cried out 'God save Queen Katherine!' but had also called Anne 'a goggle-eyed whore'.

The King was determined that those who spoke out against him would be silenced, and the government made strenuous efforts to eradicate seditious talk. In May, it issued the first of a series of propaganda tracts designed 'to inform his Grace's loving subjects of the truth'. His Grace's loving subjects were not impressed.

Abroad, news of Anne's elevation met with little enthusiasm. Cromwell's agents in Antwerp informed him that a cloth picture of the new Queen had been pinned obscenely to a portrait of Henry VIII; and in Louvain, students were scratching scurrilous slogans about Henry and Anne on the walls and doors.

On 15 April, Katherine's chamberlain, Lord Mountjoy, received a message from the King, bidding him warn the Princess Dowager that she would soon be retired to a smaller house, there to live on a reduced allowance which Chapuys feared would not be enough to cover the expenses of her household for three months. Chapuys was, in fact, very anxious about Katherine's future, having perceived that her very existence posed a threat to Anne Boleyn's security. The ambassador realised that the King's subjects were too frightened to intervene on Katherine's behalf, while he knew that Anne could be vindictive and that her influence over the King was enormous. If Chapuys was not mistaken, malignant forces were already at work against Katherine, and on 16 April he warned Charles V that the King was 'in great hope of the Queen's death. Since he was not ashamed to do such monstrous things, he might, one of these days, undertake some further outrage against her.' It was a well-founded conclusion, given Anne's rumoured involvement in the poison plot against Fisher. Katherine and Mary now posed the most serious threat to her future, and that of her unborn child. What might she not do to them? Katherine herself was aware of the danger threatening her and Mary, and from now on would keep a careful vigil, wary of anything that might be an attempt on her life.

Henry soon learned from Chapuys that the Emperor would neither recognise Anne Boleyn as Queen of England, nor accept any judgement of Cranmer's on his marriage to Katherine. The King remained unmoved, and told the ambassador he would 'pass such laws in my kingdom as I like'. Cranmer, meanwhile, had summoned various divines and canon lawyers to a specially convened ecclesiastical court in the twelfth-century priory at Dunstable, not far from Ampthill. At the end of April, Katherine was cited to appear before this court in May, but ignored the summons because she did not recognise Cranmer's competence to judge her case. Although the recently passed Act of Restraint of Appeals prevented any person from appealing to Rome for any cause whatsoever, Katherine maintained that she was Henry's wife, not his subject, and not bound by his laws. Cranmer declared her contumacious, and proceeded without her.

Six miles from where Katherine now lived the clergymen gathered on 10 May to decide her fate. Several days of debate followed, then – at last – on 23 May, the Archbishop finally reached his decision, and with the assent of the learned divines in the court, pronounced Henry VIII's union with Katherine of Aragon to be 'null and absolutely void' and 'contrary to divine law'. The Pope, said Cranmer, had no authority to dispense in such a case.

Cranmer then dealt with the King's marriage to Anne Boleyn, and on 28 May 1533, from a high gallery at Lambeth Palace, he announced that he had found it to be good and valid. The Dunstable court was then closed. After six long years, Henry finally had what he wanted: Anne was now legally his, and their child would be indisputably legitimate.

Cranmer's pronouncement had come not a moment too soon, for on that very day, Queen Anne was escorted by barge by the Lord Mayor of London and his brethren from Greenwich to the Tower, where she would spend the night before her civic reception and coronation. Norfolk, as Earl Marshal, had been put in charge of the arrangements, but so fraught was the relationship between himself and his niece that by the time Anne left Greenwich they were barely on speaking terms. On that day, the much tried Duke confided to Chapuys that he had always opposed the King's marriage to Anne – which was a lie – and had tried to persuade the King therefrom – an even bigger lie. He even went so far as to praise Katherine of Aragon for her 'great modesty, prudence and forbearance, the King having been at all times inclined to amours'. Anne, of course, was neither modest, prudent, nor forbearing, but she had arranged brilliant marriages for two of Norfolk's children – his heir, Surrey, married the daughter of the Earl of Oxford, and his daughter, Mary, married the King's natural son, Henry FitzRoy – and she had persuaded the King to waive a dowry in the case of his son's bride. This went a long way towards endearing her to Norfolk's estranged Duchess, who stopped plotting the restoration of Queen Katherine and returned to court.

In spite of the antipathy of the Earl Marshal towards the Queen, the coronation festivities went as planned. When Anne came to the Tower, the river was full of gaily decorated barges, many of them filled with musicians. Crowds lined the riverbanks to see the water pageants and the Queen's own barge, hung with cloth of gold and heraldic banners, making its stately way along the Thames. At the Tower, Anne was greeted by the King who displayed a 'loving countenance' and kissed her heartily before leading her into the newly refurbished royal apartments where they would spend the next two nights. On the Friday evening, Henry dubbed eighteen gentlemen Knights of the Bath, an ancient ritual normally performed only at the coronations of reigning monarchs.

On Saturday, 31 May, wearing a surcoat of white cloth of tissue and a matching mantle furred with ermine, with her hair loose beneath a coif and circlet set with precious stones, Anne rode in a litter of white cloth of gold drawn by two palfreys caparisoned in white damask through the City of London to Westminster. Before and behind her streamed a great procession of courtiers and ladies, said to have extended for half a mile, and over her head the Barons of the Cinque Ports held aloft a canopy of cloth of gold with gilded staves and silver bells.

Anne's civic reception and the route she followed were much the same as at Katherine of Aragon's welcome to London thirty-two years earlier, and the pageants – staged at great cost to the citizens – were on similar themes. As was customary, free wine ran in the conduits for the crowds lining the streets, children made speeches, and choirs raised their voices in honour of the new Queen. The verses recited in one pageant were composed by Nicholas Udall, Provost of Eton College from 1534 to 1541, and ended in the chorus:

'Honour and grace be to our Queen Anne!' She was wished 'hearty gladness, continual success and long fruition'. 'Queen Anne, prosper, go forward and reign!' she was told and in St Paul's Churchyard the choristers sang an anthem, 'Come, my love, thou shalt be crowned!' The City of London had spared no expense in honouring a queen who was not popular, even commissioning Hans Holbein to design triumphal arches for the processional route, and regilding the Eleanor Cross in Cheapside for the occasion. But although the crowds had turned out in their hundreds, perhaps thousands, their reception of their new queen was cold. They came to stare, not to cheer, and as Anne passed by, smiling and greeting the people on either side, she counted less than ten people who called out 'God save your Grace!' as they had once called to Queen Katherine. Anne's fool, who rode in the procession, was angered by the sparsity of uncovered heads in the crowds, and yelled, 'Ye all have scurvy heads and dare not uncover!' Worst of all, when the people saw the intertwined initials of the King and Queen amongst the decoration, they roared with laughter, crying out 'HA! HA!' When Anne finally arrived at Westminster Hall, to be greeted by Henry, she was upset at the hostility shown her by the crowds. 'How liked you the look of the City, sweetheart?' enquired the King. 'Sir, the City itself was well enow,' Anne answered, 'but I saw so many caps on heads and heard but few tongues.' Chapuys too had sensed the hostility, although he had not been part of the procession. 'All people here cry murder on the Pope for his procrastination in this affair,' he told the Emperor.

Sunday, 1 June 1533 was Anne's coronation day. Dressed in a gown of crimson velvet edged with ermine beneath a purple velvet mantle, and with her hair loose beneath a caul of pearls and a rich coronet, Anne walked in procession from Westminster Hall to Westminster Abbey beneath a glittering canopy of cloth of gold. Following her went a great train of lords and ladies, the yeomen of the King's Guard, the monks of Westminster, bishops and abbots richly coped and mitred, and, finally, the children of the Chapel Royal with the two archbishops. The red carpet along which they proceeded extended right up to the high altar of the abbey, where Anne sat enthroned upon a raised platform. Cranmer performed the ceremony of anointing, then he placed the crown of St Edward upon her head, a sceptre of gold in her right hand, and a rod of ivory in her left, thus effectively crowning her as queen regnant, as no other queen consort has been before or since.

A fanfare of trumpets announced the Queen's return to the Palace of Westminster. 'Now the noble Anna bears the sacred diadem!' enthused the future Bishop of Ely, Richard Cox, an eyewitness, but his enthusiasm was shared by few of his fellow Englishmen. Chapuys thought the coronation was 'a cold, meagre and uncomfortable thing', and the London crowds evidently agreed with him, for again they watched in silence, few bothering to cheer or uncover.

Anne's coronation banquet in Westminster Hall was a lavish affair that lasted several hours. She was seated alone at the centre of the top table, with two countesses behind her, ready with napkin and fingerbowl. She ate three dishes (out of twenty-eight served) at the first course, and twenty-three at the second. As the Knights of the Bath served the food, trumpeters played. When the feast ended, Anne was served wine, comfits and sweets, and gave the Lord Mayor of London her gold cup, thanking him and the citizens of London for their efforts on her behalf. The King also gave them his hearty thanks on the day following. Court festivities continued for some days after the coronation with tournaments, hunting expeditions, banquets and dancing, the courtiers falling over themselves to do honour to their new mistress. Yet, as the French ambassador observed, this was not because they approved of her, but because they wished to gain favour with the King.

Henry had done for Anne all he had promised to do: he had married her and had her crowned with as much pomp as if she were a reigning monarch. It was now up to her to seal her part of the bargain by presenting him with the son which Henry, at forty-two, now needed more desperately than ever, not only to ensure the succession, but also to justify the risks he had taken to marry Anne and break with Rome. The birth of a male heir would bring many waverers and dissidents over to his side, and, he was well aware, it would silence once and for all that infuriating woman at Ampthill.

On the day of Anne Boleyn's coronation, the Nun of Kent was publicly prophesying doom for the King and his new wife, something she had been doing effectively for the last two years. This time the authorities acted, and in July she was brought before Cranmer to be examined. He let her go with a warning not to incite the people with her so-called prophecies, but in August, the Privy Council received a report that she had ignored this, and she was brought before Cranmer again. This time, she admitted she had never had a vision in her life. In September, she and her associates were arrested, having confessed that their visitations and revelations were fraudulent, and in September, the Nun was sent to the Tower. Chapuys applauded Katherine's repeated refusals to see Elizabeth Barton: there could be no suspicion of collusion, although the Council was doing its best to unearth evidence of it, and so incriminate her in the Nun's treasonable activities. But there was nothing to find, and even Cromwell told Chapuys he admired Katherine's prudence: 'God must have given her her wit and senses,' he said. Yet Elizabeth Barton had now said enough to convince the Council that she and her associates were guilty of high treason, and they were made to do public penance at Paul's Cross before being sent back to the Tower.

Others had also expressed their disapproval of Anne Boleyn's coronation. The Marquess of Exeter, the King's cousin, and his wife stayed away, pleading sickness. Henry was not fooled: both were known to be supporters of the Princess Dowager and associates of the Nun of Kent. When the Nun was arrested, Lady Exeter wrote a grovelling letter to the King protesting that she had never meant to offend him, and the Exeters escaped Henry's wrath for the time being. Bishop Fisher had also believed in the Nun of Kent; he was now under house arrest, having been placed there on Palm Sunday, 'the real cause of his detention being his manly defence of the Queen's cause', according to Chapuys. In fact, Henry had wanted Fisher silenced when Cranmer came to pronounce judgement.

In Spain, the Emperor was outraged at the way in which his aunt had been treated, though Chapuys was forced to admit to the Council that his master had no intention of declaring war on Katherine's behalf. At this, Cromwell openly expressed his relief. It was as well the Princess Dowager was a woman, he reflected: 'Nature wronged her in not making her a man. But for her sex, she would have surpassed all the heroes of history.'

The Pope, meanwhile, having heard the shocking news from

England, was realising at last that he ought to act swiftly, and on 11 July, he declared the marriage between Henry and Anne null and void, and threatened Henry with excommunication if he did not get rid of Anne by September. He also annulled all the proceedings of the Dunstable court, and in August issued a brief of censure when he realised that Henry meant to ignore his decrees. Henry continued to take no notice. 'God, who knows my righteous heart, always prospers my affairs,' he told Chapuys loftily.

In May, the Princess Mary was officially informed by a deputation of the Privy Council of Cranmer's judgements. She bravely told them that she would accept no one for queen except her mother, whereupon the councillors forbade her to communicate in any way with Katherine, and would not allow even a note of farewell. For Mary, the long, sad years of trial had begun. Her defiance, inspired by Katherine's courage, had the effect of fanning Anne Boleyn's smouldering resentment into bitter hatred, and also caused an open rift between Mary and her father. Anne tried at first to bribe Mary into submission by sending cordial letters and inviting her to court, asking her to honour her as queen, and promising it would be a means of reconciliation with her father. Mary replied curtly that she knew of no queen of England save her mother, but if 'Madam Boleyn' would intercede for her with the King, she would be much obliged. Anne was furious, but she sent Mary another invitation. Again, Mary rebuffed her, so she moved to the next stage in her campaign, threats. These had no effect either, and from then on it was open war, with Anne publicly vowing to bring down the pride born of Mary's 'unbridled Spanish blood'.

Katherine was not officially informed of the Archbishop's two judgements until 3 July. On that day, another deputation of lords of the Council, headed by Lord Mountjoy, arrived at Ampthill and presented her with a parchment advising her that the King was lawfully divorced and married to the Lady Anne, who was now queen. 'As the King cannot have two wives, he cannot permit the Dowager to persist in calling herself queen,' she was informed. It would be better for her if she accepted this new marriage and recognised Anne as Queen of England – better for everyone, in fact. But Katherine took a pen and, to the horror of Mountjoy, scored through the words 'Princess Dowager' with such vehemence that the nib tore the parchment, which still survives today bearing the marks of its mutilation. 'I am not Princess Dowager but the Queen and the King's true wife!' she cried angrily. 'And since I have been crowned and anointed queen, so I will call myself during my lifetime.' When Mountjoy ventured to remind her that the rightful queen was now Queen Anne, Katherine retorted with scorn that 'all the world knoweth by what authority it was done,' and declared she would abide by no judgement save that of the Pope.

The lords, who had heard her out with growing irritation, then delivered an ultimatum from the King. If she persisted in her obstinacy, he might withdraw his fatherly love from their daughter. Katherine blanched at this, but remained resolute and said she would not yield for her daughter's sake or anyone else's, notwithstanding the King's displeasure. Warned that she was putting herself in danger of the King's anger and its consequences, she replied: 'Not for a thousand deaths will I consent to damn my soul or that of my husband the King.'

Henry was furious at the failure of Mountjoy's mission, and took his revenge by ordering, at the end of July, that Katherine be moved to the Bishop of Lincoln's thirteenth-century palace at Buckden in Huntingdonshire. Part of this building still survives today. When Katherine stayed there, the newer Great Tower assigned to her was already fifty years old, and rendered chilly and uncomfortable by the damp that rose from the Fens upon which it was situated. Katherine and her much reduced household were lodged in a corner turret of the three-storyed red-brick building, which was, by intention, more comfortless than the rest. Buckden was also very remote, and a long way from London and the court. It was surrounded by a secure moat, and located in a wild and desolate area, overlooking the Great Fen. Few people lived in the district, a fact that had not escaped Henry's attention. But if he had hoped to bring Katherine to submission by exiling her to such a place, he was destined to be disappointed. As the former queen's cortège wound its way to Buckden on 30 July, the country people ran after it in hordes, wishing Katherine comfort and prosperity, and professing themselves ready to serve her and, if need be, die for her.

At Buckden visitors were forbidden, by the King's express command, and there was very little money. What Katherine could spare she gave in alms to local poor folk. Nor was food plentiful, and she fasted often, usually for religious reasons. Beneath her clothes, she wore the hair shirt of the third order of St Francis, to remind her of the frailty of the flesh. Her leisure hours were spent on embroideries with her women, fashioning altar-cloths for the churches in the district, but the greater part of her days was devoted to prayer, and it was prayer that sustained her. At Buckden, a room with a window adjoined the chapel, and Katherine would kneel here, day and night, praying at the window. When she had gone, her ladies would find the sill wet with her tears, for she shed many for the loss of both husband and child. Yet her forbearance was remarkable. When one of her women began to curse Anne Boleyn, Anne's greatest rival bade her hold her peace and 'pray for her', for the time would come when 'you shall pity and lament her case'.

Chapuys relates how in August, Anne demanded that Katherine surrender the rich triumphal cloth and christening gown she had brought from Spain. These were in fact Katherine's personal property, and she refused to let Anne have them: 'God forbid I should ever give help in a case so horrible as this!' she exclaimed. Nor did the King press the point. The christening robe remained at Buckden.

In August, the Pope drew up a sentence of excommunication against Henry VIII. Katherine, appalled, wrote to Clement, begging him not to put it into effect, and Clement, for once, heeded her plea. But by September, she was feeling desperate about her predicament. The Pope must be made to give judgement, and soon.

> There is no justice for me or my daughter [she wrote to Chapuys]. It is withheld from us for political considerations. I did not ask His Holiness to declare war – a war I would rather die than provoke – but I have been appealing to the vicar of God for six years and I cannot have it! Write to the Emperor, bid him insist that judgement be pronounced!

She had also heard malicious gossip, designed to scare her, that the next Parliament would decide if she and her daughter were to 'suffer martyrdom'. Bravely, she declared she did not fear it, but what was ominous to Chapuys was that Katherine's keepers had been instructed to break her resistance with such threats.

The Queen's pregnancy progressed well. It was made public in May, when her increasing girth obliged her to add a panel to her skirts. Being Anne, she complained bitterly about the loss of her figure, but her father told her bluntly to thank God she found herself in such a condition. In July, she went with Henry to Hampton Court to rest, and was reported to be in good health and spirits. Normally at that time of year Henry would be preparing to go on progress, but in 1533 he stayed near London, hunting, so as to be on hand. He also ordered prayers for her safe delivery to be said in churches. Astrologers and seers were consulted by the future parents about the baby's sex. Only one dared predict it would not be a boy: William Glover, famous throughout the kingdom for foretelling the future, told Anne he had had a vision of her bearing 'a woman child and a prince of the land'. This was not well received.

In August, the first cracks in the relationship between Henry and Anne began to appear. With his wife fully occupied with preparations for the coming child, and perhaps no longer inclined to want his sexual attentions, the King, who had now settled down in his marriage to a point where he could be complacent about it, had been unfaithful. The identity of this fleeting inamorata is not known, although Chapuys thought her 'very beautiful', and reported that many nobles had promoted the affair, doubtless to spite Anne. Whoever she was, the liaison was quickly over. However, Anne found out. Unlike Katherine, she was not reticent about such matters, and made a fuss. Henry was irritated to find her upbraiding him for a passing infidelity; now that they were married, he expected her to be as meek, docile and submissive as Katherine had been, and he did not take kindly to her censure. Worse still, he was hurt, for he had just presented her with a great French bed, part of the ransom for the Duke de Longueville in 1515, and he made it clear that it was as well it had already been delivered, for she would not have had it now, having used displeasing words and shown herself so full of jealousy. This only made Anne angrier, but Henry cut her short. Chapuys says he told her she must shut her eyes, 'and endure as more worthy persons. She ought to know that it was in his power to

humble her again in a moment, more than he had exalted her before.'
After this, he avoided her for three days, and then there was much
'coldness and grumbling' between them. Chapuys dismissed this as a
'love quarrel, of which no great notice should be taken', but there
was more to it than that. The wheel had come full circle: not a year
before, Anne had been the mistress and Henry the servant. Eight
months of marriage had changed all that. Henry was now dominant,
and he expected Anne, as his wife, to play a subservient role, though,
after seven years of having the upper hand, this did not come easily
to her. It would be foolish to read into Henry's remarks much more
than the bluster of a man caught straying, but all the same they are an
indication that he was mentally comparing Anne with Katherine and
finding her wanting. Anne had now been queen for five months,
long enough for him to realise that she lacked the dignity and
circumspection required for success in that capacity, and long
enough for her arrogance to begin to irritate him. This is not to say
that her spell was wearing thin, merely that marriage had altered the
balance of their relationship. Henry was still in love with her, but that
did not now preclude sex with other women when he felt the need.

In the middle of August, the King and Queen went to Windsor,
then to Greenwich, where Anne took to her chamber to await the
birth. 'I never saw the King merrier than he is now,' commented a
courtier, Sir John Russell, as Henry occupied himself during the last
tense weeks of waiting with his favourite sport, hunting. At last, on
the morning of 7 September 1533, in a bedchamber hung with
tapestries depicting St Ursula and her 11,000 virgins, Anne went into
labour, just as the Duke of Suffolk, whose wife Mary Tudor had
died in June, was being married in another part of the palace to
thirteen-year-old Katherine Willoughby, daughter of Maria de
Salinas, Katherine's close friend. On the face of it, the bride was a
strange choice, but the 48-year-old Duke had wanted her when she
had been betrothed to his son, and had broken the betrothal to marry
her himself. He must have set out with every intention of avoiding
his formidable mother-in-law whenever possible, for he had already
suffered a conflict of loyalties during his first marriage. As it turned
out, though, he forged a satisfactory friendship with Lady Willoughby.
His young wife grew up to be an ardent reformist and one of the
early luminaries of the Protestant faith.

Suffolk's marriage, however, was completely eclipsed by the events taking place in the Queen's apartments. All went well, the mother-to-be being sustained by the assurances of the physicians and astrologers that her child would be male. A vain fancy, as it turned out, for the infant born to her shortly after three o'clock that afternoon was a girl.

According to Chapuys, both Henry and Anne were disappointed at the child's sex, and Henry was angry that he had been so misled by those paid to make predictions about it. Yet his new daughter was strong and healthy, with Tudor red hair and her mother's features, and her arrival surely presaged a long line of sons. When Henry came to see his wife and child for the first time after the birth, he had had time to reflect on this, and was philosophical when Anne expressed regret at not having given him a boy. 'You and I are both young,' he told her, 'and by God's grace, boys will follow.' It was not perhaps the most tactful remark to make to a woman who had just experienced childbirth for the first time, particularly when he went on to assure her he would rather beg from door to door than forsake her. Their child, he announced, would be called Elizabeth, which by happy coincidence was the name of both his mother and Anne's.

Reaction to the birth was predictable. Chapuys spoke for the Emperor and the rest of Europe when he concluded that God, by sending a daughter, had entirely abandoned the King. The Princess Mary, who had been forced against her will to attend Anne's confinement, was secretly triumphant, knowing that as far as Catholic Europe was concerned Elizabeth would never be regarded as anything other than a bastard begotten and borne in sin by an infamous courtesan. In England too, there was unfavourable comment. The Bishop of Bath's secretary, John Erley, made insulting remarks about the King's apparent inability to sire male heirs. 'I would have gotten a boy,' he boasted, 'or else I would have so meddled with the Queen till my eyes did start out of my head!'

Letters announcing the birth of a prince had already been prepared; now, with an 's' added, they were dispatched abroad. The King ordered a *Te Deum* to be sung in churches, and went ahead with the splendid christening he had already planned for the hoped-for son. On the Wednesday after her birth, the Princess Elizabeth was wrapped in a purple mantle with a long train furred with ermine, and, escorted by the Dukes of Norfolk and Suffolk, was carried in the arms of the Dowager Duchess of Norfolk under a canopy of estate to her baptism in the chapel of the Observant Friars. Neither Henry nor Anne attended, and the central figures at the christening were the baby's godparents, Archbishop Cranmer, the Dowager Duchess of Norfolk, the Dowager Marchioness of Dorset, and the Marquess of Exeter – who, as a supporter of the former Queen, told Chapuys he really wanted to have nothing to do with the ceremony, but did not wish to displease the King.

Inside the chapel, a vast throng had gathered. The font was of solid silver, three steps high, and covered with a fine cloth. Around it stood many gentlemen with aprons on and towels over their shoulders, who received the baby when she was lifted, naked and dripping wet, out of the font by the Archbishop. A brazier burned in a nearby cubicle where she was dressed after the ceremony. Then Garter King of Arms cried: 'God, of His infinite goodness, send prosperous life and long to the high and mighty Princess of England, Elizabeth!' The trumpets blew a fanfare, and the child was brought to the altar, where the Archbishop confirmed her. Then refreshments were served to the guests, and the godparents presented the Princess with gifts, standing cups of gold and gilt bowls with covers.

Now, with the trumpets sounding before them, the procession re-formed and made its way back through corridors lit by 500 torches to the Queen's apartments, where Anne, robed and lying on her great French bed with the King at her side, received her daughter joyfully, and offered the guests more refreshments.

Elizabeth had been baptised with all possible ceremony, yet there were no attendant celebrations. The tournament planned by the King was cancelled, as were the fireworks, and no bonfires were lit in the City of London. Two friars were arrested for saying they had heard that the Princess had been christened in hot water, 'but it was not hot enough'. Chapuys thought 'the little bastard's' christening had been 'cold and disagreeable', but he was viewing it through prejudiced eyes. The fact remained, however, that although Elizabeth was Henry's recognised heir, she had not been welcomed like one.

Anne quickly conceived a deep and protective love for her child, and to begin with hated to let her out of her sight. When she returned to take her place at court, there, by her throne under the canopy of estate, lay her baby on a velvet cushion. She had wanted to breastfeed Elizabeth herself, but Henry was shocked at the notion: queens never suckled their own offspring. A wet-nurse was engaged, and Anne was forced to endure the first break in the bond between herself and her child. In December, when she was three months old, Henry assigned to Elizabeth her own household, and established it at Hatfield Palace, which was convenient for London yet well away from its unhealthy, plague-infested air. Lady Margaret Bryan, who had formerly cared for the Princess Mary, was appointed Lady Governess to Elizabeth, and had the command of a veritable army of nursemaids, laundresses, officials and servants. Chapuys noticed that the child was taken to Hatfield from Greenwich by a roundabout route, via Enfield, 'for the sake of pompous solemnity', and the better to impress upon the people the fact that she was the King's heiress.

The Princess Mary's trials began in earnest after Elizabeth was born. She was deprived of the title of princess, and her household was disbanded. Then, in December, she was sent to Hatfield – not without protest – to act as a maid of honour to her half-sister, whose title she refused to recognise. Her beloved Lady Salisbury was dismissed, and in her place were appointed Lady Anne Shelton and Lady Alice Clere, two female relatives of Anne Boleyn, who had been set to spy on her and generally make her life a misery. Anne, commented Chapuys, had alienated the King from his former humanity and was doing her utmost to break Mary's resolve.

She began her persecution by demanding Mary's jewels, on the grounds that the King's bastard daughter could not be permitted to wear what was meant for his heiress. Nor did Anne approve of the King visiting Mary, and would throw a tantrum whenever he suggested doing so. Once she even sent Cromwell after him to Hatfield, to dissuade him from seeing Mary, but when Henry was leaving, he chanced to look up and saw his daughter on a balcony, kneeling in supplication to him. Deeply moved, he bowed and touched his hat, at which all the members of his retinue followed suit; then he rode away, not daring to defy his wife by actually speaking to Mary. When Anne heard about the incident, she was not pleased.

By this time, Mary was perilously near to breaking-point, and her health had suffered, though four months of misery in Elizabeth's household had only strengthened her determination to defend her rights and those of her mother. This took courage, however, in such a hostile environment. She missed her mother intolerably, and thought of little but escaping from England, though Katherine forbade it, bidding her obey her father in all things save those that touched her conscience.

Henry strayed again sexually while Anne was lying-in after the birth of Elizabeth. At the same time, rumours were circulating in the court that he was beginning to tire of her. In November 1533, the French ambassador noticed that 'the King's regard for the Queen is less'. Disappointment in not having a son may have accounted for this; for all his brave words at Elizabeth's birth, Henry must have felt that Anne had failed him. In less than a year of marriage the magic had worn off to some degree and the King had leisure to wonder why he had risked so much for her, though he would not have admitted as much. He still maintained he had been right to put away Katherine and marry her, but he could see for himself how unpopular Anne was. 'There is little love for the one who is queen now, or any of her race,' reported the French ambassador in November, and in January 1534 there were more outbreaks of treasonous talk, with Henry accused of being a heretic living in adultery and Anne of being a mischievous whore who would one day be burned at the stake. Even the Duke of Northumberland, Anne's former admirer, was overheard by Chapuys saying to a friend that the Queen was a bad woman, which effectively demolishes the myth that he loved her to the end of his days. And when Lord Dacre was tried for treason, having long supported Katherine of Aragon and been one of Anne's most bitter enemies, twenty-four peers and twelve judges, having heard him speak for seven hours in his defence, unanimously acquitted him. The Queen's anger knew no bounds when she heard of this, yet both she and Henry were aware that Dacre's acquittal was symbolic of the general mood.

By Christmas 1533, all was well again on the surface between the royal couple. They exchanged gifts, Anne giving Henry a splendid gold basin encrusted with rubies and pearls and containing a diamond-studded fountain with real water issuing from the nipples of three solid gold naked nymphs. Yet the same festive season saw quite a drama being acted out at Buckden. Early in December, the Princess Dowager had sent a message asking the King if she might move to a healthier house, as her present lodging was hopelessly damp and cold, and her health was beginning to suffer. Of course, this was what Anne Boleyn had intended should happen, and she suggested that her rival be moved to Somersham Castle, near Ely. Henry agreed to this, but when Chapuys protested that Somersham was 'the most unhealthy and pestilential house in England, surrounded by deep water and marshes', he changed his mind and said Katherine should go to the old Yorkist stronghold Fotheringhay Castle in Northamptonshire instead. Unknown to Chapuys, Fotheringhay was in an even worse condition than Somersham, and Henry knew it. Katherine knew it too, and when she was informed of the proposed move, she refused to go there. Henry, goaded by Anne, was equally adamant that she should, and dismissed yet more of her servants, insisting that those remaining must not address their mistress as queen, but as Princess Dowager, the title she refused to acknowledge. To enforce her obedience, the Duke of Suffolk was sent to Buckden with a detachment of the King's guards.

Suffolk did not relish his task. It was December, and he was reluctant to leave the warmth and splendour of a court preparing for Christmas and his bride of three months for a damp, lonely house on the Fens and a mission he found distasteful: harrying a sick woman. He told his mother-in-law, Lady Willoughby, that he hoped he would meet with an accident on the way that would prevent him from carrying out his orders. Unfortunately for the Duke, he arrived at Buckden on 18 December safe and sound, and entered almost immediately into a heated exchange with Katherine, who told him she would rather be torn in pieces than admit she was not the King's wife. This set the tone for the visit. Suffolk told her he had come to escort her to Fotheringhay, at which – without further argument – she withdrew to her chamber and locked herself in. 'If you wish to take me with you, you will have to break down the door!' she cried, and no threats or entreaties could persuade her to come out.

Suffolk dared not force the door, or seize Katherine by force: she was the Emperor's aunt, and there would be repercussions. So he proceeded to the business of dismissing her servants, leaving only a few to care for her needs. Those remaining were ordered in the King's name to refer to their mistress in future as the Princess Dowager, but her chaplains, Father Abell and Father Barker, insisted that as they had both sworn their oaths of service to Queen Katherine, they could not perjure themselves by calling her anything else. Suffolk placed the two priests in custody in the porter's lodge, and wrote to the King, asking what he should do with them.

While he waited for a reply, Suffolk was reduced once again to standing outside Katherine's door and pleading with her to come out. She would not listen, either to him, or to Lord Mountjoy, or to her almoner, Father Dymoke. Suffolk wrote again to the King, telling him her defiance was 'against all reason'; unless he bound her with ropes and 'virtually enforced her', there was no hope of her compliance. He was heartily sick of his mission, having seen for himself how the years of anxiety and sorrow had taken their toll of Katherine's health. Nevertheless, he thought her 'the most obstinate woman that may be'.

Meanwhile, word had reached the local people, via Katherine's departing servants, of what was going on in the castle, and men from the surrounding district began to gather silently outside the walls, armed with scythes, pitchforks and other implements. They did nothing, but watched and waited for any sign of ill-treatment of the woman they still held to be their queen. Suffolk grew uneasy, and wished he had never heard of Buckden. As it was, he was obliged to remain there until 31 December, when he received instructions from the King bidding him leave Katherine where she was and return to court. Henry would graciously allow the Bishop of Llandaff, who spoke Spanish, to remain as Katherine's chaplain. When Suffolk had gone, the labourers dispersed, and Katherine emerged from her chamber to find her rooms stripped of most of their furniture, and the majority of her servants gone.

Suffolk was not entirely an unfeeling man, and when he returned to Greenwich, he warned the King about Katherine's precarious health. Later, Henry told Chapuys she had dropsy, and would not live very much longer. 'I think he would be glad,' commented the ambassador. In fact, Katherine did not have dropsy, but Henry was right on one point: she was already in the first stages of the cancer that would eventually kill her. Henry, who could not have known this, thought her environment was responsible for her ill health, and he callously left her at Buckden in the hope that she would soon succumb to her malady.

Queen Anne conceived again soon after the birth of Elizabeth. At the beginning of December 1533, her family knew she was pregnant for the second time, and her cousin, Lord William Howard, made the news public while on an embassy to Rome, for which he had left England early in December. Care was taken not to weary the Queen, and Archbishop Cranmer warned the reformist preacher Hugh Latimer not to make his sermons longer than an hour and a half, as Anne tired easily. Nor did disturbed sleep help the exhaustion of early pregnancy. Henry had just been presented with a peacock and a pelican, but unfortunately these birds made such a clamour outside Anne's windows from dawn onwards that she could not rest in the mornings. The King therefore found the birds another home at Sir Henry Norris's house in Greenwich – Lady Norris's broken nights were not a matter of state importance. Birds of a different sort found more favour with Anne when, in May 1534, Lady Lisle, wife of the Governor of Calais – who was anxious to ingratiate herself with the Queen as she had daughters she wished to place at court – sent her a brace of dotterels (a species of game bird) and a singing linnet in a cage. 'The Queen liked them very well,' reported Lady Lisle's London agent, especially the songbird, 'which doth not cease at no time to give her Grace rejoicing with her pleasant song'.

In April, Anne and Henry visited their daughter, who had moved to Eltham Palace, and there inspected the preparations that were in hand 'against the coming of the Prince'. That month, Anne's receiver-general reported that she was already showing 'a goodly belly', and she made it known that her chief desire was to present the King with a son who would be the living image of his father.

In March 1534, the King paid Anne the supreme compliment of providing for her to be regent and 'absolute governess of her children and kingdom' in the event of his early death. Then, on 23 March, Parliament passed one of the most controversial pieces of legislation of Henry's reign: the Act of Succession, which vested the succession to 'the imperial crown of England' in the children of Henry and Anne. On 1 May, the contents of this Act were proclaimed in all the shires of England, and the King's subjects were warned that anyone saying or writing anything 'to the prejudice, slander or derogation of the lawful matrimony' between the King and 'his most dear and entirely beloved wife Queen Anne', or against his lawful heirs, would be guilty of high treason, for which the penalty was death and forfeiture of lands and goods to the Crown. Furthermore, it was proclaimed that the new Act required all the King's subjects, if so commanded, to swear an oath 'that they shall truly, firmly, constantly, without fraud or guile, observe, fulfil, maintain, defend and keep the whole effect and contents of this Act'. The oath also required recognition of the King's supremacy. Those refusing to take it would be accounted guilty of misprision of treason and sent to prison. The Crown had thrown down the gauntlet, and it remained to be seen how the people of England would react to the challenge.

Nothing now could save the Nun of Kent. She had been attainted, with her accomplices, of high treason on 20 March, and on 20 April, all five were drawn on hurdles to the gallows at Tyburn and there hanged, cut down while still alive, and beheaded before great crowds. Theirs was the first blood spilt as a result of the 'great matter'. It would not be the last.

Most people, including members of the religious orders, took the oath required by the Act of Succession without demur. Although Anne Boleyn herself was unpopular, the new order in England was welcomed by many, and people flocked to the churches on Easter Day to hear, in the words of Chapuys, 'the most outrageous and abominable things in the world', which presumably included the bidding prayers for Anne and Elizabeth. On 5 May, Convocation met at York and formally renounced its allegiance to the Pope.

Thomas Cromwell, promoted in April to be Secretary to the King, was now in a position that involved him in increasingly confidential business; he was also able to advise Henry on decisions on policy. Though Henry never had the affection for Cromwell that he had had for Wolsey, nevertheless 'Mr Secretary' was to prove extremely useful to him, having successfully planned the break with Rome, and the King congratulated himself on having discovered the man's undoubted ability and potential. Most important of all was the fact that Cromwell was prepared to deal with those tasks that called for a certain flexibility of conscience, and that made him invaluable. Those who wanted to communicate with Henry generally had to go through Cromwell, and hence, though outwardly on good terms with most people, he became both envied and greatly resented. The old nobility despised him for his lowly origins, much as they despised Wolsey, and many feared him, knowing his lack of scruple. His spies were known to be everywhere, and with the King so touchy about his marriage and the royal supremacy, even chance remarks, heard by the wrong ears, might be construed as treason.

Some brave souls were defiant, and refused to take the oath to the Act of Succession. One was John Fisher who was still under house arrest, and had received letter after letter from the King containing 'terrible' words about his opposition to Henry's remarriage. In January 1534, Henry had deprived Fisher of his bishopric, and in March, he was attainted of misprision of treason for having supported the Nun of Kent, and sent to the Tower. Chapuys thought him to be 'in great danger of life', even though Fisher had written to the King protesting his loyalty. In April, Fisher refused to take the oath, and when, in May, Henry learned that the Pope had made the former bishop a cardinal, and was sending his red hat to England, he observed tartly that Fisher would have to wear it on his shoulders, for by the time it arrived he would not have a head to put it on.

Thomas Abell, Katherine's chaplain, was also attainted in March 1534, and sent to the Tower, where he would suffer dreadful privations during his imprisonment. And in April, the King's wrath reached Sir Thomas More, who had likewise refused to swear the oath. More, who had declared himself the King's loyal subject and had denied he had ever been against Anne Boleyn, 'this noble woman really anointed Queen', was arrested, and asked again if he would take the oath. For the second time he refused, and no amount of persuasion could make him reveal his objections. By then, Queen Anne was crying out for his blood, and on 17 April, he too was sent to the Tower, and lodged in a cell above Fisher's in the Bell Tower. His arrest shocked many, given his standing as lawyer, scholar and statesman, and his former friendship with the King. Finally, the Princess Mary's former tutor, Richard Fetherston, went to the Tower in December 1534.

In March 1534, the Pope gave judgement at last on Henry VIII's nullity suit, after seven years of procrastination. As a result of the pressure brought to bear upon him by the Emperor, Clement had reluctantly convened the consistory in January finally to resolve the problem. Katherine, hearing of this from Chapuys, wrote to the Emperor in February: 'Beg His Holiness to act as he ought for God's service. There is no need to tell you of our sufferings. As long as I live, I shall not fail to defend our rights.' For weeks, Clement dithered and prevaricated, until his cardinals lost patience with him and urged him to proceed to sentence. Finally, on 23 March, he pronounced that the marriage between Henry VIII and Katherine of Aragon 'always hath and still doth stand firm and canonical, and the issue proceeding standeth lawful and legitimate'. Henry was ordered to resume cohabitation at once with 'his lawful wife and Queen, to hold her and maintain her with such love and princely honour as becometh a loving husband and his kingly honour so to do'. If he refused, he would be excommunicated. As a final indignity, Henry was required to pay the costs of the case.

When Henry heard the sentence, from the French ambassador, he was visibly shaken, but undeterred. The Pope, he declared, no longer had any authority over English affairs. News of Clement's judgement spread rapidly, and here and there public celebrations were held to herald Katherine's expected return to favour. At Buckden, there was a loyal demonstration of goodwill towards her, and Katherine herself went down on her knees and thanked God. After seven long and bitter years, she was at last vindicated, and now trusted that the King would restore her to her lawful place. Patiently, she waited for a message from him, summoning her back to court, her heart brimming with forgiveness. But no such message ever came, and gradually the bitter truth dawned: nothing had changed so far as Henry was concerned, nor would change. In deep sorrow, Katherine wrote to Chapuys, and came as near as she ever would to urging the Emperor to use armed force to deal with her husband. 'She now realises that it is absolutely necessary to apply stronger remedies to the evil,' wrote the ambassador, but 'what they are to be, she durst not say.' When the Emperor realised that Henry meant to ignore the Pope's judgement, he told his advisers he would not fail 'in what is necessary for the execution of the sentence'. What was necessary, Chapuys told Katherine, was armed force, but Charles had not meant to imply this. He meant to compel the Pope to excommunicate Henry, in the hope that that would bring the English king to his senses. Charles also instructed Chapuys to advise Katherine and Mary to take the oath required by the King, protesting that they were taking it out of fear; 'it cannot prejudice their rights,' he wrote.

From April 1534, Chapuys's reports are full of unspecified dangers threatening Katherine and her daughter. Henry might not countenance the outright murder of his wife and child, but he was not above hounding them to their deaths by ill-treatment, and in this Anne Boleyn aided and abetted him. She also urged the King to put them to death by judicial process, but Henry was too concerned about the consequences to agree to that, although he made threats often enough. There remained poison, and many people, among them Chapuys, believed Anne to be quite capable of using it to achieve her end, while Dr Butts, Henry's physician, believed that unless the King fell ill – when he might be persuaded to listen to the advice of someone other than Anne – the lives of Katherine and Mary were in danger.

Anne's hostility was on a personal level. It was based on jealousy of Katherine's breeding and virtues, which showed up Anne herself in none too favourable a light, on rage that Katherine had dared defy Henry for so long, and on fear, because Katherine and her daughter appeared to be doing their best to oust her own daughter from the succession and herself from the throne. 'Neither the Queen nor the Princess will be safe for a moment while the Cuncubine still has power; she is desperate to get rid of them,' warned Chapuys. He alerted Katherine to the danger threatening her, and told her bluntly that he had heard Anne saying she 'would not be satisfied until both the Queen and her daughter had been done to death by poison or otherwise'.

Katherine exercised constant vigilance to ensure that her food was prepared only by those servants she trusted. At any time now the King's commissioners would come and demand that she take the oath. Failure to do so could mean imprisonment. But when the Archbishop of York arrived to administer the oath to her and her household, Katherine stood firm and, ignoring the Emperor's advice, refused to swear. The Archbishop, who had been briefed 'not to press very hard', was dismayed by the hostility shown him by Katherine's servants, who either refused to take the oath or pretended not to understand English, and in exasperation he dismissed those who proved obdurate.

Katherine's obstinacy provoked the King, at the end of April 1534, to order her removal to Kimbolton Castle in Huntingdonshire, a house built in 1522 of wood and stone. It was a secure residence, access being gained only through an archway on the western side, and would be, in effect, Katherine's prison. Today, the Tudor house is encased in a Georgian exterior, and Katherine's rooms have been entirely remodelled. Two officers of the Crown were appointed her governors, Sir Edmund Bedingfield and Sir Edward Chamberlayne. Her small household would accompany her, and would only remain subject to Bedingfield's approval. Katherine asked if she could be allowed to keep her confessor, her physician, her apothecary, two menservants, and 'as many women as it should please the King's Grace to appoint. I am often sickly,' she told Bedingfield, 'and I require their attendance for the preservation of my poor body.' Her request was granted; fortunately, most of her people were Spaniards who had not been naturalised and were therefore exempt from taking the oath.

Katherine was taken to Kimbolton early in May 1534, and found herself housed in two rooms on the opposite side of the courtyard to the governors' apartments and the great hall. Bedingfield and Chamberlayne kept very much to their side of the house, and Katherine's household of twenty servants had as little communication with them as possible. Bedingfield was not the kindest of gaolers, and he was later to report to Cromwell that 'my fidelity in executing the orders of the King renders me no favourite with the Princess Dowager, therefore she conceals everything from me'. In fact, he hardly ever saw her. A division was apparent in the household from the first, as Katherine refused to speak to anyone who did not address her as queen.

She had been at Kimbolton for three weeks when the Bishop of Durham was sent by the King in another attempt to make her swear the oath. She told him she would never relinquish the title of queen, but retain it till death. The Bishop then threatened her, as he had been authorised to do, with the penalty required by the law for persons who refused the oath, but at this her anger flared. 'Hold thy peace, Bishop!' she cried. 'These are the wiles of the devil! I am Queen, and Queen I will die! By right, the King can have no other wife. Let this be your answer.' The Bishop warned her she might be sent to the scaffold if she persisted in her obstinacy. 'And who will be the hangman?' she retorted. 'If you have permission to execute this penalty on me, I am ready. I ask only that I be allowed to die in sight of the people.' At this, the Bishop backed down, for he had rather exceeded his brief. The penalty for refusing to swear the oath was imprisonment, not death, and Katherine could be said to be suffering that already.

When the Bishop came to administering the oath to Katherine's household, he was neatly outwitted, for the naturalised Spaniards readily swore, in their native tongue, as Katherine had bidden them: '*El Rey se ha heco cabeza de la Iglesia.*' The Bishop had expected considerable opposition, and was surprised at such co-operation. He did not know, however, that, instead of acknowledging the King to be head of the Church, they had merely acknowledged that he had made himself head of the Church!

When the King heard that Katherine had again refused to take the oath, he grumbled bitterly to Chapuys that 'the Lady Dowager is being well-treated in everything, but has very disobediently behaved herself to us'; although he had sent bishops to give her advice 'in the most loving fashion', she had disobediently and wilfully resisted and 'set at naught and condemned our laws and ordinances'. Chapuys, who had his own secret links with Katherine, knew that Henry was lying. It was an alarming situation, and Chapuys was not alone in his concern. He told the Emperor: 'Everybody fears some ill turn will be done to the Queen, seeing the rudeness to which she is daily subjected.' He considered her loyalty to Henry to be superhuman: 'She is so scrupulous, and has such great respect for him, that she would consider herself damned if she took any way tending to war.'

In the spring of 1534, Mary became very ill. Her sickness was undoubtedly the result of sorrow and stress. The ambassador begged the Council to allow Katherine to nurse Mary herself, but they refused. Henry trusted no one these days, and believed that together mother and daughter would hatch a plot with the Emperor to depose him. Cromwell told Chapuys that Mary's present predicament was her own fault, 'and that if it pleased God . . .'. He did not finish, and Chapuys concluded that the King 'really desires the Princess's death'.

In July 1534, recovered from her illness and fortified by a letter from her mother secretly conveyed by Chapuys, Mary refused to take the oath. Lady Shelton, who was present, shook the girl violently in front of the Earl of Wiltshire, who had been sent to administer the oath. 'If I were the King,' she cried, 'I would kick you out of the house! I would make you lose your head!' But Mary stood firm, and when Anne heard what had happened, she wrote suggesting Lady Shelton administer 'a good banging' to 'the cursed bastard'.

By this time, Anne was well advanced into her pregnancy. In June, she was reported to be in good health. The baby was due around the end of July, but before the Queen could take to her chamber, something went wrong and it was born prematurely; it was either stillborn, or died very soon after birth. Such was the secrecy surrounding the event that even the sex of the infant is not recorded – it was probably a girl, and Henry could not afford to lose face a second time. Anne made a quick recovery, but the loss of her child had been a bitter blow and she was very difficult to live with for a time. Late in July, the King and Queen went on their annual summer progress without any official announcement of the end of her pregnancy being made.

During that summer, Chapuys became increasingly concerned about Katherine's health. He had heard that her condition had deteriorated. In July, Henry agreed he might visit her, but had second thoughts about it and sent a messenger after the ambassador, commanding him to return to court, where he was informed by Cromwell that at no time in the future would he be permitted access to the Princess Dowager. In mid-September, when Katherine's illness grew worse, and it was thought for a time that she was dying, Lady Willoughby begged Cromwell for leave to see her, but it was likewise refused. Hearing of his aunt's illness, Charles V questioned the English ambassadors closely about reports that she had been badly treated. Henry personally instructed his envoys to say that the reports lied, and that the Lady Katherine had an honourable establishment with her own servants and money to meet her needs;

as for his daughter, he would deal with her 'as we think most expedient'. Charles was not deceived by all this; he had, after all, read the dispatches of Chapuys, which told an entirely different story.

In September 1534, Anne thought she was pregnant again. Yet her hopes were premature, for on 23 September, Chapuys informed the Emperor that 'the Lady is not to have a child after all.' Relations between the royal couple were not at all satisfactory just then. Once again, at the end of Anne's last pregnancy, the King had been unfaithful. Chapuys reported that the object of Henry's desire was 'a very beautiful and adroit young lady for whom his love is daily increasing'. She was probably one of the Queen's ladies, but her name is unknown. However, the ambassador had hopes that the affair would serve to diminish Anne's influence with Henry. The young lady was known to be sympathetic towards Katherine and Mary, and that could only be to their advantage. The course of the affair was interrupted by the summer progress, but when Henry returned, he renewed his attentions more ardently than before, and without bothering to conceal what was going on from the Queen, whose sexual attraction had begun to pale; Chapuys noted triumphantly that Henry was 'tired to satiety of her'. Thus, when Anne remonstrated with him, and threatened to send the girl away from court, he turned on her and angrily told her that she had good reason to be content with what he had done for her, which he would not do now if he were to begin again. Chapuys did not attach too much importance to these remarks, 'considering the changeable character of the King and the craft of the Lady, who well knows how to manage him'. But Anne did.

With the loss of her second child, she realised she had lost much of her influence, and some good measure of Henry's love. Her French ways of love-making were beginning to repel him and drove him into the arms of other women, while Anne was left facing the bitter fact that only by bearing a son could she revive her husband's love and respect. The diminishing of Anne's influence, noted Chapuys, 'has already abated a good deal of her insolence'. Her gradual fall from favour meant that some courtiers now deemed it safe to visit the Lady Mary; even Anne herself wrote her a conciliatory letter, telling Mary to be of good cheer for her troubles would soon be at an end. She perhaps feared she might one day be in need of Mary's clemency, given the insecurity of her own position.

Anne's discontent and unhappiness were made worse in the autumn of 1534 by the appearance of a pregnant Mary Boleyn at court. It transpired that Mary had secretly married – for love – a young man of little standing and no fortune called William Stafford. This was a highly unsuitable match for the Queen's sister; Wiltshire, learning of it, immediately cut off Mary's allowance, and Anne banished her and her husband from court. It was three months before Mary attempted a reconciliation, and when she did it was by means of a letter to Cromwell, in which she confessed that 'love overcame reason'. Yet while she begged Mr Secretary to help her recover the 'gracious favour of the King and Queen', her letter had a sting in its tail, which perhaps holds a clue as to the true nature of the relationship between the sisters, who had never been close, for it ended:

For well I might a' had a greater man of birth, but I assure you I could never a' had one that loved me so well. I had rather beg my bread with him than be the greatest queen christened.

The letter, unfortunately, came into the hands of the Queen, and her reaction to it shattered any hopes of a reconciliation, for Anne, naturally, did not take kindly to the obvious comparison with herself. The taunt went too deep. Mary Stafford and her husband were never again received at court, and retired to William's modest house in the country, where they lived together in peaceful obscurity until Mary's death on 19 July 1543.

On 26 September 1534, Pope Clement died, and three weeks later the College of Cardinals elected his successor, Paul III. The new pontiff was infinitely more resolute than his predecessor, and one of his first acts was to threaten to put into effect the sentence of excommunication on Henry VIII drawn up by Clement but never published. Though Henry ignored this, there still remained the ever-present threat that Paul would publish his Bull and incite the Emperor to war: Henry, as an excommunicate ruler standing alone, could not expect aid from the other Christian princes of Europe.

The King tired of his unnamed mistress by the end of October 1534, although Anne knew by now that there were sure to be others. There are hints in contemporary letters that Henry kept several young girls for his pleasure at Farnham Castle, and Norfolk, who knew Henry well, told Chapuys that his master had always been 'continually inclined to amours'. A man called William Webbe was out on his horse near Eltham Palace one day, with his pretty sweetheart riding pillion, when he chanced to encounter his sovereign on the road. The King pulled the girl from the horse and kissed her in front of the aghast Webbe, then took her straight back to the palace with him. Such encounters were purely sexual and did not last, yet there was a strong anti-Boleyn faction at court that would dearly have loved to see Anne displaced, and who did their best to encourage any amorous intrigues of the King.

Anne was now ageing visibly. The portrait of her painted at around this time shows she had already lost her looks. Her once vivacious eyes now regard the world with suspicion, her smiling lips are pinched tight shut, and her cheeks are beginning to sag. The frustration, sadness and stress she had suffered had left their marks on her face, and Henry's desire for her had cooled, leaving him susceptible to the charms of younger women. Anne had bitterly resented Henry's last affair, and had conspired with her sister-in-law Lady Rochford to have the girl removed from court, but the King found out and banished Lady Rochford instead. When Chabot de Brion, the Admiral of France, came to England on a state visit in November 1534, the King made a point of inviting a number of beautiful ladies to court to take part in the festivities. 'He is more given to matters of dancing and ladies than he ever was,' observed Chapuys hopefully. A great banquet was given in the Admiral's honour. The Queen was present; she had for some time been trying to bring about a marriage between the Princess Elizabeth and the Duke of Angoulême, third son of Francis I. If the French were to agree to it, then Anne would have manoeuvred Francis I into recognising her as Queen – which, to her chagrin, he had never done – and her daughter as lawfully born.

Chapuys records that at the banquet, the Admiral sat talking to the Queen while they watched the dancing. Then the King arrived and told Anne he would fetch the Admiral's secretary and present him to her. Moments after his departure, de Brion realised that Anne was no longer taking part in their conversation: she was glancing about the hall furtively. Then, to his consternation, she suddenly burst out laughing. The Admiral, ever conscious of his dignity, asked if she were amusing herself at his expense, but she shook her head, still laughing, although tears were in her eyes as she pointed across to where the King was standing. 'He went to fetch your secretary,' she said, 'but he met a lady, who made him forget the matter!' And she laughed again, but without mirth.

Christmas 1534 was not a happy one. Anne's favourite dog Little Purkoy (from the French word *pourquoi*, presumably because of his enquiring expression), a gift from Lady Lisle, died. A great dog lover, the Queen had 'set much store' by him, and no one dared tell her the sad news until, in the end, the King broke it to her. Yet he was feeling less than sympathetic towards her at the time. She had quarrelled again with Norfolk, exercising her peculiar talent for alienating her supporters; Norfolk told the King she had used words to him that should not have been used to a dog; he, however, had retaliated by calling her 'a great whore'. Once upon a time, Anne might have expected Henry to avenge such a gross insult, but not any more. Henry's view was that she had provoked Norfolk beyond endurance, and he sympathised with the Duke.

Chabot de Brion's secretary, Palmedes Gontier, met Anne at a court banquet on 2 February 1535, and recorded his impressions in a letter to his master sent three days later. He perceived that all was not well. She seemed extremely apprehensive. Three days later he saw her again, and noted how her face fell when she saw that there was no reference in the letters he brought from the Admiral (who had returned to France) to her daughter's proposed betrothal. When the King was out of earshot, she complained to Gontier of the long delay in receiving word on this matter, saying it had 'caused and engendered in the King her spouse many strange thoughts, of which there was great need that a remedy should be thought of'. She could only conclude that King Francis intended her to be 'maddened and lost, for she found herself quite near to that, and more in pain and trouble than she had been since her espousals'. She dared not speak as openly as she would have liked, she went on, 'for fear of where she was and of the eyes that were watching her countenance'. She told

Gontier 'she could not write, could not see me, and could no longer talk with me.' She then left with the King, leaving Gontier to conclude that she was 'not at her ease' and that she had 'doubts and suspicions' of her husband.

It seems Henry had finally realised that marrying Anne had been a mistake. No longer did he see her through a lover's eyes: after two years of marriage, he was well able to regard her objectively, and could see little to impress him. Her arrogance, vanity and hauteur all proclaimed her inadequacy as a queen, and her public displays of emotion and temper were embarrassing. She had succeeded in making enemies of those who might have been her friends, and had displayed an unbecoming eagerness to wreak vengeance upon her enemies. She had probably lied about her virginity, and – worst of all – she had failed as yet to produce a son. Not only did Henry regret having married her, he had also brutally acquainted her with the fact. Yet, given any sign that he was contemplating her removal, the imperialists would be urging him to take Katherine back, something he could never contemplate. For the time being, therefore, Anne must remain; she might yet give him an heir. A son would still solve all her problems, as she well knew, but she told Henry early in 1535 that God had revealed to her in a dream that it would be impossible for her to conceive a child while Katherine and Mary lived. They were rebels and traitresses, she said, and deserved death. Henry failed to rise to her bait, another sign that her power was diminishing.

In February 1535, Mary fell gravely ill, and there were fears she might die. Even the King was alarmed, although he refused to heed his physicians' advice, and Chapuys's pleas, that she should go to her mother for whom she was pining. Katherine, in desperation, wrote to Cromwell, begging him to urge the King to let her nurse Mary herself at Kimbolton: 'A little comfort and mirth with me would be a half health to her.' She would 'care for her with my own hands and put her in my own bed and watch with her when needful'.

In March, Mary's condition worsened, and Katherine's anguish deepened, for she knew her own sickness to be mortal, and once again she begged Henry to let her see Mary. Yet still he refused. 'The Lady Katherine,' he told Chapuys, 'is a proud stubborn woman of very high courage. She could easily take the field, muster a great army, and wage against me a war as fierce as any her mother Isabella

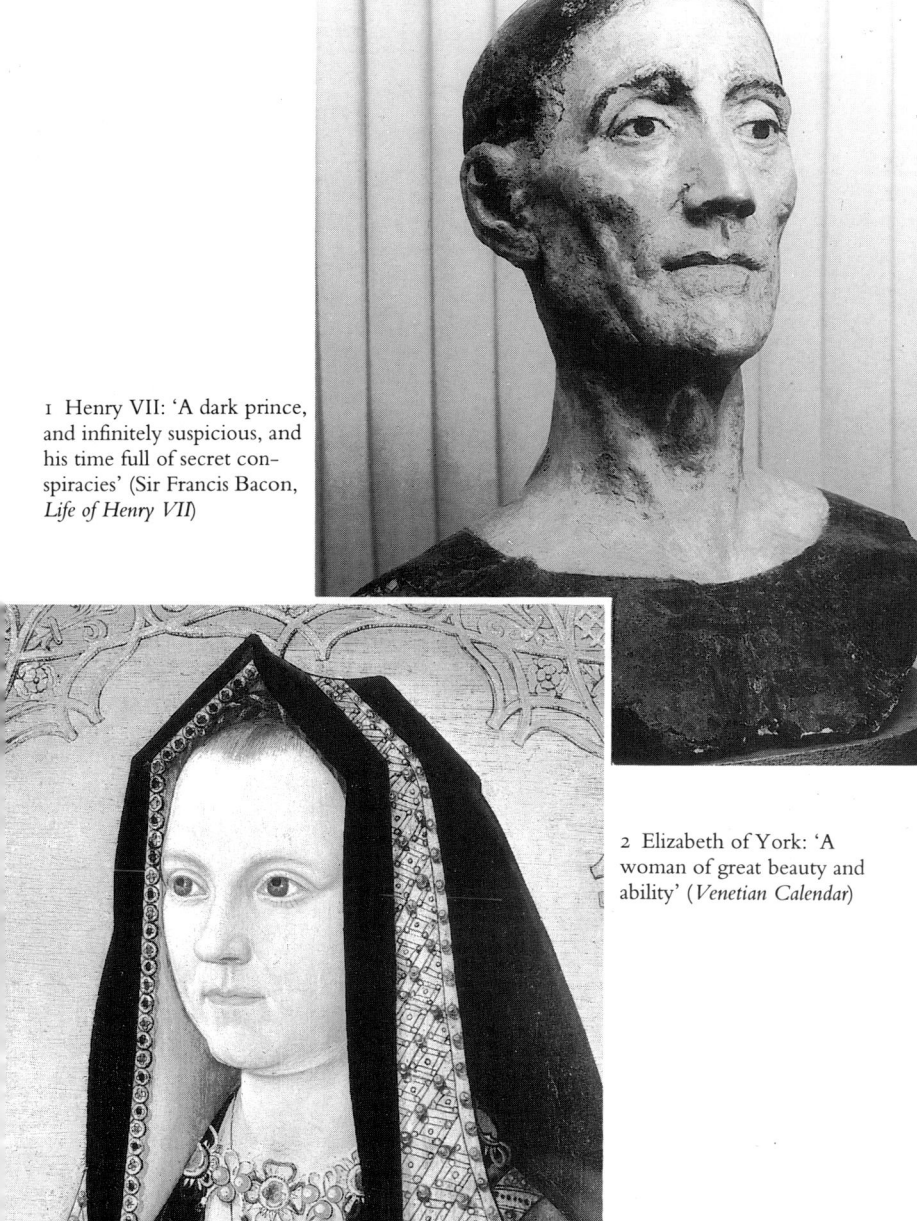

1 Henry VII: 'A dark prince, and infinitely suspicious, and his time full of secret conspiracies' (Sir Francis Bacon, *Life of Henry VII*)

2 Elizabeth of York: 'A woman of great beauty and ability' (*Venetian Calendar*)

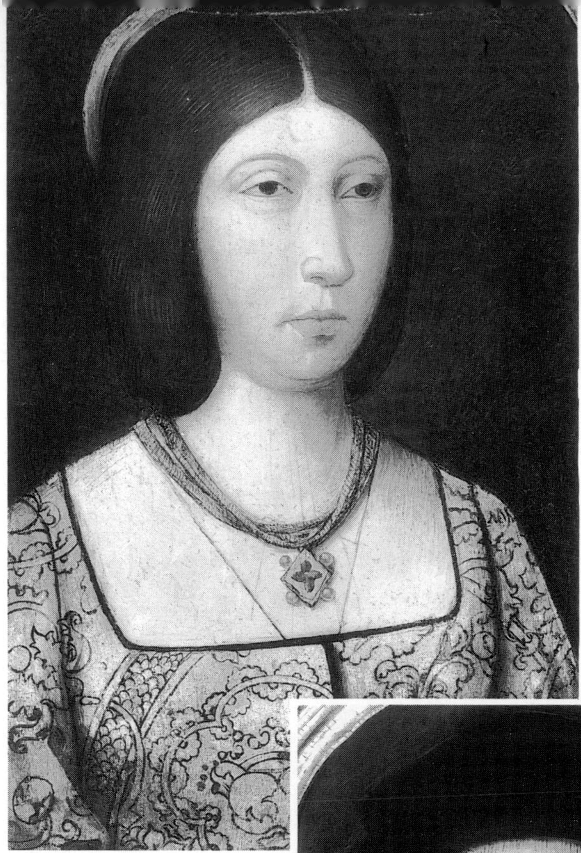

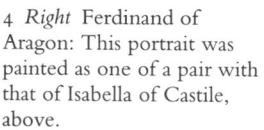

5 *Right* Katherine of Aragon by Miguel Sittow: 'She thrilled the hearts of everyone. There is nothing wanting in her that the most beautiful girl should have' (Thomas More, 1501)

6 *Below right* Katherine of Aragon (portrait in Buccleuch Collection): 'My good brother of England has no son because, although young and virile, he keeps an old and deformed wife' (Francis I of France, 1518)

3 *Left* Isabella of Castile: 'She was a very good woman, both clever and sensible' (Pulgar's *Chronicle*)

4 *Right* Ferdinand of Aragon: This portrait was painted as one of a pair with that of Isabella of Castile, above.

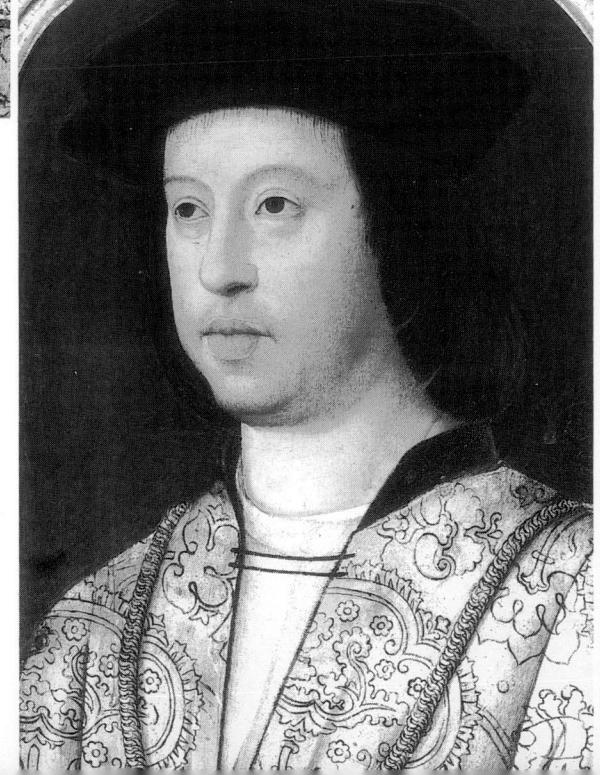

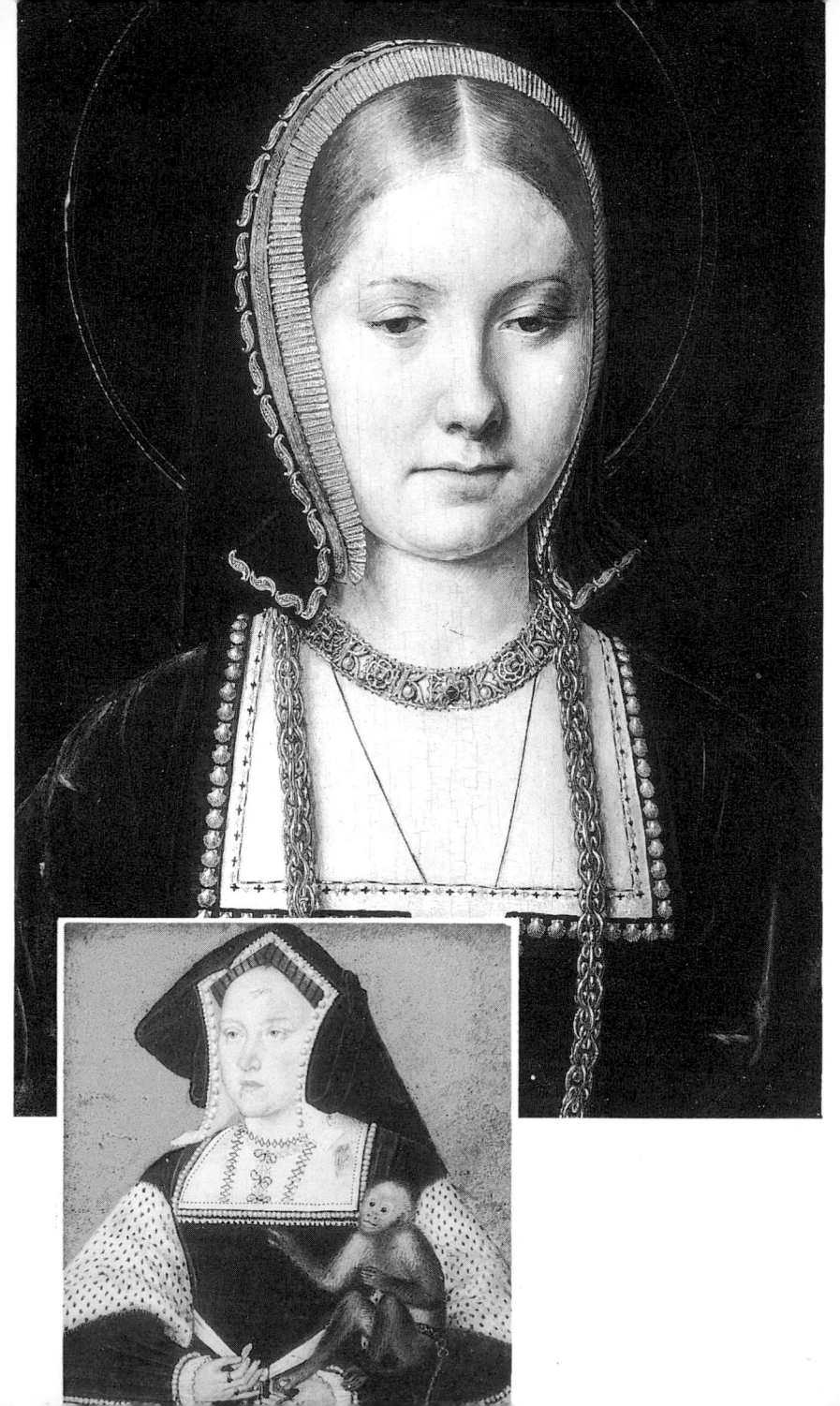

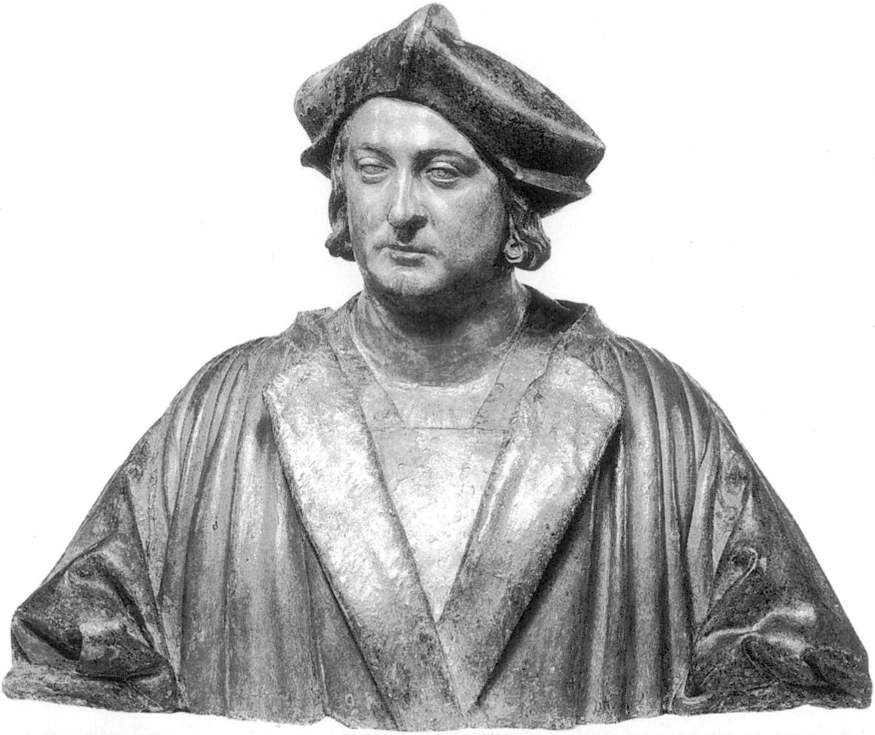

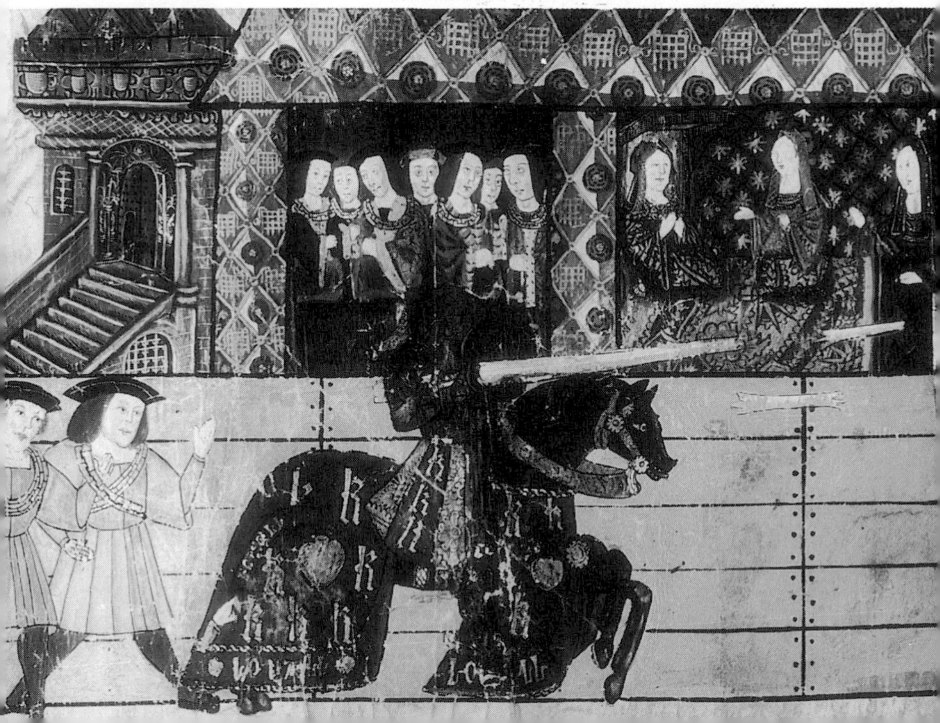

7 *Left* Henry VIII: 'Our natural, young, lusty and courageous king, entering into the flower of pleasant youth' (George Cavendish)

9 *Right* Thomas Wolsey: 'The Cardinal is the person who rules both the King and the kingdom' (Sebastian Guistinian, *Venetian Calendar*)

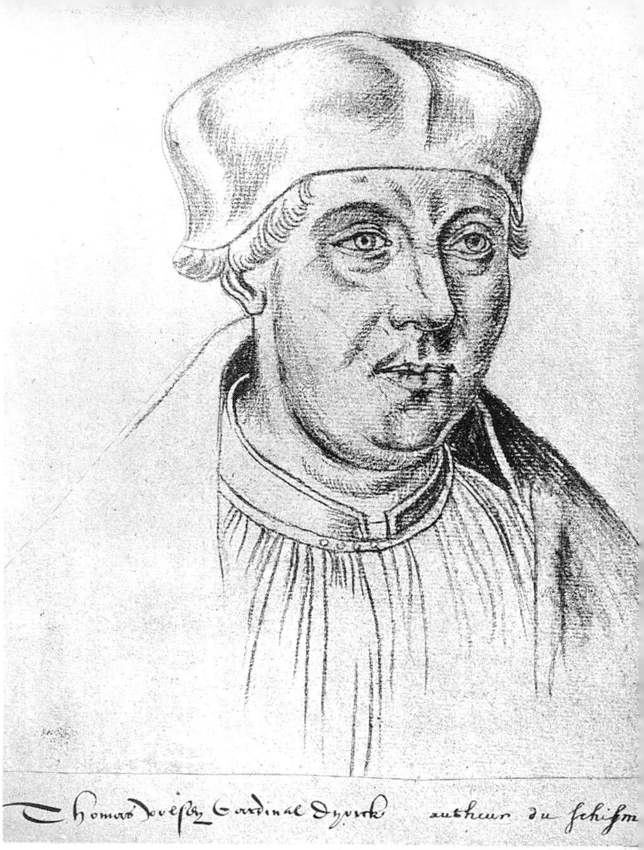

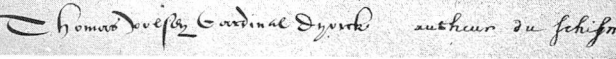

10 *Right* Francis I of France: 'He is a Frenchman, and I cannot say how far you should trust him' (Henry VIII, *Venetian Calendar*)

8 *Left* The Great Tournament Roll of Westminster: 'A solemn joust in honour of the Queen, the King being called "Coeur Loyal"' (Hall's *Chronicle*, 1511)

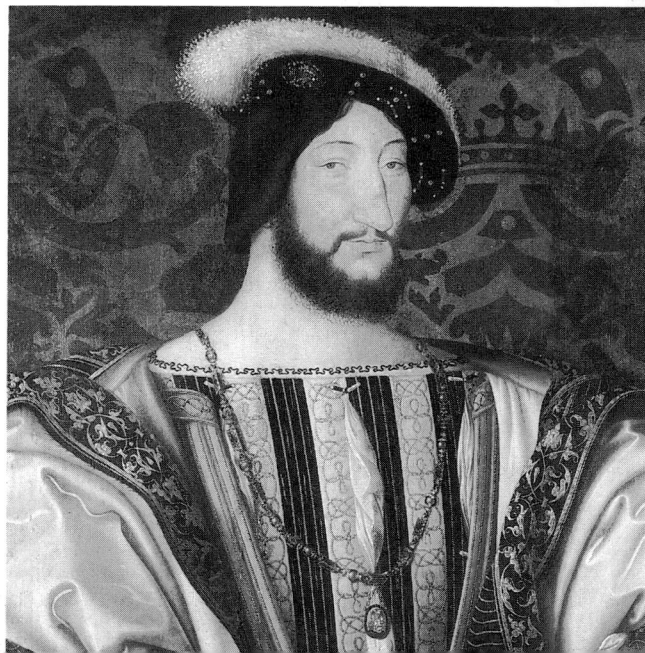

11 Love letter from Henry VIII to Anne Boleyn, 1528: 'I now think the
King so much in love that only God can get him out of this mess'
(Letter from Jean du Bellay to Francis I)

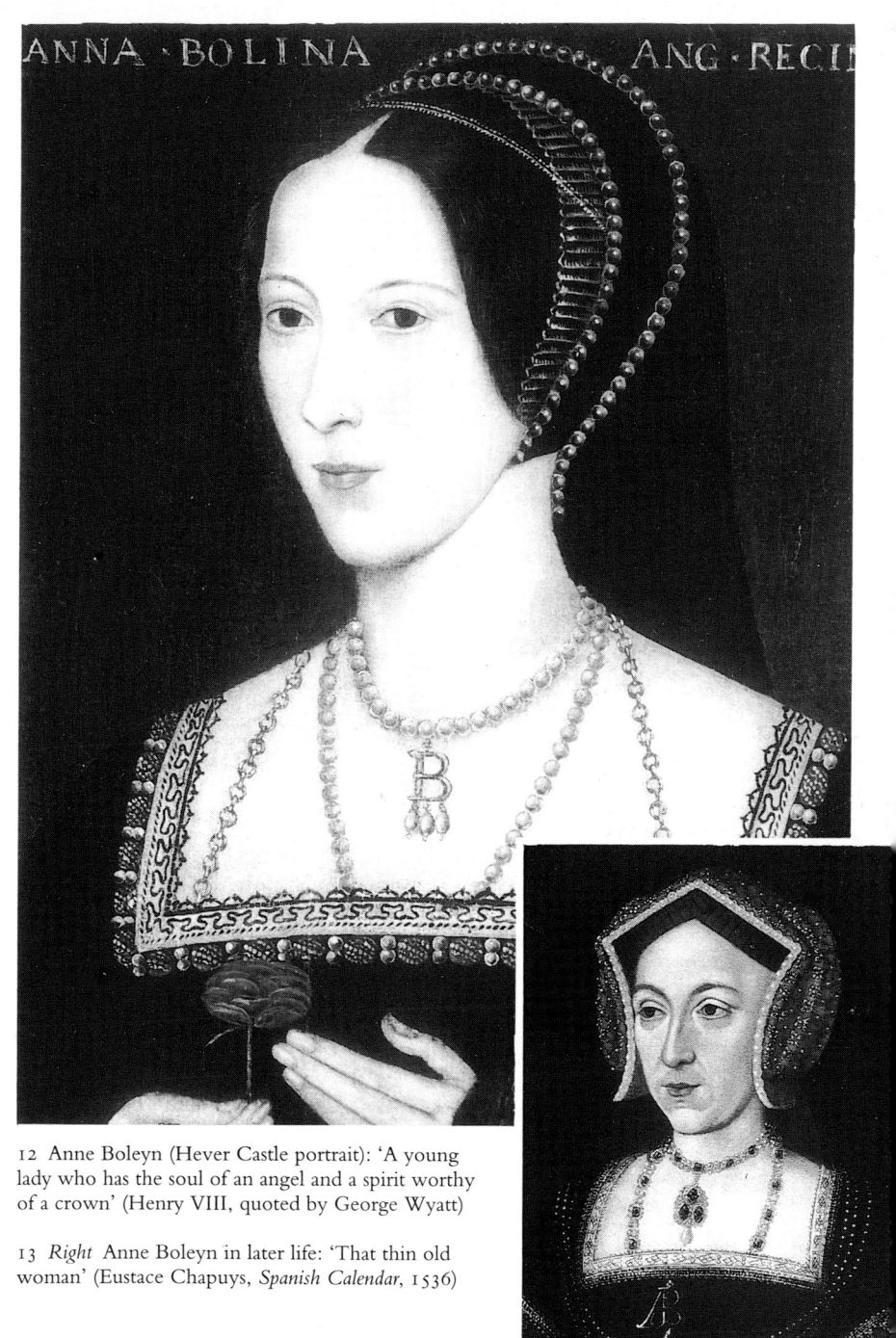

12 Anne Boleyn (Hever Castle portrait): 'A young lady who has the soul of an angel and a spirit worthy of a crown' (Henry VIII, quoted by George Wyatt)

13 *Right* Anne Boleyn in later life: 'That thin old woman' (Eustace Chapuys, *Spanish Calendar*, 1536)

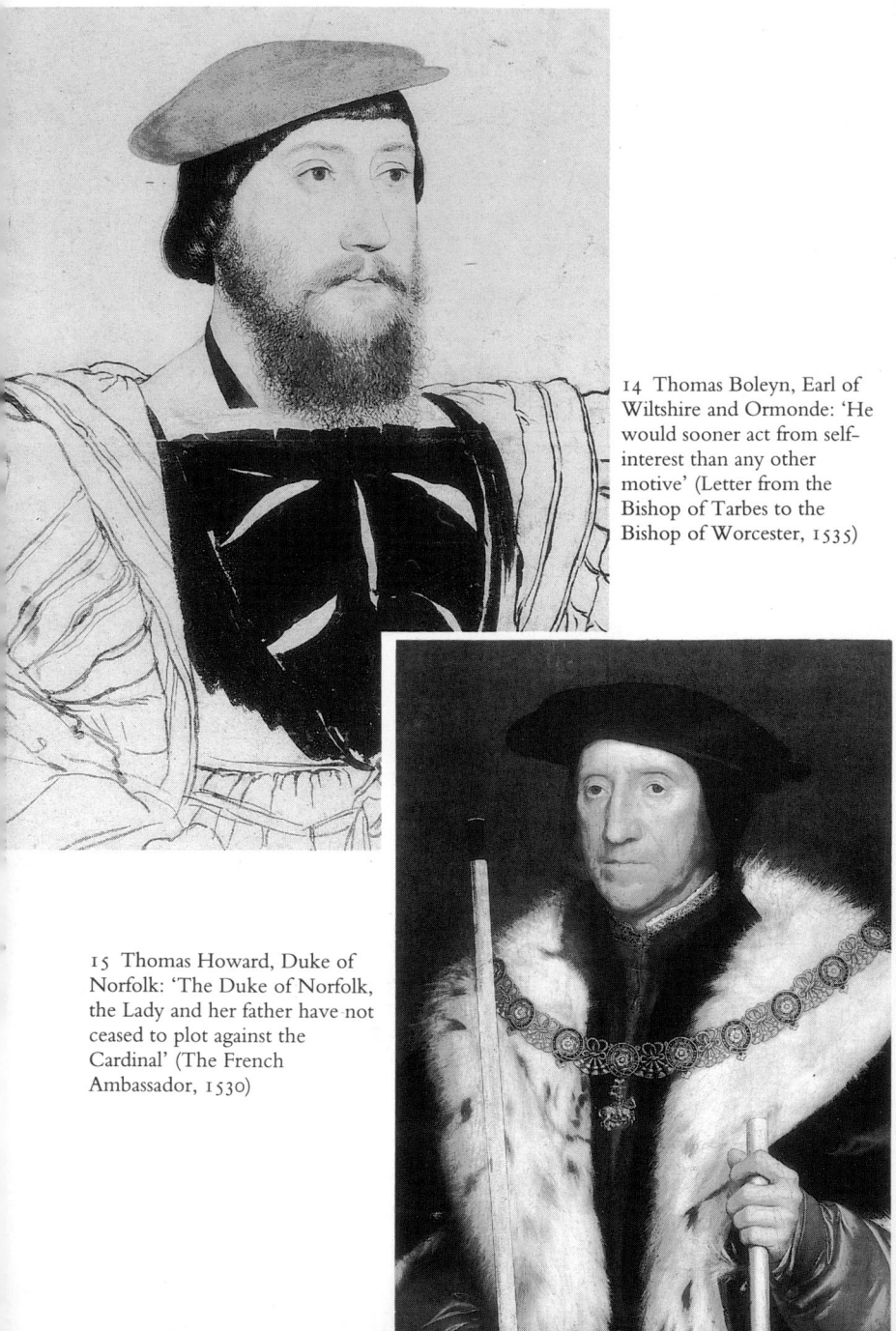

14 Thomas Boleyn, Earl of Wiltshire and Ormonde: 'He would sooner act from self-interest than any other motive' (Letter from the Bishop of Tarbes to the Bishop of Worcester, 1535)

15 Thomas Howard, Duke of Norfolk: 'The Duke of Norfolk, the Lady and her father have not ceased to plot against the Cardinal' (The French Ambassador, 1530)

ever waged in Spain.' His remarks are proof that he knew very little about Katherine's illness. Fortunately, Mary recovered, and by April she was well enough to rejoin Elizabeth's household which was then at Eltham.

In February 1535, the King found a new mistress, thanks to his wife, who had now come to terms with the inevitable and reasoned that, if Henry had to have an affair, it should be with someone sympathetic to her, and not a member of the imperialist faction. She had therefore deliberately selected her cousin and lady-in-waiting Madge Shelton, who was the daughter of Lady Shelton; Anne persuaded Madge, who seems to have been quite amenable to the arrangement, to encourage Henry's advances. In no time at all, Madge was in the King's bed, where Anne hoped she would use her influence to make Henry a little kinder to his long-suffering wife. However, the short affair resulted, predictably, in Anne once more suffering pangs of jealousy; nor did it improve her situation at all.

By mid-March, though, she was in an altogether happier frame of mind, for she had discovered she was pregnant again. By 24 June, her condition was obvious, and Sir William Kingston remarked that 'she hath as fair a belly as I have seen'. But after that no more is heard of this pregnancy, and it is safe to assume it ended in a stillbirth at around the sixth month at the end of June. Again, details of the confinement were kept secret: Henry did not wish to parade another failure before the world. Nor was Anne's disappointment helped by news brought from France by her brother that Francis I would not agree to Elizabeth's betrothal to his son. Her mood now swung from hopeful anticipation to despair, and then to anger. 'She has been in a bad humour,' wrote Chapuys, 'and said a thousand shameful words of the King of France and the whole nation.' Sometimes she managed to hide her chagrin and grief under a façade of gaiety. Margaret More, visiting her father in prison, told him that there had been nothing else at court but sporting and dancing, and that the Queen 'never did better'.

Alas, it pitieth me to remember into what misery, poor soul, she will shortly come [mused More]. These dances of hers will prove such dances that she will spurn our heads off like footballs, but it will not be long ere her head will dance the like dance.

None knew better than he how easily the King's favour could turn to wrath.

Around this time, Cromwell, earning the approval of the reformists and the Queen, was preparing an enquiry into the abuses said to be rife within the religious houses. Closure of minor houses, or badly run ones, had been commonplace since the days of Henry V, and had accelerated under Wolsey, but this was something of quite a different order. Cromwell meant to have every monastery and convent visited and reported upon, with a view to its possible closure and the appropriation of its wealth by the Crown.

It was a masterful plan, and it had great appeal for a king who had long since squandered his father's fortune and was now desperately in need of funds, and who as its supreme head, was trying to divest the Church of England of the kind of abuses that had corrupted the Roman Church as well as any lingering allegiance to the papacy. It is doubtful if either Henry or Cromwell foresaw the far-reaching social consequences that would result from the closure of a large number of religious houses, nor that they envisaged much opposition from the English people, who had not protested overmuch about the break with Rome. Cromwell was made Vicar General in January 1535, and given permission to arrange for the visitation of every religious house in England. His report on the wealth of the Church – the *Valor Ecclesiasticus* – was compiled by July 1535, and in that month the King's commissioners began their visitations, starting with minor establishments.

Queen Anne vigorously supported the reforms. After she became queen, she had become the focus of all the hopes of those who had secretly embraced the Lutheran faith; they imagined she shared their views, which was not so, although she did constrain the King to be tolerant with heretics. One Protestant, Robert Barnes, who had once fled from England for fear of persecution, was able to return, thanks to Anne's protection, and preached openly in London, unmolested. In 1534, Anne secured the freedom of another convicted heretic, Richard Herman, whom Wolsey had sent into exile for having advocated the translation of the Bible into English, something of which Anne herself was strongly in favour. Not for nothing did Miles Coverdale, in 1536, dedicate his English translation of the Bible to both Henry VIII and 'your dearest wife and most virtuous Princess, Queen Anne': this book, with Anne's initials beautifully embossed on the cover, is now in the British Library. It is a fact that not a single heretic was burned while Anne was queen. Her tolerance was unusual in an age that favoured rigid religious practice. However, it also lent ammunition to her detractors, for, to many, it was proof that she was herself a heretic.

In 1533, Anne had tried to save Catesby Priory from closure at the request of the nuns, and even offered to buy it herself. However, when the King learned that the nuns were unable to support themselves, he was compelled to refuse her request. Two years later, Anne would not have been so anxious to help. In 1535, she sent her officers to examine the famous phial of the Holy Blood at Hayles Abbey in Gloucestershire, which had been revered for centuries; back came the report – it was the blood of a duck, renewed as necessary by the monks who charged pilgrims to see it. The Queen ordered it to be removed from public view, but as soon as her men had gone, the monks put it back, and people still flocked to see it. In December 1535, Anne visited Syon Abbey, and harangued the nuns about their popish forms of worship.

Of the ten bishops preferred to sees while she was queen, seven were of the reformist persuasion, and in this her influence was plain. 'What a zealous defender she was of Christ's Gospel!' John Foxe would write many years later; and the Scots reformer, Alexander Aless would one day tell Elizabeth I that 'true religion in England had its commencement and its end with your mother'. Elizabeth's first Archbishop of Canterbury, Matthew Parker, began his career as Anne Boleyn's chaplain, even though Anne knew he favoured the teachings of Luther.

She was also a patron of the new learning. In 1533, Erasmus dedicated two books to her father, and referred in each preface to 'the most gracious and virtuous Queen Anne'. She also assisted the French humanist Nicholas Bourbon, who had been imprisoned in France for his religious views – Anne earned his undying gratitude for securing his release, and even after her death, when her name was never uttered, he would boldly dedicate one of his treatises to her memory.

As she grew older, Anne consciously cultivated a new image for herself, that of godly matron. She rarely appeared in public without a book of devotions in her hands. She aided scholars, particularly poor ones, and provided money for their education, maintaining several at the University of Cambridge, and she entrusted her nephew and ward, Henry Carey, to the fine tutelage of Nicholas Bourbon. She also helped Wolsey's bastard son, Thomas Winter, when he returned penniless from his studies at the University of Padua, which had been paid for by the King.

Anne's charities were widespread, yet little publicised during her lifetime. She had begun them in 1532, when she had, among other good deeds, sent money and medicine for the relief of the mother of Richard Lyst, a lay brother in the convent of the Observant Friars at Greenwich. Lyst had at one time been much against her, but her kindness softened his heart, and he became such a staunch supporter that other members of the community scathingly referred to him as Anne's 'chaplain'.

Anne gave alms weekly to the poor to the value of 100 crowns, together with clothing sewn by herself and her ladies. Throughout her reign, she discreetly provided also for widows and poor householders, sometimes giving out £3 or £4 for cattle or other livestock. When visiting a town or village, she sent her almoner ahead to find out from the parish authorities if there were any needy families in the district. A list would be drawn up, and the Queen would make grants of money towards their support. After her death, there was found among her papers a list of grants she intended to use for the relief of poor artisans. At the end of the sixteenth century, George Wyatt estimated that her charities had amounted to at least £1,500 yearly for the poor alone. He also commended her work for the poor in providing them with garments she had sewn herself; he had seen with his own eyes examples of her needlework in the fine tapestries on display at Hampton Court; yet, in his opinion, far more precious in the sight of God 'were those works which she caused her maidens to execute in shirts and smocks for the poor'.

In the spring of 1535 the shadow of treason, real or imagined, and the King's wrath with those who opposed his marriage and his policies hung over England. In April, an Oxford midwife was jailed for calling the Queen a 'goggle-eyed whore and a bawd', and a priest, Robert Feron, was also imprisoned for saying that 'the King's wife in fornication, this matron Anne, be more stinking than a sow'. But these were just the little fish. To snare more influential traitors the King would unleash a minor reign of terror, as he demonstrated to his subjects just how terrible his justice – and his vengeance – could be.

In May, the Prior of the London Charterhouse and four Carthusian monks, having denied the royal supremacy, suffered traitors' deaths at Tyburn. Sir Thomas More watched the men being tied to hurdles at the Tower, and noticed that they were 'as joyful as bridegrooms going to their marriages'. Wearing their habits, they were dragged by horses through the streets of London, strung up on the gallows, and left to hang until half-choked. Then they were cut down and revived with vinegar, so that they might suffer the full horrors of the punishment required by the law for treason: castration, disembowelling, and decapitation. After their deaths, their bodies were cut into quarters, which were publicly exhibited. The monks died bravely, before a shocked audience, and news of their end was greeted with horror throughout Catholic Europe. Of course, it was Anne who was blamed for the atrocity. She herself considered that justice had been done, and remained unmoved: one of the condemned men had had the effrontery to allege that Henry had once had an affair with her mother.

On 7 May, for the last time, Fisher and More refused to take the oath. Anne was constantly urging the King to put them to death, and 'when the Lady wants anything, there is no one who dares contradict her, not even the King himself,' wrote Chapuys. Anne was then pregnant, and must be humoured, since when Henry 'does not want to do as she wishes, she behaves like someone in a frenzy'.

In June, more Carthusian monks were executed for refusing to acknowledge the King's supremacy. They were chained upright to stakes and left to die, without food or water, wallowing in their own filth – a slow, ghastly death that left Londoners appalled. In the King's view, such measures were necessary to bring his subjects to heel, and while the monks suffered, he feasted with Anne at Hanworth, and allowed himself to be persuaded that Fisher, too, ought to die for his obstinacy. Two days later, the former bishop was put on trial for treason and sentenced to death, and two days after that, three more monks of the Charterhouse suffered at Tyburn. Fisher himself was beheaded on 22 June 1535 on Tower Hill at the age of seventy-six. A shocked populace blamed Anne for his death, and it was partly for this reason that news of the stillbirth of her child was suppressed – people would very clearly have seen the hand of God in it. Anne herself suffered pangs of conscience on the day of Fisher's execution, and attended a mass for the repose of his soul, though by the evening of the next day she had composed herself sufficiently to stage for the King's entertainment a masque depicting divine approval of recent events in England. Henry was so pleased to see himself cutting off the heads of the clergy that he told Anne she must have the performance repeated on the Eve of St Peter, a day formerly dedicated to honouring the Pope.

The political executions of 1535 gave Chapuys fresh cause for concern over the future safety of Katherine and Mary, who had also refused to take the oaths or acknowledge the royal supremacy. One Monday in June the King sent a deputation of his Council to Kimbolton to search Katherine's rooms for anything incriminating that might be hidden there. The councillors made no secret of their anger at not finding what they were looking for, and at court the advantages her death would bring were spoken of quite openly. On 30 June, Cromwell told Chapuys that 'if God had taken to Himself the Queen, the whole dispute would have been ended, and no one would have doubted or opposed the King's second marriage or the succession.' Fortunately for Katherine, the fear of Charles V, bent upon vengeance, was enough to stay Henry's hand.

Others were not so fortunate. On 1 July, Sir Thomas More was tried for treason in Westminster Hall and condemned to death. He mounted the scaffold on Tower Hill on 6 July, and died bravely by the axe, saying he was 'the King's good servant, but God's first'. If there had been tremors of horror at Fisher's death, there were shock waves now, and they reverberated around Europe, where the consensus of opinion was that Henry had gone too far this time. Even Henry had serious doubts that he had been right, and characteristically he blamed Anne Boleyn for More's death.

Then there was Father John Forrest, a member of the Order of Observant Friars at Greenwich, and a former confessor to Katherine of Aragon, who had been imprisoned for espousing her cause in 1533. In 1535, he was attainted and sentenced to be burned at the stake. Katherine, hearing this news, wrote offering what comfort she could to Forrest, signing herself 'your very sad and afflicted daughter, Katherine'. He replied promptly, saying her words had 'infinitely comforted me', and asking for her prayers, 'that I may fight the battle to which I am called. In justification of your cause, I am content to suffer all things.' However, on the following day, the King was graciously pleased to commute his sentence to life imprisonment. For some years to come Forrest would continue to assert that Katherine had been the King's true wife, and by May 1538 Henry had had enough, sending him to an agonising death at Smithfield: he was suspended by chains about his arms and waist above a slow-burning fire, and slowly roasted to death. His execution provoked murmurs of protest, and the French ambassador complained to Francis I that he had 'to deal with the most dangerous and cruel man in the world'. Mary's former tutor, Richard Fetherston, and Katherine's former chaplain, Thomas Abell, were also condemned to death in July 1540, their crimes being described as high treason. Even after both the women involved in it were dead, his 'great matter' remained a sensitive issue with the King for the rest of his life.

One person who escaped Henry's clutches was Reginald Pole, who had condemned the King's marriage to Anne Boleyn in 1533 after choosing exile on the Continent. Still hoping to gain his support, however, in February 1535 Henry asked Pole if he would set out in writing his opinions on the King's marriages. It was an invitation that Pole could not resist, and he spent several months working on a reply. When it came, it would be so damning, so offensive to the King, and so provocatively treasonous that Henry's suppressed dislike of Pole grew overnight into pathological hatred, and his reaction was ultimately so savage that Pole's friends knew he would never be able to return to England while the King lived.

With the loss of Anne's child around the end of June, Henry ceased playing the doting husband. In the summer of 1535 the Venetian ambassador reported that he was 'tired to satiety' of Anne, and there were rumours at court that he wished to put her away. Once he accused her of having been responsible for the recent executions, and for having been the cause of all the present troubles in his kingdom. Anne retaliated swiftly, reminding him he was more bound to her than man could be to woman. Had she not delivered him from a state of sin? Had she not helped to make him the richest prince in Christendom? Without her, he would not have reformed the Church, to his own great profit and that of all his subjects. Henry ignored her: Anne had done all these things and more, but she had failed to bear a living son.

Anne's chief consolation nowadays was her little daughter, and she often visited her at Eltham or Hatfield. Sir William Kingston thought Elizabeth to be 'as goodly a child as has been seen', and 'much in the King's favour, as should be, God save her!' Henry too was proud of his red-haired daughter, and liked to show her off to visiting ambassadors, sometimes dressed in rich clothes, and sometimes naked, so that they could see how well formed she was. Elizabeth had been weaned off breast milk at the age of one, at the King's express command, and with the Queen's assent. Orders were relayed from the royal parents through Cromwell to Lady Bryan, who had instructions to approach Mr Secretary on any matter relating to her charge. This meant that Cromwell's duties now ranged from overseeing the closure of the monasteries to approving nursery routines.

Anne was delighted when, in July 1535, King Francis at last agreed to enter negotiations for the marriage of Elizabeth to his third son. Yet it was Mary to whom people were looking when they considered the future. Elizabeth was not yet two, and if anything should happen to the King, Mary would have an infinitely better chance of holding the throne. Even Cromwell decided at this time to lend Mary his support, and discussed with Chapuys the possibility of altering the Act of Succession with a view to naming Mary the King's heir. The Queen got to hear of this, and her anger knew no bounds, but although she threatened Cromwell with execution, he paid little heed: 'She cannot do me any harm,' he told Chapuys.

Only five days after More's execution, Chapuys noted that his Majesty was happily dancing and flirting once again with the ladies of his court. When William Somers, Henry's fool, proclaimed to the court: 'Anne is a ribald, the child is a bastard!', Henry was angry – so angry, in fact, that Somers had to leave court for a while – but he did nothing more, whereas once he would have acted swiftly to punish anyone who slandered his wife.

In the summer of 1535, the King and Queen set off on a progress westwards towards Wales. There was, however, little of the usual holiday atmosphere, for Henry was troubled by news lately arrived from the Continent that the Emperor was about to take Tunis from the Turks, thereby depriving them of a great naval base and stemming the tide of their encroachment upon the eastern reaches of the Empire. What concerned Henry was that, if Charles were successful in this enterprise, his armies would be free to fight elsewhere, and England might be a prime target for invasion. Henry knew he was regarded as a schismatic rebel, and he feared Charles would make this the excuse to interfere on his aunt's behalf.

Late in July, the royal party arrived at Winchcombe; from thence they rode into Wales, and then back through the south-west of England, and so into the county of Wiltshire. On 4 September, Henry and Anne arrived at Wulfhall, a half-timbered manor house on the outskirts of Savernake Forest, where they were to stay for six days. Wulfhall was the home of the Seymour family, hereditary rangers of Savernake Forest, and its present owner was Sir John Seymour, whose daughter Jane was one of the Queen's maids of honour. There is no evidence that Henry VIII's courtship of Jane Seymour began during this visit, yet it is significant that mention was made of it in diplomatic reports within two months, and it may well be that the traditional assumption that it began at Wulfhall is the correct one.

Wulfhall has long since disappeared. In the sixteenth century, it was a substantial house that had already been standing for at least 300 years. The manor of Ulfhall (probably derived from 'Ulf's hall', after a Saxon or Danish thane) was recorded in the Domesday Book in 1086. The house Henry stayed in was built along traditional lines around a courtyard, with a chapel and a recently incorporated innovation, a long gallery, which was quite novel in the 1530s. Surrounding the house were three gardens.

Sir John Seymour was well known to his royal visitor. A man with a sound reputation for being a capable administrator, he had at one time carried out diplomatic missions abroad on the King's behalf. He had been Sheriff of Wiltshire since 1508, and Sheriff of Dorset and Somerset since 1518. He was also a Justice of the Peace for Wiltshire, and an extensive landowner in that county. The Wulfhall estate itself comprised 1,270 acres, most of which had been converted to pasture for sheep, conforming to the prevailing agricultural trend. For all this, however, Sir John ranked quite low on the aristocratic scale, and for him this royal visit was a signal honour.

Sir John, then nearing sixty, was the father of a large family. His wife was Margaret, the daughter of Sir Henry Wentworth of Nettlestead in Suffolk; as a young girl at Henry VII's court she had been a celebrated beauty, and the poet laureate, John Skelton, had written in her honour a poem entitled 'To Mistress Margery Wentworth', praising her maidenly virtues and her 'benign, courteous and meek' qualities. Mistress Margery had been married to Sir John Seymour around 1500 and for him it was a brilliant match, for although the Seymours were said to have been descended from one of William the Conqueror's Norman knights, surnamed St Maur after his birthplace in Touraine, they had never been more than country gentry. Their first certain ancestor came from Monmouthshire; a branch of the family was already established in Wiltshire at the end of the fourteenth century, and provided a Member of Parliament for Bedwyn Magna, the village near Wulfhall. The manor of Wulfhall had come to the Seymours by marriage to the heiress of the Esturmi family in the early fifteenth century, through which they also acquired the hereditary guardianship of Savernake. Thereafter, they proudly displayed in the manor house the great ivory hunting-horn, bound with silver, that was the symbol of their office. Gradually, by lucrative and advantageous marriages, they had, like the Boleyns, increased not only their land and wealth, but also their social standing. The marriage of Sir John Seymour to Lady Margaret Wentworth, however, was the most prestigious of them all, for Lady Margaret was descended from Edward III and Henry 'Hotspur' Percy, the hero of Shrewsbury. She was, in all respects, a most desirable wife for a man like Sir John, who was considered to be one of the foremost in the rising class of gentry known as 'new men', solid, respectable, loyal to the crown, and owing their status to wealth rather than breeding. Such men were greatly favoured by Tudor monarchs distrustful of the ancient blood of the older nobility.

Of the ten children born of the marriage, four died young, probably of plague. Two of the surviving sons, Edward and Thomas, were to play prominent parts in English history. The other son, Henry, shunned public life and led the existence of a country gentleman. The eldest daughter, Elizabeth, was a widow in 1535, her husband having died the previous year. The other daughters were Dorothy, later the wife of Sir Clement Smith, and Jane.

Unhappily, there had been a rift in the Seymour family some five years before the royal visit, and the ensuing scandal had shocked even Henry VIII's courtiers. Young Edward Seymour had been sent to court at an early age, and had served as page to both Mary Tudor when she was Queen of France, and the King himself. When still quite young, he had been married to Katherine, the daughter of Sir Edward Fillol. Very little is known about the marriage apart from the fact that Katherine bore two sons, John and Edward, in 1528 and 1529. A year later, Edward was shattered to discover that his wife and his father had for some time been lovers, and that there was every possibility that Sir John had fathered Katherine's two children. Edward's retaliation was swift. Katherine was bundled into a nunnery, where she died within five years. For a time, Edward spoke of divorcing her, though he did not do so, but he disinherited her two boys, and would have nothing to do with them. After his wife's death, he remarried immediately, his bride being the formidable Anne Stanhope, a lady who would rule both her husband and her family with a will of steel, and whose pride would be notorious.

By the time Henry VIII arrived at Wulfhall in 1535, the scandal had died a natural death, and a truce had been called between Edward and his father; Edward's new marriage had done much to mellow his bitterness. The King certainly knew of the affair, but probably felt that the family had suffered enough without his censure. As for Sir John, he must have seen his sovereign's visit as a sign that the past was done with and forgotten.

Although royal visits to private subjects were at this date by no means as crippling financially as they were to become under Elizabeth I, entertaining one's king and queen of necessity called for a substantial outlay to pay for the special fare provided for the royal table, for not only did the royal guests have to be accommodated but their retainers also, and that could mean a good many people. However, the King's charm and courtesy, especially towards the ladies, were well known; Henry VIII was invariably an appreciative and genial guest, laying aside formality and conversing with his host and the family as if they were his equals.

Despite the brooding presence of the Queen, Henry must have enjoyed his stay at Wulfhall, where the excellent hunting to be found in Savernake Forest provided a welcome respite from the cares of state. Sir John was a good host, and Lady Margaret typified all that the King thought a wife should be: meek, decorous, well bred, and, above all, fruitful – unlike Anne in every way.

Jane Seymour was probably the second daughter of Sir John and Lady Margaret. The date of her birth is nowhere recorded, and has until now been estimated as 1509–10. This calculation has been based on two things: a report of the Spanish ambassador, dated May 1536, stating that Jane was then more than twenty-five years old, and a miniature of her painted in the 1580s by Nicholas Hilliard, which gives her age as twenty-five in 1536. The miniature may be discounted as reliable evidence: it was based on one of Holbein's portraits of Jane Seymour, none of which give her age. A far more likely date of birth, based upon sound evidence, would be between October 1507 and October 1508. When Jane was buried with the full honours due to a queen of England in November 1537, twenty-nine ladies walked in he funeral procession: seemingly an odd number until one discovers that it was customary at medieval funerals to mark the age of the deceased in such a way, just as it was traditional to ring the passing bell once for every year the departed soul had spent on earth. On this assumption, Jane was twenty-nine when she died, and a birthdate of 1507–8 would accord with Chapuys's statement that she was over twenty-five in 1536.

This means that Jane was around twenty-seven when the King visited Wulfhall, a very late age to remain single in an era when most girls were married by fifteen or sixteen. There had, at an unspecified date, been talk of a betrothal between Jane and Sir Robert Dormer's son William; Sir Francis Bryan, who was connected by marriage to the Seymours, did his best to promote the match, but met with opposition from Lady Dormer, who seems to have felt that Jane was not a good enough match for her son. Eventually William Dormer was betrothed elsewhere, and it was probably this that precipitated Bryan into securing a position at court for Jane; thus she came to join the household of Katherine of Aragon as a maid of honour sometime during the 1520s.

Jane greatly admired Queen Katherine, and later used her as her own role model when she herself became queen. Katherine's court provided a kind of finishing school for young women of good family, and it was in this learned and pious atmosphere that Jane Seymour grew to maturity. Of her education, we know very little. During her childhood there had been a salaried priest, Father James, at Wulfhall, who may have given Jane some rudimentary lessons along with her brothers. As an adult, she could read and sign her name, but she was not learned as both Katherine of Aragon and Anne Boleyn were, nor was she as intelligent as they. For Jane, an education of a traditional sort had been provided, and it was doubtless her mother – as was customary – who taught her the usual feminine skills such as household management, needlework, and cookery. Jane's expertise as a needlewoman became legendary, and examples of her work still survived a century after her death to testify to her skill. Yet she also enjoyed outdoor sports, having been taught to ride at an early age, and as queen she would enjoy following the hunt.

Jane was just one of many aspiring young women in Queen Katherine's household. She grew to know and like the Princess Mary, eight years her junior, and she would also have known Anne Boleyn well, for she was a fellow maid of honour for a time. By virtue of her position, Jane would have been a witness to the events leading up to the legatine court hearing in 1529, and would have observed at first hand the downfall of the Queen and the rise to power of Anne Boleyn. She certainly saw enough of these things to make her decide that her sympathies lay with Katherine, and, later on, when Katherine was beyond all human help, Jane would extend her friendship to the Lady Mary, in an attempt to make up to her for what she and her mother had suffered.

When the Queen was exiled from the court in 1531, Jane may have been one of those who went with her to The More and ultimately to Ampthill. Yet it is more likely that she transferred to the household of Anne Boleyn at this time: she had certainly joined it by Christmas 1533, and Anne would hardly have accepted someone who had chosen to share Katherine's exile. Like Anne, Jane was ambitious; her family, too, were ambitious for her. To remain in the service of a fallen queen, however much admired, would not have done much for Jane's chances of making her way in the world and contracting an advantageous marriage. Anne Boleyn was at that time amassing a huge train of female attendants, and it would have been easy for Jane, with her experience of the court, to secure a place with her.

At Christmas 1533, Henry VIII presented gifts to several ladies in his wife's household, among them Jane Seymour, whom he had known since she first arrived at court; he would certainly have approved of her timely transfer to Anne's service. Yet it was not until September 1535 that he began to take particular notice of her. This probably came about as a result of the visit to her family home. Far from being in residence at Wulfhall at the time of the King's arrival, which is the traditional version of events, Jane was in the Queen's train and travelling on progress with her.

Henry was no longer the athletic young man who had married Katherine of Aragon. After 1533, he had begun to put on weight, and became less active than in his youth; he had also had recurrrent trouble with one leg after being wounded by a fall from his horse in 1528. Yet he continued to hunt regularly and rode with skill, and people still thought him handsome, in spite of the fact that his red hair had receded, leaving the crown of his head bald. Although in recent years his latent ruthlessness and cruelty had become more evident, and his subjects now feared rather than loved him, he could be charming when he pleased, and he was being charming now.

For her part, Jane presented a welcome contrast to the Queen. She concealed her ambition beneath a veneer of placid gravity, and where Anne's eyes had once flashed an invitation, Jane's were kept modestly lowered. Her manner was pleasing, her temperament calm. The King was very taken with her, and before long his courtiers were aware, as was his wife, that he was pursuing the plain Mistress Seymour, and that – as Anne had once done to great advantage – the lady was holding him off while protesting a chaste devotion for her king. There were those at court who had been waiting for an opportunity like this to unseat Anne from Henry's affections, not only because she was unpopular and had not borne a male heir, but also because they resented her promotion of the reformist cause. Foremost among them was Chapuys, who desired nothing more than Anne's fall, and who, at a very early stage, saw in Jane Seymour the means by which this might be achieved.

Jane must have given the King some indication that his advances were welcome; his courtship presented her with an opportunity that was too good to miss. With Anne Boleyn's example before her to prove that a maid of honour could successfully aspire to queenship, she does not seem to have considered that by encouraging the King she was betraying the mistress to whom she had sworn an oath of service. The Seymours belonged to the faction which despised Anne and all that she stood for, while secretly reserving their allegiance to Katherine of Aragon and her daughter; thus they abetted Jane from the beginning, urging her to encourage the King's courtship and seeing it as a means to several ends. It is likely that, as the King prepared to leave Wulfhall after a good week's hunting, some of the courtiers were already predicting the imminent downfall of the Queen. Among them was Sir Francis Bryan, the son of Lady Margaret Bryan, a member of the King's immediate entourage, and one of his friends. Bryan had paid lip-service to Queen Anne, but he privately disapproved of her, and he was perhaps the first person to see in Jane Seymour a means of toppling Anne from her throne. Certainly, he did his best to encourage Henry's affair with Jane from the beginning.

When Henry and Jane were both back at court after the progress, their affair continued, gaining in intensity. In November, the French ambassador saw them together and concluded that the King was in love again. So open was the affair that courtiers were falling over themselves to win the friendship of the new favourite, leaving the Queen to sit alone in her empty apartments. History was repeating itself.

Jane's brothers, Edward and Thomas, were both with her at court, and they prudently warned her not to yield her virginity to Henry: she must create the impression of a modest and virtuous gentlewoman who wished to preserve her virtue until she was married. Jane played her part perfectly, knowing full well that she was employing the same tactics Anne Boleyn had used years before – and, once again, Henry took the bait. A man who set much store by female virtue, he was enchanted, if frustrated, and set about laying siege to this virtuous citadel. Jane's resolve withstood this, but her virtue did not prevent her from accepting the expensive gifts that Henry gave her. Indeed, her calculated campaign to ensnare her mistress's husband shows her to have been a woman of ruthless determination. It is true that she enjoyed the vigorous support of her family, but it is impossible to believe that she was a mere tool of the imperialist party which was encouraging the affair: any woman setting out on the course Jane Seymour would follow over the next few months would have had to be possessed of both strength and resolution, as well as driving ambition and a flexible conscience. Jane had all these, hidden beneath a demure manner that deceived many. Yet, to her credit, she aimed to use her talents and her growing power to persuade the King to return to the fold of Rome and restore the Lady Mary to her rightful place in the succession. These were matters about which she felt strongly, although she knew she could only broach them once she had firmly established herself in the King's affections. Like Anne Boleyn before her, she had set her sights high.

In October 1535, Cromwell brought the King devastating news: Tunis had fallen to the Emperor, and the Turks had been crushed. Chapuys told his master that Henry and Anne looked 'like dogs falling out of a window', so dismayed were they by the news. And as if this was not enough, there were reports of a ruined harvest, due to the bad weather that year. Anne was even blamed for this by the common people: they saw it as a sign from God that He was displeased with the King for marrying her. General unrest was mounting, and there were still murmurs of disapproval about the executions that had taken place earlier in the year. It was not a happy homecoming when Henry and Anne ended their progress at Windsor on 26 October.

That same month, Katherine was writing to the Pope, begging him to find a remedy for what was happening in England; by so doing she was putting herself in grave danger, for, if intercepted, her letter could have been used as evidence that she had tried to incite a foreign power to make war upon the King, and that was treason. Henry suspected that Katherine was up to something of the sort, and in November he told his Privy Council that he would no longer remain in 'this trouble and fear and suspicion' engendered by Katherine and Mary, and insisted that proceedings be taken against them in the next session of Parliament, 'or, by God, I will not wait any longer to provide for this myself!' Seeing the dismay on the faces of his councillors, he told them it was nothing to cry or make wry faces about. 'If I am to lose my crown for it, I will do what I have set out to do,' he warned. When Chapuys reported this to Charles V, and told him that 'the Concubine has for some time conspired for the death of the Queen and her daughter,' Charles replied, 'The threats of which you speak can only be designed to frighten them, but if they really are in danger you may tell them from me that they must yield.' He did not share Katherine's professed enthusiasm for martyrdom, and he was in fact beginning to find the whole affair rather tiresome. 'I cannot believe what you tell me,' he wrote to Chapuys. 'The King cannot be so unnatural as to put to death his own wife and daughter,' even though Henry's treatment of them had been 'cruel and horrible'. But if the King would not go so far, Chapuys feared that Anne Boleyn would, for she 'is the person who manages and orders and governs everything, whom the King does not dare to oppose'. Anne believed – mistakenly, as it turned out – that while Katherine lived, her own life was in danger. 'She is my death and I am hers,' she said at this time, 'so I will take good care that she shall not laugh at me after my death.' It was a supreme irony that Katherine's existence was later shown to have guaranteed Anne's safety, rather than having threatened it, for while Katherine lived, Henry dared not set Anne aside.

Anne's influence was to some degree restored during November because she had found herself to be pregnant with a child conceived during the autumn progress. Nevertheless, she was depressed during the first months of her pregnancy because she was fearfully aware that her whole future depended on its outcome: the King would not tolerate another failure. Outwardly, he was being solicitous, but George Wyatt tells us that he 'shrank from her' in private, 'at this time when most she was to have been cherished', which did not help Anne's frame of mind. The Bishop of Tarbes, visiting the English court, noticed that 'the King's love for his wife is less than it has been, and diminishes every day because he has new amours'. Anne was well aware of his pursuit of Jane Seymour, which was another reason for her depression.

Anne Boleyn's pregnancy brought Katherine and Mary nearer than ever to being put to death by judicial process or less lawful means. Anne, with the interests of her coming child to protect, now began a campaign to eliminate them both; Chapuys heard how Henry had not only promised to disinherit Mary, but also to kill her, and Anne had also let it be known that if Henry did not make an end of the girl, she herself would. 'If I have a son, as I hope shortly, I know what will become of her,' she declared. Yet Mary stood firm.

> God [she told Chapuys] had not so blinded her as to confess for any kingdom on earth that the King her father and the Queen her mother had so long lived in adultery, nor would she contravene the order of the Church and make herself a bastard.

She had no sense of self-pity: 'Her grief is about the troubles of the Queen her mother.'

Yet Katherine's troubles would soon be mercifully at an end. She fell dangerously ill on 1 December 1535, having grown weaker and weaker during recent months, suffering pains in her chest. Unable to eat very much, she was now confined to her bed, and her physician doubted she would ever rise from it. Katherine herself realised that time was running out for her, even though she rallied after a few days and was able to get up and sit in a chair. Queen Anne, thinking she was recovering, went flying to the King and begged him once more to have the former Queen and her daughter put to death. But Henry had read the reports of Katherine's illness, and knew he need do nothing to expedite her end, although Anne, whom Chapuys called 'this she-devil', declared she would not rest 'until he is freed from these poor ladies'. From Spain, the English ambassador reported that 'people expected to hear every day of the execution of Queen Katherine, and that the Princess Mary was expected soon to follow her.'

Katherine had more mundane matters on her mind. Her funds were depleted, and on 14 December she was forced to beg the

Emperor to pay her servants: 'I am as Job, waiting for the day when I must sue for alms, for the love of God.' Three days later, she celebrated her fiftieth birthday. It would be her last. On 26 December, she suffered a relapse, and was forced, in great pain, to take to her bed again, although she could not sleep. Her doctors, Dr de la Saa and Dr Balthasar Guersye, both knew her condition was grave, and de la Saa warned Bedingfield in writing that 'if the sickness continueth in force, she cannot remain long'. As the days dragged by, the pain grew worse, but Katherine refused to let Dr de la Saa call in other doctors, saying she had 'wholly committed herself to the pleasure of God'. This dismayed him, for he privately feared that his mistress was being poisoned, and did not wish to bear the responsibility of that diagnosis alone.

By then, Chapuys had heard that Katherine had 'fallen into her last sickness'. His immediate impulse was to go to her; he had espoused her cause with a zeal beyond the requirements of his brief, and he felt it important that someone who cared for her should be there when the end came. On 30 December, he saw the King, and asked if Henry knew she was dying. 'Yes, I do not believe she has long to live; when she is gone, the Emperor will have no further excuses for interfering in English affairs,' was the reply. Chapuys, stung, retorted: 'The death of the Queen will be of no advantage! His imperial Majesty will never abandon her while she lives.' Henry shrugged. 'It does not matter, she will not live long. Go to her when you like.' He refused, however, to let Mary visit her mother.

Followed by Henry's spies, Chapuys rode off to Kimbolton that same evening; two days later, he arrived, and was duly admitted to the bedchamber of the former Queen, whom he had not seen for five years. He was profoundly shocked to see her 'so wasted that she could neither stand nor sit up in her bed'. Yet she was overjoyed to see him. 'Now I can die in your arms, not abandoned like one of the beasts,' she said. Then, remembering even now her duty as a hostess, she went on: 'You will be weary from your journey. We will speak further another time. I myself shall be glad of sleep. I have not slept two hours these past six days; perhaps I shall sleep now.'

Later that day, another visitor arrived, but this one had no permit from the King. Lady Willoughby, formerly Maria de Salinas, forced her way into the castle before Bedingfield and his men could stop her, so determined was she to be with the mistress she had served and loved for thirty-five years. Her arrival meant that Chapuys's presence was no longer necessary, and after three days he prepared to leave. 'In our last conversation,' he recorded, 'I saw the Queen smile two or three times, and after I left she was willing to be amused by one of my people whom I left to entertain her.' Before his departure on 4 January, he saw Katherine's physician and arranged with him that, if her health deteriorated further, he would make her swear before she died that she 'had never been known of Prince Arthur'. Chapuys, knowing well that his contemporaries set much store by death-bed confessions, realised that this was the last, and the only thing he could do now for the woman whose cause he had so ably championed for more than six years.

Two days later, Katherine made her will. She asked that her debts be cleared and her servants recompensed 'for the good service they have done for me'. She wished to be buried in a convent of Observant Friars, little realising that their Order had recently been suppressed in England. She asked that 500 masses be said for her soul and that someone should go to the shrine of Our Lady of Walsingham – soon to be demolished – on her behalf. To her daughter Mary she left 'the collar of gold which I brought out of Spain' and her furs. Her other bequests were to members of her household, including her tailor, laundress and goldsmith. Lastly, she asked the King, 'my good lord', if he would 'cause church garments to be made of my gowns', a request he would refuse; nor did he honour Katherine's bequests to their daughter.

On the last evening of her life, Katherine felt herself growing weaker, yet before the end came, she would make one last effort to heal the rift between herself and the man she firmly believed to be her husband. Almost at the point of death now, her thoughts turned to Henry, whom she still loved, and who had once loved her long ago. Remembering their life together, she dictated a last letter to him, even though he had expressly forbidden her to communicate with him. The words came from her heart, in that quiet bedchamber, as darkness settled upon the castle:

My lord and dear husband,
I commend me unto you. The hour of my death draweth fast on,

and my case being such, the tender love I owe you forceth me with a few words to put you in remembrance of the health and safeguard of your soul, which you ought to prefer before any consideration of the world or flesh whatsoever; for which you have cast me into many miseries and yourself into many cares. For my part, I do pardon you all, yea, I do wish and dearly pray God that He will also pardon you. For the rest, I commend unto you Mary our daughter, beseeching you to be a good father unto her, as I have hitherto desired. . . . Lastly, I vow that mine eyes desire you above all things.

Supported by her maids, the dying woman painfully traced the signature that symbolised all she had stood for and fought for during the last bitter years of her life. It was her final defiance: 'Katherine the Queen'.

Shortly afterwards, she fell asleep, with Lady Willoughby sitting beside her, who later would relate to Chapuys the details of Katherine's last hours. On the next day, 7 January 1536, she awoke at 1.0 a.m., anxious to hear mass, but not before dawn, even though her confessor was ready to allow it; he had to wait until daylight came. Katherine received her last communion 'with a fervour and devotion that it was impossible to exceed', praying God that He would pardon the King the wrong he had done her, and that divine wisdom would give him good counsel and lead him to the true road.

She was sinking fast. At ten that morning, she received extreme unction, then drifted off again into sleep, while her household gathered about her. Early in the afternoon she woke, and there were more prayers, but the end was obviously at hand. Shortly before 2.0 p.m., Katherine of Aragon, sometime Queen of England, said clearly: '*Domine, in manuas tuas commendo spiritum meum*', and rendered her spirit to God.

After Katherine's death, Sir Edmund Bedingfield informed Cromwell of her passing and arranged for the wax chandler to carry out an autopsy and then embalm the body and 'cere' it in a waxed shroud. A plumber was also engaged to seal the corpse in a leaden coffin, 'for that may not tarry'. The autopsy was carried out that evening by the chandler and his assistant; Bedingfield would not allow either of Katherine's doctors or her confessor, the Bishop of

Llandaff, to be present. The autopsy showed that most of the internal organs were normal, save for the heart, 'which had a black growth, all hideous to behold, which clung closely to the outside' and which did not change colour when washed in water; cut open, the heart was black inside. Modern medical opinion accepts this as conclusive evidence that Katherine died of a malignant tumour of the heart, yet to her contemporaries it appeared consistent with the symptoms of poisoning, and for this reason the autopsy report was suppressed. Later, Chapuys was suspicious when Dr de la Saa told him that Katherine's condition had worsened after she had drunk 'a certain Welsh beer': both men believed it had been tampered with, and Chapuys thought that if the body were properly examined 'the traces will be seen'. The bishop managed to obtain sight of the secret autopsy report, and told the ambassador about the growth on the heart. Chapuys concluded that Katherine had certainly been poisoned, and in view of the threats made by Anne Boleyn during the weeks preceding her death, this was a reasonable assumption to make. Nor was Chapuys alone in making it, for it was widely believed both in England and abroad that Anne had murdered her rival. Even King Henry had his suspicions.

The former Queen's death excited little comment in the chronicles and letters of the period, yet she was sincerely mourned by many, and it was with great sadness that Chapuys informed the Emperor of the death of his aunt, 'her, who for 27 years has been true Queen of England, whose holy soul is in eternal rest. There is little need to pray for her.' Many came to regard Katherine as a veritable saint, and an anonymous hand added a halo to one of her early portraits. Roman Catholics saw her as one of the great pillars of the old faith in England, and her death was regarded as the end of everything she had stood for. That she was in some measure responsible for what was now happening in England occurred to none of her apologists, as it had not occurred to her during her lifetime.

Katherine's devotion to the King, her single-mindedness, her strength of character, and her courage still inspire admiration, however misplaced they may seem to modern eyes. They were certainly misplaced in the view of some of her contemporaries: when Bishop Gardiner heard of Katherine's death, he announced that by taking her to Himself God had given sentence, a sentiment echoed by other reformists. Yet the people of England, who had taken Katherine to their hearts from the first, mourned her sincerely, remembering only her personal virtues, her many charities, her selflessness, and those five dead heirs to England.

It was Chapuys who broke the news of her death to the King. Henry displayed neither grief nor distress, only joyful relief – to the disgust of the ambassador – saying, 'God be praised that we are free from all suspicion of war!' Naturally, the Boleyn faction rejoiced: 'Now I am indeed a Queen,' declared Anne triumphantly, while Lord Rochford thought it a pity the Lady Mary did not keep company with her mother. The King had the Princess Elizabeth conducted to mass to the sound of trumpets, as if to underline her undoubted right to succeed him. Yet in private, the Queen showed herself troubled, perceiving with awful clarity that now only the fragile life in her womb stood between her and disaster. She had the full measure of Henry, and to her ladies expressed the fear that he might do with her as he had with Katherine, for she was perceptive enough to realise that, in the eyes of almost everyone, Henry was now a widower and free to remarry. If she were to lose this child, there was every reason to believe he would set her aside and do just that.

However, in public she showed herself confident. On 9 January, she and the King presided over a magnificent court ball held to celebrate England's liberation from the threat of war. Both Henry and Anne wore yellow, the colour of royal mourning in Spain, as a mark of respect for the woman whom Henry insisted had been his sister-in-law. The Princess Elizabeth was paraded round the room in the arms of her father, who took great pleasure in showing off the precocious child.

Henry chose Peterborough Abbey as Katherine's final resting-place, and gave orders that she was to be buried with all the honours due to a Dowager Princess of Wales, 'our dearest sister, the Lady Katherine'. He was so relieved that he spared no effort in providing her with a magnificent state funeral, at which a great train of ladies was to be present. The King himself provided black cloth for their apparel, as well as linen for the nun-like mourning veils and wimples then customary on such occasions. He also declared that it was his intention to raise to Katherine's memory a fine monument, and he kept his word, although nothing remains now of the beautiful tomb he had built over her remains: it was destroyed by parliamentary troops during the Civil War. Over the matter of a memorial service Henry was less lavish, deeming it an unnecessary expense, and he also confiscated all Katherine's remaining personal effects to meet her funeral expenses. Most of these were still in the Royal Wardrobe at Baynard's Castle, and included a clock set in a bejewelled and enamelled book of gold, a double portrait of Henry and Katherine, seven pairs of Spanish slippers, and even necessaries provided for the former Queen's confinements.

On 29 January, the body of Katherine of Aragon was conveyed to Peterborough with all the trappings of a medieval royal funeral. The chief mourners were Lady Bedingfield, the young Duchess of Suffolk and the Countess of Cumberland, Eleanor Brandon, the King's niece. Chapuys did not attend by choice, 'since they do not mean to bury her as Queen'. The funeral sermon was preached by John Hilsey, who had replaced Fisher as Bishop of Rochester; he was a staunch King's man, and alleged, against all truth, that Katherine had acknowledged at the end that she had never been the rightful Queen of England. Then the woman who had in reality stoutly maintained to the last that she had been the King's wife was buried as Dowager Princess of Wales in the abbey church, later the cathedral. Henry VIII was at Greenwich on that day, and he observed the funeral by wearing black mourning clothes and attending a solemn mass. Anne, however, donned yellow once more, and grumbled because nothing was spoken of that day but the Christian deathbed of her rival.

For more than 200 years, it was believed that Lady Willoughby was afterwards laid to rest in the same tomb as Katherine, and in 1777 an attempt was made to prove this. The grave was opened, yet only one coffin lay within. It was strongly fastened, and to open it was thought sacrilegious. Nevertheless, one curious witness bored a hole through the coffin lid and slid a wire through it, hooking out a fragment of the black and silver brocade robes in which Katherine had been buried. This smelt strongly of embalming fluid, but disintegrated upon exposure to the air. The coffin was then reinterred and has remained undisturbed ever since. Four centuries after Katherine's death, another queen, Mary of Teck, the wife of

George V, gave orders that the symbols of queenship were to be hung above Katherine's resting place, and they may be seen there still, two banners bearing the royal arms of England and Spain. Thus, Katherine has been accorded in death the honours of which she was so cruelly deprived when she was alive.

Mary's reaction to her mother's death is not recorded, but may well be imagined, for in January 1536 she again fell gravely ill, and her life was thought to be in danger. Queen Anne wasted no time in extending an olive branch, and by 21 January had thrown the first bait by inviting her to court, where she would be exempt from carrying the Queen's train and would always walk by her side – but only if she submitted to her father's laws. Mary, however, had no intention of dishonouring her mother's memory by accepting such an offer: there could never be any question of a reconciliation with Anne Boleyn. She intended to take up the cause her mother had been forced to lay down, and carry on the fight to restore herself to her rightful place in the succession. She little knew it, but fate was already on her side.

After Katherine's death, Henry VIII told Chapuys that he desired to renew his former friendship with the Emperor 'now that the cause of our enmity no longer exists', and even asked if Charles V would use his influence to have the papal sentence in Katherine's favour revoked. Charles, of course, would never accede to such an outrageous request, but he too wanted to renew the Anglo-Imperial alliance. However, there were difficulties while Anne Boleyn lived, for the Emperor was reluctant to recognise her as Queen of England, though he might soon have no choice if she were the mother of a male heir to the throne.

On 24 January 1536, during a joust at Greenwich, the King was thrown from his horse and lay for two hours without regaining consciousness. When the Duke of Norfolk broke the news to the Queen, she showed very little concern, even though the Duke told her that most people thought it a miracle that her husband had not been killed. Inwardly, however, Anne must have trembled at the thought of what would become of her if Henry died and left her to fend for herself in a hostile world in which civil war would be a near certainty.

Fortunately the King's strong constitution triumphed, and he was soon up and about again. He would never, however, be a fit man afterwards. The old wound on his leg had reopened and an abscess had formed, which would remain open and suppurating for the rest of his life, in spite of the strenuous efforts of his physicians to heal it. From now on, he would have to wear a dressing and have the leg bound up. At first he adapted well to the disability, refusing to allow it to prevent him from riding and hunting, yet in time it severely curtailed his enjoyment of the sporting activities and dancing that had hitherto meant so much to him. For an active man, it was a cruel blow, and the effect upon Henry's already uncertain temper was disastrous. As his frustration at his enforced inactivity grew, along with the pain he suffered, he would become increasingly subject to savage and unreasonable rages. He was nearly forty-five now, growing bald, and running to fat; as he grew older, he would become more and more addicted to the pleasures of the table, and more and more gross. He would also, with each passing year, become more egotistical, more sanctimonious, and more sure of his own divinity, while still seeing himself as a paragon of courtly and athletic knighthood. The discrepancy between image and reality was one he could not bring himself to face.

In January 1536, this transformation was only just beginning, and the King's self-esteem was such that he regarded himself as the epitome of masculine charm, beauty and virility. He would have been shocked to learn that that virility was shortly to be publicly called into question.

11
Shall I die without justice?

On the day of Queen Katherine's funeral, Chapuys noticed Henry paying marked attention to 'Mrs Semel [*sic*]' and giving her 'very large presents'. During the afternoon, the Queen caught her husband with Jane on his knee, and flew into a frenzy, according to the account given years later by the English Duchess of Feria, who learned of the episode from her mistress Mary Tudor, who, in turn, probably learned of it from Jane Seymour herself. Henry, seeing his wife hysterical and fearing for their child, sent Jane out of the room and hastened to placate Anne. 'Peace be, sweetheart, and all shall go well with thee,' he soothed.

But the damage had been done. That evening, Anne aborted a foetus of about fifteen weeks' growth that had all the appearance of a male. 'She has miscarried of her saviour,' wrote Chapuys. The King in disappointment and sorrow commented, 'I see that God will not give me male children.' In a cold and unforgiving mood he stalked into the Queen's bedchamber, where Anne was sobbing fearfully, and complained about 'the loss of his boy' with many harsh words. Anne burst out that the fault lay with him, because he had been unkind to her, at which Henry flung back that she 'should have no more boys by him'. Seeing him so implacable, Anne forgot all caution, and cried desperately that he had no one to blame but himself for this disappointment, which had been caused by her distress of mind about 'that wench, Jane Seymour'. Breaking down again, she told him, 'Because the love I bear you is so much greater than Katherine's, my heart broke when I saw you loved others.' But she had gone too far. 'I will speak with you when you are well,' said Henry icily, and walked out of the room.

When he had gone, Anne bravely told her ladies it was all for the best: 'I shall be the sooner with child again, and the son I bear will not be doubtful like this one, which was conceived during the life of the Princess Dowager.' Yet she was being over-optimistic, for when Henry had closed the door of her room behind him, he had also closed the door on his second marriage.

There was great speculation at court as to what had caused the Queen's miscarriage. Anne herself blamed Norfolk, claiming the mishap was due to the shock she received when he told her of the King's fall from his horse. Some thought it the result of a defect in her constitution, while others, more perceptive, guessed it had been caused by fear that Henry would treat her as he had Katherine. Chapuys thought this 'not unlikely, considering his behaviour towards a damsel of the court, called Miss Seymour'; Anne's ladies knew that she was temperamentally incapable of ignoring this, as Katherine would have done.

The real reason for the miscarriage may have been that Anne was one of the small minority of people who are rhesus negative and who, during a first pregnancy which results in a healthy child, may produce in the bloodstream a substance called agglutinogen, which destroys rhesus-positive red cells in any subsequent foetus, usually with fatal results. Such a condition was of course unknown in the sixteenth century – it was not identified until 1940 – and could well account for Anne's three miscarriages after the birth of Elizabeth. If so, then she would never have borne another living child.

Cromwell had a secret interview with Chapuys on the evening of 29 January. He was anxious to promote an alliance between England and the Empire, but realised that Anne was a stumbling-block to it. However, he saw the ambassador as a necessary ally in his plan, and was eager to confide in him that the King had just said to him

that he had made this marriage seduced by her witchcraft, and for that reason he considered it null and void, and that this was evident because God did not permit them to have male issue, and that he believed he might take another wife.

'This is incredible!' wrote Chapuys to his master, adding that the Queen had already repented of her hasty words and was 'in great fear'.

Anne's chief concern was that Henry would divorce her, believing this was the worst he could do. But the truth was that Henry did not want any more protracted legal proceedings to end yet another marriage, nor any more disputes about the succession. There had to be another way of removing the Queen. That Henry was accusing Anne of witchcraft, then a capital crime, as early as January 1536, suggests that even then he was probably contemplating her death. Anne's enemies had always made political capital out of her extra fingernail and the moles on her body, calling them devil's teats, and the people of England had long believed her guilty of using the black arts to seduce the King. Yet there was, apart from that, no other evidence, and Henry seems to have abandoned the idea of accusing Anne of witchcraft almost as soon as he had conceived it. However, the seed had been sown, both in his mind and in Cromwell's, and – had Anne but known it – her life was already in danger.

In early February, the estrangement between the royal couple was common knowledge, and speculation was rife. Chapuys thought Jane would make an excellent Queen of England; she was known to have imperialist sympathies, and had openly expressed her support for the Lady Mary. With Jane as queen, there was every hope that Mary might be restored to her former position and to the succession. This was what the ambassador had been told to work towards, and now he saw his chance. He was not without influence or friends at court, and he knew a great many people who secretly supported Mary and who would have been gratified to see the downfall of the Queen. Chapuys now made it his business to form a faction with them and to cultivate a friendship with the ambitious Seymour brothers, who were advising their equally ambitious sister on all her dealings with the King. And as Anne's influence waned, so did this faction brought together by Chapuys gain in strength and confidence.

The King was no fool: he could see which way the wind was blowing, having been told by Chapuys that the Emperor wanted peace in order to preserve the mutually profitable trading links between his people and Henry's. He had also been made aware, by implication, that the removal of Anne would facilitate this. Were she to be sacrificed to pro-imperialist policy, few would speak out in protest, for she was almost universally disliked. The imperialists were aware of this too, and thus Jane Seymour found herself courted, not only by Henry VIII, but also by Anne's enemies and Chapuys's faction. The ambassador advised her to drop heavy hints about Anne's heretical leanings in Henry's ear, and to say that the people of England would never accept her as their true Queen. She must say these things in the presence of her supporters, who would all then swear, on their allegiance to the King, that she spoke the truth. Jane certainly acted upon this advice, and it had the desired effect upon the King, who was now receptive to criticism of his wife. Jane also followed her own instincts, and the advice of her friends, by not admitting Henry to her bed. Instead, she dropped heavy hints about marriage, which fell on fertile ground, and before long Henry began to behave towards her with great circumspection, leading others to believe that he was already considering her as a future wife. From this time on, he took care to avoid any hint of scandal attaching itself to her name; her family and adherents were quick to notice this new deference on the part of the King, and Sir Francis Bryan told Jane's parents that they would shortly see their daughter 'well bestowed' in marriage.

Henry VIII finally made up his mind to rid himself of Anne Boleyn sometime in February 1536. Apart from the fact that their marriage was in ruins, the political situation in Europe made its dissolution highly desirable. Relations between Francis and Charles were deteriorating, and Henry was anxious to secure Charles's friendship. Anne was a bar to this, and would have to go. Chapuys, who had intimated as much to Henry, sounded out Cromwell as to what might happen, and though Cromwell was noncommittal, the ambassador concluded that something was afoot.

It was indeed. Henry left Greenwich for London for the Shrovetide celebrations, taking the unprecedented step of leaving Anne behind. Jane was left behind also, for Henry wanted her out of the way while he plotted the fate of her mistress. A month after her miscarriage, Anne was still grieving over the loss of her son, realising full well that she had lost not only a child but also her husband. Her company consisted of her ladies and her female fool, whose antics did little to alleviate her wretchedness. For the first time, she could appreciate how Katherine had suffered, and she expressed the view that her fate would be the same as the former queen's. She had guessed that Henry was thinking of taking another wife.

Jane Seymour was a continual thorn in Anne's side. Presents and messages from Henry arrived regularly for her, to Anne's disgust, and jealousy made her shrewish. She kept a continual watch on Jane's activities, and on more than one occasion lashed out and slapped her rival, using her prerogative as mistress. When Jane received a locket containing the King's miniature from Henry, and made a great show of opening and shutting it in front of Anne, the Queen reacted violently, ripping the locket from Jane's neck so roughly that she cut her own finger. Anne would dearly have loved to dismiss Jane from her service, but she dared not do so.

On 29 February, Charles V formally instructed Chapuys to begin negotiating an alliance with Henry VIII, and in early March war broke out between Spain and France. The removal of Queen Anne was now a matter of urgency. Chapuys had told the Emperor much about Jane, 'the young lady whose influence increases daily', saying she was a lady of great virtue and kindness, who was known to be sympathetic towards the Lady Mary. 'I will endeavour by all means to make her continue in this vein,' he wrote, although he expressed in the same letter his concern that 'no scorpion lurks under the honey'. Chapuys, too, had sensed that Jane's meek appearance hid an inner toughness.

Henry was finding his absence from Jane unbearable, and it was at this time that an incident occurred that was to change the course of their affair. The King had sent Sir Nicholas Carew from London with a love-letter and a purse of gold for her. Until now, Jane had not scrupled to accept expensive gifts, but even she drew the line at accepting money. Instead, she seized her opportunity to drop a timely hint, hoping to provoke the King into declaring his true intentions. She kissed his letter with great reverence, then handed it back unopened to Sir Nicholas. Then, falling to her knees, she asked him to beg the King on her behalf to consider that she was a prudent gentlewoman of good and honourable family, a woman without reproach who had no greater treasure in this world than her honour, which she would not harm for a thousand deaths. If the King wished to send her a present of money, 'she prayed him to do so when God might send her a husband to marry'.

Henry was delighted with this calculated show of maidenly propriety. 'She has behaved herself in this matter very modestly,' he said, 'and in order to let it be seen that my intentions and affection are honourable, I intend in future only to speak with her in the presence of her relatives.' When he returned to Greenwich, he turfed Cromwell out of his suite of rooms that were connected to Henry's own apartments by a secret gallery and installed there Sir Edward Seymour (who had recently been made a gentleman of the privy chamber) and his wife Anne. It was arranged that Jane would share these rooms with her brother and sister-in-law, and that they would act as chaperons when the King came to pay court to her. But the secret gallery did not remain a secret for long – Chapuys already knew of it by 1 April.

The imperialists supported the idea of a royal divorce, believing that the dissolution of the King's marriage to Anne would mean recognition of the Lady Mary's right to the succession. Charles V urged Chapuys to press for Mary's restoration as her father's heiress: 'It matters not what the wrong done to her late mother may have been.' The ambassador was also to find out Anne Boleyn's views on the matter: the Emperor wanted the alliance with England so much that he was prepared to accept Elizabeth's right to a place in the succession after Mary. Above all, Chapuys was not to dissuade Henry from marrying again. Chapuys, of course, would never have dreamed of doing so. In fact, on 1 April, he learned from Cromwell that Henry was certainly contemplating taking another wife, and that it would not be a Frenchwoman. He guessed then that the King meant to marry Jane Seymour. Jane left Greenwich in April; not only was she distressed by the rumours and lewd ballads about her affair with the King then circulating in London, but Henry also wanted her away from the court while plans were laid for the elimination of the Queen. So Jane returned to Wulfhall, travelling with her brother and his wife.

Anne had spent the early months of 1536 at Greenwich, occupying herself with charitable works, playing with her dogs, and ordering new clothes, including embroidered caps and leading reins, for her little daughter. Her accounts show that she kept the child sumptuously dressed, taking a personal interest in Elizabeth's attire. She rarely saw the King now, and no one would tell her anything while rumours of divorce and annulment abounded. Fear was closing in on her, and her inner turmoil may easily be imagined.

Henry had been pondering the problem of what to do with Anne for some weeks now. He was eager to commit himself without further delay to the proposed imperial alliance, and feared that the Emperor might think him lukewarm if he did not act soon. Then Cromwell's agile mind came up with a solution as fantastic as it was atrocious, which he presented to the King some time in April. He told Henry he had certain suspicions of the Queen as a result of information laid by his spies. His intention was to accuse Anne of a capital crime, such as high treason, and institute proceedings against her. The crime must be such as to inspire not only revulsion for Anne but also sympathy for Henry, and it must be something that would merit divorce as well as death. Given Anne's love of flirtation and her encouragement of the fashioniable cult of courtly love, few would find it hard to believe that, desperate for a child, she had resorted to adultery and even to plotting the death of the King in order to save her own skin.

Adultery in a queen was not high treason at that date: according to the Statute of Treasons of 1351, 'violating the King's companion' was the treasonable act, and therefore only Anne's putative lovers would stand guilty of it. But compassing the death of the King was high treason, and it attracted the death penalty. In presenting this as a possible solution to the King, Cromwell took a risk that Henry would be angry at the suggestion that he had been cuckolded, and at the implied insults to the woman who was still, after all, his wife and the Queen of England. But Henry, spurred by his passion for Jane Seymour, his need of the Spanish alliance, and his desire for vengeance upon Anne, who had promised so much and failed to deliver, accepted the allegations at face value, merely asking Cromwell to find evidence to support them. How seriously the King took the allegations is difficult to judge; outwardly, he behaved as if he were convinced of Anne's guilt. He believed she had lied to him over her chastity before marriage, and he was well aware that she encouraged courtly flirtations with the young men in her circle. But he was also a master of the art of dissimulation, and what is more likely is that he and Cromwell, without ever acknowledging the fact to each other, both knew that they were parties to a plot to do away with an innocent woman for the sake of expediency, and that – for it to succeed – they must appear convinced of her guilt.

All that Henry asked was that the business be over and done with as soon as possible, so that he would be free to marry Jane and make peace with Charles V. Anne must be kept in the dark as much as possible until the last moment: she must not be given time to muster support. Above all, she must be prevented from appealing to Parliament, the supreme court, and accordingly Parliament was dissolved on 14 April. Two days later, Mr Secretary intimated to Chapuys that his master would soon be ready to conclude the alliance with the Emperor. Not knowing what was going on, and having heard nothing more about a divorce, the ambassador steeled himself to make friendly overtures to Queen Anne, as the Emperor had instructed, and on the Tuesday after Easter, when Anne went in procession to chapel, Chapuys bowed low to her, something he had never done before. It was a bitter moment for him, but Anne was gracious, and sank into a deep reverence. Having as a result grounds for hope that Charles V was prepared to acknowledge her title, she went about for the rest of the day loudly proclaiming that she had abandoned her friendship with King Francis and was on the side of the Emperor. But when Chapuys did not appear at a public dinner that evening she grew worried, and asked Henry why he was absent. 'It is not without good reason,' replied her husband sourly. Chapuys did not speak to Anne again: the Lady Mary and others of his faction had been astonished by his behaviour in the chapel, and he felt ashamed.

Meanwhile, Cromwell retired to his house at Stepney, ostensibly because he was ill, but in reality to give him time to compile the 'evidence' against the Queen. He returned to court on 23 April, the same day that Chapuys was telling the Emperor that Henry was 'sick and tired of that she-devil'. The King had also refused Anne's request to admit Rochford to the Order of the Garter.

Cromwell's plans were now complete, and from then on events moved swiftly. On 24 April, the Lord Chancellor appointed a commission of oyer and terminer, consisting of himself, Cromwell, Norfolk, Suffolk and others, which would hold an enquiry into every kind of treason. The King, emphasising his innocence of what was afoot, now behaved as if he meant to continue in his marriage, and on 25 April he wrote to his ambassador in Rome, saying he felt it likely that 'God will send us heirs male [by] our most dear and most entirely beloved wife the Queen'. By now several people were involved in the proceedings against that same dear and most entirely beloved wife. Norfolk had long since been alienated from his niece by her arrogance, and he was prepared to dissociate himself from her: she was too big a liability. Suffolk had never liked her, and Cromwell knew she must go. He alone knew how false the allegations were; the other commissioners were required to accept them at face value, which they did without difficulty.

Anne suspected that something was going on, and on 26 April she charged her chaplain, Matthew Parker, with the care of her daughter Elizabeth if anything happened to her. What she feared she did not say, but her plea made a profound impression upon Parker, and years later, when Elizabeth was queen, he would say he owed her allegiance, not only as her Archbishop of Canterbury, but also because 'he cannot forget what words her Grace's mother said to him not six days before her apprehension'.

Ostensibly, life went on as normal. The King was planning to go with Anne to Calais on 4 May. But before 29 April, the Privy Council had already been informed of the proceedings against the Queen, and there were rumours at court of her imminent disgrace. The Bishop of London, when asked outright if Henry meant to abandon Anne, would say nothing, but his silence was eloquent.

Cromwell's net now closed in around his victims. For some time he had been busy collating the gossip brought to him by his agents, and secretly interviewing the women in the Queen's household. One spy had heard one of the Queen's maids say that Anne 'admitted some of her court to come into her chamber at undue hours', and named Lord Rochford, Sir Henry Norris, Sir Francis Weston, William Brereton and Anne's musician Mark Smeaton in this connection. One young woman, reprimanded by the Countess of

Worcester for flirting, retorted that she was 'no worse than the Queen'. On the basis of such evidence as this Mr Secretary constructed a case. Anne was to be charged with adultery with the five men named, and also with conspiracy to murder the King. The charge of incest with her brother, which was the result of evidence maliciously laid by Lady Rochford, who was jealous of the close bond between Anne and George Boleyn, had been included to make the Queen's crimes seem all the more abominable.

We should pause here to consider Anne's so-called accomplices and ask the question: what were these men to her? Sir Henry Norris was a prominent courtier who had long enjoyed the King's favour, holding the office of Groom of the Stole, which required his attendance when Henry performed his natural functions; Norris was also Chamberlain of North Wales, a position he would not have held had he not enjoyed the King's confidence and trust. William Brereton is more obscure, but he too was a gentleman of the King's privy chamber, and may have been a witness at Anne Boleyn's wedding. Sir Francis Weston was twenty-five, and came from an honourable family whose seat was at Sutton Place in Surrey. Like Brereton, he was a gentleman of the privy chamber, and in 1533 had been one of those admitted to the Order of the Bath at Anne Boleyn's coronation. He was friendly with Henry, Anne and Rochford, played tennis with the King, and cards with Anne and Henry. He was married with a baby son.

The most remarkable inclusion in the list of Anne's supposed lovers was the musician, Mark Smeaton, whose name excited the most comment when the charges were made public. Anne's contemporaries wondered how she could ever have stooped so low. Hence we may conclude that Smeaton was not of gentle birth and had risen so far only on account of his musical talent. Of all the men accused, he would be the only one to admit his guilt, almost certainly under duress: it is possible, but not provable, that he suffered torture. Catholic writers would later make much of Anne's supposed intrigue with Smeaton, and Mary Tudor herself believed that the musician was Elizabeth's real father.

Anne certainly knew all these men except Smeaton well. Yet before April 1536, there is nothing in the records to suggest that her relations with them were anything other than circumspect. She knew her movements were watched, and she was no fool: it is inconceivable that she would have risked her crown and her life for the sake of casual sex with any man who took her fancy. The argument that she was so desperate to conceive a male heir, that she would go to any lengths to become pregnant – the implication being that the King was incapable of siring healthy children – fails when set against the fact that Anne conceived by him four times during their marriage without any difficulty, and that he expressed no doubt at any time that these children were his. As for plotting his death, Anne was well aware that, with Henry dead, her enemies would be out for her blood, and that at the very least she would suffer imprisonment or exile with her child disinherited.

Cromwell, however, felt that he had prepared a watertight case, and on 29 April he laid all the charges, with the accumulated evidence, before the King. As Henry read, he grew livid with fury – as if in fact he believed that Anne's betrayal was genuine. The evidence was enough to arouse jealous anger in any man, but Henry was also King of England and Supreme Head of the Church. He was about to be publicly proclaimed a cuckold – and it was all Anne's fault. He had suspected something of this nature, he said, and now here was proof of it, enough to convince him that he had been right all along to order an investigation. When he calmed down, he gave orders for the arrest of all those named in the charges, including Queen Anne.

Nothing is known of Jane Seymour's involvement in the plot against the Queen. She had been active for months in nurturing Henry's antagonism towards Anne, and she must have known that Henry intended to get rid of his wife before she retired from the political arena. Henry had made it clear he wanted to marry her, and she must have accepted as a necessary preliminary the removal of her rival. Yet even when it became clear that this would not be by divorce or annulment, she did not flinch. All too often Jane Seymour has been seen merely as a willing tool, yet it is clear that she was in fact quite as ambitious and ruthless as her predecessor. She was perceptive, and knew when to speak her mind, a mature woman who knew what she wanted and pursued it with steely single-mindedness. For her former mistress she had no pity whatsoever, and the most charitable thing that can be said about Jane Seymour in this context is that, given that she was ignorant of what the charges for the proceedings against Anne would be, she accepted them as justified when they were laid. Whether it occurred to her that such charges were a little too conveniently timed is another matter.

On Sunday, 30 April, the King – still smarting with anger and humiliation – spent several hours closeted with Cromwell and the Council. The Queen walked her dogs in Greenwich Park, and when she returned to the Palace in the afternoon, she saw crowds gathered outside: word had spread that the Council was meeting that evening to discuss a matter of the utmost urgency, and people had flocked to Greenwich to await news. This alarmed Anne and, sure that the matter about to be debated concerned herself and that it boded ill for her, she gathered up her daughter in her arms for maximum emotional impact and went to find her husband. Alexander Aless, a Protestant divine from Scotland, witnessed their confrontation through a window of the palace, and in 1559 recorded his memories of it in a letter to Elizabeth I:

Alas, I shall never forget the sorrow I felt when I saw the sainted Queen, your most religious mother, carrying you, still a little baby, in her arms, and entreating the most serene King your father in Greenwich Palace, from the open window of which he was looking into the courtyard when she brought you to him. The faces and gestures of the speakers plainly showed the King was angry, though he concealed his anger wonderfully well.

Aless, unfortunately, was out of earshot of the conversation, so we do not know what was said between Henry and Anne; what is certain is that it resolved nothing. And when the Council meeting broke up that evening at eleven o'clock, it was announced that the King would not be going to Calais. No reason was given.

Cromwell was still gathering evidence against his victims. He found out that Smeaton, who only earned £100 per annum, had just spent a great deal of money on horses and liveries for his servants, and that people were wondering where he got the money, the implication being that the Queen had given it to him in return for services rendered. But Smeaton never had the opportunity to flaunt his horses and liveries, for on 30 April he was arrested and taken to Cromwell's house at Stepney for questioning.

One of the best sources for this crucial period is the account of George Constantine, the personal servant of Sir Henry Norris who would share his imprisonment in the Tower. Constantine tells us that Smeaton confessed his guilt, but only, it was thought, after he had been 'grievously racked'. There was no rack at Cromwell's house, but there was one at the Tower, even though torture was illegal. It is likely that Smeaton was racked on arrival at the Tower later that day or the next, and that this provoked his confession. The tale that he was tortured with a knotted cord round his eyes comes from the Spanish Chronicle, which is notoriously inaccurate, written as it was by a Spanish merchant living in London who relied heavily on gossip. His account probably reflects the kind of rumours that would shortly be circulating in the capital rather than what actually happened.

Anne had not noticed Smeaton's absence, and on May Day she took her seat with the King in the stands to watch a great tournament at Greenwich. Two of the contestants were Rochford and Norris, both named in the charges as the Queen's lovers. According to one late and hostile Catholic source, the account of the Jesuit Nicholas Sanders in his book on the origins of the English Reformation, Anne dropped a handkerchief to Norris to wear as a favour, which seemed to confirm the King's suspicions, but this incident is nowhere related in contemporary sources. Henry was in a thunderous mood, and hardly acknowledged Anne's presence; suddenly, without saying anything, he got up and left, leaving her to preside alone over the event, doubtless bewildered and afraid. She could not know it, but she would never see Henry again.

When the jousting ended, the King gave orders for Henry Norris to be arrested; he then departed for Whitehall, with Norris riding beside him so that Henry could question him. Norris was promised a full pardon if he would tell the truth. He had been horrified to learn he was accused of criminal intercourse with the Queen, and vowed to Henry that he would rather die a thousand deaths than be guilty of confessing to a crime he had not committed. Henry was not impressed, and Norris was sent to the Tower the following morning. The King, hearing that he had again protested his innocence to his chaplain, cried, 'Hang him up then!' On that same day, 2 May, Lord Rochford was arrested and also taken to the Tower. This took place so discreetly that few people were aware of it, and certainly not the Queen. When the blow fell, therefore, it took her almost completely by surprise.

On the morning of the 2nd she was watching a game of tennis, vexed with herself for not having laid a bet since her champion was winning, when a messenger arrived with a summons to present herself before the Privy Council. When she arrived in the council chamber, she was confronted by her uncle, Norfolk, Sir William FitzWilliam and Sir William Paulet, all grim-faced. They formally charged her, without preamble, with having committed adultery with Norris, Smeaton and one other, who was not named, and told her that both the men cited had already confessed their guilt, which was not true in the case of Norris. A stunned Anne failed to reply to the charges, and was escorted back to her apartments, there to remain under guard while the Council decided what was to be done with her. Anne did not panic at this stage: queens in the past had been found guilty of adultery, and none had suffered worse than honourable confinement. Besides, she was innocent of the charges. What did concern her was that blameless men were suffering on her account: for herself, she feared nothing worse than divorce, imprisonment or exile, but these men might face death.

Anne was still at dinner when, at two o'clock that afternoon, the door opened to admit Norfolk, Cromwell and Lord Chancellor Audley, accompanied by several lords of the Council. They all bowed. Norfolk held a scroll of parchment in his hand, the warrant for the Queen's arrest. Anne rose and asked why they had come. Her uncle replied that they came by the King's command to conduct her to the Tower, 'there to abide during his Highness's pleasure'. She answered steadily: 'If it be his Majesty's pleasure, I am ready to obey.' There was no time to change her clothes or pack anything – money would be provided for her needs while in the Tower, she was told. She committed herself to the custody of the Privy Council, and was conducted to her barge.

The conveyance of state prisoners to the Tower of London usually took place under cover of darkness, but Anne was taken in broad daylight. It was a nightmare journey. Norfolk took great pleasure in telling her with a good deal of virtuous tut-tutting that her paramours had confessed their guilt. Anne did not respond, but when, at five o'clock, the barge was rowed through the Court Gate – not the Traitors' Gate, as has traditionally been asserted – she was almost at breaking-point, and as she entered the grim fortress, her self-control gave way. At the top of the steps waited the Constable of the Tower, Sir William Kingston, and its Lieutenant, Sir Edmund Walsingham. Kingston would have charge of Anne during her sojourn; he was in his sixties, and knew her well, having often been at the court. He was not an unkind man, but he was somewhat hardened by the duties of his office, and made a point of distancing himself from the prisoners in his care. Towards Anne, he would behave with unfailing courtesy and humanity, becoming, despite his belief in her guilt, secretly impressed by her courage. He had received instructions from Cromwell that everything she said was to be recorded, in the hope that she would incriminate herself, and his reports are preserved in the Cotton MSS. in the Cottonian Library in the British Library, and are a valuable source of information about Anne's stay in the Tower.

When the Queen, in a state of near collapse, had been assisted from her barge and up the steps, she sank to her knees on the cobblestones, praying God to help her as she 'was not guilty of her accusement'. She begged the Privy Councillors, before they departed, to 'beseech the King's Grace to be good unto her'. Then she cried, 'Mr Kingston, do I go into a dungeon?' 'No, Madam,' he replied, 'you shall go into the lodging you lay in at your coronation.' 'It is too good for me!' sobbed Anne. 'Jesu, have mercy on me!' And she sank to her knees again, 'weeping a great pace, and in the same sorrow fell into a great laughing', behaviour she would exhibit many times during the early days of her imprisonment. Kingston helped her up once more, but she was distraught, repeating again and again, 'I am the King's true wedded wife! Oh, my mother, my mother!' Then, calming down, she declared: 'My God, bear witness there is no truth in these charges. I am as clear from the company of man as from sin.' She asked Kingston if she might have the Holy Sacrament placed in her bedchamber, 'that I may pray for mercy'. Already, she was beginning to suspect the worst.

Kingston now led her away. 'I was received with greater

ceremony the last time I entered here,' she remarked. The royal apartments were on the east side of the inner ward between the Lanthorn Tower, the White Tower, and the Wardrobe Tower. Very little is known about them. The Tower had been a royal palace since Norman times, but by the reign of Henry VIII it was considered old-fashioned and uncomfortable. Cromwell put in hand renovations in the early 1530s for Anne Boleyn's coronation, and the works carried out then are shown on a plan of the Tower dated 1597, by which time the old great hall would be crumbling. The royal apartments did not long survive it, which suggests that Cromwell's improvements were mainly cosmetic. The Queen's lodging comprised a presence chamber, a dining chamber, a bedchamber, and a garden. It was to these rooms that Anne was conducted on 2 May 1536.

There, she found waiting for her three ladies-in-waiting, one of whom was Margaret Wyatt, Lady Lee, the poet's sister, who had probably known Anne since childhood; her old nurse, Mrs Orchard, and a Mrs Stonor; two male servants and a boy. There were also four ladies whose duty was to inform on her: her aunt Elizabeth, wife of Sir James Boleyn; Lady Shelton, another aunt, who had formerly had charge of the Lady Mary; Mary, Lady Kingston, wife of the Constable; and Mrs Cosyn, wife of Anne's master-of-horse, William Cosyn. There was no love lost between Anne and these ladies, and she realised at once why they were there, telling Kingston she thought it 'a great unkindness in the King to set such about me as I never loved. I would fain have had mine own Privy Chamber, whom I favour most.' Kingston replied that 'the King took them to be honest and good women.' Privately, he agreed with Henry's choice, for these ladies could tell Anne nothing of her father or brother, or anything else; the King wanted her kept in ignorance of the evidence against her in the hope that she would reveal information that could be used to incriminate her.

Left alone with her attendants, Anne could not stop talking. She ate 'a great dinner', and soon afterwards called for supper. Lady Boleyn taunted her that her love of intrigue had brought her where she was, and at the end of the evening Lady Kingston and Mrs Cosyn made their report to the Constable. Anne, meanwhile, was working herself into another frenzy, saying she was 'cruelly handled at Greenwich'. She summoned Kingston, and asked him outright if he knew why she was there. He reminded her of the charges against her, saying that another name had been added to the list of her accomplices, but she answered, with spirit, 'I hear I shall be accused with four men, and I can say no more but Nay, without I should open my body!' And, with a dramatic gesture, she opened wide the overskirt of her gown: 'They can bring no witnesses.' Kingston lied that Norris had confessed his guilt. 'Oh, Norris, hast thou accused me?' she wailed. 'Thou art in the Tower with me, and thou and I shall die together! And Mark, thou art here too.' And she wept, 'Oh, my mother, thou wilt die with sorrow.' Then she turned to Kingston, and her next question showed that she understood very well how grave her situation was: 'Master Kingston, shall I die without justice?' He replied: 'The poorest subject of the King hath justice.' Anne laughed hysterically at this, knowing well that those charged with capital offences were rarely acquitted.

Anne would have been even more horrified had she known just how desperate Henry was to be rid of her. Not only was he planning to have her executed for high treason, but he had ordered Cranmer on the day of her arrest to find grounds for annulling his marriage to her. Once Anne was dead, there must be no impediment to Jane's children taking precedence in the order of succession.

News of the Queen's arrest had spread around the court by the evening of 2 May. Chapuys learned of it with relief, seeing Anne's fall as a manifestation of divine vengeance for all the wrongs she had inflicted upon Katherine and Mary. Nor did he have any difficulty at this stage in believing the charges against her, predicting that the outcome of the affair would be her execution. Indeed, there was little doubt in anyone's mind that this would be Anne's fate. When the people learned she was in the Tower, they were unmoved, believing her guilty as charged. No one spoke up in her favour. Nevertheless, Henry refrained from going out in public while Anne was in the Tower. His only sorties out of the palace were into the gardens and on evening trips by barge to visit Jane, who had just returned from Wulfhall and was temporarily staying at an unknown lodging.

By now Henry had convinced himself that Anne had been a monster of lechery. He remembered her ruthlessness in hounding Wolsey to his death, how she had more or less admitted her involvement in the plot to poison Fisher, and how she had urged him to have Katherine and Mary executed or murdered. Henry had heard the rumours that Katherine had died of poison, and was now convinced that Anne had been responsible. When Henry FitzRoy, Duke of Richmond came to bid his father goodnight on the evening after Anne's arrest, Henry embraced him and wept as he told him that he and his half-sister Mary ought to thank God for escaping 'that cursed and venomous whore, who tried to poison you both'. There was no evidence for this, but Henry was prepared to believe that no crime was too monstrous to have been committed by Anne. And when Richmond died of consumption the following July, Henry and most other people would believe that Anne had administered a slow-working poison which caused his death.

The Lady Mary learned of the Queen's arrest on the following day from Chapuys, who boasted that he had been instrumental in bringing it about. Mary instructed him to join forces with Cromwell and the many other people who were working for the advancement of Jane Seymour; Chapuys had, of course, been doing this for months already.

One person who did feel sorrow on behalf of Anne was Cranmer, who wrote to the King to express his sorrow and loyalty.

> My mind is clean amazed [he wrote], for I never had better opinion of woman, but I think your Highness would not have gone so far if she had not been culpable. I loved her not a little for the love which I judged her to bear towards God and the Gospel. Next unto your Grace, I was most bound unto her of all creatures living.

He hoped and prayed she would declare her innocence. 'I am exceedingly sorry that such faults can be proved by the Queen,' ended Cranmer, 'but I am, and ever shall be, your faithful subject.' He would now go on to do exactly as the King bade him: against his sense of self-preservation, his long-standing affection for Anne counted for very little.

In the Tower, Anne learned of her brother's arrest, and declared that Norris and Rochford would vindicate her. After a night in prison she still veered from black despair to buoyant confidence and back again, as panic took her: 'One hour she is determined to die, and the next hour much contrary to that,' Kingston told Cromwell. Anne could not stop talking about the men accused with her. She told Mrs Cosyn she had made Norris swear to her almoner that she was a good woman, for she had teased him about delaying his marriage, saying he looked for dead men's shoes, 'for if aught came to the King, you would look to have me!' Norris, shocked, had denied this, but Anne had feared that her remarks had been overheard and could be misconstrued, so she made him swear to her virtue. Mrs Cosyn then deliberately let slip that Sir Francis Weston was being questioned by the Privy Council about his relationship with the Queen. Anne expressed some apprehension about what he would say, as he had told her on Whit Monday that Norris 'came more into her chamber for her sake than for Madge Shelton's [his mistress]'. Weston himself had been asked teasingly by Anne if he loved Madge, and he had replied that 'he loved one in her house better than [Madge or his wife]', which was the correct courtly answer to such a question. 'Who?' the Queen had asked. 'It is yourself,' he replied. This was all grist to Cromwell's mill, for, taken literally, it could prove very damaging indeed.

Anne's fragile confidence would have been shattered had she known that her husband was already planning his wedding to Jane Seymour. On 4 May, Jane took up temporary residence at Beddington Park, the Surrey home of Sir Nicholas Carew, a magnificent house built in 1500 and set in a large park; the great hall, on which the one at Hampton Court is said to have been modelled, still survives today. Here, Henry could visit Jane discreetly. His visits took place under cover of darkness, though nothing improper occurred; the royal swain had insisted on Jane's parents and brother Edward being present when he came courting. He was taking no chances with Jane's reputation: no one would ever be able to accuse her of light behaviour in the years to come.

Chapuys tells us that it was during one of these visits that Jane brought up the delicate subject of Mary, daring to say that when she was queen she hoped to see Mary reinstated as heir apparent. This irritated Henry, who told her she was a fool, who 'ought to solicit the advancement of the children they would have together, and not any others'. Jane replied that she did think of them, but also of Henry's peace of mind, for unless he showed justice to Mary,

Englishmen would never be content. Jane intended to have her own way over Mary, and she would not give up easily.

On the day that Jane arrived at Beddington, Sir Francis Weston and William Brereton, having failed to convince the Council of their innocence, were taken to the Tower, Brereton having previously confided to George Constantine that 'there was no way but one with any matter alleged against him', meaning that he was innocent. The next day, Friday, 5 May, saw the last arrests, those of Sir Thomas Wyatt and Sir Richard Page. Neither was ever charged, and it is probable that Cromwell had never intended that they should be: if two of those accused with the Queen were allowed to go free, it would underline the guilt of the rest. Wyatt was a natural choice, as his earlier love for Anne was well known. As for Page, nothing is known of him.

Of the prisoners in the Tower, Rochford showed the most agitation. 'When shall I come before the King's Council?' he asked Kingston. 'I think I shall not come forth till I come to my judgement.' Then he burst into tears. Anne was glad that she and her brother were under the same roof. Yet when she was told of the arrests of Weston, Brereton, Wyatt and Page, she burst out laughing uncontrollably at the absurdity of it all. She showed no compassion for Smeaton when told he was manacled in irons, saying only that he 'was a person of mean birth, and the others were all gentlemen'. Smeaton, she said, had only once been in her chamber, and that was at Winchester the previous year, when she had sent for him to play the virginals for her; nothing improper had happened then, and the only other time she could remember having spoken to the musician was the previous Saturday, when she had chided him for aspiring to a courtly flirtation with her: 'You may not look to have me speak to you as I would do to a nobleman, because you are an inferior person.' 'No, no, a look sufficeth!' Smeaton had protested, and that was the end of the matter.

Anne told Kingston that if her bishops were with the King, they would all speak for her. In fact, their silence had been deafening. Of her imprisonment she said, 'I think the King does it to prove me,' and according to Kingston, 'did laugh withal, and was very merry'. But the merriment did not last, and she was soon weeping again, saying, 'My lord my brother will die!'

Henry VIII moved to Hampton Court on Saturday, 6 May, and set in train preparations for his wedding to Jane Seymour. In a high good humour, he had his hair cropped, where hitherto he had worn it long over his ears; Anne had liked him clean-shaven, thus he was also growing a beard, which he would never again shave off.

The legal process against the Queen began on 10 May when the Grand Jury of Middlesex found a True Bill against the accused on all the charges. On the following day, the Grand Jury of Kent did likewise. The case could now proceed to trial. The indictment drawn up by Cromwell was formidable. It asserted that Queen Anne, 'despising her marriage and entertaining malice against the King, and following daily her frail and carnal lust', had procured by various base means many of the King's servants to be her adulterers. Rochford, Norris, Weston, Brereton and Smeaton were named as those who had succumbed to her 'vile provocations'. Twenty separate offences were listed, yet the indictment also mentioned other unspecified ones, 'on divers days before and after 6 October 1533', something that Anne would have found very difficult to disprove – or the Crown to prove, for that matter. Nor had Cromwell checked his facts: some of the offences could not have been committed at all, because Anne was nowhere near the man in question at the time, or, on at least five occasions, was heavily pregnant. Mark Smeaton is described as 'a person of low degree', as if to emphasise how far the Queen had stooped for her pleasure, and over her alleged incestuous affair with Rochford, said to have begun in November 1534, the indictment bristled with righteous outrage, saying that Anne had 'procured her own natural brother to violate her, alluring him with her tongue in his mouth, and his tongue in hers, against the commands of Almighty God and all laws human and divine'. The charge of incest was meant to inspire horror and revulsion, but thanks to George Boleyn's testimony at his trial, it failed; it was the alleged affair with Smeaton that captured the public's imagination, and provided endless copy for writers throughout the sixteenth century.

The indictment also alleged that, from October 1534 onwards, the Queen and her lovers, jointly and severally, had plotted the King's death, Anne having promised to marry one of them afterwards; she had also told them 'she would never love the King in her heart'.

Henry, it concluded, had taken the news of this treachery so badly that 'certain harms and perils have befallen his royal body'. It must be said that none of these harms and perils was at all evident.

No mention had been made in the indictment of Wyatt and Page. In fact, Cromwell had already secretly informed Wyatt's father that his son would not be harmed, for the old man wrote to him on 11 May, saying that neither he nor his son would ever forget Mr Secretary's kindness.

On Friday, 12 May, the Duke of Norfolk, as High Steward of England, presided over the trial of Norris, Weston, Brereton and Smeaton at Westminster Hall. The Queen and Lord Rochford would be tried separately by their peers, a privilege reserved for the aristocracy only; their trials were set for the following Monday.

The accused men were brought by river to Westminster. Few details survive of the proceedings. Witnesses were called, and one member of the jury, Sir John Spelman, related that some were ladies of the court who testified to such promiscuity on the part of the Queen that it was said in court that there was 'never such a whore in the realm'. One witness repeated the words of a deceased Lady Wingfield, which was hearsay. At the end of it all, the jury returned a verdict of guilty, and the four men were condemned by Lord Chancellor Audley to be drawn, hanged, castrated and quartered. Chapuys says that Brereton was 'condemned on a presumption, not by proof or valid confession, and without any witnesses'. Most courtiers reacted to the verdict with sorrow, especially on behalf of Norris and Weston, both popular and respected men. Weston's family made frantic attempts to save his life, and on 13 May it was rumoured that he might escape the death sentence. But Lord Hussey, writing to Lord Lisle on 12 May, was of the opinion that all would suffer death, even the Queen and Rochford; Anne, he said, deserved it, for her crimes had been 'so abominable' that he prayed God would give her grace to repent.

The condemnation of the four men could not but presage an unfavourable outcome of Anne's own trial and that of her brother. Her reaction to the news of their sentence is unrecorded. Equally ominous was the dissolution of her household at Greenwich, by the King's command, on Saturday, 13 May, when her servants were discharged from their allegiance. Obviously her trial would be a mere formality.

On 14 May, Cromwell wrote to all England's ambassadors abroad, informing them of the action taken against the Queen and the judgement on the men accused with her: 'She and her brother shall be arraigned tomorrow,' he wrote, 'and will undoubtedly go the same way. I write no particularities, the things be so abominable.' Abroad, it was shrewdly concluded by some that the King had invented the whole thing to get rid of Anne, though her reputation was so poor that there were also a great many people who believed Henry's actions justified.

On the same day, Henry decided he could no longer live without Jane, and recalled her to London, where he installed her in the house of Sir Francis Bryan on the Strand, one mile from Whitehall, where he himself was now in residence. Here, Jane had her first taste of what it would be like to be a queen, being housed in great splendour, attired in rich garments, and waited on by the King's officers and servants, all wearing splendid liveries. She seems to have accepted her sudden elevation with complacent calm, wasting no pity on the woman she would shortly supplant. Indeed, she was awaiting the result of Anne's trial with barely concealed impatience.

Preparations for that trial, which would be held in the great hall of the Tower, had been made over the weekend. A raised platform was erected in the centre, around which were placed rows of benches, enough to accommodate the estimated 2,000 spectators who would be present. Chairs were provided for the twenty-six peers who would act as judges, and the Duke of Norfolk, as High Steward of England, was given a throne under a cloth of estate, for he represented the King. The hall has long since been demolished, but the seating placed there for the trial was still in existence in 1778.

This was the scene that greeted Anne when she was escorted into the court by Sir Edmund Walsingham, Sir William Kingston, Lady Boleyn, and the chief executioner, with his axe turned away from her. Her entry was impressive; she presented herself at the bar with considerable dignity, curtsying to the judges and looking about her without any sign of fear, as if she had been attending some great state occasion. Gone was the hysteria, the violent mood swings; Anne was now reconciled to the inevitability of death, but she was resolved not to go down without a fight. Cromwell, knowing this, was very tense before the trial, fearing that Anne's wit and courage would undermine his case and even secure an acquittal, something he found too awful to contemplate. Far too much was at stake, including his own neck.

When Anne was seated in a chair on the platform in the centre of the court, the indictment was read in all its detail. Her face, however, betrayed no emotion, even when another charge was added, that of having poisoned the late Queen Katherine and attempting to do the same to the Lady Mary. Instead, she listened patiently, then answered clearly to each charge, refuting them all firmly, and arguing her case with such clarity and good sense that her innocence, which she protested vehemently, seemed manifest to many of those watching her.

Nevertheless, when the twenty-six peers were asked to give their judgement upon the Queen, every one pronounced her guilty. Anne stood unmoved as they each rose in turn to give their verdict, carrying herself as if she was receiving some great honour. Outside, the people in the crowds that had gathered were telling each other incorrectly that Anne had cleared herself by a wise and noble speech.

Norfolk now pronounced sentence. However poor relations between him and his niece had been in recent months, family feeling took precedence at this point, and he wept as he addressed her:

> Because thou hast offended our sovereign lord the King's Grace in committing treason against his person, the law of the realm is this: that thou shall be burnt here within the Tower of London on the Green, else to have thy head smitten off, as the King's pleasure shall be further known of the same.

There was a shriek from the gallery as Anne's old nurse, Mrs Orchard, gave way to hysterics. The Earl of Northumberland fainted, and had to be helped out – he was already mortally ill, and died some months later. But Anne received the sentence calmly, raising her eyes and saying, 'O Father, O Creator, Thou who art the Way, the Life, and the Truth, knowest whether I have deserved this death.' She said she was prepared to die, but was extremely sorry that others, innocent as she, should die through her. She believed she had been condemned for reasons other than the causes alleged, and swore she had always been faithful to the King, although

> I do not say I have always shown him that humility which his goodness to me merited. I confess I have had jealous fancies and suspicions of him, which I had not discretion enough, and wisdom, to conceal. But God knows, and is my witness, that I have not sinned against him in any other way. Think not I say this in the hope to prolong my life. God hath taught me how to die, and He will strengthen my faith. As for my brother, and those others who are unjustly condemned, I would willingly suffer many deaths to deliver them, but since I see it pleases the King, I shall willingly accompany them in death, with this assurance, that I shall lead an endless life with them in peace.

Finally, she asked for time in which to prepare her soul for death. An anonymous Frenchman who was present recorded that her speech made even her bitterest enemies pity her.

Anne was then escorted from the court by the Constable, attended by Lady Kingston and Lady Boleyn, and the executioner with his axe turned towards her, signifying that she was condemned to die. After her departure, a buzz of conversation broke out, and the Lord Mayor expressed the opinion that 'he could observe nothing in the proceedings against her but that they were resolved to make an occasion to get rid of her'. Even Chapuys felt that Anne had been condemned upon a presumption and 'without valid proof or confession', and George Constantine told Cromwell 'there was much muttering of Queen Anne's death'.

After her condemnation, Anne was not taken back to the royal apartments, but was lodged instead in rooms in the Lieutenant's house (afterwards known as the Queen's House), a half-timbered building between the Bloody Tower and the Bell Tower. It was much altered in 1540, and has been restored since, but the first floor bedroom occupied by Anne still exists, with its linenfold panelling and stone fireplace, dominated by a great four-poster bed, and overlooking Tower Green (or East Smithfield Green, as it was then known) and the Royal Chapel of St Peter ad Vincula, which had not then acquired the reputation Macaulay gave it as 'the saddest spot on earth'.

There was no longer any need for the women to inform on Anne, and Mrs Cosyn was discharged at this point. She was replaced, at Anne's request, by her own niece, Katherine Carey, who was seven years old; it was not thought unsuitable in those days to expose such a young child to the realities of suffering and death.

Jane Seymour did not show herself in public on the day of the trial. She was much agitated about its outcome, and waited with her parents for news. Chapuys, who attended, had promised to tell them about it. In the morning, Jane had received a note from the King, telling her that at three o'clock she would hear of the condemnation of the Queen from Sir Francis Bryan, and this was exactly what did happen, to Jane's intense relief.

Rochford's trial followed that of his sister. The evidence for incest rested solely upon the fact that he had once been closeted for a long time alone with Anne. Chapuys says that Rochford's 'wicked wife' supplied this information, and the French poet Lancelot de Carles, a witness at the trial, quotes Rochford as saying, 'On the evidence of only one woman, you are prepared to believe this great evil of me.' Other witnesses felt that Lady Rochford had acted more out of envy and jealousy than loyalty to the King.

Rochford was also charged with having expressed doubts that Elizabeth was the King's daughter. He made no answer to this, but to the other charges he replied so well that bets were being laid on his acquittal. And he would perhaps have escaped the death penalty, had it not been for a letter from his wife, produced in court at the last minute and containing details of the 'accursed secret' he shared with the Queen. Again he denied these allegations eloquently and sensibly, confessing to nothing. There was one tense moment when he was handed a piece of paper on which was written a statement he had allegedly made to the effect that the King was impotent. This was too sensitive to be read out in court, and Rochford sealed his fate when he declared that he would not 'create suspicion in a manner likely to prejudice the issue the King might have from a second marriage', thereby implying what had been written and creating a sensation in court. 'I did not say it!' he cried, but it was too late. The twenty-six peers found him guilty by a unanimous decision, and Norfolk sentenced him to the full horrors of a traitor's death. Had he not been so proud, wrote Sir Thomas Wyatt, every man would have bemoaned his fate, if only for his great wit, but Rochford had alienated so many with his arrogance that few spoke up in his favour, although there were many who admired his courage at his trial.

The King, and most of his subjects, thought the sentences entirely justified. Told of Anne's spirited defence, Henry replied, 'She hath a stout heart, but she shall pay for it!' To celebrate the verdicts, he held a lavish river pageant, then went to supper at the house of the Bishop of Carlisle, where he produced a book he had written entitled *The Tragedy about Anne*. 'For a long time I foresaw this,' he said. Chapuys was present at that supper, and offered Henry his commiserations on the Queen's treachery. Henry answered complacently that many great men had suffered from the arts of wicked women, and he did not appear unduly upset. Then he left for the Strand, where he dined late with Jane on food prepared by his own cooks.

On 16 May, Chapuys noticed more and more courtiers going to pay their respects to Jane, while in the Strand the common people waited to catch a glimpse of her. Yet the ambassador was cynical: he thought the King 'may well divorce her when he tires of her'. Nor was Jane universally popular, for scurrilous ballads about her were circulating in London, which the King tried in vain to suppress; a letter he sent to her at this time, the only one to survive from their courtship, refers to this:

My dear friend and mistress,
The bearer of these few lines from thy entirely devoted servant will deliver into thy fair hands a token of my true affection for thee, hoping you will keep it for ever in your sincere love for me. There is a ballad made lately of great derision against us; I pray you pay no manner of regard to it. I am not at present informed who is the setter forth of this malignant writing, but if he is found out, he shall be straitly punished for it. Hoping shortly to receive you into these arms, I end for the present
Your own loving servant and sovereign,

H. R.

On the day after Anne's trial, Kingston wrote to ask Cromwell, 'What is the King's pleasure touching the Queen, as for the preparation of scaffolds and other necessaries?' Neither he nor Anne knew as yet whether she was to be burned or beheaded, or even when. In fact, Henry was waiting for Cranmer to declare his marriage to Anne null and void. The Archbishop had been studying the relevant documents, but had faced severe difficulty in finding grounds for an annulment. Northumberland had angrily reaffirmed that there had never been a precontract between him and Anne. Nor dared Cranmer imply that the King's marriage to Katherine of Aragon had not been lawfully annulled. In the end, he seems to have found a legal loophole in connection with the King's liaison with Mary Boleyn, which had placed Henry and Anne within the forbidden degrees of affinity. The Pope had issued in 1528 a dispensation permitting them to marry when Henry was free, yet the 1534 Act of Supremacy had decreed that existing papal dispensations would no longer be held as valid if they were contrary to Holy Scripture and the law of God. Cranmer probably applied this ruling to the bull dispensing with Henry's relationship with Mary Boleyn, which meant that his marriage to Anne was incestuous and invalid; and in July 1536, Parliament would declare it void because of 'certain just, true and unlawful impediments' that were not known of when it was contracted.

On 16 May, Cranmer visited the Tower to offer some spiritual consolation to Anne and administer the Holy Sacrament. He also required the Queen's consent to the annulment of her marriage; she had her daughter's rights to consider, and had she disputed it the proceedings could have been very protracted. It may be that Cranmer offered her the easier death in return for her co-operation; even more probable is the likelihood that he held out the possibility of her being reprieved and sent into exile as bait, for when he left she was much more cheerful and told her ladies that 'she was to be banished', and thought she might be sent to a nunnery at Antwerp. This in itself would have been enough to make her agree to everything Cranmer asked of her, even to abandoning her child's claim to the succession and condemning her to a lifetime marred by the stigma of bastardy.

The King had commuted the sentence on the condemned men to decapitation; the *Lisle Letters* make it clear that all of them, even

Smeaton, died by the axe on the scaffold on Tower Hill, and not at Tyburn. They were told by Kingston on the evening of 16 May that they must prepare for death on the morrow. Rochford took it well, although he was worried that his debts had not been cleared. Kingston promised to raise the matter with Cromwell. Weston spent his last evening writing a farewell letter to his parents, asking them and his wife to forgive him all the wrongs he had done them, and calling himself 'a great offender to God'. Brereton's wife certainly believed her husband to be innocent, and kept the gold bracelet he sent her as a parting gift for their son in memory of his father.

The executions of the men took place early in the morning of Wednesday 17 May before large crowds. The Queen was taken beforehand to the Bell Tower, whose windows overlooked Tower Hill, so that she might watch them die; according to Chapuys, this greatly 'aggravated her grief'. The condemned men all died 'charitably'. Rochford mounted the scaffold first, and made a long and pious speech of which there are three versions. According to the chronicler Charles Wriothesley, he said, 'Trust in God, and not in the vanities of the world, for if I had so done, I think I had been alive as ye be now.' He prayed that God would give the King a long and good life, then submitted to the axe. Weston followed: 'I thought little I would come to this,' he lamented. Then it was Norris's turn: he bravely declared that, 'in his conscience, he thought the Queen innocent of these things laid to her charge, and he would die a thousand deaths rather than ruin an innocent person.' Brereton died next. 'If any of them were innocent,' wrote George Constantine, 'it was he.' Only Smeaton was left. 'Masters,' he faltered, from a scaffold awash with blood, 'I pray you all pray for me, for I have deserved the death.' Within seconds, his head and body had joined the others in a cart standing beside the scaffold, which carried them back to St Peter ad Vincula within the Tower. Rochford was buried inside the chapel, and the rest in the adjacent churchyard, Weston and Norris in one grave, Brereton and Smeaton in the other. The heads were buried with the bodies, for the King had decided not to display them on poles above London Bridge, as was usually the case with those executed for treason.

Meanwhile, the Queen, much shaken, had returned to the Lieutenant's house. There was now no doubt in her mind that she would shortly follow the men to the scaffold, and all that concerned her now was to clear her name and prepare her soul for death. When Kingston came to tell her she must die the following morning, she asked him if any of those just executed had protested her innocence, and he told her that only Smeaton had confessed he deserved death. This upset Anne, and she cried,

> Alas! Has he not then cleared me of the public shame he has brought me to? Alas, I fear his soul suffers for his false accusations! But for my brother and those others, I doubt not but they are now in the presence of that Great King before whom I am to be tomorrow.

Kingston was now able to tell Anne that she would not die at the stake, but suffer a quicker death by decapitation, and that the King, to ensure a swift and painless end for the woman he had once loved, had sent to St Omer in France for a headsman whose expertise in cutting off heads with a sword was renowned. The man was already on his way.

During the afternoon of 17 May, Archbishop Cranmer convened a court at Lambeth for the purpose of annulling the King's marriage to Anne Boleyn. Anne was represented by her proctor, Dr Nicholas Wotton, and it was he who heard Cranmer pronounce that her union with the King was invalid and therefore null and void, and her daughter a bastard. Afterwards, it was announced publicly that Anne had never been the lawful Queen of England. She would go to the scaffold as Lady Marquess of Pembroke.

On the green outside her window she could see workmen erecting a high scaffold, for which they would be paid £23. 6s. 8d. They continued working through the night in order to have it ready by nine o'clock the next morning, the time set for Anne's execution. It was practically impossible for Anne and her ladies to sleep. At 2.0 a.m. Anne's chaplain arrived, and she spent the rest of the night praying with him. Cranmer came to the Tower soon after dawn on 18 May, as he had promised, to hear Anne's last confession and administer Holy Communion. She sent for Kingston, that he might be present when she 'received the good Lord', and also so that he could hear her declare her innocence before God. He later informed the King that, both before and after receiving the Sacrament, Anne swore on the damnation of her soul that 'she had never been unfaithful to her lord and husband'. Her ladies, who were also present, repeated this to Chapuys, who reported to the Emperor that 'the Concubine' had affirmed that she had 'never offended with her body against the King'.

Shortly before nine o'clock, Kingston received word from Cromwell that the headsman had been delayed on the Dover road and would not be at the Tower until noon. Anne, who had steeled herself to face death that morning, was 'very sorry' to hear this, 'as I thought to be dead before this time, and past my pain'. Kingston told her 'it should be no pain, it was so subtle', to which she replied, 'I have heard say the executioner was very good, and I have a little neck.' And she put her hands around it, 'laughing heartily'. Kingston told Cromwell he had seen many men and women executed who had been in great sorrow, 'but, to my knowledge, this lady hath much joy and pleasure in death'. Kingston then cleared the Tower of foreigners, since the King would allow only his own subjects to witness Anne's execution. The Constable advised Cromwell to keep the time of the event a secret in order to avoid crowds of Londoners coming to watch, for he supposed 'she will declare herself to be a good woman for all men but the King at the hour of her death'.

When noon came, the executioner had still not arrived, and Kingston had to tell Anne that her ordeal would be prolonged until nine o'clock the next morning. She was visibly shaken by the news. It was not that she desired death, she said, but she thought herself prepared to die, and feared the delay might weaken her resolve. But somehow she got through the next hours, spending most of the time at prayer and the rest in conversation with her ladies, telling them she blamed Chapuys for what had befallen her. Chapuys later said he was glad to know that 'the English Messalina' had held him accountable for her doom. 'I was flattered by the compliment, for she would have cast me to the dogs!'

Meanwhile, at Lambeth, on 18 May, Cranmer issued a dispensation permitting the King's marriage to Jane Seymour even though the parties were within the forbidden degrees of affinity, for Jane's grandmother, Elizabeth Neville, was a cousin of Henry's great grandmother Cicely Neville, Duchess of York. Henry's behaviour during the days leading up to Anne's execution astonished everybody. Displaying great *joie de vivre*, he was, Chapuys tells us, 'Out to dinner, here, there and everywhere with the ladies,' returning along the river after midnight to the sound of music and singing. The Bishop of Carlisle, who had once again hosted a dinner for his king, afterwards told Chapuys that Henry had 'behaved with almost desperate gaiety'. The ambassador thought that the King's rejuvenation sprang from 'hope of change, a thing especially agreeable to this king', and the prospect of 'getting soon a fine horse to ride'. Regarding Anne, whom Chapuys referred to as 'that thin old woman', Henry now believed that more than a hundred men had slept with her, 'but you never saw a prince or husband make greater show or wear his horns more patiently and lightly than this one does. I leave you to imagine why.'

Chapuys noted that Wyatt and Page were still in the Tower, but once Anne had been disposed of they would be freed, Wyatt upon his father's surety of his good behaviour, and Page on condition that he never again came near the King or the court.

Henry spent the evening of 18 May at the Strand with Jane Seymour, who was richly dressed and already carrying herself like a queen. Chapuys thought her behaviour 'very commendable' at this time. It is tempting to wonder how often her thoughts dwelt upon her predecessor, who was now languishing only a mile away downriver, waiting for death.

Anne could not sleep that night. She prayed, and talked with her ladies. She was quite calm, and at times almost cheerful, saying that those people who thought up nicknames for royalty would be able to call her Queen Anne Lackhead after her death, managing to laugh as she spoke. Chapuys was later gratified to hear that Anne thought her execution was a divine judgement upon her for having treated the Lady Mary so badly, and for having conspired her death. 'No person ever showed greater willingness to die,' the ambassador wrote. Robbed of everything she held dear in the world, Anne was now eager to leave it, placing her hope and trust in the deity she so firmly believed in.

Alexander Aless, the Scots reformer, was still in London. For some days, he had remained indoors, so knew nothing of the outcome of Anne's trial. On the night of 18–19 May, he had a terrible nightmare, dreaming that he beheld the severed head of Queen Anne with its vertebrae, arteries and veins exposed in all their bloody horror. Much troubled by this, he rose early in the morning and made his way to Lambeth Palace, where he encountered the Archbishop in the gardens. Cranmer looked unutterably sad, and Aless asked what was troubling him. 'Do you not know what is to happen today?' asked Cranmer, sighing. 'She who has been the Queen of England on earth will today become a queen in Heaven.' And he sat down on a bench and wept, as Aless realised with a jolt what his dream had foretold.

At nine o'clock on Friday, 19 May 1536, Kingston appeared at the door to Anne's rooms. 'Madam, the hour approaches,' he said; 'you must make ready.' Anne answered fearlessly: 'Acquit yourself of your charge, for I have been long prepared.' He gave her a purse containing £20.00, so that she could pay the headsman for his services and distribute alms for the poor, then escorted her, her ladies following, down the stairs and out into the May sunshine where a small contingent of the Yeomen of the King's Guard awaited to conduct the prisoner to the scaffold.

A crowd of two or three thousand people had gathered around the scaffold, which was now draped with black cloth and strewn with straw. Cromwell, his son Gregory (soon to marry Jane Seymour's widowed sister Elizabeth), Lord Chancellor Audley and the ailing Duke of Richmond were all present, as was the Duke of Suffolk, but Norfolk had stayed away.

A great murmur rose from the crowd as Anne Boleyn advanced on her short walk to Tower Green. She wore a robe of dark grey or black damask, trimmed with fur, with a low square neck and a crimson kirtle; from her shoulders flowed a long white cape. She looked exhausted and dazed, which was partly the result of two sleepless nights and partly from apprehension; she also kept looking behind her, as if she expected at any moment to see the King's messenger come galloping into the Tower to bring word of a reprieve. If so, it was a vain hope.

On the scaffold the headsman, black-garbed and hooded, his sword hidden in the straw, waited with his assistant and a priest beside the low wooden block. Anne mounted the steps with great composure, and smiled as she gazed down on the people below her. She asked Kingston not to give the signal for her death until she had spoken 'that which she had a mind to say'. Then, with an untroubled countenance and a firm voice, she delivered a carefully prepared speech:

Good Christian people, I am come hither to die, according to law, and therefore I will speak nothing against it. I come here only to die, and thus to yield myself humbly to the will of the King, my lord. And if, in my life, I did ever offend the King's Grace, surely with my death I do now atone. I come hither to accuse no man, nor to speak anything of that whereof I am accused, as I know full well that aught I say in my defence doth not appertain to you. I pray and beseech you all, good friends, to pray for the life of the King, my sovereign lord and yours, who is one of the best princes on the face of the earth, who has always treated me so well that better could not be, wherefore I submit to death with good will, humbly asking pardon of all the world. If any person will meddle with my cause, I require them to judge the best. Thus I take my leave of the world, and of you, and I heartily desire you all to pray for me.

She then turned to her ladies, who had ascended the scaffold with her, and told them not to be sorry to see her die, begging their pardon for any harshness towards them, praying them to take comfort for her loss, and admonishing them to 'be always faithful to her whom with happier fortune ye may have as your queen and mistress'. Anne then gave her prayer book to Lady Lee; entitled *The Hours of the Blessed Virgin Mary*, it had been made and illuminated for Anne in France around 1528, and she had inscribed it: 'Remember me when you do pray, that hope doth lead from day to day.' The prayer book still survives, and is now at Hever Castle.

Her farewell speeches done, Anne knelt with the priest for some final prayers. Then, she rose and took off her French hood, beneath which she had on a coif over her long dark hair, bound high so as not to impede the headsman, who now knelt to ask her forgiveness for what he must do. This she granted, and gave him his fee. Then she unclasped her necklace and knelt before the block. One of her maids tied a blindfold round her eyes, then withdrew to join the other ladies, who were weeping in a corner of the scaffold. The crowd also knelt, out of respect for the passing of a soul. Then, as Anne prayed aloud, saying over and over again, 'Jesu, receive my soul! O Lord God, have pity on my soul! To Christ I commend my soul!', the executioner retrieved his sword and cut off her head 'before you could say a Paternoster', according to Sir John Spelman, who was present. Then the headsman picked up the head and held it aloft, crying, in heavily accented English, 'So perish all the King's enemies!' At this moment, the onlookers saw the dead woman's eyes and lips move, a reflex action resulting from the shock of decapitation to the nervous system, yet to Tudor eyes an almost supernatural phenomenon.

'The Queen died boldly,' Kingston wrote to Cromwell later. 'God take her to His mercy.' Quickly, the crowd dispersed, and soon Tower Green was deserted, save for the broken body on the scaffold and the four weeping ladies who kept vigil beside it. No coffin had been provided, but an arrow chest lay waiting beside the steps. Reverently the ladies lifted the pathetic remains into it, and covered them with a sheet. The chest was then carried into the Royal Chapel of St Peter ad Vincula, where it was buried in the choir that afternoon, Lady Lee being chief mourner.

As Anne's head fell in the straw, the guns on the Tower wharf signalled, in a resounding report, her end to the world. Few mourned her passing, yet within two weeks of her death there were circulating in London ballads portraying her as a much wronged heroine, thus giving birth to a legend that has persisted, with gathering momentum, ever since.

Thomas Boleyn, Earl of Wiltshire, a broken man, now retired to Hever with his countess. She died in 1538 and was buried in the Howard Aisle in Lambeth Church; Wiltshire died a year later, and was laid to rest in Hever Church beneath a fine brass. Their grandson, Henry Carey, was created Viscount Hunsdon by Elizabeth I, and was much favoured by her. His sister Katherine married Sir Francis Knollys, another of Elizabeth's courtiers, and George Boleyn's son, named after his father, became Dean of Lichfield.

In the royal palaces, carpenters, masons and sempstresses were set to work removing Anne's initial wherever it occurred, and replacing it with Jane's. Portraits of Anne were taken down and hidden away. It was as if she had never existed. And not once, during the years that were left to him, would the King be heard to utter her name again.

12
Like one given by God

Henry VIII was at Whitehall Palace when the Tower guns signalled that he was once more a free man. He then appeared dressed in white mourning as a token of respect for his late queen, called for his barge, and had himself rowed at full speed to the Strand, where Jane Seymour had also heard the guns. News of Anne Boleyn's death had been formally conveyed to her by Sir Francis Bryan; it does not seem to have unduly concerned her, for she spent the greater part of the day preparing her wedding clothes, and perhaps reflecting upon the ease with which she had attained her ambition: Anne Boleyn had had to wait seven years for her crown; Jane had waited barely seven months.

It was common knowledge that Henry would marry Jane as soon as possible; the Privy Council had already petitioned him to venture once more into the perilous seas of holy wedlock, and it was a plea of the utmost urgency due to the uncertainty surrounding the succession. Both the King's daughters had been declared bastards, and his natural son Richmond was obviously dying. A speedy marriage was therefore not only desirable but necessary, and on the day Anne Boleyn died the King's imminent betrothal to Jane Seymour was announced to a relieved Privy Council. This was news as gratifying to the imperialist party, who had vigorously promoted the match, as it would soon be to the people of England at large, who would welcome the prospect of the imperial alliance with its inevitable benefits to trade.

Although the future Queen had rarely been seen in public, stories of her virtuous behaviour during the King's courtship had been circulated and applauded. Chapuys, more cynical, perceived that such virtue had had an ulterior motive, and privately thought it unlikely that Jane had reached the age of twenty-five without having lost her virginity, 'being an Englishwoman and having been so long' at a court where immorality was rife. However, he assumed that Jane's likely lack of a maidenhead would not trouble the King very much, 'since he may marry her on condition she is a maid, and when he wants a divorce there will be plenty of witnesses ready to testify that she was not'.

This apart, Chapuys and most other people considered Jane to be well endowed with all the qualities then thought becoming in a wife: meekness, docility and quiet dignity. Jane had been well groomed for her role by her family and supporters, and was in any case determined not to follow the example of her predecessor. She intended to use her influence to further the causes she held dear, as Anne Boleyn had, but, being of a less mercurial temperament, she would never use the same tactics. Jane's well-publicised sympathy for the late Queen Katherine and the Lady Mary showed her to be compassionate, and made her a popular figure with the common people and most of the courtiers. Overseas, she would be looked upon with favour because she was known to be an orthodox Catholic with no heretical tendencies whatsoever, one who favoured the old ways and who might use her influence to dissuade the King from continuing with his radical religious reforms.

Jane was of medium height, with a pale, nearly white, complexion. 'Nobody thinks she has much beauty,' commented Chapuys, and the French ambassador thought her too plain. Holbein's portrait of Jane, painted in 1536 and now in the Kunsthistorisches Museum, Vienna, bears out these statements, and shows her to have been fair with a large, resolute face, small slanting eyes and a pinched mouth. She wears a sumptuously bejewelled and embroidered gown and head-dress, the latter in the whelk-shell fashion so favoured by her; Holbein himself designed the pendant on her breast, and the lace at her wrists. This portrait was probably his first royal commission after being appointed the King's Master Painter in September 1536; a preliminary sketch for it is in the Royal Collection at Windsor, and a studio copy is in the Mauritshuis in The Hague. Holbein executed one other portrait of Jane during her lifetime. Throughout the winter of 1536–7, he was at work on a huge mural in the Presence Chamber in Whitehall Palace; it depicted the Tudor dynasty, with the figures of Henry VII and Elizabeth of York in the background, and Henry VIII and Jane Seymour in front. This magnificent work was one of the first to depict full-length likenesses of royal personages in England (although a late sixteenth-century inventory of Lord Lumley's pictures records a full-length portrait of Anne Boleyn, which has either been lost or cut down). Sadly, the Whitehall mural no longer exists, having been destroyed when the palace burned down in the late seventeenth century. Fortuitously, Charles II had before then commissioned a Dutch artist, Remigius van Leemput, to make two small copies, now in the Royal Collection and at Petworth House. His style shows little of Holbein's draughtsmanship, but his pictures at least give us a clear impression of what the original must have looked like. The figure of Jane is interesting in that we can see her long court train with her pet poodle resting on it. Her gown is of cloth of gold damask, lined with ermine, with six ropes of pearls slung across the bodice, and more pearls hanging in a girdle to the floor. Later portraits of Jane, such as those in long-gallery sets and the miniature by Nicholas Hilliard, all derive from this portrait or Holbein's original likeness now in Vienna, yet they are mostly mechanical in quality and anatomically awkward.

However, it was not Jane's face that had attracted the King so much as the fact that she was Anne Boleyn's opposite in every way. Where Anne had been bold and fond of having her own way, Jane showed herself entirely subservient to Henry's will; where Anne had, in the King's view, been a wanton, Jane had shown herself to be inviolably chaste. And where Anne had been ruthless, he believed Jane to be naturally compassionate. He would in years to come remember her as the fairest, the most discreet, and the most meritorious of all his wives.

Her contemporaries thought she had a pleasing sprightliness about her. She was pious, but not ostentatiously so. Reginald Pole, soon to be made a cardinal, described her as 'full of goodness', although Martin Luther, hearing of her reactionary religious views, feared her as 'an enemy of the Gospel'. According to Chapuys, she was not clever or witty, but 'of good understanding'. As queen, she made a point of distancing herself from her inferiors, and could be remote and arrogant, being a stickler for the observance of etiquette at her court. Chapuys feared that, once Jane had had a taste of queenship, she would forget her good intentions towards the Lady Mary, but his fears proved unfounded. Jane remained loyal to her supporters, and to Mary's cause, and in the months to come would endeavour to heal the rift between the King and his daughter.

Henry and Jane dined together in the Strand on the evening of 19 May; afterwards, the King took his barge and went straight to Hampton Court, where he would stay for a week. At six o'clock on the following morning, Jane followed him there, and at nine o'clock, they were formally betrothed in a ceremony lasting a few minutes. It is likely that Jane's family were present, for after the ceremony she returned with them to Wulfhall, there to await her marriage.

The next day, Henry wore white mourning once more, and gave orders for his daughter Elizabeth to be taken from Greenwich to Hatfield in the care of Lady Margaret Bryan, and kept out of his sight. There was an outstanding account to settle in respect of money outlayed by Sir William Kingston in respect of necessities provided for Elizabeth's mother. And there remained the problem of Mary. In spite of Jane's entreaties on the girl's behalf, Henry's attitude was unchanged: unless she acknowledged his laws and statutes, he would proceed against her. Mary was still in very grave danger.

Yet, even knowing her peril, she remained obdurate. Her father wanted her to abandon her deepest-held convictions and beliefs, and swear that her mother's marriage had been incestuous and unlawful, and that she accepted him as Supreme Head of the Church of England – something she could not bring herself to do. It seemed that coercion or force might be necessary if the King were to have his way, and several of the King's advisers thought that now would be a good time to put pressure on Mary. She was known to be weak and sickly. Seven years of insecurity and misery had made her a martyr, at twenty, to headaches, menstrual problems, and nervous depression, as well as vague, ill-defined illnesses, and she was still grieving for her mother.

The news of Anne Boleyn's death had revived Mary's spirits considerably, for she hoped the way might now be clear towards a reconciliation with her father. She knew she could count upon the support of Jane Seymour and the imperialist party, and prayed that the time had come to forget the unhappy past. She wrote to the King, begging to be taken back into his favour, humbly beseeching him to remember that she was 'but a woman, and your child'. Henry did not reply. The war of nerves had begun.

Mary, on the advice of her friend Lady Kingston, next tried approaching Henry through Cromwell, whom she had been told was secretly sympathetic towards her and might well use his very considerable influence on her behalf. On 26 May, Mary wrote to Mr Secretary, begging him to intercede for her with the King. Yet before her letter had time to arrive, Henry sent a deputation of the Privy Council to see Mary and make her submit to her father over the matter of her mother's marriage and the royal supremacy. She refused to do this, even though Norfolk told her that if his daughter had offered such 'unnatural opposition', he would have beaten and knocked her head against the wall until it was as soft as baked apples. This reduced Mary to floods of tears, but even the threat of violence was not sufficient to move her. When Henry learned of her defiance, he became more determined than ever to break her will. Nor was the Emperor inclined to interfere; Mary was not his subject, and he was more concerned about establishing the new alliance and reluctant to offend Henry VIII. Mary was on her own now.

Preparations for the royal wedding were now almost complete. Like all Henry VIII's marriages, it would be a private ceremony, although there would be public festivities to mark it. In the Queen's apartments, Anne Boleyn's falcon badge had been replaced by Jane's personal emblem, a phoenix rising from a castle amid flames and Tudor roses painted in red and white; this emblem would surmount the motto chosen by Jane, 'Bound to obey and serve'. Her initials had now replaced Anne's, although this had been done in such a hurry that at Hampton Court, the As are still visible underneath the Js. The monograms on the royal linen had been similarly altered, and at Zürich, where Coverdale's Bible with its dedication to Henry and Anne was being reprinted, the printers had to superimpose Jane's name on the frontispiece.

Both Henry and Jane returned to a transformed Whitehall Palace before 29 May. They were married there the following day in the Queen's Closet by Archbishop Cranmer. After the wedding ceremony Jane was enthroned in the Queen's chair beneath the canopy of royal estate in the great hall, where she presided over the court for the first time. Later that day, the King made her a grant of 104 manors in 4 counties, as well as a number of forests and hunting chases, for her jointure, the income that would support her during her marriage. One London estate, Paris Garden, was an unusual choice, for it was situated on the insalubrious Surrey shore of the Thames and its rents came from bear pits and brothels. Henry's personal wedding gift to his bride was a gold cup designed by Hans Holbein and engraved with the initials of the royal couple entwined with a love-knot; the Queen's motto appeared three times in the design. A drawing of this cup exists in the Ashmolean Museum in Oxford; the original was pawned by Charles I in 1625 and melted down four years later.

On 1 June, the King and Queen went by barge to Greenwich. The tradition that they spent their honeymoon at Wulfhall is based on an incorrect interpretation of a letter written by Sir John Russell in early June, in which he mentions a visit by Henry and Jane to Tottenham Parish Church. There exists today a Tottenham House not far from the site of Wulfhall, and a building called Tottenham Lodge seems in the sixteenth century to have been a dower house in the grounds of the Seymour estates; Lady Seymour lived there during her widowhood. Nevertheless, it is not feasible to suppose that this was the Tottenham referred to in Sir John Russell's letter, for the time-scale dictates that it must have been Tottenham Church, north-east of the City of London, that was honoured by a royal visit at this time.

Within a week of his wedding, the King was optimistically speaking of 'the Prince hoped for in due season', leaving no doubt in the minds of his courtiers – who had, after all, heard of the slur on Henry's virility raised at George Boleyn's trial – that the royal marriage had been successfully consummated. Soon afterwards, prayers were being offered up in churches for the quickening of the Queen.

When Jane arrived at Greenwich, she was attended by a bevy of ladies. On that Friday, she dined in public with her husband for the first time. Sir John Russell was impressed by her demeanour on that occasion, and told Lord Lisle she was

> as gentle a lady as ever I knew, and as fair a queen as any in Christendom. I do assure you, my lord, the King hath come out of hell into heaven for the gentleness in this, and the cursedness and the unhappiness in the other. When you write to the King again, tell him that you do rejoice that he is so well matched with so gracious a woman as she is.

After dinner on that Friday, the new Queen's servants were all sworn in. There had been a great rush for places in Jane's household. In Katherine of Aragon's day the Queen's retinue had numbered 168; Anne Boleyn had increased the number, and Jane increased it further still, to 200. The King did not attend the long and tedious ceremony of oath-taking; he was busy listening to the reports of the privy councillors who had visited his daughter at Hunsdon. What they told him made him seethe with anger, and he was all for having Mary put on trial for treason, but when Queen Jane learned of his intentions, she begged him not to proceed. Her prayers fell on deaf ears, however, for the King, forgetting he was a bridegroom, told her she must be out of her senses. Thus early in her married life did Jane learn to tread warily with her husband.

Yet fate was on her side. The royal justices were reluctant to proceed against Mary, and suggested that instead of being tried for treason she be made to sign a paper of submission, recognising her father as head of the Church and her mother's marriage as incestuous and unlawful. Cromwell supported this idea, and persuaded the King to agree. He already regretted lending Mary his support, and in early June wrote her a scathing letter in which he deplored her unfilial stand against her father; with it, he enclosed the list of articles she was to sign, warning her he would not vouch for her safety if she refused. Mary, however, was still determined not to risk her immortal soul for the favour of an earthly king, however much she craved her father's love and approval. She ignored Cromwell's letter, and waited for a reply to a letter she had written to the King on 1 June, congratulating him on his marriage and begging leave to wait upon Queen Jane, 'or do her Grace such service as shall please her to command me'. Her letter had ended with the fervent hope that 'God would send your Grace shortly a prince, whereof no creature living would more rejoice than I'.

Henry did not bother to reply; and for the time being, the Queen, who had been put firmly in her place on the issue of Mary, deemed it wise to hold her peace.

Jane was proclaimed Queen of England on 4 June 1536 at Greenwich. On that day, she went in procession to mass, following the King with a great train of ladies, and in the evening she dined alone in her presence chamber under a canopy of estate before a large audience of courtiers. It appears she had clearly defined ideas of what she hoped to achieve as queen. First and foremost, she hoped to remain queen, and to this end she modelled her behaviour from the first upon that of Katherine of Aragon, whom she had greatly admired. Her other aims were threefold: to give the King a male heir, to work for the reinstatement of the Lady Mary, and to advance her family. She knew her power to be limited, and wisely concluded that it was essential not to misuse what influence she did have. Yet her quiet dignity – which endeared her to king and commons alike – hid a strong will and a determination to succeed within her chosen sphere.

Henry VIII, it must be said, was not an ideal husband, and cannot have been an easy man to live with at this stage of his life. His irritability stemmed from Mary's behaviour and from the pain of the suppurating wound on his leg. His autocracy extended to his private life, his word being law in the domestic sphere. Now that he could no longer indulge so much in the sporting pastimes he had loved in his youth, he had turned to theology for solace, and religion was now one of his chief preoccupations. He saw himself as the spiritual father of his people, appointed by God to lead them; and, as time passed, he grew increasingly pedantic and dogmatic, so that few dared argue with him. With his intimates he could be rude, intolerant, scathing and brutal; at other times, he was his old, genial self, but it was a side of him seen less and less as age and ill health encroached upon his once-splendid constitution. As he grew older, he became subject to bouts of savage temper, while at the same time a curiously sentimental streak in him became more pronounced. When he wanted to, he could exert great charm, and he was to the end of his life a man who enjoyed flirting with the ladies, much to the dismay of his successive wives and their supporters. But after his experiences with Katherine and Anne he would never again allow any woman to have it in her power to rule him. Jane Seymour, and his later wives, knew very well that to retain his favour they must adopt an attitude of adoring and respectful submission.

Henry VIII's marriage to Jane Seymour was a success, although as usual Henry's passion abated somewhat once he had secured his quarry; this had happened with Katherine, and even more dramatically with Anne. Yet it appears that he genuinely loved Jane for herself, and he accorded her the respect due to her, even though he could be very abrupt with her. In later life, he would convince himself that he had loved her the best of all his wives, and he was fond of declaring that he considered her to be his first lawful one. Jane was weighed down by jewels given to her by the King (her favourite seems to have been a fashionable IHS pendant); then there were the rich gowns with trains a statutory three yards long, the furs, and the head-dresses. There still exists an inventory of furniture provided by Henry for his wife's sojourn in the Tower prior to her coronation (which never took place), which lists such items as silk fire-screens and an elaborate inlaid box in which to keep legal documents. In all material respects, Henry was an indulgent husband.

We know very little about Jane's charitable enterprises, though fragments of information survive. For example, she offered a place in her household to Elizabeth Darrell, Sir Thomas Wyatt's destitute mistress, who had once served with her under Queen Katherine. But as for other charities, hardly anything is known of them, though had she been queen for longer, more information might have been recorded about them.

The King was now preparing for the forthcoming session of Parliament, which would confirm his marriage and settle the succession on Jane's children. He was also occupied with the advancement of the Queen's family, as he had been with the Boleyns a decade earlier. On 5 June, Sir Edward Seymour was created Viscount Beauchamp of Hache in the county of Somerset, and was appointed Chancellor of North Wales and Lord Chamberlain to the

King. His brother Thomas was made a gentleman of the privy chamber, and his other brother Henry was knighted. All three were given extensive grants of land. Edward and Thomas were now embarking on brilliant careers in public life, careers that would, in both cases, come to a tragic end on the block many years later. Sir John Seymour, the Queen's father, received no lands or titles, but he was already a sick man, and after his daughter's marriage he seems to have retired to Wulfhall with his wife.

The Seymour family certainly exercised a certain amount of patronage within the Queen's household, but mainly in the lower ranks. Some of Anne Boleyn's principal officers had been retained for their experience, and by Christmas 1536, Anne's treacherous sister-in-law, Lady Rochford, was back at court as Lady of the Bedchamber to Queen Jane. Some of the former Queen's servants had been transferred to the employ of the Lord Steward, but most had been retained, and in fact, the new Queen's household was very much as it had been in Anne's time.

On 6 June, after mass, Chapuys was personally conducted to the Queen's apartments by the King and formally presented to her. He kissed her hand, congratulated her on her marriage, and wished her prosperity, adding that, although the device of 'the lady who had preceded her on the throne' had been 'Happiest of Women', he had no doubt that she herself would realise that motto. He was certain, he said, that the Emperor would rejoice – as her husband had done – that such a 'virtuous and amiable' queen now sat upon the throne, and told her that it was impossible to comprehend the joy and pleasure which Englishmen in general had expressed on hearing of her marriage, especially as it was said that she was continually trying to persuade the King to restore Mary to favour. Jane promised Chapuys that she would continue to show favour herself to Mary, and would do her best to deserve the title of Peacemaker with which he had gallantly addressed her. The ambassador replied extravagantly by saying that, without the pain of labour and childbirth, Jane had gained in Mary a treasured daughter who would please her more than her own children by the King, to which she responded by saying again that she would do all she could to make peace between Henry and his daughter. Then she seemed at a loss as to what to say next, until the King came to her rescue and led Chapuys away, saying that he was the first ambassador Jane had received, and that she was not yet used to such audiences; he also remarked that his wife was by nature kind and amiable and 'much inclined to peace'; she would, he said, strive to prevent him from taking part in a foreign war, if only to avoid the pain and fear that separation would cause. After this Chapuys was obliged to revise his earlier, more cynical assessment of Jane, and now wrote of her virtue and her intelligence; later, he would commend her discretion, saying that she would not be drawn into discussions about religion or politics, and that she bore her royal honours with dignity.

On the following day, 7 June, Jane made her state entry into London at the King's side. They came by river, in the royal barge, from Greenwich to Westminster, and were escorted by a colourful procession of smaller boats, all gaily decked out for the occasion. Behind them sailed a great barge carrying the King's bodyguard in their scarlet and gold uniforms. As the royal procession passed along the river, the people cheered from the crowded banks, and warships and shore-guns sounded salutes. At Radcliffe Wharf, the royal barge halted so that the King and Queen could watch a pageant mounted by Chapuys in their honour: the ambassador, resplendent in purple satin, awaited them under a marquee embroidered with the imperial arms, and when they approached the quayside, gave the signal for two small boats, one carrying trumpeters, the other a consort of shawms and sackbuts, to leave their moorings and act as a musical escort for the royal barge, as it resumed its stately progress towards Westminster. The walls of the Tower had been festooned with banners and streamers, and the barges paused again to take the salute from the 400 guns lined up along its wharf, those same guns that had announced Anne Boleyn's death three weeks earlier. It is unlikely, however, that Henry and Jane allowed their triumph to be clouded by morbid thoughts; Anne was best forgotten, a conviction strongly reinforced by the loud approval voiced by the citizens of London for their new queen.

At Westminster, the royal couple came ashore and walked in procession to Westminster Abbey, where they heard high mass before returning to Whitehall Palace. In comparison to the ceremonies at the civic receptions for Katherine of Aragon and Anne Boleyn, Jane's entry into the capital was a very quiet affair. Katherine and

Anne had also been crowned within weeks of becoming queen, but Henry's Exchequer was so depleted that he could not now afford the expense of another coronation. It was his intention to have Jane crowned later in the year, when hopefully his financial situation would have improved; by then, the funds and treasures of several dissolved religious houses would have been diverted to the Crown. Indeed, Henry had already set a provisional date in late October, and had made some preliminary plans. Jane would come to the Tower by river from Greenwich in a great barge fashioned to look like the Bucentaur, the ceremonial vessel used by the Doges of Venice. She would then make a progress through London to Westminster, and be fêted with pageantry and music. Her crown would be the one worn by her two predecessors, an open coronal of heavy gold set with sapphires, rubies and pearls; sadly, it no longer exists, having been melted down on the order of Oliver Cromwell.

Next morning, on 8 June, Jane came to the gallery above the new gatehouse at Whitehall and waved goodbye to Henry as he rode in procession to open Parliament. In the House, when Lord Chancellor Audley in his opening speech praised the Queen and declared that her 'age and fine form give promise of issue', there was resounding applause, and the King departed, smiling benignly, confident that his ministers could be left to deal satisfactorily with the question of the succession. Soon afterwards, a new Act of Succession decreed that the crown should pass on Henry's death to the children of Queen Jane, 'a right noble, virtuous and excellent lady', who, 'for her convenient years, excellent beauty, and pureness of flesh and blood, is apt, God willing, to conceive issue'. The Act also acknowledged the 'great and intolerable perils' which the King had suffered as a result of two unlawful marriages, and drew attention to the 'ardent love and fervent affection' for his realm and people that had impelled him, 'of his most excellent goodness', to venture upon a third marriage, which was 'so pure and sincere, without spot, doubt or impediment, that the issue procreated out of the same, when it shall please Almighty God to send it, cannot be lawfully disturbed of the right and title in the succession'. It was also enacted that the King's first two marriages had been unlawful, and that the Ladies Mary and Elizabeth were illegitimate and unfit to inherit the throne. Failing any issue by Queen Jane, the King was granted the unprecedented power to appoint anyone he chose to be his successor, and that included the issue of 'any other lawful wife'.

The problem of Mary still had to be resolved. When she realised that Henry was not going to answer her letter, Mary also perceived, with terrible clarity, that the only way to earn his clemency was by submitting to his demands, hateful though they were to her. Both Chapuys and the Emperor were constantly urging her to do as her father required, assuring her of the Pope's absolution should she be compelled to sign against her will the articles sent by Cromwell. Yet Mary could be as stubborn as her father. She wrote to him again, begging him of his 'inestimable goodness' to pardon her offences, and saying she would never be happy until he had forgiven her. 'Most humbly prostrate' before his noble feet, she craved the favour of an audience, for she had humbly repented of her faults. Again, Henry refused to reply, and to Jane and Cromwell he expressed doubts about Mary's sincerity, which none of their reassurances could dispel. Nothing less than her signature on those articles would persuade him that she meant what she said and Cromwell, knowing his master to be implacable on this issue, privately urged her to sign at once, hinting at terrible consequences if she did not.

For the next day or so, Mary wrestled with her conscience, then she gave way. On 13 June, fortified by Chapuys's assurance that the Pope would absolve her from all responsibility for what she was about to do under duress, she finally acknowledged her father to be supreme head of the Church of England and her mother's marriage 'by God's law and man's law incestuous and unlawful'. Thus, by a few strokes of the pen, did Mary repudiate in the eyes of the world everything she had hitherto held sacred; she had capitulated for worldly reasons, where others had stood firm and suffered for their principles, and she would never, as long as she lived, forgive herself for this betrayal.

But the deed had been done, and the articles were already on their way to the King with a covering letter begging his forgiveness and stating that the writer was so conscious of having offended him that she dared not call him father. Chapuys thought she had never done a better day's work, and cheerfully assured the Emperor that he had relieved Mary of every doubt of conscience. There now remained, ostensibly, no bar to Mary's reconciliation to her father, but the King, who was certainly gratified to learn of his daughter's submission, was irritated that he had been made to wait so long for it. Instead of replying personally to her, he sent Sir Thomas Wriothesley, one of his 'new men', to Hunsdon, with orders to obtain a fuller declaration of her faults in writing. In return, Wriothesley was to ask Mary to name those ladies she would like appointed to her service should his Majesty decide to increase her household pending a return to favour. Such instructions could only have come from the King himself, and Mary was pathetically grateful; she wrote a long and abject letter to Cromwell, acknowledging her faults and thanking him for his kindness in furthering her cause with the King. When Henry read it, he allowed his long-suppressed paternal feelings to revive: it would not be long before he was ready to play once more the part of a loving father.

No one was more delighted than the Queen when Mary signed her submission. Jane had worked for months towards a reconciliation, and she now looked forward to receiving her stepdaughter at court. There were few ladies in her household with whom she could associate on virtually equal terms; in order to emphasise her rank, she had set herself apart from those with whom she might have been familiar, and the truth was that she was now feeling rather lonely. Mary would be a friend and companion to her, for she ranked high enough to enjoy the privilege of the Queen's friendship. Many other people at court welcomed the prospect of Mary's return to favour, as did the common people when news of its likelihood spread.

The King made his first friendly move towards Mary at the end of June, when he sent his officers to Hunsdon to see she had all she required and to advise her that it would not be long before he brought the Queen to visit her. In the meantime, Henry prepared to enjoy his first summer with his new wife, having just made Cromwell Lord Privy Seal in place of Anne Boleyn's father, who had retired from court, and sent to jail an Oxfordshire man called John Hill for saying that Anne had been put to death only for the King to take his pleasure with Jane Seymour. It is a fact that Master Hill was the only person on record as having spoken out against the King's new marriage, a sure indication of how popular it was.

During the long summer days there were jousts and triumphs in honour of the Queen, as well as pageants on the river. Jane was an accomplished horsewoman, and shared to some extent the King's passion for hunting, a sport in which they frequently participated. On 29 June, St Peter's Night, they visited the Mercers' Hall in Cheapside, and stood at a window to watch the annual ceremony of the setting of the marching watch of the City. It was a stirring occasion, the procession being illuminated by torchlight. Throughout that summer, Henry and Jane commuted between Whitehall and Greenwich, travelling in the royal barge, which was frequently filled with minstrels playing a variety of instruments. The royal couple watched a firework display, and went on a short progress. On 3 July, they presided over the magnificent celebrations that graced the triple wedding of the Earl of Westmorland's son and two daughters, and were guests of honour at the banquet which followed, when Henry came in procession from Whitehall wearing Turkish costume. It was, almost, like old times.

Jane, meanwhile, had sent her brother, Lord Beauchamp, to visit Mary, with instructions to obtain a list of the clothing she would need when she returned to court. Beauchamp himself, possibly at the Queen's suggestion, presented Mary with a superb horse, and told her that the King's 'gracious clemency and merciful pity' had overcome his anger at her 'unkind and unnatural behaviour'. When he had gone, Mary wrote again to the King, declaring that she would never vary from her confession and submission, and prayed that God would send him and the Queen issue. After receiving this, Henry let it be known that he would shortly be reconciled to his eldest daughter, whereupon several influential courtiers rushed to Hunsdon to ingratiate themselves with her.

Mary's health had been poor for months, and the strain of all this was almost too much for her. The King therefore decided to defer her official reception at court for a time, and visited her privately with Jane on 6 July at a house in Hackney. It was an emotional reunion, with Henry speaking affectionately to his daughter for the first time in six years. He was gentle, kind and patient with her, and told her how deeply he regretted having kept her so long from him. This much was overheard by his retinue, but the rest of the conversation took place in private. Afterwards, though, it was obvious that the meeting had been conducted with 'such love and affection, and such brave promises for the future, that no father could have behaved better towards his daughter'. Jane gave her stepdaughter a diamond ring; Henry's gift was 'a thousand crowns for her little pleasures'; he did not wish her to be anxious about money and in future, he told her, she should have as much as she wished. The King and Queen left after vespers, promising to see Mary again soon.

Two days later, Chapuys was happy to report to Charles V a great improvement in Mary's circumstances: she had more freedom than ever before, and was now being served with great solemnity and honour. All she lacked was the title Princess of Wales, but that, said Chapuys, was of no consequence, because it had been announced that she was from henceforth to rank as second lady at court after Queen Jane. On 8 July, Mary wrote to thank her father for the 'perfect reconciliation' between them, and ended by once more expressing the hope that 'my very natural mother, the Queen' would shortly have children. She also wrote to Cromwell, who responded by sending her a ring inset with portrait miniatures of Henry, Jane and herself, made specially for her; the bearer of this gift was none other than the King himself, who had been so impressed with it that he insisted on presenting it in person when he and Jane next visited Mary at Richmond later in July.

So far, Jane had displayed little interest in Henry's younger daughter, who was now nearly three. The imperialist party had all along supported the restoration of the Lady Mary, but there was no political faction prepared to act in the interests of the bastard child of a convicted traitor. The King had banished Elizabeth from his sight, and wanted nothing to do with her. Yet she was an intelligent child, and highly precocious. 'Why, Governor,' she had asked Sir John Shelton, who had charge of her household, 'how hath it, yesterday Lady Princess, and today but Lady Elizabeth?' We do not know how Elizabeth found out about her mother's death, but it is likely to have been early on, as the arrival of a new stepmother on the scene would certainly have provoked awkward questions in one so forward. What is certain is that the knowledge of what had happened to Anne Boleyn had a traumatic effect on Elizabeth, and may well have crippled her emotionally for life; it is a fact that she made a point of avoiding marriage and any other serious commitment to a man. In the meantime, though, she was just a little girl who was fast outgrowing her clothes, much to the dismay of Lady Bryan, who had great trouble persuading Cromwell to replace such necessary items as nightgowns and underclothing.

Yet now, conscious of her own good fortune, Mary found time to spare a thought for her half-sister, of whom she had always been fond, for all that Elizabeth was Anne Boleyn's child. Deprived of a child of her own, Mary lavished all her frustrated maternal affection on Elizabeth, and on 21 July paid a visit to her at Hatfield. Afterwards, she wrote to their father, telling him that Elizabeth was in good health and that he would have cause to be proud of her in time to come, and ending by sending her usual felicitations to 'the Queen, my good mother'. Already, a bond of friendship had sprung up between the two women.

Late in July, the King and Queen, with the court, spent a weekend in Dover; this was the visit postponed from May, when Anne Boleyn's arrest had intervened. According to Chapuys, Henry was feeling low, not only because of his bastard son's death, but also because he was disappointed that the Queen had as yet shown no signs of being pregnant. Chapuys gained the impression that her coronation was being postponed until she had proved she could bear children, but this was not the real reason. The progress did little to restore the King's former good humour, and on 12 August he confided to Chapuys that he felt himself growing old and doubted whether he would have any children by the Queen. It would be reasonable to suppose that advancing infirmity was affecting Henry's potency, especially in view of the fact that none of his wives after Jane conceived a child by him, except, perhaps, Katherine Howard; it may even be that what had been said at George Boleyn's trial had had some basis in truth. Because Jane took so long to conceive a child, it would appear that there was a difficulty, and the likelihood is that it lay with Henry. Yet outwardly, the royal couple showed no signs of tension; indeed, they gave the impression of being harmoniously and happily married.

Henry still managed to go hunting, and on 9 August led a party out with Jane – on that day, twenty stags were brought down. Later in August the King visited Mary at Hunsdon and told her that her return to court would not be long delayed. Her health was improving steadily, and Henry was anxious to stage a public reunion. Jane had complained that she felt lonely, for there were 'none but my inferiors' with whom to make merry, and had pleaded that she might 'enjoy the company of my Lady Mary's Grace at court'. 'We will have her here, darling,' Henry had promised, 'if she will make thee merry.' Early in September, he wrote to his daughter, commanding her to prepare for a move to court in the near future, and shortly afterwards he proclaimed her his heir, in default of any issue by Queen Jane. As news of this spread, crowds gathered around the royal palaces, where apartments were being prepared for Mary, in the hope of seeing her, and Lady Salisbury, Mary's former governess, was cheered when she visited the court at the King's invitation.

Plague returned to London in September, so the court moved to Windsor. Jane was looking forward with pleasure to Mary's arrival, and was also happily involved in planning her coronation with the King and his ministers. It was due to take place on the Sunday before All Hallows' Day, and funds were now available for it, thanks to the efforts made by Cromwell and the King's commissioners to divert the wealth of dissolved monasteries into the royal coffers; the dissolution was now gaining momentum. Henry, who had read some of the reports, professed himself scandalised that the word of God was not being observed as it should have been in some houses. There were allegations of lechery, sodomy and over luxurious living, though it is hard to estimate how much corruption there actually was in the monasteries of England at that time, and how much was fabricated by the royal officials, who knew that the King meant to close them and appropriate the spoils.

The economic and social consequences of the dissolution are beyond the scope of this book, but by 1540 the wealth of the religious houses had been swallowed up by the Exchequer, and their buildings and lands had been sold at a profit to supporters of the King's reformist policies. The dissolution resulted in the secularisation of the Church, and, in many areas, notably the south, it was popular, there being a tangible resentment of the riches hitherto enjoyed by the religious houses. In addition, the heretical teachings of Luther and others had come, through closer contact with Europe, to find

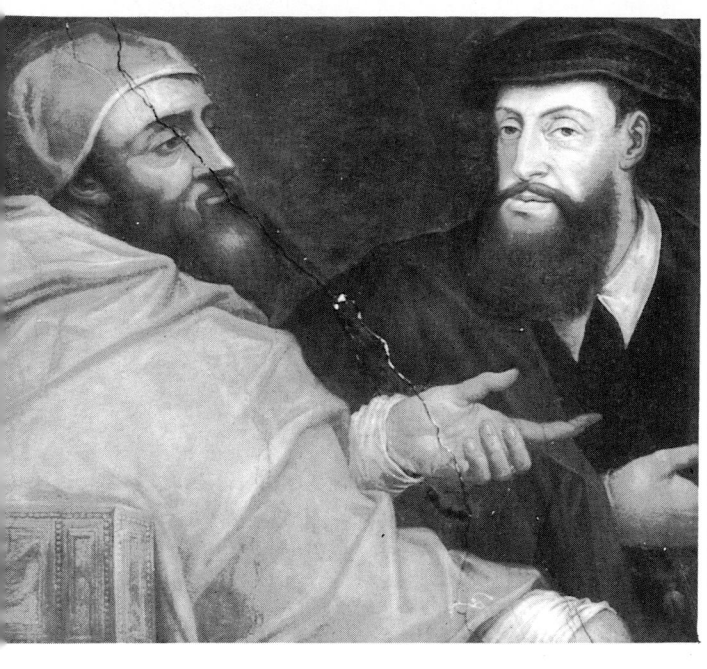

16 Pope Clement VII and the Emperor Charles V: 'The Emperor is determined to maintain the rights of his aunt, and will never consent to the divorce' (Charles V's ambassador to Pope Clement, 1527)

17 *Below* Petition from the English nobility to the Pope, 13th July 1530: 'We beg your Holiness without delay to assist these his Majesty's most just and reasonable desires'

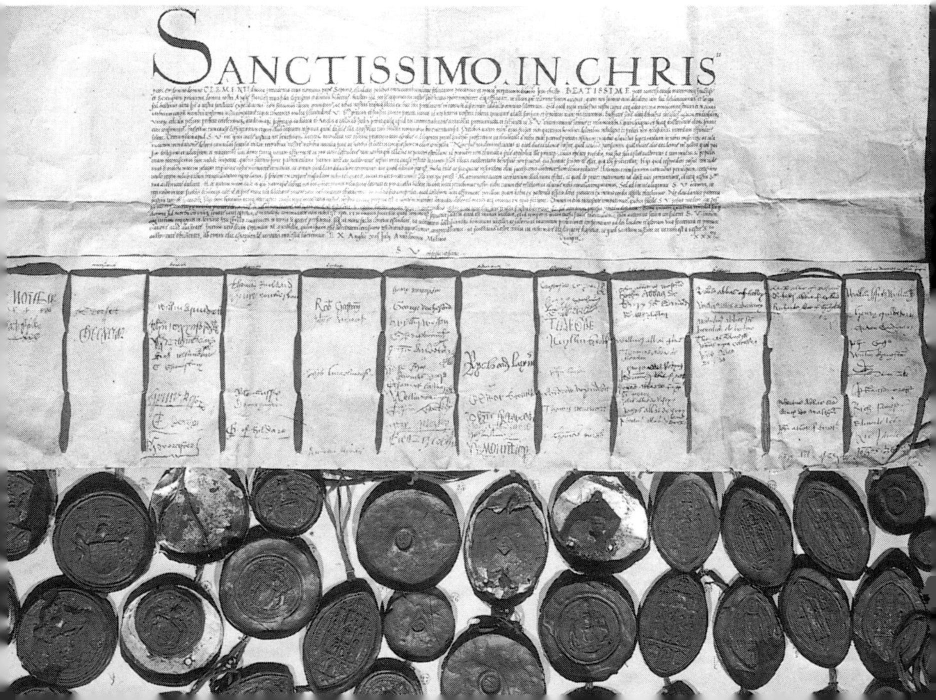

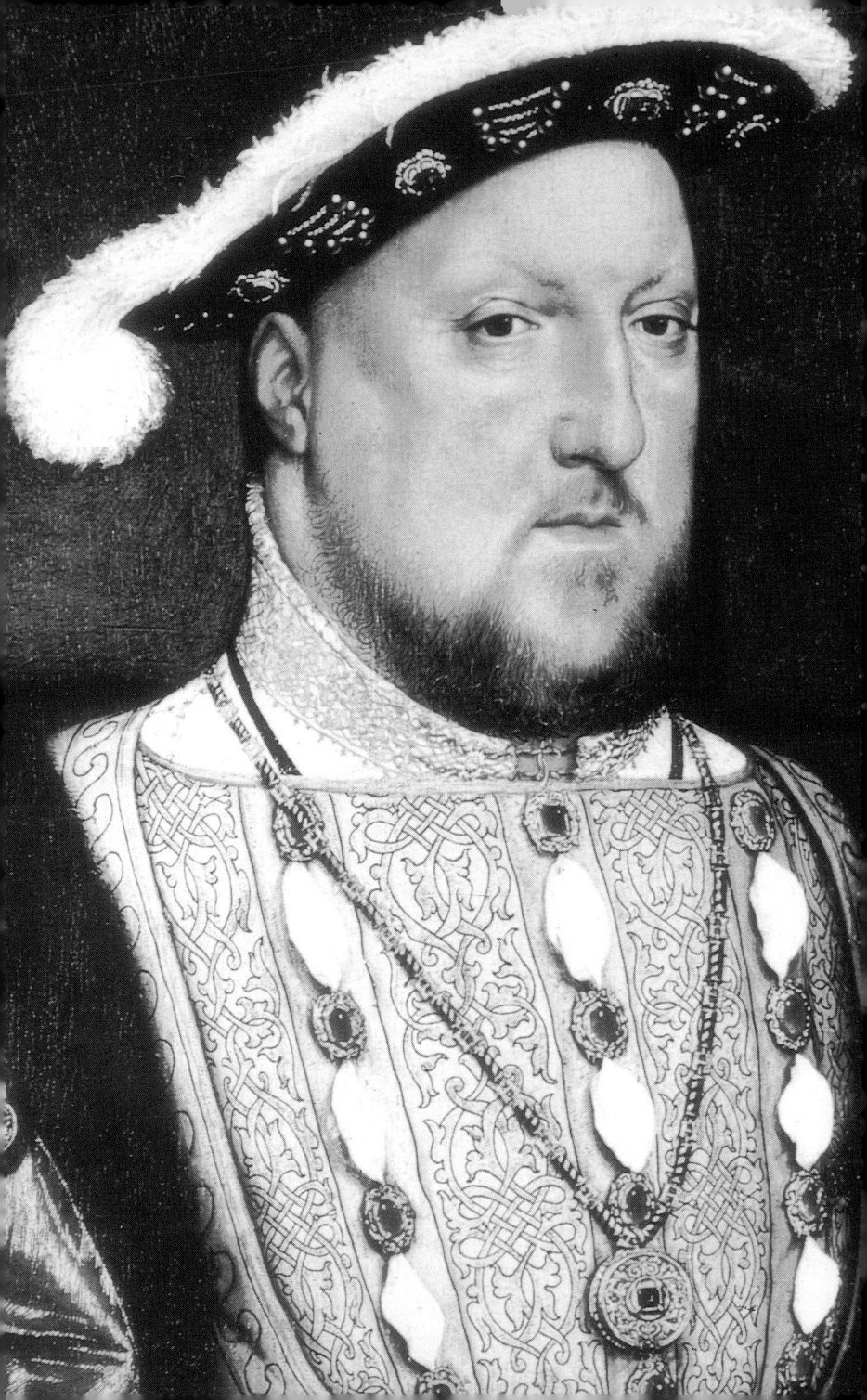

18 *Left* Henry VIII: 'Nature, in creating such a prince, has done her utmost to present a model of manly beauty' (*Venetian Calendar*, 1531)

19 *Right* Thomas Cranmer: 'He is a servant of Anne's, and at least should be required to take a special oath not to meddle with the divorce' (Eustace Chapuys, *Spanish Calendar*)

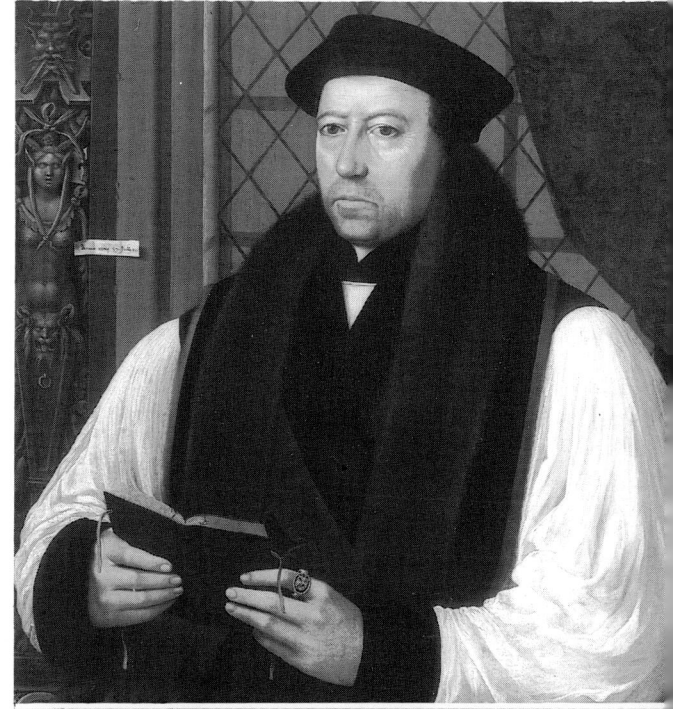

20 *Right* Thomas Cromwell: 'Ready at all things, evil or good' (Eustace Chapuys, *Spanish Calendar*)

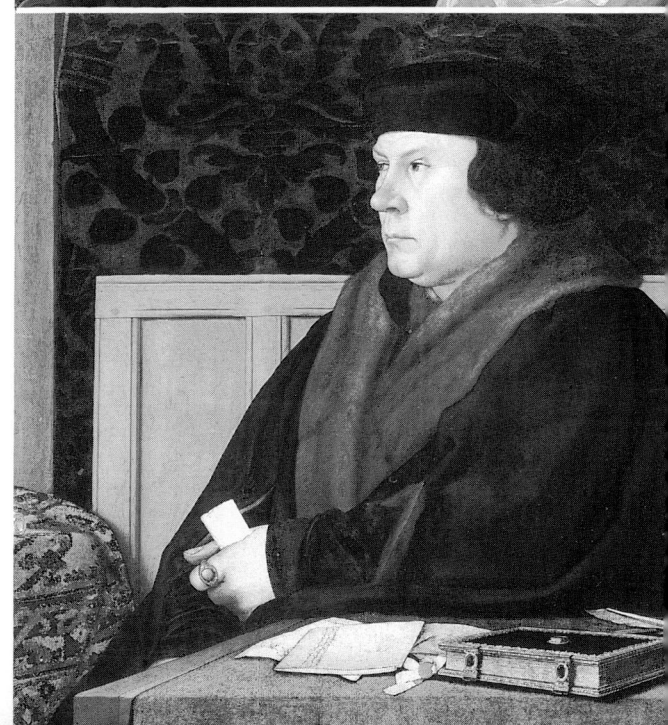

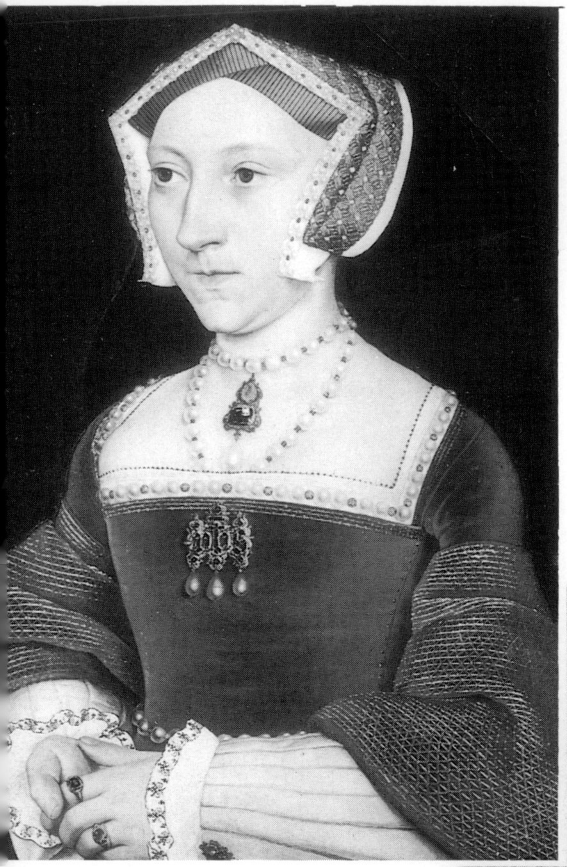

23 *Right* Whitehall Palace: both Anne Boleyn and Jane Seymour were married to Henry VIII there

24 *Below right* The Hampton Court dynastic group portrait. In this picture Jane Seymour appears posthumously

21 *Above* Jane Seymour: 'She is as gentle a lady as ever I knew, and as fair a queen as any in Christendom' (*The Lisle Letters*, 1536)

22 *Right* Prince Edward: 'The goodliest babe that ever I set mine eyen upon' (*The Lisle Letters*)

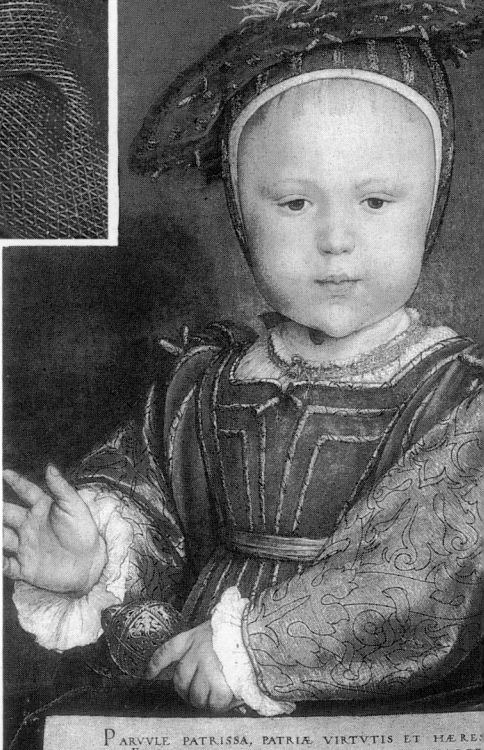

PARVVLE PATRISSA, PATRIÆ VIRTVTIS ET HÆRES
ESTO, NIHIL MAIVS MAXIMVS ORBIS HABET
GNATVM VIX POSSVNT COELVM ET NATVRA DEDI
HVIVS QVEM PATRIS, VICTVS HONORET HON
ÆQVATO TANTVM, TANTI TV FACTA PARENTIS

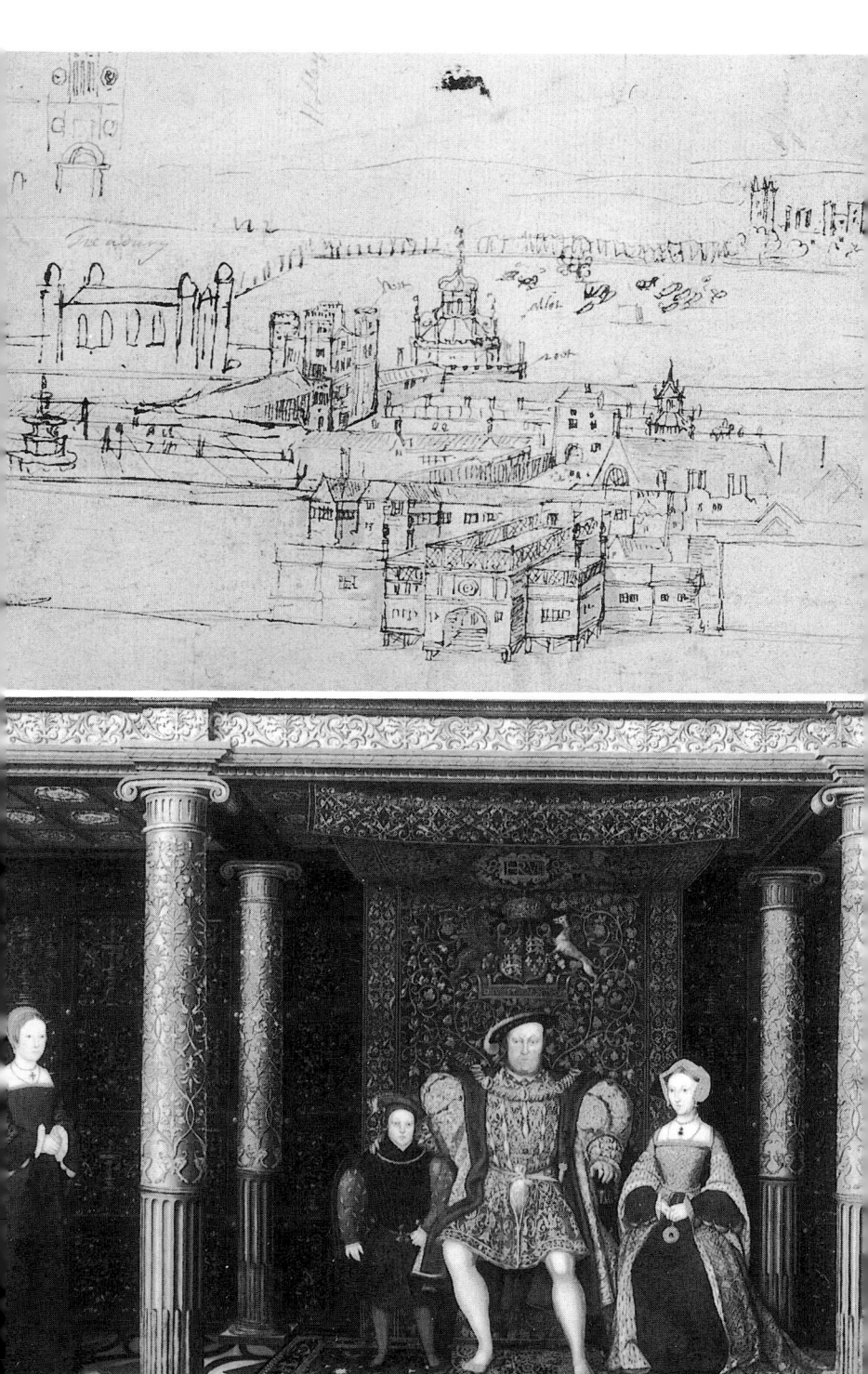

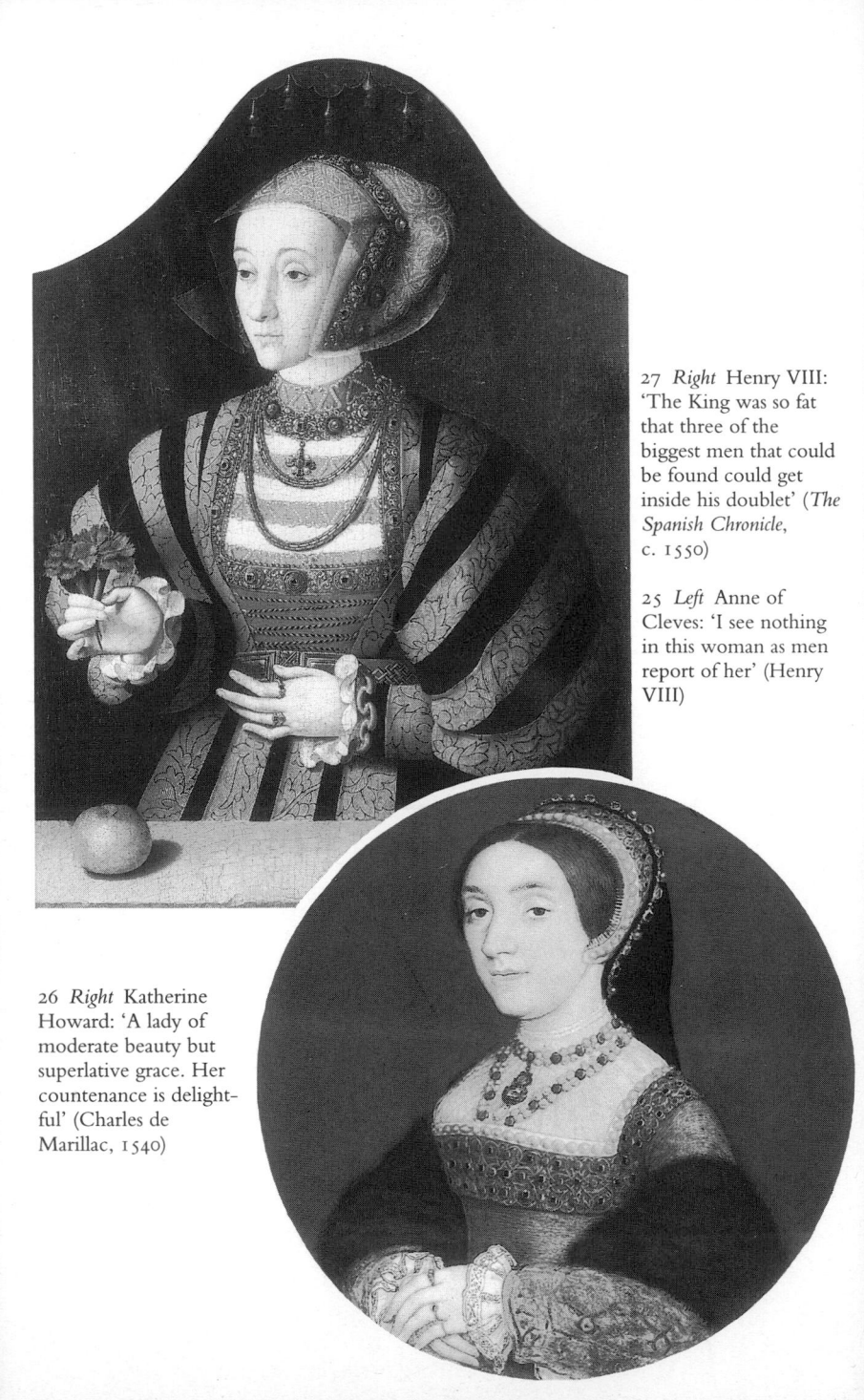

27 *Right* Henry VIII: 'The King was so fat that three of the biggest men that could be found could get inside his doublet' (*The Spanish Chronicle*, c. 1550)

25 *Left* Anne of Cleves: 'I see nothing in this woman as men report of her' (Henry VIII)

26 *Right* Katherine Howard: 'A lady of moderate beauty but superlative grace. Her countenance is delightful' (Charles de Marillac, 1540)

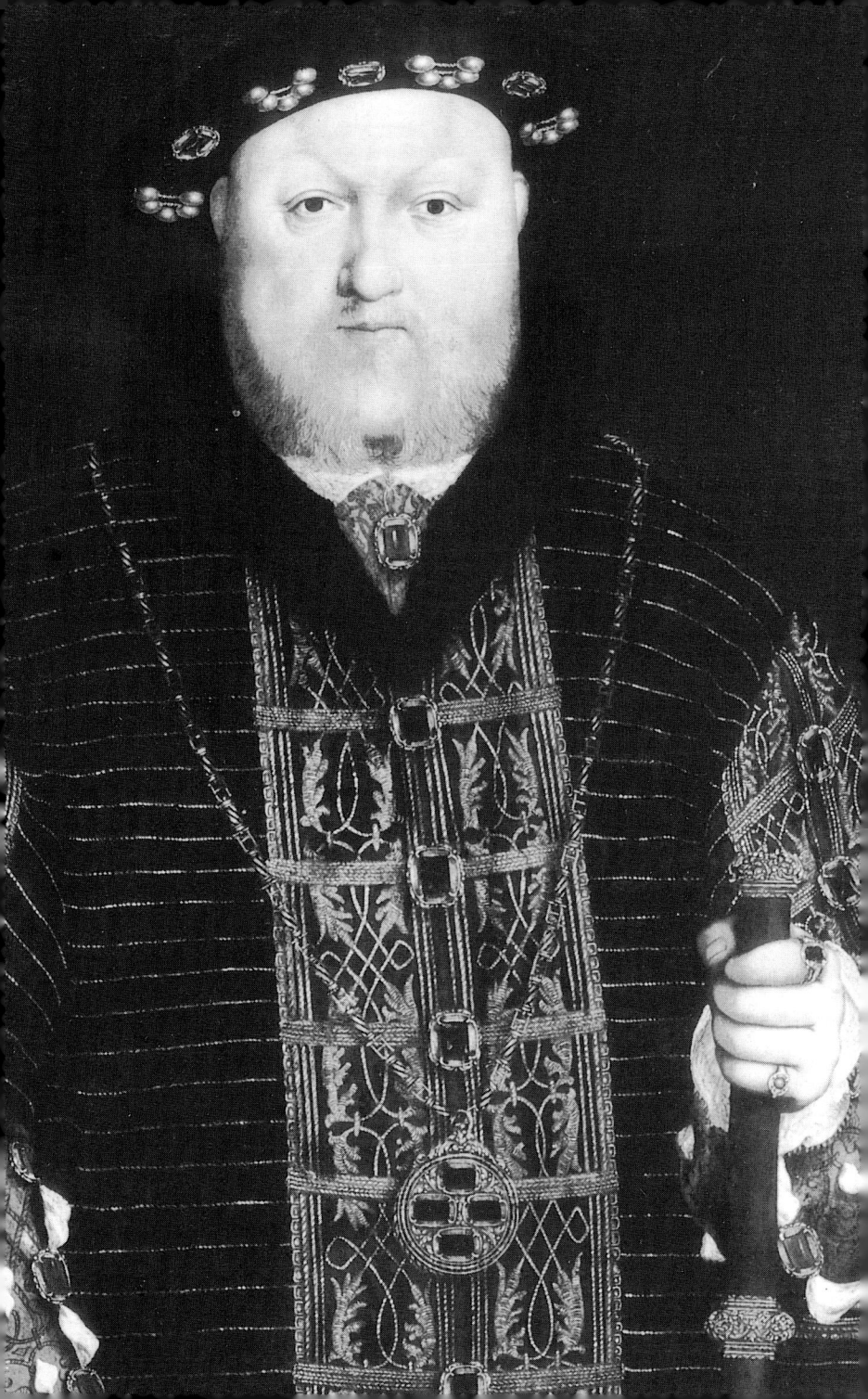

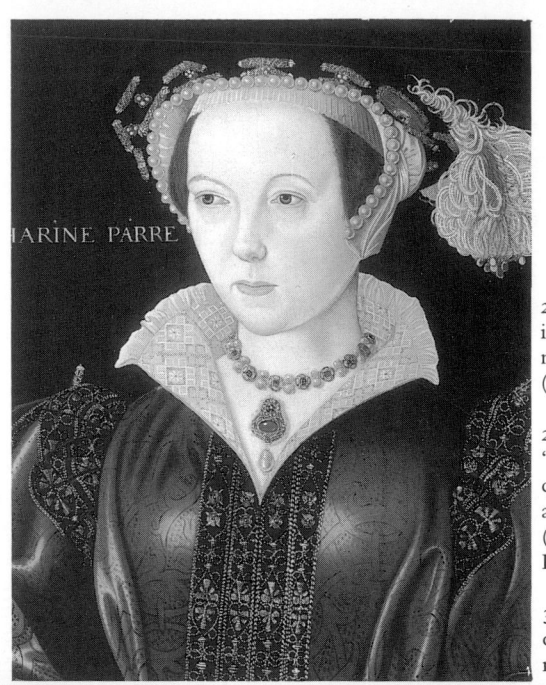

28 *Left* Katherine Parr: 'The Queen is graceful, and of cheerful countenance, and is praised for her virtue' (Eustace Chapuys, *Spanish Calendar*)

29 *Below left* The Lady Elizabeth: 'Your beauty and other excellent qualities have so bewitched me that I am no longer master of myself' (Letter from Thomas Seymour to the Lady Elizabeth, 1548)

30 *Below* Thomas Seymour: 'A man of much wit, but very little judgement' (The Lady Elizabeth, 1549)

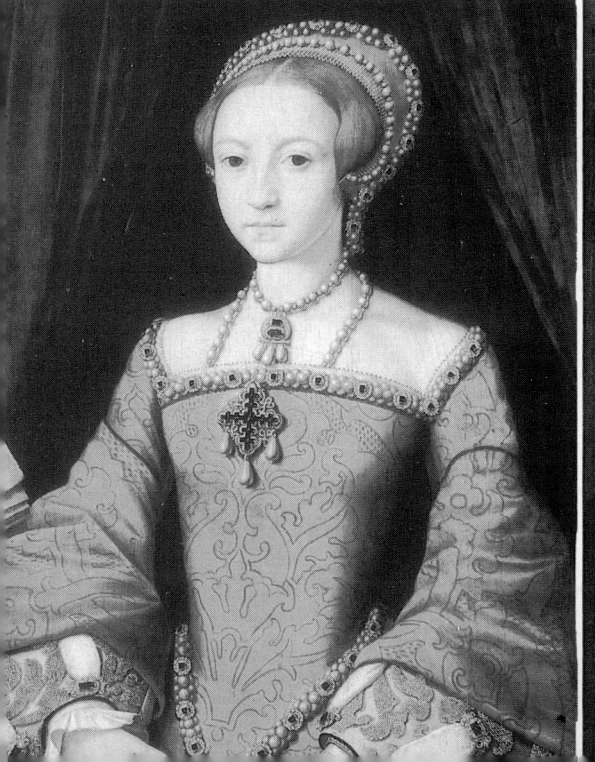

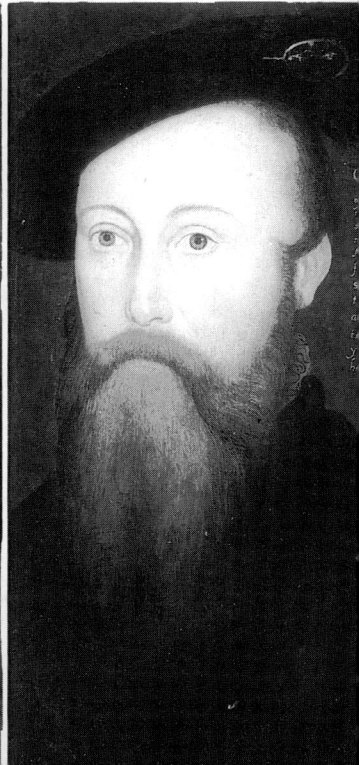

favour with a growing number of people, while many bishops actively encouraged reform.

But gradual closure of many of the smaller monasteries meant that hordes of monks and nuns were being turned out into the world with only inadequate pensions to live on. They therefore became dependent upon the succour provided by local parishes and charitable persons. In the past, the monasteries themselves had looked after vagrants and the destitute, but those same monks and nuns who had taken in the poor were now themselves reduced in many cases to begging, a problem the government had not anticipated and did little to address.

Public outrage at the growing number of beggars whom local communities were forced to support was further exacerbated in many areas by the curtailment of ancient religious traditions occasioned by the break with Rome and the dissolution. Dissatisfaction was greatest in the northern and eastern counties where, away from the influence of London, disapproval of the King's measures was strong and religious sensibilities outraged. Conservatives were appalled to see churches and monastic buildings destroyed; they watched aghast as the King's men broke up images of the Madonna and saints, took axes to stained-glass windows, and carried away vestments and altar plate to the treasury. The King meant to purge his Church of England of all its superstitious and popish facets: holy shrines were desecrated – many being exposed as fakes – and the seeking of miracles was forbidden. Public grievance over the changes was made even more acute by the levying of heavy taxes to finance the programme of ecclesiastical reform.

Such was the social and political backdrop against which the King hoped to stage Jane's coronation. In September, carpenters were set to work in Westminster Hall, preparing it for the coronation banquet. Henry and Jane were then at Windsor. On 27 September, Sir Ralph Sadler, the Queen's secretary, arrived there with letters from Cromwell in London, and tried to see Henry before he joined the Queen in her chamber for supper; but although he said he had urgent news to impart, the King made him wait until he had eaten. Afterwards, he summoned Sadler and read the letters he had brought. The news was bad. There was plague at Westminster, even in the Abbey itself. Henry told Sir Ralph that the coronation would have to be put off for a season. As it turned out, plague was not the only delaying factor. Within days, there was worse news from London: the King now had a rebellion on his hands.

The rebellion known as the Pilgrimage of Grace began with a riot in the town of Louth in Lincolnshire, where the inhabitants felt that the King had gone too far with his religious reforms. This was no ordinary riot, however, but was organised by determined men. Others flocked to join them, and soon a contingent of the men of Norfolk had swelled their ranks; by 13 October, the rising had spread to Yorkshire, where three days later a rebel army occupied York. It was at this point that one of the burghers of York, a man named Robert Aske, set himself up as the rebels' leader. Then they were joined by the men of Hull under their leader John Constable.

Before very long this army of the people was marching south, its leaders carrying banners depicting the Five Wounds of Christ, which gave the rebellion its name; they saw their cause as nothing less than a crusade, their aim being to persuade the King to heal the breach with Rome and leave the monasteries alone.

At first, the King considered leading an army himself against them, and, acknowledging his trust in his queen, he announced that she would be regent in his absence, with Cranmer and the Privy Council acting as her advisers. But the Pilgrimage of Grace posed a personal dilemma for Jane, who was herself a religious conservative and had a certain amount of sympathy with the rebels. She ventured to voice her doubts to the King, choosing to do this in public and hoping, by her intervention, to diffuse his anger against the rebels. One day in late October, when Henry was sitting beneath his canopy of estate, surrounded by his court, she fell on her knees before him and begged him to reconsider the fate of the monasteries, asking him to restore some of the smaller ones. Henry said nothing, but his face registered his irritation; Jane ignored this, and went on, daring to suggest that perhaps God had permitted the rebellion as a punishment for the deliberate ruin of so many churches. At this, the King's patience gave way, and he exploded with anger, brutally ordering her to get up and attend to other things, and reminding her that the last queen had died as a result of meddling too much in state affairs. Jane took Henry's warning to heart, and never again interfered in politics. Those like the Prioress of Clementhorpe, who asked for her aid in saving her convent, met with disappointment, for Jane could do nothing. Her first duty, as she saw it, was obedience to her husband, and she took his advice, busying herself with domestic affairs, estate business and matters concerning her servants.

In November 1536, she was writing from Windsor to Cromwell, requesting his help in assisting a former retainer who had fallen into poverty: 'Ye could not do a better deed for the increase of your eternal reward in the world to come,' she told him. Then she was commanding her park keeper at Hampton Court to send venison to the gentlemen of the King's Chapel Royal; her warrant still survives, bearing one of only two extant examples of her signature. She also ordered a survey to be made of her lands and property, and her officers were eventually able to report to her that they found all her tenants and farmers 'as glad of her Grace as heart could be'; the year that had seen her marriage to the King was viewed by them as a year of peace in England.

Sadly, it was not to end that way. For two months, the rebellion flourished, the pilgrims being joined by more and more supporters. Henry gave up the idea of confronting them himself since he did not relish the idea of a winter campaign, and, in order to gain time in December, he sent word to Aske that he would meet his demands, promising 'with comfortable words' to send Norfolk north to ratify the agreement. He himself, he declared, would follow later. He also agreed to the rebels' demand that the Queen be crowned at York Minster. Henry was nothing if not a practised dissembler, and Aske accepted his assurances in good faith, joyfully disbanding his army in the confident belief that his sovereign would be true to his word. On 8 December, Aske was formally pardoned, and peace was restored.

The King's public rebuke to his wife caused no lasting damage to their marriage; in November, they were reported to be well and merry, and they were at Windsor in early December, planning their first Christmas together at Greenwich. The winter of 1536–7 was bitterly cold, and the roads were iced up, but this did not deter the King from summoning Mary to court for their public reconciliation. She arrived at Windsor on 17 December, richly dressed and with a train of gorgeously attired ladies, and proceeded through the ranks of courtiers in the presence chamber to where her father and Queen Jane awaited her by a roaring fire at the far end of the room. After curtsying twice, the small, spare girl with red hair and a *retroussée* nose made a sweeping obeisance to the King, fell on her knees, and asked for his blessing. He took her hand, raised and kissed her, then presented her to the Queen, who also kissed her and warmly bade her welcome. Then Henry turned to the Privy Councillors standing near by, gave them a menacing stare, and declared, with superb tactlessness, 'Some of you were desirous that I should put this jewel to death!' There was an embarrassed silence until the Queen spoke up: 'That were great pity, to have lost your chiefest jewel of England.' Henry smiled. 'Nay, nay!' he replied, patting Jane on the belly, an indication that he thought she might be pregnant, 'Edward! Edward!' Already, he had decided upon a name for the hoped-for son, though within a week or so he would know Jane was not pregnant this time.

The excitement was proving too much for Mary, and to Henry's consternation she suddenly fainted at his feet. Both he and Jane stooped to assist her, with the courtiers crowding round; when Mary regained her senses a few moments later Henry bade her be of good cheer, as nothing would go against her. When she had revived sufficiently, he took her hand and walked her up and down the room.

After this, Mary was often at court. She quickly became close to the Queen and was accorded precedence immediately after her. And it was thanks to Mary's intercession that the King invited Elizabeth to court for the Christmas season. Foreign visitors to Greenwich would have been astonished to see the royal family together; it seemed that at last the King was settling down to something resembling family life. At table, the King and Queen sat together, with Mary opposite Jane a little further along the table. Elizabeth was too young to sit at table with the adults, but those who saw Henry playing with her during the festivities observed his affection for her.

Just before Christmas, the Thames froze in London. On 22 December, Henry, Jane and Mary, warmly wrapped in furs, rode on horseback from Westminster to the City, which was gaily decorated in their honour with tapestries and cloth of gold; priests in copes with crosiers stood at every street corner waiting to bless the royal party and, in spite of the bitter cold, the people turned out in large numbers to watch the procession, cheering loudly. After a service in St Paul's to mark the beginning of the Christmas celebrations, Henry and Jane then spurred their horses across the frozen river and galloped to the Surrey shore, Mary following with the rest of their retinue. Then they rode to Greenwich Palace, where they would stay for Christmas, when Jane would preside for the first time over the glittering Yuletide court. Yet the season was marred for her by news of the death of her father on 21 December at Wulfhall. He had never lived in the public eye, so there was no observance of court mourning for him, nor did the Queen attend the funeral at Easton Priory in Wiltshire (the body was later moved to Bedwyn Magna Church). It may be that she had never been close to a father she had rarely seen in recent years; there is certainly no record that she was unduly affected by his death.

On New Year's Day, gifts were exchanged. Both Henry and Jane gave Mary costly presents, as did Cromwell, and Mary, among other gifts, gave some money to Elizabeth's chaplain because she was concerned about the child's religious education.

But this peaceful lull could not last. Robert Aske had been the King's guest at court over Christmas, and after it had ended he and his followers began to realise that the King had no intention of honouring his promises. The dissolution of the monasteries had resumed, taxes were still heavy, and there were as yet no definite plans for a royal visit to York, much less a coronation in that city. Disillusioned and bitter, the rebels regrouped, but this time, Henry was not prepared to send them fair words. Instead, he sent that redoubtable commander the Duke of Norfolk into Lincolnshire at the head of a great army, to teach those in revolt that they must not presume to question the will of their king. It was a terrible lesson. Norfolk hanged as many traitors as he could lay his hands upon, and in March 1537 presided over a Grand Assize that condemned a further thirty-six men to death. Their bodies, left rotting on gibbets for months, served as a grim warning to all those who dared contemplate further rebellion. Constable was arrested and condemned to death in June, being hanged alive in chains over the gates of Hull, where he shortly perished of exposure and starvation, and Aske was captured in July, and suffered the same fate at York. By then, the rebellion had long since been effectively crushed.

Having successfully dealt with the worst crisis of his reign, Henry VIII discovered that he had another cause for rejoicing, for in the early spring of 1537, Queen Jane discovered that she was pregnant; she had conceived around the middle of January. Shortly afterwards, Henry took her on a progress through Kent, visiting Rochester and Sittingbourne before going on to Canterbury as pilgrims and making their offerings at the shrine of St Thomas à Becket. It was characteristic of Henry that he was already planning the dissolution of the great Abbey of St Augustine there – within a year, Becket himself would have been denounced as a traitor to his king, his shrine broken up, and his bones destroyed.

From Canterbury the King and Queen rode to Dover to see the newly constructed pier. Then it was back to Hampton Court where, on 20 March, Jane granted the master of the Hospital of St Katherine-by-the-Tower, an institution serving as both church and hospice under the traditional patronage of successive queens of England, exemption from all annual tithes in consideration of the burden borne by the hospital from the increasing numbers of poor people. And, at around the same time, Jane stood sponsor at the christening of her brother Edward's child, who bore her name; Mary and Cromwell also attended the ceremony.

Jane's pregnancy was announced at the beginning of April, when the King conveyed the happy news to the Privy Council. In the minutes of this meeting, the councillors recorded that they trusted in God that the Queen's Grace would bring forth many fair children, 'to the consolation and comfort of the King's Majesty, and of his whole realm'. News of Jane's condition spread quickly, and soon there were celebrations, not only in England, but as far away as Calais, where Lady Lisle, wife of the Governor, was not only copying the gold and silk embroidered caps and nightgowns worn and popularised by Queen Jane, but was also doing her best to place one of her daughters in Jane's service. She thought the news to be 'merry tidings'.

Throughout that spring, Henry was merry himself, and cheerful, even though his leg pained him and kept him indoors for much of the time. Late in May the Queen appeared at Hampton Court in the open-laced gown of a pregnant mother, and it was announced that the child had moved in her womb. 'God send her good deliverance of a prince, to the joy of all faithful subjects,' wrote one courtier. When news that the baby – 'like one given by God' – had quickened reached London on Trinity Sunday, a special mass was celebrated in St Paul's Cathedral in thanksgiving that 'our most excellent lady and mistress, Queen Jane, hath conceived and is great with child'. On the same day a *Te Deum* was sung in churches throughout the realm, 'for joy of the Queen's quickening', and in London that evening the citizens were provided with free wine and bonfires were lit. The King abandoned plans for a summer coronation; that could wait until after October, when the child was due.

Throughout the summer, prayers were offered in churches for Jane's safe delivery. She undertook no public engagements, and led a relatively quiet life, being attended by the royal physicians and the best midwives in the kingdom. To please her, the King had her brother Edward admitted to the Privy Council on 22 May. He also made sure she lacked for nothing. Her condition had given her a craving for quails, a great delicacy at that time, but unfortunately out of season. Henry went to considerable trouble to have the birds shipped over from Calais, commanding Lord Lisle to provide 'fat quails which her Grace loveth very well, and longeth not a little for'. If none was to be found in Calais, then a search must be made in Flanders. On 24 May, a large consignment of quails arrived, a welcome sight to the Queen and her relieved husband; they ate a dozen roasted at dinner, and a further dozen for supper. Jane's craving for quails persisted right through her pregnancy; the Lady Mary sent her some in June, and Lord and Lady Lisle dispatched a constant supply from Calais, for which the Queen sent her grateful thanks.

The King was still in excellent spirits, and Sir John Russell found him behaving 'more like a good fellow than a king'; it was said he had never been merrier. Early in June, after a brief visit to Guildford, the court moved to Windsor because there was plague in London. The King hunted daily in Windsor Great Park, and the game he shot was served to the Queen along with her favourite quails. By the middle of July, Jane was very large and had unlaced her gowns to their fullest extent. As a token of appreciation to Lady Lisle, she agreed to find a place in her household for one of her two daughters, Anne and Katherine Bassett. Lady Lisle had been unsuccessful in securing places for them the previous year, and was desperate to have at least one accepted. Jane commanded her to send both girls over from Calais, so that she could decide which one she liked best. They must bring two changes of clothes, one of satin, the other of damask. The sister not chosen by the Queen would be offered a place in the household of the Duchess of Suffolk. Once the choice was made, Jane would provide wages and food only: Lady Lisle must see that her daughter was properly kitted out, and must exhort her girls to be 'sober, sad, wise and discreet, lowly above all things, obedient, and willing to be governed and ruled by my Lady Rutland and my Lady Sussex, and to serve God and be virtuous, for that is much regarded'.

It is pure speculation to suggest that, had she lived, Jane Seymour might well have been the most formidable of Henry's wives, yet this is certainly indicated by the standards she set for her household and by her warning, sent through Lord Hussey to Lady Lisle, that the court was 'full of pride, envy, indignation, mocking, scorn and derision'. She had succeeded in ridding her household of Anne Boleyn's wayward influence, and was vigorously re-establishing the virtuous precepts set by Queen Katherine. Beneath her outward show of humility, there was steel, even though it was confined to the domestic sphere only. A year on the throne had transformed Jane into a pious and godly matron who was fully conscious of her rank and dignity, and who carried the knowledge that she might well be nurturing the heir to England in her womb.

Jane's chief companions at this time were her sister Elizabeth, now the wife of Cromwell's son Gregory, and the Lady Mary. At the end of August, wagers were laid on the sex of the royal baby and the date of its birth, and the doctors and soothsayers were all confidently predicting a boy. 'I pray Jesu, an [if] it be his will, send us a prince,' prayed a courtier fervently. The birth was to take place at Hampton Court, and the court moved there early in September. On the 16th, Jane took to her chamber. Anne Boleyn had once occupied the magnificent rooms assigned to her; they were near the Silver Stick Gallery, and had linenfold panelling and gilded ceilings, much like the recently restored suite known as 'Wolsey's Rooms', except that Jane's long-vanished apartments would have been bigger.

Here Lady Lisle's daughters came. Jane picked the elder, Anne Bassett, who was sworn to her service on 17 September. Anne would become a popular figure at court during the years to come, even attracting the King's amorous attention at one time, yet she kept her good reputation. For the present, however, she was dismayed to find that her attire did not meet the Queen's exacting standards. Jane insisted her French hood would have to go, and Lady Sussex hurriedly found a suitable gown of crimson damask and a gable hood for Anne to wear when in the Queen's presence. Jane ordered the girl to obtain two new hoods with stiffened frontlets, as well as two good gowns of black velvet and black satin, and insisted that she replace her coarse linen undergarments with ones of fine lawn. Finally, to her dismay, the Queen learned that there were far too few pearls stitched to Anne's girdle, and warned her that if she did not appear at court in the proper clothes, she would not be allowed to attend the royal christening when the time came.

Jane was nevertheless a generous mistress; she gave Mary Zouche, one of Holbein's sitters whose portrait survives at Windsor, a gift of jewelled borders for a hood or gown, and after Jane's death the King granted Mary a pension of £10 per annum in consideration of her good service. The Queen also gave some jewellery to Mary, Lady Monteagle, one of her ladies-in-waiting. But she was not over-familiar with her ladies, and nor would they have expected her to be. She had the company of the Lady Mary during these last weeks of her pregnancy, and that was enough for her.

In London, the plague raged. Henry was alarmed for the safety of his wife and unborn child; as for Jane, she was horribly afraid. The King gave orders that no one who had been in London was to approach the court, but even this did not dispel her fears. 'Your ladyship would not believe how much the Queen is afraid of the sickness,' wrote Anne Bassett to her mother. To further minimise the risks, Henry moved with his household to Esher, in order to reduce the number of people staying at Hampton Court. He did not apparently consider his presence there necessary for his wife's peace of mind, but he told Norfolk that he would not travel far from her at this time,

considering that, being a woman, upon some sudden and displeasant rumours that might by foolish or light persons be blown abroad in our absence, she might take to her stomach such impression as might engender no little danger or displeasure to that wherewith she is now pregnant, which God forbid.

The Council had advised him not to travel more than sixty miles from Hampton Court, 'especially as she being, as it is thought, further gone by a month or more than she thought herself at the perfect quickening, remembering what dependeth upon the prosperity of that matter'.

It was obvious by early October that the birth was imminent, and the courtiers were telling each other to 'look daily for a prince'. The King was so certain that his child would be a boy that he gave orders for a Garter Stall to be made ready in St George's Chapel for 'the Prince hoped for in due season'. On 7 October, as the Queen showed no signs of going into labour, the Lady Mary went briefly back to Hunsdon to attend the christening of the child of one of her tenants; when she returned, Jane was still up and about. In Leicestershire, at Bradgate Manor, the King's niece, Frances Brandon, Marchioness of Dorset, gave birth to a baby girl and named her after the Queen; this child grew up to be the ill-fated Lady Jane Grey, who would lose her head before her seventeenth birthday. And in London, the young Duchess of Suffolk bore a healthy son.

At last, on the afternoon of 9 October, the Queen's labour pains began. As soon as they were well established, the King sent the royal heralds to London with the news. In the City, the response was overwhelming: bells were rung, masses sung in every parish church with congregations spilling out into the street in some places, and, on 11 October, a solemn procession walked from St Paul's Cathedral to Westminster Abbey, headed by the Lord Mayor and his aldermen, and including representatives of the guilds and livery companies of the City, and the clergy in their ceremonial copes. All offered prayers for the Queen's safe delivery.

Jane's ordeal lasted three days and three nights. It was rumoured in London that she would have to be cut open to facilitate her infant's safe delivery, a rumour that would in later years be embroidered by Catholic writers hostile to Henry VIII. Their lurid accounts give graphic – and entirely fictional – details of Jane's labour, alleging that her limbs were stretched to ease delivery, and that at length the King was asked who should be saved, the mother or the child. He is said to have opted for the child, as other wives could easily be found. A Caesarean operation is then said to have been performed. None of this is true. There is no evidence for a Caesarean operation being performed on a living mother before 1610 and, if it had, the result would have been a speedy and agonising death. Not until the twentieth century could this procedure be safely carried out.

Nevertheless, Jane Seymour's sufferings were great, and the labour prolonged and painful. But, finally, at two o'clock in the morning of Friday, 12 October 1537, it came to an end when she was safely delivered of a healthy, fair-haired boy. The King, after a wait lasting twenty-seven years, finally had his heir. It was, said a courtier, 'the most joyful news that has come to England these many years'.

Henry was at Esher when his son was born, but when he was informed that the Queen had been happily delivered of a prince, he rode to Hampton Court to see her and to welcome the child. The royal father was delirious with pride and joy, and named the child Edward; by a happy coincidence he had been born on St Edward's Eve. He became Duke of Cornwall at the moment of his birth, and it was confidently expected that his father would create him Prince of Wales and Earl of Chester, though this never came to pass. He was healthy, and bore resemblances to both his parents, having his father's features and his mother's fairness.

Henry wasted no time in informing the world of the glad tidings. Within minutes of his arrival at Hampton Court, his heralds had been dispatched to every part of the country with instructions to spread the news. In London, a *Te Deum* was sung in every parish church, and the bells in the City began a joyful pealing which would continue all day and all evening. There were bonfires in the streets, and the Tower guns shot off 2,000 rounds of ammunition in honour of the Prince. Banners were set up, and impromptu banquets given by prominent citizens. The messengers bearing the news were given costly gifts, and at the Steelyard the merchants of the Hanseatic League lit a hundred torches and generously provided free wine and beer for the citizens. Everywhere, housewives were hanging garlands above their doors and balconies and preparing food for the Tudor equivalent of street parties, while before the great doors of

St Paul's many bishops gathered to provide a feast for the people before celebrating mass. A holiday mood prevailed, and very little work was done that day; the feasting and carousing continued until the evening, when the Lord Mayor rode through the crowded streets thanking the people on the King's behalf for their demonstrations of love and loyalty. The conduits were still flowing with ale and wine, and there were many who woke with sore heads the next day, or found they had been robbed, thieves and pickpockets being certain of the King's pardon on such an occasion.

London's bells ceased their clangour at ten o'clock in the evening. At around the same time, the Queen was sitting up in bed writing to Cromwell to inform him that 'we be delivered and brought in childbed of a prince conceived in most lawful matrimony between my lord the King's Majesty and us,' and commanding him to convey the news to the Privy Council. Her letter was signed 'Jane the Queen'. Her triumph was now complete. Letters of congratulation came pouring into the palace, and the royal secretaries were kept busy announcing the royal birth to foreign princes and other dignitaries. The Prince was not the only baby born at Hampton Court on 12 October; in another suite, the Queen's sister-in-law, Lady Beauchamp, gave birth to a son who was also called Edward. In all, it was an auspicious day for the Seymours.

Overjoyed as he was with his 'fine boy', Henry was concerned for the infant's safety as there was still plague in the capital, and the first months of life were always hazardous. With these considerations in mind, he gave orders that every room, hall and courtyard in the Prince's apartments was to be washed down with soap and swept daily. Everything that came near the child – clothing, bed-linen, toys – was to be scrupulously clean. It is doubtful whether Jane saw much of her son after his birth. He had his own apartments, where he was cared for by wet-nurses, nursemaids and other servants. Unlike Anne Boleyn, Jane would not make a fuss about suckling her own child.

The Prince was christened on Monday, 15 October. Because of the risk of plague, the numbers attending were severely restricted, yet nearly 400 persons were present at the midnight ceremony in the Chapel Royal at Hampton Court, which had recently been completed and which still boasts its splendid Tudor ceiling. The guests had all gathered beforehand in the Queen's apartments, where Jane received them lying on a day bed of crimson damask lined with cloth of gold. Around her shoulders she wore a crimson mantle edged with ermine, over which flowed her loose blonde hair. Beside her sat the King in a richly upholstered chair. Her son was carried in procession through torchlit corridors just before midnight by Lady Exeter, with Norfolk holding his head steady and Suffolk supporting his feet. The King had chosen Archbishop Cranmer, Norfolk and Suffolk, and the Lady Mary as godparents. The Lady Elizabeth was in the procession too, carried in the arms of Lord Beauchamp, the Queen's brother, and holding the chrysom tightly in small fists. In the Chapel, the Prince was proclaimed heir to the King and, after he had been baptised by the Archbishop, he was conveyed back to the Queen's apartments with great pomp; this time, Elizabeth walked, holding Mary's hand. Jane took her son and gave him her blessing, then the King gathered him into his arms and, with tears of joy streaming down his face, blessed Edward in the name of God, the Virgin Mary and St George. The Prince was then carried off by the Duchess of Suffolk to his own apartments, followed by his household of 400 persons. Afterwards, refreshments were served for the guests, hippocras and wafers for the nobility, bread and sweet wine for the gentry. Then, when everyone present had kissed the hands of the King and Queen, the company dispersed. Jane had played her part to perfection; no one had noticed that anything was amiss with her.

On the afternoon of the following day, Jane suffered a bad attack of diarrhoea, which left her feeling rather ill, but by the evening she was better. During the night, however, she was sick, and early on Wednesday morning her condition was giving cause for concern. It was obvious that she was suffering from puerperal fever, a common hazard for women in childbed in those days. It is quite likely that Jane had suffered a tear in her perineum during delivery, which had become infected. Very little was known about hygiene in that period, and midwives did not understand the need for clean hands. Moreover, Jane's regime since the birth had been quite irregular, and she had been over-indulged by her attendants who were accused of having given her too rich a diet.

The Queen rapidly became so ill that it was feared she would die;

her confessor, the Bishop of Carlisle, was sent for, and he administered the last rites shortly before eight o'clock in the morning, before issuing a bulletin about the Queen's illness. Then, just as the Bishop was about to administer extreme unction, Jane rallied, and on Thursday she was so much restored that the King, who had been very anxious about her, felt able to continue with the celebrations in honour of the Prince's birth. On that day, he created Edward Seymour Earl of Hertford. On Friday, London was still celebrating, and the rest of the kingdom was following suit. The Bishop of Gloucester reported from the West Country that there was 'no less rejoicing in these parts than there was at the birth of John the Baptist'. Later that day, however, the Queen grew feverish again, and the King ordered a solemn intercession of the clergy; this took place in St Paul's, with the Bishop of London officiating.

For three days, she lay in delirium. On Monday night, her condition worsened, and the Bishop of Carlisle wrote to inform Cromwell that she was dying. The King had intended to return to Esher for the start of the hunting season on Tuesday, 23 October, but 'could not find it in his heart' to leave Jane in such a state. On that Tuesday, however, she seemed a little better, although she had been in great danger during the night. Her doctors told the King that, if she survived the next night, they 'were in good hope' that she would live. The Chapel Royal was full that day: 'If good prayers can save her, she is not like to die,' people were saying. 'Never was lady more popular with every man, rich or poor.'

At eight o'clock that evening, Henry was summoned urgently to his wife's bedside; she was failing fast. Norfolk wrote a hurried note to Cromwell, urging him to come to Hampton Court at once 'to comfort our good master, for as for our mistress, there is no likelihood of her life, the more pity, and I fear she shall not be alive at the time ye shall read this'. The King remained at Jane's side throughout the evening and into the night. In the early hours of Wednesday, 24 October, the Bishop of Carlisle was summoned to administer the last rites, and at about two o'clock, Jane slipped quietly from sleep into death.

Henry VIII could not bear anything to do with death. On the following morning his horror of remaining in the same house as

Jane's corpse got the better of him, and he fled to Windsor, leaving the Duke of Norfolk to look after the funeral arrangements. Once at Windsor, Henry went into seclusion for a time, refusing at first to see anyone, which was perhaps as well, for his ministers had already begun debating whether or not they should urge him to marry again for the sake of his realm. Surprisingly, when this suggestion was tentatively put to the King a few days later, he agreed that a fourth marriage might be wise, in view of the fact that his sole male heir was just an infant who might at any time succumb to a multitude of childhood ailments. 'He has framed his mind to be indifferent to the thing,' recorded one councillor. Despite his natural grief, as soon as Jane was buried he would be considering possible brides.

Jane was given a magnificent funeral. Her body was embalmed on 25 October, the entrails being removed and buried in the Chapel Royal at Hampton Court. The corpse was then dressed in a robe of gold tissue with the crown on its head and some of the Queen's jewels. It lay in state in the presence chamber for a week from 26 October, surrounded by tapers and with an altar beside it, at which masses were sung night and day for the soul of the departed. The obsequies began when Lancaster Herald charged those gathered to honour Jane's memory: 'Of your charity, pray for the soul of the Queen!' The body was then moved to a catafalque set up in the Chapel Royal, where the Queen's ladies would keep vigil beside it for a further week. The Lady Mary was chief mourner. She and the other ladies wore mourning habits of black with white head-dresses to signify that the Queen had died in childbed. Mary paid for thirteen masses to be sung for Jane's soul, and took charge of the late Queen's household, which would shortly be disbanded. It was probably Mary who carried out the King's command that Jane's beautiful diamonds and pearls were given to the wife of Sir Nicholas Carew, as Jane had wished.

Early in November, the Lord Mayor ordered 1,200 masses to be sung in the City 'for the soul of our most gracious Queen', and a solemn service was held in his presence in St Paul's. Alms were also given in the Queen's name to the poor.

On 8 November, Jane's coffin was taken to Windsor, where the King had decided she should be buried. It went in procession on a horse-drawn hearse followed by 200 poor men all wearing Jane's badge and bearing aloft lighted torches. The Lady Mary rode a horse draped in black velvet, and was attended by twenty-nine mourners, one for every year of the late Queen's life. At Colnbrook, Eton and Windsor, the poor men went ahead and lined the streets, while behind them stood the sorrowing crowds, hats in hands, watching silently as the funeral cortège wound its way past them. At the entrance to St George's Chapel, within the precincts of Windsor Castle, the coffin was received by the Dean and College, and was carried inside by six pallbearers. At the high altar, Archbishop Cranmer waited to receive it. The Lady Mary followed the coffin, her train borne by Lady Rochford. After prayers, the body was left to lie in state overnight, while the Lady Mary kept a grief-stricken vigil beside it. The next day, masses and dirges were sung, and the late Queen's ladies laid velvet palls upon the coffin, as was customary. Upon the palls was set a lifelike wooden effigy of the Queen that had been carried in the funeral procession but which has long since disappeared.

On Monday, 12 November, Queen Jane was finally laid to rest with great pomp and ceremonial 'in the presence of many pensive hearts', including those of her brothers, who would from now on enjoy enormous influence as uncles to the Prince. After the coffin had been lowered into a vault in the choir before the high altar the officers of the Queen's household broke their staves of office over it, thus symbolising the termination of their allegiance and service. On that day, the bells in London tolled for six hours, and on 14 November, a requiem mass was held in St Paul's Cathedral, thus bringing to an end the Queen's obsequies.

Etiquette precluded the presence of kings at their wives' funerals. After three weeks spent 'passing his sorrows' at Windsor while the funeral rites took place, Henry moved to Whitehall, where he once more took up the reins of government, but he was in very low spirits. The Bishop of Durham tried to alleviate his sufferings by reminding him that although God had taken from him 'that most blessed and virtuous lady', He had given him 'our most noble Prince, to whom God hath ordained your Majesty to be mother as well as father. God gave to your Grace that noble lady, and God hath taken her away as pleased Him.' Gradually, the King pulled himself together, and before very long his 'tender zeal' towards his subjects overcame his sad disposition, and he 'framed his mind' to a fourth marriage. By 3 November, he was reported to be in good health and 'merry as a widower may be'. He was now beginning to accept the tragedy that had befallen him, and to cope with his loss. He would wear full mourning, in deepest black, in Jane's memory, for three months, and court mourning would last until Easter 1538.

Jane's short, successful career and her tragic end caught the public's imagination, and she was celebrated in popular ballads long after she was dust. She had achieved nearly everything she set out to do: she had given the King the son he so desperately needed, she had helped to restore the Lady Mary to the succession and her father's affections, and she had used her influence to bring about the advancement of her family. She had provided the King with a family life for the first time in years, and had meddled hardly at all in matters of religion or politics. His grief at her death is testimony of his love for her. It was, in every respect, the most successful of his six marriages, and it was the only one to result in a surviving male heir.

In 1543, when Henry was married to Katherine Parr, he commissioned from an unknown artist a painting of himself, his wife, and his three children, which may still be seen at Hampton Court. Henry is shown seated on his throne in one of his palaces, with Mary and Elizabeth standing at either side of him. The six-year-old Edward stands at his father's knee, and sitting beside the King is not Katherine Parr, as might have been expected for she was an admirable stepmother, but Jane Seymour, wearing the gown in which Holbein had portrayed her in his Whitehall fresco. This inclusion of Jane in what was not so much a family group as a brilliant piece of Tudor propaganda is proof that Henry VIII wished to promote her image as one of the founding matriarchs of his dynasty. For Jane, this represents a considerable achievement, considering that her career, from her meetings with the King at Wulfhall in the autumn of 1535 to her death at the height of her triumph in 1537, had lasted just two short years.

When Henry VIII died, he left instructions that he was to be buried with Jane. His will gave detailed directions for the erection of a joint tomb surmounted by effigies of them both, carved 'as if sweetly sleeping'. But it was never built, and today the vault is marked only by a brass plate in the choir pavement. For a time, there was a Latin inscription to Jane's memory on the brass plate marking the grave, which, roughly translated, read as follows:

> Here lieth a Phoenix, by whose death
> Another Phoenix life gave breath:
> It is to be lamented much
> The world at once ne'er knew two such.

In 1813, the tomb of Henry and Jane was opened by order of the Prince Regent. Inside were found two coffins, one very large, of antique form, and another very small, as well as the coffin of Charles I and that of one of Queen Anne's infants. Henry's coffin was opened, revealing a skeleton 6'2" in length, with red hairs still adhering to the skull. The coffin containing the remains of Jane Seymour was left undisturbed.

Part III

How many wives will he have?

13
I like her not!

Had they ventured out of doors on New Year's Day 1540, country folk in Kent would have seen a party of horsemen, muffled to the ears in furs, galloping full tilt along the road that led to Rochester. Few would have guessed that this was the King, accompanied by eight gentlemen of his privy chamber, on his way to greet his new bride.

The visit had not been planned. After two years and two months without a wife, Henry VIII could no longer contain his eagerness to meet the lady in question, and had set out on the spur of the moment the night before, leaving behind the New Year festivities at Whitehall. His intention was to forestall the official ceremony of welcome and to meet his bride in private in order 'to nourish love'. With this in mind, the royal wooer hastened towards his destination, joyful anticipation in his heart.

The Princess whom he was contracted to marry was lodged with her retinue in the Bishop's Palace in Rochester, having disembarked at Deal some six days before. She was now awaiting a summons to London where her official reception was to take place. She was surprised, therefore, when the King was announced, and a party of men clad in coats of moire was ushered into her presence; in fact, she was trembling with nervousness.

Henry VIII had long been impatient for this moment, having a very natural desire to come face to face with the woman whose portrait he had fallen in love with. But when he entered the room where she awaited him with trepidation, he took one look at her, and his face fell.

Negotiations for the marriage had dragged on for more than a year by the time of that ill-fated meeting. Nor was this the first princess upon whom Henry had set his sights since Jane Seymour's death. It has often been said that Henry paid Jane the compliment of remaining a widower for two years, but it must be remembered that he did not do this through choice. With only one son, he still needed to ensure the succession by siring others, and therefore remarriage was of paramount importance. This apart, there were advantages to be gained by an alliance with a foreign power, and this Cromwell was eager to arrange. Henry himself, although approaching forty-seven, was still one of the most eligible men in Europe, even if, in view of what had happened to his first three wives, there were few princesses who could contemplate marrying him without a shudder. He was of course unaware that any lady might have such reservations, yet it does seem that at that time there was a dearth of suitable royal brides on the marriage market, due not only to the reluctance of some of those that were available, but also to religious barriers and to the constant shifting of continental political alliances.

Fortunately, the King's son was thriving in the care of his wet-nurse, Mother Jack, who had suckled him since his birth. By the time he was a month old, he was sucking vigorously, and at this age he was also given his own separate establishment at the old royal manor house at Havering in Essex. Here, rigorous standards of hygiene were still imposed by the King: the rooms were to be swept and cleaned twice a day, and – once the child was weaned – all his food was to be tested for poison. The capable Lady Bryan was once again appointed Lady Governess, and Edward would remain in her care until he was six.

His royal father visited him frequently. In May 1538, when Edward was seven months old, Henry spent a whole day at Havering, playing with the child and making him laugh. He carried the boy around in his arms for a long time, and held him up at the window so that the assembled crowds could see their future King. That summer, Edward was brought to Hampton Court to be with his sisters; Lady Lisle saw him then, and told her husband that he was 'the goodliest babe that ever I set mine eyen upon. I think I should never weary of looking on him.' The Prince grew fast, and could stand alone before his first birthday, a sturdy little boy with a loving nature and an earnest expression on his face. After his birthday, Mother Jack's services were dispensed with, and in her stead Mrs Sybil Penne was appointed chief nurse under Lady Bryan. The latter was very fond of her charge, and delighted in recounting his progress in her regular reports to Cromwell. One reads:

> Would to God the King and your lordship had seen him last night, for his Grace was marvellously pleasant disposed. The minstrels played, and his Grace danced and could not stand him still, and was as full of pretty toys as ever I saw child in my life.

When Edward was summoned to court to see his father, Lady Bryan made it her business to see he was suitably dressed, and badgered Cromwell constantly for clothing and jewellery for him. Unlike his sister Elizabeth, Edward had few problems with teething, and had four teeth by the time he was one. Before he was eighteen months old, his household had been expanded and the security around him tightened. No effort or expense was spared to protect this 'most precious jewel', and it was generally agreed by all that the sooner Edward was provided with a brother the better.

Mary Tudor, of course, was next in line of succession, despite her illegitimate status. After Queen Jane's death, she returned to Hunsdon, where she settled down to a quiet and peaceful life such as any lady of rank might enjoy in the country. At Easter 1538, she visited the court, wearing white taffeta edged with velvet, for the King had already discarded mourning for Queen Jane, and had given Mary special permission to do so for her visit. Thereafter, Mary was only at court infrequently, there being no lady of sufficient rank to act as her chaperon.

As for Elizabeth, she too went to Hunsdon, where she was looked after by Mary, since Lady Bryan had been transferred to Prince Edward's household. The child was brought to court by her sister for the Easter celebrations in 1538; she was then four and a half, and even Chapuys described her as being 'certainly very pretty'. She was a sharp, precocious little girl, and under Mary's tutelage she was rigidly schooled in good behaviour. Taught at an early age to wield a needle, she was able to complete a shirt of cambric as a New Year gift for her brother Edward in 1539. Yet for all her intelligence and ability, she was still excluded from the succession, even though her father had decided to treat her as one of the family.

Henry's obsessive desire to protect his heir made him more than usually sensitive to any hint of treason. As well as crushing opposition to the Acts of Succession, he was particularly concerned about the activities of the Pole family, and at the end of August Cardinal Pole's brother Geoffrey was sent to the Tower for aiding and abetting the exile. Henry had not forgiven or forgotten Pole's shattering diatribe against him, and his hatred of his former protégé bordered sometimes upon mania. Because of this, he now viewed every member of the Pole family with suspicion, remembering that Plantagenet blood ran in their veins. Understandably, the Poles reacted with antagonism. In the autumn of 1538, Lord Montagu, Reginald's eldest brother, and the Marquess of Exeter, another Plantagenet descendant, were both executed as a result of their suspected involvement in a plot to kill the King. Exeter's son, young Edward Courtenay, was left in the Tower, where he would remain for another fifteen years. Thus, in one stroke, Henry VIII eliminated most of the remaining members of the House of York.

There remained only Margaret Pole, the Countess of Salisbury, former governess to the Princess Mary and the mother of Lord Montagu, Cardinal Pole and Geoffrey Pole. During the enquiry into the activities of her sons, the King's officers had searched the old lady's house and found a banner embroidered with the royal arms of England: it lacked any of the differences appropriate to any member of the royal house of lower rank than the sovereign. The Countess, a respectable dowager of sixty-six, denied that she had ever intended to dispute the right of the King to the throne, but her staunch protests could not save her, and she too was committed to the Tower in March 1539. Her imprisonment would be rigorous: she was put in a cold cell without adequate food or clothing. Nor was there any hope of release. The King wanted her out of the way because, obsessively, he feared that, even at her age, she might be made the focal point of a revolt against the Crown. Added to the supposed treason of her sons and herself was an old score the King meant to settle: the Countess's championship of Queen Katherine. On 12 May 1539, Parliament passed an Act of Attainder against Margaret Pole, whereby she forfeited all rights to her life, title, estates and goods. The King immediately appropriated all her property, but he did not order her execution, leaving her to languish in prison, perhaps in the hope that death would intervene before long.

With the future of his dynasty assured by only one little boy, who was subject to all the ills that carried off children in that age of high infant mortality, Henry needed to remarry, and soon. He had begun his search for a bride in November 1537, one month after Queen Jane's death. Initially, he and Cromwell had decided to opt for a marriage alliance with France in order to counterbalance the extensive power of the Emperor, and also because Henry did not want another Spanish bride. King Francis had marriageable daughters, and it was said that there were other beautiful ladies of high rank available in France. Late in November, Henry approached the French ambassador, Castillon, and confided his preference for a French marriage. The ambassador obligingly suggested a few possible brides, but Henry was being cautious, fearing that his personal requirements might be brushed aside in the interests of politics. He told Castillon he wished to see the ladies in question and get to know them a little before making a decision. Castillon, who had never heard of such a preposterous and insulting idea, replied caustically, 'Perhaps, Sire, you would like to try them one after the other, and keep the one you found the most agreeable.' Henry, he recorded, blushed at this, and did not pursue the matter any more at that time. But a few days later he saw Castillon again and, undeterred, suggested that potential French brides be brought to Calais for his inspection. When King Francis was told, he laughed, and said 'It would seem they meant to do with women there as with their geldings: collect a number and trot them out to take which goes best!' However, he was not having his daughters or the ladies of his court being taken like prize animals to market, and he refused to sanction the suggestion.

Henry VIII was not to be put off. Although he preferred the idea of a French marriage, his ambassadors abroad were instructed to report on other likely brides. John Hutton, the English envoy in Brussels, reported that the Duke of Cleves had a daughter 'but there is not great praise either of her personage or her beauty'. He then went on to say that the Duchess of Milan, who had been born Christina of Denmark, had just arrived in Brussels; she was the Emperor's niece, sixteen years old, very tall and 'of excellent beauty'. Her speech was soft, and she had a gentle face; in Hutton's opinion, she resembled Lady Shelton 'that used to wait on Queen Anne'. The young Duchess had only recently been widowed, her elderly husband having died in Italy, and she was still wearing black mourning clothes.

> There is none in these parts for beauty of person and birth to compare with the Duchess; she is not so pure white as the late Queen, whom God pardon, but when she chanceth to smile, there appeareth two pits [dimples] in her cheeks and one in her chin, the which becometh her right excellently well.

Hutton's missive was sent to a member of the Privy Council, Sir Thomas Wriothesley, who showed it to the King. When Henry read of the charms of the Duchess of Milan, he was tempted to abandon his plans to make a French marriage in order to pursue the lovely Christina. After all, she had excellent connections. Born in 1521, she was the daughter of King Christian of Denmark by Isabella of Austria, the Emperor's sister. At the age of fourteen, she had been married to Francesco Maria Sforza, Duke of Milan, who had died in November 1535. She had now come to live with her aunt, Mary of Hungary, Regent of the Netherlands, in Brussels, until another husband could be found for her.

Everyone agreed that the Duchess of Milan was beautiful, and her extreme youth was in her favour, since her character could be more easily moulded to suit her husband. But Henry had reservations; he was growing fat and preferred buxom women like Katherine and Jane had been, not slim ones like Anne Boleyn, and Christina was reported to be of slender build. 'I am big in person and have need of a big wife,' the King declared, abandoning for the present any ideas of courting her. He had heard of the charms of a French noblewoman, Mary of Guise, and was 'so amorous' at the prospect of allying himself to her that he was now disinclined to consider anyone else, even though he was bound to concede that Christina of Milan was eminently suitable in most respects.

Mary of Guise was the eldest daughter of Claude, Duke of Guise, one of the most powerful men in France, being related to the royal house of Valois. Like Christina, Mary was also a widow; she had been married to Francis, Duke of Longueville, until his death in June 1537; but unlike Christina, she was of mature age, being twenty-two, and – more importantly – had borne two sons. Rumour had it that she was as buxom as the King could desire. Henry thought she was a highly suitable candidate for the vacant consort's throne, and in January 1538, after a very quiet Christmas at Greenwich, he put out a feeler for Mary's hand. The lady, however, being given advance warning of his imminent proposal, hurriedly accepted that of her other suitor, Henry's nephew, James V of Scotland, whom she married the following May.

Henry was disappointed but undaunted, and Cromwell tried to alleviate his master's sense of rejection by suggesting that he return to his earlier intention of paying court to the Duchess of Milan. In March 1538, the King sent his court painter, Hans Holbein, to Brussels to paint Christina's portrait, and at around this time the merry widower discarded his mourning garments for Jane Seymour. Yet although his grief for her had abated, he was in constant pain from his bad leg, and in May 1538 he was forced to submit to the attentions of the barber surgeons and have his abscess lanced. This relieved the pain somewhat, but it did not cure it. The King's sporting activities were now more or less curtailed: no longer could he ride in the lists, but was forced to sit and watch the galling spectacle of younger, fitter men doing what he had once done better. And, to make matters worse, increasing immobility was making him more and more obese, and his once splendid head of red-gold hair was thinning. To mask the ravages of advancing age and ill health, Henry dressed himself more sumptuously than ever before, and set a new fashion for the men of his court of a square look with built-up shoulders and bulky sleeves: the larger the man, the better the style suited him. No longer did the King's increasing girth look conspicuous, for every man of fashion was doing his best to emulate his sovereign.

Henry's temper was less easily controlled, and constant pain and envy of others did not serve to improve it. Those that were closest to him, especially Cromwell, suffered the most from his irascibility. Henry turned on his Lord Privy Seal at least twice a week, bawling him out and calling him a knave and other derisory names, and sometimes he hit him on the head, pounding him soundly, so that Cromwell would leave the King's chamber shaking with fright and with rumpled hair, albeit with a smile on his face that acknowledged that this was the price he had to pay for his privileged position. Others, like the Poles and the Exeters, experienced the more deadly consequences of the King's anger.

By the middle of 1538, England's relations with both Spain and France had deteriorated; at the same time, Charles V and Francis I had drawn closer together. In June 1538, they signed the Treaty of Nice, which was intended to bind them in friendship for ten years, and although this was not an offensive treaty against Henry VIII, it did leave him in political isolation. Nevertheless, he had received Holbein's finished portrait of the Duchess of Milan and been enchanted with it, and in September an English embassy led by Wriothesley was sent to Brussels to convey the King's proposal of marriage. On 6 October, they saw the Regent Mary, who gave them permission on the Emperor's behalf to approach Christina, who agreed to see them the following day.

The young Duchess was very outspoken. The idea of marrying Henry VIII did not appeal to her, and she declared as much with candour. She said, reported the ambassadors,

> that the King's Majesty was in so little space rid of the queens that she dare not trust his Council, though she durst trust his Majesty; for her council suspecteth that her great-aunt was poisoned, that the second was innocently put to death, and the third lost for lack of keeping in her childbed.

If she had two heads, she said, 'one should be at his Grace's service!' She then told Sir Thomas Wriothesley that he should not labour any further 'for I mind not to fix my heart that way,' saying she thanked God she was not 'of so light sort'.

When Wriothesley asked her what her real inclination was, she would only say that she was at the Emperor's command.

Marry! [replied Wriothesley] Then I may hope to be among the Englishmen that shall be first acquainted with my new mistress, for the Emperor hath instantly desired it. Oh, Madam, how happy shall you be if it be your chance to be matched with my master! You shall be matched with the most gentle gentleman that liveth, his nature so benign and pleasant that I think to this day no man hath heard many angry words pass his lips!

These lies did not deceive Christina, who stood her ground and refused to commit herself. Later, she confided her reluctance to the Emperor, who was sympathetic, with the result that the imperial Council made it obvious to Henry VIII that his suit was hopeless.

By that time Henry was only too pleased to withdraw. For some time, Cromwell had been urging him to forget his religious scruples and ally himself to one of the Protestant German Princes, a move which he predicted would tip the balance of power in Europe in England's favour once more. The King was well aware of the cool wind blowing in his direction from France and the Empire, and also aware that the Protestant states of Germany were a permanent thorn in the Emperor's side. An alliance between England and one of these states might well divert Charles from any thought of joining with France to make war upon England. Cromwell now remembered that, back in November 1537, Sir John Hutton had mentioned that the Duke of Cleves had an unmarried daughter. In fact, he had two.

John III, Duke of Cleves, was fifty-eight, and a Protestant; his marriage to Mary of Jülich-Berg-Ravensberg had produced four children. His son, William, born in 1516, would succeed him in 1539 as Duke of Cleves. His eldest daughter, Sybilla, an auburn-haired beauty whose charm has been immortalised in a portrait by Lucas Cranach, had been married in 1526, at the age of twelve, to John Frederick, Elector of Saxony, one of the most zealous Lutheran rulers in Europe. The two younger daughters, Anne, born on 22 September 1515 in the ducal capital of Düsseldorf, and Amelia, born in 1517, were as yet unmarried. Henry VIII was now toying with the idea of taking one or other as his bride. When the Duke of Cleves learned of this, he rightly perceived that it would be a brilliant match for whichever girl was chosen, and immediately offered his elder daughter to Henry.

When, in late 1538, the Pope learned of the executions of Montagu and Exeter, and reissued the Bull of Excommunication of 1534 against Henry, the attitude of France and the Empire hardened towards England, and an alliance with Cleves seemed more attractive. Naturally, as a Protestant, the Duke of Cleves could be counted upon to remain friendly in the face of papal hostility.

On 12 January 1539, Charles V and Francis I signed a new treaty at Toledo, by the terms of which both agreed not to make any fresh alliances without the consent and knowledge of the other. This sealed the estrangement between Henry and his former allies and his resolve to make an alliance with Cleves. In February, the King told Wriothesley that his Council were urging him daily to arrange a fourth marriage in order to beget more heirs to ensure the succession. They had warned him that age was 'coming fast on, and that the time flyeth and slippeth marvellously away'. For this reason, he was not minded to waste any more time. Cromwell, whose brainchild the Cleves match had been, was appointed Lord Great Chamberlain by way of reward, and in March, Henry sent Nicholas Wotton and Robert Barnes, a well-known Protestant who would be likely to find favour with Duke John, as envoys to Cleves, to arrange a marriage with either the Lady Anne or the Lady Amelia.

The English ambassadors were well received in Düsseldorf, but not by Duke John. He had just died, and in his place was his serious-minded, Protestant son William, a young man of twenty-three. William had strong ideas about feminine modesty, and when his sisters were brought in to be introduced to Wotton and Barnes, they were so well covered with 'a monstrous habit and apparel' that the ambassadors could see very little of their faces, let alone their figures. Later, when the sisters had withdrawn, Wotton complained about this to the Duke, who retorted, 'Would you see them naked?' He had no high opinion of moral standards in England.

Wotton turned to Cromwell for help. As a result, on 23 April 1539, Cromwell dispatched Hans Holbein to Cleves, as well as another envoy, Christopher Mont, who carried instructions to the envoys to procure portraits of Anne and Amelia. Mont arrived ahead of Holbein, and in due course Wotton and Barnes appeared before Duke William and requested permission for portraits to be made. The Duke said he would consider the matter, and then kept them waiting for days. Mont intervened, and persisted in repeating the request each day, while Wotton and Barnes, in a state of great agitation, wrote to Cromwell and begged him to excuse the delay to the King, adding that by all reports the Lady Anne was the better favoured of the two princesses. At length, William said he was happy for his sisters' likenesses to be painted, but only by his own court painter, Lucas Cranach, who happened to be sick just then. When Cranach had recovered and was able to complete the portraits, William would send them on.

Cromwell reported all this to Henry, adding,

> Every man praiseth the beauty of the said Lady Anne, as well for her face as for her person, above all other ladies excellent. She as far excelleth the Duchess of Saxony as the golden sun excelleth the silver moon. Every man praiseth the good virtues and honesty with shamefacedness which plainly appeareth in the gravity of her countenance.

Undoubtedly, Cromwell was exaggerating what he had been told. Few had actually seen very much of Anne of Cleves's charms, for she was always well swathed in cumbersome clothing when she appeared in public, and such occasions were rare. Her upbringing had been very strict, and anything approaching frivolity had been frowned upon. Yet Cromwell had good reason to exaggerate: this match had been his idea from the first, and it was vitally important to him that it should be successfully concluded. It would not be an exaggeration to say that his whole future depended upon that, nor is it beyond the bounds of reason to suppose that Cromwell had sent Hans Holbein off with instructions to make the lady look as attractive as possible in her portrait.

When the King read Cromwell's letter he was entranced. This princess, it seemed, was a paragon of beauty and womanly modesty, though it appeared that her brother was reluctant to let her go. He kept raising objections to the marriage: he said his sisters had been raised in a narrow environment of virtuous industry – how then would either of them fare as queen in a court known for its licentious habits? He said he was too poor to afford a dowry. He said that, in view of what had happened to the King's other wives, he felt that any woman marrying Henry VIII would only know insecurity and unhappiness. These objections were all duly conveyed to Cromwell, and a reply came back speedily. The King had decided he would take the Lady Anne without a dowry if her portrait pleased him. This was a very generous offer, and one that an impoverished ruler could not afford to turn down. The young Duke quickly capitulated, agreed to the marriage, and gave Holbein permission to paint Anne's likeness.

Holbein set to work at once, and the result was one of the most exquisite portrait miniatures ever painted, which may be seen today in the Victoria and Albert Museum in London. Anne smiles out demurely from an ivory frame carved to resemble a Tudor rose. Her complexion is clear, her gaze steady, her face delicately attractive. She wears a head-dress in the Dutch style which conceals her hair, and a gown with a heavily bejewelled bodice. Everything about Anne's portrait proclaimed her dignity, breeding and virtue, and when Henry VIII saw it, he made up his mind at once that this was the woman he wanted to marry. Cromwell breathed a sigh of relief, and the marriage negotiations went ahead.

The choice of a Protestant bride for the King of England led to avid speculation in Europe, and especially in Lutheran circles. Christopher Mont wrote to the Elector of Saxony, Anne's brother-in-law, to say that the Protestant cause would be greatly advanced once Anne became Queen, 'for the King is so uxorious that the best way of managing him is through his wives'. English Protestants believed that their new Queen might well be another Anne Boleyn, and that they would once again have a friend and champion upon the throne. Yet Mont was inaccurate in his assessment of Henry VIII, who was never uxorious, expected unquestioning obedience from all his wives, and reacted brutally when he did not get it. Henry assumed that Anne of Cleves would be happy to conform to the Catholic form of worship when she became Queen of England, and there is no evidence to show that she did otherwise from the time of her arrival. When she died, she died a professed Catholic, and it seems that the transition from one faith to another had been fairly effortless. Lutherans in England were therefore destined to be disappointed in her.

Now that his proposal had been accepted, Henry deemed it the proper time to find out more about his future bride, and wrote to Wotton, asking him to make discreet enquiries. On 11 August 1539, the ambassador reported that the Lady Anne had been brought up by her mother, 'and in a manner never far from her elbow'. The Duchess Mary was 'a wise lady', and had been very strict with her children. Anne was of a humble and gentle disposition, and the Duchess was so fond of her that she was loath to see her depart. As for her education, the future Queen of England was an expert needlewoman, could read and write her own language, and was very intelligent. However, she had no knowledge of French, Latin, English or any other tongue; nor could she sing or play a musical instrument, 'for they take it here in Germany for a rebuke and an occasion of lightness that great ladies should be learned or have any knowledge of music.' Nevertheless, Wotton believed that Anne was bright enough to learn English fairly quickly. He added that Holbein was painting full-scale portraits of Anne and Amelia: that of Amelia is now either lost or unidentified, but his masterpiece of Anne of Cleves hangs nowadays in the Louvre in Paris.

When the King read Wotton's description of Anne's accomplishments, he may well have felt a little disconcerted, especially when he learned that his wife-to-be spoke only High Dutch, a language of which he had no knowledge whatsoever. Moreover, she came from a court that scorned music, which was one of Henry's passions, and it seemed she knew nothing of dancing or fashion either, so narrow had been her upbringing. Nevertheless Henry felt that these were all minor obstacles which could be overcome by love, that supreme blessing which he felt sure would make this marriage a crowning success. Already, he was growing impatient for his bride's arrival in England.

At the end of August, however, the Duke of Cleves remembered that there might well be an impediment to the marriage. His father had once opened negotiations with the Duke of Lorraine for a marriage between the Duke's son, the Marquess of Pont-à-Mousson, and Anne, and it was just possible that a precontract had been entered into, in which case it would have to be dissolved in the ecclesiastical courts in order to facilitate the more advantageous marriage with the King of England. Enquiries were duly made both in Cleves and in Lorraine. Happily, no evidence of any precontract was unearthed, and at the end of September Wotton was able to inform the King that he found the Duke of Cleves and his Council 'willing enough to publish and manifest to the world that my Lady Anne is not bounden, but ever hath been and yet is at her free liberty to marry wherever she will'.

On 4 September 1539, the marriage treaty was signed by the Duke of Cleves at Düsseldorf, and the Lady Anne thanked her brother and the people of Cleves 'for having preferred her to such a marriage that she could wish for no better'. Duke William then sent his representatives to England where the treaty would be ratified; they arrived at Windsor on 23 September, and were entertained by the King with hunting and feasting for the next eight days, before moving to Hampton Court, where the marriage treaty was concluded on 4 October. Great preparations then commenced for the reception of the bride and the wedding to follow. Some noblemen had already ordered their wedding clothes, and there was the usual stampede for places in the new Queen's household. Katherine Bassett, whose sister Anne had gone to court to serve Jane Seymour and remained there ever since as a great favourite of the King, was now urging her mother, Lady Lisle, to 'be so good lady and mother to me as to speak that I may be one of the Queen's maids'.

The religion of the bride provoked some comment. The Lady Mary was at first dismayed to learn that her father was marrying a Lutheran heretic; yet in time she would become firm friends with Anne of Cleves, and would be partly responsible for Anne's conversion to the Catholic faith. The King saw his marriage as paving the way for a 'softening of the asperities which are now distracting Germany', and hoped to use his influence, and that of the Duke of Cleves, to 'find some honourable middle course' which would put an end to the religious problems of the German principalities. He told Marillac, the French ambassador, that, because he had but one son, he was marrying for the sake of children, and considered he could do no better than Anne of Cleves, who at twenty-four was 'of convenient age', in sound health, and of good stature, 'with many other graces which his Majesty says she possesses'.

In Cleves, discussions were taking place as to the best route for Anne to take to England. There were two ways of making the journey: one was by ship from one of the Baltic ports, and the other was overland to Calais. Duke William and his advisers were of the opinion that Anne should travel by land, as she had never before been on a ship, and might well suffer dire consequences as a result of a voyage across the Baltic during winter. There were even fears that the ordeal might 'alter her complexion' and make her unattractive to her new husband. It was decided, therefore, that Anne should travel by land along the north coast of Europe to Calais, and there take ship for England. In late October, news of her imminent departure from Cleves was sent by fast messenger to the English court, and on 5 November the eager bridegroom was informing his Council that he expected Anne's arrival in about twenty days' time, saying he intended to go to Canterbury to receive her.

Anne left Cleves early in November; she had been provided with a retinue of 263 attendants and 228 horses. Her progress was slow and, when she did not arrive at Calais on the expected date, Henry sent a courier to find out what was happening. The man returned with the news that Anne would be there on 8 December. To welcome her, Henry dispatched the Duke of Suffolk across the Channel, together with the Lord Admiral, Sir William FitzWilliam, Earl of Southampton, whose duty it would be to escort the future Queen safely to England. With them went many other lords and court officials. Norfolk and Cromwell were told to make their way to Canterbury in due course in order to greet Anne and welcome her to England on the King's behalf.

Henry planned a Christmas wedding at Greenwich, to be followed by twelve days of festivities, while Anne's official entry into London was scheduled for 1 January, to be followed by her coronation on Candlemas Day, 2 February, in Westminster Abbey. From Hampton Court, the King issued a stream of orders concerning the reception of his bride and the preparations for their wedding. Two splendid royal beds were sent to Dartford and Rochester, places where Anne was to stay en route to London, so that she would be as comfortable as possible. Plans were drawn up for the formation of the new Queen's household, since those who had served Jane Seymour had long since been discharged. The chief officers were appointed in November, as well as several ladies-in-waiting and maids of honour. Once again, Anne Basset was chosen to serve a queen of England; her mother

Lady Lisle was so grateful to the King for the appointment that she sent him some quince marmalade and damson conserve made by herself, which he so enjoyed that he asked for more. Henry had a soft spot for Anne Bassett; in 1539, he presented her with a horse and saddle. Later, when she was older, there would be rumours of an affair between them, though for the present Henry had no interest in any woman save Anne of Cleves.

He was in the best of spirits. His leg was troubling him less for the moment, he was eager to see his bride, and his gaiety was infectious. He had heard from Dr Wotton, who was part of Anne's escort, that she was tall and thin, of medium beauty, and of 'very assured and resolute countenance'; on the face of it, these were all attributes that the King admired least in women, but he was so blinded just then by what he was pleased to call love that he could only read into Wotton's description the highest praise. He was now more impatient than ever to meet the lady, and had convinced himself she would surpass his three previous wives a hundredfold.

Others were not deceived by Wotton's words. Of course, Holbein's miniature had been displayed at court, but Holbein was an artist who painted what his inner eye saw, and he had after all had his instructions from Cromwell. Several people at court were already privately expressing doubts that Anne of Cleves was as attractive as she was depicted in that portrait, and early in December, a scurrilous little rhyme was secretly circulating:

> If that be your picture, then shall we
> Soon see how you and your picture agree!

One doubts that this ever came to the King's notice; no one would venture to destroy his illusions.

Meanwhile, Anne had arrived in Antwerp, having been met four miles outside the city by a company of fifty English merchants wearing velvet coats and gold chains. She then went in procession along streets lit with torches, until she came to the English-owned house where she would spend just one night before travelling on. The house was thrown open to the public, and many came to see the future Queen of England.

Anne reached Calais on 11 December, and was given a magnificent welcome. Just past Gravelines, she was met by Lord Lisle, Governor of Calais, who greeted her on the King's behalf and escorted her towards the town. A mile from its gates, the Admiral was waiting to pay his respects, clad in a coat of purple velvet and cloth of gold, and wearing a seaman's whistle set with gems. With him were the Duke of Norfolk's brother, Lord William Howard, Sir Francis Bryan, 400 gentlemen in coats of satin damask, and 200 yeomen wearing coats of red and blue cloth, the colours of the royal arms of England. Southampton bowed low, then escorted Anne into Calais by the Lantern Gate. Here, she could see the ships in the harbour, all gaily bedecked with banners in her honour.

Anne was at last on English soil. At her entry through the gate, a salute was fired from the cannon along the harbour wall, and she was presented by the Mayor of Calais with a solid gold 'C' (for Cleves) as a compliment. On the other side of the gate, Lady Lisle and a host of ladies and gentlewomen sank into deep curtsys as Anne appeared. In front of the hall of the merchants of the Staple the town burgesses were lined up in formation, and they offered their new queen a rich purse containing 100 golden sovereigns, for which she heartily thanked them. Anne then went to view the King's ships that were in port, the *Lyon* and the *Sweepstakes*, after which she progressed through the narrow streets, while 150 rounds of ordnance were let off from those ships in her honour. Her retinue, unaccustomed to such things, were wide-eyed with astonishment at the splendour of her reception, and Anne herself took a refreshingly unaffected pleasure in it all. Finally, she passed through two lines formed by the merchants of the Staple to the entrance to the Exchequer Palace, where she was to lodge during her stay. The next morning, there was another salvo from the guns, followed by jousting in her honour.

Southampton was pleasantly impressed by Anne. On the day of her arrival, he wrote to Henry VIII to apprise him of it, saying how glad he was his Grace had decided to marry again and that he prayed that the Almighty would bless the union with children, so that 'if God failed us in my lord Prince, we might have another sprung of like descent and line to reign over us in peace'. These were very proper sentiments, but the Admiral also confessed that he had had misgivings about Anne of Cleves's suitability to be Queen. However, 'hearing great report of the notable virtues of my lady now with her excellent beauty, such as I well perceive to be no less than was reported', he had wholeheartedly revised his opinion. Lady Lisle was also impressed, and wrote to her daughter, Anne Basset, to say that her future mistress was 'so good and gentle to serve and please'. Anne thought this would be a great comfort to the Queen's servants, as well as to the King himself, who was by then 'not a little desirous to have her Grace here'.

Anne's stay in Calais was to last considerably longer than had been anticipated because bad weather prevented a Channel crossing. The King soon realised that his bride would not be with him in time for Christmas, and kept himself busy with negotiations for a proposed marriage between the Lady Mary and Duke Philip of Bavaria, another Protestant ruler, though Mary declared she would rather remain unmarried than enter into such an alliance. The King was sympathetic, but determined to press on with the negotiations, and when Philip came to London, Mary was obliged to go to court to greet him. Unwillingly, she obeyed, and the Duke afterwards told her father that he wished to proceed with the marriage. Shortly afterwards Mary fell ill – or feigned illness – and retired from court. She was away for some time, and even missed attending her father's wedding. Philip of Bavaria was therefore advised to remain in England until her return, but by then the King's enthusiasm for the German alliance would have been dramatically doused, and Philip would find that his waiting had been in vain.

The weather remained bad until Christmas Day. Anne was entertained with more banquets and jousts, and the Admiral – finding she did not play cards, which was one of the King's favourite pastimes – took it upon himself to teach her, reporting to his master that she was an apt and willing pupil, eager to please. Southampton found himself liking Anne very much, and exerted himself to make her enforced stay in Calais as enjoyable as possible. Anne obviously returned his liking: one evening, she invited him and a few other gentlemen to supper in her apartments, which was not thought by the English a seemly thing for a woman betrothed to another man to do, although Anne in her innocence was unaware of this. Southampton was worried about how the King would react when he found out, but at the same time too embarrassed to refuse the invitation. In the end he went, and was relieved to find that her 'manner, usage and semblance was such as none might be more commendable, nor more like a princess.'

On 26 December, a fair wind was blowing, and the Admiral judged it prudent to set sail for England without any further delay. He himself conducted Anne on board ship at midday; the voyage took seventeen hours, and she disembarked at Deal at five o'clock the next morning. Sir Thomas Cheyney, Lord Warden of the Cinque Ports, was waiting to receive her and escort her to Deal Castle, a fortress recently built on Henry VIII's orders as part of a chain of coastal defences. While she was resting there, the Duke and Duchess of Suffolk arrived with the Bishop of Chichester and a multitude of other notable people to pay their respects and to accompany Anne that night to Dover Castle, where she was to stay for a day or so. Then the weather turned bitterly cold, with freezing storms. Nevertheless, Anne insisted upon pressing on towards London, so 'desirous was her Grace of reaching the King's presence'. On Monday, 29 December, with hail and sleet blowing continually in her face, she journeyed with her retinue to Canterbury, where Archbishop Cranmer, accompanied by 300 gentlemen, bade her welcome, as did the Bishop of Ely. The two prelates then brought her to the great monastery of St Augustine, where she was lodged in the guesthouse. In spite of the bitter weather, crowds came out to see her, as she made her way along the streets of the ancient city. As it was evening, torches had been lit, and the Mayor had arranged for a gunfire salute to be sounded at Anne's entry. In her bedchamber, she found fifty gentlewomen in velvet hoods waiting to attend her, which especially pleased her. Suffolk told Cromwell she was 'so glad to see the King's subjects resorting to her so lovingly, that she forgot all the foul weather and was very merry at supper'.

Cromwell was relieved and gratified to hear of Anne's rapturous reception by her future subjects. She had behaved very well indeed, justifying his earlier praise of her virtues. Several people who had seen her were impressed with her looks and her manner, and she seemed eager to make up for her lack of accomplishments by learning as quickly as possible how to please the King. Cromwell now allowed himself to relax a little; all seemed set fair for a successful royal marriage, and he could look forward to the rewards he would receive from a grateful king.

Anne left Canterbury on 30 December and rode to Sittingbourne, where she stayed that night. On New Year's Eve, she went on towards Rochester; the Duke of Norfolk, accompanied by 100 horsemen in velvet coats and gold chains, met her on Reynham Down and escorted her to the Bishop's Palace in the city, where she was to stay for two nights. Here awaited Lady Browne, wife of Sir Anthony Browne, a stern matron who was to supervise the new Queen's maids of honour. When Lady Browne was presented to the Lady Anne, she could barely conceal her dismay, and later confided in a letter to her husband that Anne was wearing such dreadful clothes and was obviously the product of so gross an upbringing that everything about her was 'far discrepant from the King's Highness' appetite'. In Lady Browne's judgement, 'the King should never heartily love her.' Others perhaps shared her misgivings, but were more discreet about it, and the royal bridegroom remained blissfully unaware of such undercurrents. So eager was he to see Anne that on New Year's Eve he set out on that fateful journey to Rochester 'to nourish love'.

When Henry greeted Anne in her presence chamber in the Bishop's Palace, he gave no sign of what he was thinking. He welcomed her to England with great courtesy, while she in turn, 'with most gracious and loving countenance and behaviour', sank to her knees to receive him. Henry raised her up gently and kissed her on the mouth, as was customary in England. He stayed for the afternoon, engaging in a rather halting conversation with the aid of an interpreter, and had supper with Anne in the evening. However, inside him anger and disappointment were boiling to fever pitch. He had known, when he first looked at her, that he could never love Anne of Cleves. In fact, he now realised, she revolted him. She was so different from the image portrayed by Holbein and described by Cromwell that he felt betrayed, ill-used and deceived. He had brought with him a present of furs, but he was in such a state of agitation that he forgot to give them to Anne, and Sir Anthony Browne later presented them to her.

Someone had made a very grievous mistake, and they were going to suffer for it. Part of the fault lay with Holbein, who had so cunningly misrepresented Anne in his portrait of her. Yet Holbein

Henry could forgive: he was an artist, with an artist's conception of things, something the King understood very well. But Cromwell had suggested this marriage and manoeuvred Henry into it; Cromwell had extolled the lady's charms and her beauty. Cromwell, had he but known it, was doomed from the very moment Henry set eyes on Anne of Cleves.

When the visit was over, the King left his unsuspecting bride and found Sir Anthony Browne waiting in the corridor. Sir Anthony could see he was in a terrible temper, and was quickly enlightened when Henry told him he had been 'so struck with consternation when he was shown the Queen' that he had never been 'so much dismayed in his life as to see a lady so far unlike what had been represented'. Scowling ferociously, he said, 'I see nothing in this woman as men report of her, and I marvel that wise men would make such report as they have done!' And with that he stumped off.

As soon as Henry got back to court, he sought out the Lord Admiral, who had given him such glowing reports of Anne. 'How like you this woman?' demanded Henry aggressively. 'Do you think her personable, fair and beautiful, as report hath been made unto me? I pray you tell me true.' 'I take her not for fair,' replied the Admiral cautiously, 'but to be of a brown complexion.' 'Alas!' wailed the King, 'Whom shall men trust? I promise you I see no such thing as hath been shown me of her, by pictures and report. I am ashamed that men have praised her as they have done – and I love her not!' Years before, he had written in his book against Martin Luther of 'the fate of princes to be in marriage of far worse sort than the condition of poor men. Princes take as is brought them by others, and poor men be commonly at their own choice.' He was now for the first time experiencing the painful reality of this.

From eager anticipation, Henry had quickly descended to the depths of gloom. 'I like her not! I like her not!' he kept saying, and it was thought by his courtiers, not incorrectly, that he would do his best to extricate himself from the betrothal contract. Yet on 2 January, he departed with the court for Greenwich, as arranged, to prepare for the wedding that was supposed to take place in a few days' time. With him he took a cherished New Year's gift, the only thing that cheered him in his disappointment – a portrait by Holbein of the two-year-old Prince Edward, in a red satin gown and bonnet, and bearing a strong resemblance to his father. There was no likelihood after that of Holbein falling from the King's good graces.

Anne of Cleves was then at Dartford, where she would remain until summoned to London for her official reception. Cromwell was still receiving messages congratulating him on his sound judgement in choosing Anne as the future Queen, but the senders of these messages had not yet seen the King. However, it was not long before word of Henry's discontent spread, and it soon became apparent that he was 'very melancholy', as well as being 'nothing pleasantly disposed' towards Cromwell. As soon as Henry arrived at Greenwich, he sent for Cromwell and accused him, before the Council, of having deceived him over Anne of Cleves. For a moment or two, an alarmed Cromwell floundered, trying to think of a way to excuse himself, then he vainly tried to shift the blame on to the shoulders of the Admiral, saying that,

> When that nobleman found the Princess so different from the pictures and reports which had been made of her, he ought to have detained her at Calais till he had given the King notice that she was not so handsome as had been represented.

Southampton, who was present, reacted angrily to this, and protested that he 'was not invested with any such authority; his commission was to bring her to England, and he had obeyed his orders.' Cromwell then admitted that he had spoken of the lady's beauty 'in terms of commendation which had misled his Highness and his Council', but protested that this was not his fault, because he had received false reports. As he said this, he looked meaningfully at the Admiral, who blustered and said that 'as the Princess was generally reported for a beauty, he had only repeated the opinions of others, for which no one ought reasonably to blame him, especially as he had supposed she would be his queen'. The King agreed that the Admiral could not have acted in any other way, but he was furious with Cromwell. Cromwell had got him into this mess, he now expected Cromwell to get him out of it, and he put this to his minister in no uncertain terms.

Cromwell, still strongly convinced that the alliance with Cleves was necessary to England, stood his ground. If Henry alienated the Germans, he pointed out, he would stand alone without allies, with France and the Empire possibly poised for a joint offensive against him. Besides, Anne herself had done no wrong, and it would be most unchivalrous of the King to reject her at this late stage and send her home disgraced; no man would consider her after that. More to the point, her brother, impoverished though he was, might well retaliate by declaring war on Henry. There was no way out, in fact: the King must marry Anne of Cleves and make the best of it.

Henry stalked out of the council chamber in a rage, but even he knew that Cromwell was right, and that he must go through with the marriage. Yet he was consumed with anger against the man for having involved him with Cleves in the first place; but for Cromwell's insistence that he ally himself with these German heretics he would not now be faced with the prospect of taking a wife so repugnant to him. For all his reluctance Henry forced himself to continue with the wedding preparations. His messengers had already 'made public outcry in London that all who loved their lord the King should proceed to Greenwich to meet and make their devoir to my Lady Anne of Cleves, who would shortly be their queen,' and even now crowds were gathering around the palace and along the banks of the Thames. Many noblemen had brought their wives to court to be received by the future Queen. It was too late to back out now.

Yet Henry was not giving in gracefully. He grumbled to Cromwell that Anne was 'nothing so well as she was spoken of', declaring vehemently that 'if I had known so much before, she had no coming hither. But what remedy now?' Cromwell replied firmly that there was no remedy, and said he was sorry that his Grace was 'no better content'. Even now, Henry had not given up hope of being freed from his obligation to honour the marriage contract. When, on 3 January 1540, the Lord Chamberlain asked which day his Majesty would be pleased to name for the coronation of his queen, Henry replied tartly, 'We will talk of that when I have made her my queen!' All the same, on that same day he left Greenwich with a great train to receive his bride and her retinue at Shooter's Hill, near Blackheath, and welcome them to London.

'Blackheath hath borne some gorgeous and pleasant spectacles,' wrote the Elizabethan antiquary William Lambard many years later, 'but none so magnificent as that of King Henry VIII, when he brought in the Lady Anne of Cleves.' It was one of the last great spectacles of Henry's reign, and if the King was feeling less than enamoured of his bride he concealed it well in public. He went by barge to Greenwich on that Saturday, accompanied by all his nobles and the Lord Mayor and aldermen of London; every barge was decorated with streamers and banners. At the same time, the Lady Anne was travelling to Blackheath from Dartford. At the foot of Shooter's Hill a rich pavilion of cloth of gold had been set up; surrounding it were other, smaller pavilions. Inside them were braziers containing scented fires at which Anne and her ladies could warm themselves. Anne was accompanied by what remained of her retinue from Cleves, which now consisted of a hundred persons on horseback, as well as the Dukes of Norfolk and Suffolk, the Archbishop of Canterbury, and other bishops, lords and knights. At twelve o'clock, she led her train down Shooter's Hill, and was received in front of the pavilions by her Lord Chamberlain, the Earl of Rutland, and Sir Thomas Denny, her Chancellor, and all her other councillors and the newly appointed officers of her household. Dr Kaye, her almoner, then made a short address in Latin, and formally presented to Anne all those sworn to serve her: as she could speak no English, Duke William's secretary replied to the address on her behalf. The great ladies of her household then came forward and curtsied to her: Lady Margaret Douglas and the Marchioness of Dorset, the King's nieces, his daughter-in-law the Duchess of Richmond, the Countess of Hertford, the Countess of Rutland, and Lady Audley; sixty-five ladies of lesser rank followed them. Anne then alighted from her chariot and 'with most goodly demeanour and loving countenance' thanked everyone most heartily, and kissed the chief ladies of her household; her councillors and officers then knelt in turn to kiss her hand, after which she retired with her ladies into the main pavilion to get warm.

Word was then sent to the King, waiting at Greenwich, that Anne had arrived, and he at once set off with a great train across Greenwich Park. He had dressed himself magnificently for the occasion, in a coat embroidered with cloth of gold, diamonds, rubies and Orient pearls, with a jewelled sword and girdle and a velvet bonnet adorned with precious stones, 'so rich of jewels that few men could value them'. About his neck hung a collar of such gems and pearls 'that few men ever saw the like'. He was attended by ten footmen attired in rich liveries of goldsmiths' work. Not once did his face betray his inner feelings: his behaviour in the public eye was as usual impeccable, conveying the impression that he was an eager and satisfied bridegroom. Indeed, he would never show anything other than courtesy towards Anne of Cleves in public, and he played his part so well that it was not until weeks after their wedding that she realised she did not please him.

Yet even as Henry rode out to welcome Anne, his lawyers were examining the marriage contract to see if there were any flaws in it, and also investigating the circumstances of Anne's supposed betrothal to the son of the Duke of Lorraine. As she waited in her tent for the King to appear, Anne was happily innocent of this. She had changed into a taffeta gown embroidered with raised cloth of gold; it was in the Dutch fashion, with a round skirt, and lacked the courtly train worn by ladies of rank in England. Nevertheless, it drew flattering comments from onlookers. A caul held her hair in place, over which was 'a round bonnet or cap set full of Orient pearls', surmounted by 'a coronet of black velvet'. Around her neck she wore a parure of rich stones that glittered in the winter sunlight. In this attire, she sallied forth when word came that the King was half a mile away. At the door of the pavilion, she mounted her richly caparisoned horse, and with her footmen in liveries embroidered with the Black Lion of Cleves rode to meet her future husband. Henry, seeing her approach, reined his horse to a standstill and waited until she drew level with him. He then doffed his bonnet, 'and with most lovely countenance and princely behaviour saluted, welcomed and embraced her, to the great rejoicing of the beholders'. Whereat the Lady Anne, 'not forgetting her duty, with most amiable respect and womanly behaviour received his Grace with many sweet words and great thanks and praise'. Certainly, she was making strenuous efforts to familiarise herself with the English language.

For a while, the royal couple chatted and exchanged pleasantries; then, with Anne on the King's right hand, they rode back towards the pavilions and the vast crowds waiting to see them.

Oh! What a sight was this, to see so godly a prince and so noble a king to ride with so fair a lady of so goodly a stature and so womanly a countenance! I think that no creature could see them but his heart rejoiced!

So gushed the chronicler Hall for whom Henry VIII could do no wrong. With the trumpets going before them, King and Princess proceeded through the assembled ranks of knights and esquires, followed by the lords of the Privy Council, the gentlemen of the privy chamber, the men of Cleves in velvet coats, the Lord Mayor, the barons, bishops, earls and dukes, Archbishop Cranmer, Duke Philip of Bavaria (still waiting for an answer to his proposal to the Lady Mary), the foreign ambassadors, Lord Privy Seal Cromwell, and the Lord Chancellor. With the King rode Sir Anthony Browne, while Sir John Dudley, newly created Master of her Horse, accompanied the future queen, leading a spare palfrey for her.

For the processional journey back to Greenwich Palace, Anne rode in a carved and gilded chariot bearing the ducal arms of Cleves. With her sat 'two ancient ladies of her country', while the next chariot held six young German ladies dressed in ornate gowns, who were reckoned by the English to be very good looking. A chariot bearing Anne's chamberers followed, and then one carrying her laundresses. Behind that was drawn an empty litter of cloth of gold and crimson velvet, a gift from the King to his bride. Anne's serving men, all clad in black and riding great horses, brought up the rear of the procession. Thus they rode through the park, while the citizens of London were crowding the Thames in their boats, straining to catch a glimpse of the German princess who would soon be their queen. The guilds of London were also there in their barges, many of which had been painted with the royal arms of England and the ducal arms of Cleves, and from every barge issued the melodious sounds of minstrels and the voices of men and children singing in honour of the occasion. Henry and Anne paused on the wharf to see and hear the pageant and were lavish in their praise of it.

Soon afterwards, Anne was alighting from her chariot in the inner courtyard of Greenwich Palace. As the royal pair arrived, a great peal of guns let off a salute from one of the towers. Henry embraced and kissed his bride, and bade her welcome to her own house; then taking her by the arm, he led her through the great hall, where the King's guards were standing to attention before the hearth, and on to her privy chamber, where he left her to rest for a while.

That evening there was a sumptuous banquet in Anne's honour, after which she changed into a taffeta gown with long flowing sleeves gathered above the elbow into armlets; it was trimmed with rich sables – probably those presented to her on the King's behalf at Rochester – and the tight undersleeves were made of very costly material. On her head, she wore a lawn cap in the Dutch style, adorned with pearls and precious stones, which was judged to be of great value by those who saw it. Cleves might have been a poor duchy, but it had done its princess proud in sending her to England with such a splendid trousseau.

Later, when Anne had retired to bed, the King sought out Cromwell. 'How say you? Is it not as I told you?' he demanded. 'She is nothing fair. Her person is well and seemly, but nothing else.' Cromwell, trying to make the best of the situation, replied, 'By my faith, you say right, but me thinketh she hath a queenly manner withal.' Henry had to admit that was so, but he was not at all happy and made no secret of the fact. On the following day, Sunday, 4 January, he was complaining that he was 'not well handled', and declared that,

> If it were not that she had come so far into my realm, and the great preparations and state that my people have made for her, and for fear of making a ruffle in the world and of driving her brother into the arms of the Emperor and the French King, I would not now marry her. But now it is too far gone, wherefore I am sorry.

Cromwell was sorry too. He was filled with anxiety, for Henry was in what he recognised to be a dangerous mood. It now wanted but two days until the date set for the wedding ceremony. The King's lawyers had found no evidence at all of a precontract between Anne of Cleves and the son of the Duke of Lorraine, nor could they find any fault with the marriage contract. Every avenue of escape was closed to the King: he would have to go through with the wedding. Cromwell was staking all his hopes on Henry growing to like Anne better once he had established a sexual relationship with her; should she become pregnant, then the King might well view her with very different eyes.

Henry, however, had no intention of trying to make this marriage a success. He was desperate to be free of his obligations, and on the day before the knot was to be tied, he besought a worried Cromwell to help him. 'Is there no remedy, but that I needs must put my neck into the yoke?' he cried. Once again, Cromwell patiently explained why it was too late to back out, and after a while Henry calmed down and agreed to go ahead with the wedding on the following day. In the evening, he duly informed the Privy Council that that was his intention, while his bride-to-be was making her own preparations in blissful ignorance of the controversy raging around her.

It is difficult now to pinpoint exactly what it was about Anne of Cleves that aroused so much distaste in the King. Henry was realist enough to accept that a monarch had to marry for the good of his realm, and that this might mean a union with someone with whom he might be ill matched, yet in this case he professed to feel such revulsion that he was on the brink of putting his own needs before the benefit of his kingdom. There can be no doubt that Holbein exaggerated Anne's charms, and therefore it may be concluded that looks were not her strong point. Because Anne was queen for such a short time, there was little demand for portraits of her. Apart from Holbein's work, only one other portrait type survives, being a likeness by a Flemish artist, Barthel Bruyn the Elder, which today hangs in St John's College, Oxford. This picture may well hold the clue to Anne's looks, for it depicts a more angular face than that in the Holbein portraits; it also, being a side-facing portrait, shows that Anne had a long pointed nose and heavy-lidded eyes. Figure-wise, her tall stature may well have made her seem ungainly to a man who had been married to three petite women. Furthermore, she suffered from excessive body odour, according to the King. Taken together, all these things could well account for his distaste, and he could only deplore her lack of education, wit and musical ability, three things he greatly esteemed in women. Anne's other personal qualities, and her earnest desire to please, meant little when compared with all her drawbacks. Others had been impressed by her, but then they did not have to marry her and sleep with her. Henry did, and he was so revolted at the prospect that he had even forgotten the urgent need to beget more sons.

The wedding day, Tuesday, 6 January 1540, was the Feast of the Epiphany and the last day of the Yuletide celebrations at court. The King was up early, and dressed in his wedding clothes: a gown of cloth of gold, embroidered with great flowers of silver and banded with black fur, a coat of crimson satin slashed and embroidered and fastened with huge diamonds, and a rich collar of gold about his neck. At eight o'clock, accompanied by his nobles, he paused in the gallery leading to the chapel where the marriage ceremony would take place, and declared, 'My lords, if it were not to satisfy the world and my realm, I would not do what I must do this day for any earthly thing.' And he looked pointedly at Cromwell. However, there was no time for further recriminations, as the bride was coming, escorted by the lords sent to fetch her.

Anne was wearing a gown of cloth of gold embroidered with large flowers of great Orient pearls; again, it was cut in the Dutch fashion, having a round skirt without a train. Her long fair hair was hanging loose, in token of her virginity, and she wore a coronet of gold set with precious stones, with trefoils resembling bunches of rosemary. About her neck was a costly necklace, with a matching belt around her slim waist. Walking between the Count of Overstein and the Grand Master of Cleves, with her face composed and her expression at once demure and serious, she followed the lords into the King's chamber, out the other end, and into the gallery where Henry awaited her. There, she made three deep obeisances, and together they then proceeded to the Chapel Royal, where Cranmer would marry them.

Anne was given away by the Count of Overstein. On her finger the King placed a ring engraved with the motto 'God send me well to keep.' When the ceremony was over, the King and Queen went hand in hand into Henry's closet to hear mass, and offered their tapers, Anne obediently following the rituals of the established faith to please her new husband. After mass, the bridal party was served spiced wine. The King then went to his privy chamber to change into a gown of tissue lined with embroidered crimson velvet, while Anne went with her ladies to her own chamber, escorted by the

Dukes of Norfolk and Suffolk. A little after nine, the King and Queen met in Anne's room, where a procession formed, Anne's serjeant-at-arms and all her other officers going before her, and thus in stately fashion the bridal pair passed through the palace to their wedding banquet.

Later, in the afternoon, Anne changed into a gown of rather masculine cut, with sleeves gathered above the elbow; her ladies donned gowns with the abundance of chains so popular in Germany and the Low Countries. Thus attired, they accompanied the Queen to evensong, after which she had supper with the King. A programme of masques and other entertainment followed, until it was time for the newly wedded pair to be put to bed.

Henry was in no mood by then to consummate the marriage. It was fortunate therefore that Anne's mother had not considered it appropriate to acquaint her daughter with the facts of life: the King's bride was entirely ignorant of sex, and had little idea of what to expect in the marriage bed. So she lay there, while her new husband ran his hands all over her body and then, it must be assumed, rolled over and went to sleep, leaving her undoubtedly bewildered and embarrassed.

When morning came, the King was up early. He was in a very bad mood. While he was dressing, Cromwell – who had probably not slept at all – arrived, and anxiously enquired, 'How does your Grace like the Queen?' Henry glowered at him. 'Not so pleasant as I trusted to have done,' he muttered ominously. Cromwell, with understandable apprehension, asked why his master was so dissatisfied, at which the King's temper flared, and he retorted:

Surely, my lord, I liked her before not well, but now I like her much worse! She is nothing fair, and have very evil smells about her. I took her to be no maid by reason of the looseness of her breasts and other tokens, which, when I felt them, strake me so to the heart, that I had neither will nor courage to prove the rest. I can have none appetite for displeasant airs. I have left her as good a maid as I found her.

Hearing this, Cromwell knew himself beaten, and that Henry was already smoothing the way towards having the marriage annulled.

Cromwell could not foresee how this would be done, but he knew the King, and he had little doubt as to what would be the outcome. As for himself, he could only hope that his master would not exact too terrible a revenge.

The King was in a dangerous mood. Few men would gladly admit to having failed to consummate their marriage, yet by the end of that day Henry had told most of the influential people at court of his inability to make love to the Queen, saying that 'he had found her body disordered and indisposed to excite and provoke any lust in him'. He even sought out his physician, Dr Butts, and explained that his failure to have sexual intercourse with Anne was not due to impotence on his part; indeed, he boasted that he had experienced wet dreams twice during the wedding night, and thought himself able to perform the sex act with others, but not with his wife. 'Surely,' he said mournfully, 'I will never have any more children for the comfort of the realm.' Before very long, the whole court was laughing behind closed doors at the royal-marriage farce. Fortunately, the new Queen could speak very little English, and failed to realise that she was the butt of so many cruel jokes.

It says a great deal for Anne of Cleves that she managed to settle into her position with dignity. Many people liked her and admired her courage and common sense, and the common people were impressed with what they had seen and heard of her. On 11 January, she attended a tournament held in honour of her marriage, and for the first time appeared dressed in English costume, with a French hood that everyone agreed much became her. Yet her efforts to please had little effect upon her husband. Three days later, Cromwell told the Council that the new Queen remained a virgin because the King's Highness 'liked not her body, and could not be provoked or stirred to that act, though able to do the act with other than with her'. This selective impotence posed a grave problem for the state: if there were no heirs from the marriage, its whole purpose was in vain. Yet the Privy Councillors agreed that for the moment there was no way out, for fear of reprisals from the Duke of Cleves. Anne must remain queen, and Henry must make the best of it.

Not long afterwards, the new Queen received a courteous little note from the Lady Elizabeth, her younger stepdaughter. Elizabeth was still at Hertford Castle, and was impatient to come to court and meet her father's new wife.

> Permit me to show, by this billet [she wrote in this the first of her letters to survive], the zeal with which I devote my respect to you as queen, and my entire obedience to you as my mother. I am too young and feeble to have power to do more than felicitate you with all my heart in this commencement of your marriage. I hope that your Majesty will have as much goodwill for me as I have zeal for your service.

Touched by this letter from a very accomplished and erudite six-year-old, Anne showed it to the King, and asked if Elizabeth might come to court. But Henry was in no mood to grant anyone any favours, and would not hear of it. He took the letter and gave it to Cromwell, then ordered him to write a reply. 'Tell her,' he said brutally, 'that she had a mother so different from this woman that she ought not to wish to see her.'

At this point there came about a significant change in the shifting scene of European politics. Both the Emperor and the King of France began to make friendly overtures to Henry VIII because their mutual pact was beginning to go the way of many others and deteriorate into barely concealed hostility. There were signs that both were looking for a renewal of friendship with England, and it soon became obvious to Henry that his position had strengthened immeasurably. A German alliance was now neither attractive nor necessary. In fact, in this new situation, it was positively undesirable, being not only unpopular with the Emperor and the French, but also with the strong Catholic faction at the English court headed by the Duke of Norfolk and the conservative Stephen Gardiner, Bishop of Winchester.

Henry did not hasten to rid himself of Anne of Cleves immediately, however. He realised that it was wiser to wait until the Emperor's true intentions were revealed; if Charles continued to show himself friendly, then Henry would reciprocate, in the hope that Charles would stand as a bulwark between him and Cleves when the time came for him to end his marriage. In the meantime, he got rid of

Philip of Bavaria, who left England on 27 January, much to the relief of the Lady Mary, who was now recovered from her illness. While he was about it, the King also dismissed most of Anne's German attendants and packed them off to Cleves. Before they left, he gave a sumptuous feast in their honour, and sent them away laden with gifts. As a special favour to the Queen, a few of her people were allowed to stay in England, but Henry meant to send them home too, once she had grown accustomed to English ways.

Tradition dictated that a new queen made a state entry into London prior to her coronation, but the King had abandoned his plans for a February crowning, without offering Anne any explanation as to why. Instead, he grudgingly arranged for the civic reception to take place. On 3 February, the Privy Council issued orders requiring the 'commons of London' to put on their best clothes and take to their barges on the following day in order to do honour to their queen. King and Council were united in their determination to give the Duke of Cleves no grounds for criticism.

On 4 February, the King and Queen took the royal barge from Greenwich to Westminster; with them, in other barges, sailed the nobility of England and the bishops. As they passed the Tower, a great peal of guns saluted them. The citizens of London were cheering from the riverbanks, and the guildsmen were passing in their decorated barges. The City's welcome was warm and encouraging, and Anne must have been gratified by this. At Westminster, the King helped her out of the barge, and together they walked with their attendants to Whitehall Palace, where they were to stay for a time.

It was while the court was at Whitehall that Anne Bassett, who had been appointed one of Anne's maids of honour back in December and was now reporting for duty, was informed that the Queen had brought with her so many German attendants that, even allowing for those who had been sent home, there was no place for her, or for several other English ladies, in her household. Naturally, Anne Bassett was very put out and she complained to her mother Lady Lisle, who in turn wrote expressing her grievance to Lady Rutland, wife of the Queen's Lord Chamberlain. Lady Rutland replied that the King would not allow any more maids to be appointed until there was a vacancy created by someone leaving the

Queen's household. However, she advised, it might be as well to lay her daughter's case before Mother Lowe, the strict German mistress of the Queen's maids, as she was in the best position to find a place for Anne Bassett. Lady Lisle did write to Mother Lowe and was gratified to hear from Anne, only a week later, that she was now waiting upon the Queen.

It was well known among the ladies of the Queen's household that their mistress was a wife in name only. Inhabiting a sophisticated court where intrigue and adultery were commonplace, they found it scarcely believable that Anne of Cleves should be so innocent. One day, around late February, the Queen told her senior ladies-in-waiting, Lady Rutland, Lady Rochford, and Winifred, Lady Edgecombe how kind and solicitous her husband the King was. 'Why,' she said in her guttural, halting English, 'when he comes to bed he kisseth me, and taketh me by the hand, and biddeth me "Good night, sweetheart"; and in the morning kisseth me and biddeth "Farewell, darling."' The ladies present exchanged furtive glances: was that all? After a significant pause, they told Anne they hoped she would soon be with child, to which she replied that she knew very well she was not. Lady Edgecombe asked how it was possible for her to know that: 'I know it well, I am not,' answered Anne. 'I think your Grace is a maid still,' ventured Lady Edgecombe with some daring, not to say impudence. Anne laughed at this; 'How can I be a maid, and sleep every night with the King?' she said, and repeated what she had said earlier of their nightly routine. 'Is this not enough?' she queried. It was Lady Rutland who spoke: 'Madam, there must be more than this, or it will be long ere we have a duke of York, which all this realm most desireth.' Anne's face registered dismay. 'Nay,' she said, 'I am contented I know no more.' Nevertheless, her ladies proceeded to enlighten her, and afterwards asked her if she had acquainted Mother Lowe with the King's neglect of his marital duties. By this time, Anne had had enough of being interrogated, and replied firmly that 'she received quite as much of his Majesty's attention as she wished'.

Nevertheless, the seeds of anxiety had been sown in her mind. She now knew that something was very wrong with her glittering marriage; in one stroke her illusions about the King had been effectively shattered. What was the meaning of his neglect? Did he not love her? Did he intend to set her aside, as he had done Queen Katherine? Or, even worse, do away with her, as he had done with Anne Boleyn? We shall, of course, never know exactly what Anne's private feelings were at this time, but it is certain that from then on she was watchful, alert for the first signs of anything adverse, and careful to conduct herself with the utmost decorum.

In March 1540, the King's conscience reared its righteous head once more. He told his Council that it would not permit him to consummate his marriage as he felt sure he was not entitled to do so, being convinced that there had in fact been a precontract between Anne and the Duke of Lorraine's son. 'I have done as much to move the consent of my heart and mind as ever man did,' he said piously, 'but the obstacle will not out of my mind.' The Council realised they were being ordered to supply grounds for dissolving the marriage, and after some discussion they told the King it was their opinion that non-consummation was in itself grounds for annulment. There was no need to rake up the precontract with Lorraine; it was a dubious pretext at best. Nevertheless, they would have the matter investigated once more. This seemed to satisfy Henry.

The spring of 1540 saw the surrender of the abbeys of Canterbury, Christchurch, Rochester and Waltham. With this closure, the dissolution of the monasteries was complete. Henry was now wearing on his thumb the great ruby that had, since the twelfth century, adorned the shrine of Becket at Canterbury. On his orders, the saint's body had been exhumed and thrown on a dung heap, because Becket had been a traitor to his King. Not all the monastic wealth found its way into the royal coffers in the Tower. Vast tracts of abbey land were bestowed upon noblemen loyal to the crown: Woburn Abbey was given to Sir John Russell, Wilton Abbey to Lord Herbert, and so on. Many stately homes surviving today are built on the sites of monastic establishments, sometimes with stones from the abbeys themselves. This redistribution of land from church to lay ownership served the purpose of binding the aristocracy by even greater ties of loyalty and gratitude to the King: they were hardly likely to oppose radical religious reforms when they had benefited so lavishly as a result of them.

Although Henry had retained most of the old Catholic rituals when he broke with the Pope, Lutheranism had gained a foothold in

England in recent years, and was growing in popularity, even though the penalties for heresy were severe. The King's marriage to a Protestant princess had made not one whit of difference to religious practice in England; Anne of Cleves was happy anyway to conform to all the outward forms of Catholic worship. Nevertheless, she was regarded as being a figurehead for the reformist party at court, especially by the strong Catholic faction, headed by the Duke of Norfolk and Bishop Gardiner. This party was firmly opposed to any religious changes that tended towards Lutheranism, and it was very much in favour of the dissolution of the royal marriage. Thus while Cromwell was doing his best to promote the excellent qualities of the Queen, Norfolk and Gardiner were urging the King to divorce her. 'Cromwell is tottering,' reported Charles de Marillac, the French ambassador, on 10 April. It was the opposition's hope that, once rid of Anne of Cleves, Henry would marry a more orthodox bride who would represent their own interests. It must also be said that, as with Wolsey's enemies a decade before, jealousy was one of their guiding motives.

On 17 April, Henry surprised everyone by creating Cromwell Earl of Essex. This looked like a setback for the Catholic party, but in reality it was no such thing, being another example of the King's subtle cruelty. By lulling Cromwell into a sense of false security, he hoped to exact a more satisfying revenge, which would be as unexpected as it was deadly. Nor was it long before the Catholic faction suspected what would be the outcome, and realised that it was imperative to concentrate their energies on hastening the fall of the new Earl.

The King had confided to Norfolk that he meant to force Cromwell to bring about the dissolution of the marriage he had worked so hard to create before he destroyed him. Henry was still telling people that he could 'not overcome his aversion to the Queen sufficiently to consider her as his wife'; he was sure, he said mournfully, that God would never send him any more children if he continued in this marriage, and declared that 'before God, he thought she was not his lawful wife'. His councillors remembered having heard all this on another occasion, and were praying that this queen proved not so obdurate as the first had been. Everyone knew from bitter experience that a royal divorce could be a messy and fraught business that could drag on for years, and it was not surprising that the Council shrank from the prospect.

There now emerged, however, the strongest possible incentive for the King to end his marriage. In April 1540, it was noticed that he had 'crept too near another lady'. Her name was Katherine Howard, and she was the niece of the Duke of Norfolk and a first cousin to Anne Boleyn. The Catholic party had timed her entrance well. She had been deliberately placed in the Queen's household as a maid of honour with detailed instructions as to how to attract the King's attention. Norfolk had already seen one niece attain the consort's throne, and saw no reason why another should not aspire to the same dignity. Besides, this one was younger, more malleable, and much prettier than the first.

Katherine was about fifteen. She was the eldest daughter of Norfolk's younger brother, Lord Edmund Howard, who had died, aged sixty-one, in 1539. Lord Edmund had been Comptroller of Calais; being a younger son, he had very little by way of inheritance from his father, the second Duke of Norfolk, and had spent the greater part of his life shouldering heavy debts. Little is known about him; one of his few surviving letters relates how a medicine prescribed for him by Lady Lisle had caused him to 'bepiss my bed'. He had first married Joyce Culpeper, widow of Mr Ralph Legh, to whom she had borne five children. She presented Lord Edmund with another five, of whom Katherine was perhaps the fourth. There were three sons: Charles, Henry (who died young) and George, and two daughters, Katherine and Mary, who later married Thomas Arundel, who was executed for treason in 1552.

As with Anne Boleyn, Katherine Howard's date of birth may only with difficulty be determined. All contemporary writers are agreed that she was very young when she married the King. She was certainly born before 1527, as in that year, in a letter to Wolsey, her father stated he had ten children, 'my children and my wife's'. But as the date of Lord Edmund's marriage is not known, it is not possible to estimate a date of birth for their eldest son, Charles. We do know, however, that Charles, Henry and George were born before 1524, for in that year they are mentioned in the will of John Legh, their mother's former father-in-law. Katherine and her sister Mary are not mentioned in this will at all, although they are named in the will of

John Legh's wife Isabella in 1527. It may therefore be safely assumed that they were not yet born in 1524, and that the evidence contemporary to the period of Katherine's birth argues a date of c. 1525.

This must now be compared to later evidence dating from the time of her marriage to the King in 1540. The 1525 date is corroborated by the admittedly dubious Spanish Chronicle, which states that Katherine was fifteen when she first met Henry VIII. We have seen that this source is generally unreliable, although it has been credited with accuracy in places. Mr Richard Hilles, a London merchant, writing in 1540, referred to Katherine as 'a very little girl', and although this may refer to her diminutive stature, it could also refer to her age, as it conveys a distinct impression of extreme youth. Marillac stated in 1541 that Katherine's relationship with her admirer, Francis Dereham, lasted from the age of thirteen until she was eighteen. As their affair ended in 1539, this would place her date of birth in or around 1521, a date many historians have accepted without examining the other evidence. But if Katherine had been alive in 1524, how then do we explain the omission of her name from John Legh's will? Moreover, it must also be stressed that Marillac was frequently inaccurate in his diplomatic reports, and was not above inventing facts of his own. From other evidence, which will be examined in detail in the next chapter, it appears that Katherine's relationship with Dereham was of short duration only, much less than the five years alleged by Marillac, and probably lasting no longer than two years. Her earlier liaison with her music master, Henry Manox, was of even shorter duration. Thus, if she was born in 1525, she was twelve when she became sexually active, and we must remember that many girls were married at that age in the Tudor period.

The date of 1519 has sometimes been given as Katherine's birthdate because of an inscription on a portrait by Holbein of a lady long identified as Katherine Howard. However, it has now been proved that the portrait in question has no connection with her, and probably represents Jane Seymour's sister Elizabeth, the wife of Gregory Cromwell. Taking all the other evidence into account, there is a strong case to be made for Katherine having been born in 1525, or thereabouts, which made her, indeed, a 'very little girl' at the time she attracted the attention of Henry VIII. And Henry, of course, was just at that susceptible age when a man likes to prove to himself and others that he is still an attractive proposition to young girls.

Katherine's mother died when she was no more than a toddler, and her father quickly remarried. Her new stepmother was Dorothy, daughter of Sir Thomas Troyes and widow of Sir William Uvedale. However, the new Lady Howard was to play very little part in Katherine's life, for she was sent at that time to live in the household of her step-grandmother, the Dowager Duchess of Norfolk, widow of the second Duke; such an arrangement was customary with daughters of the nobility. Here, she received some rudiments of education, although the Duchess was a lax guardian and allowed her charge to run wild, something that would have grave repercussions for both of them in the future. Katherine remained with the Duchess, commuting between the Dowager's town house at Lambeth and her country estate at Horsham in Sussex, until her uncle Norfolk arranged for her to go to court in the spring of 1540. Meanwhile, her father, who had lost his second wife and married yet a third time, to Mrs Margaret Jennings, had died in 1539. This left Katherine bereft of any close relatives with genuine concern for her welfare, for her uncle saw her merely as a tool with which to achieve his political ends, and her step-grandmother was not very interested in her.

Several portraits said to be of Katherine survive, but only one may be said to be authentic, and that is a miniature by Holbein, of which two versions exist, one in the Royal Collection and another in the collection of the Duke of Buccleuch. These are very similar, showing the subject seated, half-length, against a celeste-blue background. She wears a very low-cut dress of tawny brocade with furred over-sleeves and green damask false sleeves, and an ornate French hood rests on her auburn hair. The face of the sitter is faintly impudent, tilted at an angle, wearing an imperious expression, although plump and round with the rather large Howard nose. Recent research, undertaken by Dr Roy Strong, former Director of the National Portrait Gallery, has shown that the miniature's identification as Katherine Howard, dating from 1756, is probably based on sound foundations. The sumptuous costume, and the fact that the sitter was painted at all, would indicate also that here, indeed, is one of Henry VIII's unfortunate queens, and the only possible identification is with Katherine Howard. Other portraits once claimed to represent her, such as the Holbein half-length in Toledo, Ohio, copies of which are in the National Portrait Gallery, London, and Trentham Hall, a Holbein sketch of dubious authenticity in the Royal Collection, and a portrait at Hatfield House showing a lady wearing the gable hood of the 1520s, have all been shown to be spurious.

It was not long before Katherine attracted the attention of the King. By April 1540, he was said to be very enamoured of her, and before the month was out had made her substantial grants of lands confiscated from convicted criminals. Katherine's youthful charm rejuvenated Henry, and she seems to have responded warmly to his advances, having no doubt been well primed by her family. It was certainly a dazzling experience to be courted by the King, and Katherine was not without ambition – Norfolk and Gardiner had explained what their purpose was in pushing her into the spotlight. Yet she was no Anne Boleyn, being a good deal younger than Anne had been, and far more empty-headed, although she was precocious enough when it came to experience of men. It had already therefore occurred to her that she might become queen of England, and this was no doubt enough to compensate for the fact that, as a man, Henry had very little to offer a girl of her age. He was now nearing fifty, and had aged beyond his years. The abscess on his leg was slowing him down, and there were days when he could hardly walk, let alone ride. Worse still, it oozed pus continually, and had to be dressed daily, not a pleasant task for the person assigned to do it as the wound stank dreadfully. As well as being afflicted with this, the King had become exceedingly fat: a new suit of armour, made for him at this time, measured 54″ around the waist. He was frequently irascible, quick to burst out in temper, and given to bouts of black depression as the years advanced. Yet on occasion he could still exert himself to be charming, especially to the ladies, and he was doing that now for Katherine's benefit, behaving as if he were the magnificent specimen of manhood who had vanquished so many women in his youth. Katherine flattered Henry's vanity; she pretended not to notice his bad leg, and did not flinch from the smell it exuded. She was young, graceful and pretty, and Henry was entranced. The Catholic faction watched with satisfaction as their affair progressed. The Queen, not now so naïve as formerly, watched too; she bore Katherine no rancour on a personal level, for she was not in love with her husband, yet this new development made her fearful. If Henry believed she stood in the way of his future happiness, what might he not do to rid himself of her?

May Day was celebrated that year with all the usual festivities at court. The King remembered that, in the eyes of the world, he was still a married man, and appeared with his queen at the jousts that were given for five days at Westminster to mark the occasion. They also attended the banquets that were held in Durham House, which had been thrown open in order to admit the public, who were eager to view the festivities. Here, the King entertained those who had been victorious in the jousts and gave them gifts, 100 marks each and houses to live in. Cromwell, meanwhile, was watching the royal couple closely, and learned to his discomfort that they were no better acquainted than before. On 6 May, he sought out Sir Thomas Wriothesley, and told him how troubled he was. 'The King liketh not the Queen, nor ever has from the beginning; I think assuredly she is as good a maid for him as she was when she came to England.' Wriothesley said he was sorry to hear it, and urged Cromwell to 'devise how his Grace may be relieved'. Cromwell agreed that this was the only course to take. 'But how?' he asked. Wriothesley would not be drawn, or did not know, yet he too had urged the King to ally himself with Cleves, and like Cromwell, he feared for his own skin. 'For God's sake, devise relief for the King, or we shall both smart for it!' he begged. A few days later, he brought up the matter of the King's marriage in Council, lamenting 'the hard case in which the King's Highness stood, in being bound to a wife whom he could not love'. Of course, there were many men similarly afflicted, but their unwillingness to have relations with their wives did not affect the succession to the throne. The Council, to a man, agreed that something must be done to extricate his Grace from this match that was so repugnant to him.

Henry continued to complain about the Queen to Cromwell, saying she 'waxed wilful and stubborn with him'. She was probably tense with anxiety and hurt by his inexplicable neglect, but it was characteristic of Henry to shift the blame for what had happened on to her shoulders, and to take offence at her tactical withdrawal. She probably could not help herself; worry about what might happen to her resulted in her being less amiable towards her terrifying spouse than she had been hitherto. Cromwell saw fit to warn her against antagonising the King, and reminded her of 'the expediency of doing her utmost to render herself more agreeable'. None knew better than he the wisdom of this advice, yet Anne was too bewildered and uneasy to heed it; in fact, she took this friendly warning to be a preamble of worse things to follow. Nor was she even aware of how she had given offence.

What with his inept minister and his difficult wife, the King was going about feeling very sorry for himself. He let it be known that he was 'in a manner weary of his life', although this was belied by his behaviour with Katherine Howard. Before very long, this assumed woefulness had given way to anger, directed chiefly against Cromwell, who was responsible for his present predicament. Once aroused, Henry's anger would not abate until he had exacted his revenge.

On 10 June 1540, Cromwell entered the council chamber as usual, in readiness for the day's business, but before he could be seated, the Duke of Norfolk stepped forward and arrested him in the King's name. Before he knew where he was, Cromwell was being transported by barge to the Tower, whither he had himself sent so many others. There were those who were sad to see him toppled, although the majority rejoiced, chief among them the members of the Catholic faction, who rightly saw in Cromwell's fall the triumph of their own ambitions. On that same day, a Bill of Attainder against Cromwell was drawn up and laid before Parliament; the charges included both treason and heresy. Such an Act, the instrument that Cromwell himself had used so often to bring others down, ironically was being employed in the same way against him. On 19 June, the Bill received the approval of the upper House, and was sent down to the Commons.

The King now laid plans for the annulment of his marriage to Anne, which would inevitably follow. He sent her to the old palace at Richmond on 24 June, on the pretext that there was plague in London and that the country air would benefit her health. Anne left without question, but with forebodings. Charles de Marillac heard 'talk of a diminution of love and a new affection for another lady'. Henry had promised to join Anne in two days, but did not do so; Marillac told his master that, had there been any truth in the story that there was plague in the City, the King would not have remained for any considerations, 'for he is the most timid person that could be in such cases'. Rumours were flying fast around court and City, and people began to be aware that there was a new love in the King's life. His intention to put away the Queen was known of in the City before 24 June, as was his affection for Katherine Howard. The citizens watched the King being rowed in a small boat, in broad daylight, to visit her on many occasions at Lambeth, whither she had retired once the Queen had left court, and Bishop Gardiner entertained Henry and Katherine to banquets at his palace in Southwark. However, the cynical Londoners regarded this not so much as evidence that the Queen was about to be divorced, but as adultery. Before long, the royal barge was to be seen every night on its way to Lambeth, so that the King could pass the evening there; ostensibly, he was visiting the Dowager Duchess of Norfolk, but few were deceived by this excuse.

Far from being impotent, Henry was now laying siege in earnest to Katherine's virtue. Her family, unaware of the fact that she was already sexually experienced, had warned her to maintain her 'pure and honest condition', although she was to make it obvious that she would welcome the royal advances once a wedding ring was on her finger. Both Anne Boleyn and Jane Seymour before her had reached the consort's throne by deploying such tactics, and Katherine was wise enough to realise that her family's advice was sound. As for the King, blissfully unaware that he was being manipulated, he was, for the last time in his life, passionately in love.

It was now the end of June. As Anne of Cleves waited apprehensively at Richmond for a husband who never came, and as the King pursued Katherine Howard in London, events were moving speedily towards a climax. On 29 June, the Bill of Attainder against Cromwell passed successfully through the Commons and became law, which meant that he was adjudged a traitor and would forfeit both life and honours, as well as all his possessions. Told of this, the condemned man wrote to the King from the Tower, hoping that his master would be merciful and at least spare his life: 'To me, you have been most bountiful, more like a father than a master. I ask mercy where I have offended, but I have done my best, no one can justly accuse me of having done wrong wilfully.' His best had not been enough; even though the charges against him made no mention of his having caused the King to be bound in an unsatisfactory marriage, it was this that sealed his fate. Although Archbishop Cranmer interceded on his behalf, the King was adamant that Cromwell must die, although he was pleased to defer the execution so that he might use Cromwell to help him dissolve the Cleves marriage. When Cromwell realised that he was indeed to suffer the extreme penalty, he grew frantic, and on 3 July, sent Henry another letter of supplication, which ended with the plaintive cry: 'Most gracious Prince, I cry for mercy, mercy, mercy!' Henry was not listening.

By 5 July, some inkling of what was afoot had reached Queen Anne at Richmond; her chamberlain, the Earl of Rutland, acting on the King's orders, made a point of assuring her that Henry would 'do nothing but that should stand by the law of God, and for the discharge of his conscience and hers, and the quietness of the realm, and at the suit of all his lords and commons'. Whether this put Anne's mind at rest is debatable; what is probable is that the prospect of a divorce was not unwelcome to her. She would not be a second Katherine of Aragon.

In Parliament on 6 July the lords petitioned the King to have the legality of his marriage investigated by a convocation of the clergy, saying they were concerned about the likelihood of a disputed succession should Anne of Cleves bear children. They pointed out that if the Duke of Lorraine's son stood by his alleged precontract, the King's marriage would be null and void. However, if – as was supposed – the King and Queen were married in name only, then the Church had power to annul their union. The King readily agreed that the clergy should look into the matter; lamenting the fact that he had been 'espoused against his will', he told Parliament that he could refuse nothing to his people, and was ready to answer any questions that might be put to him, for he had no other object in view but 'the glory of God, the welfare of the realm, and the triumph of truth'. Moreover, Henry was now sure enough of the Emperor's goodwill to risk angering the Duke of Cleves, though he had decided to make generous financial provision for Anne in an attempt to avert this.

That afternoon saw the Privy Council making its way to Richmond to see the Queen and obtain her consent to the institution of divorce proceedings. When they had explained the situation to her at length, Anne answered 'plainly and frankly that she was contented that the discussion of the matter be committed to the clergy as judges competent in that behalf'. The King, hearing this, was delighted that she should be so reasonable.

On 7 July, Henry made a written declaration to be laid before the clergy appointed to investigate his marriage. He assured them that he had no ulterior motive in seeking a divorce. When the Cleves marriage had been suggested, he had been anxious to proceed, 'because I heard so much both of her excellent beauty and virtuous behaviour'. But when he saw her at Rochester, he 'liked her so ill that I was woe that ever she came into England, and deliberated with myself that, if it were possible to find some means to break off, I would never enter yoke with her'. Both Admiral FitzWilliam and Sir Anthony Browne would bear this out, and Cromwell also, 'since he is a person knowing himself condemned to die, and will not damn his soul'. Cromwell, in particular, could testify that the King had gone into the marriage protesting that he did not consent to it. Moreover, went on the King, he himself had 'lack enough of the will and power' to consummate the marriage, as both his physicians could testify.

This they were glad to do. Dr Chambers confirmed what his master had said, and related how he had advised the King 'not to enforce himself', for to do so might result in an inconvenient debility of the sexual organs. He recalled that Henry had said 'he thought himself able to do the act with other, but not with her'. And Dr Butts gave evidence that the King had had nocturnal emissions of semen in his sleep during the period of his marriage to Anne of Cleves – in the good doctor's view, this was proof that intercourse had not taken place. The King himself reaffirmed later that Anne had come to him a virgin – he was perhaps mindful that remarks made by him at the time of their marriage had cast doubt on this – and said he had shared her bed every night for four months and 'never took from her by true carnal copulation'.

While the King was drafting his declaration to the clergy, his marriage was being debated in the House of Lords, where three good reasons were given for its dissolution: Anne's probable precontract with Lorraine, Henry's lack of consent to the marriage, and its non-consummation. This last was seen as most important since 'the whole nation had a great interest in the King's having more issue, which they saw he would never have by this queen'.

On 9 July 1540, the convocations of both Canterbury and York reached a decision. They announced that they found the King's marriage to Anne of Cleves to be null and void on the three grounds put forward by Parliament. Both the King and the Lady Anne were at liberty to remarry. Thus, with a minimum of fuss, was the King's fourth marriage ended.

On that day, a deputation of the Privy Council waited upon the ex-Queen at Richmond to inform her of the annulment of her marriage, and to tell her that from henceforth it was the King's pleasure that she call herself his sister. Anne must have felt considerable relief when she heard this, but her outward manner was calm. She did not faint, as some later apocryphal sources allege, but declared her consent to the annulment, and 'showed herself amenable to it'. The lords then informed her that the King had settled upon her a handsome annuity of £4,000 per annum, as well as the manors of Bletchingly and Richmond, with Hever Castle, Anne Boleyn's childhood home, which had reverted to the Crown on the death of the Earl of Wiltshire. Anne would now be a woman of means, with the added status of being the King of England's honorary sister. The world also knew she was still a virgin: Henry had made it as easy as possible for her to remarry if she so wished. There now opened before Anne such a vista of new-found freedom that she positively welcomed the dissolution of her marriage, and in this mood she declared to the lords her eagerness to co-operate in any way the King should wish.

Henry immediately despatched Dr Wotton to Cleves to break the news gently to Duke William. Wotton was also charged, on the Lady Anne's orders, with informing the Duke that she would not be returning to the land of her birth, as the grants of land made to her were only hers on condition that she remained in England. What was more, she liked it in England, and meant to stay for good. The Duke took the news mildly, merely commenting 'he was glad his sister had fared no worse'. All the same, as he explained in a letter to Henry VIII, he was sorry for what had happened, although he

would not depart from his amity for his Majesty for any such matter. He could have wished that his sister should return to

Germany, but if she was satisfied to remain, he had confidence that the King would act uprightly towards her, and he would not press it.

Privately William thought Henry's behaviour was deplorable, and he was fearful that Anne might be persecuted for her faith if she stayed in England. His fears would prove unfounded.

Soon, the news was buzzing around the courts of Europe. Both Francis I and Charles V approved of the annulment. Martin Luther was not so charitable. 'Squire Harry wishes to be God, and do as he pleases!' was his scornful comment, prompted no doubt by disappointment that the Protestant cause had been deprived of a potential champion in England.

On 11 July, at the request of the Council, the Lady Anne wrote a tactful letter to the King, formally acknowledging the dissolution of their marriage. In it she affirmed that, 'though this case must needs be both hard and sorrowful for me, for the great love which I bear to your most noble person,' she accepted and approved the decision of the clergy, 'whereby I neither can nor will repute myself your Grace's wife, considering this sentence and your Majesty's pure and clean living with me.' For all this, she hoped that she would sometimes have the pleasure 'of your most noble presence, which I shall esteem for a great benefit'. She was comforted, she went on, 'that your Highness will take me for your sister, for the which I most humbly thank you accordingly'. And, beseeching the Almighty to send the King long life and good health, she signed herself, 'Your Majesty's humble sister and servant, Anne, the daughter of Cleves.'

It is likely that this masterpiece of diplomacy was drafted for Anne by members of the Privy Council. While acknowledging the justness of the clergy's decision to annul the marriage, it yet manages to convey a poignant sense of loss, calculated to flatter the King. In reality it seems unlikely that Anne can have felt much distress at their separation: from a humiliating bondage she had suddenly been translated into a life of luxurious freedom, finding herself to be, for the first time, her own mistress. As the King's sister, she would take precedence over most of the ladies of the kingdom, and a place at court would always be reserved for her. There is no doubt that she had grown to appreciate her adopted land, and she was now fortunate enough to own three of the most charming houses it could boast. It was not such a bad bargain when all was said and done.

Anne's marriage was formally annulled by a specially introduced Act of Parliament on 12 July 1540. Immediately after it was passed, the Privy Council humbly petitioned the King to

> frame his most noble heart to the love and favour of some noble personage to be joined with him in lawful matrimony, by whom his Majesty might have more store of fruit and succession to the comfort of the realm.

Katherine Howard's name was not mentioned, yet the lords were in little doubt as to who their next queen would be. The only people at court who were dissatisfied at the prospect were those who supported the reformist cause and the ex-Queen's German attendants and their mutterings were predictably ignored.

Word that Katherine Howard might soon be Queen of England quickly spread. In Yorkshire, it came to the notice of Joan Bulmer, who had known Katherine well in her Lambeth days, prior to 1540. Joan had been a serving woman in the Duchess of Norfolk's household, and had at one time acted as Katherine's secretary since the future Queen was barely literate, her education having been largely overlooked. Then Joan married and moved to Yorkshire, where she now lived, and Katherine had doubtless assumed she would never see her again. She was wrong: Joan Bulmer was an ambitious woman, who did not enjoy being isolated in her north-country fastness. She wanted to come to court, where there was excitement to be had, and power to be gained by subtle means. So she wrote to Katherine on 12 July, begging to be accepted into her household once she was queen, 'as it is thought that the King of his goodness will put you in the same honour that [Anne of Cleves] was in which no doubt you be worthy to have.' She reminded Katherine of 'the unfeigned love that my heart hath always borne towards you', and confided that her changed circumstances had brought her 'into the utmost misery of the world and most wretched life'. There was no way out of it, either, unless Katherine, of her goodness, could find the means to invite Joan to London. If she were to command Joan's unpleasant husband, he would have to obey and send his wife. On and on the letter went, the writer pleading, cajoling, and flattering; she ended by beseeching Katherine

> not to be forgetful of this my request, for if you do not help me, I am not like to have worldly joys. Desiring you, if you can, to let me have some answer of this for the satisfying of my mind; for I know the Queen of Britain will not forget her secretary, and favour you will show.

Katherine was a kind-hearted girl, and she was happy to oblige. She was too inexperienced to perceive the rather menacing undertone in the letter, the sinister reminder of things better forgotten, and the underlying threat implicit in such a reminder. Before long, Mistress Bulmer had been given a place in her growing entourage, but it was a favour Katherine would live to regret.

Meanwhile, the Lady Anne of Cleves was astonishing everyone by her exemplary conduct. To a court accustomed to redundant queens creating havoc, her behaviour was remarkable, and on 13 July the King in gratitude sent her gifts of great value and richness, as well as letters from her brother and Dr Wotton. Anne opened and read these with pleasure, and then sent Henry her humble thanks for having let her see them. Afterwards, in response to Dr Wotton's hint that the Duke of Cleves and his ministers were concerned about how she was being treated in England, Anne dutifully wrote herself, in German, to Duke William, to reassure him. Nor was that all. In the presence of Norfolk and Wriothesley, she spoke to her brother's emissary and stressed that she was 'merry and honourably treated', and so cheerful did she appear that the man could not doubt it. Afterwards, Anne dined with the lords of the Council, and promised them that she would never deviate from her acceptance of the annulment of her marriage. She had, she told them, returned her wedding ring to the King in token of this. After listening to the report of his Councillors, Henry wrote to Anne, on 14 July, to thank her for being so conformable to his 'wise and honourable proceedings'. If she continued in this way, he assured her, 'you shall find us a perfect friend content to repute you as our dearest sister.'

On 17 July, Sir Thomas Wriothesley arrived at Richmond to disband the former Queen's household, and to see her new servants, selected by the Privy Council, sworn in. Anne said farewell publicly to those who were leaving her service, and cordially welcomed the newcomers, many of whom were merely transferring, being her compatriots. Afterwards, she told Wriothesley that she knew herself to be under a great obligation to the King, and that she would never oppose him in any way, not even for her brother or her mother or anyone else. She also promised to let Henry see any letters she received from abroad, and to be bound by his advice concerning matters raised in them.

To the King, this seemed almost too good to be true, and he found himself searching for flaws in Anne's conduct. Being of a suspicious nature and devious in his own actions, he could not conceive that anyone could be so candid and straightforward. Indeed, after his nine-year battle with Katherine of Aragon over the validity of their marriage, he found it hard to believe that Anne had capitulated without any kind of fight. His suspicions were therefore aroused, and they centred upon the correspondence to which Anne had unwittingly drawn his attention, namely the letters that were to pass between her and Duke William. What Henry feared was that Anne might secretly incite her brother to make war on her behalf.

Having persuaded himself that this was a very real possibility, the King instructed his Council to visit Anne again and instruct her to write one further letter to William in German, 'to the intent that all things might more clearly appear to him'. However well Anne had behaved, she was a woman, and might choose to 'play the woman' rather than keep her promises. She was therefore to persuade her brother not to listen to 'tales and bruits', and reassure him also that she was entirely content with her lot. Unless she wrote such a letter, warned the King,

> all shall remain uncertain upon a woman's promise, viz. that she will be no woman; the accomplishment whereof, on her behalf, is as difficult in the refraining of a woman's will, as in changing her womanish nature, which is impossible.

So much for Henry's opinion of the integrity of the fair sex, though he did order the Council to say to Anne, 'for her comfort, that howsoever her brother may conduct himself, or her other friends, she (continuing in her uniformity) shall never fare the worse for their faults'. The Council dutifully returned to Richmond, where Anne was happy to comply with their request. Hopefully, the King would now be satisfied, and she deemed it the appropriate time to make a request.

Anne had by now come to know all the King's children. Mary was of an age with her, and the two had established a warm friendship. Yet, of the three, it was Elizabeth, that bright perceptive child, of whom she was most fond. Anne had a kind heart, and she undoubtedly felt sorry for this little girl who had been so cruelly deprived of her mother. Unlike Prince Edward, Elizabeth was not fussed over by an army of governesses and nurses and even Lady Bryan had been taken from her. Anne herself had no desire to remarry, and knew it was unlikely that she would ever have children of her own. Elizabeth could help to fill that empty space in her life, and she, in turn, could supply the child with something of a mother's love. She was charmed by Elizabeth's beauty, wit and demonstrative nature, and felt it would be a pleasure to have her company sometimes. So she now asked the King if she might be permitted to invite Elizabeth to visit her on occasion, saying 'that to have had [her] for her daughter would have been greater happiness to her than being queen'. The King readily granted her request, and thereafter, it may be assumed, the Lady Elizabeth was a frequent guest at Richmond.

The French ambassador, Marillac, writing on 21 July to his master, was astounded at the ease with which the King had obtained an annulment of his marriage.

The Queen appears to make no objection [he wrote with disbelief]. The only answer her brother's ambassador can get from her is that she wishes in all things to please the King her lord, bearing testimony of his good treatment of her, and desiring to remain in this country. This, being reported to the King, makes him show her the greater respect.

The ambassador had learned how Henry had decreed that Anne was from henceforth to be regarded as a private person. No ministers were to trouble her or visit her. The people of England, went on the report, much regretted her divorce, for she had won their love, and they esteemed her as

> one of the most sweet, gracious and humane queens they have had, and they greatly desire her to continue their queen. Now it is said that the King is going to marry a young lady of extraordinary beauty, a daughter of a deceased brother of the Duke of Norfolk. It is even reported that this marriage has already taken place, only it is kept secret. The Queen takes it all in good part.

Anne was, indeed, quite reconciled to the prospect of Henry's remarriage. She now thought it politic to retire for a short time from public life, and took herself off to the country, living at either Bletchingly, Richmond or Hever, and enjoying her freedom as a lady of means.

Henry had not yet married Katherine Howard, although so much secrecy surrounded his affair with her that rumours were rife at court. In late July, Marillac heard that she was with child, although this proved to be false. It was only after he had dissolved Parliament for the summer recess on 25 July that Henry began to make plans for his wedding. On 27 July, he sent for the Bishop of London to come and marry him at the palace of Oatlands, whither he had just gone with the court. The ceremony would take place in secret on the following day.

There remained just one other formality to be dispensed with and that was the execution of Cromwell. On 28 July 1540, the former minister was taken from his prison in the Tower and brought to the public scaffold on Tower Hill, where a large crowd had gathered. Among them was Cromwell's old friend, Sir Thomas Wyatt. Cromwell noticed him there, weeping, and cried out, 'Oh, Wyatt, do not weep, for if I were not more guilty than thou wert, when they took thee [i.e. to the Tower after Anne Boleyn's arrest], I should not be in this pass.' The King had commuted the sentence to decapitation, even though the condemned man was of lowly birth. But Cromwell suffered, none the less: the executioner bungled his work, and it took two strokes to sever the neck of the prisoner. The King's evil genius died in the manner of so many of his own victims, because the marriage he had arranged to bring joy to his master and profit to himself had proved his ruin.

Anne of Cleves might well have ended up as another of Cromwell's victims. It is to her credit that she did not. Her handling of a difficult and potentially dangerous situation shows that she was, perhaps, the wisest of Henry VIII's wives. She was certainly the luckiest.

14
Rose without a thorn

Today, what remains of Henry VIII's palace of Oatlands lies beneath the foundations of a council estate in Weybridge, Surrey. Much of it was pulled down in the seventeenth century, yet it was a favoured retreat of the King and his children, and Henry spent a great deal of money on it. He had acquired the manor, with its moated red-brick house, in 1537; thereafter he set about enlarging and beautifying it, adding façades, new wings, an arched bridge over the moat, and an octagonal tower. He then had the moat filled in and extended the building over it, creating a new courtyard in the process. The hunting in the nearby park was excellent, and the palace was convenient for Hampton Court. By 1540, most of the improvements had been completed, and it was because it was such a pleasant place that the King decided to take Katherine Howard there for their wedding.

The marriage ceremony, on 28 July, was conducted in private by Bishop Bonner. For ten days, absolute secrecy was maintained about it. The King was infatuated with his bride, and wished for time to spend alone with her before surrounding her with all the paraphernalia of court etiquette and the lack of privacy this entailed. At last, it seemed to him, he had found a wife who embodied all the qualities he most admired in women: beauty, charm, a pleasant disposition, obedience and, he believed, virtue. He considered himself blessed indeed. Whether Katherine was so elated with her husband is a matter for conjecture, but to all appearances the new Queen suffered her wifely duties with commendable fortitude, displaying at all times a cheerful and loving manner towards her august spouse.

This marriage represented the triumph of the conservative faction at court, which meant that the Howards were once again the most powerful family in the kingdom. The changed order was to have immediate repercussions, even before the King's marriage was made public. On 30 July, Richard Fetherston, former tutor to the Lady Mary, Edward Powell, who had once championed the cause of Katherine of Aragon, and Thomas Abell, Katherine's former chaplain, were all dragged on hurdles from their prison in the Tower to Smithfield, where they were executed for high treason. On that same day, Robert Barnes, the Lutheran scholar who had helped to arrange the King's marriage to Anne of Cleves, was burnt as a heretic. The message was clear: the King would not tolerate opposition, nor was he prepared to countenance heresy. Henceforward he would be ruthless in eradicating it, and the latter years of his reign would be very dangerous times for English Protestants. Henry was to be ably assisted in his crusade against these heretics by Bishop Gardiner, an energetic opponent of Lutheranism.

While the martyrs for both faiths suffered, and the King honeymooned with his young bride, the former Queen was making the most of her new freedom. Early in August, Marillac described 'Madam of Cleves' as being 'as joyous as ever'. Far from lamenting the ending of her marriage, she was holding court at Richmond and wearing new dresses every day. The ambassador thought this either showed prudence or 'stupid forgetfulness of what should so closely touch her heart'. His report is borne out by Anne's household accounts for that month, which record payments for new gowns, among them a dress of black velvet edged with fur. Anne had not only adopted English fashions but also English food. 'There is no place like this England for feeding right well!' she declared, and her table at Richmond became renowned. Indeed, she often played hostess to guests from the court. When she was not doing that, she spent all her time at 'sports and recreation'.

The King himself was one of her visitors. After his marriage, he and Katherine left Oatlands and moved to Hampton Court. From here, Henry rode over alone to Richmond, with only a few attendants, on 6 August. Marillac reported that he and Anne were on 'the best possible terms, and they supped so pleasantly together that some thought she was to be restored to her place'. However, this was not entirely a social call. Three members of the Privy Council were present to witness Anne's signature on a document thought to have been the deed of separation. It was noticed, moreover, that Henry was treating Anne with less distinction than when she was queen. Then, she had been seated beside him at meals. Now, she sat apart, at some distance, at a corner of an adjoining table. Marillac concluded, quite rightly, that there was no likelihood of Henry taking her back.

Nevertheless, there were rumours, and on 8 August the King instructed the Privy Council to inform all his ambassadors abroad that he had remarried. On the same day, Katherine Howard appeared as queen at Hampton Court, dining publicly under a cloth of estate.

Henry's envoys were told that the King had been attracted to Katherine

upon a notable appearance of honour, cleanness and maidenly behaviour . . . [and that] his Highness was finally contented to honour that lady with his marriage, thinking in his old days – after sundry troubles of mind which had happened to him by marriage – to have obtained such a perfect jewel of womanhood and very perfect love towards him as should have been not only to his quietness but also to have brought forth the desired fruits of marriage.

The whole realm, they were told, 'did her honour accordingly'.

The month of August was given over to banquets and hunting in honour of the King's bride. Katherine revelled in her new-found importance, for her doting husband was happy to gratify her every whim: every day, she wore new gowns, and appeared laden with the jewellery with which Henry had showered her. He had rarely been so extravagant with his previous wives. Each day, Katherine discovered some new caprice, and her greed earned her the disapproval of many of the older people at court, including the Lady Mary, who did not treat her with the same respect as she had Jane Seymour and Anne of Cleves. Mary may have found it discomfitting to have a stepmother nine years her junior, for all that she came from a Catholic family, and there may well have been an element of jealousy in her attitude, for she herself was still unmarried at twenty-four. Marillac commented that the pure atmosphere that surrounded Mary was in 'marvellous contrast to the tainted air of the court'.

Whether Marillac was referring to the new Queen is not known, yet it was not long before Katherine Howard revealed herself as a frivolous, empty-headed young girl who cared for little else but dancing and pretty clothes. This seems not to have bothered the King, who looked on lovingly as his pert little wife capered through the boisterous dances of the period, dances in which he could no longer join. Instead, he encouraged the young men of the court to partner her, and watched benignly as they led her out.

Nothing in Katherine's early life had prepared her for her present position. Her youngest years had been spent in impoverished gentility, for her father had found it hard making ends meet on his limited income. She had then gone to live with the Dowager Duchess of Norfolk for the rest of her formative years; the Duchess had neglected her charge in every respect, so that she was often obliged to resort to servants and people of lowly rank for company. It was a life, moreover, devoid of luxury. But now she had the King as her husband, what seemed like unlimited riches at her disposal, power at her fingertips, and an army of servants at her beck and call. Not unnaturally, it all went to her head. However, she had a pleasing manner and a sunny personality; there is no hint that she ever displayed the arrogance shown by her cousin Anne Boleyn. Katherine had a kind heart, and was willing to use her influence on occasion to assist those in trouble. But she was also incapable of resisting the facile charm of sycophants. She had virtually no understanding of the intrigues and pitfalls surrounding her, and her obvious innocence would lay her open to compromising situations.

The King, nevertheless, found her the perfect wife in every respect. All he asked of her was that she give him more sons. She was fifteen, and ripe for this in a period when girls were married off very young. However, although Henry was visiting her bed nearly every night for the first few months of their marriage, she did not conceive, and it may be that he, with his huge bulk and advancing infirmity, was no longer capable of fathering a child.

In mid-August, the Queen's household was re-formed. The ladies appointed to serve Katherine included the Lady Margaret Douglas, the King's niece, the Duchess of Richmond, the Dowager Duchess of Norfolk, the Countess of Sussex, Lady Margaret Howard (Katherine's stepmother, now a widow), and Lady Clinton, who was not Elizabeth Blount, the King's former mistress and first wife of Lord Clinton, but his second wife, Lady Elizabeth FitzGerald whom he married after Elizabeth's death in 1539. The ladies of the Queen's Privy Chamber were the Countess of Rutland, Lady Rochford, and Lady Edgecombe, who had all served Anne of Cleves, and Lady Baynton. Other ladies and gentlewomen in attendance included Lady Arundel (Katherine's sister) and Lady Cromwell (Queen Jane's sister Elizabeth), while Mrs Stonor, who had waited upon Anne Boleyn in the Tower, was a maid of honour.

On 18 August, a new bidding prayer was said in every church in the kingdom when the new Queen's name replaced that of her predecessor. Four days later the King left Windsor to go on his usual late-summer progress, and the Queen went with him, travelling to Reading, and then through Oxfordshire. While they were away, a priest was brought before the magistrates at Windsor, accused of having 'spoken unbefitting words of the Queen's Grace', words which cast aspersions upon Katherine's moral integrity. The Privy Council was duly informed, and on their orders the priest was commanded to remain within his own diocese and admonished to be 'more temperate in the use of his tongue'.

On 29 August, Henry and Katherine arrived at the manor of Grafton in Northamptonshire, where nearly eighty years before Henry's grandparents, Edward IV and Elizabeth Woodville, had secretly married, and where, only eleven years before, Henry had parted from Wolsey for the last time. Yet there were no ghosts to trouble the happy couple on this occasion, for Marillac observed that:

> The King is so amorous of her that he cannot treat her well enough, and caresses her more than he did the others. The new Queen is a lady of moderate beauty but superlative grace. In stature she is small and slender. Her countenance is very delightful, of which the King is so greatly enamoured, and he

knows not how to make sufficient demonstrations of his affection for her.

Katherine, added Marillac, was dressed in clothes that followed the French fashion, like all the other ladies at the English court, and bore her device embroidered in gold thread around her arms: *Non aultre volonté que le sienne* ('No other will than his'). In fact Henry was so besotted with Katherine that he ordered a medal to be struck in commemoration of their marriage. It was of gold, embossed with Tudor roses and true lovers' knots entwined, and it carried the inscription: HENRICUS VIII: RUTILANS ROSA SINE SPINA, a pretty reference to the King's rose without a thorn, his perfect bride.

The royal pair remained at Grafton until 7 September before riding south into Bedfordshire, where they stayed at Ampthill for a fortnight. Katherine of Aragon had been exiled here after being banished from court. Henry, however, was more concerned about the behaviour of the Queen's vice-chamberlain, Edward Baynton, who, with others, had been drunk and disorderly in the King's presence, and Henry, fearing that their bad example might contaminate the purity of his queen, now issued stern orders 'concerning the sober and temperate order that his Highness would have them to use in his Highness' chamber of presence and the Queen's'.

The King's train left Ampthill on 1 October and travelled to Wolsey's old house, The More in Hertfordshire, before returning to Windsor on 22 October. There, Henry was astonished to learn that rumour was currently crediting him with having made Anne of Cleves pregnant while on his visit to Richmond in August. He was relieved when further investigations revealed that Anne had merely been confined to bed with a stomach upset, which some mischievous persons had whispered was morning sickness. Marillac sneered at the rumours, for the King was so openly affectionate towards Katherine Howard, and 'bestows so many caresses on her, with such singular demonstrations of affection', that it was impossible to believe he had belatedly contemplated seducing Anne of Cleves. Henry's love for his wife was further proved in October when the Queen Consort Act was passed by Parliament; this Act set out in plain terms the rights and privileges of the Queen, giving her the power to act as 'a woman sole, without the consent of the King's Highness'. Immediately after the Act was passed, Henry granted to Katherine Howard all the lands and manors that had once been in the possession of Queen Jane.

It was around this time that a crisis arose in the Queen's household. Her chief lady-in-waiting, Lady Margaret Douglas, the King's 25-year-old niece, was a young woman of strong and determined character. Some four years earlier she had clandestinely married Lord Thomas Howard, an affair that ended with his imprisonment and death in the Tower, whither he had been sent for daring to marry Margaret without the King's permission. It had taken her a long time to recover from his death, but now she was learning to enjoy life again, for, during the summer progress, she had fallen in love with the new Queen's brother, Charles Howard. So indiscreet were the lovers that, by the time the court returned to Windsor, the King had heard the gossip about them. His wrath was terrible. He packed his niece off to Syon Abbey, recently vacated by the dispossessed nuns, and forbade Howard to contact her. Katherine had wisely refused to have anything to do with the intrigue, and therefore remained in the King's good graces.

People were still expressing pious hopes that the Queen might be pregnant. In November, Richard Jones dedicated his book *The Birth of Mankind*, a treatise on reproduction and midwifery, to 'our most gracious and virtuous Queen Katherine', with a warning to all men to 'use it godly'. Although Katherine had as yet no need of such a book, being married to her had rejuvenated the King. On 4 December, Marillac reported that Henry had adopted a new daily routine: he rose between five and six, heard mass at seven, then rode out hawking until dinner, which was at 10.0 a.m. He and Katherine were staying at Woking just then, and Henry told Marillac he felt much better in the country than when he was forced to stay in London during the winter. Even his leg had temporarily improved, enabling him to ride at will.

Henry and Katherine were again at Oatlands from 7 to 18 December, and then moved on to Hampton Court for the Christmas season. The King's New Year's gifts to his wife were lavish, and included two pendant laces with 26 'fair table diamonds' and 158 'fair pearls', as well as a rope of 200 large pearls. She also received from him a square pendant containing 27 diamonds and 26 clusters of pearls, as well as a muffler of black velvet edged with sable fur into which were sewn 38 rubies and 572 pearls. At least some of these gems had belonged to the King's previous wives, for the treasury was so depleted that he could not have afforded to buy them all. Indeed, Henry was so short of funds just then that he could not spare the expense of having the Queen crowned; possibly he had decided that the coronations of queen consorts were from now on conditional upon the production of an heir.

The New Year revels of 1541 brought together a family gathering. The Lady Mary had come up from Hunsdon to be present, although she had little in common with the giddy young Queen, and relations were very stilted between them. Katherine did not worry unduly about this, however, for Anne of Cleves was also at court, and she got on famously with both of them. Anne had sent the King and Queen two great horses with violet velvet trappings before arriving at Hampton Court on 3 January. That evening, the King retired early, but Anne stayed up dancing with the young Queen, and the next day dined with her and Henry. When Henry gave Katherine yet more presents, this time a ring and two small dogs, she generously passed them over to the Lady Anne.

From 7 to 10 February 1541 Henry was in London alone, attending to business with the Council while Katherine remained with the court at Hampton; this was the first time they had been apart since their marriage. On the King's return, or soon after, his leg began to pain him once more, causing him to become virtually chair-bound for a time. By Shrove Tuesday, he was sunk in apathy, and not interested in any kind of recreation, even music. Marillac described him as suffering from *mal d'esprit*, and at one point his doctors were in fear for his life. There was little they could do to alleviate his pain, or his depression, and for some weeks it was left to Queen Katherine to preside over a court that felt strangely empty. There were masques on 21 and 22 February, but the King did not attend them.

In private, the Queen was dutiful in attending to her husband's needs, yet he was not an easy person to live with at this time. He was melancholy and irascible. It was felt that his great bulk only made matters worse, and Marillac observed that the King was 'marvellously excessive in eating and drinking', adding that 'people say he is often of a different opinion in the morning than after dinner'. He could not bear people near him during those weeks, and kept to his rooms, so that it was said that the court 'resembled more a private family than a King's train'. Kings were expected to live their lives publicly, but Henry had had enough. He could not accept this latest setback to his health, or face the fact that he was now a prisoner of his ageing, sickly body. Queen Katherine could not arouse him from his depression, and he shut his door even against her.

Although Katherine was alarmed by the King's behaviour, which was contrary to all she knew of him, her fears were soon to be allayed for by 19 March Henry was much his old self again. His leg was now a little better, and this enabled him to muster his inner resources to help him face the future.

That spring saw Katherine stirred to action by the plight of three people imprisoned in the Tower. One was Margaret Pole, Countess of Salisbury, who had languished there for nearly two years with inadequate clothing and heating to protect her aged body from the bitter winter weather. When she learned of this, the Queen saw her tailor on 1 March and ordered him to make up garments which were to be sent to Lady Salisbury: a furred night-gown, a kirtle of worsted, a furred petticoat, a satin-lined night-gown, a bonnet and frontlet, four pairs of hose, four pairs of shoes and one pair of slippers. With the King's permission, Katherine paid for all these items out of her privy purse.

The second prisoner in whom the young Queen took an interest was Sir Thomas Wyatt, who was again in the Tower on a minor charge. When the King recovered from his malady, Katherine pleaded for Wyatt's release. Chapuys, who had recently returned to court, told Charles V that this was a very courageous act on her part, and that Henry had only grudgingly consented after laying down certain conditions, namely that Wyatt confessed his guilt, and undertook to resume conjugal relations with his wife, from whom he had been estranged for fifteen years. For a week, Katherine worked to persuade the King to leave out this latter condition, but Henry was in a prim and virtuous mood, and insisted upon it. Wyatt was duly released, it being given out that 'at the great and continual suit of the Queen's Majesty, the King, being of his own most godly nature inclined to pity and mercy, hath given him his pardon in large and ample sort'. Katherine also obtained the release of a third prisoner, Sir John Wallop, confined to the Tower for some petty misconduct.

The pardoning of Wyatt was a very popular move at court, and for weeks both King and Queen basked in the approval and applause of those around them. Henry was impressed by his wife's tender compassion for the prisoners, feeling it an appropriate attribute in the consort of a ruler such as himself. It was very gratifying being able to play the role of indulgent husband and merciful sovereign, and flattering to the King's vanity.

In early April 1541, Katherine thought she might be pregnant at last. This, Marillac told Francis I, 'would be a very great joy to the King, who, it seems, believes it, and intends, if it be found true, to have her crowned at Whitsuntide'. Sadly Katherine's hopes came to nothing: it may have been a false alarm, or she may even have suffered an early miscarriage. What is certain is that disappointment cast the King once more into a black mood, and in early May the Queen herself was visibly in low spirits owing to a rumour that Henry planned to get rid of her and take back Anne of Cleves. There was no foundation to this tale, as Henry hastened to reassure his wife, but his disappointment certainly affected their happy relationship for a time, and it may well have made Katherine dissatisfied with her marriage.

Life at court was mundane and quiet that spring. None of the King's children was there and there was little in the way of entertainment. The young Queen was bored. Then news arrived of an uprising against the King in Yorkshire. Headed by Sir John Neville, a fervent Catholic, its purpose was to depose Henry VIII's Lord President of the North and restore the old forms of religion in England. Henry also seems to have feared that disaffection among his subjects would lead to plots for the reinstatement of the Plantagenets. A few sprigs of that ancient royal house still lived: one was Margaret Pole, who had a valid claim to the throne, although she herself had never expressed any desire to occupy it. Indeed, for years, she had rendered loyal and devoted service to the Tudors, and it was mainly because of her sons' disaffection that she had been imprisoned in the Tower. Yet now, with a rebellion on his hands, the King behaved as if the Countess was a threat to his security, and – in spite of the Queen's protests and pleas for mercy – he ordered that the death sentence provided for in the Act of Attainder passed against Lady Salisbury be put into effect immediately.

On the morning of 28 May 1541, there occurred one of the worst atrocities of Henry's reign. The 68-year-old Countess was awakened by the Constable of the Tower with the news that she was to die that day. She was given a short while to prepare her soul for death, then led out to the scaffold on Tower Green, where Anne Boleyn had died, and where a crowd of spectators awaited her. The executioner was not the usual one employed on such occasions and was young and inexperienced. Faced with such a prisoner, he panicked, and struck out blindly, hacking at his victim's head, neck and shoulders, until he had finally butchered her to death.

The cruel end of Lady Salisbury sickened even the Tudor court, but the King was unrepentant. The northern uprising was speedily put down, and its leaders executed at the end of July. The peace of the realm had been preserved, and the security of the dynasty maintained, although Henry's reputation had suffered in the process. He was now more feared than beloved by many of his subjects.

On 30 July 1541, the King left London to go on a progress with the Queen and a great train of courtiers to the Eastern counties and the North, the centres of so much recent disaffection. He believed that his presence there might inspire loyalty and also act as a deterrent against any thought of future revolts. There were also two other matters to be accomplished. One was the collection of the huge fines levied on the cities that had supported Neville's rebellion, and the other was a meeting between Henry VIII and his nephew, James V of Scotland, who had promised to ride down to York to greet his uncle.

The royal cavalcade travelled via Dunstable, Ampthill, Grafton, Northampton, and Stamford to the city of Lincoln. Here, after formally pardoning the citizens for their part in the Pilgrimage of Grace and the recent uprising, the King went with the Queen into the cathedral, where they heard mass. During their stay, they were lodged in the adjacent Bishop's Palace. After leaving Lincoln, they journeyed to Boston, then a flourishing port, where Henry was able to indulge his passion for ships. From Boston, the progress wound its way into Yorkshire, passing into Northumberland as far as Newcastle – the furthest north Henry had ever been during his reign – and then south again to Pontefract, whose castle had been in 1400 the scene of the murder of Richard II. The court arrived there at the end of August.

Meanwhile, disturbing news from abroad had reached England. The Emperor and the King of France were on the brink of war with each other, and both wanted Henry's support. In August, Francis I proposed a marriage between the Lady Mary and his heir, the Duke of Orléans (the Dauphin had died in 1536); but Henry was reluctant to commit himself and so offend Charles. Thereafter, relations between England and France, never very good of late, deteriorated steadily. Since his excommunication in 1539, Henry VIII had been building elaborate defences along the south coast of England, in anticipation of a possible French invasion, and his castles still stand today at Deal and Walmer. He did not trust Francis, suspecting him of plotting an invasion of his kingdom, and for this reason he wanted the Emperor as a friend and ally, bearing in mind also the vital trade links between England and the Low Countries.

Henry did not let matters of state affect his enjoyment of the progress; as for the Queen, she was in high spirits, revelling in the warmth and approval emanating from the people who lined the roads and lanes to see her. Yet in Pontefract, she came face to face with her past when a young man who had once lived in the Dowager Duchess's household presented himself at court. His name was Francis Dereham, and he came with a recommendation from the Duchess, whose distant relative he is thought to have been, and who had led him to believe that the Queen would be pleased to have him in her household. But Katherine feared there was another reason that had prompted Dereham's appearance at court, the same reason that had inspired Joan Bulmer to press to be taken into her service. Dereham possessed information that could cause untold harm to Katherine's reputation, and he might well mean to exploit that knowledge, and use it to gain preferment. Hence, when he too requested employment, she dared not refuse, and on 27 August he was appointed her private secretary. 'Take heed what words you speak,' Katherine warned him. When the King asked why she had employed Dereham, she told him that the Duchess of Norfolk had asked her to be good to him – 'and so I will.'

Dereham proved to be a most unsuitable addition to her

household. He had a fiery temper, and was over-familiar with his royal mistress, arousing the dislike of many who felt that Katherine was giving him preferential treatment. One of the Queen's gentlemen ushers, a Mr John, fell out with Dereham when the latter remained seated at dinner or supper after the Queen's council had risen, an action that seemed deliberately disrespectful. Mr John sent a messenger one evening with orders for Dereham to rise with every-one else, but Dereham refused. 'Go to Mr John and tell him I was one of the Queen's counsel before he knew her, and shall be there after she hath forgotten him!' he said insolently. This provoked a brawl between the two men with Dereham emerging the victor. It was as well the King did not hear of it, for there were severe penalties for violent behaviour within the court, though Dereham could be discreet when he wanted to, and he kept in the background when Henry was around. Others noticed his proprietorial and somewhat familiar manner with the Queen. Katherine was always susceptible to male flattery and attention, and there were those in her household and at the court who were strongly attracted to her, and jealous of Dereham's influence. She did not know it, but she was standing on the edge of a precipice.

In the middle of September, the King's train arrived in York, where Henry was due to rendezvous with James V. James, being distrustful of his uncle, did not turn up. Relations between England and Scotland had never been very good during Henry's reign, but from now on they would be plainly antagonistic. After waiting with mounting anger for several days for the King of Scots, Henry gave up and went off to Hull, arriving there on 1 October, and staying for five days. Henry was feeling much restored and in a holiday mood, though the progress was now drawing to an end. During October, the royal cavalcade moved slowly south, passing through Kettleby and Collyweston and Ampthill, before reaching Windsor on the 26th.

Two items of bad news awaited the King on his return. One concerned the death of his sister, Queen Margaret of Scotland, on 8 October at Methven Castle, and the other was a report from Prince Edward's doctors that the four-year-old heir was ill with a fever. Marillac told Francis I that Edward was 'too fat and unhealthy' to live long, but he was clearly being malicious. Fortunately, the King's initial panic upon hearing the news of his son's illness was soon alleviated by tidings that the child was making a good recovery. Continuing reports of Edward's progress put Henry into a good mood, and he seems at this time to have become even fonder of his queen, if that were possible. He could not bear to be without her for long, calling her the jewel of his age, and continually thanking God for sending him such a wife. He was even planning a public service of thanksgiving. But his idyll was soon to be abruptly and tragically shattered.

While the King was away on progress, a Protestant called John Lascelles came and confided to Archbishop Cranmer that he knew things about the Queen's past that would reflect upon her marriage with the King. He vowed he would rather die declaring the truth, since it so nearly touched the King, than live with the concealment of the same. Cranmer asked why he had not come forward before, to which he replied that he had been wrestling with his conscience.

Cranmer was not an unkind man, but he preferred to do whatever was expedient, and he was, it must be remembered, a secret Protestant himself, as well as an advocate of reform. He had never approved of the King's marriage to Katherine Howard, although he held nothing personal against her: it was what she represented that he privately and passionately opposed. He therefore saw in John Lascelles a catalyst for change: if anything could be proved against the Queen, it might be possible to remove her from the political scene and discredit her supporters, the powerful Catholic faction. The way would then be clear for the King to marry a bride put forward by Cranmer and his partisans who would be as energetic as Anne Boleyn in the reformist cause.

Cranmer therefore listened patiently and courteously to what John Lascelles had to say. He heard that Lascelles's sister Mary had, before her marriage to a Mr Hall, lived with Katherine in the ladies' dormitory in the Duchess of Norfolk's house at Lambeth, and had known her well. Later, when it was announced that Katherine was to become Queen of England, Mrs Hall had been prompted by her brother to seek service with her. 'I will not,' she answered, 'but I am very sorry for her.' Lascelles had asked why. 'Marry, for she is light, both in living and in conditions [i.e. behaviour],' was the answer. Lascelles did not elaborate on this, but told the Archbishop that his sister could supply more details if she was required to.

When Lascelles had gone, Cranmer pondered for a long time. Anne Boleyn had been found guilty of misconduct after marriage; was it possible that the same thing might be proved against Katherine Howard? Fornication before marriage was not a crime, but it argued a lightness of morals that might lead a young and impressionable girl into an adulterous relationship after the knot was tied. The possibility was there. Yet Cranmer knew he was treading on very dangerous ground. Anne Boleyn's fall had come about because the King was desperate to be rid of her: he was deeply in love with Katherine, and likely to react violently to any inference that she was not as virtuous as he believed her to be. It would not be wise to act until a solid case of incontrovertible fact had been established. Indeed, it might be wiser not to do anything at all.

There was much at stake. Cranmer knew Henry well enough to predict that he would sacrifice his personal needs in the interests of the state; adultery in a queen jeopardised the succession and was insulting to the King. Henry's vast pride would not permit him to retain a wife who had cuckolded him, or made a fool of him. He would be devastated, but he would not be stupid. It was essential, however, for Cranmer to get his facts right beforehand, for it would be death to incur the King's displeasure over such a matter.

He summoned Mary Hall. Her information was far more precise than her brother's. She told Cranmer that some years before, when she was living in the household of the Dowager Duchess of Norfolk, it was common gossip that the Queen, then a very young girl, had been encouraging the attentions of her music master, Henry Manox. One of the ladies of the household, Dorothy Barwike, had told Mary that Manox was troth-plight to Katherine Howard, 'with whom he was much in love'. Manox, of course, had no business to be affiancing himself to a daughter of the Howards, and Mary Hall took it upon herself to reprove him for his behaviour.

Man [she had said sharply], what mean thou to play the fool of this fashion? Know not that if my lady of Norfolk knew of the love betwixt thee and Mistress Howard, she will undo thee? She is come of a noble house, and if thou should marry her, some of her blood would kill thee!

Manox had sneered and replied,

Hold thy peace, woman! I know her well enough. My designs are of a dishonest kind, and from the liberties the young lady has allowed me, I doubt not of being able to effect my purpose. She hath said to me that I shall have her maidenhead, though it be painful to her, not doubting but I will be good to her hereafter.

Mary had been appalled by his cynicism, and the fact that he was leading Katherine on with empty offers of marriage, but she was a charitable woman and excused him on the grounds that he 'was so far in love with her that he wist not what he said'. Which says far more about Mary Lascelles's ignorance of the ploys of the male sex than it does about Manox's true intentions.

But Katherine could also be fickle. Shortly afterwards she transferred her affection to Francis Dereham, without having granted Manox the ultimate favour. Their affair progressed quickly and soon, according to Mrs Hall, they became lovers. For a hundred nights and more, Dereham had crept into the ladies' dormitory and climbed, dressed in doublet and hose, into Katherine's bed. The other women and girls in the room were left in little ignorance of what was going on by the noises that issued from beyond the drawn bed-hangings, and one maid refused to sleep nearby because Katherine 'knew not what matrimony was'. At the same time, Manox, full of spite, was going about boasting that he knew of a private mark on Katherine's body. He told Mary Hall that he would speak to Katherine about her behaviour with Dereham, but Mary told him to keep quiet. 'Let her alone,' she said, unable to contain her disgust at Katherine's behaviour 'for if she holds on as she begins, we shall hear she will be naught within a while.'

Cranmer listened to all this with interest, giving due attention to his informant. He could find nothing amiss in her character, and later reported to the Council that 'she did from the first opening of the matter to her brother seem to be sorry, and to lament that the King's Majesty had married the Queen'. Now he dismissed her after taking a written statement, and retired to think about what she had told him.

On 30 October, the King and Queen came to Hampton Court. Henry now gave orders for the special service of thanksgiving for his marriage to take place on 1 November. On that day he publicly thanked God in the Chapel Royal for blessing him with so perfect a companion: 'I render thanks to Thee, O Lord, that after so many strange accidents that have befallen my marriages, Thou hast been pleased to give me a wife so entirely conformed to my inclinations as her I now have.' At the same time, in churches throughout the land, every good subject paid similar honour to the Queen's virtues.

While Henry was giving thanks, Cranmer softly entered the Chapel, not without apprehension. He had decided, after much deliberation, that he ought to lay what information he had before the King now, although he had agonised for hours over how best to do it. In the end, he had decided to summarise the facts in a letter, which he now laid by the King's side before retiring from the service.

Back in his chamber, Henry read what Cranmer had written: that his cherished Katherine was accused of 'dissolute living before her marriage with Francis Dereham, and that was not secret, but many knew it'. His first reaction was one of astonished disbelief. He summoned Cranmer at once and demanded an explanation. Cranmer repeated all that had gone before, and ended by saying he had been forced to convey the news by letter 'as he had not the heart to tell him by mouth'. Henry was stunned, but he kept his composure. He told the Archbishop he did not think there was any foundation in these malicious accusations; nevertheless, Cranmer was to investigate the matter more thoroughly. 'You are not to desist until you have got to the bottom of the pot,' said Henry. At the same time, he gave orders that the Queen was to be confined to her apartments with just Lady Rochford in attendance until her name was cleared, as he was confident it would be. He himself would stay away from her until then. In fact, he never saw her again.

Katherine and her ladies were practising dance steps when the King's guards arrived and said it was 'no more the time to dance'. When they dismissed most of her servants, Katherine – who had more on her conscience than pre-marital romps with Manox and Dereham – became extremely agitated, and demanded to know the reason for her confinement, but the guards could not enlighten her. She thought she knew already, and in the days to come the knowledge prevented her from eating and sleeping. In fact, she was not, as yet, in such a bad case as she feared, for the King was inclined to believe in her innocence because, in his view, the evidence provided by John Lascelles and Mary Hall was a malicious fabrication. On 2 November, he told Sir Thomas Wriothesley and Sir Anthony Browne that:

> He could not believe it to be true, and yet, the accusation having once been made, he could not be satisfied till the certainty hereof was known; but he would not, in any wise, that in the inquisition any spark of scandal should arise against the Queen.

On the following day, Cranmer questioned John Lascelles again, but the man only repeated and confirmed what he had said earlier, affirming it to be the truth. Cranmer sat on this knowledge for two days before passing it on to the King. In the meantime, he discovered that the Queen had taken Francis Dereham into her service. On 5 November, he and the Council informed the King that they believed the allegations against Queen Katherine had a sound basis in fact: that she now employed one of her former lovers was seen as very sinister indeed. 'She has betrayed you in thought,' Cranmer told his master, 'and if she had an opportunity would have betrayed you in deed.'

It should be remembered that at this stage Cranmer had not one jot of evidence beyond what he saw as his own logical conclusions that Katherine had ever committed adultery. But Henry's suspicious mind had also jumped to that same logical conclusion. He slumped in his chair, pierced to the heart; for some time he could not speak. Finally, he broke down in tears in front of the Council, weeping copiously and pouring out his heartbreak. They marvelled at this, thinking it 'strange in one of his courage' to show such emotion. 'The King has wonderfully felt the case of the Queen,' reported Chapuys. Indeed, from that moment onwards, Henry was an old man. The semblance of youth had gone for ever. On the same day, he left Hampton Court with a few attendants and galloped to Oatlands, even though the house was full of poignant memories. He remained there for some days, away from the public gaze and the court gossip, his pride broken, and his heart. He did not want to air his shame.

Chapuys thought the King might well be more merciful towards Katherine than her relatives, who had already abandoned her in an attempt to save their own skins. Only Norfolk, who perhaps felt to a degree responsible for what had happened, showed some compassion towards his niece. He was present when Katherine was informed of the charges of misconduct laid against her, and witnessed her hysterical reaction. He told Marillac that she was refusing to eat or drink anything, and that she did not cease from weeping and crying 'like a madwoman, so that they must take away things by which she might hasten her death'. Norfolk had already assumed that his niece would end on the block as her cousin had done, and it is obvious that Katherine herself expected it.

The Queen was not the only person affected by what had happened. Lady Rochford, who was guilty of aiding and abetting crimes the Council did not yet know about, suddenly realised the danger she was in and 'was seized with raving madness'. Since the two women were confined together, it was thought by many that the same fate would befall the Queen. Earlier on, before Henry left Hampton Court, Katherine had dashed past her guards and tried to reach him while he was at prayer in the Chapel Royal, but she had been intercepted by her pursuers and dragged screaming back to her rooms. She knew, as well as everyone else, that if she could see Henry she stood a good chance of being forgiven. But Henry knew his own weakness in this respect, and kings must not be seen to be weak. He had removed himself, and Katherine knew her case was hopeless.

At Lambeth, the Dowager Duchess of Norfolk heard reports of the Queen's misconduct, and realised that it was under her roof that that misconduct had taken place. She also recalled certain incidents that tended to confirm what was being said. Nevertheless, she took a more rational view of what was happening than most of her clan. 'If there be none offence sithence the marriage, she cannot die for that was done before,' she reasoned. Yet she began searching the house for incriminating evidence, knowing that, if Katherine fell, the Howards would topple with her.

Cranmer was now certain that he could uncover evidence of adultery after marriage. When he visited the Queen in her apartments on 6 and 7 November, it was in the hope of wringing a confession of this from her. Without it, no one could proceed against her, for pre-marital fornication was neither a crime nor acceptable grounds for annulling a marriage. Knowing that much depended upon the outcome of the interview, Cranmer assumed his most paternal and solicitous manner. Afterwards, he wrote an account of what had happened for the King.

He found the Queen 'in such lamentation and heaviness as I never saw no creature, so that it would have pitied any man's heart in the world to have looked upon'. It was impossible to speak rationally with her in this state, and therefore he did not stay long. Katherine remained in 'a vehement rage' all night, and was still quite frenzied when he returned the next morning. Even Cranmer was shaken by her behaviour, and feared for her sanity. Yet he brought her hope, in the form of a letter from her husband, promising her mercy if she would confess her faults. When this letter was read to her, she calmed down a little, although Cranmer feared it was only a temporary lull. But at least they were able to converse sensibly for a while, Katherine telling him she was willing to do all he asked of her and that she would reply to his questions 'as truly and faithfully as she would answer at the Day of Judgement and by the Sacrament which she received on All Hallows Day last past'. Cranmer himself admitted later that he meant to frighten her by exaggerating the grievous nature of her offences as well as 'declaring to her the justness of your Grace's laws, and what she ought to suffer by the same'. Only then did he intend to extend the offer of mercy to her.

Yet Katherine was so distraught that he felt constrained instead to stress the 'benignity and mercy' of the King in an attempt to comfort her, sensing that any mention of the law might drive her 'into some dangerous ecstasy, or else into a very frenzy, so that the words of comfort, coming last, might have come too late'. When Katherine at last understood that Henry really did mean to deal gently with her, 'She held up her hands and gave most humble thanks to your Majesty, who had showed her more grace and mercy than she herself could have hoped for.' After that, she became 'more temperate and moderate', even though she did not cease sobbing and weeping, and at one point, when panic hit her once more, she started screaming. The Archbishop was becoming familiar with this pattern, and tried hard to reason out the cause, doing his best to allay her fears while at the same time trying to glean more information. If she had 'some new fantasy come into her head', he said gently, she could confide it to him.

Gradually, Katherine pulled herself together. When she could speak coherently, she cried,

Alas, my Lord, that I am alive! The fear of death did not grieve me so much before as doth now the remembrance of the King's goodness, for when I remember how gracious and loving a Prince I had, I cannot but sorrow. But this sudden mercy, more than I could have looked for, maketh mine offences to appear before mine eyes much more heinous than they did before. And the more I consider the greatness of his mercy, the more I do sorrow in my heart that I should so misorder myself against his Majesty.

And she wept so bitterly that nothing Cranmer could say would comfort her. Eventually, she calmed down, and he left her to rest until the evening.

When he returned, she was still relatively calm, and they talked awhile, he giving her words of comfort, but at six o'clock she again grew hysterical, remembering that at that hour Master Heneage usually brought her news of the King and a loving message from him.

Cranmer did not obtain a great deal of information from Katherine about her liaison with Dereham before her marriage, but he did learn enough to conclude that there had probably been some kind of precontract between them that would invalidate Katherine's marriage to the King, even though Katherine herself 'thinks it to have been no contract'. The Archbishop obtained a written declaration or confession from her, describing what had passed between her and Dereham, but, after he had left, she sent word to say that she wished to change it. On Cranmer's return, she insisted that Dereham had in fact raped her with 'importunate force', and that she had not at any time freely consented to intercourse with him. Cranmer knew, of course, that she was lying, and suspected she might well have lied about other things, such as whether or not she had betrayed the King after her marriage. He warned her that her life was forfeit – although there was no legal basis for this statement – and reminded her again that the King was prepared to be merciful. Her written confession of her fault and her plea for her husband's forgiveness might soften Henry's heart. It was her only hope.

The Queen's confession did not satisfy Cranmer. In it, Katherine declared that Dereham had 'many times moved me unto the question of matrimony', but she had never accepted any of his proposals. She had neither willingly indulged in illicit intercourse with him, nor had she said the words alleged by Mary Hall to have been spoken by her to Dereham, 'I promise you I do love you with all my heart.' She was also sure she had never promised by her faith and troth that she would have no other husband but him. She was too naïve to realise that by admitting to a precontract she could have saved her life, for if she had never been the King's legal wife, she could not be accused of adultery, which she now realised they were trying to prove. Instead she seems to have felt that confessing to the existence of a precontract would somehow prejudice her case. She had certainly been affectionate towards her lover, for she had given him a collar and sleeves for a shirt, which had been made by 'Clinton's wife of Lambeth', as well as a silver bracelet, although she accused him of snatching the latter from her and keeping it in spite of her protests. A ruby ring found by the King's men in Dereham's possession was 'none of hers'.

The news that Dereham, Manox and other members of the Duchess of Norfolk's household had been arrested a day or so previously and imprisoned in the Tower was enough to send her into another paroxysm of hysterical panic, yet it also constrained her to be more truthful. Dereham, she continued, had given her presents, mainly lovers' tokens. 'He knew of a little woman in London with a crooked back, who was skilled in making flowers of silk,' who made him a French fennel to give to Katherine, and later a heart's-ease for a New Year's present, although the Dowager Duchess returned it to him, considering it a most improper gift. Yet Dereham was not put off. He bought some sarcenet, which Katherine had had made up into a quilted cap by the Duchess's embroiderer, a man surnamed Rose. Although Katherine had not specified any particular pattern, Mr Rose decorated the cap with friars' knots, which were a symbol of true love. When Dereham saw it, he exclaimed, 'What, wife, here be friars' knots for Francis!' The fact that he was used to addressing her as 'wife' was taken to be strongly indicative of a precontract between them.

These, then, were the only gifts that passed between the lovers, except for £10.00 that Dereham gave to the Queen during the recent progress – for what purpose is not specified. There was also the matter of £100 he left with her when he went away from the household at Lambeth to seek his fortune in Ireland, where he is thought to have turned to piracy. This money was the bulk of his savings, and he entrusted it to Katherine, saying that, if he did not return, 'I was to consider it as my own.' To Cranmer and others, this argued an established relationship based on a firm understanding that the young couple would marry some day.

When Katherine was asked whether she had called Dereham husband and he had called her wife, she answered that it was common gossip in the household that they would marry; some of Dereham's rivals – a reference to Manox, perhaps – were very jealous of him, and it pleased him to flaunt his conquest in their faces. He had asked Katherine if he might have leave to refer to her as his wife; she agreed, and promised to call him husband. Thus they fell into the habit of using these terms.

Dereham seems to have been quite a ladies' man: he kissed Katherine openly and often, and did the same to many other women in the house. On one occasion, he kissed Katherine so passionately that those watching them observed 'that he would never have kissed me enough'. Dereham retorted, 'Who shall let [prevent] me to kiss my own wife?' Then the others teased him, saying the day would surely come when 'Mr Dereham will have Mrs Katherine Howard.' 'By St John!' said Dereham, 'You may guess twice and guess worse!' Katherine inwardly cringed at such talk, and asked Dereham what would happen 'an [if] this should come to my lady's ear?' But it never did. The Duchess was a neglectful guardian, and was either deaf to the rumours or deliberately ignored them. If she was confronted with something not to her liking, then she dealt with it, but otherwise she seems to have cared little for the moral welfare of those in her charge.

Katherine's confession next dealt with the delicate matter known as 'carnal knowledge', and dealt with it honestly and frankly. She confessed that on many occasions Dereham

> hath lain with me, sometimes in his doublet and hose, and two or three times naked, but not so naked that he had nothing upon him, for he had always at the least his doublet, and as I do think his hose also; but I mean naked, when his hose was put down.

On the nights he visited her bed, he would bring with him wine, strawberries, apples, 'and other things to make good cheer, after my lady was gone to bed'. He never attempted to steal the Duchess's keys, and nor did Katherine; the door to the ladies' dormitory was frequently left unlocked at night for a variety of reasons, so they had no need. Sometimes, he would arrive at Katherine's bedside early in the morning, and behave 'very lewdly', but never, she insisted, was this at her request or with her consent.

There was always the fear of discovery. 'What shift should we make if my lady should come in suddenly?' asked Wilks and Baskerville, two of the women sharing the dormitory. Katherine told them she would send her lover into a nearby gallery, and on one occasion was obliged to do this. When Dereham learned that Katherine might be going to court, he said he would not remain for long in the Duchess's household, to which she replied that he might do as he liked. She had felt little grief at the prospect of being parted from him, and had not shed a tear over it; nor had she told him – as alleged by Mary Hall – he would never live to say, 'Thou hast swerved.' Everyone that knew her was aware how glad she was to be going to court, and once she had left the Duchess's household and Dereham had gone to Ireland, she had not written to him. As far as she remembered, the last conversation between them prior to their parting had concerned Katherine's distant cousin, Thomas Culpeper. Dereham had heard a rumour that she was going to marry Culpeper, and asked if it were true, but she denied it, saying, 'What should you trouble me thereabouts, for you know I will not have you; and if you heard such report, you know more than I.'

In mentioning Thomas Culpeper in her statement, Katherine unwittingly played into Cranmer's hands, for Culpeper was now at court, one of the most highly favoured gentlemen of the King's privy chamber. He was a cousin of the Queen on her mother's side, and Katherine had been fond of him since childhood. In fact, in recent months, that fondness had developed into something far deeper and more dangerous. Cranmer did not know this, but his suspicions were now aroused – he was, it must be remembered, searching for evidence of adultery – and he persuaded the Council to order Culpeper's arrest and detention for questioning.

Thus the evidence against the Queen built up. Cranmer sent her confession to the King on 7 November, along with the further statement alleging that Dereham had raped her by force. In the meantime, Katherine received a visit from some of the lords of the Council, who helped her to draft a plea for forgiveness to send to the King. It read:

I, your Grace's most sorrowful subject and vile wretch in the world, not worthy to make any recommendations unto your Majesty, do only make my most humble submission and confession of my faults. And where no cause of mercy is given on my part, yet of your most accustomed mercy extended to all other men undeserved, most humbly on my hands and knees do desire one particle thereof to be extended unto me, although of all other creatures most unworthy either to be called your wife or subject. My sorrow I can by no writing express, nevertheless I trust your most benign nature will have some respect unto my youth, my ignorance, my frailness, my humble confession of my faults and plain declaration of the same, referring me wholly unto your Grace's pity and mercy. First at the flattering and fair persuasions of Manox, being but a young girl [I] suffered him at sundry times to handle and touch the secret parts of my body, which neither became me with honesty to permit, nor him to require. Also Francis Dereham by many persuasions procured me to his vicious purpose, and obtained first to lie upon my bed with his doublet and hose, and after within the bed, and finally he lay with me naked, and used me in such sort as a man doth his wife, many and sundry times, and our company ended almost a year before the King's Majesty was married to my Lady Anne of Cleves, and continued not past one quarter of a year, or a little above.

This dates the liaison with Dereham to the autumn and winter of 1538–9, when Katherine was about thirteen; her affair with Manox belongs to the period immediately prior to that.

Now that she had declared the whole truth to the King, she humbly besought him to consider

the subtle persuasions of young men and the ignorance and frailness of young women. I was so desirous to be taken unto your Grace's favour, and so blinded with the desire of worldly glory, that I could not, nor had grace, to consider how great a fault it was to conceal my former faults from your Majesty, considering that I intended ever during my life to be faithful and true unto your Majesty after; nevertheless, the sorrow of mine offences was ever before mine eyes, considering the infinite goodness of your Majesty towards me from time to time ever increasing and not diminishing. Now I refer the judgement of all my offences with my life and death wholly unto your most benign and merciful Grace to be considered by no justice of your Majesty's laws but only by your infinite goodness, pity, compassion and mercy, without the which I acknowledge myself worthy of extreme punishment.

When Henry read this abject plea, he was somewhat cheered. His beloved wife had not been unfaithful to him after all. Then Cranmer arrived, to inform him that, in his opinion, the Queen had in fact been precontracted to Dereham, and that her marriage to the King was therefore invalid. An annulment now seemed inevitable, but at least it would spare Henry from having to execute another of his wives.

In more buoyant mood, Henry returned to Hampton Court, where he 'socialised with the ladies, as gay as ever I saw him', wrote Marillac. He did not, however, see his wife. Then, on 10 November, on the pretext that he was going hunting, he returned to London, picnicking in a field on the way. At Whitehall, he sat in council from midnight until 4.0 or 5.0 a.m., and again the following day, remaining closeted for some time and only breaking for meals. Obviously a matter of great importance was under discussion, as the

King did not often attend Council meetings, nor stay so long when he did. When they emerged, the councillors seemed troubled, especially Norfolk, who was not normally a man to show in his face what he was feeling. The court, which had now arrived from Hampton, was seething with rumours, not least of which was that Henry wanted to change his queen yet again. Marillac's master, Francis I, was anxious for Henry to take back Anne of Cleves, as he had already allied himself with the German princes and hoped that by such a connection Henry would see fit to join forces with him against the Emperor. Marillac was therefore working for a reconciliation between Henry and Anne, a sure indication that it was being taken for granted by most people that the King would soon be a free man. Marillac also reported a rumour that the Queen's physicians had told the King she would never bear children. This is unlikely to have been true, and was probably one of the wilder rumours current at that time. Not so wild was his supposition that Katherine would follow Anne Boleyn, her cousin, to the block.

She, meanwhile, was still confined to her chamber, and was permitted no entertainment; there she would remain until the Council had determined what to do with her. Cranmer was playing for time. He was still trying to uncover evidence of adultery, although as yet there was none. He was also worried that Henry would break his resolve and see Katherine: the chances that a reconciliation would then take place were high. Cranmer therefore suggested that the Queen be sent to a private house until her fate was decided. He had yet, he said, to question Dereham, Culpeper and others who had been involved in the affair. Henry agreed. On 11 November, the Archbishop went to Hampton Court and informed Queen Katherine that she was to be sent to the former Abbey of Syon at Brentford in Middlesex, where she would be under house arrest but 'yet served as queen'. In two days' time she would be taken by river to her new lodging. Lady Rochford, who was believed to know more than she would divulge about her mistress's behaviour, was sent to the Tower to await questioning.

While he was at Hampton, Cranmer learned from the Council that the King had decided to lay before Parliament, as the supreme court, the matter of the Queen's 'abominable behaviour'; Henry meant to arouse Parliament's indignation and disgust at her conduct and therefore her precontract with Dereham would not be referred to, as it constituted her only defence.

> No man would think it reasonable that the King's Highness (although his Majesty doth not yet take the degree of estate utterly from her) should entertain her so tenderly in the high degree and estate of a queen, who for her demerits is so unworthy of the same.

It seems that what Henry wanted from Parliament at this stage was a divorce.

On 13 November, while Katherine prepared to leave Hampton Court, Sir Thomas Wriothesley arrived, paid his respects, then summoned her household into the great chamber, where he 'openly declared certain offences she had done', urging those in possession of useful information to divulge it. Then he discharged everyone present except those few ladies who were to accompany Katherine to Syon Abbey. These were given clothes for their mistress: six French hoods with edges of goldsmiths' work, six pairs of sleeves, six gowns, and six kirtles of satin damask and velvet. On the King's orders, all were of sober design, and unadorned with precious stones or pearls, such as a queen would usually wear. Katherine was obliged to leave all her other clothes, her gorgeous court dresses and jewelled hoods, at Hampton Court, as well as her jewellery, which was delivered into the keeping of Sir Thomas Seymour, who took it, with other valuables, back to the King. Katherine was then taken by barge to Syon Abbey, which had recently been vacated by Lady Margaret Douglas, who had been sent to Kenninghall in Norfolk.

15
Worthy and just punishment

At Syon, Katherine was treated with respect. She lacked neither food nor warmth, and was served by her own ladies. Yet, from her point of view, she had been deprived of all the trappings of queenship that mattered to her and consigned to a seclusion that did little to alleviate her depression or allay her fears. She had no idea of what was to happen to her, nor was she informed of what was being said about her by those under questioning. She was certainly not aware that the interrogation of all the suspects had begun that very day, nor that letters had already gone out to all English ambassadors at foreign courts, relating her offences – her name would soon be a byword in Europe for immorality.

She was left to wander around the three chambers assigned to her. They were furnished in moderate comfort, but the hangings were of 'mean stuff'. There was no cloth of estate. Edward Baynton, her chamberlain, dined in one room with the rest of the staff, while Katherine kept to the other two. She had four gentlewomen and two chamberers in attendance, as well as her confessor. Lady Baynton was chief lady-in-waiting. Katherine had certainly fared better than Anne Boleyn. There were no spies listening to her every word, and she was not yet in the Tower. There was, perhaps, still hope.

Archbishop Cranmer was not a cruel man, but he was determined that the Queen should be sacrificed in the cause of reform. If she was allowed to live, there was always the possibility that the King might relent and take her back. It was therefore imperative that a charge of adultery be brought against Katherine, even though there was as yet no evidence for it. It was hoped by the Archbishop and his supporters that the interrogations of the prisoners in the Tower would yield enough information to send the Queen to the block.

The musician, Henry Manox – said by Mrs Hall to have taken sexual liberties with Katherine – was the first to be questioned. He said that he had been engaged by the Dowager Duchess of Norfolk to teach Katherine music and singing. He admitted having tried to seduce her, and divulged how the Duchess had unexpectedly come upon them both one day while they were indulging in intimate foreplay. She had beaten them both for it, and commanded them never to be alone together again. This had not deterred Manox, and he had continued to lay siege to Katherine until she had agreed he might caress her private parts – in his own words, he had 'felt more than was convenient'. However, he swore on the damnation of his soul that he had never enjoyed full intercourse with her. Eventually, he said, Katherine had tired of him, and transferred her affections to Dereham. He, Manox, had been extremely jealous, and had waylaid her one day, saying, 'Let me perceive by some token that you love me.' 'What token shall I show you?' Katherine had retorted, 'I will never be naught with you, and able to marry me you be not.' Manox had then sought to be revenged on his former sweetheart, and had gone straight to the Duchess with a friend surnamed Barnes and warned her that, if she were to rise again half an hour after retiring to bed, and go to the ladies' dormitory, 'you shall see that which shall displease you'. He did not know whether she had acted upon his advice. The Council, seeing that he had committed no crime and could help them no further, then released him.

They next called Katherine Tylney, one of the Queen's chamberers, as it was believed that she might help to prove adultery against the Queen. Knowing that Katherine had engaged Dereham as her secretary during the recent progress – an action that now seemed damning in the light of what had been discovered about her past – Sir Thomas Wriothesley questioned Mrs Tylney about the Queen's behaviour on that progress. Had she left her chamber any night at Lincoln or elsewhere? Tylney recalled that at Lincoln Katherine left her room late at night on two occasions and went to Lady Rochford's chamber, which was up two short flights of stairs. On the first occasion, Mrs Tylney and Margaret Morton had accompanied their mistress, but Katherine had sent them both downstairs again. Tylney went to bed, but Morton had later returned upstairs, and did not come to bed until around two o'clock. Tylney woke then, and said, 'Jesus, is not the Queen abed yet?', to which Margaret replied, 'Yes, even now.' On the second night, Katherine made all her other ladies go to bed, and took only Tylney upstairs with her. She remained in Lady Rochford's chamber as long as before, and Tylney was obliged to wait outside with Lady Rochford's waiting woman, so she never saw 'who came unto the Queen and my Lady Rochford, nor heard what was said between them'. Tylney was certain that Katherine had gone to Lady Rochford's room to meet someone. She also remembered taking 'sundry strange messages' from her mistress to Lady Rochford, so strange that she 'could not tell how to utter them'. This had gone on after the court returned to Hampton. There, one day, Katherine had told Tylney to go to Lady Rochford and ask her 'when she should have the thing she promised her'. Lady Rochford had answered that 'she sat up for it, and she would the next day bring her word herself.'

Wriothesley was pleased with Tylney's evidence, and told Sir Ralph Sadler that she 'hath done us worthy service' and that he was 'picking out anything that is likely to serve the purpose of our business'. Certainly Tylney's evidence pointed at something very odd going on, and the Council had little difficulty in concluding that the Queen had gone to meet a lover – possibly Dereham – in the room of Lady Rochford, who had acted as her bawd. If this were true, then Tylney's evidence would be damning.

In a mood of grim anticipation, the Council summoned Margaret Morton, Tylney's companion on the nights in question. She deposed that Lady Rochford had definitely been a party to some intrigue being carried on by the Queen, not only at Lincoln, but also at Pontefract and York. At Pontefract, the Queen had had angry words with herself and another chamberer, Mrs Luffkyn, and had forbidden them to enter her bedchamber. Morton was implying here that Katherine had an ulterior motive for keeping them out. Lady Rochford had also conveyed letters between the Queen and a third party, whom Morton supposed to have been Thomas Culpeper. One night, while the court was at Pontefract, Katherine was in her bedchamber with no attendant other than Lady Rochford – which, in itself, was unusual; Lady Rochford had not only locked the chamber door, but also bolted it on the inside. Consequently, when the King came unexpectedly to spend the night with his wife, he found the door fastened, and there was some delay before Lady Rochford opened it to admit him.

The Council now questioned Morton closely about Thomas Culpeper. Hitherto, they had suspected Katherine of intriguing with Dereham, but it now appeared that she might have been even more profligate with her favours. Morton confirmed their suspicions when she declared that she 'never mistrusted the Queen until at Hatfield I saw her look out of her chamber window on Master Culpeper, after such sort that I thought there was love between them'. Once, Katherine had been alone in her closet with Culpeper for five or six hours, and Morton thought 'for certain they had passed out' (a Tudor euphemism for orgasm). All the while, she remembered, Katherine had 'been in fear that somebody should come in'.

Katherine had not only been playing with fire, but she had also been indiscreet about it, and incredibly stupid. The Council now wasted no time in searching through Culpeper's effects, and found a letter, signed by the Queen (and appallingly spelt, for she was barely literate), which confirmed what everyone had begun to suspect, that she had, indeed, been conducting a love affair with her cousin. It read:

Master Culpepper,
I heartily recommend me unto you, praying you to send me word how that you do. I did hear that ye were sick, and I never longed for anything so much as to see you. It maketh my heart to die when I do think that I cannot always be in your company. Come to me when Lady Rochford be here, for then I shall be best at leisure to be at your commandment. . . . And thus I take my leave of you, trusting to see you shortly again. And I would you were with me now, that you might see what pain I take in writing to you.
Yours as long as life endures,
                                                      Katherine

Katherine's letter, although undated, was the most telling evidence against her, supported as it was by a weight of incriminating allegations by Tylney and Morton.

The Council continued its relentless quest for evidence: it was now hot on the trail. Alice Restwold, one of the inmates of the Duchess's household at Lambeth, gave an account of the time Dereham came into Katherine's bed when she herself was sharing it. She had got out 'for shame' and refused to sleep there again, for she was a married woman, and knew 'what belonged to that puffing and blowing'. This might have brought a touch of humour into the otherwise grave enquiry, but it did not assist a charge of adultery. Joan Bulmer also gave evidence, but her statement is no longer extant. It appears that she had at some stage abetted the Queen's intrigues.

The Council decided to call Lady Rochford next. Jane Rochford, who was later described as 'the principal occasion of the Queen's folly', had by now calmed down a little, and was lucid enough to be questioned. Thinking only of saving her own skin – for she, more than anyone, had cause to know the penalties for adultery in a queen – she abandoned Katherine to the wolves and admitted that Culpeper had had sexual intercourse with her mistress – she could not think it otherwise, 'considering all things that she hath heard and seen between them'. She testified that their intrigue had begun back in the spring, probably at the time when the King was suffering from depression and had left his wife to her own devices. Apparently, Culpeper had always cherished an affection for his pretty cousin, and it was he who had made the first advances. At first, they had not been welcome. 'Will this never end?' Katherine had sighed irritably to Lady Rochford, and had asked her to 'bid him desire no more to trouble me, or send to me.' But Culpeper had been persistent, and eventually the Queen had admitted him into her chamber in private. Before very long, they were meeting in Lady Rochford's rooms, with Lady Rochford standing guard in case the King came. It is likely that Culpeper had been there on the occasion described by Morton when Henry had come to sleep with his wife.

According to Lady Rochford, Katherine was well aware of the risks she was taking. 'This will be spied one day, and then we will all be undone,' she had said. Marillac later told Francis I that Katherine had used Dereham to incite Culpeper's jealousy, telling Lady

Rochford to say to Culpeper that, if he would not listen to Katherine's side in the petty arguments they frequently engaged in, 'there was behind the door another'. Lady Rochford, however, said nothing of this, but her evidence was of vital importance, because it was that of an eyewitness and a participant. She was also guilty of aiding and abetting acts of treason, and the King was not known to be merciful to such offenders. Thus, for all her willingness to co-operate, she found herself back in the Tower after her examination. It was then that madness took its final hold on her.

Thomas Culpeper was the next to be interrogated. He was 'a beautiful youth', and had stood high in the King's favour. He confessed to having fallen in love with the Queen some months before, and admitted that she would at first have nothing to do with him. Later, she had grown warmer towards him. He was aware of her past, for she told him that, had she remained in the maidens' chamber at Lambeth, she would have 'tried' him. But her high rank had, he said, precluded any intimacy between them. Nevertheless, according to Culpeper, she was before very long 'languishing and dying of love for him', and would call him her 'little sweet fool'. He admitted that he had visited her in private, saying that Lady Rochford had contrived the interviews. Yet it was Katherine who, at every house she visited on the progress, would 'seek for the back door and back stairs'. At Pontefract, she was fearful that the King had set a watch on the back door, so Lady Rochford made her servant watch the courtyard to see if this was so.

As the affair progressed, so the Queen's fear of discovery deepened, although it was not sufficiently acute for her to abandon her lover. She warned him to

beware if he went to confession, lest he should shrive him of any such things as should pass betwixt her and him; for if he did, surely the King, being Supreme Head of the Church, should have knowledge of it.

Culpeper had promised not to say anything compromising.

At this stage, the Council wanted to know if Culpeper had committed adultery with the Queen. He answered that, although Lady Rochford had 'provoked him much to love the Queen, and he intended to do ill with her and likewise the Queen so minded to do with him, he had not passed beyond words'. This, of course, was not what the assembled lords had been expecting to hear. Lord Hertford spoke for them all, therefore, when he told Culpeper that his intentions towards Queen Katherine were 'so loathsome and dishonest' that in themselves they could be said to constitute high treason. By this, it became apparent to Culpeper that he was doomed, and Katherine with him, and, the interrogation being at an end, he was taken back to prison.

The privy councillors deliberated. At length, they concluded that they 'vehemently suspected' the Queen of adultery with Thomas Culpeper, especially in view of his having been brought by Lady Rochford to her chamber at Lincoln during August, and having stayed there alone with Katherine from eleven o'clock at night until four o'clock in the morning. It was also considered significant that the Queen had, around this time, given him a gold chain and a 'rich cap'. 'You may see what was done before marriage,' reasoned Cranmer; 'God knoweth what has been done since!' The Council thought it might be expedient for the Archbishop to examine the Queen again, 'for she hath not, as appeareth by her confession, so fully declared the circumstances of such communications as were betwixt her and Culpeper'. It was felt that Cranmer, by careful questioning, 'might get of her more information'. A signed confession of adultery was what was really required, and the councillors had few doubts that the young Queen could be bullied or coerced into making one. Accordingly, Cranmer and Wriothesley went to visit Katherine at Syon to question her 'with respect to her intimacy with Culpeper'. They promised her mercy if she would make full confession of her faults, but Katherine, under their interrogation, strenuously denied intimacy with Culpeper, and persisted in her denial, even though she was probably lying to save her own skin and her lover's.

Meanwhile, the rumourmongers were once again busy. Two London housewives had been hauled before the Council and reprimanded for their unthinking *lèse-majesté*. One, Elizabeth Bassett, had wondered if 'God is working His own work to make the Lady Anne of Cleves queen again'. Her friend, Jane Ratsey, had replied that 'it was impossible that so sweet a queen as the Lady Anne could be utterly put down', and Mrs Bassett had exclaimed, 'What a man the King is! How many wives will he have?' Speculation that Henry might take back Anne of Cleves was widespread, since it was understood by many that the reformist party was working to bring down the Queen and the conservative Howard faction. But such an idea had never crossed the King's mind, and the Bishop of Winchester was obliged to be quite blunt with an eager German diplomat, saying that Henry 'would never take back the said lady'.

The Queen's fall was now common knowledge. Instinctively, her Howard relations banded together, fearful in case her disgrace should reflect upon them. They guessed that Cranmer would bring down the whole clan if he could. The Dowager Duchess's servant, Pewson, had broken the news to her that the Queen had played the King false (he said, incorrectly, that it was with Dereham), and that Katherine Tylney, the Duchess's relative, was privy to her guilt. This rather inaccurate version of the truth so frightened the Duchess that she ordered the immediate burning of all Dereham's papers and effects remaining at Lambeth House. At the same time she made it known that she did not believe the tales about the Queen to be true; however, if they were, then Katherine and her lovers 'deserved to be hanged'.

The Duchess also took it upon herself to question William Damport, a friend of Dereham's who still remained in her household. She told him she had heard that Dereham and Queen Katherine had been arrested, and asked if he knew why. Damport said he thought the evidence was based upon 'some words spoken by a gentleman usher'. The Duchess confided to him that she was greatly alarmed 'lest any harm should befall the Queen in consequence of evil report'. She was also worried that the King would point the finger of blame at her for having neglected her duties in respect of Katherine's moral welfare. She realised now that she had been very remiss, and it was far too late to do anything about it.

Contrary to what the Duchess had heard, Katherine was as yet suspected of adultery with Culpeper only, and not with Dereham, though rumour was doing its best to magnify her crimes. The Duke of Norfolk, having washed his hands of his niece, told Marillac that she had 'prostituted herself to seven or eight persons'. Norfolk was in fact making sure that his own neck was safe by publicly slandering

Katherine at every opportunity, in case people remembered who it was that had first brought her to the King's notice, and his voice spoke louder than any in denouncing her.

Henry now knew the worst, that Katherine had cuckolded him with Culpeper, whom he had favoured. He took the news relatively calmly, yet it must have been a dreadful blow to him. On 16 November, Chapuys told the Emperor that the King would be more likely to show mercy to Katherine than her own relatives, especially Norfolk, who said, 'God knows why, that he wished the Queen was burned.' Yet whether the King wished to show mercy or not, the law would take its course. Nor could he permit someone so unsuitable to enjoy the rank of Queen of England. On 22 November, a proclamation made at Hampton Court announced that Katherine had forfeited her honour and should be proceeded against by law; henceforth, she would no longer be called Queen, just plain Katherine Howard.

The Council was still collecting evidence. Norfolk was sent to search his stepmother's household at Lambeth and to interrogate its occupants. William Ashby, one of the Duchess's servants, revealed how his mistress had searched Dereham's coffers and removed all his papers, saying she would 'peruse them at her leisure, without suffering any person to be present'. She had declared, in the presence of her comptroller, that 'she meant not any of these things to come to revelation'. The Duchess, he added, had been 'in the greatest fear' lest her servants tell her son, Lord William Howard, about the 'familiarity' between the Queen and Dereham. She had wondered whether the King's promised pardon would extend to 'other persons who knew of their naughty life before the marriage'. Finally, Ashby told Norfolk that the Duchess had rifled through the papers of Damport, who by now was also a prisoner in the Tower, suspected of misprision of treason. The picture Ashby presented was one of a very frightened woman with an overburdened conscience, who was almost certainly guilty of that same crime. Her failure to disclose what she knew of Katherine's early life, and her attempts to destroy all evidence of it, pointed convincingly to this.

After the Duke had left, the Duchess began to realise what a nasty predicament she was in. Feigning illness, she took to her bed, but this did not prevent the lords of the Council, among them

Wriothesley and Southampton, from coming to Lambeth to arrest her. She sent word down to them that she was 'not well enough to be moved', yet they insisted on seeing her, 'the better to perceive whether she were indeed as sick as she pretended'. They quickly perceived she was not, and informed her that the Lord Chancellor wished to question her. At this, the old lady pretended to suffer a relapse, but the lords, 'with much ado, got her to condescend to her going'. The Duchess's fears were not unfounded. By nightfall on the day of her arrest, she too was a prisoner in the Tower, after a most unsatisfactory session of interrogation by Lord Chancellor Audley, in which she said enough to incriminate the whole Howard family.

Towards the end of November, the Council decided to question the Dowager Duchess again. Wriothesley and Southampton visited her in the Tower, where they found her in bed, and genuinely ill this time. They assured her 'on his Majesty's behalf of her own life if she would in some sort make us her ghostly confessors'. She replied that 'she would take her death of it, that she never suspected anything wrong between them'. She had indeed 'perceived a sort of light love and favour between them more than between indifferent persons, and had heard that Dereham would at sundry times give [Katherine] money', but she had thought this all 'proceeded from the affection that groweth of kindred, the same Dereham being her kinsman'. She begged the King's forgiveness for not having disclosed what she knew before his marriage to Katherine, and the lords were able to assure Henry that she appeared 'wondrous sorrowful, repentant and sickly'.

They then asked her a long list of questions: How did she educate and bring up Mistress Katherine? What changes of clothing had she given her? When had she first realised that the King favoured her? Had they discussed the King's courtship? What advice had she given the girl? The Duchess's answers revealed nothing that could point to the continuation of the liaison between Katherine and Dereham after the former's marriage to the King. In fact, she said Katherine herself had admitted later that she had no idea where Dereham was. It was obvious that the Duchess could help no further with the enquiry, so she was left alone to brood upon her shortcomings as a guardian.

Living with the knowledge of Katherine's infidelity was no easy task for the King. On 26 November, Sir John Dudley told the Earl of

Rutland that Henry was 'not a little troubled with this great affair'. To spare him further pain, therefore, the Council was carrying out the investigation on its own, while he sanctioned further action as necessary. It was all too obvious that the King was a broken man: this tragedy touched him too closely.

Thus the arraignment of Culpeper and Dereham on 1 December in Westminster Hall was arranged entirely by the Privy Council. Dereham was to be tried for 'presumptive treason', according to the indictment, which accused both the Queen and her accomplices of having led 'an abominable, base, carnal, voluptuous and licentious life'; Katherine, who was not being tried, was described as 'a common harlot'. While 'maintaining an appearance of chastity and honesty', she had led the King on to fall in love with her 'by word and gesture', he believing her to be 'pure', and had 'arrogantly contracted and coupled herself in marriage' in spite of being a harlot before and an adultress after.

A separate indictment was brought against Culpeper, who was charged with having had criminal intercourse with the Queen on 29 August 1541 at Pontefract, and at other times, before and after that date. Katherine was accused in the indictment of having insinuated to Culpeper 'that she loved him above the King and all the others', and Culpeper was accused of inciting her to adultery. Jane Rochford was named as their go-between, who contrived meetings in the Queen's lavatory and 'other suspect places' and 'falsely and traitorously aided and abetted them'.

The two men were tried together. Dereham was accused of joining the Queen's service with 'ill intent', traitorously imagining that he and she might continue their wicked behaviour. He was further accused of having concealed the precontract between them to facilitate Katherine's marriage to the King; her acquiescence to this was taken as proof of her intention to continue in her abominable life. Of course, Dereham pleaded not guilty to all these accusations, although there was little he could say in his defence. Likewise Culpeper, although realising that the evidence was heavily weighted against him, changed his plea to guilty during the course of the trial and thus sealed his fate. A verdict of guilty was given against both prisoners, and the Duke of Norfolk, grim faced, sentenced them to be drawn on hurdles to Tyburn 'and there hanged, cut down alive, disembowelled, and, they still living, their bowels burnt; the bodies then to be beheaded and quartered'. Such was the terrible penalty meted out to those who had dared to be intimate with the Queen of England.

Marillac quickly scribbled down news of the outcome of the trial to send to Francis I, saying he felt that Culpeper especially deserved to die, even though he would not admit to having full intercourse with Katherine, 'for he confessed his intention to do so, and his confessed conversations, being held by a subject to a queen, deserved death'. Many people had been disgusted by the unsavoury details of the Queen's intrigues that had been made public at the trial, and some felt that they should not have been divulged, but, as Marillac said, 'the intention is to prevent it being said afterwards that they were unjustly condemned'. As for the fate of the Queen, the ambassador held out little hope, predicting that 'the end of these tragedies will be no less scandalous than pitiful'. Pitiful indeed, for Katherine was not yet seventeen years old. Nor did it seem that the King would be merciful, for he had 'changed his love for the Queen into hatred, and taken such grief at being deceived, that of late it was thought he had gone mad'. On one occasion, he had

> called for a sword to slay her he had loved so much. Sitting in Council, he suddenly called for horses without saying where he would go. Sometimes he will say irrelevantly that the wicked woman had never such delight in her incontinence as she should have torture in her death.

On one occasion, Henry was so distressed that be burst into tears, 'regretting his ill-luck in meeting such ill-conditioned wives, and blaming the Council for the last mischief'. A few days later, Marillac recorded that the King had gone 'twenty-five miles from here with no company but musicians and ministers of pastime, and spent most of his time hunting, seeking to forget his grief'. Yet for all his anger, all his sport, and all his efforts to cheer himself up, Henry had never been so miserable in his life. Apart from the wound to his heart, there was the wound to his pride – he had been made to look a fool.

Not everyone sympathised. Chapuys, who had had long experience of the King's ways, told Charles V on 3 December that Henry had shown more sorrow at Katherine Howard's misdemeanours than he had at the treason, loss or divorce of any of his previous wives. As Chapuys put it,

> It is like the case of the woman who cried most bitterly at the loss of her tenth husband than at the death of all the others together. Though he had been a good man, it was because she had never buried one of them before without being sure of the next; and as yet this King has formed neither a plan nor a preference.

The Council was still trying to wring a confession of adultery from Dereham, or at least uncover evidence of it. They tortured his friend, William Damport, but although they used the brakes to force out his teeth, he would not or could not say anything to incriminate Dereham. All he would say was that, just prior to Katherine's marriage to the King, Dereham had boasted that, if Henry were dead, he would marry her. And, some months later, he had seen the Duchess of Norfolk point out Dereham to a gentleman in the Queen's chamber, saying, 'This is he, who fled away to Ireland for the Queen's sake.'

On 6 December, Dereham himself was tortured. Asked if he had said he was sure he might marry the Queen if the King were dead – it was treason to predict the death of the King – he denied it, until told that Damport had confessed it. Then he admitted it, although, as Wriothesley later told Sadler, 'no torture could make him confess this before.' Afterwards, the condemned man was made to sign a written confession, which set forth all the circumstances of his affair with Katherine. In it, he admitted that they had exchanged 'a promise of marriage', that they had lived together as man and wife while he was in the service of her grandmother, and that they were regarded as betrothed by their friends in that household. He had been accustomed to call her wife, and she had often called him husband before witnesses; they had exchanged gifts and love-tokens frequently in those days, and he had given her money whenever he had it. At Lambeth, he had haunted her chamber nightly, and they were then so far in love that they would 'kiss and hang by their bellies together as they were two sparrows'. Onlookers would joke, 'Hark to Dereham, broken winded!' to which he would reply, 'Who should hinder him from kissing his own wife?' He recalled that the Duchess had once caught him kissing her granddaughter, for which she beat him, also giving Joan Bulmer a blow for having allowed it. Dereham stated that he had been brought into the royal household by the Queen's desire, 'who told the Duchess of Norfolk to bring him'. It seems unlikely, however, that Katherine would have suggested such a thing: she was at the time involved with Culpeper, of whom Dereham was very jealous. It is more likely that it was Dereham, anxious for preferment, who wormed his way into the Queen's household, by means of the good offices of the Dowager Duchess, knowing Katherine dared not refuse him. He knew too much about her past, and her long-standing affection for Culpeper, for her to risk offending him.

In his confession, Dereham vehemently denied committing adultery with Katherine. Nevertheless, the Council felt that his applying to join the Queen's household, and her acceptance of him into it, was proof in itself of evil intent; it was said by some that 'they were worthy to be hanged one against the other'.

Later that day, the King was asked if he would remit the sentence against Dereham. He read the confession, and was angered that the prisoner had not admitted adultery with the Queen, declaring that he thought Dereham 'hath deserved no such mercy at his hand, and therefore hath determined that he shall suffer the whole execution'. On the following day, the Council, having also read Dereham's confession, wrote to Sir John Gage, the new Constable of the Tower, and Richard Rich, who had supervised the torturing, with instructions to proceed to the execution of the prisoners, if they felt that no more was to be gained from them by further interrogation. The condemned men must of course be allowed time to prepare to meet their God for the salvation of their souls, but unless the King decreed otherwise, the executions would take place on 9 December.

In the meantime, the families of both Dereham and Culpeper had been making frantic pleas to the Council to have the sentences commuted to beheading only. On 9 December, Gage was advised, early in the morning, that, though Culpeper's offence was considered 'heinous', he was to be drawn to Tyburn on a hurdle, but would be spared the full rigours of a traitor's death, and suffer only decapitation, 'according to his Highness's most gracious determination'. Culpeper was, after all, a gentleman born, unlike Dereham, and those of gentle birth were usually spared the full sentence.

The executions, however, did not take place on the 9th, as the Council was too busy with another urgent matter to issue the final order authorising them. This other matter concerned Anne of Cleves: the Council's attention had been drawn to a rumour, probably spread by Protestants, that she was expecting the King's child, and had also had a son by him, born at one of her country houses during the summer of 1541. The matter was debated all day by the lords, who felt they had quite enough on their hands with one immoral queen and that they could well do without another. After deliberating, they consulted the King, who thought it expedient to order a full enquiry into the matter. Members of the Privy Council were immediately despatched to Richmond to question the members of the Lady Anne's household, and the Lady Anne herself if needs be. The questioning was to take some time, but eventually, two members of Anne's household, Frances Lilgrave and Richard Taverner, admitted having slandered the Lady Anne, and were committed to the Tower for their impudence.

Dereham and Culpeper were put to death at Tyburn on 10 December. Culpeper died first, after exhorting the crowd to pray for him. No block had been provided: he knelt on the ground by the gallows, and was decapitated with one stroke of the axe. Dereham then suffered the full horror of being hanged, disembowelled, beheaded and quartered, after which both heads were set up on pikes above London Bridge.

There was no hope now for the Queen, although it was the King's wish that she should not stand open trial. Instead, an Act of Attainder was to be brought against her when Parliament reassembled in January. This would allow her a few weeks in which to prepare for death.

Even now, the reformist party was doing its best to bring further evidence against her and her family; it was imperative to them that the whole Howard faction be neutralised, thus paving the way for Cranmer and his partisans to gain ascendancy over the King. The Duchess of Norfolk was already in custody, 'so enmeshed and tangled up' in the affair that 'it will be hard for her to wind out again'. She was questioned again by Wriothesley on the day Katherine's lovers died, when she admitted having pushed Katherine into the King's way even though she knew of her previous affairs, and confessed to having persuaded the Queen to take Dereham back into her service. She also admitted to having destroyed all his letters.

In the middle of December, other members of the Howard clan were arrested by Wriothesley in the King's name. Lord William Howard and his wife, and Anne Howard, the Dowager Duchess's daughter, were committed to the Tower; Lord William had had hardly anything to do with Katherine Howard, and 'stood as stiff as his mother and made himself most clear from all mistrust and suspicion'. His arrest was absurd anyway, as he had been acting as Governor of Calais for the past year or so, and could not have been a party to Katherine's adultery. But the lords of the Council were determined to bring him down with the rest of his family, and had summoned him home in foul weather, so foul that some of his staff had been swept overboard during the voyage from France. Lord William's sister, another Katherine Howard, the Countess of Bridgewater, was also put in the Tower, and her children sent with Lord William's to be cared for by Archbishop Cranmer and others. When, on 14 December, the Duke of Norfolk learned of these arrests, he was fearful for his own safety – he had, after all, more cause than they to fear the King's justice – and wrote at once to Henry, excusing himself from all guilt and abandoning his family. He was sure, he said, that the arrests were justified. After the

abominable deeds done by my two nieces, I fear your Majesty will abhor to hear speak of me or my kin again. Prostrate at your Majesty's feet, I remind your Majesty that much of this has come to light through my own report of my mother-in-law's [*sic*] words to me when I was sent to Lambeth to search Dereham's coffers. My own truth, and the small love my mother-in-law and my two false traitorous nieces bare me, make me hope, and I pray your Majesty for some comfortable assurance of your royal favour, without which I will never desire to live.

But no comfortable assurance came. Henry was displeased with all the Howards, including the Duke. He was no fool, and remembered vividly how Norfolk had furthered his intrigue with Katherine in the first place. He had placed a viper in his sovereign's bosom, and he should pay for it. He did not reply to the letter, and hearing nothing, the Duke deemed it politic to maintain a low profile, hoping that the King's displeasure would not last. After a time, he was received back, but Henry never fully trusted him again.

As for the rest of the Howard family and their servants, King and Council had decided on a highly profitable solution. Lord William and his wife, Katherine Tylney, Joan Bulmer, Alice Restwold, William Ashby, William Damport, and Elizabeth Tylney and Margaret Bennet, the two other witnesses to the Queen's misconduct, were all, on 22 December 1541, arraigned for misprision of treason 'for concealing the evil demeanour of the Queen, to the slander of the King and his succession'. All pleaded guilty, and were sentenced to perpetual imprisonment and loss of goods and lands; however, not long afterwards, the King pardoned most of them and had them freed. The old Duchess of Norfolk was also included in the indictment, but she was not brought to trial as she was 'old and testy' and 'may die out of perversity to defraud the King's Highness of the confiscation of her goods'. She too was sentenced to loss of liberty and lands, and the King ended up somewhat richer as a result.

This did not, however, provide a panacea for his misery. He knew now that the illusion of youth he had enjoyed with Katherine had gone for ever; all he had to look forward to were encroaching illness, old age and death. To begin with, he had meant to be merciful towards Katherine, but now he found he had no desire to save her from the headsman, and wished her to suffer as he was suffering. The law would take its course and he would not lift a finger to stop it. Then the world would see how he dealt with those who made a fool of him.

Francis I had reacted to the news of Katherine's fall with sympathy. 'She hath done wondrous naughty!' he exclaimed, when Sir William Paget informed him of the Queen's misconduct. And to Henry he wrote:

I am sorry to hear of the displeasure and trouble which has been caused by the lewd and naughty behaviour of the Queen. Albeit, knowing my good brother to be a prince of prudence, virtue and honour, I do require him to shift off the said displeasure and wisely, temperately, like myself, not reputing his honour to rest in the lightness of a woman, but to thank God of all, comforting himself in God's goodness. The lightness of women cannot bend the honour of men.

Comforting words indeed from Henry's greatest rival and Europe's most debauched monarch. Henry must have squirmed when he read them.

The festive season passed gloomily that year, with the King making no effort to join in the half-hearted revels staged by his courtiers. Marillac described him as 'sad, and disinclined to feasting and ladies'. He was putting on even more weight, and looked very old and grey. His ministers, however, were begging him to marry again, reminding him that he had only one son, but there was not one among the court ladies that he fancied: the wound left by Katherine Howard's infidelities was too raw as yet. The Council could only hope that time would heal it. With 'such an exceptional prince', all things were possible.

Parliament reconvened on 16 January 1542, and the Lords and Commons combined to urge the King 'not to vex himself with the Queen's offence, and that she and the Lady Rochford might be attainted'. To make this easier for him, it was suggested that he give his royal assent to the proceedings under the Great Seal, which could then be done by the Lord Chancellor. The King agreed to this, and the Lords at once began debating the fate of the Queen. The Lord Chancellor, recounting her 'vicious and abominable' deeds, urged that a Bill of Attainder be drawn up without delay, which was done that same afternoon. It was in the form of a petition, from the Lords and Commons, requesting the King to consent to the conviction of 'Mistress Katherine Howard, late Queen of England' and Lady Rochford for high treason, the penalty being death and confiscation of goods. The Act received its first reading that evening. Shortly afterwards, another Act would be passed, ruling that 'an unchaste woman marrying the King shall be guilty of high treason'. Anyone concealing any flaw in the character of a putative queen of England would likewise be guilty of high treason. And if any woman presumed to marry the King without admitting she had been unchaste, she would merit death.

Henry seems to have been concerned that Katherine had as yet had no chance to defend herself in public. 'Wishing to proceed more humanely', he sent some members of his Council to see her on 25 January; they invited her, in the King's name, to 'come to the Parliament chamber to defend herself'. She declined, however, saying she submitted herself to the King's mercy and good pleasure, and confessed she had deserved to die. Her humility did much to soften the hearts of the privy councillors, and three days later the Lord Chancellor reminded the peers in the House of Lords

> how much it concerned them not to proceed too hastily with the Bill of Attainder for the Queen, that she was no mean or private person, but a public and illustrious one. Therefore her cause ought to be judged in a manner that should leave no room for suspicion of some latent quarrel.

He proposed that a second deputation, comprising members of both Houses, should go to see her, 'partly in order to help her womanish fears', and partly to advise her 'to say anything that makes her cause the better'. It was only just, he concluded, that such a princess should be 'tried by equal laws with themselves', and he assured his listeners that 'her most loving consort' would find it acceptable if she cleared herself in this way, even now.

Katherine, however, knew she had no plausible defence, and was resigned outwardly to her fate. She told the second deputation that her only care was to make a good death and 'to leave a good opinion in people's minds now at parting'. Gone was the hysterical girl of a few weeks past, and in her place was one who even found the courage to be gay. Chapuys reported on 29 January that she was

> very cheerful, and more plump and pretty than ever; she is as careful about her dress and as imperious and wilful as at the time she was with the King, notwithstanding that she expects to be put to death, that she confesses she has deserved it, and asks for no favour except that the execution shall be secret and not under the eyes of the world.

Chapuys thought that if the King did not intend to marry again he might show mercy to her, or even divorce her on a plea of adultery. Learned theologians had debated the possibility of a divorce, but had as yet not made public their conclusions. But Chapuys was still pessimistic, and even as he was writing his letter news came to him that the Commons had debated the Queen's fate and had come to the same conclusion as the Lords, and the Queen, he feared, 'will soon be sent to the Tower'.

The Council, however, felt that Parliament was being too humane towards Katherine; the reforming faction felt there had been no need to give her any opportunity to defend herself, as the case against her had already been proved. Accordingly, the privy councillors petitioned the King that the Bill of Attainder be put through its second and third readings without delay so that the case could be concluded and judgement given. Henry gave his assent, and Parliament was urged to speed up the passing of the Bill. Its second reading took place on 6 February and, on the following day, after its third and final reading, it became law, which meant that the Queen and Lady Rochford were both sentenced to death and loss of goods and lands. All that was needed now was the royal assent. On that same day, the King went into the House of Commons and thanked them 'for that they took his sorrow to be theirs'.

Henry was feeling a little better now, more himself. Since November, he had hunted daily to divert his 'ill humour' and would not attend to much business. Now, however, he was again seeking the company of the ladies of his court. After the Act of Attainder against the Queen was passed, Chapuys told Charles V that Henry had 'never been so merry since first hearing of the Queen's misconduct'. On 29 January, he had given a banquet attended by sixty-one ladies, and was particularly attentive to the estranged wife of the poet Wyatt, 'a pretty young creature with wit enough to do as badly as the others if she were to try'. Yet Elizabeth Brooke was a notorious adultress, and the King did not pursue the matter. He also showed a marked preference for Anne Bassett, for whom he had long cherished a soft spot. 'The common voice,' went on Chapuys, 'is that this King will not be long without a wife, because of the great desire he has to have further issue.'

The passing of the Act of Attainder seemed to satisfy Henry, although he complained that there was as much reason to convict the Duchess of Norfolk of treason as there had been to convict Dereham. In her case the Council urged the King to leniency, and he relented, agreeing that the old lady might live. She was eventually released on 5 May 1542, and died three years later. But he was not so merciful towards his wife or Lady Rochford, and on 9 February sent the Duke of Norfolk to Syon Abbey with his fellow deputies to inform Katherine of her sentence. The only comfort the Duke brought was the promise that it would be carried out in private, as she had wished: she would die on Tower Green, as Anne Boleyn had.

Katherine took the news bravely. She again confessed to and acknowledged 'the great crime of which she had been guilty against the most high God and a kind prince and lastly the whole English nation', and begged Norfolk 'to implore his Majesty not to impute her crime to her whole kindred and family', asking instead that Henry extend his 'unbounded mercy and benevolence to all her brothers, that they might not suffer for her faults'. Lastly she asked if the King would kindly bestow her clothing upon her maidservants after her death, as she had no other means of rewarding them for their loyalty. Norfolk promised to convey her requests to the King, and then left without having been able to tell her the date set for her execution.

Her suspense did not last long, however. On Friday, 10 February, the lords of the Council returned to Syon with orders to convey the Queen to the Tower of London. As soon as she learned what they had come for, Katherine knew a moment of blind panic, finally realising in that instant that Henry did mean to have her executed. All her calm deserted her, and she refused to go. The lords tried persuasion and then bullying, but to no avail. Eventually, they bundled her, shrinking with fear, into the waiting barge, which was then escorted along the river by a barge containing the Lord Privy Seal, other members of the Council, and those servants who were to look after the Queen in the Tower. The barge carrying Katherine was enclosed; this was as well, for the rotting heads of Culpeper and Dereham were still to be seen above London Bridge. The Queen, wearing a black velvet dress, sat with four of her ladies and three or four members of the Privy Council. Behind came the Duke of Suffolk's barge, crowded with his retinue. At the Tower stairs, the lords disembarked first and the Queen followed. The same forms of respect were shown to her as in happier days. She was greeted by the Constable of the Tower, Sir John Gage, who 'paid her as much honour as when she was reigning', but he was concerned to find that his prisoner was in a state of such abject distress that she seemed on the verge of collapse. 'She weeps, cries and torments herself miserably without ceasing,' he wrote to the Privy Council, after having conducted Katherine to her lodging. It is uncertain where this was, but likely that it was the rooms in the Lieutenant's house once occupied by Anne Boleyn.

In the evening, John Longland, Bishop of Lincoln, came to hear the Queen's confession and to offer her spiritual comfort. She swore to him, 'in the name of God and His Holy angels, and on the salvation of my soul', that she was innocent of the crimes for which she stood condemned. She had never 'so abused my sovereign's bed'. She did not seek to excuse the faults and follies of her youth; God would be her judge, and she looked for His pardon. She asked the Bishop to pray with her for divine mercy, and fell to her knees beside him, beseeching the Almighty for strength to cope with her coming ordeal.

The Act of Attainder against Katherine still lacked the King's signature, and the execution could not go ahead without it. To spare Henry any further distress, the Council arranged for the royal assent to be signified by attaching the Great Seal; and at the top of the Act was written the time-honoured phrase: '*Le Roy le veut*' – 'The King wills it.' On Saturday, 11 February, the Act was read in Parliament to the assembled members of both Houses, and the royal assent proclaimed.

The Queen's execution could now take place, but not on a Sunday, so Katherine had a day's reprieve. On the evening of that Sunday, she was visited by Sir John Gage and instructed to 'disburden her conscience' to her confessor, for she was to die the following day. Calmer now, she spoke of her anxiety about making a good impression on the scaffold, and asked if the block might be brought to her room, so that she might learn how to place herself. Gage thought this a strange request, but he did not refuse it. The block was brought and Katherine spent the evening coming to terms with her fate.

The Tower was a hive of activity that weekend, for the Constable's staff were busy caring for the illustrious prisoners then lodged within the fortress. But at least Katherine's last night on earth was not disturbed, as Anne Boleyn's had been, by the noise of workmen erecting the scaffold.

Monday, 13 February 1542 was cold and dull, with a ground frost. At seven o'clock, every member of the King's Council except Norfolk, who had been excused this final duty, and Suffolk, who was ill, presented themselves at the Tower with a number of other lords and gentlemen, among them the Earl of Surrey, who was Norfolk's son and the Queen's cousin. All were conducted to Tower Green, where the scaffold had once again been hung with black cloth and strewn with straw. When Katherine was led out of her lodgings by Sir John Gage and a detachment of yeomen warders, she appeared so weak that she could hardly stand or speak. Nevertheless, she made what one onlooker, Otwell Johnson, in a letter written to his brother the next day, described as a 'godly and Christian end'. She asked

> all Christian people to take regard unto her worthy and just punishment with death, for her offences against God heinously from her youth upward in breaking of all His commandments, and also against the King's Royal Majesty very dangerously.

She admitted she had been justly condemned and that she merited a hundred deaths, and required the people to look to her as an example and amend their 'ungodly lives', urging them to obey the King in all things. She prayed for her husband, and willed everyone present to do the same, before commending her soul to God and 'earnestly calling for mercy upon Him'. Not for Katherine the elegant sword that had beheaded her cousin, but – as the chronicler Hall confirms – an axe, that severed her pretty auburn head in a single stroke just moments after she had made her last speech.

Lady Rochford followed her to the block. She was still 'in a frenzy', according to Chapuys, and the King had had to order the passing of a special Act enabling him to have insane persons executed before he could dispose of her. Yet, at the last, faced with the axe and the spectacle of the Queen's blood-soaked remains being wrapped in a black blanket by her sobbing ladies, she recovered her reason sufficiently to enable her to make an edifying speech before submitting to the executioner.

Katherine's attendants laid her remains in a waiting coffin and carried it into the nearby Chapel of St Peter ad Vincula. There, later that day, she was buried near Anne Boleyn. Then her name was tactfully forgotten by all until, in 1553, the Act of Attainder against her was among those reversed by Queen Mary; because they did not bear the royal signature, such Acts were no longer recognised as legal.

16
*Never a wife
more agreeable
to his heart*

The marriage of Henry VIII and Katherine Howard was never formally annulled, even though there were good grounds for so doing, and consequently the King became a widower on her death. For a time, though, he was anything but a merry one, and it was eighteen months before he found the woman he wanted to make his sixth wife and before he recovered fully from the blow dealt by Katherine's adultery.

On 25 February 1542, a fortnight after Katherine's execution, Chapuys reported him to be in better spirits; he had presided over three court banquets prior to the onset of Lent, and was now following a new rule of life: 'Sunday was devoted to the lords of his Council, Monday to the men of law, and Tuesday to the ladies.' On the previous Tuesday he had gone from room to room ordering and arranging the lodgings prepared for those ladies still remaining at the court, and had 'made them great and hearty cheer, without showing special affection to any particular one'. It soothed his hurt vanity to be once more the centre of female attention, yet he was in no hurry to remarry, and Chapuys thought he would not do so unless Parliament pressed him to it. Anyway, there were few ladies at court who would aspire to such an honour, the ambassador added wryly, because of the new Act requiring 'any lady the King may marry, on pain of death, to declare any charge of misconduct that can be brought against her'. This rather narrowed down the field, since the ladies of Henry's court were not known for their virtue.

There remained, as ever, the problem of the succession. Prince Edward was still thriving, but in May 1542, there were fears – fortunately unfounded – that he was once more ailing, and this prompted both Privy Council and Parliament to remind the King of the need for more sons for the future peace of the realm. But Henry was not ready to face marriage again, though his health had improved. The physician and scholar, Andrew Boorde, who saw the King at this time, noted that his hair was still plentiful and red, if a bit thin on top, and his pulse strong and regular. His digestive system was in perfect working order, and he was better able to curb his temper than in former years. A huge man in height and girth, he sweated a lot, and overate, but Boorde ignored this last fact. The King's leg was still troubling him, but it was better than it had been. His contemporaries thought him fit enough to remarry and sire children, and ignored his mental state. Chapuys sagely concluded that the next queen would be one of Henry's own choosing – 'When he takes a fancy for a person or a thing he goes the whole way.'

The Duke of Cleves, however, hearing the news of Katherine Howard's fate, had other ideas. He was hoping that Henry would take back his sister, and in the spring of 1542 instructed his ambassadors to use their influence to promote a reconciliation. One German envoy visited Cranmer at Lambeth and asked him outright to bring this about. Cranmer replied that he thought it 'not a little strange' that the Duke of Cleves should ask him, of all people, as he was the one person who knew all the 'just causes' for the annulment of the Lady Anne's marriage. The King, hearing of this from his Archbishop, instructed Cranmer to inform the Duke of Cleves most firmly that there could never be a reconciliation between Anne and himself.

It could not be denied, however, that there was a significant dearth of likely candidates to fill the empty consort's throne. Most ladies saw queenship as fraught with insecurity, for the King 'either putteth away or killeth his wives', and it was generally conceded among them that the woman he eventually married would need nerves of steel and sharp wits, not to mention virtue beyond question.

For the present Henry concentrated on possible matches for his children. Elizabeth had been deeply affected by Katherine Howard's end, and stated there and then that she would never marry, a resolution she never broke. Marriage, for her, had too close an association with death to ever seem safe. As for Mary, her opinion of Katherine Howard had never been particularly high, so she was not as shocked as her young sister when she heard the news. That spring, the King reopened negotiations with France for a marriage between Mary and the heir to the French throne, the Duke of Orléans, though these came to nothing as neither side could agree on the dowry, and the already fragile relationship between England and France suffered a further buffeting. The King now made it a priority to reinforce his country's defences against a possible attack by the French, and continued with his programme of coastal fortifications.

The other thorn in his side was Scotland. There had been an alliance between the French and the Scots for centuries, both nations being hereditary enemies of England, and James V of Scotland had consistently frustrated Henry's hopes of arranging a treaty of friendship advantageous to England. Understandably, the King did not want the Scots pouring over his northern border – as they had done in 1513 – while he was occupied with repulsing a French attack in the south. He was furious with James, and had retaliated by sending a military force against him; on 24 November 1542, James V's army was utterly defeated by the English at the Battle of Solway Moss. When Henry received news of the victory, he showed some of his old jubilation, and Chapuys remarked that the habitual sadness he had displayed since learning of the conduct of Queen Katherine had gone. He now confidently expected his nephew of Scotland to treat with him in more deferential terms, terms that would give Henry some control over Scottish affairs. But King James was in no position to treat with his uncle. When he learned of the defeat of his army, he took to his bed at Falkland Palace and died on 14 December, the day he learned his wife had just presented him with a daughter, Mary, who was now Queen of Scots in her own right.

Nothing could have suited Henry VIII better. With its monarch dead and a baby occupying the throne, Scotland no longer posed a threat to England's security. The nobles would be too busy fighting among themselves for power to concern themselves with England, and the Queen Regent, Mary of Guise, would have her hands full controlling them. It was the infant Queen of Scots who interested the

King most, though: he wanted her as a bride for Prince Edward. Such a union would necessarily unite the two countries under Tudor rule, a very attractive prospect to Henry, who wasted no time in sending envoys to the Queen Regent to lay his proposal before her. And on New Year's Day, 1543, Prince Edward, now five, performed his first public duty, entertaining at Enfield a party of noble Scotsmen captured at Solway Moss. They ended up warmly praising the little boy, calling him 'so proper and towardly an imp'. Already, he had beautiful manners and was well behaved. He was fair like his mother, and had something of her retiring, unexuberant manner, but facially he resembled his father, and he had inherited Henry's formidable intellectual powers. Already the child was learning the rudiments of theology and other disciplines, and his father was excessively proud of him.

After Solway Moss, Henry livened up considerably. He spent a good deal of time 'feasting ladies', and began eyeing one or two as prospective wives. He seemed to have forgotten Katherine Howard, and the court recovered some of its gaiety. His good mood was further enhanced by his satisfaction at having concluded a new alliance with the Emperor Charles, whereby both sovereigns had pledged themselves to invade France within two years and to assist each other when called upon to do so. Now, with his new fortifications and his new alliance, Henry could rest assured that he had done all that was needful for the defence of his kingdom.

There was, however, another reason for his new-found contentment: he had at last, to the relief of his advisers, found a lady he could both love and respect. But this was no grand passion – he was done with that. Besides, the lady was married, although her husband was very ill and not expected to live long. She was virtuous and attractive, and Henry wanted her: even as her husband lay on his sick-bed, the King was sending her gifts to signify his esteem. He was certain that in the fullness of time his suit would be accepted, and that the object of his affection would be honoured and delighted to join with him in holy wedlock. He was wrong. She was dismayed at the prospect.

Katherine Parr had been born around the year 1512, the eldest child of Sir Thomas Parr, a descendant of Edward III, by Maud, daughter of Sir Thomas Green of Green's Norton, Northants. She was born either in her father's castle at Kendal in the county of Westmorland, where she spent her childhood, or in his London house at Blackfriars. Kendal castle dated from Norman times, and Katherine's ancestors had lived in it since the fourteenth century. The fabric of the building was much decayed in 1586, according to the antiquarian William Camden, although some rebuilding had taken place in early Tudor times. The Parrs were respected gentry, not very rich but connected to all the noble families of the north, such as Vaux, Throckmorton, Neville, FitzHugh and Dacre.

Lady Parr was only seventeen when she gave birth to Katherine. Shortly afterwards she presented her husband with a son, William, and later on a second daughter, Anne. But on 11 November 1517, when Katherine was five, her father died, and was buried in the monastery of the Black Friars in London, leaving Lady Parr to bring up her three children single-handed. This was a task she undertook conscientiously and with commendable ability, disdaining all offers for her hand in order to devote her full attention to their education. She was a very religious woman and she inspired in them from the first a simple yet reverent love of God, whose word permeated every aspect of her teaching. She was something of a disciplinarian, and expected her daughters to learn proficiency in the traditional feminine skills. There is a tale, probably apocryphal, that Katherine Parr did not take kindly to her mother's strictures and protested that her hands were destined to touch crowns and sceptres, not needles and spindles. Yet she grew up with a great respect for learning and an appreciation of the more sober pleasures in life; of all the wives of Henry VIII, she was the most erudite and the most intellectual.

When Katherine was nearly twelve, her mother entered into negotiations with Lord Dacre for her marriage to Henry Scrope, Lord Scrope's son and heir. Lord Scrope was Lord Dacre's son-in-law, and the marriage had been proposed by Lord Dacre himself, who was a cousin of Sir Thomas Parr, and felt that the young Katherine would be a good match for his grandson. Lady Parr was agreeable, but later ran into difficulties with Lord Scrope over the amount of dowry and jointure to be settled upon her daughter. A series of letters survives which shows that not only was Lord Scrope offering a paltry sum, but he was also unwilling to return Katherine's dowry if she died before the marriage could be consummated, or if it was not consummated for any other reason. Lord Dacre was sympathetic to Lady Parr, and tried to persuade Scrope to change his mind, reminding him that he could save money by sending young Henry to live with Lady Parr until such time as the young couple were of an age to live together, when they would both return to Lord Scrope's house. He reminded his son-in-law that Lady Parr was of the 'good wise stock of the Greens', and warned him that his demands were so 'far asunder that it is impossible ye can ever agree'. If Henry went to stay with Lady Parr he would not only be kept by her but would 'learn with her as well as in any place that I know, as well nurture as French and other languages'. Even after this, however, Lord Scrope persisted in his demands, and early in 1525 Lady Parr informed Lord Dacre that she had decided to abandon the project. This was as well, for young Henry Scrope died on 25 March that year.

Katherine was by then nearing thirteen and growing into a comely girl with auburn hair and a *retroussée* nose; her family background ensured that she did not lack for suitors, yet when it came to choosing her a husband, Lady Parr opted for a man old enough to be Katherine's grandfather. Around 1526 she married her daughter to the Lord Borough. Some confusion exists as to the identification of this gentleman, some sources naming him as Sir Edward de Burgh, who died before April 1533. He was, in fact, Sir Edward's grandfather, another Edward de Burgh, second Baron Borough of Gainsborough in the county of Lincolnshire. He was a member of a distinguished family, and had been born in 1463 or thereabouts, making him sixty-three in 1526, old even by modern standards to marry a girl of fourteen. Such matches, however, were not uncommon in Tudor times, particularly among the aristocracy. Lord Borough had been married before, in 1477, to the daughter and heiress of Lord Cobham, and by her he had had three children. Anne Cobham died early in 1526 and Lord Borough lost no time in seeking a replacement.

After her marriage, Katherine was taken by her new husband to live in the house he had inherited around 1496, the charming Old Hall in Gainsborough, with its magnificent timbered great hall with a stone oriel window, which had been erected by his father on the site of an earlier dwelling in 1484. Lord Borough himself had added to the house, and two kings had visited it, Richard III in 1485 and Henry VIII in 1509. A year after Henry's visit, Lord Borough had been described as being 'distracted of memory'; it is not clear whether or not he ever recovered, nor was mental disturbance considered in the sixteenth century to be an impediment to marriage. Nevertheless, there are indications that the Borough household was a happy one.

Like many girls in her position, Katherine found herself a stepmother to children older than herself. Lord Borough had two sons: his heir, Thomas, was a man of thirty-eight, who was married to Agnes Tyrwhitt, whose brother Sir Robert was married to Lord Borough's daughter. This lady, whose first name is unknown, quickly became firm friends with her young stepmother, a friendship that would endure throughout their lives. Completing the family was Henry de Burgh, whose wife, Katherine Neville, was – at twenty-seven – the member of it nearest to Katherine Parr in age. Then there were Thomas's children, Edward, Thomas and William, who of a certainty would have commanded much of Katherine's attention, for she was fond of children.

Katherine's marriage to her ageing husband did not last long. He died in 1528, leaving her a widow at sixteen. Whether she stayed on at the Old Hall is not known. All that is certain is that her mother died the following year leaving Katherine virtually independent and her own mistress. Around the year 1530 she received an offer of marriage from Lord Latimer of Snape Castle in the north riding of Yorkshire, which she accepted. A woman on her own could not live comfortably without a male protector in those days, when marriage or the conventual life were the only acceptable options open to her if she wished to guard her reputation – only old women ruled their estates alone. And Lord Latimer was, after all, a good matrimonial catch. He was in his late thirties, a more suitable age for marriage to a young woman of eighteen. Born John Neville, he was a member of the great medieval house of Neville that had been so closely related to the Plantagenets. Like Lord Borough, he had been married before, twice in fact: firstly to Dorothy de Vere, daughter of the Earl of Oxford – she had borne him one daughter and his heir, John. Lady Dorothy died on 7 February 1527 and was buried at Wells in

Yorkshire. After her death, Lord Latimer took as his second wife, on 20 July 1528, Elizabeth Musgrave, but she bore him no children and died soon afterwards. Lord Latimer and Katherine Parr were married before 1533: the date of their wedding is not recorded.

Thus Katherine came to live in Snape Castle, described by the antiquarian John Leland as 'a goodly castle in a valley with two or three good parks well-wooded about it'. It was Lord Latimer's chief residence, and was sited two miles from the village of Great Tanfield, near Bedale. Today, it is a ruin, only the perpendicular chapel with its Dutch carvings of the life of Christ surviving intact. Here Katherine Parr, the new Lady Latimer, settled down to her first experience of mature married life, ordering her household and accompanying her husband on his occasional trips to London, where he also had a house conveniently situated for attending the court.

Little of note marked the early years of this marriage and there were no children. In 1534, Katherine's sister Anne married Sir William Herbert. Then, in 1536–7 occurred the Pilgrimage of Grace, in which Lord Latimer, coming from a Catholic family, fought on the side of the rebels, for which he later received the King's pardon. It may have been around this time that Katherine first became interested in Protestantism, a leaning she would be forced to conceal for many years; it was not until much later that she would be able to embrace openly the Lutheran faith. At this date she could merely sympathise in private with the reformist cause. Being intelligent, forthright and having sound common sense, it was perhaps natural that she should favour the tenets of the new religion above the mysteries and intricacies and, it must be said, contemporary abuses of Catholicism. Yet, for the duration of her marriage to Lord Latimer and for some time afterwards, she would be obliged to conceal her true religious inclinations beneath a facade of conventional observance.

In the late 1530s, Lord and Lady Latimer were often at court, where they were on good terms with Henry VIII, who had fortunately decided to overlook Latimer's part in the Pilgrimage of Grace. In 1540, Katherine interceded with the King for the release of her cousin, Sir George Throckmorton, who had been imprisoned in the Tower by Cromwell because of his open criticism of the royal supremacy. Spurred on by the pleas of Throckmorton's wife, Katherine Vaux, another of her cousins, who was very distressed at the plight of her husband, Katherine sought out the King when he was in a good mood and humbly asked him to free Sir George. This was a good moment to appeal to Henry, for he was just then plotting the downfall of Cromwell, and was happy to agree to Lady Latimer's request, being doubtless impressed by her integrity and sincerity. However, there was no question of his feelings for her at that time being anything other than affectionate, for he was deeply in love with Katherine Howard and planning to marry her.

A year after Katherine's execution, however, Henry was looking at Lady Latimer through different eyes, and very much liking what he saw. She was then thirty-one, and still attractive, and on 16 February 1543, Henry made her a gift of 'pleats and sleeves'; his exchequer accounts also record that he ordered gowns in the Italian style for her. It was known by then that Lord Latimer was failing in health and would not live long; he had been ill since the previous autumn, having made his will on 12 September. It was highly unusual for the King to give rich gifts to a married woman, and Katherine, doubtless concerned about her husband's state of health, was disconcerted at receiving them, although she did not dare return them. Then, on 2 March 1543, Lord Latimer died, and the King was obliged to bide his time out of respect for the widow. After the funeral in St Paul's Cathedral, Lord Latimer's will was proved, and Katherine inherited the manors of Nunmonkton and Hamerton with an annuity for four years to finance the upbringing of her step-daughter, Margaret Neville. Thus Katherine became an independent woman of substance.

She seems to have remained at court after her husband's death. What kept her there was not so much having to finalise the details of her husband's estate, nor the interest of the King, but the very obvious admiration of Sir Thomas Seymour, brother of the late Queen Jane. Sir Thomas was about six years older than Katherine Parr, and very handsome. He was also impetuous and extremely ambitious, and he saw in the rich and attractive widow a means of increasing his fortune. He had been working on her emotional susceptibilities since January, when he had returned to court after a diplomatic mission to Nuremberg in Germany, and after Lord Latimer's death, Katherine began to encourage this dashing and unscrupulous adventurer as a suitor. She was both physically and emotionally attracted to him, and it was not long before the two were discussing marriage.

At the same time, a scandal erupted in the Parr family. Just as the King was also beginning to nurture an amorous interest in the widowed Lady Latimer, her brother William, Lord Parr, applied to Parliament for a divorce from his wife, on the grounds of her adultery with an unidentified lover with whom she had eloped in 1542. She was Anne Bourchier, daughter and heiress of the last Earl of Essex of the Bourchier line, whom he had married in February 1526. Furthermore, Lord Parr was so incensed at his wife's infidelity that he was pressing the King to authorise the highest penalty for her offence, which in those days was death.

Her brother's action shocked Katherine Parr, who refused to stand by and allow her sister-in-law to suffer execution. According to the chronicler Hall, she went straight to the King and threw herself at his feet, nor would she rise until he had promised to spare Lady Parr from the headsman's axe. At first, Henry remonstrated with her: 'Madam, you know that the law enacts that a woman of rank who so forgets herself shall die unless her husband pardon her.' Katherine answered, 'Your Majesty is above the law, and I will try to get my brother to pardon.' Eventually, Henry agreed that 'if your brother can be content, I will pardon her'. At this, Katherine went to William and told him that the circumstances of the case were not as he had been given to believe by false witnesses; she would use her influence with the King to have them tortured, she said, 'and then by God's help we shall know the truth'. Parr was already, it seems, aware of the King's interest in his sister, and he knew himself defeated. He forgave his wife, and was rewarded for his clemency when, on 17 April, Parliament granted him a divorce. Lady Parr's adultery was established in law, and an Act passed at the same time declared her children bastards and unfit to inherit. Her Essex estates were then entailed upon her husband, who was created Earl of Essex the following December.

The King, it appears, was following his time-honoured custom of advancing the relatives of the woman he meant to marry. Although there is no evidence that Henry had as yet declared himself to Katherine Parr, he admitted Lord Parr to the Privy Council in March 1543, and made him a Knight of the Garter on 23 April following.

This alone should have warned Katherine that the King's intentions were serious, but she either did not notice or affected to ignore the fact, being too involved emotionally with Seymour. Henry saw this and was jealous: Seymour was a younger man who epitomised many of the things Henry had been in his youth, and this in itself did not exactly endear him to his sovereign. His courtship of the comely widow was not to be borne. Henry wanted her, and Henry meant to have her.

Until this time, around late April or early May 1543, Katherine had been unaware of the King's true feelings and intentions towards her. Yet now it began to dawn on her that he too was a suitor, not in an aggressive way, but by appearing 'sad, pensive and sighing' whenever she was around. He was lonely and feeling sorry for himself, and only Lady Latimer's presence could ease him. Katherine responded correctly and respectfully, but she had no desire to be Queen of England or wife to a man who had already gone through five spouses. Her heart was given to Thomas Seymour; as she was to write to him, referring to this time, five years later, 'As truly as God is God, my mind was fully bent the other time I was at liberty to marry you before any man I know.' Henry sensed that this might be the case, and – seeing that Katherine showed no sign of becoming anything more than friendly towards him – decided on a course of rather more drastic action. In May, he dealt with the problem of Thomas Seymour by simply removing him from the scene and sending him on a permanent embassy to the court of the Regent of the Netherlands in Brussels. This must have been a blow, for different reasons, to both Katherine and Sir Thomas, yet Katherine was obliged to hide her true feelings because the King now began to pursue her in earnest, and she had no alternative but to let him think his advances were welcome.

On 1 July 1543, negotiations for the future marriage between Prince Edward and Mary, Queen of Scots were concluded with the signing of the Treaty of Greenwich. With the marriage of his heir so satisfactorily provided for, Henry felt that he might now marry for his own comfort, and it was at this time that he proposed to Katherine Parr. Her initial reaction was one of dismay. The King was not Katherine's idea of a desirable bridegroom, being, according to an eyewitness, the author of the Spanish Chronicle, 'so fat that such a man had never been seen. Three of the biggest men that could be found could get inside his doublet.' At fifty-two, he was already an old man, with an old man's set ways and uncertain temper. His bad leg sometimes rendered him immobile and needed constantly redressing; on occasions it stank. There was grey in his red hair and beard. All the same, he presented himself as a prospective bridegroom with all the assurance he had displayed to Anne Boleyn nearly twenty years before, and it was obvious that he would not brook any refusals. Katherine knew she had little choice in the matter, and when Henry, sensing her reluctance, became insistent, she capitulated.

Katherine was no giddy girl, and she was more suited than most for the task facing her, having been once before married to an old man, and having nursed Lord Latimer through his final illness. She was steady and she was sensible, and, having had the care of grown stepchildren before, all of whom seem to have got on well with her, she was uniquely fitted for the role of stepmother to the King's three children, whose interests she would protect with her customary efficiency.

She was not a pretty woman, or a beauty, but rather comely with red-gold hair and hazel eyes. For many years, portraits of various widely differing ladies were identified as Katherine Parr: these include one at Lambeth Palace, one by Ambrosius Benson in the collection of the Earl of Ashburnham, and a miniature at Sudeley Castle. There is only one portrait that can be said with certainty to depict Katherine, and that is the half-length painted by William Scrots in 1545, which is now in the National Portrait Gallery. The sitter wears a rich costume of scarlet damask banded with cloth of gold; the gown is loose fitting and has the upturned collar that became popular in the 1540s. She is past the first flush of youth, and appears rather plain. On her head is a jaunty cap atop her pearly hood, from which hangs a feather. William Scrots replaced Hans Holbein as Henry's court painter after Holbein's death, but his work lacks the draughtsmanship of Holbein's, and is somewhat mechanical in quality.

There is also, in the Royal Collection, a Holbein drawing that may well portray Katherine Parr. Inscribed 'The Lady Borough', it is a very faint sketch of a face, but enough remains to show a striking resemblance to the lady in Scrots's portrait. Holbein painted most of his English portraits after his return from Germany in 1532, yet some had been executed earlier, during the years 1526 to 1528, when Katherine Parr was married to Lord Borough. It could be argued that the drawing represents Katherine Neville, who married Lord Borough's son Henry in 1528, but comparison with the Scrots portrait, especially in the line of the nose and the slant of the eyes, lends credence to the likelihood that this is in fact an early portrait by Hans Holbein of Katherine Parr.

Katherine's looks, however, were not her chief attraction. People were drawn more to her warm and amiable personality and her intellectual qualities; she exuded goodwill. She was a good conversationalist, and loved a friendly argument, especially on matters of religious doctrine. She found favour with Cranmer and his reformist party because she was known to be 'very zealous towards the Gospel', according to the Elizabethan author of *The Book of Martyrs*, John Foxe, and they perceived that, like themselves, she might secretly nurture Protestant views. Foxe also remarked of Katherine that she was 'but a woman accompanied with all the imperfections natural to the weakness of her sex', yet in spite of this prejudiced masculine view, typical of that period, Katherine was seen by the reformers to be the perfect instrument whereby they could influence the King. They put heart and soul into encouraging the marriage, grateful that the King's inclinations at last coincided with their hopes.

Katherine proved to be popular with most people, mainly because she had a pleasant manner with both nobility and servants alike. Her chaplain, John Parkhurst, who later became Bishop of Norwich, remembered in his latter years that she was 'a most gentle mistress'. Perhaps the most outstanding thing about her was her formidable intellect, which had been cultivated to an unusual extent by her mother and by the people with whom she had associated in later life. She was perceptive, articulate, thirsty for knowledge, both general and religious, and industrious. Her virtue, a female quality always suspect in an age that believed that teaching women to write would encourage them to pen love-letters, was beyond question. After her marriage to the King, she made a point of 'avoiding all occasions of idleness and condemning vain pastimes'. No one would have cause to believe that she had ever been loose like Katherine Howard.

In many ways Katherine was a rather austere woman, who may be cited as the perfect example of the Renaissance ideal of the godly matron. However, far from being an early feminist, she used her intellectual powers to promote her own strong views, which were strictly conventional, on the conduct of the female sex. She believed, she wrote in her treatise *The Lamentations of a Sinner*, published in 1547, that women should 'learn of St Paul to be obedient to their husbands, and to keep silence in the congregation, and to learn of their husbands at home'. She herself, however, did not always practise what she preached, for she was to grow fond of disputing with her royal husband – who liked to think himself far superior to her on such topics – and was not above telling him what he ought to think, especially on religious matters. Naturally the King resented this, and there would be clashes. For all this, though, Henry admired her learning, and still more her virtue. She was, in every way, a woman he could respect, and she made the perfect companion for his later years. She was quieter and more staid than most of his previous wives, nor did she display the caprices of Anne Boleyn and Katherine Howard.

Katherine's chief interest was theology; 'godly matters' fascinated her. Like a true subject of Henry VIII, she detested the Pope, and once compared him to Pharaoh, saying 'He hath been, and is, the greater persecutor of all true Christians than ever was Pharaoh of the Children of Israel.' She was so anxious to promote her religious views that she wrote and published two books, proof indeed of her intellectual ability. This was the first time a queen of England ever aired her personal views to her subjects, and we are fortunate in having these works as testimony to the workings of the mind of this remarkable queen. Of course, much of what she wrote reflected the political ideology of the day. Of Henry VIII, Katherine was, naturally, lavish with praise:

> Thanks be to the Lord that He hath sent us such a godly and learned King in these latter days to reign over us, King Henry VIII, my most sovereign, favourable lord and husband: one, if Moses had figured any more than Christ, through the excellent grace of God, meet to be another expressed verity of Moses' conquest over Pharaoh.

She wholeheartedly approved of the King's reforms within the Church, and loved to discuss them with him, putting forth her own views without reserve. Fortunately, they usually coincided with his.

Katherine could also speak and write fluent French, which her mother had taught her. There exists today in the Cecil Papers at Hatfield House a poem said to have been written by her in that language. There is good reason to believe that, had Katherine lived in an age when women were encouraged to develop their intellectual powers, and had she not been hampered by the conventions of her time, she would have turned out to be a very successful and formidable lady in her own right.

With all her excellent qualities, there can be little doubt that the King 'deigned to marry' her for the companionship she could give him rather than for sensual pleasure or assuring the succession. It may well be that Henry was now impotent, and had been since he was married to Katherine Howard, which would account for the fact that neither union produced any children. It is true that Katherine's previous marriages had been childless, yet she did later conceive and bear a child by her fourth husband, so it is unlikely that the fault was hers.

On 10 July 1543, Archbishop Cranmer issued a special licence for the marriage of his sovereign lord King Henry with Katherine Latimer, late the wife of Lord Latimer, 'in whatever church, chapel or oratory he may please, without publication of banns, and dispensing with all ordinances to the contrary for reasons concerning the honour and advancement of the whole realm'. Henry was not minded to wait, and wanted to be married with as little fuss as possible. Accordingly, two days later, on 12 July, the wedding took place privately in the Queen's closet at Hampton Court. The Lady Margaret Douglas, lately returned to court after being pardoned for her illicit love affair, was chief bridesmaid. When the King was asked if he would take Katherine Parr to be his lawful wife, he answered 'Yea', with a 'joyful countenance', and the ghost of Katherine Howard was laid to rest at last.

One of the witnesses to the marriage was the Lady Anne of Cleves, who showed not the slightest annoyance at her former husband uniting himself to another lady; indeed, she seemed very pleased about it. She knew, more than anyone else, what Katherine was letting herself in for: 'A fine burden Madam Katherine has taken upon herself!' she later remarked, though Chapuys understood her dismissive attitude to mean that she was bitter because the King had not returned to her. He reported that she wanted to return to Cleves, but that was because her mother was ill, and not because she had 'taken great grief and despair at the King's espousal of his new wife, who is not nearly so good looking as she is'. Moreover, after the Duchess of Cleves died later that year, there was no more talk of Anne returning home.

Nearly everyone approved of the new Queen. Wriothesley, writing to inform the Duke of Norfolk of the marriage, described her as

a woman, in my judgement, for certain virtue, wisdom and gentleness, most meet for his Highness. And sure I am that his Majesty had never a wife more agreeable to his heart than she is. The Lord grant them long life and much joy together.

Chapuys told the Emperor that Katherine was 'praised for her virtue'; he added that she was 'of small stature, graceful, and of cheerful countenance'. The King, it was said presently, was very satisfied with her. The people of England, too, rejoiced when news of the marriage was made public. Sir Ralph Sadler sent a letter of congratulations to Lord Parr, saying it had

revived my troubled spirits and turned all my cares to rejoicing. I do not only rejoice for your lordship's sake, but also for the real and inestimable benefit and comfort which thereby shall ensue to the whole realm, which now with the grace of God shall be stored with many precious jewels.

One of Katherine's first acts as queen was to write to her brother, that same Lord Parr, informing him of her advancement, 'it having pleased God to incline the King to take me as his wife, which was the greatest comfort that could happen to me'. Thoughts of Sir Thomas Seymour had been resolutely banished out of her head. She went on:

I desire to inform my brother of it as the person who has most cause to rejoice thereat. I pray you to let me know of your health, as friendly as if I had not been called to this honour.

For Lord Parr, as for other members of Katherine's family, there was now the heady prospect of continual advancement and the acquisition of wealth and status. The Queen's sister and her husband, Sir William Herbert, came to court, as did members of the Throckmorton family, one of whom, Clement, became Katherine's cupbearer. And her former stepdaughter, Lady Tyrwhitt, was taken into her household, as was the Queen's cousin Maud, the widow of Sir Ralph Lane.

Once the Queen's household had been organised, the King took his bride to Windsor, where he celebrated his marriage by having three Protestant heretics burned to death in the Great Park. Conservatives such as Bishop Gardiner, who already suspected the Queen of having Lutheran sympathies, were watching her closely at this time to see how she reacted to the burnings, but she made no attempt to intercede for the victims and settled down afterwards to enjoy her honeymoon.

The court stayed at Windsor throughout August. Katherine had already resolved to be a loving stepmother to the King's three children, and she was determined to provide for them a happy and stable domestic life. It concerned her that all three lived away from the court and rarely saw their father, so, in August, with the King's approval, she wrote to them all, expressing the wish that they should come and visit her at court, as it was the King's pleasure and hers. The Lady Elizabeth responded promptly, and expressed – in very eloquent terms – her appreciation of Katherine's kindness, which she was sure she did not deserve. She promised that she would so conduct herself that Katherine would never have cause for complaint, and that she would be diligent in showing obedience and respect: 'I await with much impatience the orders of the King my father for the accomplishment of the happiness for which I sigh, and I remain with much submission, Your Majesty's very dear Elizabeth.'

Before long, both Elizabeth and her sister Mary arrived at court. Their new stepmother must have been a very welcome presence in their lives, especially to Elizabeth, who had for most of her young life lacked a mother's love and guidance. The King had never felt comfortable in the company of Anne Boleyn's precocious daughter, but now, under Katherine Parr's benign influence, he softened and unbent towards her.

Elizabeth was nearly ten. Her early promise had been fulfilled, and she was now as intelligent and sharp-witted as many an adult. Already she showed signs of having inherited her mother's love of flattery and her coquettish manner, as well as her courage. But, although she was temperamental, Elizabeth was not as volatile as Anne Boleyn had been, and her insecure childhood had taught her the value of discretion and dissimulation. Already she spoke several languages and was well grounded in the classics. This impressed Queen Katherine, and she immediately took upon herself the duty of supervising Elizabeth's education; indeed, she was to make such a good job of it that the King would later ask her advice when it came to appointing a suitable tutor for Prince Edward.

Henry's eldest child, the Lady Mary, was again finding it a pleasure to visit the court. She and Katherine Parr soon became great friends, and it is certain that Katherine did much to ease Mary's frustration by according her all the respect due to a princess. She became her confidante in everything except matters of religion, and – being near in age – they shared similar interests.

That left Edward. His visits to court would be less frequent than his sisters', for the King feared he might catch some mortal disease from too great a contact with the world beyond the rigorous standards of hygiene in his nursery. However, this did not prevent Katherine from overseeing his progress or being watchful of those who looked after him. In time, Edward would come to love his stepmother as much as his cold nature allowed him to love anybody; she was perhaps the most gentle influence he knew in his short life. At last there was a degree of harmony in the King's family.

On 12 October 1543, Edward celebrated his sixth birthday, and his royal father decided it was time to begin his formal education. Prior to this date, Edward had been 'brought up among the women', as he later recorded in his journal. Now he was to be handed over to male tutors and governors, chief of whom was a man with reformist views, Dr Richard Cox, a fellow of King's College, Cambridge, and the future Bishop of Ely. On the King's orders, the child was to be taught the usual curriculum of the period: classics, theology, languages, mathematics, grammar, and the known sciences, as well as sports and gentlemanly pursuits. Barnaby FitzPatrick, the son of an Irish nobleman, was shortly afterwards appointed Edward's whipping-boy, for it was unthinkable that the heir to the throne be chastised by lesser mortals. Fortunately, the boys became firm friends.

So absorbed was the King in plans for his heir's education and for an invasion of France scheduled for the following summer, that he did not notice fresh trouble brewing in Scotland. Thus the revocation of the Treaty of Greenwich by the Scottish Parliament in December 1543 came as an unpleasant shock to him, as did news that the 'auld alliance' between Scotland and France had been renewed. Henry's rage was terrible indeed. Gone were his hopes of a united Britain, gone his ambition to rule Scotland. Worse still, it had been intimated that his precious son was not good enough for the Scottish Queen. Such insults were not to be borne.

In retaliation, Henry sent an army to Scotland under Lord Hertford with the intention of subduing his rebellious neighbour. He could not afford to leave his northern border open when he took the offensive against the French the following year, and he wished, above all, to teach the Scots a lesson they would never forget. The English army set off just before Christmas to begin its 'rough wooing' of the Queen of Scots, and Hertford executed his master's orders with devastating thoroughness. Leith, Edinburgh and Holyrood were burned, and then he blazed on to Berwick, leaving a trail of destruction and misery along the borders; even today, in such towns as Jedburgh and Melrose, the results of his depredations may still be seen.

The campaign wore on throughout the spring and summer of 1544, while the young Queen Mary was hidden by her mother in a remote abbey. Nor did reports of the destruction appease Henry; in 1545, Hertford was again commanded to attack the Scots, and this time he wrought havoc by sacking, among others, the great abbeys of Dryburgh and Coldingham. At this point, any Scottish nobles who might have been sympathetic to an alliance with England had been alienated, and the Scots had been driven further into the arms of the French. All internal struggles ceased as the aristocratic factions united against England. English raids persisted until Henry's death, and eventually the Scots were obliged to send Queen Mary to France, for fear she might be abducted by the English. There, she would be brought up by the French royal family, and marry into it.

Katherine Parr's first Christmas season as queen was overshadowed by events in Scotland, yet the festivities at Hampton Court were much as usual. On the Sunday before Christmas Lord Parr was created Earl of Essex and the Queen's uncle, another Sir William Parr, was created Lord Parr of Horton and appointed chamberlain to the Queen. After Christmas, however, Henry's leg began to give him trouble, and in January 1544 he suffered several agonising attacks of pain. Chapuys, who was by now himself a virtual invalid and hoped to be going home to Savoy soon, thought that Henry's 'chronic disease' and 'great obesity' were endangering his life and needed careful attention. The King, he reported, was so weak on his legs he could hardly stand. Yet no one dared remonstrate with him about the amount he was eating, nor did they try to prevent him from going about his daily duties as if nothing were wrong with him. His one comfort was the kindness of his wife, who proved as devoted a nurse as she was a companion. He could not praise her enough: evidently the first six months of their marriage had been a success.

On 7 February 1544, as a mark of his esteem, the King passed a new Act of Succession. 'Forasmuch as his Majesty, sithence the death of the late Queen Jane' – Queen Anne and Queen Katherine are not mentioned, for as far as the King was concerned they did not count – 'hath taken to wife Katherine, late wife to Lord Latimer, by whom as yet his Majesty hath no issue, but may full well, when it shall please God,' it was provided that, 'if their union might be blessed with offspring', such offspring would be placed after Prince Edward in the order of succession. Failing any issue of the King's present marriage, the Act optimistically – and alarmingly, as far as Katherine was concerned – invested the succession in 'the children [the King] might have by other queens'. After them, would come the Lady Mary and then the Lady Elizabeth. The new Act was generally approved of by the King's subjects, and many hoped that the Queen might yet have a child, although she had now been married for seven months with no sign of pregnancy. As Sir William Paget wrote, 'We trust in God, which hath hitherto preserved his Majesty to his glory and honour and our comfort, to preserve him longer and send him time enough to proceed' to the siring of heirs. It was to prove a vain prayer.

That February, the Queen entertained the Spanish Duke of Najera, who arrived at court on the 17th, and the Lady Mary, who could speak Spanish, was there to assist her. When Eustache Chapuys, the Spanish ambassador, escorted the Duke into the Queen's presence, both royal ladies asked courteously for news of the Emperor. Unfortunately, Katherine was not feeling very well, but she put on a brave face and danced 'for the honour of the company'. Chapuys was impressed by her manner towards Mary, and he told the Emperor that she had constantly urged the King to keep Mary as second in line to the throne after Edward in the new Act of Succession.

Also present on that occasion was the Duke of Najera's secretary, Pedro de Gant, who left an account describing how the Duke kissed the Queen's hand on being presented, and of her leading him to another room where he was entertained with music and 'much beautiful dancing'. Katherine danced first with her brother, 'very gracefully', and then the Lady Mary partnered Lady Margaret Douglas and then some of the gentlemen of the court. A Venetian from the King's household danced galliards 'with such extraordinary activity that he seemed to have wings upon his feet – never was a man seen so agile!' The dancing went on for several hours, after which the Queen signalled to a nobleman who spoke Spanish to present some gifts to her guest. Najera again kissed her hand and she retired to her chamber. Pedro de Gant thought her 'graceful', and said she had a 'cheerful countenance; she is praised for her virtue'. On this occasion, she wore an underskirt of cloth of gold beneath a sleeved overdress of brocade lined with crimson satin, the sleeves being lined with crimson velvet, and the train being two yards long. Hanging around her neck were two crosses and a jewel of very magnificent diamonds; there were 'a great number of splendid diamonds in her head-dress' also.

After Najera had left the court, Mary stayed on. She had been occupying her time lately with translating Erasmus's *Paraphrases of the Gospel of St John*, an exercise of which the Queen heartily approved, for she felt that it became a woman of rank to undertake intellectual pursuits. Also, around this time, Mary sat for her portrait by a certain Master John, who charged her £4.00 for it. This same artist was also commissioned by Katherine Parr to paint another portrait, now in the National Portrait Gallery, and said to be of the King's great-niece, Lady Jane Grey, who in 1548 lived in the Queen's household. For a long time this second portrait was thought to be of Katherine herself, but the identification with Jane is said to be proved by the similarity of a brooch worn by the sitter to a brooch on an authenticated engraving of Jane. It is probable that Katherine gave Jane this piece of jewellery, and that the portrait is after all one of the Queen. The lady in the portrait looks more than ten years old, as her figure is quite developed and her jowls sag slightly; facially, she bears a striking resemblance to the Scrots portrait of Katherine Parr and she also wears an identical pendant.

On 22 April 1544, Lord Chancellor Audley died, and the indefatigable Wriothesley replaced him on 3 May. Wriothesley, for all his flattery, did not like Katherine Parr, and later did his best to bring about her downfall. He was not a man of great religious bias, but one who adapted his views to suit the times. His antipathy may have been purely personal. He had helped to bring down both Anne of Cleves and Katherine Howard, and seems to have enjoyed political intrigue for its own sake. For the present, he was the political ally of the staunchly conservative Stephen Gardiner, Bishop of Winchester, who suspected the Queen of heresy and was awaiting his opportunity to unseat her. Together, Wriothesley and Gardiner posed a potential threat to Katherine's future as Queen, although fortunately she was aware of their suspicions and careful to give them no cause for complaint.

One of the chief pleasures of queenship, Katherine found, was the ability to help others. To her mind, it was the chief duty of a queen to assist those who came to her in need. Thus, when Lady Hertford grew anxious about her husband, who was absent in Scotland and engaged on a very dangerous mission, Katherine spoke to the King on her behalf, and was able to inform Lady Hertford, in a letter written on 3 June 1544, that her husband would be recalled before Henry set sail for his planned invasion of France. The King's children and some of his other relatives had good reason to be grateful to her also, as did her servants and the humble people who benefited from her charity.

At the end of June, the King and Queen were present at the wedding of the Lady Margaret Douglas to the Earl of Lennox, one of the few remaining Scottish nobles with Anglophile sympathies. This took place in the chapel of Henry's new London palace, which had been built on the site of the old leper hospital of St James, not far from Whitehall. It had been intended as a residence for Anne Boleyn, but she had not lived to see its completion, and it was Katherine Parr who stood by Henry's side when St James's Palace was first used for a state occasion.

Preparations for the invasion of France were now so far advanced that the King decided to set out in early July. Before then, however, he accorded his wife the highest honour of all, in token of his trust in her and his respect for her integrity. On 7 July, it was announced in Council that she was to be regent in his absence, and Archbishop Cranmer, Lord Chancellor Wriothesley, Lord Hertford, Dr Thomas Thirlby and Sir William Petre were designated her advisers.

Prior to his departure, Henry also gave instructions about the education of his son. Dr John Cheke, a fellow of St John's College, Cambridge, and a famous academic with secret Lutheran tendencies, was appointed to supplement Dr Cox 'for the better instruction of the Prince'. Sir Anthony Cooke was also engaged to teach sports and recreational activities. Henry's choice of Cheke was applauded by all the great minds of his day and we may be certain that Katherine Parr had either urged or approved of it. Roger Ascham, who later became tutor to the Lady Elizabeth, called Cheke 'an excellent man, full of learning'.

When Cheke arrived upon the scene, he and Cox drew up a new curriculum of study for the Prince, to include languages, philosophy and 'all liberal sciences' in addition to his usual studies. Already, Edward was an extremely precocious and solemn child; so serious was he that he is known to have laughed out loud in public only once during his life. No doubt this was due to the fact that he was very early on made aware of the great destiny awaiting him, and whose shoes he must one day fill. From birth, he was isolated from the hubbub of court life and over-protected by an anxious father; he had never known the security of a mother's love, and hence grew into a self-contained child. His father was an affectionate yet distant, glittering figure, who must have inspired awe in his son whenever they met. It was left to Katherine Parr to alleviate the little boy's loneliness; it was slow progress, but she eventually won his affection, although it was too late to repair all the damage that had been caused by his early upbringing.

With Elizabeth, Katherine had initially had more success, for this child was eager and able to reciprocate the warmth emanating from her stepmother, even though she was inclined to use it as a stepping-stone to the King's favour. Through Katherine's good offices, she too had a new tutor at this time, William Grindal. Yet, early in 1544, a rift occurred between Elizabeth and her father. The cause is not known, yet it was enough to make Henry banish his younger daughter from the court. Queen Katherine did all she could to effect a reconciliation between father and daughter, but the King proved obstinate, and her efforts were in vain. Now he was going abroad with the rift unhealed, and there was nothing that Katherine could do about it.

By the second week in July, the English fleet was ready to sail, and the royal army was mustered at Dover. The Queen accompanied her husband to the port and kissed him farewell on 14 July, when he embarked for France. She then led the whole country in a prayer of intercession for his safety and success which she had composed herself to be read in churches:

O Almighty King and Lord of Hosts, which by Thy angels thereunto appointed dost minister both war and peace . . . our cause now being just, and being enforced to enter the war and battle, we most humbly beseech Thee, O Lord God of Hosts, so to turn the hearts of our enemies to the desire of peace that no Christian blood be spilt. Or else grant, O Lord, that with small effusion of blood and little damage of innocents, we may to Thy glory obtain victory; and that, the wars being ended, we may all with one heart and mind knit together in concord and amity, laud and praise Thee, who livest and reignest, world without end, Amen.

After the King's departure, Katherine returned to Greenwich, there to attend to her duties as regent and await news of her husband

and his campaign. She wrote to him regularly throughout their time apart, gentle, touching letters that testify plainly to the lively affection that had grown between them. In the first, she spoke of how much she was missing him:

> Although the distance and time and account of days neither is long nor many of your Majesty's absence, yet the want of your presence, so much desired and beloved by me, maketh me that I cannot quietly pleasure in anything until I hear from your Majesty. The time seemeth to me very long, with a great desire to know how your Highness hath done since your departing hence, whose prosperity and health I prefer and desire more than mine own. And whereas I know your Majesty's absence is never without great need, yet love and affection compel me to desire your presence. Again, the same zeal and affection forceth me to be best content with that which is your will and pleasure. Thus love maketh me in all things set apart mine own convenience and pleasure and to embrace most joyfully his will and pleasure whom I love.

She acknowledged herself greatly indebted to God for His benefits bestowed upon her:

> even such confidence have I in your Majesty's gentleness, knowing myself never to have done my duty as were requisite and meet for such a noble prince [is this, one wonders, a reference to her seeming inability to conceive a child?], at whose hands I have found and received so much love and goodness that with words I cannot express it.

This said, the Queen concluded, 'lest I should be too tedious to your Majesty,' committing Henry to God's care and governance.

Shortly afterwards, she received a letter from the Lady Elizabeth, bewailing her exile from the court and thanking Katherine for her hitherto fruitless intercession with the King. She had not dared to write to her father, she confessed, and begged her stepmother to send a letter on her behalf, 'praying ever for his sweet benediction' and beseeching God to send him victory over his enemies, 'so that your Highness and I may as soon as possible rejoice in his happy return'.

Absence from his wife had made Henry all the fonder, and when Katherine wrote again, begging him to forgive Elizabeth for her unknown offence and receive the child again at court, he relented, and gave his permission for her to go to Greenwich to keep Katherine company. Mary was already there, which meant that the Queen could extend her own special brand of kindness to both of Henry's daughters at once.

Meanwhile, the King had arrived in France and had laid siege to the city of Boulogne. The campaign had worked wonders for his health, as Chapuys noted in August, saying that he 'works better and more than I would have thought'. In fact, Henry was in his element, and was enjoying himself as much as he had on his earlier campaign in France, more than thirty years before. It was a relief to find that, despite encroaching age and infirmity, he could still mount a horse and bully the French. If he could not recapture his youth, he could at least enjoy this Indian summer.

On 9 August, the Queen wrote to Henry to tell him that she had dispatched the Earl of Lennox to Scotland in the hope that he would be able to seize the reins of government there, and she imputed the enthusiasm and speed with which he was carrying out his mission to serve a 'master whom God aids'. God, unfortunately, was not disposed to aid this particular venture, which was doomed to end in failure since Lennox's feeble efforts to grasp power were ineffectual. Not knowing this as yet, Katherine set out on a short progress in order to avoid the plague which was raging in London just then. News of her coming sent local gentry into hasty flurries of preparation; the Countess of Rutland, learning that Katherine was at Enfield and would be staying with her two nights hence, wrote to her father, Sir William Paston, asking him to send her some fresh fish, as 'here is small store, and the court is merry!'

Katherine was still worrying about the King, and she had not had news of him for some time. Even her enemy, Lord Chancellor Wriothesley, was moved by her concern.

God is able to strengthen His own against the devil [he told her] and therefore let not the Queen's Majesty in any wise trouble herself, for God shall turn all to the best; and sure we be that the King's Majesty's person is out of all danger.

Feeling somewhat cheered at his words, Katherine wrote yet another letter, which is now lost, to her husband, and sent him some venison, which he loved. At last, on 8 September, he wrote to her in response to her enquiries about certain domestic matters:

Most dearly and most entirely beloved wife,
We recommend us heartily unto you, and thank you as well for your letter as for the venison which you sent, for the which we give unto you our hearty thanks, and would have written unto you again a letter with our own hand, but that we be so occupied, and have so much to do in foreseeing and caring for everything ourself, as we have almost no manner rest or leisure to do any other thing. And whereas you desired to know our pleasure for the accepting into your chamber of certain ladies in places of others that cannot give their attendance by reason of sickness, albeit we think those whom you have named unto us as unable almost to attend by reason of weakness as the others be, yet we remit the accepting of them to your own choice, thinking nevertheless that though they shall not be meet to serve, yet you may, if you think so good, take them into your chamber to pass the time sometime with you at play, or otherwise to accompany you for your recreation. . . . No more to you at this time, sweetheart, both for lack of time and great occupation of business, saving we pray you to give in our name our hearty blessings to all our children, and recommendations to our cousin Margaret [Douglas] and the rest of the ladies and gentlewomen, and to our Council also.
Written with the hand of your loving husband,
                                                          Henry R.

Three days after this letter was written, the King realised that the inhabitants of Boulogne would not withstand the siege for very much longer. Wrote Chapuys: 'I never in my life saw the King so joyful and in such good spirits and so elated.' Henry told one of the Emperor's generals that he had vowed to bring France to submission and was now fulfilling that promise. 'I have been all my life a Prince of honour and virtue,' he said sanctimoniously, 'who never contravened my word, and am too old to begin now, as the white hairs in my beard testify.' His elation was justified, at least for the time being. On 14 September 1544, Boulogne fell to him; four days later he entered it in triumph, riding through the streets at the head of his army. On the same day, the King of France was forced to sign a peace treaty with the Emperor at Crêpy.

In the meantime, Katherine Parr had been staying with the Countess of Rutland at her medieval castle at Oakham; the Queen had brought with her all three of her stepchildren, to keep them safe from the plague. From Oakham, she issued strict orders to the Council, commanding them to make a proclamation that no person who had been in contact with a plague victim was to come near the court nor was anyone to allow any courtier into a house where there had been infection, 'under the Queen's indignation and further punishment at her pleasure'. These sensible measures effectively eliminated any threat of danger to the Prince and his sisters, and to Katherine herself. Fortunately, by late August the epidemic was on the wane, and the Queen deemed it safe to return to Greenwich, where she was when she heard news of the fall of Boulogne.

Katherine was well aware of the importance of her husband's victory, and she immediately ordered that a general thanksgiving be offered up in all the towns and villages throughout England, in gratitude for the taking of the city. These special services were held on 19 September. And to her husband, Katherine wrote: 'I thank God for a prosperous beginning of your affairs, and I rejoice at the joyful news of your good health.'

Late in September, the Queen went to Hanworth for a short break from state duties. There, she read the Lady Mary's translation of Erasmus's *Paraphrases*, and was very impressed with it; at the end of the month she returned the manuscript with a letter full of warm praise, suggesting that Mary have it published, as it was a 'fair and useful work'. Mary declined to do so, but Katherine replied that she did not see 'why you should reject the praise which all deservedly would give you; yet I leave all to your own prudence, and will approve of that which seems best to you.' Mary responded by saying she was willing to have the work published, but only under a pseudonym, to which Katherine answered that in her opinion Mary would 'do a real injury if you refuse to let it go down to posterity under the auspices of your own name'. Her words made Mary relent. The translation was printed and widely read, receiving high praise from scholars such as Nicholas Udall, Provost of Eton College.

After leaving Hanworth, the Queen returned to Greenwich, there to await the King's homecoming. On 30 September, a triumphant Henry disembarked at Dover, and travelled as fast as possible to see the wife from whom he had been parted for three months. It was a happy reunion, the King and Queen openly showing their affection for each other, and their pride in each other's achievements during the past weeks. Katherine may well have reflected at this time that, if she had given up the chance of a marriage more to her liking with Thomas Seymour, she had at least achieved a measure of contentment with the King, who had been consistently loving and kind to her.

For the remainder of the autumn, Henry diverted himself with his favourite pastime, hunting. His recent burst of energy had not yet spent itself. This was, however, the last time he would ever engage in such pursuits.

In October that year, Sir Thomas Seymour's embassy to the Low Countries came to an end and he returned to court. The King knew very well how things had once stood between Seymour and Katherine, and once again appointed Seymour to an office that would necessitate his being away from court for long periods, that of Lord High Admiral of England. Evidently Henry was still suspicious of Seymour's intentions towards the Queen, although no breath of scandal or hint of impending infidelity tainted her good name. Whatever her private feelings were, she hid them well, and paid no more attention to Seymour than to anyone else, while he, following her lead, betrayed by no sign that there had ever been anything more than friendship between them.

At Christmas, Chapuys took the opportunity to thank the Queen, on behalf of the Emperor, for all that she had done for the Lady Mary, to which she 'replied very graciously that she did not deserve so much courtesy. What she did for the Lady Mary was less than she would like to do, and was only her duty in every respect.' As to maintaining the friendship between England and Spain, Katherine told the ambassador that she 'had done and would do nothing to prevent its growing still further, and she hoped that God would avert the slightest dissension, as the friendship was so necessary and both sovereigns were so good'. Chapuys could not help admiring her. She was, in his opinion, a very pleasant and well-meaning person, whose goodwill could be used to advantage when it came to preserving the alliance between his master and Henry VIII. Yet Chapuys feared he would not be there to use this advantage: he was growing old and nearing retirement, and was so infirm that he was now confined to a kind of wheelchair on occasions. He had already applied for his recall, and was awaiting the Emperor's assent.

New Year arrived, the beginning of 1545. The Lady Elizabeth sent her stepmother her own translation, neatly written in fine italic script, of Margaret of Navarre's book, *Le Miroir de l'Ame Pécheresse*, a devout meditation on the love of a Christian soul towards God and His Christ. Elizabeth hoped that there was nothing in it 'worthy of reprehension', and begged that no other person than Katherine be allowed to see it, 'lest my faults be known of many' as 'it is all imperfect and incorrect' and 'in many places rude', with 'nothing done as it should be'. This was the kind of gift Katherine liked best, and she was deeply touched that her young stepdaughter should have gone to such trouble. And when she turned to the first page of the work, she read the dedication: 'To the most noble and virtuous Queen Katherine, Elizabeth, her humble daughter, wisheth perpetual felicity and everlasting joy.'

In March, the King's health took a turn for the worse, and he was down with 'a burning fever' for several days; this seems to have affected his leg, and he suffered more bouts of agonising pain. His illness did not improve his temper, which was further aroused by reports of heresy within his realm, which was spreading at an alarming rate. Henry himself had never approved of Lutheranism. In spite of all he had done to reform the Church in England, he was still Catholic in his ways and determined for the present to keep England that way. Protestant heresies would not be tolerated, and he would make that very clear to his subjects. As a result of his enquiries, twenty-three people were arrested and examined at this time, among them a woman called Anne Askew. This Anne was twenty-three, and had not long since applied to the King for a legal separation from her husband, Thomas Kyme, who had quite literally thrown her out of doors and kept her from seeing her two children. It has often been alleged that at some time in her life Anne was acquainted with Katherine Parr, but there is no evidence to substantiate this, though Katherine was certainly sympathetic towards Anne Askew for she secretly shared the same Protestant views. Under questioning, Anne Askew admitted to being a Protestant, whereupon she was put in prison to wait further examination and lay there for many months. Queen Katherine would one day have reason to regret ever having heard of her.

The summer of 1545 was a sad one for several reasons. Katherine's ward and former stepdaughter, Margaret Neville, died, having appointed her 'dear sovereign mistress, the Queen's Highness' as her heir, since she was 'never able to render to her Grace sufficient thanks for the godly education and tender love and bountiful goodness which I have evermore found in her Highness'. Then, in May, Eustache Chapuys, who had been the Emperor's ambassador to the court of Henry VIII since 1529, informed the King that he was at last being recalled to Spain. Henry, saddened at the prospect of losing an old sparring partner, went immediately to the Queen and warned her of the envoy's imminent departure. The next morning, as Chapuys sat sunning himself in the palace gardens, he saw Katherine approaching, accompanied only by a few attendants. She told him that the King had told her he was coming to say goodbye, and said she was

> very sorry, on the one hand for my departure, as she had been told that I had always performed my duties well, and the King trusted me; but on the other hand she doubted not that my health would be better on the other side of the sea.

Chapuys could, she added, do more there to maintain the friendship between England and the Empire, which he had done so much to promote, and for this reason she was glad he was going. After more pleasantries, the Queen begged Chapuys to 'present to your Majesty [i.e. the Emperor] her humble service' and 'to express explicitly to you all that I had learned here of the good wishes of the King'. She then took leave of him. Chapuys left England shortly afterwards and died a few months later. In his place, the Emperor appointed a new ambassador, a Dutchman, Francis van der Delft.

Death also claimed, on 22 August, Charles Brandon, Duke of Suffolk, one of the King's oldest and closest friends, who left a widow with two young sons. The elder, Henry, aged ten, succeeded his father as duke, and was sent to join the household of Prince Edward. Here, the régime was tough. In fact, both the King's younger children were subject to a rigorously strict education, which – as Edward later recalled in his journal – was to 'satisfy the good expectation of the King's Majesty, my father'. This was having the effect of turning both Edward and Elizabeth into intellectual prodigies, who devoted almost every waking hour to books and religious exercises. When Edward was called out of the schoolroom for martial exercises, Elizabeth would practise the lute or viol, or occupy herself with needlework. It was the King's wish that Queen Katherine personally supervise the education of his children, a task for which she was eminently suited. Nor did she neglect her own intellectual pursuits. On 6 November 1545, she published – with the King's approval – a collection of prayers and meditations she had collated, under the excessively wordy title *Prayers and Meditations wherein the mind is stirred patiently to suffer all afflictions here, to set at naught the vain prosperity of this world, and always to long for the everlasting felicity: Collected out of holy works by the most virtuous and gracious Princess Katherine, Queen of England*.

The book was widely acclaimed. The universities of Oxford and Cambridge begged the Queen to become their patroness, an honour she gratefully accepted. In reply to her letter, Roger Ascham, then fellow of St John's College, Cambridge, wrote:

> Write to us oftener, erudite Queen, and do not despise the term erudition, most noble lady: it is the praise of your industry, and a greater one to your talents than all the ornaments of your fortune. We rejoice vehemently in your happiness, most happy Princess, because you are learning more amidst the occupations of your dignity than many of us do in all our leisure and quiet.

The Queen's book represented a real breakthrough in an age when only the most privileged women were fortunate enough to receive an education. Not even the Lady Margaret Beaufort had achieved as much, nor Katherine of Aragon. Two of the finest female minds of the century were fortunate enough to be moulded under Katherine Parr's influence – the future Elizabeth I and, later on, the Lady Jane Grey. Katherine's court was already a centre of feminine learning, and competition for places in her household was fierce. Even male scholars sought her patronage. One, Francis Goldsmith, could not find words enough to praise her, save to say that 'Her rare goodness has made every day a Sunday, a thing hitherto unheard of, especially in a royal palace.' Nor had her high rank affected Katherine's essential humanity and warmth. She was sympathetic towards poor scholars, and did her best to assist them whenever she could. Sometimes she sent them to Stoke College, of which she was patroness. Matthew Parker, who had once been chaplain to Anne Boleyn, was put in charge of them, and it was his duty to ensure also that the children of the Queen's tenants and farmers received an education 'meet for their ages and capacities'. Not surprisingly, Parker was moved to point out that all this could be done 'at no small cost and charge', but the Queen felt that no outlay was too much to pay for something she held dear. The money to fund her scholars and educational projects came entirely from her privy purse, nor would she turn away any poor scholar who came to her seeking assistance.

In the late autumn of 1545, while staying at Windsor, the King suffered some kind of attack, which laid him low for a time. On Christmas Eve, he was reported by the new Spanish ambassador to be 'so unwell that, considering his age and corpulence, fears are entertained that he will be unable to survive further attacks'. Henry was suffering terrible pain from what seems to have been venous thrombosis in his leg, and there was nothing his doctors could do to alleviate it. The Queen did her best to cheer him, and would sit by his bed and try to involve him in what he loved best, a lively dispute, preferably on some theological matter, in order to take his mind off the pain. Yet these seemingly innocent domestic interludes caused concern to the conservative faction at court, who believed that the Queen's sympathies were with the Protestant heretics and that she was being urged by the reformists to convert the King. The Seymour brothers, the widowed Duchess of Suffolk, Lady Hertford, and Lady Dudley – the last three being members of the Queen's own household – were strongly suspected of having infected Katherine with their private views, and as the King showed favour to them all, there was little anyone could do about it. Yet staunch Catholics such as Gardiner and Wriothesley believed that if the King knew the true beliefs of these people then he would deal with them as he had dealt with other Protestants. This might be one way of bringing down the Queen and removing the dangerous influence she had upon Henry VIII.

It is hardly likely that Katherine was unaware of the danger in which she stood, yet she refused to be intimidated. She knew very well that several persons in her inner circle were Protestant converts, and she also knew that heretics risked a dreadful penalty. She realised, therefore, that she should proceed with the utmost care. She had seen that the King's love could easily turn to hatred, and she did not imagine that he would react kindly to the news that his wife was a secret Protestant.

Katherine was occupied just then with a second book, *The Lamentations of a Sinner*, which was a theological discourse on faith and the proper behaviour of Christians. Its author protested, in her introduction, that she had 'but a simple zeal and earnest love to the truth, inspired of God, who promised to pour His spirit upon all flesh, which I have by the Grace of God felt in myself to be true'. The book was largely an attack on popery, and its central theme was the comparison between Moses leading the people of Israel out of Egypt and Henry VIII freeing his subjects from the iniquity of Rome. In it Katherine also put forth her views on the conduct of her own sex:

> If they be women married, they learn of St Paul to be obedient to their husbands and to keep silence in the congregation, and to learn of their husbands at home. Also, that they wear such apparel as becometh holiness and comely usage with soberness, not being accusers or detractors, nor given to much eating of delicate meats or drinking of wine; but that they touch honest things, to make the young women sober-minded, to love their husbands, to love their children, to be discreet, housewifely and good, that the Word of God may not be evil spoken of.

Such views reflected exactly the King's own opinions on the role of women within the natural order of things; he was greatly impressed by the book, and even a little jealous, taking as he did great pride in his own learning, and finding it disconcerting to wonder if a mere woman could possibly be as clever as he was.

Trouble was already brewing for Katherine. In February 1546, the King was informed that the heretic Anne Askew had implicated the Queen in a new confession. Further questioning showed that she had not even mentioned Katherine Parr, but the incident was enough to prove to Katherine that her enemies were poised to attack. There is no contemporary evidence to prove that the Queen had anything to do with Anne Askew, and the only authorities for it date from the Elizabethan era. Robert Parsons, in his *Treatise of Three Conversions of England*, published in 1603, says that Katherine received heretical books sent by Anne, and that her ladies-in-waiting, Lady Herbert, Lady Lane, Lady Tyrwhitt and others, were party to this. John Foxe, in his *Acts and Monuments*, published in 1563, tells another story, giving his source as one or more of these ladies.

Foxe gives no date for the events he describes, but if they happened at all, it must have been during the summer of 1546, probably in July. In June, the King gave his permission for Anne Askew to be examined again for heresy in the Tower. Lord Chancellor Wriothesley was in charge of the interrogation, and he saw this chance as another to incriminate the Queen. When Anne Askew proved obdurate, he ordered her to be put on the rack, and, with Sir Richard Rich, personally conducted the examination. Anne Askew later dictated an account of the proceedings, in which she testified to being questioned as to whether she knew anything about the beliefs of the ladies of the Queen's household. She replied that she knew nothing. It was put to her that she had received gifts from these ladies, but she denied it. For her obstinacy, she was racked for a long time, but bravely refused to cry out, and when she swooned with the pain, the Lord Chancellor himself brought her round, and with his own hands turned the wheels of the machine, Rich assisting. Afterwards, Anne's broken body was laid on the bare floor, and Wriothesley sat there for two hours longer, questioning her about her heresy and her suspected involvement with the royal household. All in vain. Anne refused to deny her Protestant faith, and would not or could not implicate anyone near the Queen. On 18 June, she was arraigned at the Guildhall in London, and sentenced to death. She was burned at the stake on 16 July at Smithfield, along with John Lascelles, another Protestant, he who had first alerted Cranmer to Katherine Howard's pre-marital activities. Anne died bravely and quickly: the bag of gunpowder hung about her neck by a humane executioner to facilitate a quick end exploded almost immediately.

If Katherine Parr was grieved by Anne Askew's death, she dared not show it. Like everyone else, she had been horrified to learn that the heretic had been carried to her execution on a chair as her legs were useless after the racking. Yet she kept her thoughts to herself, knowing that if it were to be discovered by her enemies that she shared Anne's views, then she too might face the flames. Foxe tells us that at this time Henry was feeling a little jaded with his marriage because the Queen had not conceived in three years; he had also heard complaints from his councillors about her interference in matters of religion. Hitherto, he had heartily approved of the strong religious bias in his wife's household. He was pleased to see Katherine spending so much time studying the Scriptures and discussing them with learned divines, and he enjoyed their debates on the subject. Now, it seemed that Katherine was going a little too far, becoming over-zealous and exhorting her husband 'that as he had to his eternal fame begun a good work in banishing the monstrous idol of Rome, so he would finish the same, purging his Church of England clean from the dregs thereof'. Where else could this lead, some were wondering, but to a Protestant state? Even Henry did not like it, and grew very stern and opinionated whenever the subject was raised. Foxe says his affection for Katherine cooled, though this is nowhere borne out by contemporary sources. Be that as it may, the Catholic party smelled a Protestant rat that was heralding the destruction of everything they held dear; until now, they had not dared to broach the matter with the King, because of his obvious love and esteem for the Queen, but now they saw their chance, and were looking daily for an opportunity to discredit her in Henry's eyes. Gardiner knew, better than most, that Henry hated being contradicted in any argument. In the past it had galled the Bishop to see the King being corrected by his wife, but now he perceived that Henry himself was becoming irritated with her arguments. Encroaching infirmity made him peevish and impatient; he ceased making his daily visits to his wife's apartments, and it was left to Katherine to decide whether or not to brave his black moods and go and sit with him after dinner or supper. At these times, her enthusiasm more often than not got the better of her, and she persisted in urging the King to carry his reforms still further.

The day came when Henry had had enough and rudely cut short what the Queen was saying and changed the subject, which left Katherine somewhat amazed. However, once the conversation had been steered to less contentious matters, Henry was his old self again 'with gentle words and loving countenance'. When it was time for the Queen to leave, he said, 'Farewell, Sweetheart', and Katherine left the room, little knowing that her enemies were about to pounce.

Bishop Gardiner had been within earshot of that conversation, and he seized his chance when the King began to grumble about her behaviour. 'A good hearing it is, when women become such clerks, and much to my comfort to come in mine old age to be taught by my wife!' he fumed. The Bishop soothed his sovereign's vanity by replying that 'his Majesty excelled the princes of that and every other age, as well as all the professed doctors of divinity', and then poured oil on troubled waters by saying that

> it was unseemly for any of his subjects to argue with him so malapertly as the Queen had just done; that it was grievous for any of his Councillors to hear it done, since those who were so bold in words would not scruple to proceed to acts of disobedience.

He added significantly that he

> could make great discoveries if he were not deterred by the Queen's powerful faction. Besides this, the religion by the Queen maintained did not only dissolve the politic government of princes, but also taught the people that all things ought to be in common.

In fact, according to Foxe, Gardiner spared no efforts in persuading the King 'that his Majesty should easily perceive how perilous a matter it is to cherish a serpent within his own bosom', and reminded him that 'the greatest subjects in the land, defending those arguments that she did defend, had by law deserved death. For his part, he would not speak his knowledge in the Queen's case,' because to do so might bring about his own destruction 'through her and her faction', unless the King agreed to give him his protection.

Henry was incredulous at the Bishop's words, but his suspicious nature allowed him to believe that the matter was indeed a serious one, otherwise Gardiner would never have dared to be outspoken. In one clever stroke, the Bishop had managed to convince him that his wife was at the centre of a heretical conspiracy to bring down traditional forms of government, and that she was supported by many influential people at court. This was enough to set all the alarm bells ringing in the King's head, and he questioned Gardiner closely on the matter, remaining closeted with him for some time. When they parted, the triumphant Bishop came away with the knowledge that Henry had consented to articles being drawn up against the Queen, with a view to putting her on trial for her life, 'which the King pretended to be fully resolved to spare'. Gardiner was to provide the proof that was needed to support his accusations.

Foxe seems to be saying here that Henry was playing a double game, and it does seem that he was reserving his judgement until all was made clear. Yet the peril in which the Queen and her ladies now stood was very real, and this was made obvious to them when the Council ordered the arrests of Lady Herbert, Katherine's sister, Lady Lane and Lady Tyrwhitt, her three favourite ladies-in-waiting. They were interrogated about the books they had, and whether the Queen kept forbidden reading matter in her closet, and their coffers were searched in the hope that proof of the Queen's heresy might be discovered. Then they were released. The King knew all this, and seemed content for it to be done.

Henry was then at Whitehall Palace with the court. Because of his health, he did not often leave his rooms, and only a few privileged members of the Privy Council were allowed access to him. Through them, he let it be known that he was agreeable to a warrant being drawn up for the Queen's arrest, should there be any suspicion of heresy. Katherine guessed nothing of this, and heedlessly continued to engage the King in religious debates. He allowed her to do this, for he was now on the alert for a sinister meaning to her arguments, and was carefully weighing every word she said. It appears he was not yet completely convinced of her guilt, and late one night, when Katherine had gone, he confided all his suspicions to his physician, Dr Thomas Wendy, who had replaced Dr Butts on the latter's death in November 1545. Henry pretended 'he intended no longer to be troubled with such a doctress as she was,' and told the Doctor what was afoot, swearing him to secrecy.

When a warrant for Katherine Parr's arrest was drawn up, the King signed it, and it was entrusted to an unnamed member of the Privy Council who fortuitously dropped it. A servant loyal to the Queen found it and brought it straight to her, and Katherine found herself confronting her doom. There was the King's signature: there could be no mistake. Her reaction was instantaneous and dramatic, her agony of mind manifesting itself in tears and hysterical screaming, which was 'lamentable to see', as her ladies remembered many years later. She was distraught with terror, recalling the fate of Anne Boleyn and Katherine Howard and realising that, on a charge of heresy, her death would be much more horrible than theirs. In her grief and fear, she took to her bed, shaking and wailing. Her cries could be heard throughout the palace, and even penetrated the King's apartments. Henry, little realising what was the matter, sent Dr Wendy and other physicians to her to try and calm her down. Wendy guessed that the Queen had somehow found out what was afoot, and sent the other doctors away. He then told her what he knew and warned her that Gardiner and Wriothesley were plotting her downfall; she should 'conform herself to the King's mind', he advised, then she might find him 'favourable unto her'.

Wendy's words afforded the Queen little comfort. Still she lay, weeping and crying, her self-control shattered. Eventually, the King, learning of her 'dangerous state', went to her himself. At the sight of him, Katherine calmed down a little, and managed to say that she feared he had grown displeased with her and utterly forsaken her. She was so obviously sincere in her grief that Henry was deeply touched and, 'like a loving husband, with comfortable words so refreshed her careful mind that she began somewhat to recover'. Henry stayed with her an hour, and when he had gone, Katherine made up her mind to cease interfering in matters of religion and to forbid her ladies to dabble in heresy. She ordered them to get rid of any forbidden books in their possession, and made it clear that from now on her chief priority was to conform to her husband's wishes.

That night, accompanied only by her sister and Lady Lane, who carried a candle before her, she made her way to the King's bedchamber, where she found Henry chatting with his gentlemen. When he saw Katherine, he welcomed her courteously, and after a while he brought up the subject of religion, 'seeming desirous to be resolved by the Queen of certain doubts'. Katherine, guessing what game he was playing, gave meek and dutiful answers, saying, 'So God hath appointed you, as Supreme Head of us all, and of you, next unto God, will I ever learn.' But Henry was not that easily mollified. 'Not so, by St Mary!' he cried. 'Ye are become a doctor, Kate, to instruct us, as oftentime we have seen, and not to be instructed or directed by us.' Katherine protested her meaning had been mistaken, 'for I have always held it preposterous for a woman to instruct her lord'. If she had ever differed with him on religion, she went on, it was only for her own information, and also because she realised that talking helped to

> pass away the pain and weariness of your present infirmity, which encouraged me in this boldness, in the hope of profiting withal by your Majesty's learned discourse. I am but a woman, with all the imperfections natural to the weakness of my sex; therefore in all matters of doubt and difficulty I must refer myself to your Majesty's better judgement, as to my lord and head.

This was a masterful speech, and a triumph of diplomacy, and the King was deeply impressed – if not a little relieved – by it. 'Is it so, sweetheart?' he replied. 'And tended your arguments to no worse end? Then we are perfect friends, as ever at any time heretofore.' Katherine's sense of relief may be imagined: a crisis had been averted and the King was once more her loving husband. Again she sat beside him as he took her in his arms and kissed her before everyone present; then he told her it did him more good to hear those words from her own mouth than if he had heard news of £100,000 coming his way. Never again, he promised, would he doubt her. It was late in the night when he finally gave her leave to depart, and when she had gone he praised her highly to his gentlemen.

Henry was shrewd enough to guess why Gardiner and his party wanted the Queen out of the way, and had known all along what game the Bishop was playing. Now that he had ample proof of the Queen's loyalty, he was very much looking forward to discountenancing them. Katherine's servant had been careful to replace the warrant for the Queen's arrest where she had found it; it was quickly retrieved by the councillor, and on the afternoon following the royal couple's reconciliation, Lord Chancellor Wriothesley prepared to use it, knowing nothing of the events of the previous night.

On that afternoon, the King made sure that the Queen joined him to take the air in the palace gardens, where he was 'as pleasant as ever he was in all his life'. Suddenly, in the midst of their laughter, the Lord Chancellor arrived, with forty of the King's guards at his heels, intending to escort the Queen to the Tower with her three ladies, who were also present. Wriothesley was nonplussed at finding his master and mistress so happily engaged, then the King, looking very stern, got up and walked off a little way, calling his Chancellor after him. Wriothesley fell to his knees and began to explain why he was there, but he was brutally cut short by Henry, who shouted 'Knave! Arrant knave! Beast! Fool!', and ordered him out of his presence. Everyone stared at the discomfited Chancellor as he and his men scuttled away. Henry strode back to the Queen; she could see he was in a fury, although he was struggling to 'put on a merry countenance', and innocently enquired what was wrong, saying charitably that she would be a suitor for the Lord Chancellor, 'as she deemed his fault was occasioned by some mistake'. To which her husband replied, 'Ah, poor soul, thou little knoweth Kate how little he deserveth this grace at thy hands. On my word, sweetheart, he hath been to thee a very knave, so let him go.' Katherine wisely held her peace. She knew very well what Wriothesley had come for, and that she had had a lucky escape.

She had learned her lesson and would from then on act the meek and dutiful wife. There would be no breath of heresy in her household, and she would comport herself with greater circumspection than ever, giving her enemies no room for criticism. She would confine herself to corresponding with men of letters such as Roger Ascham, pursuing her intellectual interests and charities, and overseeing the education of her stepchildren. Prince Edward wrote to her that August, saying that her letters and the 'excellence of your genius' made him sick of his own writing: 'But then I think how kind your nature is, and that whatever proceeds from a good mind will be acceptable, and so I write you this letter.' It seemed an age since he had seen her, he added.

August was a busy month for Katherine. On the 24th, Claude d'Annebaut, Admiral of France, visited the court as a consequence of a new treaty of peace between Henry VIII and Francis I. He was entertained with the usual banquets and hunting forays; in the evenings, rich masques were staged for his pleasure and that of Queen Katherine and her ladies, after which there was dancing in two new banqueting houses hung with rich tapestries and furnished with court cupboards containing gold plate set with precious stones.

After the Admiral had returned to France, the King and Queen went on a short progress, even though the King's health was now noticeably failing. His leg was paining him more than ever and, although he preferred to make light of his suffering, it showed in his face. He could no longer walk up or down stairs, and a mechanical hoist was needed to assist him. Norfolk told van der Delft that the King 'could not long endure'. Soon, he could barely walk at all, and an order was given for two chairs (called trams), covered in tawny velvet, 'for the King's Majesty to sit in to be carried to and from in his galleries and chambers'. His councillors believed his illness was incurable and would soon kill him, and were already plotting, each and every one, to gain control of the Prince.

Henry himself was aware that his end could not be far off, and he now made plans for the inevitable regency that would follow his death, since his heir was only nine years old. He was determined to exclude all foreign influence from the regency Council, retaining to the end his mistrust of aliens. At the same time, he was perceptive enough to realise that the general trend was towards a radical reform of the Church, and he showed himself inclined to favour those lords who supported it. As for the Prince, there was little doubt in anyone's mind that he would come to embrace the Protestant faith, and Henry wisely accepted that there was little he could do to stem the tide in this respect. Perhaps some of Katherine's arguments had taken root in his mind. He may well have sensed that his own era was dying and with it the last vestiges of medievalism: a new age was dawning, and it was his duty to lay a solid foundation for it.

But he was not dead yet; there still remained some life in that diseased body. The King's thoughts turned to his son, who had always been the chief delight in his life; now he sent the boy some presents, chains, rings, jewelled buttons, and other valuables, which prompted a stiff little note of thanks from the child.

> You grant me all these [wrote Edward], not that I should be proud and think too much of myself, but that you might urge me to the pursuit of all true virtues and piety, and adorn and furnish me with all the accomplishments which are fitting a Prince.

December arrived. Despite the King's illness, a plot to get rid of the Queen and replace her with the King's daughter-in-law, the Duchess of Richmond (daughter of the impeccably Catholic Duke of Norfolk) was uncovered. It seems to have originated with her brother, the Earl of Surrey, who had instructed her on how to win the King's favour, 'that she might rule as others had done'. On being questioned, the Duchess managed to incriminate not only her brother but also her father the Duke. On 12 December, both men were arrested on a charge of high treason and taken to the Tower. The King was in no mood to listen to pleas for mercy; since the fall of Katherine Howard he had distrusted Norfolk, and welcomed this opportunity to rid himself of him: he had suffered enough at the hands of the Howards. They could stew in the Tower until after Christmas, then he would deal with them as they deserved.

On Christmas Eve, Henry prorogued Parliament for the last time, and harangued both Houses on their attitude to religion:

> Charity and concord is not amongst you, but discord and dissension beareth rule in every place. I am very sorry to hear how unreverently that most precious jewel, the Word of God, is disputed, rhymed, sung and jangled in every ale-house and tavern. And yet I am even as much sorry that the readers of the same follow it so faintly and so coldly!

Sir John Mason said afterwards that the King had spoken 'so kingly, so rather fatherly, that many of his hearers were overcome and shed tears'. It was obvious to everyone present that this would be the King's last public speech. A Greek visitor to England in the train of the Spanish ambassador reported that the English were 'wonderfully well affected' towards their monarch; they would hear nothing disrespectful about him, and the most binding oaths were sworn on his life. He was already a legend in his own lifetime.

The court was closed to all but the Privy Council and some gentlemen of the privy chamber that Christmas, a sure indication that the King was now in a critical condition. The Queen and the Lady Mary were the only members of his family in attendance. Two days after Christmas the Spanish ambassador told the Emperor that Henry's physicians were despairing of doing anything to help their royal patient, who was 'in great danger' and 'very ill'. His leg was agony, and he was running a high temperature. Reports that he had died already were circulating in the capital.

On 30 December, Henry dictated his will. He left his kingdom and his crown to Prince Edward, and after him to any posthumous heirs that 'our entirely beloved wife Queen Katherine' might bear him. Failing those, the succession should pass to the Lady Mary and her heirs, then to the Lady Elizabeth and hers, and finally to the heirs of the King's late sister Mary, Duchess of Suffolk. His antagonism towards the Scots had ensured that he pass over the heirs of his elder sister Margaret Tudor. The King was adamant: Mary of Scotland should never rule England unless it was as Edward's consort.

With the succession provided for, Henry now made provision for his widow. As token of his appreciation of 'the great love, obedience, chastity of life and wisdom being in our wife and Queen', he bequeathed to her £3,000 in plate, jewels and household goods for the term of her life. She could also help herself to as many of the King's clothes as she pleased, and they were worth a considerable sum. She would, in addition, receive £1,000 in cash and her dower and jointure, as decided by Parliament. Katherine would find herself a very rich widow indeed when the time came.

Henry then expressed his desire to be buried beside the body of 'our true and loving wife, Queen Jane' in the choir of St George's Chapel, Windsor, and left instructions for the raising of an 'honourable tomb' which would be surmounted by effigies of Henry and Jane, fashioned 'as if sweetly sleeping'.

He rallied a little after making his will, and was well enough to leave Greenwich and travel with the Queen to London on 3 January 1547. When they were settled in Whitehall Palace, Katherine did her best to carry on as normally as possible, and tried to counteract rumours that the King was dead or dying. At New Year, she had sent her stepson portraits of Henry and herself, and on 10 January he wrote to thank her, addressing the letter to his most 'illustrious Queen and dearest mother'. He had no idea that his father was so ill, and the King and Queen were anxious to spare him the heavy knowledge that the burden of kingship would soon be his.

On 7 January 1547, an Act of Attainder against Norfolk and Surrey was passed by Parliament. Surrey was tried at the Guildhall six days later, and condemned to death. He was executed on 19 January on Tower Hill, his being the last blood to be shed on the scaffold in Henry VIII's reign. Norfolk remained in the Tower, his fate hanging in the balance, while the King fought his last struggle with mortality. On 23 January, he announced the names of those men he had appointed to serve on the regency Council: Hertford was to be Lord Protector during Edward's minority, assisted by Cranmer, John Dudley, now Lord Lisle, Lord Chancellor Wriothesley, and others including the Queen's brother, the Earl of Essex, all of whom were known to be favourable to the cause of reform. When, however, someone suggested that Sir Thomas Seymour be one of their number, Henry cried out, 'No! No!', even though his breath was failing him. He knew Sir Thomas to be a self-seeker and a scoundrel, seeing clearly through the easy charm that so deceived others, and, of course, he had other, more personal reasons for resenting the man.

What killed Henry VIII was probably a clot detaching itself from the thrombosed vein in his leg, and causing a pulmonary embolism. On 26 January, he realised he was failing fast, and summoned his wife to his bedside. Then (according to William Thomas, who wrote *The Pilgrim: A Dialogue on the Life and Actions of King Henry the Eighth* that same month) he thanked God that, 'amongst all the happy successes of his reign' and 'after so many changes, his glorious chance hath brought him to die in the arms of so faithful a spouse'. Katherine was understandably overcome with emotion, for she had become attached to this complex man who was her husband, and whom she had so unwillingly married. In spite of his appalling matrimonial history, he had on the whole been very kind and generous to her, and she had no reason to doubt the sincerity of his affection for her. Now it was time to say farewell, and she began to weep. Henry spoke gently to her, saying, 'It is God's will that we should part,' then he gestured in the direction of the lords of the Council who were waiting near his bed and said:

> I order all these gentlemen to treat you as if I were living still, and if it should be your pleasure to marry again, I order that you shall have £7,000 for your service as long as you live, and all your jewels and ornaments.

At this, Katherine broke down completely, and could not answer. Henry ordered her out of the room, not wishing to witness or prolong her distress.

On the following morning, the King saw his confessor, received Holy Communion, and commended his soul to God. He saw his daughter Mary and made her promise to be a kind and loving mother to her brother, whom he would leave as 'a little helpless child'. Mary, in floods of tears, begged him not to leave her an orphan so soon, but the King said farewell and dismissed her. On that same day, a warrant was drawn up for the execution of the Duke of Norfolk, but Henry was still incapable of signing it. Norfolk would, as a result, languish for six years in the Tower, before being released to serve yet another Tudor sovereign.

Old rivalries died hard. The King sent a message to Francis I, rumoured to be dying of syphilis – he died a month later – bidding him remember that he too was mortal. Yet Henry himself was loath to hear any mention of death, and as it was high treason to mention the death of the King, those about him were reluctant to advise him to prepare his soul for its last journey. At length, Sir Anthony Denny, one of the King's most trusted advisers, ventured to tell him that 'in man's judgement, he was not like to live', and urged him to make ready his soul for death: 'All human aid was now vain, and it was meet for him to review his past life and seek for God's mercy through Christ.' The King listened meekly, then replied, 'After the judges have passed sentence on a criminal, there is no more need to trouble him. Therefore begone.' At this, the physicians withdrew from the room. Henry spoke again: 'The mercy of Christ could pardon all my sins, though they were greater than they be.' His advisers and attendants said they doubted that so great a man could have any sins on his conscience, but Henry shook his head feebly. He refused Sir Anthony Denny's offer to send for someone to hear his final confession and administer extreme unction, saying he would have 'only Cranmer, but he not yet'. Presently, he dozed off.

Shortly after midnight, the King woke and asked for his Archbishop, and a messenger was dispatched to Lambeth. Meanwhile Henry grew weaker, before heaving a sigh and whispering, 'All is lost.' But then, just in time, Cranmer arrived. Henry was now beyond speech, and the Archbishop, speaking gently, 'desired him to give him some token that he put his trust in God, through Jesus Christ'. The King's hand lay in his, and Cranmer felt him wring it hard, proof that his master 'trusted in the Lord'.

The minutes ticked by as everyone in the room silently knelt in prayer. At two o'clock in the morning, on 28 January 1547, King Henry VIII 'yielded his spirit to Almighty God and departed this world'. He was fifty-five.

It was the end of an era. England was now to be ruled by King Edward VI, a child of nine, although few as yet knew it. The old King's death was not announced for three days, although Queen Katherine, now Queen Dowager, was told of it immediately. She seems to have gone into seclusion for a while to mourn her husband, for there is no mention of her activities at this time in contemporary sources, nor did she attend the King's funeral, but that was for reasons of etiquette – women did not attend the funerals of kings. The new King was at Hertford Castle when his uncle, the Lord Protector, arrived on 30 January to take him to Enfield, where he found his sister Elizabeth waiting for him. The two children were then informed of their father's death, at which news they wept bitterly and could not be consoled. However, when Edward had calmed down, Hertford paid homage to him as his new sovereign lord, the other lords of the Council following suit. Then the little boy was brought to London, where, on 31 January, he was proclaimed king, while the Lord

Chancellor, with tears in his eyes, informed both Houses of Parliament of the death of Henry VIII. Early in February, the Lord Protector ordered the Council to send a messenger to Anne of Cleves to break the news to her.

On 14 February, the body of the late King began its last journey, conveyed in a coffin on a rich chariot covered with a pall of cloth of gold. Resting on the coffin was a wax effigy of the King dressed in velvet adorned with precious stones. The cortège was escorted by the lords of the Council, followed by a contingent of the King's guard. Behind the hearse trotted the King's riderless charger. Banners were carried aloft in the procession, but only two of the King's six wives were represented: Jane Seymour and Katherine Parr. Henry had not considered his other marriages worthy of commemoration.

That night, the King's body rested in the ruined chapel of Syon Abbey. There the lead coffin, weakened by the motion of the carriage, burst open, and liquid matter from the body seeped on to the church pavement. A dog was with the plumbers who came the next morning to repair the coffin, and it was seen to lick up the blood from the floor, just as Friar Peto had predicted back in 1532: that if the King cast off Katherine of Aragon and married Anne Boleyn, he should be as Ahab, and the dogs would lick his blood. Those who were witnesses to this macabre scene were understandably shaken by it, for the prophecy was well known and it was a superstitious age.

Two days later, Henry VIII's coffin was carried into St George's Chapel, Windsor, where a vast concourse of black-clad mourners awaited it. There in the choir lay the open vault containing the coffin of Queen Jane. Her husband's body was laid beside her amid 'heavy and dolorous lamentation'. Gardiner preached the funeral sermon, taking as his text 'Blessed are the dead who die in the Lord'; he spoke at length on the 'loss which both high and low have sustained in the death of so good and gracious a King'. As Sir Anthony Browne said afterwards, 'there was no need to pray for him, since he was surely in Heaven.'

At the end of the service, the officers of the late King's household broke their staves over their heads and cast them after the coffin into the vault 'with exceeding sorrow and heaviness, and not without grievous sighs or tears'. Thus did they signify the termination of their allegiance and service. Then the herald cried, '*Le roi est mort! Vive le roi!*'

Far away, the young King shed bitter tears. 'This, however, consoles us,' he wrote, 'that he is now in Heaven, and that he hath gone out of this miserable world into happy and everlasting blessedness.'

It would be true to say that Henry's contemporaries saw him as something more than human. One called him 'the greatest man in the world', another 'the rarest man that lived in his time'. He certainly possessed exceptional qualities of leadership and a charismatic personality. No king of England has enjoyed such posthumous publicity as he, and no king before him or after him ever held such absolute power, nor commanded such respect and obedience. This is the measure of the man.

In his capacity as a husband Henry's worst failings were glaringly obvious. The deepest, most abiding passion in his life was for Anne Boleyn, yet it was a destructive one, souring with the familiarity of marriage and leaving the King embittered. Her death was contrived for political reasons rather than emotional ones, and Henry did not scruple to get rid of her for the sake of expediency. It is possible to feel sympathy for him after his discovery of Katherine Howard's promiscuity, yet we must remember that his sorrow did not prevent him from executing an ignorant seventeen-year-old girl as a traitor. His marriages to Katherine of Aragon and Anne of Cleves were both annulled, and Katherine was treated with appalling cruelty.

The guiding motive behind his treatment, or ill-treatment, of these four of his wives was the King's very real need for a male heir, something that was always at the forefront of his mind. It should be remembered, in his favour, that Katherine Parr showed a very genuine grief at his death, and that – apart from one occasion, when it appears that Henry kept an open mind about Katherine's activities until proof was available – they were extremely contented together, as their letters prove. Nor did Jane Seymour find Henry less than a loving, if overbearing, husband. What turned the King into the ruthless tyrant of latter years was to some extent Katherine of Aragon's stubbornness and Anne Boleyn's ambition. Taking into account the ever-present problem of the succession, it is impossible to dismiss Henry VIII as the cruel lecher of popular legend who changed wives whenever it pleased him.

His subjects certainly did not view him in that light. He never lost their affection, even during his worst excesses, nor did he ever cease to exercise that charm and common touch that came so easily to his dynasty. Out of the ruins of his marriages and the monasteries, he founded a new church and corrected abuses within it, a policy which certainly found favour with the English in the long run. Although he was a Catholic to the last and rigorous in stamping out heresy, he had the foresight to realise that religious developments in England would lead eventually to a Protestant state – there is proof of this in his choice of the men who were to sit on the regency Council. When he died, he was regarded by his subjects as 'King, Emperor and Pope in his own dominions' and as the 'father and nurse' of his people. For all his faults, he would be remembered with love by them.

17
Under the planets at Chelsea

Katherine Parr was not given a place on the regency Council by Henry VIII. He had foreseen that, being a very rich, attractive, royal widow, the chances were that she would marry again within a short while, and that the advent of a new husband upon the scene might well create discord, especially if – as Henry suspected – he was called Thomas Seymour. Added to this, she was a woman, and Henry had never approved of female rulers. Indeed, Katherine had never sought power, and she had very little to complain about. She was well provided for and, at nearly thirty-five, free to order her life as she pleased. If she remarried, she could now choose for herself, and there was, perhaps, still the possibility of her having children of her own, something she had always desired.

The only thing that pained her was that the Council quickly made it very clear that the young King was under its exclusive control; this meant that Edward was not allowed to see either his stepmother or his stepsisters, his guardians being jealous of any outside influences upon him. The boy missed their company, and consoled himself by corresponding with them, yet he was upset when he learned in early February that the Queen Dowager was planning to leave the court and retire to the Old Manor at Chelsea, one of his father's properties. 'Farewell, venerated Queen,' he wrote, knowing he would rarely see his stepmother in the future.

Very early on in the new reign, it was made clear that the sympathies of the Lord Protector and the Council were with the

Protestants, which meant that people like Katherine Parr could now practise the reformed faith openly, without fear of persecution from the government. The King, who had been educated by scholars such as John Cheke and others, who were committed if secret Lutherans, had himself already embraced the Protestant religion, and would in time become one of its most fervent exponents. Moreover, Archbishop Cranmer – who as long ago as the 1530s had been a closet Lutheran – was still Primate of the Church of England. It would only be a matter of time before the heresy laws were repealed; in fact, during Edward's reign, it would be the English Catholics who suffered persecution, the reformist party having finally gained ascendancy.

On the day of the late King's funeral, the Lord Protector conferred patents of nobility upon himself and his fellow councillors. He himself became Duke of Somerset, a title once borne by the King's Beaufort forbears, and lastly by Henry VIII's infant brother Edmund. William Parr was created Marquess of Northampton, and Wriothesley was made Earl of Southampton. Sir Thomas Seymour was back in England and able to appear at court without fear of banishment on yet another diplomatic mission. Perhaps to compensate for his exclusion from the regency Council, his brother had him elevated to the peerage as Baron Seymour of Sudeley Castle in the county of Gloucestershire, and on the next day confirmed him in his post as Lord High Admiral for life, at the same time admitting him to the Order of the Garter.

Lord Sudeley was then about forty years old, good looking, charming, and very popular. Katherine Parr had fallen victim to his looks and dashing personality before her marriage to the King, and she and Seymour had even discussed marriage at that time. During her years as queen Katherine had resolutely put Seymour out of her mind and the Admiral had played his part, though it seems that he quickly forgot about Katherine, being a rather shallow man. His contemporary and Edward VI's biographer, Sir John Hayward, described him as 'fierce in courage, courtly in fashion, in personage stately and in voice magnificent', but, he added, he was 'somewhat empty in matter'.

Lord Sudeley found it galling to be denied what he considered to be his rightful place on the regency Council; after all, he was the

King's uncle, and his brother was Lord Protector. He had also served his country both as a diplomat and on the high seas, and he was determined to get on the Council, and perhaps even supplant his brother, of whom he was very jealous. To do that, he needed power and he needed money, and the best way to gain both was by an influential marriage. With this in mind, Seymour went straight to the top. He did not at first renew his suit to Katherine Parr: she was, after all, only the late King's widow, and completely lacking in influence in a court from which she was about to depart. Real power would come with a marriage to one of the King's sisters, who were next in line of succession, a move which might, in time, bring Lord Sudeley a crown.

The Lady Mary was a staunch Catholic, so he passed her over. That left the Lady Elizabeth. She had a proud and disdainful manner which sometimes eclipsed the beauty of her red-gold hair and the flashing eyes she had inherited from her mother, yet she also had her mother's capacity for flirtation and her attraction for men, and even at thirteen, the Admiral thought her eminently desirable. In February, he began to court her, declaring his affection in flattering letters, and begging to know 'whether I am to be the most happy or the most miserable of men'.

Elizabeth did not reply at once, having a shrewd idea of what lay behind the Admiral's letters. All the same, it was flattering for a young girl to be the object of attention from such a handsome and sought-after man. Yet Elizabeth was not any young girl, and she had to have the Council's permission if she wished to marry; it was unlikely to be granted in this case. Consequently, she turned down Seymour's proposal, saying 'neither my age nor my inclination allows me to think of marriage', and that she needed at least two years to get over the loss of her father before contemplating it. She went on:

Permit me, my Lord Admiral, to tell you frankly that, though I decline the happiness of becoming your wife, I shall never cease to interest myself in all that can crown your merit with glory, and shall ever feel the greatest pleasure in being your servant and good friend.

The Admiral was crestfallen at her refusal, which had the effect of making her seem all the more desirable, but he had to recognise the fact that she was not his for the taking. It was at this point that he turned his attentions once more to Katherine Parr.

At the beginning of March the Dowager Queen was about to leave the court for Chelsea when she realised that her former lover was eager to renew their relationship. This knowledge was more than welcome to her, for she was still strongly attracted to Seymour and eager to share what remained of her youth with him. Thus their courtship proceeded, although it had, of necessity, to be conducted in secret in case the Council found out and forbade its continuance. Katherine was officially mourning Henry VIII, and could not with honour contemplate remarriage in the near future, yet so happy was she at this latest turn of events that, just before she left court, she could not resist confiding her feelings for the Admiral to her friend, Lady Paget, who replied, 'All I wish you, Madam, is that he should become your husband.' Katherine answered that she wished 'it had been her fate to have him for a husband, but God hath so placed her that any lowering of her condition would be a reproach to her'. These doubts soon receded, however, under the force of Seymour's charm, and when, that March, he proposed marriage, Katherine gladly accepted, for she was now, for the first time in her life, deeply in love. She stipulated that a suitable period of mourning must elapse before the wedding could take place, but the Admiral overruled her, urging her to marry him in secret at once. And at that, sensible, virtuous, but all-too-human Katherine Parr seized what she saw as her last chance of happiness with a man she loved; she was not, after all, so young that she could afford to waste time, and she could battle no longer with the strong emotions that were overwhelming her. Lord Sudeley was delighted; if he could not aspire to a crown, he would at least be rich, and the husband of the first lady at court accorded precedence over nearly everyone else. He would have money, prestige and a devoted wife. What more could a man want?

There were, however, obstacles: it was unlikely that the Council would approve of his marriage to the Dowager Queen, and more than probable that it would withhold its consent, if only because there might be reason to dispute the paternity of any child born to the Queen so soon after her late husband's death, which would put the succession in jeopardy. Henry VIII had, after all, only been dead for six weeks. The Admiral did not care about technicalities, and he decided to bypass the Council and go straight to the young King for permission to marry. Edward was fond of his colourful Uncle Thomas, and might well agree, and the Admiral considered it unlikely that the Council would gainsay him. In this, he showed considerable lack of judgement.

Edward, unfortunately, was kept well guarded, and not allowed to see anyone unless the Council had first sanctioned it. Sudeley therefore bribed one of the royal servants, John Fowler – a man known to be an admirer of the Queen, and trustworthy – to sound Edward out on 'whom he would have to be my wife'. Fowler saw the King later that night, and said he marvelled that the Lord Admiral was not yet married; was the King content that he should marry? 'Yea, very well,' replied Edward. Then said Fowler, 'Whom would your Grace like him to marry?' The boy considered for a minute. 'My Lady Anne of Cleves!' he piped up, but then he thought again. 'I would he married my sister Mary, to turn her opinions.' (Edward deplored Mary's adherence to Catholicism.) That was not, of course, the answer that Fowler had been hoping for, or the Admiral. But the Admiral was well aware that the Council kept the young King chronically short of money, and so he sent Fowler back the next night, well supplied with gold coins, to ask Edward 'if he should be contented I should marry the Queen'. To the Admiral's delight, Edward did not hesitate to signify his approval and consent: he was fond of his stepmother and his uncle, and did not understand the political motive behind Sudeley's proposal.

It was at this time that the Queen moved to the Old Manor House at Chelsea, which occupied an extensive site at the eastern end of what is now Cheyne Walk. It had been built by Henry VIII in 1536–7 for Jane Seymour, although she never lived there. Of red brick, it bore some resemblance to St James's Palace, which was built around the same time, although it was only two storeys in height and was built around two quadrangles. It was quite a large house, more than adequate for a queen dowager, with its three halls, three parlours, three kitchens, three drawing-rooms, seventeen chambers, four closets, three cellars, a larder, a large staircase, summer rooms (presumably without fireplaces or open on one side), and nine other rooms. It had casement windows and a water supply brought by a conduit from Kensington, and its most attractive feature was its five acres of beautiful gardens intersected by privet hedges and containing a fishpond and a variety of trees: cherry, peach, damson and nut. There were also 200 damask rose bushes.

Katherine was at Chelsea when the Admiral called to inform her of the King's consent to their marriage. Now that she was away from the public arena of the court, it would be easier to make secret preparations for her wedding, which she hoped would take place as soon as possible. Yet, while Katherine was thus happily preoccupied Sudeley's mind was on more contentious issues. He had already proved to himself that it was better to bypass the Council and go direct to the young King to get what he wanted, and he saw no reason why he should not capitalise further on Edward's admiration and affection for him. He even foresaw the day when he might ultimately rule through the King, and planned to achieve this by providing Edward with a consort who had been trained to be sympathetic to the Admiral's interests. It did not matter that the Council was already contemplating a marriage between Edward and Elisabeth of France, daughter of the new French King, Henry II; the Admiral thought he had a better candidate, one to whom Edward was close, and of whom he would thoroughly approve, for, whereas the Princess Elisabeth was a Roman Catholic, this girl was already a committed Protestant. Her name was the Lady Jane Grey, and she was the eldest daughter of the Marquess of Dorset by Henry VIII's niece, Frances Brandon, daughter of Mary Tudor and the Duke of Suffolk. Jane was almost the same age as Edward, having been born in the same month; she had been named after his mother, Jane Seymour. Her parents had arranged for her to receive a very thorough academic education from Protestant tutors, which had already developed her formidable intellect far beyond what was normal for a child of her years. As a result, she was precocious, strong willed and an intellectual snob, as well as being completely dedicated to Protestantism. Notwithstanding this, her parents demanded still more of her, and beat her when she did not come up to their expectations. As a result, her home life was desperately unhappy, and the only solace she knew was in the hours she spent with her tutors.

It was the Admiral's plan to make Jane his ward and have her join the household at Chelsea after his marriage so that the Queen could supervise her education. Sudeley saw no reason why Lord Dorset should refuse such an offer; indeed, any father with ambitions for his child would be glad of it, with its advantage of an education under the auspices of one of the most erudite women of the age, and its prospects of a good marriage for Jane when the time came – a royal one, if the Admiral had his way. Yet when Lord Sudeley's man, William Harrington, broached the matter with Lord Dorset at the latter's house at Bradgate in Leicestershire, the Marquess was unimpressed, even when informed that the Admiral hoped to match his daughter with the King. He wanted to know who would look after the child, since he had not been let into the secret of the Admiral's impending marriage, and could not see how Lord Sudeley was placed to arrange a match between the King and Jane when he was not even on the regency Council. To Dorset, it seemed a futile plan at best, and he privately doubted whether the Admiral's intentions were honourable, so he withheld his permission, and Jane stayed at home.

The Admiral was disappointed, but not unduly so, foreseeing that in time to come fathers would be queuing up to place their daughters in the household of the Queen Dowager, especially when it was known that her husband enjoyed the special favour of the King. He could afford to wait.

The Queen, meanwhile, was wondering how the news of her marriage would be received at court, and by her stepchildren. Edward would be glad for her, she knew, and perhaps Elizabeth, but in all likelihood Mary would disapprove, thinking it accomplished in indecent haste and disrespectful to her father's memory. Mary kept away from the court nowadays; there was no place for her there, and she preferred to live in the country where there was no one to censure her for following what she believed to be the true faith. At this time, she was arranging with the Duchess of Somerset, who had once served Katherine of Aragon, to reward those servants of her mother who were still living, thus fulfilling a desire she had cherished for eleven years.

Katherine Parr was still officially in mourning for the late King when she married the Lord Admiral some time before the end of

April, probably at Chelsea. Very few knew of it, for it was conducted with such secrecy that it is impossible to determine a date. Sir Nicholas Throckmorton, the Queen's cousin, may have been a witness. The King learned of the marriage in May, for he recorded it then in his journal, but the world at large did not hear of it until it was already several weeks old. Thus Katherine Parr was married for the fourth time, making her England's most married Queen. Yet, unlike her previous marriages, this was her own choice, and for a time at least she knew great happiness, unworried by the prospect of inevitable censure from the outside world. 'If the Duke [of Somerset] and the Duchess do not like the marriage, it will be of no consequence,' she told her husband, knowing that her sister-in-law would be jealous, and that it would anger the proud Duchess to have the wife of her husband's younger brother taking precedence over her, especially when the Duchess's husband was Lord Protector of England. Somerset himself was a mild and rational man and, although he would be much displeased to learn of his brother's marriage, he would in time have come to accept it with good grace had it not been for his wife, who never ceased urging him to punish the couple for their temerity. The Duchess Anne was an intolerable woman whose pride was monstrous, a termagant who exercised much influence over her weaker husband by the lash of her tongue.

Knowing that they would make a bitter enemy of the Duchess did not unduly concern the Admiral and his bride. They had flouted the authorities, defied convention, and even jeopardised the succession, but this meant little in comparison to the joy they found in each other. Initially, this was a passion that had to be indulged in secret (which undoubtedly gave it added spice), at least until Katherine invited the Lord Protector to come to Chelsea on 18 May to break the news to him. Until then, there were secret meetings at Chelsea, and love-letters between husband and wife, who had decided that the safer course was to live apart for the present. Katherine states in one letter that she had promised to restrict herself to writing once a fortnight; however, she could not restrain herself from writing more frequently, although she was happily busy and found that 'weeks be shorter at Chelsea than in other places'. Referring to her feelings for the Admiral, she went on to say:

I would not have you think that this, mine honest goodwill towards you, proceeds from any sudden motion of passion; for, as truly as God is God, my mind was fully bent the other time I was at liberty to marry you before any man I know. Howbeit, God withstood my will therein most vehemently for a time, and through His grace and goodness made that seem possible which seemed to me most impossible: that was, made me renounce utterly mine own will, and follow His most willingly. It were long to write all the process of this matter. If I live, I shall declare it to you myself. I can say nothing, but – as my Lady of Suffolk saith – God is a marvellous man. By her that is yours to serve and obey during life, Katherine the Queen, K.P.

On 17 May, Sudeley replied to his wife's letter. He was staying with her sister and Lord Herbert in London and had suffered some anxious moments there, as Lady Herbert seemed to know that he had been visiting Chelsea Old Manor at night. He denied it, yet Lady Herbert pressed the point and made it obvious that she knew very well there was something going on between the Admiral and her sister. Sudeley, blushing with embarrassment, asked her where she had heard such things, and she confessed that Katherine had confided the truth to her. The Admiral related all this in his letter to his wife, thanking her for asking her sister to invite him, 'For, by her company, in default of yours, I shall shorten the weeks in these parts, which heretofore were three days longer than they were under the planets at Chelsea.' He ended by saying he was going to take Lady Herbert's advice about how to obtain the goodwill of the Council and, more importantly, his brother. He begged the Queen to write to him every three days, and to send him one of a series of miniatures she had of herself, and signed himself as 'him whom ye have bound to honour, love and in all lawful things obey'. The letter is deferential, as to the Queen, and very formal, and shows that the Admiral was well aware of the difference between his station and Katherine's.

The Lord Protector did not turn up at Chelsea on 18 May, and sent word he would not be able to come until the end of the month. The Admiral was by now concerned about his brother's reaction to his marriage, and wrote again to Katherine, telling her that, when she saw Somerset, she must press for a public announcement of their union within two months; previously, he had thought it wise to conceal it for as long as two years, with the Protector's consent, but now, after weeks of living apart from his bride, he was reluctant to play the role of secret husband for that length of time. He confessed also to Katherine that he was worried about how to win over his brother's support. To this she replied sensibly that to deny his request to announce the marriage soon would be an act of folly on the part of the Protector, since news of it might well leak out, or the couple's clandestine meetings would be noticed. Either would cause a scandal which would touch the entire Seymour clan and discredit the family, the last thing the Protector would want.

Katherine emphasised that she did not want the Admiral to beg for his brother's goodwill if it was not given freely from the first. It would be better if he obtained letters from the King in his favour, and also the support of certain members of the Privy Council, if possible, 'which thing shall be no small shame to your brother and loving sister if they do not the like'. Next time he visited her, she said, he must come early in the morning and be gone by seven o'clock, having warned her beforehand of the time of his arrival, so that she could 'wait at the gate of the field for you'.

This state of affairs could not and did not last very much longer. At the end of May, when Somerset fulfilled his promise and came to dine with the Queen at Chelsea, she informed him of her marriage. He, in turn, broke the news to the Council. 'The Lord Protector was much offended,' noted the King in his journal, mainly because of the threat to the succession but also because he had not been consulted. The matter was debated at great length by the Privy Council, it being argued that, if the Queen was already pregnant, 'a great doubt' would exist as to 'whether the child born should have been accounted the late King's or [the Admiral's], whereby a marvellous danger might have ensued to the quiet of the realm'. Lord Sudeley was summoned to account for his actions, but at the end of the day there was little anyone could do. The marriage had been lawfully solemnised before witnesses and consummated. It was, anyway, late May: King Henry had been dead for four months, and his widow showed no signs of pregnancy, which was fortunate for the Admiral and for Katherine, for it meant that the Protector was prepared to overlook the small risk to the succession occasioned by their marriage. All the same, Somerset made his displeasure clear, and his wife was mortified at the news. The only person who remained calm was the young King, who, on 30 May, in defiance of the advice of his Council, took it upon himself to write and congratulate Queen Katherine upon her marriage, and to thank her for the many letters she had sent him since she left court. In his letter, he spoke affectionately of 'the great love' she had borne his father, her goodwill towards himself, and lastly her 'godliness and knowledge in learning and the scriptures'. If there was 'anything wherein I may do you a kindness, either in word or deed,' he ended, 'I will do it willingly.'

Katherine responded by begging the King to plead her case with the Council, which he did at the beginning of June, saying that he had known for some time that the Admiral intended marrying the Queen, and that he had sent a letter signifying his approval to Katherine. He did not divulge that the Admiral, knowing he was kept short of funds, had paid him well to do so, nor did he say that he had so phrased his letter as to request his stepmother to accept the Admiral in marriage, thus leaving her – as a loyal subject – no alternative. Against the authority of the King, Somerset was powerless; he was also a peace-loving man who loathed dissension, and he was glad enough to be reconciled with his brother and new sister-in-law. Thus he and the Council grudgingly sanctioned the marriage, giving the Admiral leave to take up residence at Chelsea with his wife.

Naturally, many people were scandalised when news of the marriage leaked out at court, and none more so than the Lady Mary, whose respect for Katherine Parr was shattered in a single blow.

Mary received a letter from the Admiral asking for her to use her influence to gain him favour with the Council, and also begging her to persuade the Queen to agree to the immediate public proclamation of their marriage. Mary was horrified at his impertinence, and dispatched a frigid reply, saying:

It standeth least with my poor honour to be a meddler in this matter, considering whose wife her Grace was of late. If the remembrance of the King's Majesty will not suffer her to grant your suit, I am nothing able to persuade her to forget the loss of him who is yet very ripe in mine own remembrance.

Where matters of the heart were concerned, she said, 'being a maid, I am nothing cunning'. By the time the Admiral received Mary's reply, he no longer needed her help and could afford to ignore her as Katherine had come round to his way of thinking and agreed that their marriage should be made public. She grieved, nevertheless, for the loss of Mary's friendship, fearing that her marriage and the widening religious gulf between them would ensure that it was never likely to be regained.

It then occurred to Mary that her sister Elizabeth might put herself morally at risk by contact with their stepmother; Mary was determined to protect her innocence and prevent her from associating with Katherine, and she wrote at once to Elizabeth, warning her against contact with such wickedness and begging her to think of her own reputation. But Elizabeth, who was fond of her stepmother and had good reason to know why she had fallen prey to the Admiral's charm, would only write a non-committal reply saying she shared Mary's 'just grief' in seeing the 'scarcely cold body of the King our father so shamefully dishonoured by the Queen our stepmother', and that she could not express 'how much affliction I suffered when I was first informed of this marriage'. However, she rationalised, neither she nor Mary were 'in such condition as to offer any obstacle thereto', and the Seymours were all powerful, having 'got all the authority into their hands'. In her opinion, the best course to take was one of dissimulation and 'making the best of what we cannot remedy'. With regard to visiting the Queen, 'the position in which I stand' and 'the Queen having shown me so much affection' obliged her to 'use much tact in manoeuvring with her, for fear of appearing ungrateful for her benefits. I shall not, however, be in any hurry to visit her, lest I should be charged with approving what I ought to censure.' In other words, she would bide her time until the furore had died down, and then do as she pleased.

Although she had married a mere baron, Katherine was yet entitled to retain and enjoy all the privileges of queenship, and now that she was known to be respectably married, she saw no reason why she should not go to court with her new husband from time to time and take her rightful place there. Accordingly, she moved the Admiral to request his brother the Protector to deliver to her the jewels traditionally worn by the queens of England, which were at that time in safe keeping in the Treasury. It was Katherine's legal right to wear them until such time as King Edward had a consort of his own, but the Duchess of Somerset had already decided that, as wife of the Lord Protector, the jewels would adorn her own person and not that of her sister-in-law. When she heard of the Queen's request, she saw the perfect opportunity to have her revenge, and wasted no time in putting pressure on her husband to make him refuse the Admiral's request.

Somerset dithered. The Admiral, impatient now, complained to the Council, saying the Protector should 'let me have mine own'. Of course, he knew very well – as did Katherine – who was causing the trouble, and when it came to a deadlock he did not hesitate to name her. From that time onwards, it was open warfare between the Duchess and the Queen. According to the Elizabethan historian William Camden, Anne Stanhope bore Katherine Parr 'such invincible hatred', and had done since the days they had sparred over 'light causes and women's quarrels'. Now the root cause of her enmity was jealousy because Katherine had precedence over her. She was to prove, in every respect, a formidable enemy.

When Katherine Parr returned to court for a visit in June, the Duchess was waiting for her. The Queen had still not been given her jewels, and was feeling annoyed. Nevertheless, she insisted on being shown every deference due to her rank, and commanded the Duchess to carry her train for her. This was a duty to which great honour was attached, but the Duchess only understood that she was being put very firmly in her place. Livid, she refused, saying 'It was unsuitable for her to submit to perform that service for the wife of her husband's younger brother.' Katherine bore the insult in silence, but she did not forget it. After that the Duchess made no secret of her animosity and did all she could to undermine the respect in which many people at court still held the Queen and to blacken her reputation. She would recall how the late King had married Katherine Parr 'in his doting days, when he had brought himself so low by his lust and cruelty that no lady who stood on her honour would venture on him.' Why, therefore, should she herself give place 'to her who in her former estate was but Latimer's widow, and is now fain to cast herself for support upon a younger brother? If Master Admiral teach his brother no better manners, I am she that will!'

While her husband was away at court, Katherine received a letter from the Lord Protector telling her she could not have the jewels. The Queen knew very well why not, and flew into a fury, only calming down to write and tell her husband the news.

> My lord your brother hath this afternoon made me a little warm! [she fumed] It was fortunate we were so much distant, for I suppose else I should have bitten him! What cause have they to fear, having such a wife? It is requisite for them to pray continually for a short despatch of that hell. Tomorrow, or else upon Saturday, I will see the King, when I intend to utter all my choler to my lord your brother, if you shall not give me advice to the contrary.

It seems, however, that either the Admiral advised his wife against such a course, or she changed her mind about going, perhaps fearing another public snub by the Duchess of Somerset.

After that supreme insult, Katherine refused to return to the court, remaining at Chelsea until she and her husband moved to the country a year later. Her reign was effectively over – that much had been made clear to her. Happy in her marriage and with time to pursue her intellectual interests, she was in fact content enough now to play the role of private gentlewoman.

On 25 June, Katherine received a letter from the King, telling her she need not fear any further recriminations regarding her marriage to Sudeley, and assuring her that 'I will so provide for you both that if hereafter any grief befall, I shall be a sufficient succour in your godly and praisable enterprises.' It gave the young King great pleasure to think of himself as the instigator of a marriage that had brought his stepmother and his favourite uncle such happiness and, although in reality he was powerless to help them further – for example, he was unable to arrange for Katherine's jewels to be restored to her – the knowledge of his goodwill was a comfort to the Queen. He wrote whenever he could, which was not often for he was rarely 'half an hour alone', and when he could not write, he sent a message of goodwill. In return, the Admiral supplied him secretly with pocket money, of which the Protector kept him very short. This only increased Edward's gratitude, and the Admiral was hopeful that, when the day came for him to propose a marriage between the King and the Lady Jane Grey, Edward would be more than amenable. The Admiral had not abandoned his master plan; he had only to wait, and in time Lord Dorset would come running.

Somerset realised he had acted unfairly, yet he dared not risk offending his wife, who was so jubilant now that victory was hers. Instead, as compensation for the loss of the jewels, he conferred upon his brother the office of Captain General and Protector's Lieutenant in the South of England, and in that same month of August made a grant to him of the manor of Sudeley, with the castle. The Admiral was delighted; situated just south of the village of Winchcombe in Gloucestershire, and set in a beautiful park, the main fabric of the castle dated from the late fifteenth century, and had been grafted on to an earlier manor house by Richard III. It had a chapel, and was in every way a residence fit for a queen with an ambitious husband. Today, much of what can be seen at Sudeley is a Victorian reconstruction, though the ruins of part of the old castle remain to give some idea of what it must have been like in Katherine's day.

The Admiral gave orders immediately for the castle to be renovated and made ready for occupation; he and the Queen hoped it would be habitable within a year, then they could escape from the hostile climate of London and the court for a while to lead the lives of wealthy country gentry. For the present, Katherine spent her time reading, writing or at her devotions. Her second book, *The Lamentations of a Sinner*, was now completed, and both her brother, Lord Northampton, and her friend, the Duchess of Suffolk, urged her to have it printed. She agreed to do so, and in November the first copies went on sale with an introduction by a young lawyer called William Cecil, who would later become Queen Elizabeth's councillor Lord Burleigh. Cecil wrote that he joined all 'ladies of estate' in following 'our Queen in virtue as in honour' in order to taste 'everlasting bliss'. The book was an even greater success than *Prayers and Meditations* had been, and was highly praised by scholars everywhere, thus sustaining Katherine's reputation as a woman of learning.

It was at this time that she invited her stepdaughter Elizabeth to join her household at Chelsea. Elizabeth had been at court, but she had not been very happy there. The introduction of rigid ceremonial required her to drop on one knee five times in front of her brother before seating herself on a mean bench far from his side. The Queen was probably aware of Elizabeth's situation, and sought to rescue her, and Elizabeth responded with enthusiasm, arriving at Chelsea early in the new year of 1548. The scandal surrounding the Queen's remarriage had long since died down, and her stepdaughter saw no reason why she should not move in with her. Katherine thought it an ideal arrangement: she could oversee Elizabeth's education once more, chaperon her through her development to womanhood, and enjoy the stimulating company of her excellent mind.

Katherine's decision to invite Elizabeth into her household was to precipitate a tragedy. She had no idea, of course, that her husband had once tried to marry Elizabeth, still less that he had seen her as an infinitely more desirable catch than a dowager queen. It never occurred to her that this slight young girl of fourteen would hold any attraction for the Admiral. From the first, the situation was fraught. In spite of herself, Elizabeth was fascinated by the handsome 'stepfather' – as the Admiral was pleased to call himself – who welcomed her with undisguised affection to her new home, and wasted no time in making it clear to her that he found her both stimulating and desirable.

He took care to conceal this from his wife, who so implicitly trusted him that she suspected nothing. She regarded Elizabeth as a child still, the orphan she had taken under her wing, an innocent whom she could guide and nurture and who would be a cherished daughter to both Katherine and her husband. The Admiral had other ideas. So did Elizabeth. As the short winter days lengthened, so did their mutual attraction develop, under the guise of an affectionate relationship between stepfather and daughter. There was no outward hint of the sexual tension between them. Both knew that if they acknowledged it they risked wounding the woman who meant a great deal to both of them.

Cocooned in her marriage, Katherine settled into her new life, a stepmother once more. On 15 January 1548, she and the Admiral attended her brother's wedding to Elizabeth Brooke, the daughter of Lord Cobham. Then, in February, the Admiral again approached Lord Dorset about the wardship of the Lady Jane Grey. To sweeten Dorset, he had installed in the Old Manor his aged mother, Lady Seymour, who would treat Jane 'as if she were her own daughter'. As for Queen Katherine, she would be only too happy to order Jane's education, and the Lady Elizabeth would provide eminently suitable companionship. It all looked very respectable, and this time Dorset leaped at the chance, as the Admiral had known he would.

Thus Jane came to join the household at Chelsea. It was a welcome change for her. She was at last out of the clutches of the parents who had made her life a misery, and of whom she strongly disapproved. There were no beatings at Chelsea, no harsh words. The Queen, the Admiral, and the Lady Elizabeth all seemed intent on enjoying their peaceful existence there, and Lady Seymour was like an affectionate grandmother. Jane could freely follow the Protestant faith to which she was devoted, and there was also freedom to study without the ever-present fear of parental criticism.

Jane was a small, thin child, yet graceful. She had small features and a well-shaped nose, with arched eyebrows darker than her hair, which was of a reddish colour. She had sparkling eyes and freckles, and to some extent resembled her cousin Elizabeth, with whom she took her lessons. The Queen herself supervised the girls' studies, and was careful to appoint tutors who would cultivate the proper attitudes to religion and learning in their minds. Katherine won so much praise for her endeavours in this respect that other ladies of noble birth did their best to emulate her, and not long afterwards Nicholas Udall, the Provost of Eton College, was writing to the Queen with the highest praise for what she had achieved through her influence.

When I consider, most gracious Queen Katherine [he wrote], the great number of noble women in this our time and country of England, not only given to the study of human sciences and of strange tongues, but also so thoroughly expert in Holy Scriptures, that they are able to compare with the best writers, as well in penning of godly and fruitful treatises to the instruction and edifying of the whole realm in the knowledge of God, as also in translating good books out of Latin or Greek into English for the use of such as are rude and ignorant of the said tongues, it is now no news at all to see queens and ladies of most high estate and progeny, instead of courtly dalliance, embrace virtuous exercises, reading and writing, and with most earnest study, apply themselves to the acquiring of knowledge.

Katherine's own household, he went on, was famous as the place 'where it is now a common thing to see young virgins so trained in the study of good letters that they willingly set all other vain pastimes at naught for learning's sake.' This much had Katherine accomplished for her own sex, whose education had by now been freed from many of the taboos formerly attached to it. Thanks to the Queen's influence, the learned female had become fashionable, and a pattern had been set for the future.

In February, Elizabeth asked her stepmother if she might have the renowned Roger Ascham as her tutor instead of Mr Grindal. Katherine, who had long corresponded with Ascham on scholarly matters, warmly approved of the change and Ascham arrived at Chelsea later that month, after Katherine and her husband had gone to stay at the London house of Lord and Lady Herbert. There was a family scandal brewing, and the Parrs were taking counsel together. It was only a month since William Parr, the Marquess of Northampton, had married Elizabeth Brooke, yet already it was being alleged by the Privy Council that his divorce from Anne Bourchier had not been legal. When this was confirmed, Northampton was ordered to put away his new wife, and never speak to her again on pain of death, as his true wife was still living. This was a blow for Parr, and a grievous disappointment for Katherine, since it was she, along with the Duchess of Suffolk, who had suggested and promoted the union with Elizabeth Brooke. Yet there was nothing that she or anyone else could do about this new situation, and before very long the Admiral took her back to Chelsea.

Then, early in March 1548, after more than twenty years of married life with four husbands, Katherine Parr discovered that she was at long last to have a child. Both she and the Admiral were delighted. Good wishes came pouring in, as well as plenty of advice and warnings to take care of herself, for she was, by the standards of her time, well into middle age and rather old to be having a first child. Nevertheless, she seems to have enjoyed good health throughout most of her pregnancy.

So wrapped up was the Queen in her personal happiness, that she failed to notice what was going on under her nose. For her husband, considering his wife to be suitably occupied with approaching motherhood, had now renewed his pursuit of the Lady Elizabeth. The Queen did not realise that while she was at her daily prayers, which took place regularly each morning and afternoon, her husband would always be elsewhere, nor did she suspect anything when Elizabeth began making excuses to be absent. The Admiral would openly romp with Elizabeth in front of members of the household, so that no one would think anything of it, and when he and the Queen stayed with Elizabeth at Seymour Place in London that spring, he went up to Elizabeth's bedroom every morning, wearing only his night-gown and slippers, and burst in, regardless of whether or not she was in bed. Her lady-in-waiting, Mrs Katherine Ashley, was present, and was immediately suspicious, thinking it 'an unseemly sight to see a man so little dressed in a maiden's chamber'. She made her feelings very clear to the Admiral, which angered him, but he did at least go away on that occasion. What really disturbed Mrs Ashley, according to her later deposition to the Privy Council, was that he only stayed if Elizabeth was in bed; if he found her up and dressed, he would just look in at the gallery door, then leave.

Lord Sudeley was irritated by Mrs Ashley's attitude, but he was undeterred by it, and it only served to make him all the more determined to have what he wanted. Elizabeth was ripe for seduction and probably willing enough; she was at a highly impressionable age, and very flattered that the dashing Admiral's attentions were focused upon her. Not for nothing was she Anne Boleyn's daughter, and male admiration was already the breath of life to her, while her budding sexuality was aroused. It is likely that she was rather frightened at the prospect of the sex act itself, and yet equally likely that her passion for the Admiral would have overcome her fear and her good sense, given time.

The morning visits continued, to Mrs Ashley's dismay. The Admiral would go into Elizabeth's bedchamber and tickle her as she lay in her bed, clad only in her night-gown. Once he tried to kiss her, but Mrs Ashley was there and ordered him out 'for shame'. However, he was back the next morning, and most mornings thereafter. What was more, Elizabeth did not rebuff him; she was thoroughly enjoying it. Soon, matters had reached the stage where the Admiral would bid her good morning, ask how she did, and smack her on the back or buttocks with great familiarity. Then he would go back to his rooms, or go to the maids' room and flirt with them.

The Queen saw nothing wrong in all this. Her husband had told her about it, knowing full well that she still regarded her stepdaughter as a child. She raised no protest when she heard that the Admiral would pull apart Elizabeth's bed-curtains and 'make as though he would come at her', causing her to shrink back giggling into the bed to avoid being tickled. The Admiral said it was harmless, and the Queen believed him. Mrs Ashley, however, was not so sure; and she was concerned about her charge's reputation. One day, when the Admiral chased Elizabeth out from behind the bed-curtains where she had hidden with her maids, the lady-in-waiting spoke to him, and said there had been complaints about his behaviour and that 'my lady was evil spoken of', presumably among the servants. The Admiral answered that he would report to the Protector 'how I am slandered,' but Mrs Ashley insisted she herself must always be present whenever he entered Elizabeth's bedchamber, and made certain from then on that she was.

But the romps continued. Sometimes, even the Queen joined in. When they were at Anne Boleyn's old manor of Hanworth in the spring, Katherine accompanied her husband to Elizabeth's room on two mornings, and joined in the tickling, amid peals of laughter. While still at Hanworth, the Admiral chased Elizabeth through the gardens; when he caught her, they wrestled together, then Seymour called for shears and cut her black gown into strips, while the Queen, in fits of laughter, held her still. Afterwards, Elizabeth fled indoors where Mrs Ashley asked in horror what had happened to her. Elizabeth told her, and received a telling off, but would only reply that 'it could not be helped'.

Elizabeth's infatuation with the Admiral was becoming quite obvious, and she was too young to have the guile to conceal it. This concerned Seymour, for obvious reasons, so, in order to divert any suspicion from himself, he told Katherine he had recently seen Elizabeth, through a gallery window, 'with her arms round a man's neck'. The Queen was shocked, and sent for Mrs Ashley, who divulged nothing of what she suspected but advised Katherine to speak to the girl herself. She did so, but Elizabeth burst into tears and denied that such a thing had ever happened, begging her stepmother to ask all her women if it were true. She had little opportunity for such things, as she was hardly ever alone, and the only men who came into contact with her, apart from servants, were her school-masters and the Admiral.

At once, the Queen's suspicions were aroused. If Elizabeth was telling the truth, her husband must be lying, and why should he do this but to protect himself? Suddenly, like pieces in a jigsaw, the truth dawned upon Katherine with terrible clarity. Everything now made sense, the morning romps, Elizabeth's behaviour, Mrs Ashley's tight-lipped disapproval. She had no proof that the affair had proceeded beyond a mere romp, but there was no doubt in her mind that her husband was after Elizabeth, and that he was the kind of man who would seduce her if the opportunity presented itself. It was therefore imperative that she take some action to protect the girl, who was, after all, under her roof and in her care.

The Queen now sent for Mrs Ashley, and confided her suspicions to her, telling her to 'take more heed, and be as it were in watch betwixt the Lady Elizabeth and the Admiral'. Mrs Ashley was relieved that Katherine was now in command of the situation, and also to know she did not suspect it to have progressed very far. Later that day she told Sir Thomas Parry, who was in charge of Elizabeth's financial affairs, that 'the Admiral had loved the Princess [sic] too well, and had done so a good while', but his bluff was about to be called. Parry, too, promised to be watchful.

Katherine's happiness was shattered. Whether or not the Admiral had actually been unfaithful to her did not matter: it was his intention that had hurt her. Yet she hid her feelings well, hoping against hope that she had been wrong. It was not long, however, before she had her worst suspicions confirmed. One day in April at Chelsea, she realised that both her husband and stepdaughter were missing. She went in search of them, throughout that vast house, until at last she came upon them, without warning, alone together, Elizabeth in the Admiral's arms. At the sight of Katherine, they fell apart at once, guilt all over their faces. But it was too late, the Queen had seen enough to tell her that her husband and the girl she had sheltered and mothered had betrayed her. She did not wait to hear their apologies, but left the room and ordered Mrs Ashley to attend her. When the woman came, the Queen told her she was displeased with Elizabeth, and why, and warned her that she would not have the girl in her house any longer than was necessary. When Mrs Ashley had gone, Katherine did not vent her sorrow in tears, nor did she indulge in a tirade of useless recriminations when once again she came face to face with her husband. Withdrawn and cold, she was sustained by her innate dignity and never betrayed by word or gesture her inner turmoil.

In May, Elizabeth left Chelsea for her manor of Cheston. Her guilt lay heavily upon her conscience, and far outweighed any attraction she had felt for the Admiral. Their affair was over, that much was obvious. He had made no attempt to see her, and she welcomed this, for it made things much easier. She told Mrs Ashley that she had 'loved the Admiral too well', and that the Queen was jealous of them both.

Before her departure, she had one last painful interview with Katherine. Her stepmother was aloof and cool, and made no reference to the reason for her going. She merely said, 'God has given you great qualities. Cultivate them always, and labour to improve them, for I believe you are destined by Heaven to be Queen of England.' Elizabeth kissed her, and was gone, unable to bear Katherine's coldness.

When she arrived at Cheston, Elizabeth was told by Mrs Ashley that the Admiral would have married her, if he had had the chance, rather than the Queen. Elizabeth asked how she knew that, whereupon Mrs Ashley told her 'she knew it well, both by herself and others'. Before very long, it was common knowledge, and caused further grief to Queen Katherine; what was worse, however, were the rumours that had suddenly sprung up regarding Elizabeth's relationship with the Admiral. There were tales of illicit meetings, criminal intercourse, even of a child born in great secrecy. Such tales, most of them fabrications, probably originated with the servants' gossip at Chelsea, yet they captured the imagination of the public. It would be another year, however, before the government took them seriously and the storm broke.

Not long after her arrival at Cheston, Elizabeth fell sick and took to her bed, which gave the rumourmongers further food for thought; however, she was up and about by July. In the meantime, she had received a letter from the Admiral, taking the blame for what had happened upon himself, and swearing to testify to her innocence if necessary. No words of love adorned his letter or her reply, in which she wrote, 'You need not to send an excuse to me', and ended 'I pray you to make my humble commendations to the Queen's Highness.' By telling the Admiral she was committing 'you and your affairs into God's hand', she was in effect telling him that all familiarity between them must cease; and while his wife lived, the Admiral took her at her word. Elizabeth saw now that she had not only caused terrible hurt to the Queen, but had also risked her reputation and her place in the succession. Never again would she be so stupid.

After Elizabeth's departure, Katherine made an effort to forget what had happened and rebuild her shaken marriage. Thanks to her determination, relations between her and her husband improved, assisted by the Queen's advancing pregnancy and the shared pleasure of anticipating the birth of their child. Early in June, the Admiral's duties called him to court, so Katherine went away to Hanworth for a few days, and while she was there, she felt her child move inside her for the first time. It was a joyful moment, and did much to erase her unhappy memories of the spring. With renewed affection, she wrote to her husband:

Sweetheart and loving husband,
I gave your little knave your blessing, who like an honest man stirred apace after and before; for Mary Odell [the midwife, who was already in attendance], being abed with me, laid her hand on my belly to feel it stir. It has stirred these three days every morning and evening, so that I trust when you come it will make you some pastime. And thus I end, bidding my sweetheart and loving husband better to fare than myself.

The Admiral replied on 9 June that Katherine's letter had 'revived my spirits'. He was still trying, with little success, to get Somerset to agree to restoring her jewels to her. Hearing that 'my little man doth shake his poll', he trusted that 'If God should give him a life as long as his father's, he will revenge such wrongs as neither you nor I can at present.' He had spoken to Somerset, he said, and had 'so well handled him' that the Duke was no longer so sure of his ground, and had said that 'At the finishing of the matter, you shall either have your own again, or else some recompense as ye shall be content withal.' He ended his letter with instructions to Katherine

> to keep the little knave [i.e. the baby] so lean and gaunt with your good diet and walking that he may be so small that he may creep out of a mouse-hole! And I bid my most dear and well-beloved wife most heartily well to fare. Your Highness' most faithful, loving husband, T. Seymour.

It is obvious from this letter that the Admiral was doing his best to regain the love and respect of his wife, especially now she was about to bear him, he hoped, an heir. And it is obvious from Katherine's letter, too, that she was happy to pretend that all was well between them. An uneasy peace had been achieved. But underneath, her wound was still raw.

Chelsea held too many painful memories, and so the Admiral had decided to take the Queen to Sudeley Castle, where their child would be born. He returned from court on 11 June, and on Wednesday, 13 June they set off for Gloucestershire. When they reached their new home, a letter from John Fowler awaited them, enclosing one from the King. Edward sent his commendations to his stepmother and to the Admiral, and informed them that the Duchess of Somerset had just given birth to 'a fine boy', to be named after the King and after her elder son, born eleven years before, who had died in childhood. This was encouraging news for Katherine, whose own confinement was now not many weeks off.

The Queen soon settled into the peaceful routine of life in the country. Then a letter arrived from Elizabeth, who wrote 'giving thanks for the manifold kindnesses received at your Highness's hand at my departure' and saying how 'truly I was replete with sorrow to depart from your Highness' and that

> I weighed it deeply when you said you would warn me of all evilnesses that you should hear of me; for if your Grace had not a good opinion of me, you would not have offered friendship to me that way at all, meaning the contrary.

There was more, in the same appealing and penitential vein, and the letter was signed 'Your Highness's humble daughter, Elizabeth'. It was undoubtedly a plea for forgiveness, and Katherine sensibly realised that Elizabeth had never intended her any real harm; she had lost her head over a handsome man who should have known better. With this in mind, Katherine could not remain angry any longer, and even though she had hurt her wrist, which was so weak that she could hardly hold the pen, she wrote a warm reply, assuring her stepdaughter of her friendship. The Admiral wrote also, at his wife's request.

Elizabeth replied on 31 July, saying Katherine's letter was 'most joyful to me', although she was concerned to hear 'what pain it is to you to write', and would have been happy to receive her 'commendations' in the Admiral's letter. She rejoiced, she said, to learn of Katherine's otherwise excellent health and enjoyment of life in the country, and was grateful to the Admiral for undertaking to let her know from time to time 'how his busy child doth; if I were at his birth, no doubt I would see him beaten, for the trouble he hath put you to!' And with the passing on of good wishes for 'a lucky deliverance' from Mrs Ashley and others, Elizabeth ended her letter, 'giving your Highness most humble thanks for your commendations'.

There was no question, of course, of Elizabeth rejoining Katherine's household. Yet the Queen did not lack for company in these final weeks of her pregnancy. Lady Jane Grey was still with her and like a daughter, and many of her old friends and acquaintances made the long journey from London to visit her; in fact, Sudeley Castle quickly became renowned as the second court in the realm because it was so well populated with the nobility and because the Admiral spared no expense in providing hospitality or in maintaining his wife's royal estate. They had, after all, more than £8,000 a year to live on, a princely sum in those days. Most welcome of all were Katherine's old friends, Sir Robert and Lady Tyrwhitt, and it was to Sir Robert that the Queen mentioned one day, when they were walking in the gardens, and Sir Robert was admiring the scenery and the castle, that when the King came of age he would ask for the return of Sudeley Castle. Sir Robert was dismayed to learn that the Queen might have to leave her beautiful home, and asked, 'Then will Sudeley Castle be gone from my Lord Admiral?' Katherine smiled, and told him that she had the King's promise that, if he recalled all the lands deeded away by the regency Council he would freely return Sudeley when that time came.

It was now August, and the Queen's child was due within the month. Most of her visitors tactfully departed, leaving only the Tyrwhitts and a few other faithful friends in attendance. Katherine spent much of her time with Lady Jane Grey, of whom she was very fond, and there had been, of late, a reconciliation with the Lady Mary, whose disapproval of Katherine's remarriage had melted as soon as she heard that her stepmother was to bear a child. Again, the two women had begun to correspond, and in the middle of August William Parr arrived at Sudeley with another letter from Mary, who was going to Norfolk and would not return until Michaelmas, 'at which time, or shortly after, I trust to hear good success of your Grace's great belly, and in the meantime shall desire much to hear of your health.' And with commendations to the Admiral, she signed herself 'Your Highness's humble and assured loving daughter.'

Katherine was therefore seemingly at peace with the world when, on 30 August 1548, her child was born at Sudeley Castle. It turned out to be no 'little knave', but a daughter, who was afterwards christened Mary, in honour of her stepsister, the Lady Mary. It was a difficult birth, and Katherine was very weak afterwards, although her physicians and the midwife, Mary Odell, were optimistic about her recovery.

The Admiral was naturally disappointed that the child was a girl, but it was not long before he was doting upon the baby, and sending the news of her birth by fast courier to the Protector. Somerset was right glad to understand by your letters that the Queen, your bedfellow, hath a happy hour, and, escaping all danger, hath made you the father of so pretty a daughter; and although (if it had pleased God) it would have been both to us and (we suppose) also to you more joy and comfort if it had, this first-born, been a son, yet the escape of the danger, and the prophecy of this to a great sort of happy sons is no small joy and comfort to us, as we are sure it is to you and her Grace also, to whom you shall make again our hearty commendations, with no less congratulation of such good success. From Syon, the 1st of Sept., 1548. Your loving brother, E. Somerset.

Of course, the Duchess of Somerset was delighted that Katherine Parr had borne a daughter; had not she herself presented her husband with a fine son, triumphing where Katherine had failed?

There was no thought of failure, or even of success, in the mind of the Queen by then. Hours after the birth, she was laid low with puerperal fever, that scourge of medieval and Tudor childbeds, and remained delirious for almost a week. With each passing day, it became more obvious that she was not going to recover. In her delirium, she spoke of her anguish over her husband's faithlessness and betrayal, which was to trouble her to the end, and which she no longer had the strength or wit to conceal. On 5 September, Lady Tyrwhitt went into the Queen's bedchamber to bid her good morning and see if there was any improvement in her condition. Katherine was half lucid, and asked Lady Tyrwhitt where she had been for so long, saying 'that she did fear such things in herself that she was sure she could not live'. Lady Tyrwhitt replied, with feigned confidence, 'that I saw no likelihood of death in her.' But Katherine was not listening; she was back at Chelsea, reliving the moment when she had found her husband and Elizabeth in an embrace. The Admiral was by the bed, and she grasped his hand, saying, 'My Lady Tyrwhitt, I am not well handled, for those that are about me care not for me, but stand laughing at my grief, and the more good I will to them, the less good they will to me.'

There was shocked silence, then the Admiral hastened to reassure her, saying, 'Why, sweetheart! I would you no hurt!' To which

Katherine replied, with heavy irony, 'No, my lord, I think so.' Then, as he leaned over her, she whispered, 'But, my lord, you have given me many shrewd taunts.' Lady Tyrwhitt remembered afterwards that she said these words 'with good memory, and very sharply and earnestly, for her mind was sore disquieted'. The Admiral pretended not to hear, and, taking Lady Tyrwhitt aside, asked her what his wife had said; 'I declared plainly to him,' she recalled. He asked if she thought he should lie down on the bed with the Queen 'and pacify her unhappiness with gentle communication'. Lady Tyrwhitt agreed this might be a good thing, whereupon the Admiral lay down and put his arms around his wife, soothing her with words of love, without regard to the presence of her ladies. He had not, however, said more than three or four words when Katherine burst out, 'My lord, I would have given a thousand marks to have had my full talk with [Dr Robert] Huicke [her physician] the first day I was delivered, but I durst not, for displeasing you.' What she actually wanted to discuss with Huicke we shall never know, but Lady Tyrwhitt guessed that it was something of a very personal nature, possibly about the resumption or otherwise of sexual relations after the difficult confinement, and because of this, and her realisation that Katherine's agony of mind was very great, Lady Tyrwhitt tactfully withdrew out of earshot: 'My heart would serve me to hear no more.' The Queen's tirade against the Admiral continued for more than an hour, and was heard by the ladies about her bedside, though they did not leave accounts of it for posterity.

Later that day, Katherine's fever subsided, leaving her with no recollection of what she had said. She was very weak, and realised, with her usual common sense, that she was dying, and that it would be best to make her will now, while she was in possession of her senses. Writing materials were brought by her secretary, and the Queen dictated:

I, Katherine Parr, etc., lying on my death-bed, sick of body but of good mind and perfect memory and discretion, being persuaded and perceiving the extremity of death to approach me, give all to my married spouse and husband, wishing them to be a thousand times more in value than they are or been.

The will was then signed by the Queen and witnessed by Dr Huicke and her chaplain, John Parkhurst, who gave her the last rites soon afterwards. We do not know if the Queen asked to see her baby daughter before the end, nor are her last words recorded, nor any details of her death, which occurred the following day, 7 September 1548, between two and three in the morning.

The Admiral was genuinely grieved at her passing, and gave orders for her body to be buried in the castle chapel. The corpse was embalmed, dressed in rich clothes, and wrapped in cerecloth, then placed in a lead coffin and left in the Queen's privy chamber until arrangements for the funeral had been completed. Young Jane Grey shed bitter tears over it, not only for the woman who had been a better mother to her than her own, but also because Katherine's death meant she would have to return home, a prospect that appalled her.

On the morning of 8 September, Katherine Parr was laid to rest. The chapel was hung with black cloth embroidered with the Queen's escutcheons; the altar rails were covered in black cloth, and stools and cushions provided for the mourners. The coffin was preceded into the chapel by two conductors in black carrying black staves, gentlemen, squires, knights, officers of the household carrying white staves, gentlemen ushers, and Somerset Herald in a tabard. Six gentlemen in black gowns and hoods bore the body, with torchbearers at either side, hooded knights walking at each corner. The Lady Jane Grey, acting as chief mourner, came next, her train borne by a young lady, then six other ladies, and other ladies and gentlemen, walking in pairs, then yeomen and lesser folk. Etiquette prevented the bereaved husband from attending.

When the coffin had been set down between the altar rails, psalms were sung in English and three lessons read; after the third, the mourners placed their offerings in the almsbox. Then Dr Miles Coverdale, the Queen's confessor, preached the sermon and led the prayers. When he was finished, the coffin was lowered into a vault beneath the altar pavement while the choir sang the *Te Deum*. After the service, the mourners went back to the castle for dinner, and then departed, leaving the Admiral to his memories in the great house that now seemed so empty. His servant Edward informed the Lady Elizabeth that 'my lord is a heavy man for the loss of the Queen his wife', but if the Admiral had hoped to find her willing to console him, he was quickly to be disappointed for there was no reply from her. For all this, his thoughts were very much with the woman who lay not far from him in her tomb, and he was heard to vow that 'no one should speak ill of the Queen, or if he knew it, he would take his fist to the ears of those who did, from the highest to the lowest.' At length, he returned to the world of men and affairs, and early in 1549 joined the English army at Musselburgh to do battle against the Scots. Yet not even his valorous performance in combat could dispel the whispers about his lack of scruples, nor the rumour, spread by Thomas Parry, 'that he had treated the late Queen cruelly, dishonestly, and jealously'.

As time passed his grief – which was undoubtedly sincere – faded. Memories grew dim. The Duchess of Somerset told him that

> if any grudge were borne by her to him, it was all for the late Queen's sake, and now she was taken by death, it would undoubtedly follow that she, the Duchess, would bear as good will to him as ever before.

With Katherine's memory daily receding, the Admiral patched up the feud and returned again to court, taking the first of many ill-considered steps that would, in 1549, lead him to the block for having schemed to gain control of the young King. When news was brought to her of his death, the Lady Elizabeth merely commented, 'This day died a man of much wit, and very little judgement.'

Lady Jane Grey mourned her benefactress most sincerely, and when she had returned to her parents' house, she wrote to thank the Admiral for 'all such good behaviour as she learned by the Queen's most virtuous instruction'. She, too, was fated to die violently, at only sixteen years of age, and her months with Katherine Parr were undoubtedly the happiest time in her short life.

Mary and Elizabeth grieved also for the loss of a stepmother who had been unfailingly kind and protective towards them. Mary could never forget what her father owed to Katherine Parr, and often spoke of 'the great love and affection that [he] did bear unto her Grace'. Her death would herald the beginning of a great divide between the sisters, who had once been close but would now gradually grow ever more suspicious of each other and end as formidable rivals in the dangerous arena of politics and religion.

When, on 20 March 1549, the Lord Admiral was executed for high treason, his seven-month-old daughter, Lady Mary Seymour, was left an orphan. Nor was this the only calamity that befell her, for later that month Parliament passed an Act disinheriting the child. The dispossessed baby was taken in by her late mother's friend, the Duchess of Suffolk, to be brought up with twelve other orphans in her care at her house at Grimsthorpe. Mary's uncle, Lord Northampton, hinted that he would be willing to have the child, but only if the Duchess of Somerset paid him the allowance she and the Duke had promised him for the infant's upkeep. The tight-fisted Duchess, however, would not pay up, and thus the burden of Lady Mary's keep fell upon the Duchess of Suffolk. Within a month, the good woman was finding it too onerous a burden, as, being the daughter of a queen, the child had to be provided with all the trappings suitable to her rank, and these were expensive. The Duchess of Suffolk wrote to William Cecil, who had been a great admirer of Katherine Parr, and asked him to use his influence with the Duchess of Somerset in persuading her to agree to paying the allowance she had promised for the Lady Mary; Lady Suffolk knew that Northampton would never take her without it, for he 'hath as weak a back for such a burden as I have'.

Despite Cecil's pleas, the allowance was not forthcoming. Anne Somerset did send her servant, Richard Bertie (who later married the Duchess of Suffolk) with a message to say that she would be forwarding some nursery plate for her niece; in turn, she wished to see an inventory of all the valuables in use in the child's nursery, so that she could decide for herself what pension was needful. Lady Suffolk was furious when she received this message, and in exasperation wrote to Cecil to say:

The Queen's child hath lain, and doth lie, at my house, with her company [i.e. servants] about her, wholly at my charge. I have written to my Lady Somerset at large; there may be some pension allotted to her, according to my lord's Grace's [Somerset's] promise. Now, good Cecil, help at a pinch all that you may help.

Enclosed was a parcel containing the requested inventory of all the valuables that had been set aside for the Lady Mary's use when she left Sudeley Castle, as well as a letter from the child's nurse, Mistress Eglonby, demanding wages for herself and her maids, 'so that ye may the better understand that I cry not before I am pricked', wrote the Duchess, whose coffers were emptying fast.

The inventory of Lady Mary Seymour's effects survives, and provides us with a fascinating account of what a well-born baby was provided with in those days. There were silver pots and goblets in her nursery, a silver salt cellar, eleven silver spoons, a porringer banded in silver, a quilt for the cradle, three pillows and one pair of sheets, three feather beds, three more quilts and sets of sheets, a tester of scarlet, embroidered, with a counterpane of silk serge, and bed-curtains of crimson taffeta, two counterpanes with embroidered pictures for the nurse's bed, six wall-hangings, four carpets to hang over the windows in cold weather, ten more hangings depicting the months of the year, two cushions of cloth of gold and a chair of the same, two stools and a gilded bedstead with tester, counterpanes and curtains (presumably for when the child was too big for a cradle), two 'milk beasts' – probably pewter jugs fashioned like animals – which were earmarked as gifts for the two maids looking after the child as and when they married, and a lute. This last may once have belonged to Katherine Parr, and was perhaps used to lull her little daughter to sleep.

The inventory was forwarded by Cecil to the Duchess of Somerset in the summer of 1549. However, not long afterwards her husband the Lord Protector was overthrown by the Duke of Northumberland – formerly John Dudley, Earl of Warwick – and she was no longer able to fulfil any of her promises, even had she wished to, for the Seymours were now in disgrace. Somerset would end his days as his brother had done, on the block, accused of high treason, in 1552. However, a few months after Somerset's fall, Parliament passed an Act restoring to Mary all her father's lands and property, though not his titles. After that, Lady Suffolk's financial troubles were at an end.

Nothing more is recorded in contemporary sources of Katherine Parr's daughter, and it is likely that she died young while still at Grimsthorpe. In the eighteenth century, most of the papers relating to Katherine Parr were destroyed in a fire at Wilton House, where they were stored, a sad loss for historians since they may have held clues to the fate of Katherine's daughter. In the nineteenth century, the historian Agnes Strickland was shown a genealogy belonging to the Lawson family of north-west England, showing that they were descended from a Lady Mary Seymour, who had grown up and married a knight called Sir Edward Bushel, who is known to have been in the household of Anne of Denmark, wife of James I. The evidence for this marriage, however, was based only on a family legend and is unsubstantiated by sixteenth-century sources; it may therefore be discounted. The sad reality was probably that Lady Mary followed her mother to the grave within a few years.

In time, a beautiful tomb was raised by the Admiral over Katherine Parr's remains within the chapel at Sudeley Castle. A marble effigy resembling the Queen was placed on it, and around the sepulchre was written an epitaph composed by her chaplain, Dr Parkhurst, who described her as 'the flower of her sex, renowned, great and wise, a wife by every nuptial virtue known'. Within a hundred years of Katherine's death, the chapel fell into decay, and the tomb was broken up by vandals. In 1782, her coffin was found amid the ruins, and opened. The body was seen to be in a good state of preservation, being clothed in costly burial garments – not a shroud, but a dress. There were shoes on the feet, which were very small. The Queen, it was noted, had been tall – the coffin measured 5' 10" in length – but of delicate build, with long auburn hair. There were traces of beauty in the dead face, the features being perfect on first exposure to the air; however, the process of decomposition began almost immediately, and the vicar insisted that the body be reinterred. This was done, but inebriated workmen buried it upside down. However, two years later, the body was to be seen outside the chapel, in the remains of the original coffin, and another vicar, Mr Tredway Nash, lamented that he wished 'more respect was paid to the remains of this amiable queen'. He wanted them put into a new coffin and buried elsewhere, so that 'at last her body might rest in peace'. The chapel was by then used for the keeping of rabbits, and was not a suitable place, as the rabbits 'scratch very irreverently about the royal corpse'. It seems, however, that the vicar's plans came to nothing, and that the coffin was merely covered with rubble.

By 1817, when the chapel was being restored, local opinion favoured a search being made for the Queen's remains, and the owner of the castle, Lord Chandos, gave his permission. Eventually, the coffin was found: it was badly damaged and found to contain only a skeleton. It was repaired, however, and finally reburied in the Chandos vault within the Chapel. During the reign of Queen Victoria the restoration of the chapel was completed, and Sir George Gilbert Scott was commissioned to design a fine new tomb in the medieval style for Katherine Parr. He made a marble effigy, copied from lost engravings of the original, which was placed on the finished monument in 1862, and this is the tomb we see there today, along with some vivid Victorian stained-glass windows, depicting Katherine Parr with her last two husbands, Henry VIII and Thomas Seymour. It is a fitting memorial to this most charming of queens.

After the death of Katherine, only one of Henry VIII's wives still lived, Anne of Cleves, who was perhaps the most fortunate, for after her divorce she had lived on in England in peace and contentment, enjoying the respect and affection of her former husband's family. Until the King died in 1547, she knew prosperity also, for her annual allowance of £3,000 was paid regularly, though after Henry's death the payments fell into arrears, and in 1550 so much was owed that Anne was driven to petitioning Edward VI about it; she was curtly informed, however, that 'the King's Highness, being on his progress, could not be troubled at that time about payments.' Nevertheless, he did authorise some of the debt to be paid soon afterwards, although Anne never received the full balance due to her for those years. In 1552 she complained again, and was granted various lands and manors, the rent from these being intended to supplement her income. Yet, as Anne pointed out, in a letter to her close friend, the Lady Mary, 'I was well contented to have continued without exchange,' to which end she had 'travailed to my great cost and charge almost this twelve months'.

This letter was written at Bletchingly in Surrey, one of the houses granted to Anne of Cleves after the annulment of her marriage. The others were Richmond and Hever, and she seems to have divided her time among all three. Richmond had once been the favourite home of Henry VII, and was by far the largest; after Anne's death,

Elizabeth I would come to love this mellow, red-brick palace on the banks of the Thames, and would die there in 1603. Bletchingly Place was also built of red brick; it had once been in the hands of that Duke of Buckingham who had been executed by Henry VIII in 1521, after which it had come into the possession of the Crown. All that remains of it today is a Tudor gatehouse at Place Farm. Hever Castle, of course, had been the home of Anne Boleyn from childhood until her marriage to the King; it had fallen to the Crown on the death of Anne's father, the Earl of Wiltshire, without heirs, in 1539. Anne of Cleves seems to have favoured it least among her houses, probably because it held too many memories of her unfortunate predecessor. Yet she did go there from time to time; in 1547, Katherine Bassett, who had entered Anne's household after the latter's divorce, was married to Mr Henry Ashley of Hever, whom she no doubt met when accompanying her mistress on a visit to the castle.

Anne was always welcome at court and therefore able to enjoy the best of both worlds, as an honourary member of the King's family and as a country gentlewoman. She was therefore a witness to the shifting vicissitudes of power and the changing fortunes of the monarchy that characterised the middle years of the sixteenth century. She saw Edward VI decline in health and learned of his death from consumption at the age of fifteen in July 1553. She heard, not long afterwards, how Northumberland had plotted to set the Lady Jane Grey – whom he had married to his son, Lord Guildford Dudley – upon the throne, that he might conserve power for himself and thus preserve the Protestant religion in England. And she learned, with sincere gladness, how the country had rallied to Mary Tudor's cause, and how Mary had overthrown Queen Jane and been herself proclaimed Queen of England. In October 1553, Anne was present at Mary I's coronation in Westminster Abbey, and occupied the same litter as the Lady Elizabeth in the procession to and from the Abbey.

Some months later, Anne was writing from Hever to congratulate Mary on her marriage to the Catholic Philip of Spain, son and heir of the Emperor Charles V, and to ask 'when and where I shall wait on your Majesty and his'. She sent also a wish that they should both enjoy 'much joy and felicity, with increase of children to God's glory and the preservation of your prosperous estates'. Sadly, Mary –

whose first legislation in Parliament had been an Act declaring her parents' marriage lawful – was never to bear a child. What was at first thought to be a pregnancy later turned out to be a malignant growth within the womb.

Mary had originally been responsible for Anne of Cleves's conversion to Roman Catholicism, and by the 1550s Anne had long since repudiated Protestantism. She would have heard, no doubt, of the coming of the Inquisition to England, and also of the burning of more than 300 heretics, among them Archbishop Cranmer, on the Queen's orders. It had been Mary's intention from the first to eradicate the Protestant heresy from her realm, and to return her kingdom to the fold of the Roman Church. This she had done, but at a price, and when she died she would be remembered, not as the saviour of the English Church, but as 'Bloody Mary', a monster of cruelty.

It appears that during these years Anne of Cleves rarely went to court, preferring to lead the life of a private gentlewoman, attending to domestic affairs and managing her estates. She seems to have become quite efficient at this, and to have converted her property into a thriving asset. The rents she received from her manors now enabled her to live in comfort, and her steward, Sir Thomas Cawarden (who had formerly been Henry VIII's Master of the Revels), assisted her so ably that when she died she bequeathed to him her manor of Bletchingly as a reward. It was Cawarden who in 1556 made her a generous loan with which to buy furniture for a small house she had recently purchased at Dartford in Kent; indeed, she seems to have relied on him implicitly in financial matters.

Anne never married again, nor did she ever leave England; her parents were dead, and her brother, a strict Protestant, did not approve of her conversion to the old faith. Thus a return to Cleves, even had she wished it, was out of the question. In fact she had grown fond of England and its people, and intended to die in her adoptive land. In her latter years, when her health began to fail, she was allowed by Queen Mary to live at Chelsea Old Manor, where Katherine Parr had once lived with Admiral Seymour, and it was here, in mid-July 1557, that she dictated her will, a document that bears witness to her kindness and compassion for others. To her brother she left a diamond ring, and to his wife a ruby ring; to her sister, the Lady Amelia, went another diamond ring, as also to the Duchess of Norfolk and the Countess of Arundel. The Lady Elizabeth was to have Anne's second-best jewel, and there was a request for her to find employment in her household for 'one of our poor maids named Dorothy Curzon'. To Mother Lovell, 'for her care and attendance upon us in the time of our sickness', there was a bequest of £10.00, likewise to 'our poor servant, James Powell'; Elya Turpin, Anne's laundress, was to receive £4.00 'to pray for us'. Each of the executors was remembered 'for their pains': the Lord Chancellor was to have a standing cup and cover of gold or a crystal glass set with precious stones; Sir Richard Preston would get 'our best gilt bowl with a cover', and Edmund Peckham a jug of gold.

The Queen, 'our most dearest and entirely beloved sovereign lady', was asked to be overseer of the will, 'with most humble request to see the same performed as shall to her Highness seem best for the health of our soul'. In token of 'the special trust and affection which we have in her Grace', Anne bequeathed to Mary Tudor her best jewel, begging her to see that her servants were well provided for, in consideration of their long service; many had been with her since 1540, and Anne reminded the Queen how her father King Henry had 'said then unto us that he would account our servants his own; therefore we beseech the Queen's Majesty to accept them in this time of their extreme need.'

Anne knew she was dying when she dictated her will, and she ended it with the requests that all those benefiting from it should pray for her soul and see her body buried 'according to the Queen's will and pleasure', and that she might be given the last rites of 'Holy Church, according to the Catholic faith, wherein we end our life in this transitory world'.

Anne of Cleves died on 16 July 1557, at Chelsea, a few weeks short of her forty-second birthday. The illness that caused her death is not named. She was buried, on 3 August, by order of the Queen, in Westminster Abbey with great ceremony. The coffin was borne from Chelsea on a hearse, and was covered with seven rich palls. Many priests and clergy walked in the procession, as well as the Bishop of London and some of the monks who had not long before been allowed to return to Westminster Abbey. With them was their Abbot, John Feckenham, with the dead woman's executors, followed by several representatives of the nobility and gentry. The late Queen's banners were carried aloft by members of her household, who also walked in the procession. At Charing Cross, the cortège was met by a hundred more of Anne's servants, all bearing torches, who joined the throng of mourners, together with her ladies, clad in black, mounted on horses, as well as twelve 'beadsmen' of Westminster and eight heralds bearing white banners of arms, who ringed the corpse.

At the Abbey door, everyone dismounted, and the Bishop of London, with the Abbot of Westminster, received the body, swinging censers of incense over it. Then the coffin was borne into the great church, covered with a canopy of black velvet, and put in position before the altar, where it remained all night while the monks sang dirges. The next morning, a requiem mass was sung, and the Abbot preached a sermon. Bishop Bonner, wearing his mitre, said mass, then the coffin was laid in its tomb in the south transept of the Abbey. The chief officers of Anne's household then came forward and broke their staves of office, casting them after the coffin. Jane Seymour's sister Elizabeth, Marchioness of Winchester, was chief mourner, and she led the ladies in making their offerings afterwards. When the obsequies were concluded, her husband, John Paulet, Marquess of Winchester, entertained all the mourners to a funeral banquet at his London home. Within a month, the monks of Westminster had despoiled the hearse left over Anne's tomb, removing all the palls and banners adorning it, and Queen Mary gave orders for Anne's countryman, the stonemason Theodore Haveus, to come over from Cleves and fashion a proper monument. In 1606, a bare marble slab decorated with the earliest example of a skull and crossbones to appear in England was placed above Haveus's tomb. Today, Anne's final resting place is obscured by two monuments dating from the late seventeenth century.

Mary I did not long survive Anne of Cleves. She died, embittered and unloved, on 17 November 1558, and was succeeded by her sister, who became Queen Elizabeth I. Mary was buried not far from Anne of Cleves, in one of the side-chapels to the great Henry VII Chapel in Westminster Abbey.

Half a century after Anne's death, the chronicler Raphael Holinshed remembered her as 'a lady of right commendable regard, courteous, gentle, a good housekeeper, and very bountiful to her servants'. There had never been, he wrote, 'any quarrels, tale-bearings or mischievous intrigues in her court, and she was tenderly loved by her domestics.'

It was an apt and well-deserved tribute.

Bibliography

General

The major sources for this book have been the monumental *Calendar of Letters and Papers, Foreign and Domestic, of the Reign of Henry VIII* (21 vols in 33 parts, eds J. S. Brewer, James Gairdner and R. Brodie, HMSO, 1862–1932), which is said to include at least one million separate facts about Henry; *State Papers of the Reign of Henry VIII*, published under the Authority of Her Majesty's Commission (11 vols, Records Commissioners, 1831–52); and, for the latter part of the reign in particular, the *Acts of the Privy Council of England* (32 vols, ed. John Roche Dasent, HMSO, 1890–1918).

Of the diplomatic sources, by far the most useful and informative, if necessarily biased, is the *Calendar of Letters, Despatches and State Papers relating to negotiations between England and Spain, preserved in the Archives at Simancas and Elsewhere* (17 vols, ed. G. A. Bergenroth, P. de Goyangos, G. Mattingley, R. Tyler et al., HMSO, 1862–1965). This incorporates ambassadors' dispatches and a large volume of the correspondence of Katherine of Aragon and the Spanish monarchs. Also very useful, especially for descriptions of pageantry and ceremonial, is the *Calendar of State Papers and Manuscripts relating to English Affairs preserved in the Archives of Venice and in the other Libraries of Northern Italy* (7 vols, eds L. Rawdon-Brown, Cavendish Bentinck et al., HMSO, 1864–1947). Other diplomatic sources for the period are the *Calendar of State Papers and Manuscripts existing in the Archives and Collections of Milan: vol. 1, 1385–1618* (ed. A. B. Hinds, 1912); the *Mémoires* of Martin and Guillaume du Bellay, French ambassadors to the court of Henry VIII (4 vols, eds V. L. Bourrilly and F. Vindry, Paris, 1908–19); *Correspondance du Cardinal Jean du Bellay* (ed. R. Scheurer, Paris, 1969); *Correspondance Politique de MM. de Castillon et de Marillac, Ambassadeurs de France en Angeleterre, 1537–1542* (ed. J. Kaulek, Paris, 1885); *Correspondance Politique de Odet de Selve, Ambassadeur de France en Angleterre, 1546–1549* (ed. G. Lefèvre-Pontalis, Paris, 1888); *Négociations Diplomatiques entre la France et l'Autriche, 1491–1530* (2 vols, ed. A. J. G. Le Glay, Paris, 1845–47); and *Papiers d'État du Cardinal Granvelle, 1500–1565* (9 vols, ed. C. Weiss, 1841–52).

Official records for the period are contained in the Rolls of Parliament, *Rotuli Parliamentorum* (7 vols, ed. J. Strachey et al., Records Commissioners, 1767–1832), in which are detailed all the Acts and Statutes, as well as parliamentary proceedings; *Household Ordinances: A Collection of Ordinances and Regulations for the Government of the Royal Household* (Society of Antiquaries, 1790); *Journals of Parliament for the Reign of Henry VIII, 1509–1536* (c. 1742); *Privy Purse Expenses of Henry VIII from November 1529 to December 1532* (ed. H. Nicolas, 1827); *Proceedings and Ordinances of the Privy Council of England* (ed. H. Nicolas, Records Commissioners, 1834–7); *The Statutes, AD 1235–1770* (HMSO, 1950); *Statutes of the Realm* (11 vols, Records Commissioners, 1810–28); *State Trials vol. 1, 1163–1600* (ed. D. Thomas, W. Cobbett and T. B. Rowell, Routledge & Kegan Paul, 1972); *English Historical Documents, 1485–1558* (eds C. H. Williams and D. C. Douglas, 1967); and, for documentary sources for the latter period of the book, the *Calendar of State Papers, Domestic Series, of the Reigns of Edward VI, Mary and Elizabeth, 1547–1580* (2 vols, ed. R. Lemon, Longman, Brown, Green, 1856) and the *Calendar of State Papers, Foreign Series, Elizabeth I* (ed. J. Stevenson et al., 1863–1950).

There are also several invaluable chronicle and narrative sources dealing with the reign of Henry VIII in general. Three are contemporary, or written by contemporaries. The first is Edward Hall's Chronicle, published in two versions: *The Union of the Noble and Illustrious Families of Lancaster and York* (first published 1542; ed.

H. Nicolas; G. Woodfall, Printer 1809) and *The Triumphant Reign of King Henry the Eighth* (first published 1547; ed. C. Whibley and T. C. and E. C. Jack, 2 vols, 1904). Hall was a lawyer; his chronicles have a strong patriotic bias in favour of Henry VIII, and he tends to gloss over compromising issues. His descriptions of state occasions have not been surpassed, and his true value is as an annalist. The second contemporary source is George Cavendish's *The Life and Death of Cardinal Wolsey* (first published 1557; ed. R. Sylvester, Early English Texts Society, 1959), which is particularly useful for the early career of Anne Boleyn. Cavendish was Wolsey's secretary and well placed to record contemporary events, yet his admiration for his master makes him a biased observer. The third, and most controversial, source is the *Cronico del Rey Enrico Otavo de Inglaterra*, written before 1552 and sometimes attributed to Antonio de Guaras, who came to England in the train of Eustache Chapuys, the Spanish ambassador. It was printed as *The Chronicle of King Henry VIII* (ed. M. A. S. Hume, George Bell and Sons, 1889), but is commonly referred to by historians as the 'Spanish Chronicle'. Much of the information in it is based on hearsay and rumour, although many writers have been fooled by a seeming authenticity of detail which is not always corroborated by other sources. This source should therefore be treated with caution.

There are several later narrative sources for the reign of Henry VIII; these may be divided into Protestant or Catholic sources, and most are accordingly biased. The Protestant sources are all English. John Foxe, in his popular *History of the Acts and Monuments of the Church* (better known as Foxe's Book of Martyrs) (published in 1563; ed. G. Townshend and S. R. Cattley, 8 vols, Seeley and Burnside, 1837–41), gives interesting details about Anne Boleyn and Katherine Parr, both of whom he represented as Reformation heroines. Raphael Holinshed's *Chronicles of England, Scotland and Ireland* (first published 1577; ed. H. Ellis, 6 vols, G. Woodfall, Printer, 1807–8) draws mainly upon Hall's chronicle. Charles Wriothesley, Windsor Herald, wrote before 1562 his *Chronicle of England in the Reigns of the Tudors from 1485 to 1559* (ed. W. D. Hamilton, 2 vols, Camden Society, 2nd series, X and XX, 1875, 1877). Wriothesley was the first cousin of Thomas, Earl of Southampton and Lord Chancellor of England, and may therefore be considered a reliable primary source, especially for the 1540s, although his work was not published until 1581. The antiquarian John Stow wrote two useful books, *The Annals of England* (1592; ed. E. Howes, London, 1631) and his celebrated *Survey of London* (1598; ed. C. L. Kingsford, 2 vols, Oxford University Press, 1908). Another valuable later work is Lord Herbert of Cherbury's *The Life and Reign of King Henry the Eighth* (published a year after his death in 1649; ed. White Kennett, 1870), which may be considered to be the first 'modern' biography of the King. Herbert used original source material, some of which has since been lost or destroyed, and he was less subjective in his approach to his subject than earlier Protestant writers.

The later Catholic sources for Henry VIII's reign, most of which were printed abroad, are all biased against the King. Nicholas Harpsfield's *A Treatise on the Pretended Divorce between King Henry VIII and Katherine of Aragon* (ed. N. Pococke, Camden Society, 2nd series, XXI, 1878) was published in 1556 when Katherine's daughter Mary I was reigning and is consequently imbued with the spirit of the Counter-Reformation. Like most later Catholic sources, Harpsfield's work contains much that is apocryphal. One of the most damaging works ever printed was Nicholas Sanders' *De Origine ac Progressu Schismatis Anglicani* (first published in 1585 in Rome; printed as *The Rise and Growth of the Anglican Schism*, ed. D. Lewis, 1877). Sanders was an English Jesuit, exiled to Rome in the reign of Elizabeth I. He had nothing but contempt for Henry VIII, but the chief object of his venom was Anne Boleyn, whom he portrayed as evil personified, the cause of the English Reformation, and the English Jezebel. Sanders is responsible for many apocryphal anecdotes about Anne – such as the tale that she was the result of an affair between Henry VIII and Elizabeth Howard, or the tale that she was raped at the age of seven – and his treatise was received with scornful scepticism in England, prompting a reply by George Wyatt (see below, under chapter 7). Another Catholic writer working at the end of the sixteenth century was Gregorio Leti, who wrote a life of Elizabeth I which was suppressed by the Catholic authorities in Italy, probably because it was too favourable to its subjects. Nearly all the original copies were destroyed, and the work only survives in a French translation of 1694, *La Vie d'Elisabeth, Reine d'Angleterre*, from which some of the original material is certainly missing. It is thought that Leti made use of contemporary sources now lost to us, and for this reason his narrative may be of some value, although parts have been shown to be apocryphal. Girolamo Pollino, another Italian Catholic, wrote his *Istoria dell' Ecclesiastica della Rivoluzion d'Inghilterra* in 1594. Although he was biased against Henry VIII, there is evidence that much of his information was drawn from reliable sources, as many of his statements are corroborated by more contemporary sources. Unfortunately, there is much that has also been shown to be fanciful. The best Catholic source is Henry Clifford's *Life of Jane Dormer, Duchess of Feria* (published 1643; ed. E. E. Estcourt and J. Stevenson, Burns and Oates, 1887). Jane Dormer was one of Mary I's maids of honour and confidantes. When the Duke of Feria came to England in 1554 in the train of Philip of Spain, he fell in love with Jane and took her back to Spain as his wife. Many years later she dictated her memoirs to her English secretary, Henry Clifford, who published them after her death. They remain one of the better late sources, although one must allow for a certain bias and lapses in an old lady's memory.

There are several collections of primary source material for the period: *Archaeologia, or Miscellaneous Tracts relating to Antiquity* (102 vols, Society of Antiquaries, 1773–1969); *The Antiquarian Repertory: A Miscellany intended to Preserve and illustrate several valuable Remains of Old Times* (4 vols, London, 1775–84, and a later edition by F. Grose and T. Astle, 1808); Thomas Fuller's *The Church History of Britain* (1655) preserves details from sources now lost to us; *Records of the Reformation: The Divorce, 1527–1533* (2 vols, ed. N. Pococke, Oxford, 1870); Thomas Rymer's *Feodera* (ed. T. Hardy, Records Commissioners, 1816–69); John Strype's *Ecclesiastical Memorials* (3 vols, 1721–33; Oxford edn, 1822); John Weever's *Ancient Funeral Monuments within the United Monarchy of Great Britain, Ireland and the Islands adjacent . . . and what Eminent Persons have been in the Same interred* (Thomas Harper, 1631); and *Excerpta Historica* (eds S. Bentley and H. Nicolas, 1831).

Of primary importance to the historian are the printed collections of correspondence. The letters of Henry VIII appear in four compilations: M. St Clair Byrne's *The Letters of King Henry VIII* (Cassell, 1936); *Lettres de Henri VIII* (ed. G. A. Crapelet, 1826); and *Love Letters of Henry VIII* (two edns: H. Savage, 1949 and Jasper Ridley,

1988). Letters written by Henry's wives appear in *Letters of Royal and Illustrious Ladies* (ed. M.A.E. Wood, 1846) and Margaret Sanders's *Intimate Letters of England's Queens* (1957). Also worth consulting are: *Lettres de Rois, Reines et autres Personages des Cours de France et d'Angleterre* (ed. J. J. Champollion-Figeac, Paris, 1845–7, vol. 2); *Original Letters illustrative of English History* (11 vols, ed. H. Ellis Richard Bentley, 1824–46); *Original Letters relative to the English Reformation* (ed. H. Robinson, Parker Society, 1846–7); *The Lisle Letters* (ed. M. St Clair Byrne, 1981), which is particularly useful for the period 1533 to 1540; *Miscellaneous Writings and Letters of Thomas Cranmer* (ed. J.E. Fox, Parker Society, 1846); *The Correspondence of Matthew Parker, 1535–1575* (ed. J. Bruce and T. Perowne, Parker Society, 1853; and the *Epistles* of Desiderius Erasmus (3 vols, trans. F. M. Nichols Russell and Russell, 1962).

The chief secondary sources for the period in general are as follows: *Handbook of British Chronology* (ed. F. M. Powicke and E. B. Fryde, Royal Historical Society, 1961), which is invaluable for details of officers of state and the peerage; the *Dictionary of National Biography* (63 vols, eds L. Stephen and S. Lee, Oxford University Press, 1885–1900) gives biographical details of the lives of most of the people in this book; *The Complete Peerage* (ed. G. H. White et al., St Catherine's Press, 1910–59) gives a wealth of genealogical data on the aristocracy; *Burke's Guide to the Royal Family* (Burke's Peerage, 1973) gives details of royal genealogy and institutions; Alison Weir's *Britain's Royal Families: The Complete Genealogy* (The Bodley Head, 1989); and C. R. N. Routh's *They Saw it Happen, 1485–1688* (Blackwell, 1956), *They Saw it Happen in Europe, 1540–1660* (Blackwell, 1965), and *Who's Who in History, 1485–1603* (Blackwell, 1964).

For general history of the Tudor period, see J. D. Mackie: *The Earlier Tudors, 1485–1588* (Oxford, Clarendon Press, 1952); G. R. Elton's *England under the Tudors* (Methuen, 1955) and *The Tudor Constitution* (Methuen, 1960); David Harrison's delightfully illustrated study, *Tudor England* (2 vols, 1953); Christopher Morris's interesting series of character portraits, *The Tudors* (Batsford, 1955); M. Roulstone's lavish *The Royal House of Tudor* (Balfour, 1974); Godfrey E. Turton's *The Dragon's Breed* (1969); G. W. O. Woodward's *Reformation and Resurgence, 1485–1603* (Blandford, 1963); and P. Williamson's *Life in Tudor England* (Batsford, 1964).

There are several books on the Reformation. J. H. Merle d'Aubigny's *The Reformation in England* (1853) is outdated and inaccurate, but there are several more modern works that are well worth consulting: Sir F. Maurice Powicke's *The Reformation in England* (Oxford University Press, 1951); Philip Hughes's *The Reformation in England* (Macmillan, 1950) – vol. 1 covers Henry VIII's reign; H. Maynard-Smith's *Henry VIII and the Reformation* (Macmillan, 1962); and, for related subjects, see Erwin Doernberg's *Henry VIII and Luther* (Stanford University Press, 1961), William A. Clebsch's *England's Earliest Protestants, 1520–1535* (Yale University Press, 1964), and James Kelsey McConica's *English Humanists and Reformation Politics under Henry VIII and Edward VI* (Oxford University Press, 1965).

Henry VIII has been the subject of many biographies. The most recent and best ones have been Jasper Ridley's *Henry VIII* (Constable, 1984), J. J. Scarisbrick's *Henry VIII* (Constable, 1968) and Carolly Erickson's brilliantly detailed *Great Harry* (Dent, 1980). Previous biographies consulted include J. J. Bagley's *Henry VIII* (Batsford, 1962), Lacey Baldwin-Smith's *Henry VIII: The Mask of Royalty* (Jonathan Cape, 1971), John Bowle's *Henry VIII* (Allen and Unwin, 1964), N. Brysson-Morrison's *The Private Life of Henry VIII* (Robert Hale, 1964), Francis Hackett's *Henry the Eighth* (1929; Chivers Edition, 1973); Robert Lacey's *The Life and Times of Henry VIII* (Weidenfeld & Nicolson, 1972), Philip Lindsay's *The Secret of Henry VIII* (Howard Baker, 1953), Kenneth Pickthorn's *Early Tudor Government: Henry VIII* (1951); A. F. Pollard's *Henry VIII* (Longmans Green and Co., 1902) and Beatrice Saunders's rather subjective study, *Henry the Eighth* (Alvin Redman, 1963). For Henry's youth, see Frank Arthur Mumby's *The Youth of Henry VIII* (Constable, 1913), which draws heavily on the Spanish Calendar, and Marie Louise Bruce's enjoyable *The Making of Henry VIII* (Collins, 1977).

All six of Henry VIII's wives are dealt with in the following works: Agnes Strickland's *Lives of the Queens of England* (8 vols, Henry Colburn, 1851, and the Portway Reprint by Cedric Civers of Bath, 1972), much outdated now but a milestone of historical research in its time; Heather Jenner's *Royal Wives* (1967); and Norah Lofts's *Queens of Britain* (Hodder and Stoughton, 1977). The last serious collective biography of the six wives was Martin A. S.

Hume's *The Wives of Henry the Eighth* (Eveleigh Nash, 1905), long out of print and out of date. Paul Rival's *The Six Wives of Henry VIII* (Heinemann, 1937) is nearer to fiction than fact, and gives no details of sources.

There have been several individual biographies of Henry VIII's wives. For Katherine of Aragon, see Garrett Mattingley's excellent *Catherine of Aragon* (Jonathan Cape, 1942), Mary M. Luke's *Catherine the Queen* (Muller, 1967), Francesca Claremont's *Catherine of Aragon* (Robert Hale, 1939) and John E. Paul's *Catherine of Aragon and her Friends* (Burns and Oates, 1966), a very useful study. (It should be noted that Katherine herself signed her name with a 'K', not a 'C'.) Anne Boleyn has attracted more biographers than any of Henry's wives: Paul Friedmann's *Anne Boleyn: A Chapter of English History, 1527–1536* (2 vols, Macmillan, 1884) was for years the standard biography, but has since been replaced by more recent works: Philip Sergeant's *The Life of Anne Boleyn* (Hutchinson, 1923); Marie Louise Bruce's *Anne Boleyn* (Collins, 1972); Hester W. Chapman's *Anne Boleyn* (Jonathan Cape, 1974); Norah Lofts's *Anne Boleyn* (Orbis Books, 1979), very much popular history, drawing on Strickland; Carolly Erickson's *Anne Boleyn* (Dent, 1984); E. W. Ives's compelling academic study, *Anne Boleyn* (Blackwell, 1986), to which this author is greatly indebted; and Retha Warnicke's controversial *The Rise and Fall of Anne Boleyn: Family Politics at the Court of Henry VIII* (Cambridge University Press, 1989). There is no separate biography of Jane Seymour, but there is a good account of her life and the fortunes of her family in William Seymour's *Ordeal by Ambition: An English Family in the Shadow of the Tudors* (Sidgwick and Jackson, 1972). Anne of Cleves also lacks a biographer, and the major account of her life is still the chapter in Strickland's *Lives of the Queens of England*. Lacey Baldwin-Smith has written a superb study of the life of Katherine Howard in *A Tudor Tragedy* (Jonathan Cape, 1961). Anthony Martiensson's *Queen Katherine Parr* (Secker and Warburg, 1973) is another excellent work.

For Henry VIII's 'great matter', see Geoffrey de C. Parmiter's *The King's Great Matter* (Longmans, 1967) and Marvin H. Albert's *The Divorce* (Harrap, 1965). William Hepworth Dixon's *History of Two Queens* (4 vols, Bickers and Son, 1873) is now greatly outdated.

There are several good biographies of Henry VIII's children, all of which have proved useful for research purposes. Mary I's early life is related by Milton Waldman in *The Lady Mary* (Collins, 1972), and there is an excellent full biography by Carolly Erickson, *Bloody Mary* (Dent, 1978). The early life of Elizabeth I is described in several books, viz.: Alison Plowden's *The Young Elizabeth* (Macmillan, 1971), Mary M. Luke's *A Crown for Elizabeth* (Muller, 1971), Edith Sitwell's *Fanfare for Elizabeth* (Macmillan, 1949), and in full biograhies by B. W. Beckinsale, *Elizabeth I* (Batsford, 1963), John E. Neale, *Queen Elizabeth I* (Jonathan Cape, 1934), Jasper Ridley, *Elizabeth I* (Constable, 1987) and Neville Williams, *Elizabeth, Queen of England* (Weidenfeld & Nicolson, 1967). For the early life of Edward VI see Hester W. Chapman's *The Last Tudor King* (Jonathan Cape, 1958) and W. K. Jordan's *Edward VI: The Young King* (Allen and Unwin, 1968).

For the royal palaces of the Tudors see James Dowsing's fascinating *Forgotten Tudor Palaces in the London Area* (Sunrise Press, no date, 1980s); Janet Dunbar's *A Prospect of Richmond* (Harrap, 1966); Ian Dunlop's *Palaces and Progresses of Elizabeth I* (Jonathan Cape, 1962); Benton Fletcher's *Royal Homes near London* (1930); Bruce Graeme's *The Story of St James's Palace* (Hutchinson, 1929); and Philip Howard's *The Royal Palaces* (Hamish Hamilton, 1960).

For the Tower of London and its history see J. Bayley's *History and Antiquities of the Tower of London* (Jennings and Chaplin, 1830); D. C. Bell's *Notices of Historic Persons Buried in the Tower* (1877), an account of the bones found in St Peter ad Vincula; *The Tower of London: its Buildings and Institutions* (ed. John Charlton, HMSO, 1978), a book that throws new light upon Anne Boleyn's imprisonment in the Tower; John E. N. Hearsey's *The Tower* (John Murray, 1960); R. J. Minney's *The Tower of London* (Cassell, 1970); and A. L. Rowse's *The Tower of London in the History of the Nation* (Weidenfeld & Nicolson, 1974).

For details of coronations and burials in Westminster Abbey, see the highly detailed *Official Guide*, Arthur Penrhyn Stanley's *Historical Memorials of Westminster Abbey* (1886) and Edward Carpenter's *A House of Kings* (Baker, 1966). For the Archbishops of Canterbury of the period, see Edward Carpenter's *Cantuar: The Archbishops in their Office* (Baker, 1971). For Scottish affairs, see Caroline Bingham's *James V, King of Scots* (Collins, 1971).

Bibliography

For pageantry and ceremonial in the Tudor period, see Sydney Anglo's *Spectacle, Pageantry and Early Tudor Policy* (Oxford, Clarendon Press, 1969) and Robert Withington's *English Pageantry: An Historical Outline* (1918). For the Tudor court, see Neville Williams's fascinating *Henry VIII and his Court* (Weidenfeld & Nicolson, 1971), Christopher Hibbert's *The Court at Windsor* (Longmans, 1964) and Ralph Dutton's *English Court Life from Henry VII to George II* (Batsford, 1963). Henry VIII's courtiers are the subject of an excellent book by David Mathew, *The Courtiers of Henry VIII* (Eyre and Spottiswoode, 1970). William Edward Mead's *The English Mediaeval Feast* (Allen and Unwin, 1931) gives interesting information about court banquets. The cultural background to the period is described in Elizabeth M. Nugent's *The Thought and Culture of the English Renaissance* (Cambridge University Press, 1966). For Tudor drama, see Frederick Boas's *An Introduction to Tudor Drama* (Oxford University Press, 1933). For poetry, see Maurice Evans's *English Poetry in the Sixteenth Century* (Hutchinson, 1967) and Philip Henderson's *The Complete Poems of John Skelton, Laureate* (1931; 2nd rev. edn, Dent, 1948). Sir Thomas Wyatt's poems are dealt with under the heading to chapter 7. Sir Roy Strong's *Tudor and Jacobean Portraits* (2 vols, HMSO, 1969) is the most exhaustive study of Tudor royal portraits so far, but Christopher Lloyd's and Simon Thurley's *Images of a Tudor King* (Phaidon Press, 1990) is useful for its descriptions of Henry VIII's iconography. Hans Holbein, the greatest painter of the early Tudor period, painted Henry VIII and at least two of his wives; the greatest authority on Holbein is Paul Ganz: *The Paintings of Hans Holbein* (Phaidon Press, 1956). For Tudor costume, the best authority is Herbert Norris's *Costume and Fashion, vol 111, The Tudors, book 1, 1485–1547* (Dent, 1928); see also Norman Hartnell's *Royal Courts of Fashion* (Cassell, 1971).

Introduction

Contemporary views of the role of women in sixteenth-century society are to be found in the following works: John Colet's *A Right*

Fruitful Monition (1515); Colet was a friend of Sir Thomas More, Dean of St Paul's and founder of St Paul's School, and his views were those of a traditional churchman; Miles Coverdale's *The Christian State of Matrimony* (1543); Desiderius Erasmus's *The Institution of Christian Marriage* (1526); Henry VIII's own view on matrimony in his *Assertio Septem Sacramentorum adversus Martinus Lutherus* (published 1521; ed. O'Donovan, New York, 1908); the Scots reformer John Knox's *First Blast of the Trumpet against the Monstrous Regiment of Women* (ed. E. Arber, The English Scholar's Library of Old and Modern Works, 1878), for an extreme view; Sir Thomas More's *Utopia* (1516) for an idealistic view; two tracts by Queen Katherine Parr, *The Lamentations of a Sinner* (1547) and *Prayers and Meditations* (1545); and William Tyndale's *The Obedience of a Christian Man* (1528). See also Doris Mary Stenton's *The English Woman in History* (Allen and Unwin, 1957).

For enlightened views on education, see Roger Ascham's *The Schoolmaster* (1570), Ascham having been tutor to Queen Elizabeth I and the Lady Jane Grey. Juan Luis Vives's rigorous plan for the education of the Princess Mary is encapsulated in *De Institutione Foeminae Christianae* (Basle, 1538; trans. R. Hyrd, and printed in London by Thomas Berthelet, 1540).

1 The princess from Spain

The negotiations for the marriage of Katherine of Aragon to Arthur, Prince of Wales, during the period 1488 to 1501 are detailed extensively in the Spanish Calendar. Katherine's presentation to the English ambassadors at the age of two is described by the herald Ruy Machado in *Memorials of King Henry VII* (ed. J. Gairdner, Rolls Series, Longman, Brown, Green and Roberts, 1858). Accounts of the reigns of Ferdinand and Isabella are given by two Spanish chroniclers, Hernando del Pulgar, in his *Crónica de los Señoras Reyes Católicas* (published 1567; to be found in the *Biblioteca de Autores Española*, vol. LXX, Madrid, 1878) and Andres Bernaldes, in his *Historia de los Réyes Católicos D. Fernando y Doña Isabel* (Seville, 1870, and a later edition by M. Gomez-Moreno and J. de M. Carriazo, Madrid, 1962). The descriptions of Ferdinand and Isabella are based on those given by Pulgar, who was Queen Isabella's secretary. An excellent secondary authority on the history of Spain in the late-fifteenth and early-sixteenth century is *The Castles and the Crown: Spain, 1451–1555* by the English historian Townshend Miller (Gollancz, 1953). The only primary source to mention Katherine of Aragon and her sisters during their childhood is Vives.

Henry VII's instructions to the City of London for the state reception of Katherine of Aragon are in the Corporation of London Records Office and also in the Harleian MS. and Cotton MS. Vitellius in the British Library. Katherine of Aragon's departure from Spain and journey to England is described by Bernaldes.

2 *A true and loving husband*

The Spanish Calendar gives details of the dispute over Katherine's dowry and Henry VII's prevarication over her accompanying Arthur to Ludlow. It also describes Katherine's reception in England, as does Leland in *Collectanea*. Henry VII's insistence on seeing Katherine at Dogmersfield is described in *Proceedings and Ordinances of the Privy Council of England* and *Collectanea*; *Collectanea* is the source for Katherine's first meeting and evening with Prince Arthur.

The description of Henry VII derives from that given by the King's official historian, Polydore Vergil, in his *Anglica Historia* (Basle, 1534; ed. D. Hay, Camden Society, 3rd series, LXXIV, 1950). Vergil is the chief primary authority for the reign of Henry VII. The first 'modern' biography of the King was Sir Francis Bacon's *History of the Reign of King Henry the Seventh* (ed. J. R. Lumby, Cambridge, 1875); today, the definitive life is S. B. Chrimes's *Henry VII* (Eyre Methuen, 1972); Eric N. Simons's *Henry VII: The First Tudor King* (Barnes and Noble, 1968) is also useful. There is a good biography of Elizabeth of York by N. Lenz-Harvey, *Elizabeth of York, Tudor Queen* (Arthur Barker, 1973), which replaces the memoir by Strickland. Both Vergil, and John Foxe, in his *Acts and Monuments*, credit Henry and Elizabeth with four sons, as does Dean Stanley. However, the contemporary Windsor altarpiece shows only three, Arthur, Henry and Edmund. Dean Stanley says that an Edward Tudor (1495?–9) was buried in Westminster Abbey; he has perhaps confused him with his brother Edmund. Details of the youth of Henry VIII are to be found in *Letters and Papers of the Reign of Henry VIII* (detailed above), hereafter to be referred to as *L & P*; for his education see Bernard André's *Vita Henrici VII* (1500–8; in *Memorials of King Henry VII*, detailed above) – André was tutor to Henry VII's two elder sons.

The major events and state occasions of the reign of Henry VII are chronicled by Polydore Vergil, Pietro Carmelianus of Brescia, in his '*Solomnes Ceremoniae et Triumphi*' (1508; ed. H. Ellis, Roxburgh Club, 1818), the London merchant Robert Fabyan in *The Concordance of Histories: The New Chronicles of England and France* (1512; ed. H. Ellis, Rivington, 1811), *The Great Chronicle of London* (eds A. H. Thomas and I. D. Thornley, Alan Sutton, 1938), *Memorials of King Henry VII*, and *The Reign of Henry VII from Contemporary Sources* (3 vols, ed. A. F. Pollard, Longmans, 1913–14). The description of Prince Arthur's manor at Bewdley comes from John Leland's *Itinerary* (5 vols, ed. L. T. Smith, London, 1906–8). Leland was an antiquary who toured England in the early sixteenth century. His other important work was *De Rebus Brittanicis Collectanea* (published 1612; ed. T. Hearne, Chetham Society, 6 vols, Oxford, 1715), an important source for the period. The best account of Katherine's state entry into London is in Hall's Chronicle, and the *Great Chronicle of London* records details of the pageants and verses performed on that occasion. For the wedding of Katherine and Arthur, see Hall's Chronicle and also William Longman's *A History of the Three Cathedrals dedicated to St Paul in London* (Longmans, Green & Co., 1973) and W. S. Simpson's *St Paul's Cathedral and Old City Life* (Elliot Stock, 1894). The wedding banquet is described in Hall's Chronicle and *Collectanea*, and the pageants to celebrate the marriage are detailed in *The Great Chronicle of London*.

Next to nothing is known of Katherine of Aragon's daily life as Princess of Wales. Accounts of her brief marriage to Prince Arthur appear in Dulcie M. Ashdown's *Princess of Wales* (John Murray,

1979), *Lives of the Princesses of Wales* by M. B. Fryer, A. Bousfield and G. Toffoli (Dundurn Press, 1983) and Francis Jones's *The Princes and Principality of Wales* (University of Wales, Cardiff, 1969). Prince Arthur's death is described by Bernaldes, and the breaking of the news of it to Henry VII by Leland in *Collectanea*.

3 *Our daughter remains as she was here*

The major source for this chapter is the Spanish Calendar, which recounts the enquiries into Katherine's virginal status, negotiations for her marriage to Prince Henry, events leading up to the signing of the marriage treaty, negotiations with the Vatican for a dispensation, the text of the dispensations obtained, Queen Isabella's doubts as to its validity, negotiations for the payment of Katherine's dowry, her finances, her ill health and depression, her chafing at the restrictions imposed on her by etiquette, and Henry VII's treatment of her. Pope Julius's prevarication over the granting of a dispensation is mentioned in *L & P*. Hall is the source for Prince Henry's creation as Prince of Wales. The Prince's repudiation of his betrothal to Katherine is described by Lord Herbert.

4 *Pain and annoyance*

The Spanish Calendar continues to be the major source for this period of Katherine's life: it describes the secret negotiations to find another bride for Prince Henry, Katherine's problems with her household and finances, the course of her illness and depression, the dispute over her dowry, her status at court, the visit of King Philip and Queen Juana to England, Henry VII's plans to marry Juana, Katherine's appointment as her father's ambassador to the English court, her relations with Henry VII, with various Spanish diplomats, and with her confessor Fray Diego Fernandez, her correspondence, her reconciliation with Fuensalida who replaced her as ambassador, and the reopening of negotiations for her marriage with Henry VIII after his father's death.

Another account of the visit of Philip and Juana is given in the Cotton MSS. in the British Library. Prince Henry's letter is quoted by Byrne. The account of Henry VII's death, and the summary of his reign and achievements is based on those given by Bacon and Carmelianus. His wealth is referred to in the Venetian Calendar. Henry VIII's love for Katherine of Aragon, his desire to marry her, and his constant reiteration of this desire before their marriage is vouched for by his cousin, Reginald Pole, in *Pro Ecclesiasticae Unitatis Defensione*, 1536, (Rome, 1698).

5 Sir Loyal Heart and the Tudor court

Hall's Chronicle mentions the doubts felt by some about the validity of Henry VIII's proposed marriage to Katherine of Aragon. The wedding ceremony, and the date on which it took place, are recorded by Bernaldes.

Descriptions of Henry VIII's appearance appear in the Spanish Calendar, the Venetian Calendar, Cavendish's *Life of Cardinal Wolsey* and the dispatches of the Venetian ambassador Sebastian Giustinian, ed. L. Rawdon Brown in *Four Years at the Court of Henry VIII* (2 vols, Smith Elder and Co., 1854). The King's sporting and musical talents are described in the Spanish and Venetian Calendars, *L & P*, Hall's Chronicle, and the Milanese Calendar; his linguistic abilities are related in the Venetian Calendar and in *L & P*; his other accomplishments in the Venetian Calendar, which also mentions his piety, his genial informality, his popularity, his hatred of the French and the clothes he wore. His reluctance to attend, and boredom at, Council meetings, and his pursuit of frivolous pleasures in his early years are attested to by the Spanish and Milanese Calendars, and John Stow in his *Annals*.

Pageants, tournaments and court festivities are described in detail in Hall's Chronicle, the Venetian Calendar and *Four Years at the*

Court of Henry VIII. The royal visit to Coventry is mentioned in the Harleian MSS. in the British Library. Henry and Katherine's inscriptions on her missal appear in the Kings' MSS. in the British Library. The plague of 1517 is mentioned by Hall. For Katherine of Aragon's visit to Merton College, Oxford, see *Registum Annalium Collegii Mertonensis* in the Library of Merton College, Oxford, and for her Chapel of Calvary see Stow's *London.* Surviving examples of Katherine's needlework were described by John Taylor in *The Praise of the Needle* (1634). The Spanish Calendar records Henry's correspondence with King Ferdinand, and Katherine's relations with Maria de Salinas, Fray Diego, and other members of her household.

6 *A chaste and concordant wedlock*

The description of Henry VIII's coronation and the succeeding celebrations is derived from Hall's Chronicle. The Spanish Calendar records Henry and Katherine's early love for each other, details of Katherine's first pregnancy, the birth of a stillborn daughter in 1510, the conduct of Fray Diego and his dismissal, the FitzWalter affair, and the Queen's fall from favour in 1514. The ordinances for royal confinements are to be found in the State Papers. The Queen's taking to her chamber in December 1510 and the Christmas festivities at Richmond are described by Hall, who also recounts the birth and death of Prince Henry in 1511, the celebrations to mark the birth, and the grief of the King and Queen at their loss. The funeral of Prince Henry is mentioned in a manuscript in the Chapter House, Westminster Abbey.

Henry's farewell to Katherine and his departure for his campaign in France in 1513 are described by Hall. Details of the Flodden campaign are given in a letter from Sir Bryan Tuke to Richard Pace in *L & P*; Katherine's speech to her troops is reported in Peter Martyr: *Opus Epistolarum Petri Martyris* (published in Alcala de Henares, Spain, 1530); the losses at Flodden are recorded in the State Papers, and the events immediately following the battle are described by Hall. Henry's conduct on the French campaign is mentioned in the Milanese Calendar, and his return to England and reunion with Katherine is related by Hall.

Hall's Chronicle also gives details of Henry's anger at the perfidy of Ferdinand and Maximilian and the collapse of their triple alliance in 1514. The betrothal of the King's sister Mary Tudor to Louis XII is related in the Spanish and Venetian Calendars and in Hall's Chronicle. Hall also tells of the early death of Katherine's son, born in 1514. Henry VIII's distrust and jealousy of the new French King, Francis I, is recounted in the Venetian Calendar. For Francis I, see Desmond Seward's *Prince of the Renaissance* (Constable, 1973) and R. J. Knecht's *Francis I* (Cambridge University Press, 1982). For Mary Tudor's marriage to Suffolk and her later life see Walter C. Richardson's *Mary Tudor, the White Queen* (Peter Owen, 1970) and Hester W. Chapman's *The Sisters of Henry VIII* (Jonathan Cape, 1969). Margaret Tudor's visit to London is recounted by Hall.

There are numerous references to Wolsey's growing power in the Venetian Calendar. For modern lives of the Cardinal, see A. F. Pollard's *Wolsey* (Longmans, Green and Co., 1929), Charles Ferguson's *Naked to mine Enemies: The Life of Cardinal Wolsey* (Little, Brown, 1958), Neville Williams's *The Cardinal and the Secretary* (Weidenfeld and Nicolson, 1975) and Jasper Ridley's *The Statesman and the Fanatic* (Constable, 1982). The birth and christening of the Princess Mary are described in Hall's Chronicle. There are several references to Henry's growing egotism in the Venetian Calendar. Sir Thomas More's friendship with the King and Queen and his rise to favour are detailed in the biography written by his son-in-law, William Roper, *The Life of Sir Thomas More, Knight* (published *c.* 1556; ed. E. V. Hitchcock, Early English Texts Society, vol. CXCVII, 1935). More's uprightness is attested to in the Spanish Calendar. Contemporary with Roper's *Life* is that by the Catholic historian Nicholas Harpsfield, *The Life and Death of Sir Thomas More* (published *c.* 1557; ed. E. V. Hitchcock and R. W. Chambers, Early English Texts Society, 1932). Selected letters of Sir Thomas More were edited by Elizabeth Frances Rogers (1961). More has attracted several biographers this century: Algernon Cecil, *A Portrait of Thomas More, Scholar, Statesman, Saint* (John Murray, 1937), Leslie Paul, *Sir Thomas More* (1953), E. E. Reynolds, *The Field is Won* (Burns and Oates, 1968), and, for revised and less sympathetic assessments, Jasper Ridley, *The*

Statesman and the Fanatic (Constable, 1982) and Richard Marius, *Thomas More* (Dent, 1984).

Katherine of Aragon's last pregnancy is detailed in *L & P* and the Venetian Calendar, the latter relating the birth of a daughter who died soon afterwards. Descriptions of the Princess Mary in childhood are to be found in the Spanish Calendar, the Venetian Calendar, Pollino, and the *Diarii* of Marino Sanuto (ed. R. Fulin, F. Stefani et al., 59 vols, Venice, 1879–1903). Hall relates the Princess's betrothal to the Dauphin, 1518. The birth of Henry FitzRoy is recorded by Hall, and public outrage at the marriage arranged by Wolsey for Elizabeth Blount is attested to in *L & P*.

For descriptions of the Field of Cloth of Gold, see Hall, Holinshed and the Venetian Calendar. A good modern account is given by J. G. Russell in *The Field of Cloth of Gold* (1969). Katherine's objections are recorded in the Spanish Calendar. Charles V's visit to England in 1520 is described by Hall, Holinshed and the Venetian Calendar. For Charles V, see *Charles the Fifth, Father of Europe* by Gertrude von Schwarzenfeld (1957). The visit of Henry and Katherine to Charles V is noted by Hall. For Thomas Cromwell's life and career, see Neville Williams's *The Cardinal and the Secretary* (Weidenfeld and Nicolson, 1975), A. G. Dickens's *Thomas Cromwell and the English Reformation* (1959), and B. W. Beckingsale's *Thomas Cromwell, Tudor Minister* (Macmillan, 1978). Henry VIII's defence of the seven sacraments, published in 1521, *Assertio septem Sacramentorum adversus Martinus Lutherus*, was edited by O'Donovan (New York, 1908). For his being awarded the title *Fidei Defensor*, see Hall. Charles V's visit to England in 1522 and his betrothal to the Princess Mary is recorded in Hall's Chronicle and the Spanish Calendar. Mary's education at Ludlow is described in the Cotton MS., Vitellius in the British Library and by Vives. The Duke of Norfolk's qualities and abilities are mentioned by Vergil and in the Venetian Calendar; the cruelty of his mistress is described in *L & P*.

The outward appearance of the marriage of Henry and Katherine is attested to by Erasmus in *The Institution of Christian Marriage* (1526). The Spanish Calendar and *L & P* both testify to Katherine's being past the age for childbearing. Henry's reluctance to send Mary to Spain is noted in Hall's Chronicle and the Venetian Calendar. Henry FitzRoy's elevation to the peerage is described in Hall's

Chronicle, *L & P*, and Stow's *Annals*. The Venetian Calendar records how Katherine took offence at it. Both *L & P* and Pollino describe Mary taking up residence at Ludlow in 1525.

Henry VIII's presence at Mary Boleyn's wedding is recorded in *L & P*. The arrival of the Spanish ambassador Mendoza is recorded in the Spanish Calendar and by Hall. The Spanish Calendar also records that he found it difficult to see Katherine, and that Katherine was against a new French alliance. The Bishop of Tarbes's doubts are explained by Hall. For the sack of Rome, see the Spanish Calendar. The King's doubts of conscience over the validity of his marriage are attested to by many sources, chiefly Hall, Cavendish, Roper, Harpsfield, various ambassadors and William Tynedale in *The Practice of Prelates* (1530).

7 *Mistress Anne*

One of the chief primary sources for Anne Boleyn's life is the biography written by George Wyatt in the late sixteenth century, *Extracts from the life of the Virtuous, Christian and Renowned Queen Anne Boleyn* (published London, 1817). Wyatt was the grandson of the poet Sir Thomas Wyatt, Anne's Kentish neighbour and admirer, and he drew his information from anecdotes handed down within his own family and the reminiscences of Anne Gainsford, who had been Anne Boleyn's maid of honour. This is a work strongly biased in favour of its subject, written as it was in answer to Nicholas Sanders's crushing attack on Anne, published in 1585. See also George Wyatt, *Memorial of Queen Anne Boleyn* (reproduced in *The Life of Cardinal Wolsey* by George Cavendish, ed. S. W. Singer, 1827) and *Papers of George Wyatt* (ed. D. M. Loades, Camden Society, 4th series, V, 1968). For hostile opinions of Anne Boleyn, see the Spanish Calendar, Reginald Pole's *Pro Ecclesiasticae Unitatis Defensione* (1536) and Sanders.

The early Boleyns are mentioned several times in the Paston Letters (ed. N. Davis, Oxford University Press, 1971), Stow's *London*, and the *Calendar of Inquisitions Post Mortem for the Reign of*

Bibliography

Henry VII. For Hever Castle, see the current Official Guide, also the pamphlet by Gavin Astor, *The Boleyns of Hever* (1971). For the character of Sir Thomas Boleyn, his children and early income, see *L & P*. Anne Boleyn's birthdate has been arrived at after considering evidence in William Camden's *Annales rerum Anglicarum et Hibernicarum, regnanto Elizabetha, ad annum salutis MDLXXXIX* (London, 1615), *The Life of Jane Dormer*, Lord Herbert's life of Henry VIII, Leti's suppressed life of Elizabeth I, William Rastell's *Life of Sir Thomas More* (fragment in the Arundel MSS. in the British Library) and the Patent of Creation of Anne Boleyn as Marquess of Pembroke (MS. in the Chapter House, Westminster Abbey); see also Ives's *Anne Boleyn*. For George Boleyn's date of birth, see George Cavendish's 'Metrical Visions' (included in *The Life of Cardinal Wolsey*, ed. S. W. Singer, 1827).

Anne Boleyn's virtues and accomplishments are described by Lord Herbert. For the duration of her stay in France, see Herbert, and also Emmanuel von Meteren's *Histoire des Pays Bas: Crispin, Lord of Milherve's Metrical History* (1618); *Epistre contenant le proces criminel fait à lencontre de la Royne Boullant d'Angleterre* by Lancelot de Carles, Clement Marot, and Crispin de Milherve (1545; included in *La Grande Bretagne devant l'Opinion Française* by G. Ascoli, Paris, 1927); *Histoire de la Royne Anne de Boullant* (MS. in the Bibliothèque Nationale, Paris; before 1550); and Charles de Bourgueville's *Les Recherches et Antiquités de la Province de Neustrie* (1583). Carles, Marot and Milherve were three great French men of letters and a valuable source of information on Anne Boleyn. Milherve was an eyewitness at her trial, and the other two, Marot in particular, knew her in France. Milherve wrote a separate metrical history. For Anne's stay in France, see the above, and also, for her accomplishments, Pierre de Bourdeille, Seigneur de Brantôme, *Lives of Gallant Ladies* (trans. R. Gibbings, 1924). For Anne's erotic experiences in France, see *L & P* and Brantôme.

Cromwell's denial of the King's having been Lady Boleyn's lover is recorded in *L & P*. For the Butler marriage negotiations, see *L & P* and the *Calendar of Ormonde Deeds, 1172–1603* (vols 3 and 4, ed. E. Curtis, 1942–3); *L & P* mentions Francis I's regret at Anne's leaving France. George Wyatt describes Anne's arrival at the English court and her success there. For her affair with Percy, see Cavendish,

L & P and the Percy MSS. at Alnwick Castle. Anne Boleyn's appearance is described by Wyatt, Sanders (a surprisingly unbiased account), Carles etc., and *L & P*. For the poet Wyatt's interest in her, see George Wyatt. The accounts by Harpsfield and Sanders are far-fetched and malicious, owing nothing to contemporary sources. For Sir Thomas Wyatt, see his *Collected Poems* (ed. J. Daalder, Oxford, 1975), Kenneth Muir's *Life and Letters of Sir Thomas Wyatt* (Liverpool University Press, 1963) and Patricia Thomson's *Sir Thomas Wyatt and his Background* (Routledge and Kegan Paul, 1964). The rise of the Boleyns is charted in *L & P*. For Anne Boleyn's early life, see J. H. Round's *The Early Life of Anne Boleyn* (pamphlet published 1885).

There are two good primary sources for Henry VIII's courtship of Anne Boleyn, those of George Wyatt and Cavendish. Henry's love letters, now in the Vatican Library, are in the collections edited by Byrne and Ridley. None of Anne's letters to Henry survives: that quoted by Leti is spurious. A letter headed 'To the King from the Lady in the Tower', purported to have been written by Anne Boleyn in 1536, is of dubious authenticity. Cavendish refers to the patience of Queen Katherine with regard to her husband's affair with Anne, and is also the chief source of evidence for Anne's deadly hostility towards Wolsey. Her cordial outward relations with the Cardinal are described in *L & P*.

8   A thousand Wolseys for one Anne Boleyn

The King's passion for Anne Boleyn is described in George Wyatt's Memorial, Cavendish, the Spanish Calendar and *Ambassades en Angleterre de Jean du Bellay, 1527–1529* (ed. V. L. Bourilly and P. de Vassière, Paris, 1905). Jean du Bellay was the French ambassador to the court of Henry VIII and a friend of Anne Boleyn. His dispatches are therefore a good source to balance against the hostile reports in the Spanish Calendar. Jewels given to Anne by Henry in August 1527 are listed in a document in the Public Record Office. For the course of their affair, and the first rumours of a divorce and of the King having found a new mistress, see Cavendish, George Wyatt and Hall. The secret hearing at Westminster is described by Cavendish, Hall and Holinshed. The Spanish Calendar describes Mendoza's activities, the Queen's apprehension and Henry's confrontation with her. It also contains details of diplomatic relations between Charles V, his ambassadors, and the Vatican, and correspondence between the Emperor, his ministers, Katherine of Aragon, Mendoza and his successor Eustache Chapuys, and the Vatican.

Bishop Fisher's opinion on the King's case is given in *L & P*. Roper is the source for the decision to refer the case to Rome; doubts about the wisdom of this are referred to in *L & P*. Wolsey's mission to France is described in *L & P*, Cavendish and Harpsfield. The Venetian Calendar includes several references to Katherine's popularity. The Felipez affair is recorded in *L & P*. Rumours of Henry's intention of marrying Anne are first mentioned in the Spanish Calendar. George Wyatt alone speaks of Anne's reluctance to marry Henry. Wolsey's resistance to the match is referred to by Cavendish and Holinshed. The embassies to Rome are described in *L & P* and in Foxe's Book of Martyrs; the Spanish Calendar includes Henry's dispensation to marry Anne. Anne's enmity towards Wolsey is attested to by Cavendish, du Bellay, the Spanish Calendar and Harpsfield. Hall is, as usual, the source for festivities at court.

The Pope's appointment of Cardinal Campeggio as legate to try the case with Wolsey in England is recorded by Hall, Cavendish, Roper and Foxe. Wolsey's solution to the Boleyn/Butler feud is found in the Ormonde Deeds. Hall and du Bellay describe Henry's treatment of Katherine. Du Bellay is the chief source for the sweating sickness epidemic of 1528; he mentions Henry's fear of catching the disease and constant moves to escape it, as does Hall's Chronicle and *L & P*. Du Bellay was the first to record that Anne Boleyn was stricken with the sweat. The Spanish Calendar reports public outrage at the King's nullity suit. Du Bellay speaks of Henry's growing disillusionment with Wolsey. William Carey's death is noted in the Spanish Calendar, and the wardship of his heir in *L & P*. The Spanish Calendar is also the source for the view that Wolsey was doing his best to prevent an annulment. Anne's letter to the Cardinal of July 1528 is in Corpus Christi College, Cambridge. Henry's staunch belief that his case was righteous is attested to in the Spanish

Calendar. Katherine's retort to Anne while playing cards comes from George Wyatt.

Campeggio's delayed arrival, and his coming to London are related by Hall and Cavendish, who both describe the legate's discussions with Henry, Wolsey and Katherine. The brief produced by Queen Katherine is discussed in *L & P*, the Spanish Calendar and the State Papers, and the Council's advice to her is contained in a document in the Public Record Office. William Tynedale, in *The Practice of Prelates* (1530), avers that Katherine's women were made to spy on her. Henry's address to the Londoners at Bridewell Palace is recorded by Hall, du Bellay and Foxe. Du Bellay refers to Anne Boleyn's unpopularity. For the Nun of Kent, see *Rotuli Parliamentorum*, *L & P*, and Alan Neame's *The Holy Maid of Kent* (Hodder and Stoughton, 1971). Anne's growing power is documented by du Bellay, Cavendish and the Venetian Calendar. Her reformist sympathies, and her reading of forbidden books are described by George Wyatt and Foxe. For Henry's piety see *L & P*.

Both Hall and du Bellay describe the preparations for the legatine hearing. Henry's gifts to Anne Boleyn are listed in *L & P*. The account of the proceedings of the legatine court is drawn from those given by Cavendish, Hall, du Bellay, Foxe, Stow's *London*, Holinshed and Herbert. Du Bellay reports rumours of Anne Boleyn's pregnancy. Wolsey's fall from favour is related by Cavendish, Hall and Roper. Campeggio's return to Rome is recorded by Foxe. Roper records Henry's sounding out of Sir Thomas More's views. For the arrival of Chapuys and his early dispatches, see the Spanish Calendar. For Thomas Cranmer, see Foxe, Cranmer's Miscellaneous Writings (see above), and the following modern works: A. F. Pollard, *Thomas Cranmer and the English Reformation, 1489–1556* (2nd edn, Cassell, 1965), Jasper Ridley, *Thomas Cranmer* (Oxford University Press, 1962) and Edward Carpenter, *Cantuar: The Archbishops in their Office* (Baker, 1971).

9 It is my affair!

The Spanish Calendar is a major source as before for relations between England and the Emperor, the fortunes of Queen Katherine, and correspondence with the Vatican. The dispatches of Eustache Chapuys are one of the major sources for this period of Henry VIII's reign. For the fall and death of Wolsey, see Cavendish, Hall, *L & P*, the Milanese Calendar, du Bellay and Holinshed. Anne Boleyn's growing power is charted in the dispatches of du Bellay, the Milanese Calendar and *L & P*; for York Place see the Spanish Calendar and Stow's *London*. For the Reformation Parliament, see *Rotuli Parliamentorum*, Hall, and Stow's *Annals*. The Venetian Calendar describes relations between Henry and Katherine and Katherine's appearance and demeanour. The ennoblement of the Boleyns is noted by Hall, who is again the chief source for court festivities for this period.

The English embassy to Bologna is related by Hall and Foxe. For the Vatican's stand on the nullity suit, see *Acta Curiae Romana in cause matrimoniale Regis cum Katherina Regina* (1531). In the same year John Stokesley, Bishop of London, Edward Foxe and Nicholas de Burgo published *The Determination of the most Famous and most Excellent Universities of Italy and France that it is unlawful for a man to marry his brother's wife, that the Pope hath no power to dispense therewith*; Hall gives details of each individual determination. For the petition of the nobility of England to the Pope, see Cavendish; Lord Herbert provides the transcript. Foxe describes Cromwell's role in the origins of the English Reformation. For Anne Boleyn's books, see William Latimer's *Treatise on Anne Boleyn* (MS. in the Bodleian Library, Oxford), a contemporary reformist source of great value.

For Katherine's confrontation with the lords of the Council in 1531, see the Spanish Calendar, Hall and *L & P*. The Princess Mary's appearance and accomplishments are described in the Venetian Calendar. Thomas Abell's book, *Invicta Veritas: an answer that by no manner of law it may be lawful for King Henry the Eight to be divorced* (Luneberg, 1532) is referred to by Hall and Foxe. Katherine's life in exile from the court is described by Hall and the Venetian Calendar.

The Venetian Calendar gives details of the banquet at Ely Place, as does Stow's *London*. The near lynching of Anne Boleyn is recorded only in the Venetian Calendar, which, with *L & P*, gives details of opposition to the King. The resignation of More from the office of Lord Chancellor is related by Roper. For the Calais trip, see Hall, the *Mémoires* of Guillaume du Bellay (see above), and the Milanese Calendar. Descriptions of Anne Boleyn's appearance are to be found in the Venetian Calendar and Marino Sanuto's *Diarii*. Her creation as Marquess of Pembroke is described by Hall and Milles's *Catalogue of Honour* (1610); the Patent of Creation is now in the Chapter House, Westminster Abbey. George Wyatt tells of Anne finding the book of prophecies. For Cranmer's request to examine the King's case, see *L & P*.

10 *Happiest of Women*

The dispatches of Chapuys are again one of the chief sources consulted. The Spanish Calendar records Anne Boleyn's first appearance as queen, as does Hall. Anne's coronation is described by several authorities, viz. the Spanish Calendar, Hall, *L & P*, Holinshed, Stow's *London* and *Annals*, Wriothesley's Chronicle, and Wynkyn de Worde's *The Noble Triumphant Coronation of Queen Anne, wife upon the most noble King Henry the VIII* (printed 1533). Evidence of Anne's unpopularity manifested on the day is given only in the Spanish Chronicle, but is hinted at by Chapuys. For Norfolk's row with Anne, see the Spanish Calendar. For Katherine of Aragon's effects, see *Inventories of the Wardrobes of Henry FitzRoy, Duke of Richmond, and of the Wardrobe Stuff at Baynard's Castle of Katherine, Princess Dowager* (ed. J. G. Nichols, Camden Society, old series, LXI, 1854). See also W. Loke's *An Account of Materials furnished for the use of Queen Anne Boleyn* (Miscellanies of the Philibiblon Society, vol. VII, 1862–3). Public opposition to the King's second marriage is detailed in *L & P*.

Cranmer's ecclesiastical court and its proceedings are described in *L & P*, Hall's Chronicle, Harpsfield's *Pretended Divorce*, and

Holinshed's Chronicle. See also *Articles devised by the whole consent of the King's most honourable Council, His Grace's license obtained thereto, not only to exhort, but also to inform his loving subjects of the Truth* (1533). The Lady Mary's obstinacy is described in the State Papers. Anne's befriending of Protestants and her reformist literature are detailed by William Latimer and Foxe. The help she gave Thomas Winter is mentioned in *L & P*; Nicholas de Bourbon records his debt to her in *Nugarum Libri Octo* (Lyons, 1538).

For Katherine's confrontation with the Council, July 1533, see the report of her chamberlain, Lord Mountjoy, in the State Papers. The King's progress is recounted by Hall; the Lisle Letters refer to the good health and high spirits of the King and Queen. Henry's adultery with an unknown mistress, with Margaret Shelton, and later his affair with Jane Seymour, are all mentioned in the Spanish Calendar. Harpsfield records that Katherine pitied Anne. Letters announcing the birth of a prince, and their alteration, are referred to in *L & P*. The birth of Elizabeth is recorded in the Spanish Calendar and Hall's Chronicle. The comment of John Erley and other disparaging remarks about Anne's child are in *L & P*. The Milanese Calendar records foreign reaction to the birth. For Elizabeth's christening, see *L & P*, Hall and Holinshed. The Spanish Chronicle mentions Anne's intense love for her child. The dispatches of Jean de Dinteville, the French ambassador, give details of Anne's unpopularity and her diminishing power. Elizabeth's household at Hatfield is described in the State Papers.

Katherine's defiance of Suffolk is recounted in the Spanish Calendar, *L & P* and Hall. Henry's New Year's gifts to Anne's ladies, including Jane Seymour, are listed in *L & P*. The order to Hugh Latimer to keep his sermons short also appears in *L & P*; for Hugh Latimer, see Harold S. Darby's *Hugh Latimer* (1953). The Lisle Letters record Lady Lisle's gifts to Anne Boleyn, details of Katherine's jointure conferred upon Anne, the execution of the Nun of Kent, and Little Purkoy's death. The involvement of Fisher and Katherine with the Nun is referred to in *L & P*. For Katherine's life at Kimbolton, see *The Kimbolton Papers in the Collection of the Duke of Manchester* (1864).

The text of the Act of Succession 1534 is given in *The Statutes* and *Rotuli Parliamentorum*. Anne's second pregnancy is documented in the Spanish Calendar and *L & P*. The oath of succession is printed in Wriothesley's Chronicle, and Fisher's and More's refusal to take it is related by Hall, Roper, and Chapuys in the Spanish Calendar. For Reginald Pole's views on the King's marriages, see *Pro Ecclesiasticae Unitatis Defensione* (1536). Katherine's defiance of Tunstall is recorded in the State Papers and the Spanish Calendar. The gifts of a peacock and a pelican are noted in *L & P*.

The Spanish Caendar, the Venetian Calendar, George Wyatt and William Roper all describe Henry's growing disillusionment with Anne. His stable of girls at Farnham and Webbe's tale are noted in *L & P*. Lancelot de Carles et al. mention Anne being blamed for the executions of 1535. Roper is the best source for More's sojourn in the Tower. Hall records the executions of the monks of the Charterhouse and Bishop Fisher. The bad harvest is mentioned in *L & P*, where there is also the sole reference to Anne's third pregnancy. Katherine's letter to Forrest, and the search of her house for incriminating evidence are related by Pollino; Hall gives a grim description of Forrest's ultimate fate. The allegation (unauthenticated) that Henry blamed Anne for More's death comes from *The Life of Jane Dormer*.

Anne's visit to Syon Abbey is described by William Latimer. Her charities, needlework, and interest in education are recorded by George Wyatt and Foxe. Her fear of being cast off as Katherine had been is noted in *L & P*. The Spanish Calendar is the chief source for Katherine's death. Pollino records Anne's jealousy of public interest in Katherine's 'good end'.

11 Shall I die without justice?

The tale of Anne catching Henry with Jane Seymour on his knee comes from *The Life of Jane Dormer* and Sanders, and may well have some basis in fact. Wriothesley's Chronical says that Anne's fright at the King's fall caused her to miscarry of a son. Anne's miscarriage is documented by the Spanish Calendar, Hall, George Wyatt, *The Life of Jane Dormer* and Sanders, and her comment to her ladies afterwards comes from *L & P*. The Spanish Calendar, in particular the dispatches of Chapuys, is a major source for the fall of Anne Boleyn. Jane Seymour's rise to prominence is noted in the Bodleian MSS. Jesus College, Oxford. Henry's courtship and the jealousy between Anne Boleyn and Jane Seymour is recorded in the Spanish Calendar and *The Life of Jane Dormer*. For Sir Nicholas Carew, see R. Michell's *The Carews of Beddington* (London Borough of Sutton Libraries and Arts Services, 1981), which also gives details of Beddington Park, where Jane stayed before her marriage. The plot against Anne Boleyn is described by Lancelot de Carles et al. and by Milherve in his Metrical History. Coverdale's Bible, with its inscription to Anne, is in the British Library. *L & P* mentions Cromwell sounding out the Bishop of London on the subject of a royal divorce. Henry's letter to Pace on the likelihood of his having male heirs is in the State Papers. The proposed trip to Calais is mentioned in the State Papers and the Lisle Letters. For Matthew Parker, see his Correspondence (mentioned above) and V. J. K. Brook's *A Life of Archbishop Parker* (1962). The Spanish Chronicle refers to Smeaton's newly acquired wealth. The torturing of Smeaton is hinted at by George Constantine, body servant to Sir Henry Norris in the Tower, in his *Memorial* (in *Archaeologia*), and the Spanish Chronicle gives unauthenticated details. For the May Day jousts, see Hall and Wriothesley.

Anne Boleyn's committal to the Tower is described in Sir John Hayward's *Life of King Edward the Sixth* (1630), but the best contemporary source for this and her imprisonment are the dispatches of Sir William Kingston, Constable of the Tower, to Thomas Cromwell, which give a day-by-day account of Anne's stay there. They are to be found in the Cotton MSS. in the British Library. Henry's nocturnal jaunts are described in the Lisle Letters. The arrests and imprisonment in the Tower of Rochford, Weston, Brereton, Norris, Wyatt and Page are described in the *Histoire de la Royne Anne de Boullant*, an almost contemporary French manuscript (Bibliothèque Nationale, Paris; before 1550). Wyatt's spurious confession is related by the Spanish Chronicle and Sanders. The information given by the Spanish Chronicle about these events is notoriously untrustworthy. George Boleyn's distress is noted in *L & P*. George Constantine avers Brereton's innocence. The King's new hairstyle is recorded in Stow's *Annals*.

The trial of Anne's so-called lovers is described by Hall and Wriothesley, and the Lisle Letters record public speculation as to the fate of the accused. Wriothesley records the breaking up of Anne's household. Anne's trial is documented by the Spanish Calendar, George Wyatt, Wriothesley, the Harleian MSS. in the British Library, the *Baga de Secretis* in the Public Record Office (in which are preserved all the surviving documents relating to the trials of Anne and her brother), Cobbett's *State Trials*, and the *Reports of Sir John Spelman* (ed. J. A. Baker, Selden Society, 93, 94, 1977–8) – Spelman attended Anne's trial. The belief of the people in Anne's innocence is attested to by Chapuys in the Spanish Calendar, George Wyatt, George Constantine, William Camden and Sir John Spelman, all of whom refer to the unfairness of the trial. For Rochford's trial, see Spelman, Wriothesley, the Spanish Calendar, George Wyatt, George Constantine, *Excerpta Historica*, Lancelot de Carles et al., Cobbett, and the *Baga de Secretis*. The sentence on Rochford is recorded in *L & P*. Thomas Fuller names Lady Rochford as a principal witness for the Crown.

Henry's announcement that he foresaw Anne's downfall is quoted in *L & P*. The execution of the male prisoners is described by Hall, Wriothesley, the Spanish Calendar, George Constantine, the *Histoire de la Royne Anne de Boullant*, the Lisle Letters, and Milherve's Metrical History. Rochford's scaffold speech appears in three versions: quoted variously by George Constantine, Wriothesley, and the Spanish Chronicle. Anne's reaction to Smeaton's confession is related by Lancelot de Carles et al. and Milherve. The case papers for the annulment of Anne's marriage to Henry have disappeared, but see Wriothesley's Chronicle and Ives's *Anne Boleyn*. The cost of erecting the scaffold and Anne's expenses in the Tower are listed in *L & P*. For Anne's execution, see the Spanish Calendar, the Lisle Letters, *L & P*, the *Histoire de la Royne Anne de Boullant*, Lancelot de Carles et al., Milherve, George Wyatt, Sir John Spelman, Hall, the Harleian MSS. in the British Library, Wriothesley, the Spanish Chronicle, Foxe. and *The Chronicle of Calais in the Reigns of Henry VII and Henry VIII, to the year 1540* (attributed to Richard Turpin; ed. J. G. Nichols, Camden Society, XXXV, 1846).

For the tomb of Thomas Boleyn, Earl of Wiltshire, see the

guidebook to St Peter's Church, Hever, Kent. For Elizabeth Howard's tomb in the Howard Aisle of Lambeth Church, see *The History of the Parish of Lambeth* by J. Nichols (1786).

12 *Like one given by God*

The Spanish Calendar, chiefly the dispatches of Chapuys, is a major source for this chapter. Jane Seymour's former service as maid of honour to both Katherine of Aragon and Anne Boleyn is recorded by Chapuys and Wriothesley. Hall notes that Henry wore mourning for Anne Boleyn. For the marriage of Henry VIII and Jane Seymour, see Wriothesley's Chronicle and the Lisle Letters. Wriothesley incorrectly gives the date as 20 May and the place as Chelsea; the Lisle Letters have the correct date and place. Wriothesley describes Jane's first appearance as queen. Chapuys and Lord Herbert describe how she looked and dressed. The Act of Succession 1536 is reproduced in *The Statutes* and *Rotuli Parliamentorum*. For John Hill see *L & P*. Stow's *London* describes the King and Queen attending the marching-watch ceremony. Henry's reconciliation with Mary is documented by the Spanish Calendar, *L & P* and Wriothesley; Wriothesley describes their meeting at Hackney. For Holbein's portraits of Jane Seymour, see *Holbein and the Court of Henry VIII* (Exhibition Catalogue, The Queen's Gallery, Buckingham Palace, 1978). Hall describes the King and Queen's trip on the ice. Mary's reception at court is recounted in the Belvoir MSS. (Historical MSS. Commission, report XII, appendix IV, vol. I, the Duke of Rutland's Papers). For Jane's patronage of the Royal Hospital of St Katherine-by-the-Tower, see Hall, and Catherine Jamison, *The History of the Royal Hospital of St Katherine by the Tower of London* (1952).

Confirmation of the Queen's pregnancy is recorded in the State Papers, and the thanksgiving services for it in *L & P*. The Lisle Letters give details of the pregnancy, Jane's fancy for quails, and details of her household and the dress of her maids of honour. The prayers for Jane when in labour are mentioned by Wriothesley. For the birth of Prince Edward, see Hall, *The Chronicle and Political Papers of King Edward VI* (ed. W. K. Jordan, Allen and Unwin, 1966), and Jack Dewhurst's *Royal Confinements* (Weidenfeld and Nicolson, 1980), which explodes once and for all the theory – quoted by Harpsfield and Sanders – that Edward was born by Caesarean section. Wriothesley describes the celebrations in London in honour of the birth, and Hall describes the christening. Both chroniclers mention the ennoblement of Jane's brothers. Prayers of intercession for the Queen's life are referred to by Wriothesley. Her death is recorded in *L & P*, Wriothesley, Hall, the journal of Edward VI, and Foxe, and her obsequies are described in the State Papers and Hall's Chronicle.

13 I like her not!

For Henry VIII's search for a fourth wife and abortive negotiations in this connection, see *L & P*. From 1537 onwards, the dispatches of the French ambassador, Marillac, are a rich source of information on the period, especially with regard to Henry's wives, but Marillac is not always a reliable source. There are few dispatches from Chapuys relating to this period: he had been recalled to Spain when relations between England and the Empire deteriorated after the Pilgrimage of Grace. The Lisle Letters offer some fascinating information about the domestic life of the court at this time: Henry's piety, his friendship with Anne Bassett, courtly festivities, Prince Edward, and the selection of ladies for the new Queen's household. For further details of the childhood of Prince Edward, see *L & P* and the Cotton MS. Vitellius in the British Library. For the Exeter conspiracy, see Horatia Durant's *Sorrowful Captives* (Griffin Press, 1960).

For the embassy to Cleves, see Hall, Foxe and the Cotton MS. Vitellius in the British Library. The *Allgemeine Deutsche Biography vols 1 and 14* (Duncker and Humbolt, Berlin, 1967–71) provides good genealogical details of the family of Anne of Cleves. Anne's journey to England is described in the State Papers, the dispatches of Marillac, and the Lisle Letters. Thomas Wriothesley's opinion of Anne is in *L & P*. Anne's reception in Calais is described in Hall's Chronicle and the Lisle Letters, and her arrival in Dover by Hall and

William Lambard in *A Perambulation of Kent* (1576); her progress through Kent is described by Hall. Henry's visit to Rochester is related in *L & P*, the State Papers, and Hall's Chronicle, and his displeasure and attempts to get out of his marriage contract are chronicled in the State Papers. Marillac describes the preparations for Anne's reception on Shooter's Hill, which event is detailed by Hall, the Lisle Letters, Lambard, and the Cotton MS. Vespasian in the British Library. For the banquet afterwards, see Hall.

Henry's decision to go through with the marriage is recorded in the State Papers. Hall describes the marriage ceremony and the events immediately afterwards. Henry's inability to consummate the marriage is attested to in the State Papers. For Anne's secretary, see *Proceedings and Ordinances of the Privy Council*. Anne's presence at the jousts is recorded by Hall, who also tells of the return of the foreign nobles to Cleves and Anne's reception in London. For Lord Edmund Howard's letter, see the Lisle Letters. Cromwell's fall is chronicled by Marillac and Hall. The May jousts are referred to in Hall and Stow's *London*. Anne's banishment to Richmond is mentioned by Hall and Marillac.

Henry's affair with Katherine Howard is detailed by Marillac and Foxe. For her date of birth, see Marillac's dispatches, the Spanish Chronicle, and *A Tudor Tragedy* by Lacey Baldwin-Smith. The petition for the examination of the validity of the King's marriage to Anne of Cleves is in the *Journals of Parliament for the Reign of Henry VIII* (published *c*. 1742), and the decision to refer the matter to the clergy is recorded in the State Papers. The debate in the Lords is described in the *Journals of Parliament*, as is the annulment of the marriage; for this, see also Hall and Foxe. The reaction of the Duke of Cleves is recorded by Lord Herbert, and his doubts over Henry's treatment of Anne are mentioned in the State Papers. Anne's request to see Elizabeth is referred to by Leti. Anne's contentment is vouched for by Marillac. The execution of Cromwell is described by Hall.

14 *Rose without a thorn*

Henry VIII's marriage to Katherine Howard is mentioned by Hall and Foxe. Hall also describes the executions of Fetherston, Powell and Abell. Henry's armour in the Tower measures 54" around the girth. Anne of Cleves's merriment and Henry's visit to her are described by Marillac. Katherine's first appearance as Queen is recorded by Hall; her new clothes and caprices are referred to in the Spanish Chronicle. For a description of the Lady Mary, see Marillac's dispatches and the Venetian Calendar. Katherine Howard's household is detailed in the State Papers. The priest's slander is reported in Acts of the Privy Council. Henry's amorous behaviour is attested to by Marillac. Richard Jonas's *The Birth of Mankind* (1540), a treatise on birth and midwifery, is dedicated to Katherine Howard. The private life of Henry and Katherine is recorded by Marillac, who also gives details of Anne of Cleves's visits to court. Henry's gifts to Katherine are referred to in *L & P*.

Henry and Katherine's separation in the spring of 1541 is deduced from information in Acts of the Privy Council; Marillac describes the King's depression and illness. The release of Wyatt is mentioned in the Spanish Calendar and the State Papers (note that Chapuys was now back in England). Rumours of a reconciliation between Henry and Anne of Cleves are reported in *L & P*. Margaret Pole's execution is described by Chapuys. Dereham's appointment as Katherine's secretary, and his row with Mr John are reported in *L & P*, as are details of the progress of autumn 1541. Marillac mentions Prince Edward's illness. For the testimonies of Lascelles and Hall, see the State Papers. Henry and Katherine's return to Hampton Court is mentioned by Hall, and the thanksgiving service for the King's marriage is referred to in the Acts of the Privy Council. Hall tells of Cranmer's letter to Henry. Henry's initiation of an enquiry into the conduct of the Queen is recorded in Acts of the Privy Council, and the investigations arising from this are recorded in the Spanish Calendar, the Acts of the Privy Council, the State Papers, and *L & P*.

15 *Worthy and just punishment*

Hall, the Acts of the Privy Council, and the State Papers describe Katherine's banishment to Syon and her life there. The discharge of her household is related in Wriothesley's Chronicle. For the Council being informed of the proceedings against the Queen, and the debates over the action to be taken, see the State Papers and Proceedings of the Privy Council. The interrogations and testimonies of the suspects and witnesses are recorded in the State Papers, *L & P*, and Hall's Chronicle. Pollino mentions Culpeper's beauty. *L & P* refers to Katherine being deprived of the trappings of queenship and degraded. The arraignment of her lovers is described in Marillac's dispatches, *L & P* and the State Papers. Marillac and Chapuys both testify to Henry's grief. His refusal to commute Dereham's sentence is recorded in the State Papers and Acts of the Privy Council. Dereham's confession, obtained under torture, is in the State Papers. Harpsfield says people were saying that Katherine and Dereham were worthy to be hanged one against the other. The State Papers report the rumours of Anne of Cleves's pregnancy. For the execution of Katherine's lovers, see Hall and Wriothesley. The account of Nikander Nucius in the Spanish Calendar (1546) is the authority for the heads of the Queen's lovers being displayed on spikes on London Bridge.

The committal of members of the Howard family to the Tower, their arraignments and their ultimate fates are all described in the State Papers, the Acts of the Privy Council, the Journals of Parliament and Hall's Chronicle. For Henry's advancing stoutness, see Marillac. Hall records the passing of the Act of Attainder for treason against the Queen and Lady Rochford; the Act is in the House of Lords Record Office. Chapuys and the Journals of Parliament report Katherine's refusal to plead before the Lords. The Spanish Calendar describes Katherine's last days at Syon and speculation as to her fate. Hall and the Journals of Parliament confirm that Henry's assent to the Attainder was given under Letters Patent. His recovery from his grief and flirtation with ladies of the court is documented by Chapuys. The Journals of Parliament record

Katherine being informed of the sentence of death passed on her. Her removal to the Tower is described by Chapuys and *L & P*; Chapuys tells how she sent for the block. For Otwell Johnson's letters, and Katherine's last days in the Tower, see Barbara Winchester's *Tudor Family Portrait* (1955), also the Lisle Letters. Katherine's execution is described by Chapuys, Marillac, Hall and Foxe; spurious details are given by the Spanish Chronicle and Leti.

16 *Never a wife more agreeable to his heart*

The dispatches of Chapuys are one of the chief sources for Henry VIII's domestic life during this period. Henry's health is described by Andrew Boorde in *A Breviary of Health* (1542; ed. F. J. Furnivall, Early English Texts Society, London, 1870), and his happier frame of mind by Chapuys. For Scottish affairs, see Hall and Byrne. For the affairs of the Lady Mary, see the dispatches of Marillac, the Venetian Calendar and the Spanish Calendar. Negotiations for the marriage of Katherine Parr to Henry Scrope are described by Strickland. For Katherine Parr's Throckmorton relations, see A. L. Rowse's *Raleigh and the Throckmortons* (Macmillan, 1962), and for Anne Parr, see Sir Tresham Lever's *The Herberts of Wilton* (1967). Snape Hall is described in *Collectanea*. For William Parr's matrimonial entanglements, see Hall, the Spanish Calendar and the Complete Peerage. Chapuys records that Henry used emotional blackmail to win Katherine's sympathy. His corpulence is described by Sir John Spelman.

Katherine Parr's religious zeal is mentioned by Foxe, and there is ample evidence for it in the two tracts published by her: *Prayers and Meditations* (1545) and *The Lamentations of a Sinner* (1547). Her character is discussed in the Spanish Calendar, the Spanish Chronicle and Foxe's Book of Martyrs. A poem by her in French is in the Cecil Papers at Hatfield House, and corroborates contemporary references to her ability to speak French. The special licence for her marriage is in the State Papers, and the ceremony itself is described by Hall.

Anne of Cleves's reaction is mentioned in the Spanish Calendar and the Spanish Chronicle.

The education of Prince Edward is described in the journal of Edward VI, Sir John Hayward's Life, and Roger Ascham's *Toxophilus* (1545). Hall refers to the ennoblement of William Parr. Chapuys mentions Henry's obesity and growing infirmity. For Najera's visit, see the Spanish Calendar, which also mentions Margaret Douglas's marriage. Henry's appointment of Katherine as Regent during his absence in France is recorded in *L & P* and the State Papers. The Spanish Calendar describes the Siege of Boulogne. Katherine's injunctions against the plague are in the Harleian MSS. in the British Library. Her farewell to Chapuys is recorded by him in the Spanish Calendar, which also refers to her reputed reformist tendencies. For her owning heretical books, see Robert Parsons's *A Treatise of Three Conversions of England* (1603); for Anne Askew, see John Bale's *The First Examination of Anne Askew* (1546) and *The Latter Examination of Anne Askew* (1547); and for the Duchess of Suffolk see Evelyn Read's *Catherine, Duchess of Suffolk* (Jonathan Cape, 1962). For Gardiner's plot against Katherine and the events that allegedly occurred in *c.* July, 1546, see Foxe. Hall records the fate of Anne Askew. The visit of the Admiral of France is described by Wriothesley.

The Spanish Calendar mentions Henry's popularity at the end of his life. His death is recorded in the Spanish Calendar, the dispatches of George de Selve, the French ambassador, Hall's Chronicle, Foxe's Book of Martyrs, and William Thomas's *The Pilgrim: A Dialogue on the Life and Actions of King Henry the Eighth* (*c.* 1547; ed. J. A. Froude, Parker, Son and Bourn, 1861). Harpsfield gives an apocryphal account. Edward VI's journal and Hayward give accounts of how the news was broken to the King's children. Hall relates the proclaiming of Edward VI as King. Henry's funeral is described by Hall and Foxe, and the summary of his life and achievements is based on those given in the Spanish Calendar, Foxe's Book of Martyrs, and William Thomas's *The Pilgrim*.

17 Under the planets at Chelsea

For the character of Sir Thomas Seymour, see Hayward. The character of the Lady Elizabeth is described in the *Life of Jane Dormer*. Hall records Katherine's wish to marry Seymour. For Katherine's house at Chelsea, see Mary Cathcart Borer's *Two Villages: The Story of Chelsea and Kensington* (W. H. Allen, 1973) and Thea Holme's *Chelsea* (Hamish Hamilton, 1972). Katherine's marriage to Seymour is mentioned by Edward VI in his journal, which also refers to the offence taken by Lord Protector Somerset and the Council; see also the indictment of Lord Sudeley, 1549, in the State Papers. William Camden relates the feud between Katherine and the Duchess of Suffolk. For a description of Lady Jane Grey, see the letter of Baptist Spinola, 10 July 1553, in the Genoese Archives. There are two excellent modern biographies of Jane: Hester W. Chapman's *Lady Jane Grey* (Jonathan Cape, 1962) and Alison Plowden's *Lady Jane Grey and the House of Suffolk* (Sidgwick and Jackson, 1985). Udall's praise is recorded in his *The First Tome or Volume of the Paraphrase of Erasmus upon the New Testament* (1548).

Details of the affair between Seymour and Elizabeth are to be found in the State Papers (Deposition of Katherine Ashley, January 1549, Deposition of Thomas Parry, January, 1549, and Deposition of the Lady Elizabeth, January, 1549). The rumours that Elizabeth bore the Admiral a child are referred to in *The Life of Jane Dormer*. Elizabeth's illness is recorded in the State Papers. Sudeley Castle is described by Leland in *Collectanea*; for Throckmorton's description of it as a second court see Rowse. Katherine's death and funeral are recorded in *A Breviate of the Interment of the Lady Katherine Parr, Queen Dowager, late wife to King Henry VIII etc.*, a manuscript in the Royal College of Arms.

For the later life of Anne of Cleves, the best sources are the State Papers and Strickland, who quotes most of the relevant documents relating to Anne. See also Fuller's *Church History*. For Anne's funeral, see the Cotton MS. Vitellius in the British Library.

The inventory of effects belonging to Katherine Parr's daughter is in the Lansdowne MSS. and is reproduced by Strickland, who also quotes all the evidence for and against the child growing to maturity. The fortunes of Katherine Parr's tomb and corpse are recounted by Treadway Russell Nash in *On the Time of Death and Place of Burial of Queen Katherine Parr* (1876), and also by Martiensson and Strickland.

Genealogical Tables

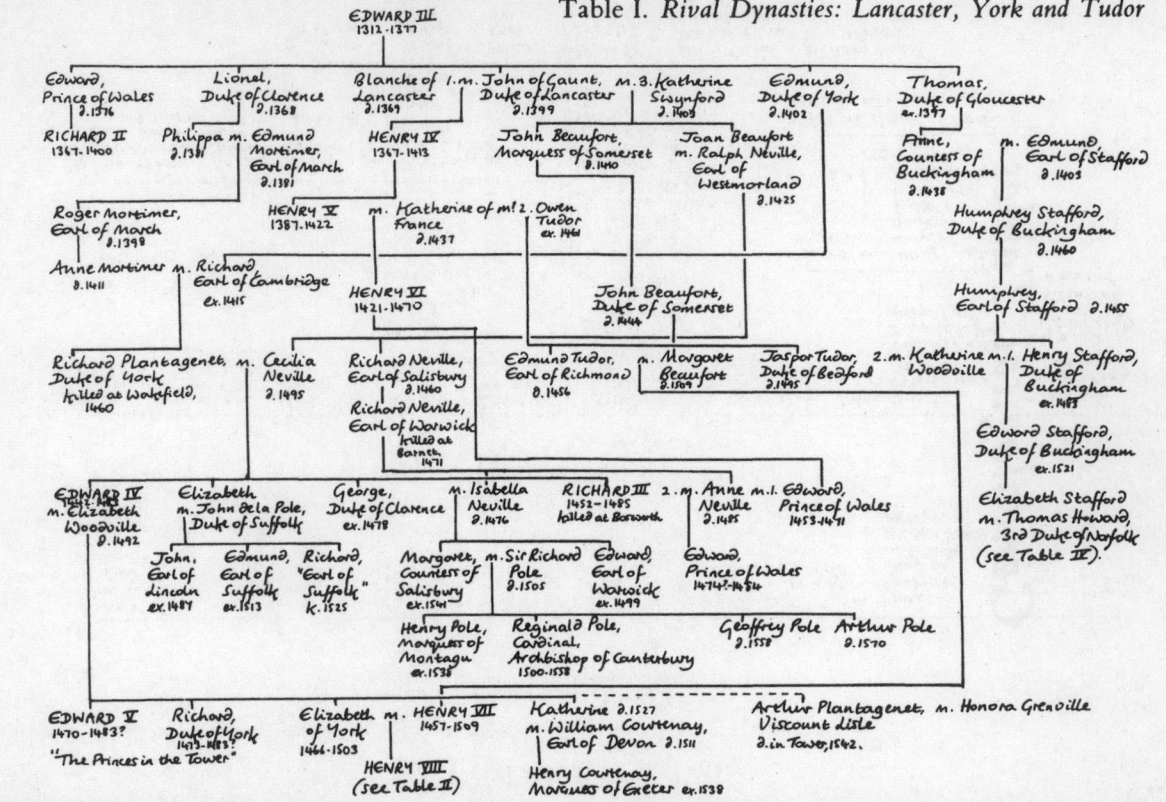

Table I. *Rival Dynasties: Lancaster, York and Tudor*

Table II. The Tudors

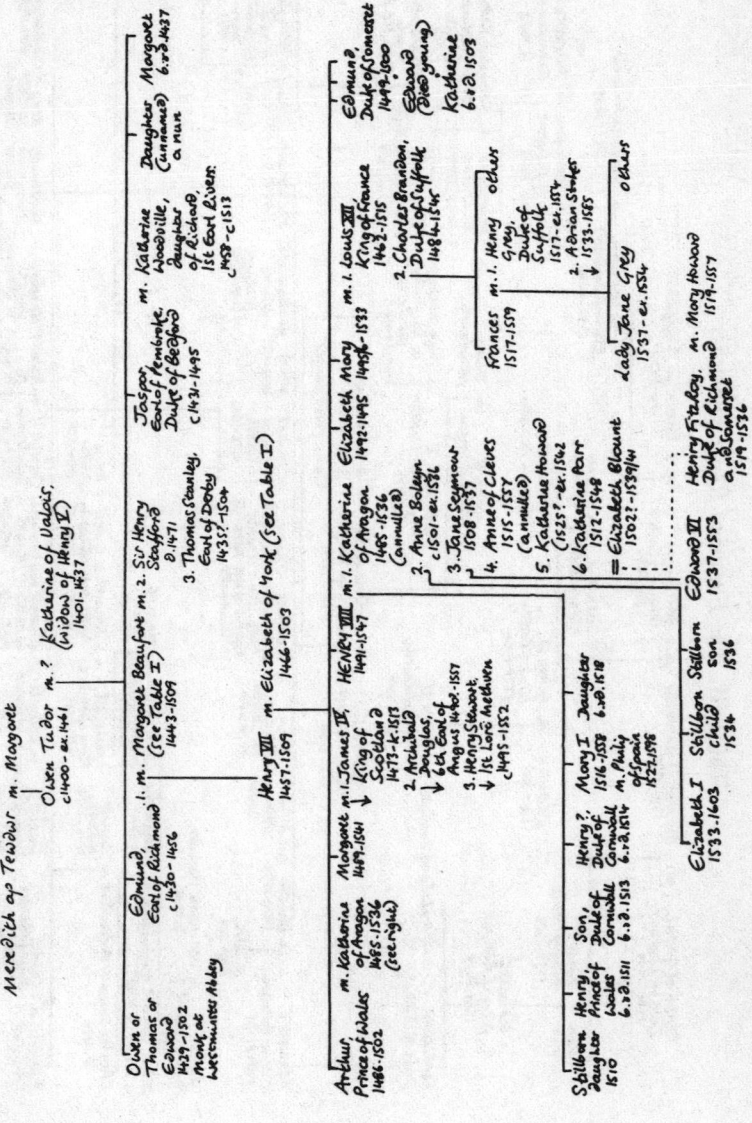

Table III. *The European Royal Dynasties*

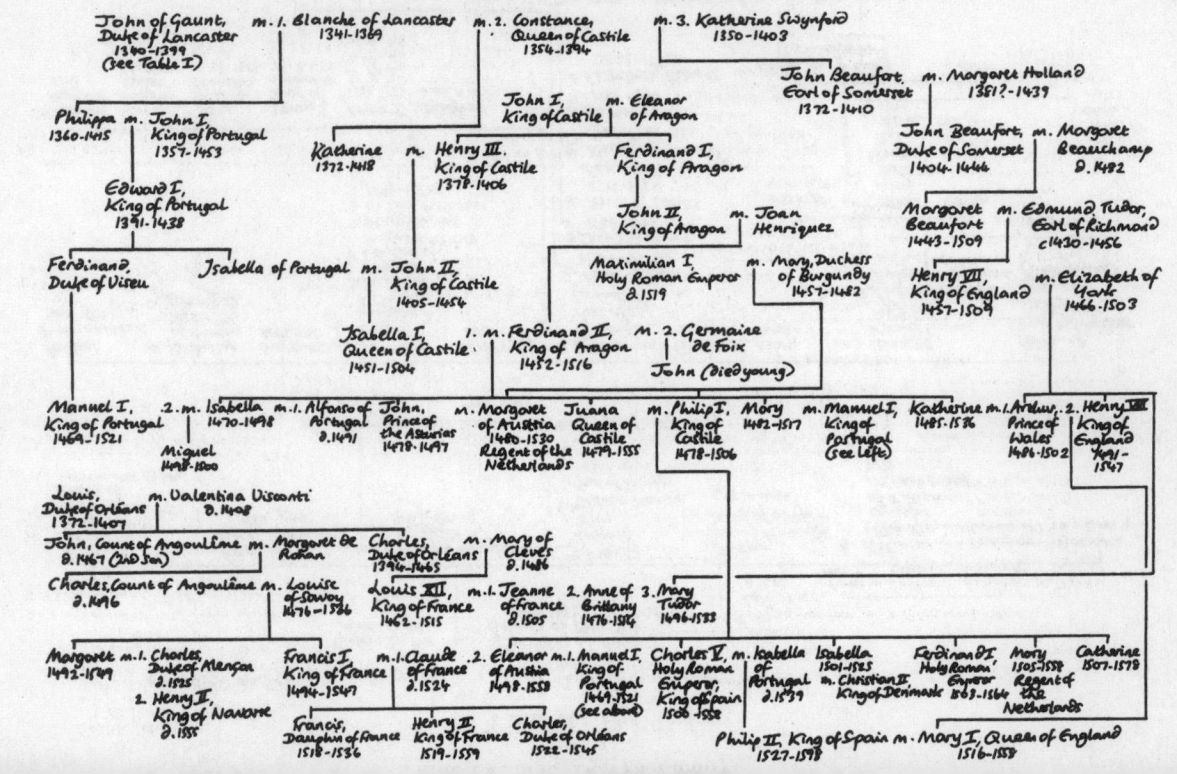

615

Ralph Boleyn
fl. 1402

John Boleyn of Salle, Norfolk

Thomas Boleyn of Salle m. Anne, dr. of
d. 1411   Sir John Bracton

Sir Thomas Hoo m. Eleanor de Felton
d. bef. 1448

Geoffrey Boleyn of Salle m. Alice   Bennid Boleyn
d. 1440   fl. 1436

Elizabeth Wychingham 1. m. Sir Thomas Hoo, m. 2. Eleanor Wells
d. bef. 1451   Lord Hoo
                             d. 1455

Anne m. Sir Roger   Eleanor m. James
1417-?   Copley   1444-1499?   Corew
                                    d. 1492

Sir Geoffrey Boleyn   m. Anne Hoo   Simon Boleyn   Cecily   3 sons,
Lord Mayor of London   1425?-1484   Chaplain of Salle   1408-1458   3 daughters
d. 1471   d. 1481

Sir Richard Corew d. 1520

Sir Nicholas Corew ex. 1539
m. Elizabeth Bryan d. 1546

Thomas   Sir William Boleyn m. Margaret Butler   Elizabeth m. Sir John   Isabella m. William   Alice m. John   Anne m. Sir Henry Heydon
1445-1471   1451?-1505   1465-1539/40   Fortescue   d. 1485   Cheyne,   Clere of   of Baconsthorpe
                                dr. of Thomas   Esq.   Ormesby   d. 1503
                                Earl of Ormonde   Sir Adrian Fortescue   Robert Clere
                                (descended from Edward I) 1476?-1536   Sir Edward Clere m. Alice

Sir James m. Elizabeth   Anne   Thomas Boleyn, m. Elizabeth,   Sir William   Edward m. Anne,   Anne m. Sir John   Anne m. 1. Sir John   Amata
of Blickling dr. of   1476-9   Earl of Wiltshire dr. of Thomas Boleyn   dr. of Sir   Sackville   Shelton   m. Sir
d. 1561   John Wood   and Ormonde   Howard, 2nd   John Tempest   d. 1554   2. Sir Thomas   Philip
                                  1477-1539   D. of Norfolk   Calthorpe   Calthorpe
                                                 d. 1538   Sir Richard Sackville d. 1566
                                                                            m. Winifred Bridges

Sir John m. Alice   Margaret
Shelton   Parker   "Madge"
                    Shelton

George Boleyn m. Jane Parker   Mary m. 1. William Corew   Anne Boleyn m. Henry VIII   Thomas Henry   Bridget m. Sir William   Dorothy m. Thomas
Viscount Rochford ex. 1542   d. 1543   d. 1528   c. 1501-1536   1491-1547   d. young   Paston   Brooke
ex. 1536   dr. of Henry,   2. William Stafford   8th Lord
               Lord Morley   Cobham
                                                            Elizabeth I Stillborn Stillborn   d. 1529
                                                            1533-1603   child   son
George,   1534   1536   George   Elizabeth m. Sir Thomas
Dean of Lichfield   Henry Corew m. Anne   Katherine   Brooke   Wyatt
d. 1603   1st Baron   Morgan   1529-1569   9th Lord   1503?-1542
                    Hunsdon   m. Sir Francis   Cobham
                    c. 1524-1596   Knollys
                                          1514?-1596   Elizabeth m. William Part,
                    George Corew   1526-1565   Earl of Essex,
                    2nd B. Hunsdon   Marquess of Northampton
                    1547-1603   1513-1571

Table V. *The Seymour Family*

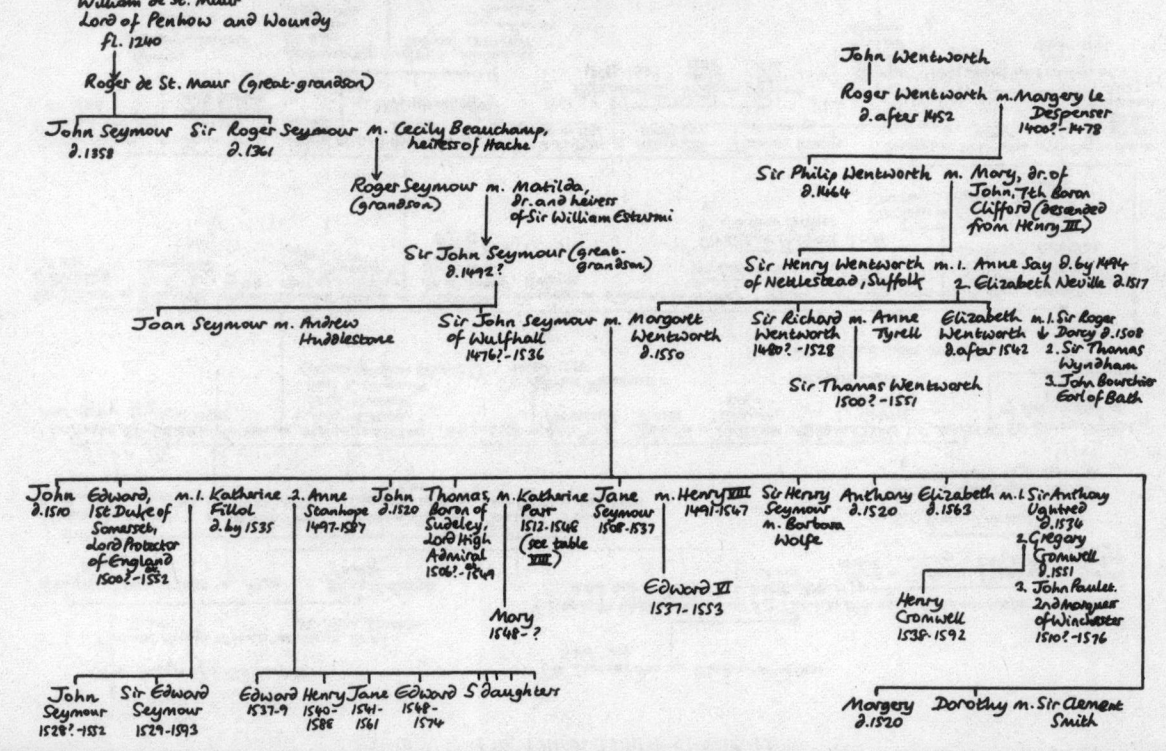

Table VI. *The Ducal House of Cleves*

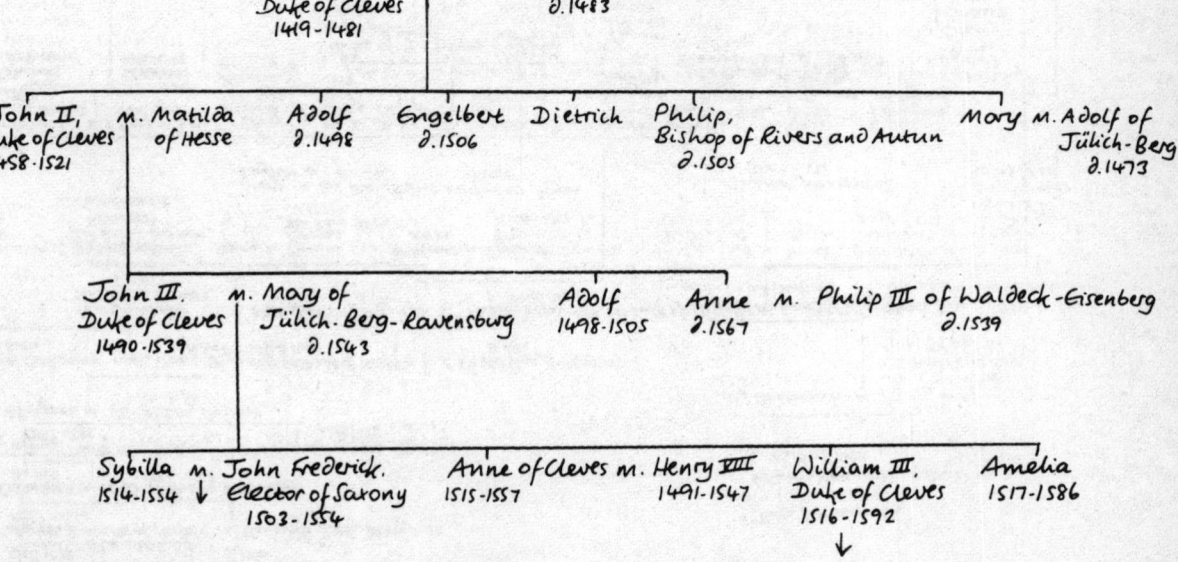

John I,
Duke of Cleves
1419-1481
m. Elizabeth of Burgundy-Nevers
d. 1483

John II,
Duke of Cleves
1458-1521
m. Matilda of Hesse

Adolf
d. 1498

Engelbert
d. 1506

Dietrich

Philip,
Bishop of Rivers and Autun
d. 1505

Mary m. Adolf of Jülich-Berg
d. 1473

John III,
Duke of Cleves
1490-1539
m. Mary of Jülich-Berg-Ravensburg
d. 1543

Adolf
1498-1505

Anne
d. 1567
m. Philip III of Waldeck-Eisenberg
d. 1539

Sybilla
1514-1554
m. John Frederick,
Elector of Saxony
1503-1554

Anne of Cleves
1515-1557
m. Henry VIII
1491-1547

William III,
Duke of Cleves
1516-1592

Amelia
1517-1586

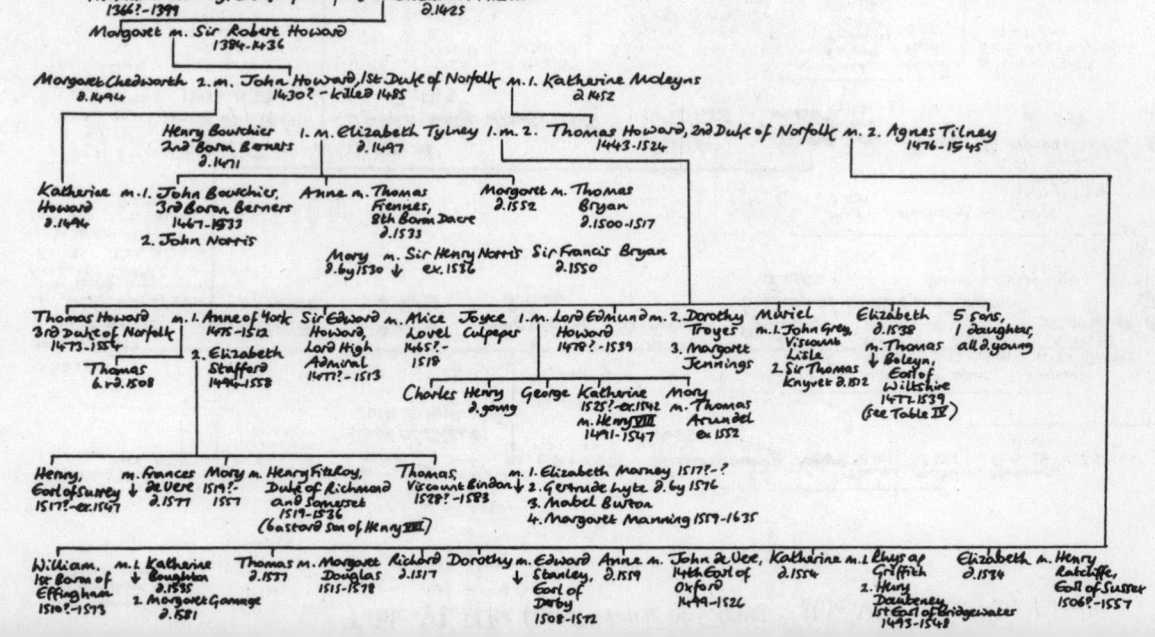

Table VII. *The Howards*

Eward I m. Margaret of France
1239-1307   1282?-1317

Thomas, Earl of Norfolk m. Alice Halys
1300-1338   d.1330

Margaret, Duchess of Norfolk m. John, 3rd Baron de Segrave
1320?-1400   d.1353

Elizabeth m. John, Baron Mowbray
d.1399   1328?-1368

Thomas Mowbray, Duke of Norfolk m. Elizabeth FitzAlan
1366?-1399   d.1425

Margaret m. Sir Robert Howard
1384-1436

Margaret Chedworth 2. m. John Howard, 1st Duke of Norfolk m.1. Katherine Moleyns
d.1494   1430? - killed 1485   d.1452

Henry Bourchier   1. m. Elizabeth Tylney   1. m. 2. Thomas Howard, 2nd Duke of Norfolk m. 2. Agnes Tilney
2nd Baron Berners   d.1497   1443-1524   1476-1545
d.1474

Katherine m.1. John Bourchier,   Anne m. Thomas   Margaret m. Thomas
Howard   3rd Baron Berners   Fiennes,   Bryan
d.1494   1467-1533   8th Baron Dacre   d.1552   d.1500-1517
        2. John Norris   d.1533

Mary m. Sir Henry Norris   Sir Francis Bryan
d. by 1530 ↓ ex. 1536   d.1550

Thomas Howard   m.1. Anne of York   Sir Edward m. Alice   Joyce   1. m. Lord Edmund m. 2. Dorothy   Muriel   Elizabeth   5 sons,
3rd Duke of Norfolk   1475-1512   Howard,   Lovel   Culpepir   Howard   Troyes   m.1. John Grey,   d.1538   1 daughter,
1473-1554   Lord High   1465?-   1478?-1539   3. Margaret   Viscount   m. Thomas   all d. young
    2. Elizabeth   Admiral   1518   Jennings   Lisle   ↓ Boleyn,
Thomas   Stafford   1477?-1513   2. Sir Thomas   Earl of
b. d. 1508   1494-1558   Knyvet d. 1512   Wiltshire
        Charles Henry   George Katherine   Mary   1477-1539
        d. young   1525?-ex.1542   m. Thomas   (see Table IV)
            m. Henry VIII   Arundel
            1491-1547   ex. 1552

Henry,   m. Frances   Mary m. Henry Fitzroy,   Thomas,   m.1. Elizabeth Marney 1517?-?
Earl of Surrey   de Vere   1519?-   Duke of Richmond   Viscount Bindon   2. Gertrude Lyte d. by 1576
1517?-ex.1547   d.1577   1557   and Somerset   1528?-1583   3. Mabel Burton
        1519-1536   4. Margaret Manning 1559-1635
        (bastard son of Henry VIII)

William,   m.1. Katherine   Thomas m. Margaret   Richard Dorothy m. Edward   Anne m. John de Vere,   Katherine m.1. Rhys ap   Elizabeth m. Henry
1st Baron of   ↓ Boughton   d.1537   Douglas   d.1517   ↓ Stanley,   d.1559   14th Earl of   d.1554   Griffith   d.1584   Ratcliffe,
Effingham   d.1535   1515-1578   Earl of   Oxford   2. Henry   Earl of Sussex
1510?-1573   2. Margaret Gamage   Derby   1443-1526   Daubeney,   1506?-1557
    d.1581   1508-1572   1st Earl of Bridgewater
                1493-1548

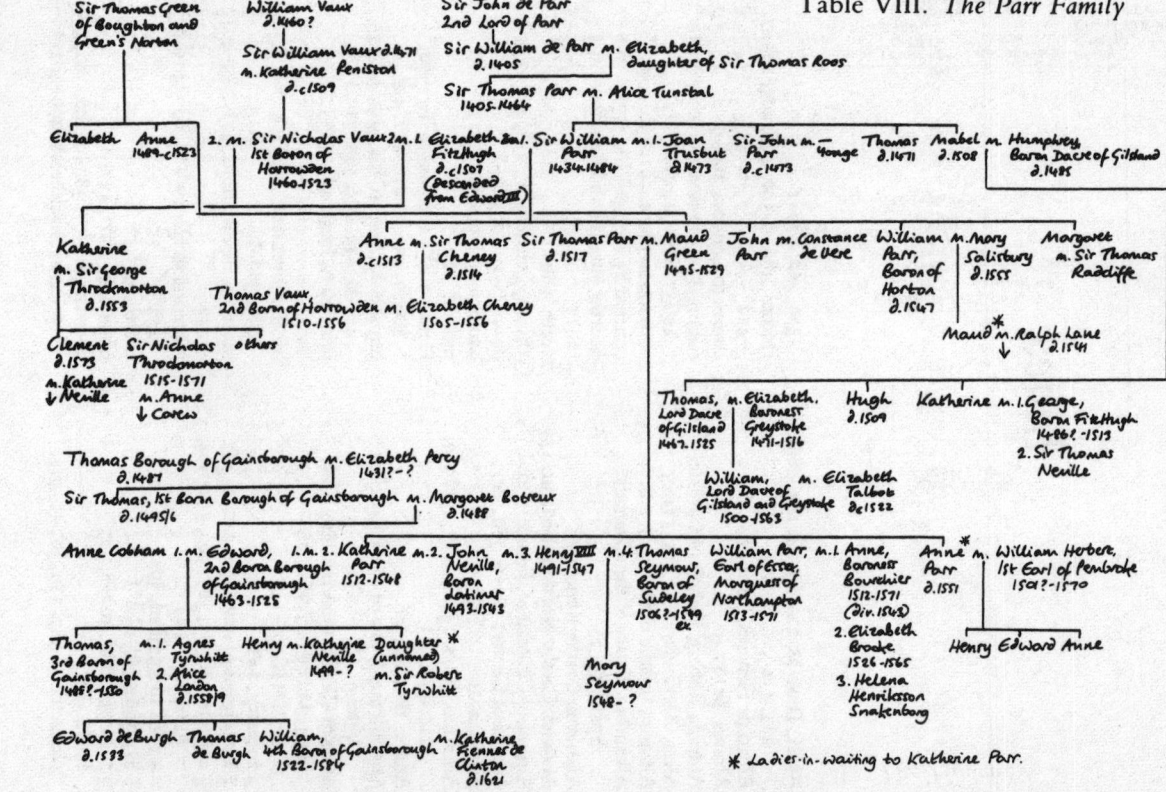

Table VIII. *The Parr Family*

619

* Ladies-in-waiting to Katherine Parr.

Index

Index

The illustrations are reproduced by kind permission of the following:

1. Wax death-mask of Henry VII, 1509, Norman Undercroft Museum, Westminster Abbey (by courtesy of the Dean and Chapter of Westminster). 2. *Elizabeth of York*, date and artist unknown, the Hamilton Collection at Lennoxlove. 3. *Isabella of Castile, c.* 1501, artist unknown, Royal Collection (by gracious permission of Her Majesty the Queen). 4. *Ferdinand of Aragon, c.* 1501, artist unknown, Royal Collection (by gracious permission of Her Majesty the Queen). 5. *Katherine of Aragon*, 1505, by Miguel Sittow, Kunsthistorisches Museum, Vienna. 6. *Katherine of Aragon, c.* 1525–6, by Lucas Hornebolte, miniature in the collection of the Duke of Buccleuch and Queensberry KT (by courtesy of the Trustees of the Victoria and Albert Museum). 7. *Henry VIII, c.* 1509–20, painted terracotta bust, probably by Pietro Torrigiano, the Metropolitan Museum of Art, New York (Fletcher Fund 1944, All Rights Reserved). 8. Henry VIII jousting before Katherine of Aragon in 1511, from *The Great Tournament Roll of Westminster* (© the College of Arms). 9. *Thomas Wolsey, Cardinal of York*, date unknown, by Jacques le Boucq, Bibliothèque d'Arras (photo Giraudon). 10. *Francis I, c.* 1525–8, by Jean Clouet, Louvre Museum, Paris (photo Giraudon). 11. Letter from Henry VIII to Anne Boleyn, *c.* September 1528, Vatican Library. 12. *Anne Boleyn*, date and artist unknown, Hever Castle, Kent (photo Woodmansterne). 13. *Anne Boleyn*, late sixteenth century, artist unknown, private collection. 14. *Thomas Boleyn, Earl of Wiltshire and Ormond, c.* 1532, drawing by Holbein, Windsor Castle Library (© 1990 Her Majesty the Queen). 15. *Thomas Howard, Duke of Norfolk, c.* 1538, by Holbein, Royal Collection (by gracious permission of Her Majesty the Queen). 16. *Pope Clement VII with the Emperor Charles V*, 1530, by Giorgio Vasari, Palazzo Vecchio, Florence (photo Scala). 17. Petition from the English nobility to the Pope, 13 July 1530, Vatican Library (photo Scala). 18. *Henry VIII*, 1536–7, by Holbein, Thyssen-Bornemisza Collection, Lugano (photo Bridgeman Art Library). 19. *Thomas Cranmer*, 1546, by Gerlach Flicke, National Portrait Gallery, London. 20. *Thomas Cromwell*, date unknown, after Holbein's lost original *c.* 1533–4 (© Frick Collection, New York). 21. *Jane Seymour*, 1536–7, by or after Holbein, Mauritshuis Museum, The Hague (photo Scala). 22. *Edward VI as a Child*, 1539, by Holbein, National Gallery of Art, Washington, D.C., Andrew W. Mellon Collection. 23. Drawing of Whitehall Palace, *c.* 1555, by Anthony van Wyngaerde, Ashmolean Museum, Oxford. 24. *The Family of Henry VIII, c.* 1543, artist unknown, Hampton Court Palace, Royal Collection (by gracious permission of Her Majesty the Queen). 25. *Anne of Cleves, c.* 1540, attributed to B. Bruyn the Elder (by courtesy of the President and Fellows of St John Baptist College, Oxford). 26. *Katherine Howard, c.* 1540–41, miniature by Holbein, Royal Collection (by gracious permission of Her Majesty the Queen). 27. *Henry VIII*, date unknown, after Holbein, Hever Castle (photo Woodmansterne). 28. *Katherine Parr*, 1545, by William Scrots, National Portrait Gallery, London. 29. *Elizabeth I as a girl, c.* 1546, artist unknown, Royal Collection (by gracious permission of Her Majesty the Queen). 30. *Thomas Seymour*, late sixteenth century, possibly after William Scrots, National Portrait Gallery, London.

THE LEGACY

Katherine Webb

WINDSOR
PARAGON

First published 2010
by Orion Books
This Large Print edition published 2010
by AudioGO Ltd
by arrangement with
The Orion Publishing Group

Hardcover ISBN: 978 1 408 48812 6
Softcover   ISBN: 978 1 408 48813 3

British Library Cataloguing in Publication Data available

BROMLEY LIBRARIES	AL
CLASS	
ACC 01958 9095	
CBS	INVOICE DATE 2 9 JUN 2011

Printed and bound in Great Britain by
CPI Antony Rowe, Chippenham and Eastbourne

To Mum and Dad

PROLOGUE

1905

Gradually, Caroline returned to her senses. The numbness inside her head receded and she became aware of myriad thoughts, darting like caged birds, too fast for her to grasp. Unsteadily, she got to her feet. The child was still there, on the bed. A slick of fear washed down her spine. Part of her had been hoping that it would not be so; that somehow he would have gone, or better still never have been there at all. He had pulled himself to the far side of the bed, struggling to crawl properly on the slippery-soft counterpane. His strong fists grasped handfuls of it and he moved as if swimming very slowly across the expanse of teal-green silk. He had grown so big and strong. In another place, in another life, he would have been a warrior. His hair was midnight black. The baby peered over the bed and then turned his head to look at Caroline. He made a single sound, like *dah*; and although it was nonsense Caroline could tell it was a question. Her eyes swam with tears, and her legs threatened to fold again. He was real; he was here, in her bed chamber at Storton Manor, and he had grown strong enough to question her.

Her shame was a cloud she could not see through. It was like smoke in the air—it obscured everything, made it impossible to think. She had no idea what to do. Long minutes passed, until she thought she heard a footstep in the hallway outside the door. It sent her heart lurching, so all she knew, in the end, was that the baby couldn't stay there. Not on the bed, not in her room, not in the manor house. He just *could not*; and neither must any of the servants, or her husband, know that he ever had been. Perhaps the staff had discovered him already, had seen or heard something whilst she had been slumped, insensible, on the floor. She could only pray that it wasn't so. She had no idea how long she had waited, her mind scrambled by terror and grief. Not long enough for the child to grow bored with its explorations of the bed, so perhaps not too long after all. There was still time to act, and she had no choice.

Wiping her face, Caroline went around the bed and picked the boy up, too ashamed to look into his eyes. They were black too, she knew. As black and inscrutable as ink spots. He was so much heavier than she remembered. She lay him down and took off all his clothes, including his napkin, even though they were coarsely made, in case they could somehow lead back to her. She cast them into the grate, where they oozed smoke and stank on the embers of the morning's fire. Then she looked around, temporarily at a loss, before her eyes lit on the embroidered pillowcase at the head of the bed. It had fine, precise needlework, depicting yellow, ribbon-like flowers. The linen was smooth and thick. Caroline stripped the pillow bare and put the struggling baby into the case. She did this tenderly, her hands aware of her love for the child even if her mind could not encompass it. But she did not use it to wrap him in. Instead she turned it into a sack and carried the baby out in it like a poacher might carry rabbits. Tears wet her face, wringing themselves from the core of her. But she could not pause, she could not let herself love him again.

Outside it was raining heavily. Caroline crossed the lawn with her back aching and the skin of her scalp crawling, feeling the eyes of the house upon her. Once safely out of sight beneath the trees she gasped for breath, her knuckles white where they gripped the pillowcase shut. Inside, the child was fidgeting and mumbling, but he did not cry out. Rain ran through her hair and dripped from her chin. *But it will never wash me clean*, she told herself with quiet despair. There was a pond, she knew. A dew pond, at the far side of the grounds where the estate met the rolling downs from which sprang the stream that flowed through the village. It was deep and still and shaded; the water dark on a cloudy day like today, matt with the falling rain, ready to hide any secret cast into it. She held her breath as the thought of it rose in her mind. It turned her cold. *No, I cannot*, she pleaded, silently. *I cannot.* She had taken so much from him already.

She walked further, not in the direction of the pond but away from the house, praying for some other option to present itself. When it did, Caroline staggered with relief. There was a covered wagon, parked in a green clearing where the woods met the lane. A black and white pony was tethered next to it, its rump hunched into the weather, and thin skeins of smoke rose from a metal chimney pipe in the roof. *Tinkers*, she thought, with a flare of desperate hope in her chest. They would find him, take him, move away with him. She would never have to see him again, never be faced with him again. But he would be cared for. He would have a life.

Now the baby began to cry as rain soaked through the pillowcase and reached his skin. Hurriedly, Caroline hoisted the sack back onto her shoulder and made her way through the trees to the other side of the clearing, further away from the house so that the trail would not point in that direction. It would seem, she hoped, that somebody coming along the lane from the south had left the child. She put him amongst the knotted roots of a large beech tree, where it was fairly dry, and backed away as his cries grew louder and more insistent. *Take him and be gone*, she implored silently.

She stumbled back into the woods as quickly and quietly as she could, and the baby's cries followed her for a while before finally falling out of earshot. When they did, her steps faltered. She stood still, swaying, torn between continuing forwards and going back. *I will never hear him again*, she told herself, but there was no relief in this, in the end. It could not be any other way, but a chill spread through the heart of her, solid and sharp as ice, because there would be no getting away from what she had done, she knew then; no forgetting it. It sat inside her like a canker, and just as there was no going back, she was no longer sure that she could go on either. Her hand went to her midriff, to where she knew a child lay nestled. She let it feel the warmth of her hand, as if to prove to this child that she was still living, and feeling, and would love it. Then she made her way slowly back to the house, where she would realise, hours too late, that having carefully stripped the baby she had then left him to be found in the fine, embroidered pillowcase. She pressed her face into

x

her bare pillow and tried to wipe the boy child from her memory.

'Tis calm indeed! so calm, that it disturbs
And vexes meditation with its strange
And extreme silentness.

Samuel Taylor Coleridge, *Frost at Midnight*

At least it's winter. We only ever came here in the summertime, so the place doesn't seem quite the same. It's not as dreadfully familiar, not as overpowering. Storton Manor, grim and bulky, the colour of today's low sky. A Victorian, neo-Gothic pile with stone-mullioned windows and peeling woodwork green with algae. Drifts of dead leaves against the walls and moss spreading up from behind them, reaching the ground-floor sills. Climbing out of the car, I breathe calmly. It's been a very English winter so far. Damp and muddy. The hedgerows look like smudged purple bruises in the distance. I wore bright jewel colours today, in defiance of the place, in defiance of its austerity, and the weight of it in my memory. Now I feel ridiculous, clownish.

Through the windscreen of my tatty white Golf I can see Beth's hands in her lap and the wispy ends of the long rope of her hair. Odd strands of grey snake through it now, and it seems too soon, far too soon. She was feverish keen to get here, but now she sits like a statue. Those pale, thin hands, folded limply in her lap—passive, waiting. Our hair used to be so bright when we were little. It was the white blonde of angels, of young Vikings; a purity of colour that faded with age to this uninspiring, mousy brown. I colour mine now, to cheer it up. We look less and less like sisters these days. I remember Beth and Dinny with their heads together, conspiring, whispering: his hair so dark, and hers so fair. I was cramped with jealousy at the time, and now, in my mind's eye, their heads look like yin and yang. As thick as thieves.

The windows of the house are blank, showing dark reflections of the naked trees all around. These trees seem taller now, and they lean too close to the house. They need cutting back. Am I thinking of things to do, things to improve? Am I picturing living here? The house is ours now, all twelve bedrooms; the soaring ceilings, the grand staircase, the underground rooms where the flagstones are worn smooth from the passage of servile feet. It's all ours, but only if we stay and live here. That's what Meredith always wanted. Meredith—our grandmother, with her spite and her hands in bony fists. She wanted our mother to move us all in years ago, and watch her die. Our mother refused, was duly cut off, and we continued our happy, suburban lives in Reading. If we don't move here it will be sold and the money sent to good causes. Meredith a philanthropist in death, perversely. So now the house is ours—but only for a little while, because I don't think we can bear to live here.

There's a reason why not. If I try to look right at it, it slips away like vapour. Only a name surfaces: Henry. The boy who disappeared, who just wasn't there any more. What I think now, staring up into the dizzying branches; what I think is that I *know*. I know why we can't live here, why it's even remarkable that we've come at all. *I know*. I know why Beth won't even get out of the car now. I wonder if I shall have to coax her out, the way one must coax her to eat. Not a single plant grows on the ground between here and the house—the shade is too deep. Or perhaps the ground is poisoned. It smells of earth and rot, velvety fungus. *Humus*, the word returns from science lessons years ago. A thousand tiny insect mouths biting, working, digesting the ground. There is a still moment then. Silence from the engine, silence in the trees and the house, and all the spaces in between. I scramble back into the car.

Beth is staring at her hands. I don't think she's even looked up yet, looked out at the house. Suddenly I doubt whether I've done the right thing, bringing her here. Suddenly I fear that I've left it too late, and this fear gives my insides a twist. There are sinews in her neck like lengths of string and she's folded into an angular shape in her seat, all hinges and corners. So thin these days, so fragile looking. Still my sister, but different now. There's something inside her that I can't know, can't fathom. She's done things that I can't grasp, and had thoughts I can't imagine. Her eyes, fixed on her knees, are glassy and wide. Maxwell wants her hospitalised again. He told me on the phone, two days ago, and I bit his head off for suggesting it. But I act differently around her now, however hard I try not to, and part of me hates her for it. She's my big sister. She should be stronger than me. I give her arm a little rub, smile brightly. 'Shall we go in?' I say. 'I could use a stiff drink.' My voice is loud in such close quarters. I picture Meredith's crystal decanters, lined up in the drawing room. I used to sneak in as a child, peer into the mysterious liquids, watch them catch the light, lift the stoppers for an illicit sniff. It seems somehow grotesque, to drink her whisky now she's dead. This solicitude is my way of showing Beth that I know she doesn't want to be back here. But then, with a deep breath, she gets out and strides over to the house as if driven, and I hurry after her.

Inside, the house does seem smaller, as things from childhood will, but it's still huge. The flat I share in London seemed big when I moved in because there were enough rooms not to have to peer through drying laundry to watch the TV. Now, faced with the echoing expanse of the hallway, I feel the ridiculous urge to cartwheel. We dither there, drop our bags at the foot of the stairs. This is the first time we've ever arrived here alone, without our parents, and it feels so odd that we mill like sheep. Our roles are defined by habit, by memory and custom. Here, in this house, we are children. But I must make light of it, because I can see Beth faltering, and a frantic look gathering behind her eyes.

'Stick the kettle on. I'll dig out some booze and we'll have tipsy coffee.'

'Erica, it's not even lunchtime.'

'So what? We're on holiday, aren't we?' Oh, but we're not. No we're not. I don't know what this is, but it's not a holiday. Beth shakes her head.

'I'll just have tea,' she says, drifting towards the kitchen. Her back is narrow, shoulders pointing sharply through the fabric of her shirt. I notice them with a jolt of unease—just ten days, since I saw her last, but she is visibly thinner now. I want to squeeze her, to make her be well.

The house is cold and damp, so I press buttons on an ancient panel until I hear things stirring, deep pipes complaining, water seething. There are rank ashes in the fire grates; there are still tissues and a sweetly rotting apple core in the waste-paper basket in the drawing room. Encroaching on

Meredith's life like this makes me feel uneasy, slightly sick. As if I might turn and catch her reflection in the mirror—an acid grimace, hair tinted falsely gold. I pause at the window and look out onto the winter garden, a mess of leggy plants falling over, unpruned. These are the smells I remember from our summers here: coconut sun cream; oxtail soup for lunch, no matter how hot the weather; sweet, heavy clouds from the roses and lavenders around the patio; the pungent, meaty smell of Meredith's fat Labradors, panting their hot exhaustion onto my shins. So different now. That could have been centuries ago; it could have happened to someone else entirely. A few raindrops skitter onto the glass and I am a hundred years away from everything and everyone. Here, we are truly alone, Beth and I. Alone, in this house again, in our conspiracy of silence, after all this time in which nothing has been resolved, in which Beth has pulled herself apart, a piece at a time, and I have dodged and evaded it all.

*   *   *

First we have to sort, to make some order of all the layers of possessions, of the items that have gathered into drifts in corners. This house has so many rooms, so much furniture, so many drawers and cupboards and hiding places. I should feel sad, I suppose, to think of it sold; the line of family history down the years to Beth and me, breaking. But I don't. Perhaps because, by rights, everything should have gone to Henry. That was when it all got broken. I watch Beth for a while, as she lifts lace handkerchiefs out of a drawer and piles them

7

on her knee. She takes them out one by one, studying the patterns, tracing the threads with her fingertips. The pile on her knee is not as tidy as the pile in the drawer. There's no point to what she's doing. It's one of those things she does that I can't understand.

'I'm going for a walk,' I announce, rising on stiff knees, biting back irritation. Beth jumps as if she'd forgotten I was there.

'Where are you going?'

'For a walk, I just said. I need some fresh air.'

'Well, don't be long,' Beth says. She does this sometimes, as well—talks to me as if I'm a wilful child, as if I might run off. I sigh.

'No. Twenty minutes. Stretch my legs.' I think she knows where I'm going.

I follow my feet. The lawn is ragged and lumpy; a choppy sea of broken brown grasses that soak my feet. It all used to be so manicured, so beautiful. I had been thinking, without thinking, that it must have got out of hand since Meredith died. But that's ridiculous. She died a month ago, and the garden shows several seasons of neglect. We have been neglectful of her ourselves, it would seem. I have no idea how she coped before she died—*if* she coped. She was just there, in the back of my mind. Mum and Dad came to see her, every year or so. Beth and I hadn't been for an age. But our absence was understood, I think; it was never tested too hard. We were never pestered to come. Perhaps she would have liked us to, perhaps not. It was hard to tell with Meredith. She was not a sweet grandmother, she was not even maternal. Our great-grandmother, Caroline, was also here while our mother grew up. Another source of discomfort. Our mother left as soon as she could. Meredith died suddenly, of a stroke. One day ageless, an old woman for as long as I can remember; the next day no longer. I saw her last at Mum and Dad's silver wedding anniversary, not here but in an overheated hotel with plush carpets. She sat like a queen at her table and cast a cold glare around the room, eyes sharp above a puckered mouth.

Here's the dew pond. Where it always was, but it looks so different in winter colours. It sits in the corner of a large field of closely grazed turf. The field stretches away to the east, woods to the west. Those woods would shed a dappled green light onto the surface; a cool colour, cast from branches that fidgeted and sang with birds. They're naked now, studded with loud rooks clacking and clamouring at one another. It was irresistible on hot July days, this pond; but with the sky this drab it looks flat, like a shallow puddle. Clouds chase across it. I know it's not shallow. It was fenced off when we were children, but with a few strands of barbed wire that were no match for determined youngsters. It was worth the scratched calves, the caught hair. In the sunshine the water was a glassy blue. It looked deep but Dinny said it was deeper even than that. He said the water fooled the eye, and I didn't believe him until he dived one day, taking a huge lungful of air and kicking, kicking downwards. I watched his brown body ripple and truncate, watched him continue to kick even when it seemed he should have reached the chalky bottom. He surfaced with a gasp, to find me rapt, astonished.

This pond feeds the stream that runs through

the village of Barrow Storton, down the side of this wide hill from the manor house. This pond is etched in my memory; it seems to dominate my childhood. I can see Beth paddling at the edge the first time I swam in it. She stalked to and fro, nervous because she was the eldest, and the banks were steep, and if I drowned it would be her fault. I dived again and again, trying to reach the bottom like Dinny had, never making it, and hearing Beth's high threats each time I popped back into the air. Like a cork, I was. Buoyant with the puppy fat on my chubby legs, my round stomach. She made me run around and around the garden before she would let me near the house, so I would be dry, so I would be warm and not white, teeth chattering, requiring explanation.

Behind me, there are distant glimpses of the house through the bare trees. That's something I've never noticed before. You can't see it through summer trees, but now it watches, it waits. It worries me to know that Beth is inside, alone, but I don't want to go back yet. I carry on walking, climbing over the gate into the field. This field, and then another, and then you are on the downs—rolling Wiltshire chalk downland, marked here and there by prehistory, marked here and there by tanks and target practice. On the horizon sits the barrow that gives the village its name, a Bronze Age burial mound for a king whose name and fame have passed out of all remembrance: a low, narrow hump, about the length of two cars, open at one end. In summer this king lies under wild barley, bright ragwort and forget-me-nots, and listens to the endless rich chortling of larks. But now it's more brittle grasses, dead thistles, an

10

empty crisp packet.

I stop at the barrow and look down at the village, catching my breath after the climb. There's not much movement, a few ragged columns of chimney smoke, a few well-swaddled residents walking their dogs to the postbox. From this lonely hill it seems like the centre of the universe. *This populous village!* Coleridge pops into my head. I've been doing the conversation poems with my year tens. I've been trying to make them read slowly enough to feel the words, to absorb the images; but they skim on, chatter like monkeys.

The air is biting up here—it parts around me like a cold wave. My toes have gone numb because my shoes are soaked through. There are ten, twenty pairs of Wellington boots in the house, I know. Down in the basement, in neat rows with cobwebs draped around them. That one horrible time I didn't shake a boot out before putting a bare foot inside, and felt the tickle of another occupant. I am out of practice at living in the countryside; ill-equipped for changes in the terrain, for ground that hasn't been carefully prepared to best convenience me. And yet when asked I would say I grew up here. Those early summers, so long and distinct in my mind, rising like islands from a sea of school days and wet weekends too blurred and uniform to recall.

At the entrance to the barrow the wind makes a low moan. I jump two-footed down the stone steps and startle a girl inside. She straightens with a gasp and hits her head on the low ceiling, crouches again, puts both hands around her skull to cradle it.

'Shit! Sorry! I didn't mean to pounce on you like

that . . . I didn't know anybody was in here.' I smile. The wan light from the doorway shines onto her, onto golden bubble curls tied back with a turquoise scarf, onto a young face and an oddly shapeless body, swathed in long chiffon skirts and crochet. She squints up at me, and I must be a silhouette to her, a black bulk against the sky outside. 'Are you OK?' She doesn't answer me. Tiny bright posies have been pushed into gaps in the wall in front of her, snipped stems neatly bound with ribbon. Is this what she was doing in here, so quietly? Praying at some half-imagined, half-borrowed shrine? She sees me looking at her offerings and she rises, scowls, pushes past me without a word. I realise that her shapelessness is in fact an abundance of shape—the heaviness of pregnancy. Very pretty, very young, belly distended. When I emerge from the tomb I look down the slope towards the village but she's not there. She is walking the other way—the direction I came from, towards the woodlands near the manor house. She strides fiercely, arms swinging.

*   *   *

Beth and I eat dinner in the study this first night. It might seem an odd choice of room, but it is the only one with a TV in it, and we eat pasta from trays on our knees with the evening news to keep us company, because small talk seems to have abandoned us, and big talk is just too big yet. We're not ready. I'm not sure that we ever will be, but there are things I want to ask my sister. I will wait, I will make sure I get the questions right. I hope that, if I ask the right ones, I can make her

12

better. That the truth will set her free. Beth chases each quill around her bowl before catching it on her fork. She raises the fork to her lips several times before putting it into her mouth. Some of these quills never make it—she knocks them back off the fork, selects an alternative. I see all this in the corner of my eye, just like I see her body starving. The TV pictures shine darkly in her eyes.

'Do you think it's a good idea? Having Eddie here for Christmas?' she asks me suddenly.

'Of course. Why wouldn't it be? We'll be staying for a while to get things sorted, so we may as well stay for Christmas. Together.' I shrug. 'There's plenty of space, after all.'

'No, I mean . . . bringing a child here. Into this . . . place.'

'Beth, it's just a house. He'll love it. He doesn't know . . . Well. He'll have a blast, I'm sure he will—there are so many nooks and crannies to explore.'

'A bit big and empty, though, isn't it? A bit lonely, perhaps? It might depress him.'

'Well, you could tell him to bring a friend. Why don't you? Call him tomorrow—not for the whole of Christmas, of course. But some of the working parents might be glad of a few extra days' grace before their little home-wreckers reappear, don't you think?'

'Hmm.' Beth rolls her eyes. 'I don't think any of the mothers at that school do anything as common as work for a living.'

'Only riff-raff like you?'

'Only riff-raff like me,' she agrees, deadpan.

'Ironic, really, since you're the real thing. Blue blood, practically.'

'Hardly. Just as you are.'

'No. I think the nobility skipped a generation in me.' I smile. Meredith told me this once, when I was ten. *Your sister has the Calcott mien, Erica. You, I fear, are all your father.* I didn't mind then and I don't mind now. I wasn't sure what *mien* meant, at the time. I thought she meant my hair, which had been chopped off short thanks to an incident with bubblegum. When she turned away I stuck out my tongue, and Mum wagged a finger at me.

Beth rejects it too. She fought with Maxwell—Eddie's father—to allow their son to attend the village primary school, which was tiny and friendly and had a nature garden in one corner of the yard: frogspawn, the dried-out remains of dragonfly nymphs; primroses in the spring, then pansies. But Maxwell won the toss when it came to secondary education. Perhaps it was for the best. Eddie boards now, all term long. Beth has weeks and weeks to build herself up, shake a sparkle into her smile.

'We'll fill up the space,' I assure her. 'We'll deck the halls. I'll dig out a radio. It won't be like . . .' but I trail off. I'm not sure what I was about to say. In the corner, the tiny TV gives an angry belch of static that makes us both jump.

*　　　*　　　*

Almost midnight, and Beth and I have retired to our rooms. The same rooms we always took, where we found the same bedspreads, smooth and faded. This seemed unreal to me, at first. But then, why would you change the bedspreads in rooms that are never used? I don't think Beth will be asleep yet either. The quiet in the house rings like a bell. The mattress sinks low where I sit, the springs have lost their spring. The bed has a dark oak headboard and there's a watercolour on the wall, so faded now. Boats in a harbour, though I never heard of Meredith visiting the coast. I reach behind the headboard, my fingers feeling down the vertical supports until I find it. Brittle now, gritty with dust. The piece of ribbon I tied—red plastic ribbon from a curl on a birthday present. I tied it here when I was eight so that I would know a secret, and only I would know it. I could think about it, after we'd gone back to school. Picture it, out of sight, untouched as the room was cleaned, as people came and went. Here was something that I would know about; a relic of me I could always find.

There's a tiny knock and Beth's face appears around the door. Her hair is out of its plait, falling around her face, making her younger. She is so beautiful sometimes that it gives me a pain in my chest, makes my ribs squeeze. Weak light from the bedside lamp puts shadows in her cheekbones, under her eyes; shows up the curve of her top lip.

'Are you OK? I can't sleep,' she whispers, as if there is somebody else in the house to wake.

'I'm fine, Beth; just not sleepy.'

'Oh.' She lingers in the doorway, hesitates. 'It's so strange to be here.' This is not a question. I wait. 'I feel like . . . I feel a bit like Alice in *Through the Looking Glass*. Do you know what I mean? It's all so familiar, and yet wrong too. As if it's backwards. Why do you think she left us the house?'

'I really don't know. To get at Mum and Uncle

Clifford, I imagine. That's the kind of thing Meredith would do,' I sigh. Still Beth hovers, so pretty, so girlish. Right now it's as if no time has passed, as if nothing has changed. She could be twelve again, I could be eight, and she could be leaning in to wake me, to make sure I'm not late for breakfast.

'I think she did it to punish us,' she says softly, and looks stricken.

'No, Beth. We didn't do anything wrong,' I say firmly.

'Didn't we? That summer. No. No, I suppose not.' She flicks her eyes over me now, quickly, puzzled; and I get the feeling she is trying to see something, some truth about me. 'Good night, Rick,' she whispers, using a familiar tomboy truncation of my name, and vanishes from the doorway.

*   *   *

I remember so many things from that summer. The last summer that everything was right, the summer of 1986. I remember Beth being distraught that Wham! were breaking up. I remember the heat bringing up water blisters across my chest that itched, and burst under my fingernails, making me feel sick. I remember the dead rabbit in the woods that I checked up on almost daily, appalled and riveted by its slow sinking, softening, the way it seemed to breathe, until I poked it with a stick to check it was dead and realised that the movement was the greedy squabble of maggots inside. I remember watching, on Meredith's tiny television, Sarah Ferguson marry Prince Andrew on the twenty-third of July—that huge dress, making me ache with envy.

I remember making up a dance routine to Diana Ross's hit 'Chain Reaction'. I remember stealing one of Meredith's boas for my costume, stumbling and stepping on it: a shower of feathers; hiding it in a distant drawer with dread in the pit of my stomach, too scared to own up. I remember reporters and policemen, facing each other either side of Storton Manor's iron gates. The policemen folded their arms, seemed bored and hot in their uniforms. The reporters milled and fiddled with their equipment, spoke into cameras, into tape recorders, waited and waited for news. I remember Beth's eyes pinning me as the policeman talked to me about Henry, asked me where we'd been playing, what we'd been doing. His breath smelt of Polo mints, sugar gone sour. I told him, I think, and I felt unwell; and Beth's eyes on me were ragged and wide.

In spite of these thoughts I sleep easily in the end, once I have got over the cold touch of the sheets, the unfamiliar darkness of the room. And there's the smell, not unpleasant but all-pervading. The way other people's houses will smell of their occupants—the combination of their washing soap, their deodorant and their hair when it needs washing; their perfume, skin; the food they cook. Regardless of the winter, this smell lingers in every room, evocative and unsettling. I wake up once; think I hear Beth moving around the house. And then I dream of the dew pond, of swimming in it and trying to dive down, of needing to fetch something from the bottom but being unable to reach. The cold shock of the water, the pressure in my lungs, the awful fear of what my fingers will find at the bottom.

LEAVING

1902

I will remain steadfast, Caroline reminded herself firmly, as she watched her Aunt Bathilda covertly through lowered eyelashes. The older woman cleared her plate with methodical efficiency before speaking again.

'I fear you are making a grave mistake, my dear.' But there was a glint in her aunt's eye that did not look fearful at all. More righteous, in fact, more self-satisfied, as if she, in spite of all protestations to the contrary, felt victorious. Caroline studied her own plate, where the fat had risen from the gravy and congealed into an unappetising crust.

'So you have said before, Aunt Bathilda.' She kept her voice low and respectful, but still her aunt glared at her.

'I repeat myself, child, because you do not appear to hear me,' she snapped.

Heat flared in Caroline's cheeks. She nudged her cutlery into a neater position, felt the smooth weight of the silver beneath her fingers. She shifted her spine slightly. It was laced into a strict serpentine, and it ached.

'And don't fidget,' Bathilda added.

The dining room at La Fiorentina was excessively bright, closed in behind windows that had steamed opaque with the vapours of hot food and exhalation. Yellow light glanced and spiked from glass and jewellery and polished metal. The winter had been long and hard, and now, just as spring had seemed poised to flourish with a tantalising week of bird song, crocuses and a green haze on the park trees, a long spell of cold rain had settled over New York City.

Caroline caught her reflection in several mirrors relayed around the room, her every move amplified. Unsettled by such scrutiny, she blushed more deeply. 'I do listen to you, Aunt. I have *always* listened to you.'

'You listened to me in the past because you had to, as I understand it. Now, as soon as you perceive yourself old enough, you disregard me entirely. In the most important decision you will ever make, at this most crucial juncture, you ignore me. Well, I am only glad my poor dear brother is not alive to see how I have failed his only child.' Bathilda heaved a martyr's sigh.

'You have not failed, Aunt,' Caroline murmured, reluctantly.

A waiter cleared their empty plates, brought them sweet white wine, to replace the red, and the pastry trolley. Bathilda sipped, her lips leaving a greasy smudge on the gilt rim of the glass, and then chose a cream-filled éclair, cut a large piece and widened her mouth to accommodate it. The floury flesh of her chin folded over her lace collar. Caroline watched her with distaste and felt her throat constrict.

'You have never made me feel dear to you,' Caroline murmured, so softly that the words were lost beneath the throng of voices and eating, drinking, chewing, swallowing. Smells of roast meat and curried soup clung to the air.

'Don't mumble, Caroline.' Bathilda finished the éclair and dabbed cream from the corners of her mouth. *Not long. Not much longer,* Caroline told herself. Her aunt was a fortress, she thought, angrily. Balustrades of manners and wealth around a space inside—a space most commonly filled with rich food and sherry. Certainly there was no heart there, no love, no warmth. Caroline felt a flare of defiance.

'Mr Massey is a good man, his family is respectable—' she began to say, adopting a tone of calm reason.

'The man's morals are irrelevant. Corin Massey will make you a common drudge. He will not make you happy,' Bathilda interrupted. 'How could he? He is *beneath* you. He is far beneath you, in fortune and in manners—in every station of life.'

'You've barely even met him!' Caroline cried. Bathilda shot her a censorious look.

'May I remind you that you, also, have *barely even met him*? You may be eighteen now, you may be independent from me, but have I earned no respect in raising you? In keeping you and teaching you—'

'You have kept me with the money my parents left. You have done your duty,' Caroline said, a touch bitterly.

'Don't interrupt me, Caroline. Our name is a good one and would have stood you in good stead here in New York. And yet you choose to wed a . . . *farmer.* And move away from everything and everyone you know to live in the middle of nowhere. I have indeed failed, that much is clear. I have failed to instil respect and good sense and propriety in you, in spite of all my efforts.'

'But I don't *know* anybody here, Aunt. Not really. I know only you,' Caroline said, sadly. 'And

Corin is not a farmer. He's a cattle rancher, a most successful one. His business—'

'His *business*? His *business* should have stayed in the wilderness and not found its way here to prey upon impressionable young girls.'

'I have money enough.' Caroline tipped her chin defiantly. 'We will not be poor.'

'Not yet, you don't. Not for another two years. We'll see how well you like living on a farmer's income until then. And we'll see how long your wealth lasts once he has his hands upon it and finds his way to the gaming tables!'

'Don't say such things. He is a good man. And he loves me, and . . . and I love him,' Caroline declared, adamantly. He loved her. She let this thought pour through her and could not keep from smiling.

When Corin had proposed to Caroline, he had said that he'd loved her from the first moment of their meeting, which was at a ball a month previously—the Montgomery's ball to mark the beginning of Lent. Since her debut, Caroline had envied the enjoyment that other girls seemed to derive from such functions. They danced and they laughed and they chatted with ease. Caroline, when forced to enter the room with Bathilda, found herself always at a disadvantage, always afraid to speak in case she caused her aunt to correct her, or to scold. Corin had changed all that.

*   *   *

Caroline chose her fawn silk gown and her mother's emeralds for the Montgomery's ball. The necklace was cool and heavy around her neck. It covered the slender expanse of her décolletage with a glow of gold and a deep glitter that sparked light in her grey eyes.

'You look like an empress, miss,' Sara said admiringly, as she brushed out Caroline's fair hair, pinned it into a high chignon on her crown and braced one foot on the stool to pull up the laces of her corset. Caroline's waist was a source of envy to her peers, and Sara always took careful pains to pull it in as far as she could. 'No man in the room will be able to resist you.'

'Do you think so?' Caroline asked, breathlessly. Sara, with her dark hair and her ready smile, was the closest thing Caroline had to a true friend. 'I fear that they will be able to resist my aunt, however,' she sighed. Bathilda had seen off more than one cautious suitor; young men she deemed unworthy.

'Your aunt has high hopes for you, miss, that's all. Of course she cares a great deal who you will marry,' Sara soothed her.

'At this rate, I will marry nobody at all, and will stay forever here listening to her disappointment in me!'

'Nonsense! The right one will come along and he will win your aunt over, if that is what he must do to have you. Just look at you, miss! You will bedazzle them, I know it,' Sara smiled. Caroline met Sara's eye in the mirror. She reached over her shoulder and grasped the girl's fingers, squeezing them for courage. 'There now. All will be well,' Sara assured her, crossing to the dresser for face powder and rouge.

Caroline, every scant inch the demure, immaculate society girl, descended the wide staircase into the incandescence of the Montgomery's ballroom. The room was alight with precious stones and laughter; ripe with the fragrance of wine and perfumed hair pomade. Gossip and smiles rippled around the room, passing like Chinese whispers; alternately friendly, amused, and vicious. Caroline saw her dress appraised, her aunt derided, her jewels admired, frank glances cast over her, and comments passed in low voices behind delicate fingers and tortoiseshell cigarette holders. She spoke little, just enough to be polite, and this at least was a trait her aunt had always approved of. She smiled and applauded with the rest when Harold Montgomery performed his party piece: the messy cascading of a champagne magnum into a pyramid of glasses. It always splashed and overflowed, wetting the stems which then stained the ladies' gloves.

The room was stuffy and hot. Caroline stood up straight, sipping sour wine that lightened her head and feeling sweat prickle beneath her arms. Fires blazed in every grate and light poured from hundreds of electric candles in the chandeliers, so bright that she could see red pigment from Bathilda's lips seeping into the creases around her mouth. But then Corin appeared in front of them and she barely heard Charlie Montgomery's introduction because she was captured by the newcomer's frank gaze and the warmth of him; and when she blushed he did too, and he fumbled his first words to her, saying, 'Hello, how are you?' as though they were two odd fellows meeting over a game of whist. He grasped her hand in its embroidered glove as if to shake it, realised his mistake and dropped it abruptly, letting it fall limply into her skirts. At this she blushed more, and dared not look at Bathilda, who was giving the young man a most severe look. 'Sorry, miss . . . I, uh . . . won't you excuse me?' he mumbled, inclining his head to them and disappearing into the crowd.

'What an *extraordinary* young man!' Bathilda exclaimed, scathingly. 'Where on *earth* did you find him, Charlie?' Charlie Montgomery's black hair was as slick as oilskin, flashing light as he turned his head.

'Oh, don't mind Corin. He's a bit out of practice at all this, that's all. He's a far off cousin of mine. His people are here in New York but he's lived out west for years now, in Oklahoma Territory. He's back in town for his father's funeral,' Charlie said.

'How extraordinary,' Bathilda said again. 'I never thought that one should have to *practise* one's manners.' At this Charlie smiled vaguely. Caroline glanced at her aunt and saw that she had no idea how disliked she was.

'What happened to his father?' she asked Charlie, surprising herself.

'He was on one of the trains that collided in the Park Avenue Tunnel last month. It was a right old mess,' Charlie said, pulling a face. 'Seventeen dead, it's now reported, and nigh on forty injured.'

'How dreadful!' Caroline breathed. Charlie nodded in agreement.

'They must run the trains with electricity. Automate the signals and remove the opportunity for sleepy-headed drivers to cause such tragedies,' he declared.

'But how could a signal work with nobody to operate it?' Caroline asked, but Bathilda heaved a gentle sigh, as if bored, so Charlie Montgomery excused himself and moved away.

Caroline searched the crowd for the stranger's bronze-coloured hair, and found herself sorry for him—for his bereavement, and for his fumbling of her hand in front of Bathilda's flat, unforgiving eye. The shocking pain of losing close family was something she could sympathise with. She sipped absently at her wine, which had gone warm in her hand and was making her throat sore. And she felt the emeralds press into her chest, felt the watery fabric of her gown on her thighs, as if her skin suddenly longed to be touched. When Corin appeared at her side a minute later and asked her for a dance, she accepted mutely, with a startled nod, her heart too high in her throat to speak. Bathilda glared at him, but he did not even look up at her to notice, giving her cause to exclaim: 'Well, *really*!'

They danced a slow waltz, and Caroline, who had wondered why Corin had chosen a dance so slow, and so late in the evening, guessed the reason in his unsure steps, and the tentative way in which he held her. She smiled uncertainly at him, and they did not speak at first. Then he said:

'You must please excuse me, Miss Fitzpatrick. For before, and for . . . I fear I am not an accomplished dancer. It has been some time since I was lucky enough to attend such a function as this, or to dance with someone so . . . uh . . .' He hesitated, and she smiled, lowering her gaze as she had been taught. But she could not look away for long. She could feel the heat of his hand in the small of her back, as if there was nothing at all between her skin and his. She felt naked suddenly;

wildly disconcerted, but thrilled as well. His face was deeply tanned, and the sun had lingered in the hair of his brows and moustache, tinting them with warm colour. His hair was combed but not brilliantined, and a stray lock now fell forward onto his brow, so that she almost reached out to brush it back. He watched her with light brown eyes, and she thought she saw a startled kind of happiness there.

As the dance ended and he took her hand to escort her from the floor, her glove snagged against the roughened skin of his palm. On impulse, she turned his hand over in her own and studied it, pushing her thumb into the callous at the root of each finger, comparing the width of it to her own. Her hand looked like a child's in his, and she drew breath and parted her lips to say this before realising how inappropriate it would be. She felt childlike indeed, and she noticed that he was breathing deeply.

'Are you quite well, Mr Massey?' she asked.

'Yes . . . I'm fine, thank you. It's a little confined in here, isn't it?'

'Come over to the window, you will find the air fresher,' she said, taking his arm to steer him through the crowd. The air was indeed close, heavy with sweat and breathing, thick with smoke and music and voices.

'Thank you,' Corin said. The long casement windows were shut against the dead cold of the February night, but that cold radiated from the glass nevertheless, providing an area of cool where the overexerted could find relief. 'I'm not used to seeing so many people under one roof all at once. It's funny, how quickly and completely a person can become unaccustomed to such things.' He hitched one shoulder in a shrug too casual for his evening coat.

'I have never left New York,' Caroline blurted out. 'That is, only for my family's summer house, on the coast . . . I mean to say . . .' but she wasn't sure what she meant to say. That he seemed foreign to her, a figure from myth almost—to have gone so far from civilisation, to have chosen life in an untamed land.

'Would you not like to travel, Miss Fitzpatrick?' he asked, and she began to understand that something had started between them. A negotiation of some kind; a sounding out.

'There you are, my dear.' Bathilda bore down on them. She could spot such a negotiation from quite a distance, it seemed. 'Do come along, I want to introduce you to Lady Clemence.' Caroline had no choice but to be led away but she glanced back over her shoulder and raised her hand in slight salute.

* * *

'Don't be ridiculous, girl!' Bathilda broke into her thoughts and returned her to the present, and the lunch table at La Fiorentina. 'You are acting like a lovesick schoolgirl! I, too, have read Mr Wister's *novel*, and it has clearly filled your head with romantic notions. I can think of no other reason why you would choose to marry a *cow-boy*. But you will learn that *The Virginian* is a work of *fiction* and bears little relation to the reality of it. Did you not also read of the dangers, and the emptiness, and the hardships of the frontier land?'

'It's not like that any more. Corin has told me all about it. He says the land is so beautiful you can see God's hand in every blade of grass . . .' At this Bathilda snorted, inelegantly. 'And Mr Wister himself acknowledges that the wild era he described is no more. Woodward is a thriving town, Corin says—'

'Woodward? Who has heard of *Woodward*? What state is it in?'

'I . . . do not know,' Caroline confessed, pressing her lips together resentfully.

'It is in no state at all, that's why you do not know. No state of the Union. It is uncharted land, full of savages and uncouth men of all kinds. Why, I heard there are no ladies to be found west of Dodge City at all—only *women* of the worst kind. No ladies! Can't you imagine how *godless* a place it must be?' Bathilda's chest swelled within the confines of her burgundy gown. A flush mottled her face all the way to her hairline, where her steel-coloured hair was gathered into a soft bouffant. She was moved, Caroline realised, incredulously. Bathilda was actually *moved*.

'Of course there are ladies! I'm sure such accounts are exaggerated,' said Caroline.

'I don't see how you can be so sure when you know nothing. How can you know anything, Caroline? You're just a child! He would tell you anything to get such a fine and wealthy wife. And you believe every word! You will leave your home and your family and all your prospects here. To live where you will have no name, no society and no comfort.'

'I will have comfort,' Caroline insisted.

A week after the ball, Corin had taken Caroline to the skating pond in Central Park, along with Charlie Montgomery and his sister Diana, who gave them a tactfully wide berth. It was late in February and the sky was an odd yellowy-white against which the spiralling snowflakes at first looked black, then turned pale against the bare trees before they reached the ground.

'As a boy I was always half afraid to skate here. I kept waiting to fall through the ice,' Corin smiled, taking small, cautious steps more akin to walking than skating.

'You needn't have worried, Mr Massey. They drain most of the water out at the beginning of the winter, to be sure that it freezes right through,' Caroline smiled. The cold was biting. It reddened their cheeks and hung their breath in ragged white clouds around them. Caroline tucked her gloved hands into her coat pockets and skated a large, smooth circle around Corin.

'You're very good at this, Miss Fitzpatrick. Much better than I!'

'My mother used to bring me here all the time. When I was a little girl. I haven't skated in a while, though. Bathilda does not care for it.'

'Where is your mother now?' Corin asked, circling his arms clumsily to keep his balance. Snow had gathered on the brim of his hat, giving him a festive look.

'My parents died. Eight years ago,' Caroline said, skating to a halt in front of Corin, who also fell still. 'There was an explosion at a factory, as they were travelling home one evening. A wall collapsed and . . . their carriage was trapped beneath it,' she told him, quietly. Corin put his hands out as if to hold her, but then let them fall again.

'What a tragic misfortune. I'm so sorry,' he said.

'Charlie told me about your father, and I'm sorry, too,' Caroline said, wondering if he noticed the similarity, as she had, in the nightmarish, claustrophobic way in which they had both lost family. She looked down at her skates. Inside them, her toes were going numb. 'Come, Mr Massey; let's move on before we cleave to the ice!' she suggested, holding out her hand to him. He took it, smiling, then grimaced as she towed him along, wobbling like a toddler.

They drank hot chocolate in the pavilion, once the ice had become so crowded with skaters that steady progress was nigh on impossible. From their table by the window they watched young boys darting recklessly between the adults. Caroline realised that she hadn't been feeling the winter weather as she normally did. Perhaps being close to Corin was enough to warm her—it seemed to make her blood run more quickly than ever before.

'You have the most extraordinary eyes, Miss Fitzpatrick,' Corin told her, smiling bashfully. 'Why, they shine like silver dollars against the snow out there!' he exclaimed.

Caroline had no idea how to reply to him. She was not used to compliments, and so she looked down into her cup, embarrassed.

'Bathilda says that I have cold eyes. She laments that I did not inherit my father's shade of blue,' she said, stirring her chocolate slowly.

But Corin reached out a finger and lifted her chin,

and she felt his touch like an electric charge. 'Your aunt is quite wrong,' he declared.

*   *   *

His proposal came a scant three weeks later, as the ice began to melt in the parks and the washed-out sky took on a deeper hue. He called upon her on a Tuesday afternoon, knowing he would find her alone, it being her aunt's custom to play bridge with Lady Atwell on that day. As Sara ushered him into the room, colour poured into Caroline's face and her throat went dry, and when she rose to greet him her legs were soft and uncooperative. A potent cocktail of joy and terror seemed to undo her whenever she saw him, and it grew stronger every time. Words vanished from Caroline's mind, and as Sara closed the door she smiled a tight, excited smile at her mistress.

'How kind of you to call,' Caroline managed at last, her voice trembling like her hands. 'I trust you are well?'

Instead of replying, Corin turned his hat around in his hands, began to speak but faltered, hooked a finger into his collar and tugged as if to loosen it. Caroline clasped her hands together to still them, and waited, watching him in astonishment. 'Won't . . . won't you sit down?' she offered at length. Corin glanced at her and seemed to find some resolve at last.

'No, I won't sit down,' he declared, startling Caroline with the gruffness of his tone. They faced each other for a long moment, at an impasse, then Corin crossed the room in two large strides, took Caroline's face in his hands and kissed her. The press of his mouth was so shocking that Caroline made no move to stop him, or to move away as she knew she ought. She was struck by the unexpected softness of his lips, and the heat of him. She could not breathe, and dizziness confounded her even as a peculiar warm ache began in her stomach.

'Mr . . . Mr Massey . . .' she stammered when he pulled away, still holding her face in his hands and studying her with quiet urgency.

'Caroline . . . come away with me. Marry me,' he said. Caroline could scarcely find the words to answer him.

'Do you . . . do you love me, then?' she asked at last. Her pulse jumped up in panic as she waited for his answer, for the words she so longed to hear.

'Do you not know? Can't you tell?' he asked, incredulously. 'I have loved you since the first moment I met you. The very first moment,' he murmured. Caroline shut her eyes, overwhelmed with relief. 'You're smiling,' Corin said, brushing his finger over her cheek. 'Does that mean you will marry me, or that you're laughing at me?' He smiled anxiously, and Caroline took his hand in hers, pressed it to her face.

'It means I will marry you, Mr Massey. It means that . . . I want nothing more than to marry you,' she breathed.

'I will make you so happy,' he promised, kissing her again.

*   *   *

Bathilda refused to announce the engagement between her niece and Corin Massey. She refused to help her assemble her trousseau, buy clothes for travelling, or pack her leather trunks for the journey. Instead, she watched her niece neatly folding away new tailoreds, gored skirts and embroidered shirtwaists.

'I suppose you consider yourself emancipated, to act so disastrously. Quite the Gibson Girl, I'm sure,' she remarked. Caroline made no reply, although the barb stuck because it was near to the mark. She rolled her jewellery into a blue velvet fold and tucked it into her vanity case. Later, she sought Bathilda out in their spacious house in Gramercy Park, finding her seated in a ray of spring sunshine, so startlingly bright it stripped years from the woman. Caroline asked again for her engagement to be announced. She wanted it to be done properly, officially, as it ought to be; but her request fell on deaf ears.

'It's hardly to be celebrated,' Bathilda snapped. 'I'm only glad I shan't be here to have to answer questions about it. I will be returning to London, to stay with a cousin of my dear late husband's, a lady with whom I have always shared great affection and regard. There is nothing to tie me here in New York, now.'

'You're going back to London? But . . . when?' Caroline asked, more meekly. Unhappily, she realised that in spite of the rift between them, her Aunt Bathilda represented her only family, her only home.

'Next month, when the weather is more clement.'

'I see,' Caroline breathed. She linked her hands in front of her, wound the fingers tightly together and squeezed. Bathilda looked up at her from the book she was ostensibly reading, her gaze

34

tempered with something almost aggressive. 'Then we shall not see each other much from now on, I suppose,' Caroline murmured.

'Indeed not, my dear. But that would have been the case even if I had remained in New York. You will be far beyond the distance I could comfortably have travelled. I will give you my address in London, and of course you must write to me. And I dare say you will find company enough on the farm. There will be other farm wives in the vicinity, I am sure,' she said, smiling faintly as she returned to her book. Caroline's lace collar seemed to choke her. She felt a jolt of fear and did not know whether to run to or from Bathilda.

'You have never shown me love,' she whispered, her voice fearful and tight. 'I do not know why you should be so surprised that I run after it when it is offered to me.' And she left the room before Bathilda could scorn this sentiment.

So Caroline married with nobody to give her away and no family to represent her. She chose a gown of diaphanous white muslin, with a wide yoke of lace ruffles across the bust and crisp frills at the neck and cuffs. Her hair was piled high on her head and held with ivory combs, and pearl drop earrings were her only jewels. She wore no make-up, and her countenance, as she took a last look in the glass, was somewhat pale. Although the weather was not warm, she carried her mother's silk fan on her wrist, fingering it nervously as she travelled to a small church on the Upper East Side, close to where Corin had lived as a boy. Sara the maid sat alone on the bride's side; and as she entered the building, Caroline longed to see her parents there. Corin wore a borrowed suit and tie,

35

his hair combed neatly back and his cheeks freshly shaven, the skin soft and slightly raw. He fidgeted with his collar as she began her approach along the aisle, but then he met her anxious gaze, and he smiled and fell still as though naught else mattered. His mother and two elder brothers were in attendance, solemn as the couple made their vows before the minister. Mrs Massey still wore her mourning dress, and although she welcomed her new daughter-in-law, her grief was too fresh for her to feel truly glad. It was another wet day, and the church was quiet and dark, smelling of damp brick dust and candle wax. Caroline did not mind. Her world had contracted to include nothing but the man in front of her, the man taking her hand, the man who looked at her so possessively and spoke with such conviction as he made his promises. With their hands joined before God, Caroline felt such an irresistible surge of elation that she could not contain it, and it spilled from her in a storm of happy tears that Corin gathered on his fingertips and kissed away. With him she would start her real life at last.

But to his new wife's dismay, Corin packed and made ready to leave New York the following day.

'We will have our wedding night in *our* home, in the house that I have built for us; not here in a place still sorrowing for my father. I came for a funeral, and I didn't bank on finding a wife,' he smiled, kissing her hands. 'I've got to sort a few things out, get the house ready for your arrival. I want it to be perfect.'

'It will be perfect, Corin,' she assured him, still unused to addressing any man by his first name alone. His kisses burned into her skin, made it hard to breathe. 'Please let me come with you now.'

'Give me a month, that's all, my sweetheart. Follow after me four weeks from today and I will have everything ready. You'll have time to say goodbye to all your friends, and I'll have time to boast to all of mine that I have married the most beautiful girl in the whole of America,' he said; and so she agreed even though his departure felt like the sky growing dark.

She called upon some of her old classmates to bid them farewell, but generally found them either occupied or not at home. Eventually, she understood herself *persona non grata,* so she spent the four weeks at home, suffering the uncomfortable silence between herself and her aunt, packing and repacking her luggage, writing letter after letter to Corin, and gazing out of the window at a view now dominated by the newly constructed Fuller Building—a wedge-shaped behemoth that towered nearly three hundred feet into the sky. Caroline had never imagined that man could build so high. She gazed at it, felt diminished by it, and the first doubts crept into her mind. With Corin gone, it almost seemed as though he had never been there at all, that she had dreamed the whole event. She turned the wedding ring on her finger and frowned, fighting to keep such thoughts at bay. But what could have been so terrible that he could not have taken her with him straight away? What had he to hide—regret for his hasty marriage to her? Sara sensed that she was troubled.

'It won't be long now, miss,' she said, as she brought her tea.

'Sara . . . will you stay a moment?'

'Of course, miss.'

'Do you think . . . do you think it will be all right? In Oklahoma Territory?' Caroline asked, quietly.

'Of course, miss! That is . . . I do not rightly know, never having gone there. But . . . Mr Massey will take good care of you, I do know that. He would not take you anywhere you would not wish to go, I am sure,' Sara assured her.

'Bathilda says I will have to work. Until I come into my money, that is . . . I will be a farmer's wife,' she said.

'That you will, miss, but hardly the common sort of one.'

'Is the work so very hard? Keeping house and all? You do it so well, Sara—is it so very hard?' she asked, trying to keep her anxiety from sounding. Sara gazed at her with an odd mingling of amusement, pity and resentment.

'It can be hard enough, miss,' she said, somewhat flatly. 'But you will be mistress of the house! You will be free to do things as you see fit, and I am sure you will have help. Oh, do not fret, miss! It may take you some while to grow accustomed to such a different kind of life to the one you have had, but you'll be happy, I am sure of it.'

'Yes. I will be, won't I?' Caroline smiled.

'Mr Massey *loves* you. And you love him—how could you not be happy?'

'I do love him,' Caroline said, taking a deep breath and holding Sara's hand tightly. 'I do love him.'

'And I'm *so* happy for you, miss,' Sara said, her

voice tightening, tears springing in her eyes.

'Oh, please don't, Sara! How I wish you were coming with me!' Caroline cried.

'I wish it too, miss,' Sara said quietly, wiping her eyes with the hem of her apron.

When a letter from Corin did finally arrive, speaking words of love and encouragement, urging her to be patient for a little while longer, Caroline read and reread it twenty times a day, until she knew the words by heart and felt galvanised by them. When the four weeks were up, she kissed Bathilda's florid cheek and tried to see some mark of regret in her aunt's demeanour. But only Sara went with her to the station, sobbing inconsolably beside her young mistress as the bay horses trotted smartly along busy streets and avenues.

'I don't know how it will be without you, miss. I don't know that I'll care for London!' the girl wept; and Caroline took her hand, winding their fingers tightly together, too full of clamouring feelings to speak. Only when confronted with the locomotive, which spat steam and soot with great vigour and filled her nose with the tang of hot iron and cinders, did she finally feel that she had found some other thing in the world as glad as she was to be making the journey. She shut her eyes as the train eased forwards, and with its loud, solemn cough of steam, her old life ended and her new one began.

2

My mother's brother, my Uncle Clifford, and his wife Mary, want the old linen press from the nursery, the round Queen Anne table from the study and the collection of miniatures that live in a glass-topped display case at the foot of the stairs. I'm not sure if this is what Meredith meant when she said her children could take *a keepsake*, but I really don't care. I dare say a few more things will find their way into Clifford's lorry at the end of the week, and if Meredith would be outraged, I will not be. It's a grand house, but it's not Chatsworth. There are no museum pieces, apart from a couple of the paintings perhaps. Just a big, old house full of big, old things; valuable, perhaps, but also unloved. Our mother has asked only for any family photographs I can find. I love her for her decency, and her heart.

I hope Clifford is sending enough men. The linen press is enormous. It looms against the far wall of the nursery: acres of French mahogany with minarets and cornicing, a scaled-down temple to starch and mothballs. A set of wooden steps live behind it, and they creak and wobble beneath me. I pull stiff, solid piles of linens from the shelves and drop them to the floor. They are flat, weighty; their landings make the pictures shake. Dust flies and my nose prickles, and Beth appears in the doorway, rushing to discover what havoc I am wreaking. There is so much of it. Generations of bed sheets, worn enough to have been replaced, not worn enough to have been thrown out. It could

40

be decades since some of these piles have been disturbed. I remember Meredith's housekeeper puffing up the stairs with laden arms; her cracked red cheeks and her broad ugly hands.

Once I've emptied the press I am not sure what to do with all the piles of linen. It could go to charity, I suppose. But I'm not up to the task of black-bagging it all, heaving it down to the car, taking it in batches into Devizes. I pile it back up against the wall, and as I do my eyes catch on one pattern, one splash of weak colour in all the white. Yellow flowers. Three pillow cases with yellow flowers, green stems, embroidered into each corner in silk thread that still catches the light. I run my thumb over the neat stitching, feel how years of use have made the fabric watery soft. There is something in the back of my mind, something I know I recognise but can't remember. Have I seen them before? The flowers are ragged looking, wild. I can't put a name to them. And there are only three. Four pillowcases with every other set but this one. I drop them back onto a pile, drop more linen on top. I find I am frowning and consciously unknit my brow.

Clifford and Mary are Henry's parents. Were Henry's parents. They were in Saint Tropez when he disappeared, which the press unfairly made a great deal out of. As if they had left him with strangers, as if they had left him home alone. Our parents did it too. We often came here for the whole of the school holidays, and for two weeks or even three, most years, Mum and Dad would go away without us. To Italy, for long walks; to the Caribbean to sail. I liked and feared having them gone. Liked it because Meredith never checked up

41

on us much, never came outside in search of us when we'd been gone for hours. We felt liberated, we tore about like yahoos. But feared it because, inside the house, Meredith had sole charge of us. We had to be with her. Eat our dinner with her, answer her questions, think up lies. It never occurred to me that I didn't like her, or that she was unpleasant. I was too young to think that way. But when Mum got back I flew to her, gathered clammy handfuls of her skirts.

Beth kept me extra close when our parents were away. If she walked ahead, it was with one hand held slightly behind her, long fingers spread, always waiting for me to take hold of them. And if I didn't she would pause, glance over her shoulder, make sure that I was following. One year, Dinny built her a tree house in a tall beech on the far side of the wood. We'd hardly seen him for days and he'd forbidden us to spy on him. The weather had been fitful, wind dimpling the surface of the dew pond, too fresh to swim. We'd played dressing up in a spare bedroom; built castles of empty flowerpots in the orangery; made a den in the secret hollow centre of the yew topiary globe on the top lawn. Then the sun came out again and we saw Dinny wave from the corner of the garden, and Beth smiled at me, her eyes alight.

'It's ready,' he said, when we reached him.

'What is it?' I demanded. 'Go on—tell us!'

'A surprise,' was all he would say, smiling shyly at Beth. We followed him through the trees, and I was telling him about the den in the topiary when I saw it and was silenced. One of the biggest beech trees, with a silvery smooth trunk and bark that wrinkled where its branches forked, like the crook of your elbow or the back of your knee. I'd seen Dinny climb it before, with a few practised swings, to sit amidst the pale green leaves far above me. Now, high up where the tree began to spread, Dinny had built a broad platform of sturdy planks. The walls were made from old fertiliser bags, bright blue, nailed to a wooden frame and belling in and out like boat sails. The route up to this fortress was marked by knotted rope loops and chunks of scrap wood, nailed to the tree to form an intermittent ladder. In the hung silence I heard the enticing rush of the breeze, the rustling snap of the tree house walls.

'What do you think?' Dinny asked, folding his arms and squinting at us.

'It's brilliant! It's the best tree house ever!' I exclaimed, bouncing urgently from foot to foot.

'It's great—did you build it all by yourself?' Beth asked, still smiling up at the blue house. Dinny nodded.

'Come up and see—it's even better inside,' he told her, moving to the foot of the tree, reaching up for the first handhold.

'Come *on*, Beth!' I admonished her, when she hesitated.

'OK!' she laughed. 'You go first, Erica—I'll give you a boost to the first branch.'

'We should give it a name. You should name it, Dinny!' I chattered, hoisting up my skirt, tucking it into my knickers.

'What about the watch tower? Or the crow's nest?' he said. Beth and I agreed—The Crow's Nest it would be. Beth hoisted me onto the first branch, my sandals scuffing welts into the powdery green algae, but I could not reach the next handhold. My fingertips crooked over the rung Dinny had nailed into the tree, so close, but too far for me to hang on safely. Dinny joined me on the first branch, let me step on his bent knee until I could reach, but from there my leg would not stretch to the next rung.

'Come down, Erica,' Beth called at length, when I was red and cross and feeling close to tears.

'No! I want to go up!' I protested, but she shook her head.

'You're too little! Come down!' she insisted. Dinny withdrew his knee, jumped down from the tree, and I had no choice but to obey. I slithered back to the ground and stared in sullen silence at my stupid, too-short legs. I had grazed my knee, but was too disheartened to be excited about the sticky worm of blood oozing down my shin.

'Beth, then? Are you coming up?' Dinny asked, and I sank inside, to be left out, to miss out on the wonderful tree house. But Beth shook her head.

'Not if Erica can't,' she said. I glanced up at Dinny but looked away again quickly, squirming away from the disappointment in his eyes, the way his smile had vanished. He leant against the tree, folded his arms defensively. Beth hesitated for a while, as if unable to choose her next words. Then her hand reached out for me again. 'Come on, Rick. We need to go and wash your leg.'

Two days later Dinny fetched us back again, and this time the trunk of the beech tree was riddled with rungs and ropes. Beth smiled calmly at Dinny and I flew to the bottom of this ramshackle staircase, staring up at the floating house as I started to climb.

'Go carefully!' Beth gasped, sucking the

fingertips of one hand as I missed my footing, wobbled. She followed me up, frowning in concentration, careful not to look down. A loose curtain of bags marked the doorway. Inside, Dinny had arranged plastic sacks stuffed with straw. There was a wooden crate table, a bunch of cow parsley in a milk bottle, a pack of cards, some comics. It was quite simply the best place I had ever been. We painted a sign, to put at the foot of the ladder. *The Crow's Nest. Trespassers will be Persecuted*. Mum laughed when she read it. We spent hours up there, adrift in whispering green clouds with patches of bright sky sparkling overhead, eating picnics, far away from Meredith and Henry. I worried that Henry would ruin it when he came to stay. I worried that he would crash through our magical place, mock it, make it seem less magnificent. But by happy, happy chance, it turned out that Henry was afraid of heights.

In my head Henry is always bigger than me, older than me. Eleven when I was seven. It seemed an enormous gap at the time. He was a *big boy*. He was loud and bossy. He said I had to do what he told me. He buttered Meredith up—she always preferred boys to girls. He went along with her on the rare occasions she came out to the woods, and more than once helped her make a nasty scheme a reality. Henry: a fleshy neck with a receding chin; dark brown hair; clear blue eyes that he would narrow, make ugly; pale skin that burnt across the nose in summer. One of those children, I see him now, who is a grown-up in miniature rather than a child, who you can look at and know, at once, what they will look like as an adult. His features were already mapped; they would grow, but not develop. He wore himself in his face, I think, charmless, obvious. But this is unfair. He never got the chance to prove me wrong, after all.

*   *   *

Eddie still has the face of a child, and I love it. A nondescript boy's face, sharp nose, tufty hair, kneecaps standing proud from skinny shanks in his school shorts. My nephew. He hugs Beth on the platform, a little sheepishly because some of his classmates are on the train behind him, banging on the glass, sticking up their fingers. I wait by the car for them, my hands puckered with cold, grinning as they draw near.

'Hey, Eddie Baby! Edderino! Eddius Maximus!' I call to him, putting my arms around him and squeezing, pulling his feet off the ground.

'Auntie Rick, it's just Ed now,' he protests, with a hint of exasperation.

' 'Course. Sorry. And you can't call me *Auntie*— you make me feel a hundred years old! Sling your bag in the back and let's get going,' I say, resisting the urge to tease him. He is eleven now. The same age Henry will always be, and old enough for teasing to matter. 'How was your train ride?'

'Pretty boring. Except Absolom locked Marcus in the loo. He screamed the place down—quite funny really,' Eddie reports. He smells of school and it starts to fill the car, sharp and vinegary. Unwashed socks, pencil shavings, mud, ink, stale sandwiches.

'Pretty funny, indeed! I had to go in and see the head a fortnight ago because he'd shut his art

46

teacher in her classroom. They pushed a block of lockers against her door!' Beth says, voice loud and bright, startling me.

'It wasn't *my* idea, Mum!'

'You still helped,' Beth counters. 'What if there'd been a fire or something? She was in there for hours!'

'Well . . . they shouldn't have banned mobile phones then, should they?' Eddie says, smiling. I catch his eye in the rear-view mirror and wink.

'Edward Calcott Walker, I am appalled,' I say lightly. Beth glares at me. I must remember not to conspire with Eddie against her, not even over something tiny. It can't be him and me against her, even for a second. She resents my help already.

'Is this a new car?'

'New-ish,' I tell him. 'The old Beetle finally died on me. Wait until you see the house, Ed. It's a monster.' But as we pull in and I look at him expectantly, he nods, raises his eyebrows, is not impressed. Then I think the manor might only be the size of one wing of his school—smaller than his friends' houses, perhaps.

'I'm so glad it's school holidays again, darling,' Beth says, taking Eddie's bag from him. He smiles at her sidelong, slightly abashed. He will be taller than her eventually—he reaches her shoulder already.

I tour Eddie around the grounds while Beth settles down with his report card. I take him up to the barrow, skirt the dreary woods, arrive at the dew pond. He has found a long stick somewhere and swishes it, beheading the weeds and dead nettles. It's warmer today, but damp. Flecks of drizzle in the breeze, and the empty branches knocking overhead.

'Why's it called a dew pond? Isn't it just a pond?' he asks, smacking the edge with his stick, crouching on supple, bony legs. Ripples fly out across the surface. The pockets of his jeans bulge with pilfered treasures. He's like a magpie that way, but they are things nobody would miss. Old safety pins, conkers, bits of blue and white china from the soil.

'This is where the stream starts. It was dug out a long time ago, to make this pond as a kind of reservoir. And *dew* pond because it traps the dew as well, I suppose.'

'Can you swim in it?'

'We used to—Dinny and your mum and I. Actually, I don't think your mum ever went all the way in. It was always pretty cold.'

'Jamie's parents have got this wicked lake for swimming in—it's a swimming pool, except it's not all chlorine and tiles and all that. It's got plants and everything. But it's clean.'

'Sounds great. Not at this time of year, though, eh?'

'Guess not. Who's Dinny?'

'Dinny . . . was a boy we used to play with. When we came here as kids. His family lived nearby. So . . .' I trail off. Why should talking about Dinny make me feel so conspicuous? Dinny. With his square hands so good at making things. Dark eyes smiling through his fringe, and his hair a thatch that I once stuck daisies into while he slept, my fingers trembling with suppressed mirth, with my audacity; to be so close and to touch him. 'He was a real adventurer. He built a fabulous tree house one year . . .'

'Can we see it? Is it still there?' he asks.

'We can go and look, if you like,' I offer. Eddie grins, and jogs a few paces ahead, taking aim at a sapling, tackling it with a two-handed blow.

Eddie's adult teeth haven't sorted themselves out yet. They seem to jostle for position in his mouth. There are big gaps, and a pair that cross over. They'll be clamped behind braces soon enough.

'What did I hear the other boys calling you from the train?' I call out to him.

He grimaces. 'Pot Plant,' he admits, ruefully.

'Why on *earth* . . . ?'

'Well, it's kind of embarrassing . . . do I have to say?'

'Yeah, you do. No secrets between us.' I smile. Eddie sighs.

'Miss Wilton keeps a little plant on her desk— I'm not sure what it is. Mum has them too—dark purple flowers, with furry leaves?'

'Sounds like an African violet.'

'Whatever. Well, she left us in there on detention at lunchtime, and I said I was so hungry I could eat anything, so Ben bet me a fiver I wouldn't eat her plant. So . . .'

'So you did?' I raise an eyebrow, folding my arms as we walk. Eddie shrugs, but he can't help but look a little pleased.

'Not the *whole* thing. Just the flowers.'

'*Eddie!*'

'Don't tell Mum!' he chortles, jogging on again. 'What was your nickname at school?' he calls back to me.

'I didn't really have one. Just Rick. I was always the youngest one, tagging along. Dinny called me

"Pup", sometimes,' I tell him.

We are closer than many aunts and nephews, Eddie and I. I stayed with him for two months while Beth recovered, while she *got help*. It was a strained time, a time of keeping going and pretending, and being normal and not fussing. We didn't have any big conversations. We didn't bare our souls, pour out our hearts. Eddie was too young, and I am too impatient. But we shared a time of extreme awkwardness, of concentrated sadness and anger and confusion. We jarred along, the both of us feeling that way; and that's what makes us close—the knowledge of that time. His father Maxwell and I holding hushed, strangled arguments behind closed doors, not wanting Eddie to hear his father call his mother *unfit*.

All that remains of the tree house are a few ragged planks, dark and green and slimy looking; like the rotten bones of a shipwreck.

'Well, I guess it's kind of had its day,' I say, sadly.

'You could rebuild it. I'll help, if you want?' Eddie says, keen to cheer me up.

I smile. 'We could try. It's more of a summer thing though—it'd be a bit cold and mucky up there now, I should think.'

'Why did you stop coming here? To visit Great-Grandma?' An innocent question, poor Eddie, to ease the moment. What a question for him to ask.

'Oh . . . you know. We just . . . went on holiday with our parents more as we got older. I don't really remember.'

'But you always say you never forget the important things that happen when you're a kid. That's what you told me, when I won that prize for speech and drama.' I had meant it to be a positive thing when I said it. But he won the prize while I was staying with him for those two months, and what we both thought, at the same time, was that what he would always remember was coming home from school and finding Beth the way he did. I saw the thought fly across his face, shut my eyes, wished I could pull my words back out of the air.

'Well, that just goes to show that it can't have been that big a thing, doesn't it?' I say lightly. 'Come on—there's loads more to see.'

We head back towards the house, ducking into the orangery as it starts to pour with rain. From there, barely getting wet, we dodge from shed to shed, through the old stables to the coach house, which is congested with junk and spattered with bird shit. Above our heads we count the swallows' nests, clinging to the beams like fungus. Eddie finds a small axe, the blade garish with rust.

'Awesome!' he breathes, brandishing it in a swooping arc. I grab his wrist, test the comprehensive bluntness of the axe with my thumb.

'Be extremely careful with it,' I say, fixing him in the eye. 'And don't bring it into the house.'

'I won't,' he says, swooping it again, smiling at the thrum of severed air.

Outside, it grows darker and the rain falls faster. A stream of muddy water bubbles past the coach house door.

'Let's go in, shall we? Your mum'll be wondering where we've got to.'

'She should come out and see the tree house, see if she thinks we could rebuild it. Do you think she would?'

'I don't know, Ed. You know how quickly she gets cold when the weather's like this,' I say. Nothing between the core of her and the winter chill. No flesh, no muscle, no thick skin.

Beth is making mince pies again when we clatter into the kitchen. She's rolling the pastry, cutting the shapes, filling them, baking them, bagging them. She started yesterday, in preparation for Eddie's arrival, and shows no sign of stopping. The kitchen table is awash with flour and scraps, empty mincemeat jars. The smell is heavenly. Flushed, she emerges from the Rayburn with another batch, slapping the trays down onto the scarred worktop. She's filled every tin and biscuit barrel. There are several bags in the ancient freezer in the cellar. I pick two up, pass one to Eddie. The filling scalds my tongue.

'These are fabulous, Beth,' I say, by way of a greeting. She shoots me a small smile, which broadens when it moves to her son. She crosses to kiss his cheek, leaving ghostly flour fingerprints on his sleeves.

'Well done, darling. All your teachers seem very pleased with you,' she tells him. I pick up the report card from the table, blow flour from it and flick through. 'With the possible exception of Miss Wilton . . .' she qualifies. She of the African violet.

'What does she teach?' I ask him, as he squirms slightly.

'French,' Eddie mumbles, through a mouthful of pie.

'She says you aren't trying nearly hard enough, and that when you do try you prove that you should be doing much better than you currently are,' Beth goes on, holding Eddie's shoulders, not letting him escape. He shrugs ambiguously. 'And—*three* detentions this term? What's that all about?'

'French is just so *boring*!' he declares. 'And Miss Wilton is *so* strict! She's really unfair! One of those detentions I got was because Ben threw a note at me! It was hardly my fault!'

'Well, just try to pay a bit more attention, OK? French is really important—no, it is!' she insists, when Eddie rolls his eyes. 'When I'm rich and I retire to the south of France, how are you going to cope if you can't speak the language?'

'By shouting and pointing?' he ventures. Beth presses her lips together severely, but then she laughs, a rich, glowing sound I so rarely hear. She can't help it, not with Eddie. 'Can I have another mince pie?' he asks, sensing victory.

'Go on. Then go and get in the bath—you're filthy!' Eddie grabs two pies and darts out of the kitchen.

'Take your bag up with you!' Beth calls after him.

'I've run out of hands!' Eddie calls back.

'Run out of inclination, is more like it,' Beth says to me, smiling ruefully.

Later, we watch a film; Beth curled with Eddie on the sofa with a huge bowl of popcorn wedged between them. When I glance at her I see that she's hardly following the film. She turns her chin, rests it on the top of Eddie's head, shuts her eyes contentedly, and I feel some of the knots inside me loosen, slipping away into the warmth of the open fire. The weekend passes quickly this way—a trip to the cinema in Devizes, school work at the kitchen table, mince pies; Eddie out in the coach house, or marauding through the deserted stables, wielding his axe. Beth is serene, if a little distracted. She stops baking when she runs out of flour, and stands for long moments, watching Eddie through the window with a faint, faraway smile.

'I might take him to France next summer,' she says to me, not breaking off this vigil as I pass her a cup of tea.

'I think he'd love it,' I say.

'The Dordogne, perhaps. Or the Lot Valley. We could go river swimming.' I love to hear her make plans. Future plans. I love to know she is thinking that far ahead. I rest my chin on her shoulder for a moment, follow her gaze out into the garden.

'I told you he'd have fun here,' I remark. 'Christmas will be excellent.' Her hair smells faintly of mint and I pull it over her shoulder, smooth it flat against her jumper with a long sweep of my hand.

*   *   *

On Sunday afternoon, Maxwell arrives to collect his son. I shout for Beth as I open the door to him, and when she does not appear I give Maxwell a short tour of the ground floor and make him a coffee. Maxwell divorced Beth five years ago, when her depression seemed to be getting worse and her weight plummeted, and he said he just couldn't cope and it was no way to raise a child. So he left her and remarried pretty much straight away—a short, plump, healthy-looking woman called Diane: white teeth, cashmere, perfect nails. Uncomplicated. Beth's depression was very convenient for Maxwell, I've always thought. But he's not all bad. He met her at a good time, that's all, when she was all grace and demure beauty. She was like a swan then, like a lily. A fair-weather friend is what Maxwell turned out to be. Now his grey raincoat is dripping onto the flagstones, but the rain can't spoil the sheen of wealth on hair, shoes, skin.

'Quite an impressive place,' he says, taking a gulp of the scalding hot coffee with a loud sound I don't like.

'Yes, I suppose it is,' I agree, leaning against the Rayburn, folding my arms. I found it hard to warm to Maxwell when he was still my brother-in-law. Now, I find it near impossible.

'Needs a lot of work, of course. But huge potential,' he declares. He made his money in property, and I wonder, with a touch of spite, how the credit crunch is working out for him. Huge potential. He said that about the cottage Beth bought near Esher, after the divorce. He sees everything with a developer's eye, but Beth kept the swollen wooden doors, the fireplaces that only draw when the windows are open. She likes it half broken. 'Have you decided what you're going to do with it?'

'No, not yet. Beth and I haven't really talked about it,' I say. A flash of irritation crosses his face. He never did like diffidence getting in the way of good sense.

'Well, this legacy could make the pair of you very wealthy women—'

'We'd have to stay here, though. Live here. I'm not sure that's what either of us wants.'

'But you needn't rattle around in the whole house. Have you thought about converting it into flats? You'd need planning, of course, but that shouldn't be a problem. You could keep an apartment and the freehold for yourselves, and sell the rest off with long leaseholds. You'd make an absolute killing, and keep to the terms of the will.'

'That would cost thousands and thousands . . .' I shake my head. 'Besides, we're having a recession, remember? I thought building and developing was at a standstill?'

'We may be in recession now, but in two years' time, three? People will always need places to live, in the long term.' Maxwell tips his head, considering. 'You'd need investors. I could help you with that. I might even be interested myself . . .' I see him look around the room with renewed attention, as if drawing up plans, measuring. It gives me a spasm of distaste.

'Thanks. I'll mention it to Beth.' My tone is final. Maxwell looks at me with a stern eye but says nothing for a while.

He fixes his eyes on a painting of fruit on the opposite wall, and at length he clears his throat slightly, so I know what he will ask next.

'And how is Beth?'

'She's fine,' I shrug, deliberately vague. Again, irritation shimmers across his features, puckers his forehead into a deeper frown.

'Come on, Erica. When I saw her last week she was looking very thin again. Is she eating? Has she been acting up at all?' I try not to think about the mince pies. About the hundreds of mince pies.

'Not that I've noticed,' I lie. It's a big lie. She's getting worse again, and though I don't exactly know why, I do know when it started—when she peaked, and started to fall again: it was when

Meredith died. When, by dying, she brought this place back into our lives.

'So where is she?'

'I've no idea. Probably in the bathroom,' I shrug.

'Keep an eye on her,' he mutters. 'I don't want Eddie spending Christmas here if she's going to have one of her episodes. It's just not fair on him.'

'She's not going to have an *episode*. Not unless you try to keep Eddie away from her,' I snap.

'It's not a question of keeping Eddie away from her. It's about doing what's best for my son, and—'

'What's best for him is that he gets to spend time with his mother. And it helps her so much to have him around. She's always much better—'

'It shouldn't be up to Edward to make his mother better!'

'That's not what I meant!'

'I only agreed to Edward coming here at all because you would be here to keep an eye on things, Erica. Beth has already shown how unpredictable she can be, how unstable. Putting your head in the sand won't help, you know.'

'I think I know my sister, Maxwell, and she is *not* unstable—'

'Look, I know you only want to stick up for her, Erica, and it's admirable. But this isn't a game. Seeing her at her worst is something that might affect Edward for the rest of his life, and I am not prepared to let that happen! Not again.'

'Keep your voice down, for God's sake!'

'Look, I just want—'

'I know what you want, Maxwell, but you can't change the fact that Beth is Eddie's mother. People aren't perfect—Beth's not perfect. But she is a great mother, and she adores Eddie, and if you could just focus on that for a change, instead of watching and waiting and crying *sole custody!* every time she gets a little bit down . . .'

'*A little bit down* is something of an understatement, though, isn't it Erica?' he says, and I can only glare at him because he is right. In the pause we hear a noise from outside the room, and exchange an accusatory glance. Eddie is in the hallway, swinging his kit bag awkwardly, left to right. It twists his skinny wrist. 'Edward!' Maxwell calls, smiling broadly and crossing to engulf his son in a brief hug.

It takes me quite some time to find Beth. The house is dark today, like the world outside. A midwinter Sunday when the sun barely seemed to rise and is now fading again. I move from door to door, flinging them open, peering in, breathing the stale smell of rooms long shut. A few hours ago we all had a late breakfast, sitting at the long table in the kitchen. Beth was bright and shiny; she made hot chocolate and warmed croissants in the Rayburn for us all. Too bright and shiny, I realise now. I didn't see her slip away. I flick at light switches as I go but a lot of the bulbs have blown. I find her at last, wedged onto the window sill in one of the top floor bedrooms. From there she can see the silver car in the driveway, streaked and scattered by the rain on the dirty window.

'Maxwell's here,' I say, pointlessly. Beth ignores me. She catches her bottom lip in two fingers, pushes it against her teeth, bites it hard. 'Eddie's going, Beth. You have to come down and see him off. Come on. And Maxwell wants to speak to you.'

'I don't want to speak to him. I don't want to see him. I don't want Eddie to go.'

'I know. But it's just for a while. And you can't let Eddie go without saying goodbye.' She rolls her head to glare at me. So tired, she looks. So tired and sad. 'Please, Beth. They're waiting . . . we have to go down.' Beth draws in a breath, unfolds herself from the sill—a slow, deliberate, underwater movement.

'Found her!' My cheerful announcement is too loud. 'This place is big enough to get lost in.' Beth and Maxwell ignore me, but Eddie smiles, at a loss. I wish Beth would put on a better act sometimes. Would show that she copes. I could shake her for not showing Maxwell a better front right now. She stands before him with her arms folded, lost inside a shapeless cardigan. She didn't fight when he left. They settled amicably—that was the word both families bandied about. *Amicable*. There is nothing amicable about Beth as she stands there now, grey-faced, raw looking. They do not touch.

'Good to see you, Beth. You look well,' Max lies.

'So do you.'

'Look, do you mind if we drop Eddie back next Saturday, rather than the Friday? Only it's Melissa's school carol concert on the Friday night and we'd all like to go together, wouldn't we, Ed?' Eddie shrugs a shoulder and nods at the same time. The poor boy could teach diplomacy. Beth's mouth pinches, her jaw knots. How she hates any mention of Max's new family, any extra second of time Eddie spends with them. But the request is reasonable, and she strives to be reasonable too.

'Of course. Of course it's no problem,' she says.

'Great,' Maxwell smiles, a quick, businesslike smile. There's a quiet pause, just the *scuff scuff scuff* of Eddie's bag, swinging to and fro. 'Have you got much planned for the week?' Maxwell asks.

'Not a lot—sorting through some of the old girl's junk, getting ready for Christmas,' I say lightly. Beth adds nothing to this summary.

'Right, well, let's get on, shall we, Ed?' Maxwell ushers his son towards the door. 'We'll see you on Saturday. Have a good week, the pair of you.'

'Wait! Eddie . . .' Beth rushes over to him and hugs him too tightly. She would go with him if she could. Keep hold of him, not let him forget her, not let him love Diane and Melissa too much. When the door is shut behind them I turn to Beth, but she won't meet my eye.

'I wish you wouldn't always be so quiet in front of Maxwell!' I burst out. 'Can't you be more . . .' I trail off, at a loss. Beth flings her arms up.

'No, I can't! I know he wants to take Eddie away from me. I can't pretend I don't know, or don't mind!' she cries.

'I know, I know,' I soothe her. She puts her hands through her messy hair. 'Eddie will be back soon,' I add. 'You know how much he loves being with you, Beth—he just adores you, and nothing Maxwell ever does will change that.' I grip her shoulders gently, try to coax a smile from her. Beth sighs, folds her arms.

'I know. I just . . . I'm going for a shower,' she says, and turns away from me.

*   *   *

With Eddie gone, the house is just big and empty again. By silent consensus we have stopped sorting through Meredith's things for now. The task is just too huge and seems pointless. The contents of this house have been here so long they've corroded in place. It would be an impossible task to remove it all now. They will have to use force, maybe bulldozers—I picture that, a metal-toothed bucket scraping through layers of fabric and carpet and paper and wood and dust. Hard work, like trying to scoop balls from an unripe melon. It will be a terrible act of violence. All the little traces of so many lives.

'I never thought, before, about what happens to a person's things when they die,' I say as we eat supper. The larder was full of Heinz tinned soups when we arrived but we're getting through them. I'll have to venture out into the village sometime soon.

'What do you mean?'

'Well . . . just that, I've never known anybody to die before. I've never had to deal with the aftermath, to . . .'

'Deal with the aftermath? You make it sound like a selfish thing to do, dying. Is that what you think?' Beth's voice is low and intense. Such a change in her, now that Eddie has left.

'No! Of course not. That wasn't what I was saying at all. I just meant that it's not something you think about, until it happens . . . who'll sort everything out. Where things will go. I mean, what will happen to Meredith's nighties? Her stockings? The food in the larder?' I am struggling; the conversation was meant to be flippant.

'What does it matter, Erica?' Beth snaps at me. I stop talking, break off a piece of bread, crumble it between my fingers.

'It doesn't matter,' I say. Sometimes I feel very lonely with Beth.

I never used to, not when we were younger, not before. We didn't antagonise each other much, or argue. Perhaps the age gap between us was big enough. Perhaps it was because we had a common enemy. Not even when we were shut inside for two whole days, two long sunny days, did we turn on each other. That was Henry's doing, and Meredith's. Meredith forbade us playing with Dinny from the word go; told us not to talk to any of his family, not to go near them, after we had innocently announced our new friendship to her at teatime.

We met him at the dew pond, where he was swimming. The day was warm but not hot. Early in the summer, I think it was; the landscape still fresh and green. A cool breeze blowing, so that when we first saw him, soaking wet, we shivered. His clothes were in a pile on the bank. All of his clothes. Beth took my hand, but we did not run away. Straight away, we were fascinated. Straight away, we wanted to know him—a thin, dark, naked boy with wet hair clinging to his neck, swimming and diving, all by himself. How old was I? I'm not sure. Four or five, no more than that.

'Who are you?' he asked, treading water. I shuffled closer to Beth, held her hand tighter.

'That's our grandmother's house,' Beth explained, pointing back at the manor. Dinny paddled a bit closer.

'But who are you?' he smiled, teeth and eyes gleaming.

'Beth!' I whispered urgently. 'He's got no clothes on!'

'Shh!' Beth hushed me, but it was a funny little sound, made buoyant by a giggle.

'Beth, then. And you?' Dinny looked at me. I lifted my chin a little.

'I'm Erica,' I announced, with all the composure I could muster. Just then a brown and white Jack Russell terrier burst from the woods and bounded over to us, yapping and wagging.

'I'm Nathan Dinsdale and that's Arthur.' He nodded to the dog. After that, I would have followed him anywhere. I longed for a pet—a proper pet, not the goldfish that was all we had room for at home. I was so busy playing with the dog that I don't remember how Dinny got out of the pond without Beth seeing him naked. I suspect that he did not.

We kept seeing him, of course, in spite of Meredith's ban, and we usually managed to keep it secret by giving Henry the slip before going down to the camp where Dinny lived with his family, at the edge of the manor's grounds. Henry usually steered clear of it anyway. He didn't want to disobey Meredith, and instead absorbed her contempt for the travellers, nurtured it, let it grow into a hatred of his own. The time she shut us in our parents had gone away for the weekend. We went into the village with Dinny, to buy sweets and Coke at the shop. I turned and saw Henry. He ducked behind the phone box, but not quickly enough, and I had a prickling feeling between my shoulder blades as we walked back to the house. Dinny said goodbye and wandered off through the trees, giving the house a wide berth.

Meredith was waiting for us on the step when we got back; Henry nowhere to be seen. But I knew how she knew. She grabbed our arms, nails cutting in, bent down, put her livid face close to ours. 'If you play with dogs, you will catch fleas,' she said, the words clipped and bitten. We were towed upstairs, made to bath in water so hot our skin turned red and angry and I wailed and wailed. Beth was silent, furious.

Afterwards, as I lay in bed and snivelled, Beth coached me in a low voice. 'She wants to punish us, by keeping us indoors, so we have to show that we don't care. That we don't mind. Do you understand, Erica? Please don't cry!' she whispered, stroking my hair back with fingers that shook with rage. I nodded, I think, but I was too upset to pay attention to her. It was still broad daylight outside. I could hear Henry playing with one of the dogs on the lawn, hear Clifford's voice, blurring through the floorboards. A wide August afternoon and we had been put to bed. Confined for the whole weekend.

When our parents got back we told them everything. Dad said, 'This is too much, Laura. I mean it this time.' I felt a flare of joy, of love for him.

Mum said, 'I'll talk to her.'

At teatime, I overheard them in the kitchen. Mum and Meredith.

'He seems like a nice enough boy. Quite sensible. I really don't see the harm in it, Mother,' Mum said.

'Don't see the harm? Do you want the girls to start using that dreadful Wiltshire slang? Do you want them to learn how to steal, and to swear? Do you want them to come home lousy and degraded? If so, then indeed, there can be no harm,' Meredith replied, coldly.

'My girls would *never* steal,' Mum told her

firmly. 'And I think *degraded* is overdoing it, really.'

'I don't, Laura. Perhaps you've forgotten how much trouble those people have caused us over the years?'

'How could I forget?' Mum sighed.

'Well, they are your children . . .'

'Yes, they are.'

'But if you want them to live under my roof, and in my care, then they will have to abide by *my* rules,' Meredith snapped.

Mum took a deep breath. 'If I hear that they have been locked up inside again, then they won't come here at all any more, and neither will David and I,' she said quietly, but I could hear the tension. Nearly a tremor. Meredith did not reply. I heard her footsteps coming towards me and I bolted out of sight. With the coast clear I went in to my mother, found her washing up with a quiet intensity, eyes bright. I put my arms around her legs, squeezed her tight. Meredith was never any less averse to us playing with Dinny, but we were never shut in our room again. Mum won on that point, at least.

*   *   *

Monday morning is leaden and wet. The tips of my fingers and toes were chilled when I woke up, and have stayed that way; and now the end of my nose too. I can't remember when I was last this cold. In London it just doesn't happen. There's the clammy warmth of the underground, the buffeting heat of shops and cafés. A hundred and one places to hide from any dip in the outside temperature. I'm in the orangery, on the south side of the house, overlooking a small lawn ringed with gnarled fruit trees. When we were playing too loudly, when we were *trying Meredith's patience*, we would be sent here, to the small lawn, while the grown-ups sat on the west-facing terrace at a white iron table, drinking iced tea and vodka. My companions in here are the skeletal remains of some tomato plants and a toad, sitting plump by the tap that drips verdigris water onto a bright green swathe of duckweed. I had forgotten the quiet of the countryside, and it unnerves me.

It's earthy and damp in here; a fecund smell, in spite of the season. One of my earliest memories of Henry, who would have been eight or nine: on the small lawn when I was five or so; a hot August day during one of those summers that seemed to last for ever; the grass baked blonde, crisping under the onslaught; the terrace stones too hot for bare feet; the dogs too fagged to play; my nose peeling and freckles on Beth's arms. They set up one of those giant paddling pools for us on the small lawn. So big that there were steps to climb over the side and an expanse of blue plastic sheet inside, so enticing even before the water went in. I can still smell that hot plastic. It was set up, smoothed out; an illicit hosepipe threaded over to it. The water from the hose came straight from the mains and it was icy on our toasted skin. Deliciously numbing. I fidgeted about in my red swimsuit, desperate for it to fill faster.

Henry climbed in straight away, with grass on his feet that floated away. He picked up the hosepipe and waved it at us, now that the grown-ups had retreated. He sprayed us and would not let us come near. I remember being so desperate to get in, to get my feet wet. But on *my* terms. I did not want to be splashed. Feet first, then the rest, gradually. Every time I got near, he sprayed me. The water was at his anklebones, his feet white and rippling. His body was white too, soft looking, nipples pouting slightly, turned down. Then he stopped, and he swore to me—he promised. He swore an oath that I could enter safely, that he had finished spraying. I made him put the hose down before I climbed in carefully. A second of ecstatic cold on my feet then Henry grabbed me, put my head under his arm, pushed the hose right into my face. Water up my nose, in my eyes, freezing, choking; Beth shouting at him from ringside. I coughed and howled until Mum came looking.

I wish Beth would come out of the house. I read somewhere that the great outdoors is just the thing for depression. A bracing walk, a communion with nature. As if depression is like a bout of indigestion, to be worked out of the system. I am not sure if it will work at this time of year, when the wind can blow right through your soul, but it has to be better than haunting that house. On the work bench I find a trug and some secateurs, and I head out towards the woods.

I walk in a loop via the dew pond. I do this most days. I can't seem to stay away. Standing on the steep edge of it, kicking over chalk and flints. Hints of something return to me when I stand here. Wherever I stand around Storton Manor, hints return to me—little snapshots that go with a view, or a smell, or a room. A ribbon tied behind a bed. Yellow flowers stitched on a pillowcase. Every step is an aide-memoire. Here at the pond there is something I should *remember*, something more than playing, than swimming, than the thrill of the forbidden. I shut my eyes and crouch down, hug my knees. I concentrate on the smell of the water and the ground, on the sound of the trees overhead. I can hear a dog barking, a long way off, in the village perhaps. There is definitely *something*, something I am trying to know. I put blind fingers forward until they touch the surface. The water bites, cold to the bone. I picture it thickening, ice crystals spinning hard threads through it. For one second I feel the old fear of being sucked down into it. For if water could come up from the bottom of it, from nowhere, like magic, then surely things could go the other way as well? A giant plughole. I would think this when I swam, sometimes. A delicious frisson, like swimming in the sea and suddenly thinking of sharks.

At the edge of the downs, where the trees disappear, the ground drops into a steep, round hollow. A giant scooping out of the earth, packed with hawthorn, blackthorn and elder, all bound up with old man's beard. The frost sets deeper here, lasts longer. I set my sights on a holly bush, right in the centre of it all, its bright berries like jewels in the colourless tangle, but I don't get far. I descend, slipping on the tussocky grass, and when I reach the thicket I can see no way in. The air is still, noticeably colder. My breath steams in front of my face as I make my way around, looking for a way in. No view but the slope up and away, the lip where it meets the sky. One attempt to force a way through and I retreat, badly scratched.

I head back into the woods, nothing in my trug so far but some tendrils of stripy ivy from the garden. These aren't public woods; they aren't managed, or criss-crossed with paths. The estate's pasture land is all leased or sold to local farmers these days, and I wonder if any of them ever come in here—take wood, raise pheasants, snare rabbits. I can see no sign of anything like that. The ground is choked with leaf fall and brambles, splintered logs mouldering into nothing. Unseen things move away from me with small rustling sounds and no other trace. Acorns, beech masts; around one tree a carpet of tiny yellow apples, rotting. I have to watch my feet to keep from stumbling and there are no birds singing above my head. Just a quiet breathing sound, as the wind sneaks through the naked branches.

I'm not watching where I'm going and I nearly step on a crouching person. I yelp in surprise. A young man with long dreadlocks and bright, mismatched clothes.

'Sorry! Hello,' I gasp. He stands up, far taller than me, and I see a large bracket fungus by his feet. Yellow and ugly. He was examining it, his nose virtually touching it. 'I . . . I don't think you can eat those,' I add, smiling briefly. The man faces me and says nothing. He is lean and rangy. His arms just hang by his sides as he stands there, watching me, and I feel the pull of unease towing me away from him. Some instinct, perhaps, or something missing from behind his eyes, tells me that all is not as it should be. I take a step back and turn left. He steps to his right to block me. I turn the other way and he follows. My heart beats harder. His silence is unsettling, he is somehow threatening even though he makes no move to reach out for me. He has a spicy smell about him, slightly sharp. I wonder if he's stoned. I turn left again and he smiles, a gummy smile that spreads across his face.

'Look, just get out of the bloody way, will you!' I snap, tensely. But he takes a step towards me and I try to step away but my heel catches in a web of brambles and I fall awkwardly, onto my side, feeling thorns punch into the heels of my hands and the air rush out of my lungs. Leaves fly up around me, the rotting smell of them everywhere. I turn my head and the tall man is leaning over me, blocking out the sky. I fight to free my foot from the undergrowth, but my movements are jerky and I make it worse. I think about shouting but the house is far behind me and there's no way Beth would hear me. She does not know I am out here. Nobody does. Panic makes me shake, makes the air hard to breathe. Then strong, heavy hands close tightly on my arms.

'Let go! Get off me! *Get off!*' I shout out wildly.

I hear a second voice and the hands release me, dropping me unceremoniously back into the mulch.

'Harry's no bother. You didn't mean to be a bother, did you, Harry?' the newcomer says, clapping the tall man on the shoulder. I peer up at them from the ground. Harry shakes his head and I see now that he is downcast, troubled; not fierce or lascivious in the slightest. 'He was just trying to help you up,' the other man says, with a hint of rebuke. Harry returns to his close scrutiny of the yellow fungus.

'He just . . . I was just . . . looking for greenery. For the house,' I say, still rattled. 'I thought . . . Well. Nothing really,' I finish. My heart slows slightly and I feel ridiculous. The stranger puts out a hand, pulls me to my feet. 'Thanks,' I mutter. There's an air rifle angled over his forearm, a dull gleam on the barrel. I kick the brambles back from around my feet and examine my stinging hands. Beads of blood are scattered there. I wipe them on the seat of my jeans and glance at my rescuer with a small, embarrassed smile. I find him watching me with an unsettling intensity, and then he smiles.

'Erica?'

'How did you . . . I'm sorry, do I know you?' I say.

'Don't you recognise me?' he says. I look again—a dark mess of hair, held back at the nape of his neck, a broad chest, a slight hook in the nose, straight forehead, straight brows, mouth a straight, determined line. Black eyes that shine. And then the world tips slightly, skews; features fall into place, and something stunningly familiar coalesces.

'*Dinny?* Is that you?' I gasp, my ribs squeezing in on themselves.

'Nobody's called me Dinny in a *long* time. It's Nathan, these days.' His smile is not quite sure of itself: pleased, as curious as I am to meet a figure from the past, yet guarded, held back. But his eyes never leave my face. Their gaze is like a spotlight on my every move.

'I can't believe it's really you! How . . . how are you? What the hell are you *doing* here?' I am amazed. It never occurred to me that Dinny grew up too, that he lived another life, that he would ever come back to Barrow Storton. 'You look so *different*!' My cheeks are burning, as if I have been caught out somehow. I can feel my pulse in my fingertips.

'But you look just the same, Erica. I saw a bit in the paper—about Lady Calcott dying. It made me think of . . . this place. We haven't been back here since my dad died. But suddenly I wanted to come . . .'

'Oh, no . . . I'm so sorry to hear that. About your dad.' Dinny's father, Mickey. Beth and I loved him. He had a huge grin, huge hands, always gave us a penny or a sweet—pulled it out from behind our ears. Mum met him, once or twice. Checking up, politely, since we spent so much time with them. And Dinny's mum, Maureen, always called Mo. Mickey and Mo. Our code name, to be used whenever Meredith might hear, was that we were going to visit Mickey Mouse.

'It was eight years ago. He went quickly, and he didn't see it coming. I suppose that's the best way to go,' Dinny says calmly.

'I suppose so.'

'What got Lady Calcott in the end?' I notice his tone, a slight bitterness, and that he doesn't commiserate with me on my loss.

'A stroke. She was ninety-nine—and must have been very disappointed.'

'What do you mean?'

'They were a long line of centenarians, the Calcott women. My great-grandmother lived to be a hundred and two. Meredith was always determined to outlive the queen. Good breeding stock, we are,' I say, and instantly regret it. Any mention of stock, of bloodlines, of breed.

There's a vibrant silence. I have so much to say to him I can't think where to start. He breaks off his intent gaze, looks away through the trees towards the house, and a shadow falls over his features.

'Look, I'm sorry I swore. At . . . Harry. He startled me, that's all,' I say quietly.

'You don't need to be afraid of him, he's harmless,' Dinny assures me. We both look down at the motley figure, crouching in the leaf mould. Dinny, standing so close to me that I could touch him. Dinny, real and right here again when he was almost a myth, just minutes ago. I almost don't believe it.

'Is he . . . is there something wrong with him?' I ask.

'He's gentle and friendly and he doesn't like to talk. If that means there's something wrong with him, then yes.'

'Oh, I didn't mean anything by it. Anything bad.' My voice is too high. I take a deep breath, let it out.

'And you were looking for . . . holly?'

'Yes—or mistletoe. Or some good ivy with berries. To decorate the house.' I smile.

'Come on, Harry. Let's show Erica the big holly tree,' Dinny says. He pulls Harry up, gently propels him into a languid walk.

'Thanks,' I say again. My breathing is still too fast. Dinny turns ahead of me and I notice a brace of grey squirrels, tied by their tails with string, slung over his back. Their black eyes are half closed, drying out. Dark, matted patches in the fur on their sides.

'What are the squirrels for?' I ask.

'Dinner,' Dinny replies calmly. He looks around, sees the horror fleet across my face and smiles half a smile. 'I guess squirrel hasn't reached the menus of smart London restaurants yet?'

'Well, some of them, perhaps. Not the ones I eat in, though. How did you know I lived in London?' He turns again, glances at my smart boots, dark jeans, soft, voluminous wool coat. The sharp ends of my fringe.

'Wild guess,' he murmurs.

'Don't you like London?' I ask.

'I've only been once,' Dinny remarks, over his shoulder. 'But generally, no. I don't like cities. I like the horizon to be more than ten metres away.'

'Well, I like having things to look at,' I shrug. Dinny doesn't smile, but falls back to walk beside me, his silence almost companionable. I search for ways to fill it. He is not much taller than me, about the same height as Beth. I can see the tie in his hair, a dark red length of leather bootlace, snapped off, knotted tightly. His jeans are muddied at the hems; he wears a T-shirt and a loose cotton jumper. I see the wind circle his bare neck and I shiver, even though I am bundled beneath layers and he does not seem to notice the cold. We walk up a shallow rise, my steps by far the loudest. Their feet don't seem to find as many snags as mine.

'Over there,' Dinny says, pointing. I look ahead, see a dark holly tree, twisted and old. Harry has picked up a fallen sprig of it, is pressing the prickles into the pad of his thumb and then wincing, shaking his hand, doing it again.

I set about cutting some branches—those with the spikiest leaves, the fattest sprays of berries. One springs away from me, snagging my face. A thin scratch under my eye that stings. Dinny watches me again, his expression inscrutable.

'How's your mother? Is she here with you?' I ask. I want to hear him talk, I want to hear everything he's done since I saw him last, I want him to be real again, to still be a friend. But I remember now—his silences. They never made me uncomfortable before. A child is unperturbed by something as harmless as a silence, oddly patient in that way.

'She's well, thanks. She doesn't travel with us any more. When Dad died she gave it up—she said she was getting too old for it, but I think she'd just had enough of the road. She would never have told Dad, of course. But when he died, she quit. She's hitched to a plumber called Keith. They live in West Hatch, just over the way.'

'Oh, well. Give her my best, when you see her next.' At this he frowns slightly and I wonder if I've said the wrong thing. He has one of those faces that can be rendered so grim, so hawkish by the slightest scowl. At twelve it made him look studious, serious. I felt as silly as thistledown then and I feel it again now.

With my trug full of holly, we walk back through the woods to the clearing where they always camped before. A broad space at the western edge of the copse, surrounded by sheltering trees on three sides, with open fields to the west and a rutted green lane that takes you back to the road. The ground here is not well drained. It squelches as we get near. In summer it's such a green place; long grasses with satin stems, the ground cracked hard and safe beneath. Harry drifts along behind us, his attention flitting from one thing to another.

'And you? Are you living here now?' Dinny asks, at length.

'Oh, no. I don't know. Probably not. For the time being; for Christmas, anyway. We've inherited the house, Beth and I . . .' How pompous I sound.

'Beth's here?' Dinny interrupts, turning to face me.

'Yes, but . . . Yes, she's here.' I was going to say *but she's different, but she won't come out*. 'You should come up to the house and say hello,' I say, knowing that he won't.

There are six vehicles in the camp—more than there used to be. Two minibuses, two campervans, a big old horse lorry and a converted army ambulance, which Dinny says is his. Coils of smoke shred away from chimney pipes, and circles of cold ash scatter the ground. Harry strides ahead to sit on a stump of wood, picking something up from the ground and setting to work intently upon it. As we approach, three dogs race over to us, barking in apparent savagery. I know this drill. I stand still, let my arms hang, wait for them to reach us, to sniff me, to see me not run.

'Yours?'

'Only two of them—the black and tan belongs to my cousin Patrick. This is Blot,' Dinny scuffs the ears of a vicious-looking black mongrel, toothy and scarred, 'and this is Popeye.' A smaller, gentler dog; a rough brown coat and kind eyes. Popeye licks the fingers Dinny offers to him.

'So . . . um, are you working around here? What do you do?' I fall back on a party stalwart, and Dinny shrugs. For a second I think that perhaps he draws endless benefits, that he steals, sells drugs. But these are Meredith's thoughts, and I'm ashamed to have them.

'Nothing right now. We follow work around the

country for most of the year. Farm work, bar work, festivals. This time of year is pretty dead.'

'That must be hard.'

Dinny gives me a quick glance. 'It's fine, Erica,' he tells me mildly. He doesn't ask me what I do. In the short walk to the camp I seem to have used up all the credit a childhood acquaintance afforded me.

'I like your ambulance,' I say, desperate. As I speak, the ambulance door bangs open and a girl climbs awkwardly out. She puts her hands in the small of her back, stretches with a grimace. I recognise her at once—the pregnant girl from the barrow. But she can only be fifteen, sixteen. Dinny is the same age as Beth: thirty-five. I look at the girl again and try to make her eighteen, maybe nineteen, but I can't.

The girl with the bubble-curls, a bright natural blonde that you rarely see these days. Her skin is pale and there are blue smudges under her eyes. In a tight, stripy jersey it is very clear how close to term she is. She sees me standing with Dinny and she comes across to us, scowling. I try to smile, to seem comfortable there. She looks fiercer than Blot.

'Who's this?' she demands, hands on hips. She talks to Dinny, not to me.

'Erica, this is Honey. Honey, Erica.'

'Honey? Pleased to meet you. I'm sorry for scaring you, up at the barrow the other day,' I say, in a cheery tone I secretly, horrified, think is my teaching voice.

Honey gazes at me with flat, tired eyes. 'That was you? You didn't scare me.' A noticeable Wiltshire burr to her speech.

'No, well. Not scare, but . . .' I shrug. She looks at me for a long moment. Such hard scrutiny from one so young. Palpable relief when she dismisses me, looks back at Dinny.

'The stove's not drawing right,' she says.

Dinny sighs, crouches down to put his hands through Popeye's coat. The first drops of rain land on our hands and faces.

'I'll see to it in a minute,' he tells her, soothingly. She stares at him then turns away, goes back inside without another glance. I am momentarily dumbstruck by her.

'So . . . when's the due date? Must be soon?' I ask awkwardly, hoping she won't hear me from inside.

'A little after Christmas,' Dinny says, looking away across the clearing.

'So close! You must be very excited. Has she got her overnight bag ready and everything? For the hospital?' Dinny shakes his head.

'No hospital. She wants to have it here, she says.' At this Dinny pauses, stands up and turns to me. 'I don't know if it's a good idea. Do you know anything about babies?' he sounds anxious.

'Me? No, not really. I've never . . . But the government are always on about the merits of home births these days. Every woman's right, apparently. Have you got a good midwife?'

'No midwife, no *home* birth—she wants to have it out there, in the woods.'

'In the *woods*? But . . . it's December! Is she mad?'

'I know it's December, Erica. But it's her right to choose, as you say,' he says flatly. There's a hint of exasperation there, beneath the surface. 'She's taking the idea of a natural birth about as far as she possibly can.'

'Well, you have a right to choose, too. The father has a right too. First babies can take their time, you know. Beth was in labour for thirty-six hours with Eddie . . .'

'Beth has a baby?'

'Had a baby. He's eleven now. He's coming for Christmas, so you'll probably meet him . . . Eddie. He's a fantastic kid.'

'So she's married?'

'Was married. Not married now,' I say shortly. He has questions about Beth, but none about me.

The rain is coming down harder again. I hunch, push my hands deeper into my pockets, but Dinny doesn't seem to notice it. I think about offering to talk to Honey, then I remember her hard eyes and I hope Dinny won't ask me to. A compromise, then.

'Well, if Honey wants to talk to somebody about it, maybe she could talk to Beth? Her experience could be a good cautionary tale.'

'She won't talk to anybody about it. She's . . . strong willed,' Dinny sighs.

'So I noticed,' I murmur. I can't stand another silence. I want to ask him about Christmas. About names for the baby. I want to ask about his travels, his life, our past. 'Well, I should be getting back. Getting out of this rain,' is all I can say. 'It was really good to see you again, Dinny. I'm glad you're back. And nice to meet Honey, too. I'll . . . well, we're up at the house, if you need anything . . .'

'It's good to see you too, Erica.' Dinny looks at me with his head on one side, but his eyes are troubled, not glad.

'OK. Well, bye.' I go, as casually as I can.

I don't tell Beth about Dinny when I find her, watching TV in the study. I'm not sure why not. There will be a reaction, I think, when I tell her. And I am not sure what it will be. I am agitated suddenly. I feel like we're no longer alone. I can feel Dinny's presence out there, beyond the trees. Like a niggling something in the corner of my eye. The third corner of our triangle. I switch off the TV, throw open the curtains.

'Come on. We're going out,' I tell her.

'I don't want to go out. Go where?'

'Shopping. I'm sick to death of tinned soup. Plus, it's about to be Christmas. Mum and Dad are coming for lunch, and what are you going to feed Eddie on Christmas day? Meredith's old Hovis crackers?' Beth considers this for a moment, then stands up quickly, puts her hands on her hips.

'God, you're right. You're right!'

'I know.'

'We need lots of things . . . turkey, sausages, potatoes, puddings . . .' she counts items off on her long fingers. Christmas is ten days away yet—we have plenty of time. But I don't say that. I make the most of her sudden animation, point to the door. 'And decorations!' she cries.

'Come on. You can make a list in the car.'

*   *   *

Devizes is prettied up for Christmas. Little fir trees lean out from the sides of shops and hotels along the High Street, strung with white lights; there's a brass band playing, and a man roasting chestnuts, plumes of acrid smoke rising from his cart. I wonder what he does for the rest of the year. Here, the darkness and the sleet draw us in, make us part of the huddled crowd. We wrap our scarves around our ears and window-shop, basking in the warm yellow light. Back in the world, the pair of us, after the solitude of the manor. It feels good, exciting, and I miss London. Inside each shop, Beth hums along to the taped carols, and as we walk I loop my arm through hers, holding her tight.

Several hours later and Beth has gone into Christmas overdrive. We have eight different cheeses, a huge ham, chipolatas, crackers—edible and the ones you pull—a turkey I struggle to carry to the car, and a cake that cost a ridiculous amount of money. We cram it all into the boot, go back for glittering baubles, strings of beads, gold paint, glass icicles, little straw angels with dresses of white muslin. There's a farm two minutes from the manor selling Christmas trees—we call in on the way back, arrange to have a tree four metres high delivered and erected on December the twenty-third.

'It can go in the hallway—they can wire it to the banister,' Beth says decisively.

Perhaps I should not let her spend when she is troubled, like now. I daren't put all the receipts together, add it all up. But Beth has money—money from Maxwell, money from her translating work. More money than I have, certainly, but it's something we never discuss. She lives small, most of the time. She squirrels it away unless Eddie needs something. All mine is absorbed by London, in getting to work, in rent, in living. Now we have enough food for ten people, when we will be five;

but Beth looks happier, her face is less drawn. Retail therapy. But that's not it—she likes to be able to give. I leave her threading garlands along the mantelpiece, with a slight frown of concentration while I put the kettle on, feeling pleased and sleepy.

There's a message from my agency on my mobile phone, about some supply work at a school in Ealing, starting on January the twelfth. My thumb hovers over the redial button, but I am strangely reluctant to press it, to have real life intrude upon me. But money must be earned, I suppose; life must resume. Literature must be crammed between deaf ears. Unless it doesn't. Unless I live here, of course. No more rent. Just the upkeep, although that would probably cost more than my rent does now. Would it be worth it for five years, even ten? Trying to live here—just long enough for the legacy to stand. Then we could sell up, retire at the age of forty, once property prices are back up. But if living here makes Beth ill? And if I will always have this feeling of something stealing up behind me? I wish I could turn and look at it, I wish I could make it out. I remember everything else that happened that summer, except what happened to Henry.

We came here the two summers after that year, and our mother watched us closely. Not to protect us, not to keep us from harm; but to assess, to see how we would react. I don't know if I was different. A little quieter, perhaps. And we stayed in the garden; we didn't want to venture further any more. Mum kept us away from Meredith, who was unpredictable by then; who flew into storms of cursing and accusation. But Beth drew further and further into herself. Our mother saw and she told our father, and he frowned. And we stopped coming.

Outside, the sun sets orange and coldly pink on the horizon. I spray the holly gold, the paint burnishing the dark leaves. It looks delicious. The fumes make me dizzy, euphoric. I am hanging it from the banisters and laying it along window sills when Beth comes downstairs, arms folded, face creased with sleep. She moves from place to place where I have hung it, touching it lightly, testing the paint with her fingertips.

'Do you approve?' I ask her, smiling. I've tuned the radio to Classic FM. They're playing 'Good King Wenceslas'. Beth nods, yawns. I sing: 'Silly bugger, he fell out; on a red hot cinder!' I've no kind of singing voice.

'You're chirpy,' Beth tells me. She comes over to the window sill I am strewing with sprigs, puts my hair behind my ear for me, touches the scratch under my eye. So rare, her touches. I smile.

'Well . . .' I say. The words teeter in my mouth. I am so tempted to say them, still so unsure if they're right or wrong.

'Well, what?'

'Well, Dinny's here,' I tell her.

LOVING

1902

The journey from New York to Woodward in Oklahoma Territory was a long one, covering a distance of nearly two thousand miles. State after state rolled out beneath the train, ever westwards. At first, Caroline was awed by the scene beyond the window. As they left behind the familiar towns of New York State, settlements became fewer and further between. They passed through woods so thick and dark that they seemed to belong to another age, closing the train in for mile after countless mile. They passed through fields of wheat and corn no less vast, no less astonishing; and towns that grew smaller and smaller, as if compressed by the wide expanses of land all around them. Beside the tracks in one station, rough dwellings had been built and children were playing, running alongside the train, waving, begging for pennies. With a start, Caroline saw that their feet were bare. She waved to them as the train eased away again, and turned to look back as their fragile homes shrank into miniature, and the land yawned away on either side. It was truly untamed, she thought, this land to the west. Men lived upon it, but they had not yet shaped it; not in the way they had shaped New York City. Caroline sat back in her seat and studied the distant purple hills with a pull of unease, feeling the once mighty train to be a mere speck, an insect crawling across the endless surface of the world.

By the time Caroline changed trains for the third and final time, at Dodge City in Kansas, she was heavy with fatigue and stale in her clothes. Her stomach felt hot and empty because the picnic Sara packed for her had run out a day and a half ago; Sara, who could not conceive of a journey so long that a half-dozen hard-boiled eggs, an apple and a pork pie would not be provisions enough. Caroline joined fellow passengers for lunch at El Vacquero, the Harvey Hotel beside the tracks in Dodge City. It was a brand new, brick building, and Caroline took this as proof of the new wealth and stability of what had recently been frontier land. She looked around discreetly, too curious about her surroundings to resist.

The unmade street outside thronged with people and ponies and buggies and wagons, making a muted noise quite unlike that of a New York street. Saddle horses were lined up along the hitch racks, resting their rumps on one tipped-back hoof. The reek of slurry was strong, drifting over the town from the nearby stock pens, and it mixed oddly with food smells and the hot bodies of people and animals. Confused, Caroline's stomach did not know whether to rumble or recoil. Men sauntered by with pistols strapped to their hips, their shirts untied at the throat, and Caroline stared at them in amazement, as if they had walked straight out of legend. Her heart beat hard with nervous energy and her throat was dry. For one instant, she almost missed Bathilda's indomitable presence at her side; missed having the barricade of her respectability to hide behind. Ashamed, she straightened her shoulders and reread the menu card.

The restaurant was busy with the lunch crowd, but a crisp girl in a neat uniform soon served her; bringing out consommé with vermicelli, and poached eggs, and coffee.

'Are you travelling far, miss?' a man asked her. He was sitting two seats away along the table, and he smiled and leaned towards her, so that she coloured, shocked to be spoken to so casually. The man was unshaven and his coat cuffs were shiny.

'To Woodward,' she said, unsure whether she should introduce herself before speaking, or indeed if she should speak to him at all.

'Woodward? Well, you've not too far to go now, I guess, considering how far you've come already— New York, if I can tell by your accent?' He smiled again, wider now. Caroline nodded quickly and concentrated on her eggs. 'You got family there you visiting? In Woodward I mean?'

'My husband,' Caroline replied.

'Your husband! Now that's a crying shame. Still, lucky this place has opened up now, isn't it? The Fred Harvey place before this was in a boxcar on stilts! Did you ever see such a thing back east?' he exclaimed loudly, and Caroline tried to smile politely.

'Ah, leave the girl alone, Doon. Can't you see she wants to eat her lunch in peace?' This was another man, sitting next to the first. He had an ill-tempered look, deep creases around his eyes. He had combed his hair fiercely to one side and there it remained, held fixed by some substance or other. Caroline hardly dared look at him. Her cheeks blazed.

'Beg pardon, missus,' the first man mumbled. Caroline ate with unseemly haste and returned to the train with her hands tucked into her fox-fur muffler, in spite of the warmth of the weather.

The country after Dodge City was wide and sparsely punctuated. Mile after gently featureless mile of prairie rolled by as the train now turned southwards on the Santa Fe line. Caroline slouched in her seat and longed to loosen her stays. Too tired to keep a ladylike posture, and since she was alone in the compartment, she tipped her head against the glass and stared into the endless, eggshell sky. The horizon had never been as wide, as flat, as far away. Gradually, the mighty span of it began to give her a slippery feeling like vertigo. She had expected to see snow-capped mountains, emerald fields of farmland, and quick rivers running. But the earth looked hot and exhausted, just as she felt. She took her copy of *The Virginian* from her bag instead and fancied herself like Molly Wood, fearlessly cutting her home ties, boldly heading to a new life in an unknown land. After a while, though, she stopped feeling like Molly Wood and started to feel afraid again, so she thought of her husband, waiting for her at Woodward, and while this seemed to slow the train and prolong the interminable journey, it did at least reassure her.

The train arrived at Woodward late in the day, as the sun began to set smeared and orange against the dusty window glass. Caroline had been dozing when the conductor strode past her compartment.

'Woodward! Woodward the next stop!' His shout woke her, sent her heart skittering. She gathered her things and stood up so quickly that her head spun and she had to sit back down again, breathing deeply. *Corin*, was all she could think. To see him again, after so many days! She peered eagerly out at the station as the train squealed to a halt, desperate to catch a glimpse of him. Catching her reflection in the glass, she hastily patted her hair into shape, bit her lips to redden them and pinched some colour into her cheeks. She could not keep calm, could not keep herself from shaking.

She climbed stiffly from the train, her skirts clinging to her legs, feet swollen and hot in her boots. She looked up and down the wooden platform, her heart in her mouth, but could not see Corin among the handful of people quitting the carriages or waiting at the station. The train exhaled with a weary sound and crept towards a siding where a water tower bulked against the sky. A warm wind greeted her, singing softly in her ears, and sand on the platform ground beneath her feet. Caroline looked around again and felt suddenly empty, suddenly unbound, as if the next rush of wind might carry her off. She straightened her hat nervously, but kept her smile ready, her eyes searching. Woodward looked small and slow. The street leading into town from the rail track was wide and unmade, and the wind had carved tiny waves into the sand all along it. She could smell the tar on the station building, hot from the sun, and the pervading stink of livestock. She looked down, sketching a line in the grit with her toe.

As the locomotive moved away a new kind of quiet settled, behind the rattle of a passing buggy and the creak of the trolley as the station man pit his back against the weight of her luggage. Where was Corin? Doubts and fears bubbled up inside her—that he regretted his choice, that she was abandoned, would have to take the next train back to New York. She turned in a circle, desperate to see him. The station porter had paused with her luggage and was trying to catch her eye, to ask, no doubt, where he should take it. But if Corin was not here, Caroline had no idea. No idea where to go, where to stay, what to do. She felt the blood run out of her face and a rush of light-headedness spun her thoughts. For a terrifying moment, she thought she might faint, or burst into tears, or both. She took a deep, trembling breath and tried desperately to think what to do, what to say to the porter to conceal her confusion.

'Mrs Massey?' Caroline did not at first register this as her name, spoken with a slow drawl. She ignored the man with his hat in his hands who had come to stand to one side of her, his body curved into a relaxed slouch. He looked to be about thirty, but the weather was wearing his face as it was fading the blue from his flannel shirt. His scruffy hair was shot through with strands of red and brown. 'Mrs Massey?' he asked again, taking a step towards her.

'Oh! Yes, I am,' she exclaimed, startled.

'Pleasure to meet you, Mrs Massey. I'm Derek Hutchinson, but everybody around here calls me Hutch and I'd be happy if you would too,' he introduced himself, tucking his hat beneath his arm and holding out a hand, which Caroline shook tentatively, just with her fingertips.

'Where is Mr Massey?' she asked.

'Corin was due back in time to come and get you, ma'am, and I know he sorely wanted to, but there's been some trouble with cattle thieves and he was called upon to ride out and see to it . . . He'll be back by the time we are, I'm sure of that,' Hutch said, seeing Caroline's face fall. Tears of disappointment blurred her vision and she gripped her bottom lip in her teeth to halt them. Hutch hesitated, unnerved by her reaction.

'I see,' she gasped, swaying slightly, suddenly longing to sit down. Corin hadn't come to meet her. In sudden terror, she began to guess at reasons he might have to avoid her.

Hutch cleared his throat diffidently and shifted his feet in an awkward manner. 'I . . . uh . . . I know it truly was his wish to meet you here himself, Mrs Massey, but when there are thieves to apprehend, it's the duty of the landowners to help one another in that mission. I have come in his stead and I'm at your service.'

'It's their duty to go?' she asked, tentatively.

'Absolutely. He was duty-bound to it.'

'Are you his . . . manservant, then?' she asked.

Hutch smiled and tipped his chin. 'Well, not quite that, Mrs Massey. Not quite that. I'm foreman at the ranch.'

'Oh, I see,' Caroline said, although she did not. 'Well. Will we be there in time for dinner, do you think?' she asked, fighting to regain her composure.

'Dinner, ma'am? Tomorrow, do you mean?'

'Tomorrow?'

'It's nearing on thirty-five miles to the ranch, from Woodward here. Now, that's not far, but too far to make a start this evening, I think. There's a room waiting for you at the boarding house, and a good dinner too, for you do look in need of a square meal, if I can be as bold as to say so.' He studied her tiny form and the pallor of her skin with a measuring eye.

'Thirty-five miles? But . . . how long will it take?'

'We'll set out early tomorrow and we should get there by noon time on the second day . . . I had not reckoned on you bringing quite so many boxes and trunks with you, and that might slow the wagon down some. But the horses are fresh, and if the weather stays this fair it'll be a good, smooth ride.' Hutch smiled, and Caroline rallied herself, finding a smile for him in return in spite of the weariness that even hearing about another day and a half of travel made her feel. Hutch stepped forward, proffering his arm. 'That's more like it. Come with me now and we'll get you settled. You look fairly done in, Mrs Massey.'

The Central Hotel on Main Street was managed by a round, sour-faced woman who introduced herself as Mrs Jessop. She showed Caroline to a room that was clean if not spacious, whilst Hutch oversaw the switching of her luggage from the station trolley to the covered wagon that would take them on to the ranch. Mrs Jessop scowled when Caroline asked for a hot bath to be drawn, and Caroline hastily produced coins from her purse to sweeten the request.

'Go on, then. I'll knock on your door when it's ready,' the proprietress told her, eyeing her sternly. The latch on the bathhouse door was flimsy and there was a knot in the wood through which a tiny glimpse of the hallway outside could be had. Caroline kept a careful eye on this as she bathed, terrified of seeing the shadow of a trespassing eye fall over it. The bath was shallow, but it restored her nevertheless. Blood eased into her stiff muscles and her sore back, and she rested her head at last, breathing deeply. The room smelt of damp towels and cheap soap. The last of the evening light seeped warmly around the shutters, and voices carried up to her from the street outside; voices slow and melodious with unfamiliar accents. Then a man's voice sounded loudly, apparently right below the window:

'Why, you goddamned son of a *bitch*! What the *hell* are you doing here?' Caroline's pulse quickened at such obscene language and she sat up with an abrupt splash, expecting at any moment to hear more cursing, or a fight, or even gunshots ringing out. But what she heard next was a rich guffaw of laughter, and the patting of hands against shoulders. She sank back into the cooling bathwater and tried to feel calm again.

Afterwards, she dried herself with a rough towel and put on a clean white dress for dinner, forgoing any jewels because she had no wish to outshine her fellow clientèle. Without Sara's help her waist was a little less tiny, and her hair a little less neat, but she felt more like herself as she descended at the dinner hour. She looked around for Derek Hutchinson and, not finding him, enquired of Mrs Jessop.

'You'll not see him again this night, I'll bet,' the woman said with a brief, knowing smile. 'He was heading over to the Dew Drop, last I saw him.'

'Heading to where, I beg your pardon?'

'The Dew Drop Inn, over Miliken's Bridge by the depot. Whatever sustenance he's taking this evening, he'll be taking it there and not here!' At this she gave a low chuckle. 'He's been riding out a good few months. A man gets hungry.' Faced with

Caroline's blank incomprehension, Mrs Jessop relented. 'Go on through and sit yourself down, Mrs Massey. I'll send Dora out with your dinner.' So Caroline did as she was bid and ate alone at the counter with no company but the inquisitive girl, Dora, who brought out a reel of questions about the east with each course of the meal. Across the room, two battered gentlemen with careworn faces discussed the price of grain at great length.

*   *   *

The morning dawned fair, the sky as clear as a bell, and there was a scent in the air that Caroline was unused to; an earthy smell of dampened ground and new-sprouting sage bushes on the prairie all around Woodward. So different to the brick and smoke and people smell of the city. The sun was strong as they began the final stretch of the journey. As Hutch helped her up into the wagon, Caroline noticed a gun belt now buckled around his hips, a six-shooter holstered into it. It gave her an odd tingling in her stomach. She tilted her bonnet forward to better shade her eyes against the bright light, but still could not help but squint. The sun seemed to be brighter here than it had ever been in New York, and when she commented on this, Hutch tipped his chin in agreement.

'I reckon that's so, ma'am. I've never been that far east myself, or that far north come to think of it; but I reckon any place with so much building and living and dying going on will wind up with its air all muddied up, just like its rivers.' A lively breeze picked up the sand from beneath the wagon wheels, whisking it around them, and Caroline flapped her hands to ward it off. The folds of her skirt were soon lined with the stuff. Hutch watched her, and he did not smile. 'Once we're clear of town there'll be less of that sand blowing, Mrs Massey,' he said.

It did not take long to pass through Woodward town. They drove down Main Street, which was flanked predominantly by wooden-framed buildings and just one or two of more permanent construction. There were several saloons, several banks, a post office, a large general store, an opera house. There was a fair bustle of wagons and horses, and a fair number of people going about their business, most of whom were men. Caroline looked back over her shoulder as they left town. From a distance she could see that many of the high building fronts were false, and had just a single storey crouched behind them.

'Is that the whole of Woodward?' she asked, incredulously.

'Yes, ma'am. Over two thousand souls call it home, nowadays, and growing all the while. Ever since they opened up the Cheyenne and Arapaho lands to the south, folks have been pouring in, starting to settle and farm. Some call it a pity, to see the open range fenced off and ploughed under. Me, I do call it progress, although I'm happy to say there's plenty of land left open to the cow herds yet.'

'Arapaho? What does that mean?'

'The Arapaho? They're Indian folks. From more northern parts originally, but settled here by the government, like so many others . . . Now, this land we're driving through right now belonged to the Cherokee until recently, although they

94

themselves lived further east. They leased it out to ranchers and cattle folk for years before it was opened up to settlers in ninety-three . . .'

'But is that safe? For civilised people to live where there are Indians?' Caroline was shocked. Hutch gave her a sidelong look, then hitched a shoulder.

'They've sold their lands and moved on east. I reckon they've as little urge to have white neighbours as some white folk have to share with Indians.'

'Thank goodness!' Caroline said. 'I could never have slept at night, knowing that such creatures were roaming around outside the window!' She laughed a little, high and nervous, and did not notice Hutch's thoughtful gaze, out over the prairie. Copying him, Caroline searched the horizon and felt her stomach flutter, to think that savages might have hunted scalps in this very place not long before. A pair of rabbits were startled from the side of the road and darted off into the brush, visible only by the black tips of their ears.

Some ten or twelve miles along the road, buildings appeared in the distance. Caroline was glad to see them. Each mile they had covered from Woodward had seemed to her another leap from safety, somehow; another mile from civilisation, even if it was also another mile closer to Corin. She shaded her eyes for a better view.

'Is that the next town?' she asked. Hutch whistled softly to the horses, two chestnut-coloured animals with hard legs and meaty behinds, and brought them to a standstill.

'No, ma'am. That's the old military fort. Fort Supply, it's called. We'll turn off the road soon, I'm afraid, so it won't be quite as smooth going.'

'Fort Supply? So there's a garrison here?'

'Not any more. It's been empty these seven or eight years.'

'But why were they here? To protect people from the Indians, I suppose?'

'Well, that was some of the reason, for sure. But more than that they was charged with keeping white folks from settling on Indian lands. So you could say, they was there to protect the Indians from the likes of you and I.'

'Oh,' Caroline said, deflating a little. She had liked the idea of soldiers guarding so close to the ranch, and had immediately pictured herself dancing a quadrille with men in neat uniforms. But as they went nearer she saw that the fort was low and roughshod, built mostly of wood and earth rather than brick or stone. The empty black gaps of its windows seemed eerily watchful and she looked away with a shiver. 'But where does this road go to now?'

'Well, not to any place, I suppose. It runs from this here down to Fort Sill, but this end of it's mostly used by odd folk like us now, to make the run into town a bit easier on the bones,' Hutch told her. Caroline looked behind them, back along the empty road. She watched the dust resettling into their tracks. She had pictured the country virgin, untouched by any hand but God's. Here already were ghostly ruins and a road to nowhere. 'We'll be crossing the North Canadian in just a short while, Mrs Massey, but I don't want you to worry about that none. This time of year it's not going to pose us any problems at all,' Hutch said. Caroline nodded, and smiled gamely at him.

The river was wide but shallow, the water reaching only halfway up the wagon wheels, and to the horses' stomachs. Hutch let the pair take the reins from him when they reached the far side, and the animals drank deeply, kicking up sprays that spattered their dusty coats and filled Caroline's nostrils with the smell of their hot hides. She wiped at some droplets on her skirt, succeeding only in making a grubby smear. They paused for lunch on the far side, where a stand of cottonwood trees curled their roots into the sandy bank and cast a dappled shade onto the ground. Hutch spread out a thick blanket, and Caroline took his hand down from the wagon, seating herself as well as she could on the ground. Her corset would not let her be comfortable, though, and she spoke little as she ate a slice of ham that required an indelicate amount of chewing, and bread that crumbled into her lap. Grains of sand ground between her teeth as she ate. The only sound was the soft hiss and clatter of the breeze through the cottonwood leaves, which twisted and trembled, flashing muted shades of silver and green. Before they moved on again, Caroline went to some lengths to extract her scalloped silk parasol from her luggage.

The wagon made slower progress over the open prairie, bumping over knots of sagebrush, dragging sometimes in patches of shifting sand or the boggy remnants of a shallow creek. Occasionally they passed small dwellings, homesteads dug in and knocked together in haste to keep a family safe, to stake a claim, to make a new beginning. But these were far apart, and grew more infrequent the further they went. As the afternoon grew long Caroline drowsed, swaying on the seat next to

97

Hutch. Each time her head began to droop some jolt brought her around again.

'We'll stop for the night soon, ma'am. I reckon you could use a hot cup of coffee and to bed down.'

'Oh, yes! I am rather tired. We must be very far from town, by now?'

'It seems further in this slow wagon. I have made the journey on horseback in a day before, without even trying too hard. All you need is a good, fast saddle horse, and your husband raises some of the finest such animals in all of Oklahoma Territory.'

'Where will we stop the night? Is there some other settlement nearby?'

'Oh, no, ma'am. We'll make camp tonight.'

'Camp?'

'That's right. Don't look so alarmed, Mrs Massey! I am a man of honour and discretion,' he said, smiling wryly at Caroline's expression of wide-eyed bewilderment. It was a moment before she realised he had imagined her scandalised at the thought of spending the night alone with him, just the two of them. She blushed and dropped her gaze, only to find it resting near the waistband of his trousers, where his shirt had pulled a little loose to reveal a small area of his hard, tanned stomach. Caroline swallowed and set her eyes firmly on the horizon. Her first fear had actually been of being outdoors all night, unprotected from animals, weather, and other savageries of nature.

Before sundown Hutch drew the wagon to a stop on a flat area where the ground was greener than it had been, and more lush. He helped Caroline down and she stood, aching everywhere, unsure of what to do. Hutch unhitched the wagon, took the bits from the horses' mouths and slapped their behinds. With glad expressions and swishing tails, they trotted lazily away to a near distance and began to crop huge mouthfuls of grass.

'But . . . won't the horses run away?' Caroline asked.

'Not far, I reckon. And they'll come miles for a slice of bread, anyway.' Hutch unloaded a tent from the wagon and soon had it built. He spread blankets on top of buffalo hides to make a bed, and put her vanity case inside for her. 'You'll be cosy as anything in there. As fine as any New York hotel,' he said. Caroline glanced at him, unsure if she was being mocked, then she smiled and seated herself inside the tent, wrinkling her nose at the smell of the hides. But the bed was deep and soft; and the sides of the tent belled in and out with the breeze, as if gently breathing. Caroline felt her heart slow, and a gentle calm come over her.

Hutch soon had a fire going and crouched beside it, tending to a large, flat pan that spat and smoked. He fed the flames with pieces of something dry and brown that Caroline did not recognise.

'What's that you're using as fuel?' she asked.

'Cow chips,' Hutch replied, offering no further explanation. Caroline did not dare to ask. The sky was a glory of pink and turquoise striations, marching away from the bright flare of the west to the deep velvet blue of the east. Hutch's face was aglow with firelight. 'I put that box there for you to sit on,' he said, gesturing with a fork. Caroline sat, obediently. In the darkness beyond the flames one of the horses snorted, and whinnied softly. Then a distant howl, high and ghostly, echoed across the flat plain to where they sat.

'What was that?' Caroline exclaimed, rushing to her feet once more. The blood ran out of her head and she reeled, flinging out an arm that Hutch caught, appearing at her side in an instant.

'Do sit, ma'am. Sit back down,' he insisted.

'Is it *wolves*?' she cried, unable to keep her voice from shaking.

'Nothing more than prairie wolves, is all. Why, they're no bigger than a pet dog, and no fiercer. They won't be coming anywhere near us, I promise you.'

'Are you sure?'

'Sure as I'm sitting right here, Mrs Massey,' Hutch assured her. Caroline pulled her shawl around her tightly, and huddled fearfully on the hard wooden box, her every fibre strung tight with alarm. Hutch seemed to sense her disquiet and began to talk. 'Coyotes, they also get called sometimes. They run around in packs and squabble over leftover bones here and there. That's all they're singing about—who's found the best old cow bones to chew. The most mischief they get up to is stealing chickens from homesteaders, but they only do that when they have to. I reckon they've learnt not to go too close to folk, unless they want to take a bullet in the tail that is . . .' And so he talked on, his voice low, and soothing somehow, and Caroline was reassured by it. Now and again the coyote song drifted over the camp, long and mournful.

'They sound so lonely,' she murmured.

Hutch glanced at her, his eyes lost in shadow. He carefully passed her a tin cup.

'Take some coffee, ma'am,' he said.

* * *

The sunrise woke her, light glowing irresistibly inside the tent. Caroline had been dreaming of Bathilda, watching over her shoulder as Caroline ran scales up and down the piano, exclaiming *Wrists! Wrists!* as she had been wont to do. For a moment, Caroline could not remember where she was. She poked her head cautiously out of the tent and was relieved to see no sign of Hutch. The eastern sky was dazzling. Caroline had never in her life been up so early. She stood up and stretched, hands in the small of her back. Her hair was in disarray and her mouth was sour with last night's coffee. She rubbed her eyes and found her brows full of sand. Her whole face, in fact, and her clothes. There was a line of dirt inside her cuffs, and she could feel it inside her collar too, rubbing at the skin. Rumpled blankets beside the cooling embers of the fire spoke of where the foreman had spent the night.

'Good morning, Mrs Massey,' Hutch called, giving her a start. He was approaching from the green expanse beyond the parked wagon, a chestnut horse held by a halter rope in each of his hands. 'How did you find your first night as a cow-puncher?' he smiled. Caroline smiled back, not really understanding him.

'Good morning, Mr Hutchinson. I slept well, thank you.'

'I'm taking these two to water at the creek over this way, then I'll get some breakfast cooking,' he said. Caroline nodded, and glanced around. 'I put a can of water there, in case you wanted to freshen up any,' he added, smiling again as he made his way past the camp.

Caroline's real want, however, was for plumbing. She dithered for a while and then realised, to her dawning horror, that she would have to relieve herself amidst the bushes, and that Hutch's ostentatious departure in the other direction was probably meant to reassure her that he would be nowhere around to witness this indignity. He had placed a wad of torn up news sheets and a thin cotton towel next to the solicitous can of water. With a horrified grimace, Caroline made as best use of these meagre facilities as she could. Upon his return, Hutch, with great delicacy, neither looked for nor asked after any of the items he had set out for her.

By midday the sun was scorching, but Caroline's arm, clutching her dusty parasol, was heavy with fatigue. She gave up and folded it into her lap. Looking up into the vast, fathomless sky, she saw two distant dark spots, circling high above.

'Are those eagles?' she asked, pointing skywards, and noticing as she did how brown with dirt her lace glove was. Hutch followed her gaze, squinting.

'Just buzzards, I'm afraid. Not really many eagles down here on the prairie. If you go up into the Rockies you'll see some beautiful birds. Those are some sharp eyes you've got there, Mrs Massey,' he told her. He looked back out over the horses' ears and sang quietly to himself: *'Daisy, Daisy, give me your answer do . . .'* Caroline let her eyes drift to the horizon, then she straightened in her seat and pointed again.

'Somebody's coming!' she exclaimed, excitedly.

'Well, we're not at all far from the ranch now, ma'am. It could be one of our own riders,' Hutch nodded, with a subtle smile.

'Is it Corin?' Caroline asked, her hands flying to her dishevelled hair. She began to tuck wayward strands of it beneath her bonnet. 'Do you think it's Mr Massey?'

'Well,' Hutch smiled again, as her frantic grooming continued, 'I know of no other man who rides a mare as black as that in this vicinity, so I think it just might be your husband after all, ma'am.'

Caroline was still brushing her skirts and pinching her cheeks, not caring if Hutch witnessed these efforts, when the rider drew near, and she at last saw Corin for the first time since she'd wed him over a month before. She let her hands fall neatly into her lap, and sat up straight even though she was bubbling with nerves inside. The black horse covered the ground in an easy lope, kicking up sprays of sand, and when at last he reached them Corin pulled the kerchief down from his face to reveal a wide grin. He was as golden and lovely as she remembered him.

'Caroline!' he cried. 'It's so good to see you!' He swung down from his horse and came to stand by her foot. There she remained, seated high on the wagon, transfixed with fear and anticipation. 'Are you well? How was the journey?' When she didn't reply Corin's face fell a little and a puzzled look came into his eyes. This was her undoing. Still lost for words, and more relieved to see him than she would ever have admitted, Caroline surrendered all propriety and toppled herself from the bench into his waiting arms. Only the sparseness of her prevented the couple ending up in the prairie sand. Behind them, reins held casually in one hand, Hutch watched with a laconic smile, and gave his boss a genial nod.

*   *   *

There was a scattering of people around the ranch house when the wagon bringing Corin Massey's new wife finally pulled up outside. They were young men mostly, with worn, dusty clothes, who seemed, nevertheless, to have made some attempts to comb their hair and tuck in their shirts. Corin smiled at the trepidation on Caroline's face as she gave her own filthy attire another despairing glance. The men nodded, tipped their hats and murmured greetings as she climbed down from the wagon, and she smiled and acknowledged them politely.

'I so want to take you on a tour of the ranch, Caroline. I'm so excited to show you everything! Unless you're too tired after your journey?' said Corin, swinging down from his horse.

'Oh, I am so tired, Corin! Of course you must show me everything, but first I need to lie down, and then take a bath,' she said. Corin nodded readily, although he looked a little disappointed. The tall, white house Caroline had envisaged was instead a low, wood-frame building; and although the front had indeed been painted white, prairie sand had blown up against it and given the bottom half a grubby look. Corin followed her gaze.

'A spring wind blew up before the paint had a chance to dry,' he told her, sheepishly. 'We'll paint over it, don't worry. Luckily we only had time to do the front, so not too much work was undone!' Caroline peered around the corner of the house, and sure enough the sides remained bare wood.

'I'll see to Strumpet. You take Mrs Massey on into the house,' Hutch said, taking the reins from Corin.

'Strumpet?' Caroline asked, bewildered.

'My mare,' Corin grinned, giving the horse's forehead a rub. Caroline knew little enough about horses, but the animal appeared to scowl. 'The most contrary, bad-tempered soul you'll find on these lands, and that's a known fact.'

'Why do you keep her, if she is so unpleasant?'

'Well,' Corin shrugged, as if this had never occurred to him, 'she's my horse.'

Inside, the walls were bare and no curtains hung at the windows. There was furniture enough but it was placed higgledy-piggledy, at odds with the angles of the room. An easy chair drawn up to the burner, with piles of livestock journals and seed catalogues beside it, was the only thing that looked to be in its right place. Many boxes and cartons stood around the floor. Caroline turned a slow circle, gazing at all this, and sand rasped beneath her boot heels. When she next looked at her husband she could not hide her dismay. Corin's smile faded from his face.

'Now, I deliberately didn't have it all fixed up because there was no point, I thought, until you'd arrived and told me *how* it should be fixed. We'll get it set up quickly enough, now that you're here,' he explained, hurriedly. Caroline smiled, drawing in a shaky breath rich with the scent of newly hewn oak. 'It just . . . it took me longer than I had planned to get the place built . . . I'm sorry,

Caroline.'

'Oh, no! Don't be!' she exclaimed, anguished to see him crestfallen. 'I'm sure it will be wonderful—I know just how we should finish it. You've done *so* well.' She turned and leant her head against his chest, and revelled in the smell of him. Corin pushed strands of hair back from her forehead and held her tightly. His touch made her warm inside, and gave her a tight feeling, like hunger.

'Come with me,' he murmured, and led her through a door in the far corner of the main room, to a smaller room where a large iron bedstead dominated. It was draped with a fine, multicoloured quilt, and Caroline ran her fingers lightly over it. The fabrics were satins and silks, cool and watery to the touch. 'I had the bed freighted all the way from New York,' Corin told her. 'It arrived right before you did; and the quilt was my mother's. Why don't you try it?'

'Oh, no! I'd dirty it. It's so lovely, Corin,' Caroline enthused.

'Well, I'm dirty too; and I say we try it out.' Corin took her hands and then her waist, and then linked his arms around her.

'Wait! No!' Caroline laughed, as he pulled them both down to land, bouncing, on the mattress.

'We never did get our wedding night,' he said softly. The sun streaming in from the window lit his hair with a soft coronet and threw his brown eyes into shadow. Caroline was very aware of the stale smell of her own unwashed body, and the dryness of her mouth.

'No. But it's not bedtime yet. And I need to bathe . . . and someone might see in.'

'We're not in New York any more, love. You

don't have to do as your aunt tells you, and we don't have to do what society tells us . . .' Corin placed his hand flat on her midriff and Caroline caught her breath, fast and shallow in her chest. He worked each button of her blouse free and smoothed it gently aside.

'But, I—'

'But *nothing*,' Corin murmured. 'Turn over.' Caroline obeyed, and Corin fumbled slightly as he undid the laces of her corset. Released, the sudden rush of air into Caroline's lungs made her head spin, and she closed her eyes. Corin turned her to face him and traced the lines of her body with the roughened palms she had noticed the first time they met. He kissed her eyelids softly. 'You're so beautiful,' he said quietly, and his voice was deep and blurred. 'Eyes like silver dollars.' Alarmed by the force of the passion she felt, Caroline kissed him as hard as she could. She had little enough idea what to expect, knowing only that Corin now had rights to her body that nobody had had before. Bathilda had hinted darkly at pain that was to be borne, and duties that were to be performed, but the press of Corin's skin against her own was a feeling more wonderful than any she had yet experienced; and the gentle insistence of his touch, the shift of his weight between her thighs, filled her with a sensation that was hot and cold and almost painful and so far beyond anything she had felt before that she cried out in astonished joy, no longer aware that there was any impropriety, or anybody else in the world to hear her.

*　　　*　　　*

Corin toured his new wife around the ranch in a buggy, since it was too far to walk and she had never ridden horseback before. He had seemed stunned by this fact, but then he'd shrugged and said, 'Don't worry; you'll learn soon enough.'

But Caroline did not trust the animals, with their ugly teeth and brute strength, and the thought of sitting atop of one did not appeal to her in the slightest. When Corin proudly introduced her to his brood mares, and to the stallion Apache, Caroline nodded and smiled and struggled to tell them apart. The creatures all looked the same to her. He drove her around the various corrals, stock pens and cattle chutes, and the low, roughly built bunkhouses where the line-riders slept. Caroline noticed how comfortable her husband seemed, without a trace of the uncertainty or diffidence he had shown in New York society. They passed a pitiful-looking hovel, half dug into the ground and then roofed with planks and sod.

'That would have been our home, if you'd come to me much sooner!' Corin told her with a smile.

'That?' Caroline echoed, appalled. Corin nodded.

'That dugout's the very first dwelling I put here when I staked my claim in ninety-three. And I wintered in it twice before I got a proper house set up—I found one out on the prairie and dragged it here—if you can believe that!'

'You stole a *house*?'

'Not stole! No, not that. I suppose it had been put up by some boomer, trying to settle the land before it was legal. Well, whoever built it had moved on, or been moved on. It was just sitting there, sheltering nothing but rattlesnakes; so I shook them out, loaded it on a flatbed wagon and dragged it back here. It was a good little house, but certainly not roomy enough for a family.' As he said this he took her hand and squeezed it; and Caroline looked away bashfully.

'A *large* family?' she queried, tentatively.

'I reckon four or five kids ought to do it,' Corin grinned. 'How about you?'

'Four or five ought to do it,' she agreed, smiling widely.

'Here, now; this is the shelter we bring the mares into when they're due to foal.'

'What's that?' Caroline asked, pointing to a conical tent beyond the mare's corral.

'That's where Joe's family lives. See the dugout beside? Joe and his wife sleep there, but his folks wanted a teepee like they'd always had, and so that's what they live in still. They're a traditional sort of people.'

'Why would . . . Joe's family live in a teepee?' Caroline asked, perplexed. Corin looked at her, as puzzled as she.

'Well, they're Indians, sweetheart. And they like to live as they ever have, although Joe himself is more forward-thinking. He's worked the trails for me since the very beginning, when I could only pay him in clothes and five-cent tins of Richmond tobacco. One of my best riders—'

'Indians? There are *Indians* here?' Caroline's heart quickened and her stomach twisted. She would not have been more shocked if he'd told her he let wolves roam amidst his cattle. 'Hutch told me they were all gone!' she whispered.

'Well, most of them have. The rest of Joe's people are on the reservation, east of here, on land that reaches the banks of the River Arkansas. Those that remained here in Oklahoma Territory, that is—Chief White Eagle leads them. But some went north again a few years back. Chief Standing Bear led them back to their Nebraska lands. I guess they were more homesick than the others . . .' he explained, but Caroline scarcely heard this brief history of the tribe. She could not believe her ears, or her eyes, that here camped on her doorstep were the savages of whose atrocities lurid stories had circulated in the east for decades. Fear froze her to the core. Wildly, she grabbed the reins from Corin and dragged the horse's head around, back towards the house.

'Hey—wait, what are you doing!' Corin exclaimed, trying to wrestle the reins from her as the horse tossed its head in protest, the bit clanking against its teeth.

'I want to go! I want to get *away* from them!' Caroline cried, shaking all over. She put her hands over her face, desperate to hide. Corin steadied the horse and then peeled her hands into his.

'Now, look!' he said seriously, eyes pinioning hers. 'Listen to me, Caroline. They are good people. *People*, just like you and me. They just want to live and work and raise their families; and no matter what you've heard back east where they like to paint Indians as the worst kind of villains, I am telling you that they don't want to trouble you or anybody else. There's been strife in the past, strife that often enough we white men brought with us, but now all any of us wants to do is get on as best we can. Joe has brought his family here to live and work alongside us, and that's taken a kind of courage you and I can't understand, I do believe. Are you listening to me, Caroline?' She nodded, although she could hardly credit what he was saying. Tears rolled down her cheeks. 'Don't cry, my darling. Nothing you've been told about Indians applies to Joe. I can guarantee you that. Come along now and I'll introduce you.'

'No!' she gasped.

'Yes. They're your neighbours now, and Joe is a firm friend of mine.'

'I can't! Please!' Caroline sobbed. Corin took out his handkerchief and wiped her face for her. He tipped her chin up and smiled affectionately.

'You poor thing. Please, don't be afraid. Come on, now. The second you meet them you'll see you've got nothing to be frightened of.'

Clicking his tongue at the beleaguered buggy horse, Corin turned it again and drove them towards the teepee and dugout. Surrounding the two dwellings was an array of washing lines and drying racks, ropes, tools and harnesses. A fire was burning outside the tent, and as they approached a small, iron-haired woman emerged with a blackened pot to place over the embers. Her back was bowed, but her eyes sparkled from deep within the creases webbing her face. She said nothing, but straightened up and nodded, eyeing Caroline with quiet interest as Corin jumped down from the buggy.

'Good morning, White Cloud, I've come to introduce my wife to you,' Corin said, tipping the wide brim of his hat respectfully at the old woman. Caroline's legs, as he helped her down, felt unsteady beneath her. She swallowed, but there remained a lump in her throat that made it hard to breathe. Her thoughts swirled inside her head like a blizzard. A man came out of the dugout, followed by a young girl, and another woman came from the teepee, middle-aged and severe looking. She said something incomprehensible to Corin, and Corin, to Caroline's utter amazement, replied.

'You speak their tongue?' she blurted out, and then recoiled when all eyes turned to her. Corin smiled, somewhat diffidently.

'Indeed, I do. Now, Caroline, this is Joe, and this is his wife Magpie, most commonly known as Maggie.' Caroline tried to smile, but she found that she could not hold the gaze of either one of them for more than a few seconds. When she did she saw a stern, dark man, not tall but broad across the chest; and a plump girl, her long hair prettily braided with coloured strings woven through it. Joe's hair was also long, and they both had high, feline cheekbones and a serious line to their brows. Magpie smiled and ducked her head, trying to catch Caroline's eye.

'I'm very pleased to meet you, Mrs Massey,' she said, and her English was perfect even if her accent was strong. Caroline gaped at her.

'You speak English?' she whispered, incredulously. Magpie gave a cheerful chuckle.

'Yes, Mrs Massey. Better than my husband, although I have been learning for less time!' she boasted. 'I'm so glad you are here. There are far too many men at this ranch.'

Caroline took a longer look at the girl, who was wearing a simple skirt and blouse, with a brightly woven blanket wrapped around her shoulders. Her feet were shod with soft slippers of a kind Caroline had never seen before. Her husband, who wore a heavy, beaded vest beneath his shirt, muttered something sharp in their own tongue, and Magpie scowled, answering him with something short and indignant. Joe did not smile as readily as his wife, and his expression seemed, to Caroline, most hostile. The blackness of his eyes alarmed her, and his mouth was a straight, implacable line.

'I have never met any Cherokee . . . people before,' Caroline said, somewhat emboldened by Magpie's cheerful demeanour.

'Still you have not.' Joe spoke for the first time, wryly. His accent was so guttural that it took a little while for her to understand him. Caroline glanced at Corin.

'Joe and his family are of the Ponca tribe,' he explained.

'But . . . Hutch told me these lands were Cherokee before . . .'

'They were. It's . . . well, put simply, there are many tribes in this country. It was Indian Territory before it was Oklahoma Territory, after all. Joe and his family are a little out of the ordinary, in that they have chosen to adopt some of the white man's ways of living. Most of his people choose to stay with their own, on reservation lands. Joe here got a taste for cattle driving and has never looked back—isn't that right, Joe?'

'Got a taste for beating you at cards, mostly,' the Ponca man said, twisting his mouth to one side sardonically.

As they moved away from the teepee, Caroline frowned.

'Joe seems an odd name for an . . . for a Ponco . . .'

'Ponca. Well, his real name, in his own tongue, is just about unpronounceable. It means Dust Storm, or something of that kind. Joe's just a lot easier for folk to say,' Corin explained.

'He does not seem to show you much respect, considering you are his employer.'

At this Corin glanced at Caroline, and a frown shaded his eyes for a moment. 'He has plenty of respect for me, I assure you; and it's respect I've had to earn. People like Joe don't give out respect because you're white, or because you've got land, or you pay their wages. They give it when you can show you have integrity and a willingness to learn, and can show respect to them where it's due. Things are a little different out here than in New York, Caroline. People have to help themselves and help each other when a flood or a freeze or a tornado might wipe out everything you have in an instant . . .' He trailed into silence. A warm wind blew off the prairie, singing through the spokes of the buggy wheels. Stinging with his rebuke, Caroline sat in unhappy silence. 'You'll soon settle in, don't you worry,' Corin said, in a lighter tone.

*   *   *

A few days later, they took their honeymoon picnic; setting out in the buggy while the sun was skirting the eastern horizon, and heading due west of the ranch for three hours or so, to a place where the land rolled into voluptuous curves around a shallow pool, fed by a slow-running creek. Silver willows leaned their branches down, shading the water's edge and touching it in places, pulling wrinkles in the wide reflected sky.

'It's so pretty here,' Caroline said, smiling as Corin lifted her down from the bench.

'I'm glad you like it,' Corin said, planting a kiss

on her forehead. 'It's one of my favourite places. I come here sometimes, when I need to think about things, or when I'm feeling low . . .'

'Why didn't you live here, then? Why did you fix the ranch over to the east?'

'Well, I wanted to fix it here but Geoffrey Buchanan beat me to it. His farmhouse is another two miles that way, but this land is in his claim.'

'Won't he mind us coming here?'

'I doubt it. He's a pretty relaxed kind of fellow but, more importantly, he won't know we're here,' Corin grinned, and Caroline laughed, crossing to the edge of the pool and dipping her fingers into the water.

'Do you come here often then? Do you get low, out here?'

'I did sometimes, when I was first here. Wondered whether I'd staked the right claim, wondered if it was too far from my family, if the land was right for the cattle. But I've not been back here for many months,' he shrugged. 'It soon became clear to me that I never did a better thing than staking the claim I did, and making those choices. Everything happens for a reason, is what I believe, and now I know that's right.'

'How do you know?' she asked, turning to him, drying her fingers on her skirt.

'Because I have you. When my father died, I thought . . . I thought for a time that I should move back to New York and look after my mother. But the second I got back there I knew I couldn't stay. And then I found you, and you were willing to come away with me . . . and if any good thing could come from losing my father, then you are that good thing, Caroline. You're what was missing from my life.' He spoke with such clarity, such resolve, that Caroline was overwhelmed.

'Do you really think that?' she whispered, standing close to him, feeling the sun's heat flush her skin. It shone brightly in his eyes, turned them the colour of caramel.

'I really think that,' he said quietly; and she stood up on her toes to kiss him.

In the shade of the willow trees they spread out their rugs, unpacked the hamper and unhitched the buggy horse, which Corin tethered to a tree. Caroline sat with her legs tucked carefully beneath her, and poured Corin a glass of lemonade. He lay down easily beside her, propped on one elbow, and undid the buttons of his shirt to let the cool air in. Caroline watched him almost shyly, still not used to the idea that he belonged to her, still not used to his relaxed manner. She had not known until her arrival at the ranch that men grew hair on their chests, and she examined it now, curling against his skin and damp with the heat of his body.

'Corin?' she asked him suddenly.

'Yes, love?'

'How old are you?'

'What? You know that!'

'But I don't! I just realised . . . I don't know how old you are. You seem so much older than me— not in appearance, I mean! Well, partly in appearance, but also in . . . in other ways,' she floundered. Corin smiled.

'I'll be twenty-seven next birthday,' he said. 'There now—are you appalled that you've married such an old-timer?'

'Twenty-seven is not so very old! I shall be nineteen in just a couple of months. But . . . you seem to have lived here for a lifetime already. You're as settled here as if you'd been here fifty years!'

'Well, I first came out here with my father, on a business trip—prospecting for new beef suppliers. My father traded in meat, did I tell you that? He sold to all the best restaurants in New York, and for a time I was destined to go into the business with him. But I knew as soon as I got out here that we were at the wrong end of that chain of supply, and I never left. I was just sixteen when I decided to stay on out here and learn about raising the beeves instead of just buying their dead flesh.'

'Sixteen!' Caroline echoed. 'Weren't you scared, to leave your family like that?' she asked. Corin thought for a moment, then shook his head.

'I've never been much afraid of anything. Until I asked you to dance,' he said. Caroline blushed happily, straightening her skirts.

'It really is hot, isn't it? Even here in the shade,' she commented.

'You want to know the best way to cool down?'

'What is it?'

'Swimming!' Corin declared, springing to his feet and pulling his shirt up over his head.

'*Swimming!* What do you mean?' Caroline laughed.

'I'll show you!' he said, sliding off his boots, kicking his pants to one side and charging into the pool, as naked as Adam, with a wild whooping and splashing. Caroline stood up and watched in utter amazement. 'Come in, sweetheart! It's the best feeling!' he called.

'Are you *crazy*?' she cried. 'I can *not* swim here!'

'Why ever not?' he asked, swimming the length

of the small pool with broad strokes of his arms.

'Well . . . well, it's . . .' she waved an incredulous arm. 'It's muddy! And it's out in the open—anybody could see! And I don't have a bathing suit.'

'Sure you do! It's right there under your dress,' Corin grinned. 'And who's to see? There's nobody around for miles—it's just you and me. Come on! You'll love it!'

Caroline walked uncertainly to the edge of the bank, unlaced her boots and hesitated. Sunlight danced prettily on the water's surface and tiny fish were lazing in the warm shallows. The sun beat down on her, scorching the top of her head and making her clothes feel tight and stifling. She bent down, pulled off her boots and stockings and put them carefully on the bank, then, gathering her skirt to her knees, she stepped in until the water lapped her ankles. The relief of cold water on her clammy skin was her undoing.

'Oh, my goodness,' she breathed.

'Now, how much better does that feel?' Corin called to her, coming over to where she stood. The white of his buttocks gleamed, distorted, beneath the surface, and Caroline laughed.

'You look just like a frog in a bucket!' she told him.

'Oh, really?' he asked, flicking a spray of water up at her. With a squeal she retreated. 'Come on, come in and swim! I dare you!'

Caroline looked over her shoulder, as if an audience might have appeared, ready to gasp in dismay at her wantonness, then she undid her dress and stays and draped them over a willow branch. She kept her chemise on, the bare skin of her shoulders crawling, feeling utterly conspicuous, then went back to the edge of the pool with her arms wrapped protectively around her. There she paused, mesmerised by the feel of the mud as it squeezed up between her toes. She had never felt anything like it, and hitched up her petticoat to look down, flexing her feet and smiling. When she looked up to remark upon it, she found Corin watching her with a rapt expression.

'What is it?' she asked, alarmed.

'You. Just look at you . . . You're so brave. And so beautiful. I've never seen anything like it,' he said simply. Water had splayed his hair across his forehead, making him younger, boyish.

Caroline had only intended to paddle, but the touch of the water and the thrill of Corin's words made her bold, and she waded in up to her waist, the water swirling the translucent folds of her chemise around her legs. With a nervous laugh she lay back and let the water buoy her up. It felt chilly as it fingered through her hair.

'Come here and kiss me,' Corin demanded.

'With regret, sir, I am far too busy swimming,' Caroline replied grandly, paddling away with an ungainly stroke. With a start, she realised she hadn't swum since childhood, at her family's summer house.

'I shall have a kiss, even if I must chase you down for it,' Corin told her. Laughing and kicking her legs Caroline tried to escape; but she did not try very hard.

*   *   *

The sun was setting as they came over the last rise

and saw the lights of the ranch house glimmering below them. Caroline's skin felt hot and raw where the sun had singed it, and her dress felt odd without the chemise underneath, which was laid out drying on the back of the buggy. She licked her lips, tasted the mineral tang of the creek water. They both carried the smell of it on their skin, in their hair. They had made love on the riverbank, and the languor of it lingered in her muscles, leaving her heavy and warm. Suddenly, she did not want to arrive back at the house. She wanted the day to last for ever; she and Corin in a shady place on a hot day, making love over and over again, without another thought or care in the world. As if reading her mind, Corin reined the horse to a halt, surveying his home for a moment before turning to her.

'Are you ready to go back?' he asked.

'No!' Caroline said fiercely. 'I . . . I wish every day could be like today. It was so perfect.'

'It truly was, sweetheart,' Corin agreed, taking her hand and raising it to his lips.

'Promise me we'll go back there. I won't go one *inch* closer to the house until you promise me.'

'We have to go back to the house! Night's coming . . . but I do promise you we'll go there again. We can go back whenever we want to—we *will* go back, and we'll have many more days like today. I swear it,' he said.

Caroline looked at the outline of him in the indigo twilight, caught the gleam of his eye, the faint shape of a smile. She put her hand out and touched his face. 'I love you,' she told him simply.

With a shake of the reins the horse began a lazy descent towards the wooden house below, and with each step it took, Caroline felt a sense of vague foreboding growing inside her. She turned her eyes to the dark ground ahead and was suddenly afraid, in spite of Corin's pledge, that no day to come would be as sweet as that which had just passed.

I have been trying to remember good things about Henry. Perhaps we owe him that, because we got to grow up, live lives, fall in love, fall out again. He liked to tell stupid jokes, and I loved to hear them. Beth was always kind, and took me with her, and helped me, but she was rather serious, even as a child. Once I laughed so hard at Henry's jokes that I nearly wet myself—the fear of it abruptly stopped the giggles, sent me scrambling for the toilet with one fist corked between my legs. *What do you call a dinosaur with only one eye? Do-you-think-he-saw-us. What do you call a deer with no eyes? No idea. Why do elephants paint the soles of their feet yellow? So they can hide upside down in custard. What's orange and sounds like a parrot? A carrot. What's small, brown and wrinkly and travels at two hundred miles an hour? An electric currant.* He could keep it up for hours, and I pushed my fingers into my cheeks where they ached.

He was telling me stupid jokes one day when I was about seven. It was a Saturday, because the remains of a cooked breakfast were still scattered on the dining room table; sunny outside but still cool. The French doors onto the terrace were open, letting a breath of air sneak in, just cold enough to tickle my ankles. I wasn't really watching what Henry was doing as he reeled out his jokes. I wasn't paying attention. I just followed him, stood close enough behind him to trip him, prompted him whenever there was a pause: *Say another one! How do you know when there's an elephant in your bed? You can see the 'E' on his pyjamas. What's brown and sticky? A stick.* He had the biscuit barrel and he was cementing two plain shortbreads together with a thick daub of English mustard. The extra strong stuff, ugly coloured, that Clifford liked on sausages. I was trying to remember a good thing about him, and now this.

I didn't think to ask why. I didn't ask where we were going. He wrapped the biscuits in a napkin, pocketed them. I followed him across the lawn like a tame monkey, demanding more jokes, more jokes. We went west, not south into the trees but to the lane instead; skirted along it, behind the hedge, until we got to Dinny's camp. Henry hunkered down in the ditch, pulled me in with him. A foaming, pungent wall of cow parsley to sink behind. At this point only did I think to whisper, 'Henry, what are you doing? Why are we hiding?' He told me to shut up so I did. A spying game, I thought; tried not to rustle loudly, checked beneath myself for nettles, ants' nests, bumble bees. Dinny's grandpa was sitting on a folding chair outside his battered white motor home, waxed hat pulled low over his eyes, arms folded, hands tucked into armpits. Asleep, I think. Deep, dark creases running from the sides of his nose to the corners of his mouth. His dogs lay either side of him, chins on paws. Two black and white collies called Dixie and Fiver, who you weren't allowed to touch until Grandpa Flag had said it was OK. *They'll 'ave those fingers, you give 'em cause.*

Henry threw the sandwiched biscuits over the hedge. The dogs were on their feet in an instant, but they smelt the biscuits and they didn't bark. They crunched them down, mustard and all. I held my breath. I said *Henry!* in my head. Dixie made a hacking noise, sneezed, put her muzzle down on one paw and rubbed at it with the other. Her eyes squinted up; she sneezed again and shook her head, whimpered. Henry had his knuckles in his teeth, his eyes bright, intent. Lit up inside, he was. Grandpa Flag was murmuring to the dogs now, awake. He had his hands in Dixie's ruff, was peering at her as she retched and snuffled. Fiver walked a small, slow circle to one side, heaved, threw up a disgusting yellow mess. A sob of laughter escaped around Henry's fist. I was strangled with pity for the dogs, boiling with guilt. I wanted to stand up and shout, *It wasn't me.* I wanted to disappear, run back to the house. I stayed, rocked on my crouched legs, hid my face in my knees.

But the worst of it was that when I was finally allowed to leave, a pinch on the arm to rouse me, we'd gone a scant twenty paces before Dinny and Beth appeared. The hems of their jeans soaked with dew, a small green leaf in Beth's hair.

'What have you two been doing?' Beth asked. Henry scowled at her.

'*Nothing,*' he said. Able to inject a world of scorn into a single word.

'Erica?' She looked at me sternly, incredulous that I should be with Henry, that I should look guilty. That I should betray them that way. But where had *they* been, without me? I wanted to shout. *They* had left *me*. Henry glowered at me, gave me a shove.

'Nothing,' I lied. I was quiet and sullen for the rest of the day. And when I saw Dinny the day after, knowing that he had been home, I couldn't look at him. I knew he knew. Because of Henry's jokes.

*   *   *

'Rick? Can we go now?' Eddie's head appears at the door to my room, where I, for once, have been skulking. Staring through the foggy glass at the white world beyond. Tiny crystals in the corners of the pane, feathery and perfect.

'The frost performs its secret ministry, Unhelped by any wind,' I quote at him.

'What's that?'

'Coleridge. Sure, Eddie, we can go. Give me five seconds.'

'One-two-three-four-five?'

'Ha, ha. Push off. I'll be down in a moment—I can hardly go out in my dressing gown.' I was defiantly still in it when I opened the door to Maxwell earlier.

'Not today,' Eddie agrees, retreating. 'It's cold enough to freeze the arse off a penguin out there.'

'Charming, dear,' I call. The frost has cast the trees in white. It's like another world out there—a brittle, albino world where white and opalescent blues have replaced dead grey and flat brown. It's dazzling bright. Every tiny twig, every fallen leaf, every blade of grass. The house is made new; no longer the ghost, or the corpse, of a place I remember. I am soaring with optimism today. It would be hard not to be. After so many overcast days, the sky seems to go up for ever. It's giddy, all that space up there. And Beth has said she'll come with us—that's how vibrant the day is.

When I told her Dinny was here she froze. I was

scared for a minute. She didn't seem to breathe. The blood could have halted in her veins, her ticking heart gone silent, such was the stillness in her. A long, hung moment in which I waited, and watched, and tried to guess what was next. Then she looked away from me and licked her lower lip with the tip of her tongue.

'We'd be strangers, now,' she said, and walked slowly into the kitchen. She didn't ask me how I knew, what he looked like now, what he was doing here. And I found I didn't mind not telling her. I didn't mind keeping it to myself. Keeping the words he had spoken in my head alone. Owning them. She was relaxed again when I went to find her, as we made mugs of tea and I dunked Hobnobs in mine. But she didn't eat that night. Not a Hobnob, not the plate of risotto I put in front of her, not the ice cream afterwards.

It's the twentieth of December today. The car steams up as I drive east through the village and then turn north onto the A361.

'One more day, guys, and then it's all downhill until spring!' I announce, flexing fingers stiff with chill inside my gloves.

'You can't wish the winter away until Christmas has been,' Eddie tells me firmly.

'Really? Not even when my hands have frozen to the wheel? Look, I'm trying to let go and I can't! Frozen on—look!' Eddie laughs at me.

'Keeping hold of the steering wheel while you drive could be considered a good thing,' Beth observes wryly from the passenger seat.

'Well then, it's a good job I'm frozen on, I guess.' I smile. I take the turning to Avebury. Eddie's been doing prehistory this term.

Wiltshire's riddled with it. We park, decline to join the National Trust, join instead the steady trickle of people going along the path towards the stones. The ground twinkles, the sun is overwhelming.

A fine Saturday and there are lots of other people at Avebury, all bundled up like we are, shapeless and dark, moving in and out of the ancient sarsen stones. Two concentric rings, not as high as Stonehenge, not as grand or orderly, but the circles far, far bigger. A road runs right through them; half the village is scattered amidst them, although the little church sits chastely without. I like this set-up. All those lives, all those years, piled up in one place. We walk all the way around the ring. Beth reads from the guidebook but I am not sure Eddie is listening. He has a stick again. He is sword-fighting somebody in his head and I wish I could see whom. Barbarians, perhaps? Or somebody from school.

'The Avebury Stone Circles are the largest in Britain, located in the third largest henge. In all, the surrounding bank and ditch and the area enclosed cover eleven point five hectares . . .'

'Beth!' I cry. She is wandering close to the edge of the bank. The grass is slick with frost-melt.

'Oops.' She corrects her course, gives a little laugh.

'Eddie, I'm going to test you on this later!' I shout. My voice blares in the still air. An elderly couple turn to look. I just want him to listen to Beth.

'The quarrying methods used include antler picks and rakes, ox-shoulder blades and probably wooden shovels and baskets . . .'

'Cool,' Eddie says, dutifully. We pass a tree

grown into the rampart, its roots cascading above ground like a knotty waterfall. Eddie scrambles down it, commando-style; crouches down, clings to it, peers up from three metres below us.

'Are you an elf?' Beth asks.

'No, I'm a woodsman, waiting to rob you,' he replies.

'Bet you can't get me before I pass this tree to safety,' Beth challenges him.

'I've lost the element of surprise,' Eddie complains.

'I'm getting away!' Beth goads, sauntering onwards. With a rebel yell Eddie scales the roots, slipping and sliding, bashing his knees. He grabs Beth with two hands, makes her squeal. 'I submit, I submit!' she laughs.

We walk out, away from the village along the wide avenue of stones that leads away to the south. The sun shines on Beth's face—a long time since I saw it lit this way. She looks pale, older, but there are blooms in her cheeks. She looks serene too. Eddie leads us, sword aloft, and we walk until our toes get too cold.

On the way back I pull up at the Spar in Barrow Storton for some ginger beer for Eddie. Beth waits in the car, quieter again now. Eddie and I are pretending not to notice. There's a horrible feeling of her teetering, being on the edge of something. Eddie and I hesitate, wanting to pull her one way, scared of accidentally nudging her, tipping her the wrong way.

'Can't I have Coke instead?'

'Yes, if you'd rather.'

'I'm really not that bothered about alcohol, to be honest. I had some vodka last term, in dorm.'

'You've been drinking *vodka*?'

'Hardly drink*ing*. Drank, once. And I felt sick, and Boff and Danny *were* sick, and it stank the place out. Gross. I don't know why grown-ups bother,' he says, airily. His cheeks have a glorious pink flare from the bite outside. Eyes bright as water.

'Well, you might change your mind later on. But for Christ's sake don't tell your mother! She'll have a fit.'

'I'm not *stupid*, you know.' Eddie rolls his eyes at me.

'No. I know.' I smile, wincing at the weight as two huge bottles of Coke go into the basket. As we approach the till, Dinny comes in. The bell rings above his head, a jaunty little fanfare. At once I don't know where to look, how to stand. He has walked right past Beth, in the car. I wonder if she saw him, if she knew him.

'Hullo, Dinny,' I greet him. I smile. Casual neighbours, nothing more, but my heart is high in my chest. He looks up at me, startled.

'Erica!'

'This is Eddie—I mean Ed—who I was telling you about. My nephew—Beth's boy.' I pull Eddie to my side, he grins affably, says *hi*. Dinny studies him closely, then smiles.

'Beth's son? It's nice to meet you, Ed,' he says. They shake hands, and for some reason I am moved, I am choked. A simple gesture. My two worlds coming together with the press of their skins.

'Are you the Dinny my mum used to play with when she was little?'

'Yes. I am.'

'Erica was telling me about you. She said you were best friends.' Dinny looks at me sharply, and I feel guilty, even though what I said was true.

'Well, we were, I suppose.' His voice calm and low, always measured.

'Stocking up for Christmas?' I butt in, inanely. The Spar is hardly bursting with seasonal fare; threadbare tinsel taped to the edges of the shelves. Dinny shakes his head, rolls his eyes slightly.

'Honey wants salt and vinegar crisps,' he says, then looks away sheepishly.

'Did you see Mum, outside? She's out there in the car—did you say hello?' Eddie asks. A flutter in the pit of my stomach.

'No. I didn't. I'll . . . I will now,' Dinny says, turning to the door, looking out at my grubby white car. His eyes are intent; he moves straight, shoulders tense, as if compelled to go to her.

I can see him, through the glass in the door. Between the spray-on drifts of fake snow in its corners. He bends down at the window, his breath clouding the air. Beth rolls the window down. I can't see her face with Dinny in the way. I see her hands go up towards her mouth and then flutter away again, drifting as if weightless. I duck; I crane my neck to see. I strain my ears, but all I can hear is Slade on the radio behind the counter. Dinny leans his bare arm on the roof of the car and I feel the ache of that cold metal on my own skin.

'Rick—it's our go,' Eddie says, nudging me with his elbow. I heave the basket onto the counter, am forced to break off my surveillance and smile at the gloomy-looking man at the till. I pay for the Coke, a Twix and some ham for lunch, and rush to get back out to the car.

'So what do you do now? You always wanted to be a concert flautist, if I remember rightly?' Dinny is saying. He straightens up from leaning on the car, folds his arms. He looks defensive suddenly, and I notice that Beth has not got out of the car to talk to him. She barely looks at him, keeps rearranging the ends of her scarf in her lap.

'Oh, that didn't quite pan out,' she says with a thin little laugh. 'I got to grade seven and then . . .' She pauses, looks away again. She got to grade seven the spring before Henry disappeared. 'I stopped practising as much,' she finishes, flatly. 'I do some translating now. French and Italian, mostly.'

'Oh,' Dinny says. He studies her, and the moment hangs, so I blunder in.

'I struggle enough with English—trying to teach it to teenagers is like trying to push water uphill with a fork. But Beth always did have a gift for languages.'

'You have to listen, that's all, Rick,' Beth says to me, and it is a reproof of some kind.

'Never was my strongest suit,' I agree with a smile. 'We've just been to Avebury. Ed was keen to see it because they've been doing it at school. Mind you, once we got there you were more interested in having a hot fudge sundae in the pub, weren't you, Ed?'

'It was *amazing*,' Eddie assures us. Dinny gives me a quizzical smile, but when Beth asks him nothing more, his face falls slightly and he steps back from the car.

'So, how long are you staying?' he asks, and he addresses this to me, since Beth is staring straight ahead.

'For Christmas, definitely. After that, we're not really sure. There's a lot of sorting out to be done,' I say. Which is honest and ambiguous enough. 'How about you?'

'For the time being,' Dinny shrugs; even more ambiguous.

'Ah.' I smile.

'Well, I'd better be getting on. Good to see you again, Beth. Nice to meet you, Ed,' he says, nodding to us and walking away.

'He didn't get the crisps,' Eddie observes.

'No. He must have forgotten,' I agree, breathless. 'I'll get some and take them over later.'

'Cool.' Eddie nods. He pulls open the back door with one hand, the other hand fighting its way into the Twix. So flippant. No idea how huge the thing that just happened is, here at the car window. I go back into the shop, buy salt and vinegar crisps, and when I get back into the car I start the engine and take us home, and I don't look at Beth because I feel too awkward, and the things I would ask I won't ask in front of her son.

*   *   *

Eddie is lying on his bed, in pyjamas, tethered to his iPod. On his front with his heels swinging over his back. He's reading a book called *Sasquatch!* and with his music on he can't hear the owls outside, calling to each other between trees. I leave him. Downstairs, Beth is making mint tea, her fingers pinching the corner of the teabag and dipping it, over and over, into the water.

'I hope Dinny didn't startle you, appearing at the car window like that?' I say. Lightly as I can.

Beth glances at me, presses her lips together.

'I saw him go into the shop,' she says, still dipping.

'Really? And you recognised him? I don't think I would have—not just from glimpsing him go by.'

'Don't be ridiculous—he looks exactly the same,' she says. I feel inadequate—that she saw something I didn't.

'Well,' I say. 'Pretty amazing to see him again after all this time, isn't it?'

'Yes, I suppose so,' she murmurs.

Now I can't think what to ask. She should not be this careless about it. It should matter more. I search her face and frame for signs. 'Perhaps we should ask them up to the house. For a drink or something?'

'They?'

'Dinny and Honey. She's his . . . well, I'm not sure if they're married. She's about to have his baby. You could talk her out of having it in the woods. I think he'd be grateful for that.'

'Having it in the woods? How extraordinary,' Beth says. 'What a pretty name though—Honey.' There is more to it than this. There has to be.

'Look, are you sure you're OK?'

'Why wouldn't I be?' she says, that same bemused tone that I don't believe. She looks at me again, and I see that her fingers are in the hot water, mid-dip. Steaming hot water, and she does not flinch.

'But you hardly spoke to him. You two used to be so close . . . didn't you want to talk to him? Catch up?'

'Twenty-three years is a long time, Erica. We're totally different people now.'

'Not *totally* different—you're still you. He's still him. We're still the same people who played together as kids . . .'

'People change. They move on,' she insists.

'Beth,' I say, eventually, 'what happened? To Henry, I mean?'

'What do you mean?'

'Well, I mean, what happened to him?'

'He disappeared,' she says flatly, but her voice is like thin ice.

'No, but, do you remember, that day at the pond? The day he vanished? Do you remember what happened?' I press. I don't think I should. I partly want to know, I partly want to move her. And I know I shouldn't. Beth's hand slips down to the worktop. It knocks her cup roughly aside, slops tea. She takes a deep breath.

'How can you ask me that?' she demands, constricted.

'How can I? Why shouldn't I?' I ask, but when I look up I see she is shaking, eyes alight with anger. She doesn't answer for a while.

'Just because Dinny's around . . . just because he's here it doesn't mean you need to go raking up the past!' she says.

'What's it got to do with Dinny? I just asked a simple question!'

'Well, don't! Don't keep asking bloody questions, Erica!' Beth snaps, walking away. I sit quietly for a long time, and I picture that day.

*   *   *

We got up early because it had been such a hot night. A night when the sheets seemed to wrap themselves around my legs, and I woke up again and again with my hair stuck in clammy rat-tails to my forehead and neck. We helped ourselves to breakfast and then listened to the radio in the conservatory, which faced north and was cool in the morning. Terracotta tiled floor, ranks of orchids and ferns on the window sill. We wallowed in Caroline's swing chair, which had blue canvas cushions that smelt faintly sharp, almost feline. Caroline was dead by then. Dead when I was five or six years old. I ran past that swing chair once, a very little girl, and did not see her in it until her stick shot out and caught me. *Laura!* she snapped, calling me my mother's name, *Go and find Corin. Tell him I need to see him. I must see him!* I had no idea who Corin was. I was terrified of the limp bundle of fabric in the swing chair, the incongruous strength behind that stick. I ducked beneath it, and ran.

We got dressed at the last possible minute, went reluctantly to church with Meredith and our parents, ate lunch in the shade of the oak tree on the lawn. A special little table laid there just for the three of us. Beth, Henry and me. Peanut butter and cucumber sandwiches, which Mum had made for us because she knew we were too hot and fractious to eat the soup. The itchy press of the wicker chair into the backs of my legs. Some small bird in the tree crapped on the table. Henry scraped it up with his knife, flicked it at me. I ducked so violently that I fell off my chair, kicked the table leg, spilt my lemonade and Beth's. Henry laughed so hard a lump of bread went up his nose, and he choked until his eyes streamed. Beth and I watched, satisfied; we did not thump him on the back. He was vile for the rest of the day. We tried everything to lose him. The heat made him groggy and violent, like a sun-struck bull. Eventually he was called inside to lie down because he was caught tying a Labrador's legs together with string while it panted, long-suffering and bewildered. Meredith would not stand for the torment of her Labradors.

But he came out again later, as the afternoon broadened. He found us at the dew pond. The three of us by then, of course. I had been swimming, pretending to be an otter, a mermaid, a dolphin. Henry laughed at my wet saggy knickers, at the bulge of water in the gusset. *Have you pissed your pants, Erica?* Then something, *something*. Running. Thoughts of the plughole at the bottom of the pond, of Henry being sucked down through it. That must have been why I said to them, again and again: *Look in the pond. I think he's in the pond. We were all at the pond*. Even though they had looked, they told me. Mum told me, the policeman told me. They had looked and he wasn't there. No need for divers—the water was clear enough to see. Meredith took me by the shoulders, shook me, shouted, *Where is he, Erica?* A tiny bubble of spit from her mouth landed warm and wet on my cheek. *Mother, stop it! Don't!* Beth and I were given dinner in the kitchen, our mother spooning beans onto our toast, her face pale and preoccupied. As dusk bloomed the evening smelled of hot grass getting damp, and air so good you could eat it. But Beth did not eat. That was the first time, that evening. The first time I saw her mouth close so resolutely. Nothing in, and nothing out.

'What's with all the crisps?' Beth asks, poking the multipack of salt and vinegar amongst the breakfast detritus on the table.

'Oh . . . they were supposed to be for Honey. I forgot to take them down to her yesterday,' I say. Eddie is sitting on the bench with his back to the kitchen table, throwing a tennis ball against the wall and catching it. The ball's flat, threadbare; it probably belonged to a Labrador once. He throws it with a maddening lack of rhythm. 'Eddie, can you give it a rest?' I ask. He sighs, aims, throws the ball into the bin in one smooth arc.

'Great shot, darling,' Beth smiles. Eddie rolls his eyes. 'Are you bored?' she asks him.

'A bit. No, not really,' Eddie flounders. The equal pull of honesty and tact.

'Why don't you deliver those crisps to Honey?' I suggest, swigging the remains of my tea.

'I've never even *met* Honey. And I only met that bloke once, yesterday. I can hardly go marching into their front yard waving crisps, can I?'

'I'll go with you,' I say, swinging my legs around and getting up. 'Do you want to come, Beth? The camp's just where it always was,' I can't resist adding. I don't know how she can not want to go back, to see.

'No. No thanks. I'm going to . . . I'm going to walk into the village. Get the Sunday paper.'

'Can I have a Twix?'

'Eddie, you're going to turn into a Twix.'

'Please?'

'Come on, Eddie. We're going. Boots on, it's

pretty muddy on the way,' I say.

I take us to the camp the long way, via the dew pond. It's becoming a daily pilgrimage. It's just a cold brown day today, none of the ice and sparkle of yesterday. I pause to walk to the edge, look into the depths of it. It's unchanged. It gives me no answers. I wonder if I just wasn't paying attention, when whatever it was happened? My mind wanders sometimes—gets snagged on a background thought, gets coaxed away. When other teachers talk to me, sometimes it happens. I don't like to think about repressed memories, about trauma, amnesia. Mental illness.

'I think you're a bit obsessed with this pond, Rick,' Eddie tells me gravely. I smile.

'I'm not. What makes you say that, anyway?'

'Every time we come near it you go all Luna Lovegood. Staring into space like that.'

'Well, *excuse* me, I'm sure!'

'I'm only *joking*,' he exclaims, pushing me awkwardly with his shoulder. 'But it does kind of look the same every time. Doesn't it?' He turns away a few paces, crouches to pick up a stone, hurls it into the water. The surface shatters. I watch him and suddenly my knees ache, sickeningly, as if I've missed my step on a ladder.

'Come on, then,' I say, turning away quickly.

'Did something happen here?' Eddie asks in a rush. He sounds tense, worried.

'What makes you ask, Eddie?'

'It's just . . . you keep coming back out here. You get that look in your eye, like Mum gets when she's sad,' Eddie mumbles. I curse myself silently. 'And Mum seems . . . she doesn't seem to like it here.' It's easy to forget how clearly a child can see things.

'Well, something did happen here, Eddie. When we were small our cousin Henry disappeared. He was eleven, the same age as you are now. Nobody ever found out what happened to him, so we've kind of never forgotten about it.'

'Oh.' He kicks up sprays of dead leaves. 'That's really sad,' he says, eventually.

'Yes. It was,' I reply.

'Maybe he just ran away and . . . I don't know, joined a band or something?'

'Maybe he did, Eddie,' I say, hopelessly. Eddie nods, apparently satisfied with this explanation.

Dinny is standing with a man I don't recognise as the dogs come charging over to us, circling proprietorially. I smile and wave as if I pop in every day, and Dinny waves back, more hesitantly. His companion smiles at me. He's a thin man, wiry, not tall. He has fair hair, cropped very close, the tattoo of a tiny blue flower on his neck. Eddie walks closer to my side, bumping me. We move nervously into the circle of vehicles.

'Hi, sorry to interrupt,' I say. I try for bright, but to my own ears I sound brassy.

'Hello there, I'm Patrick. You must be our neighbours up at the big house?' the wiry man greets me. His smile is warm and real, his handshake rattles my shoulder. At such a welcome I feel a knot in my stomach begin to loosen.

'Yes, that's right. I'm Erica and this is my nephew, Eddie.'

'Ed!' Eddie hisses at me sideways, through unruly teeth.

'Ed, good to meet you.' Patrick rattles Eddie's shoulder too. I notice Harry sitting on the step of a van behind the two of them. I think about calling out a greeting, but change my mind. Something in his hands again, something the focus of immense concentration. Most of his face is hidden behind hanging hair and thick whiskers.

'Well, uh, this might sound a little odd but we noticed you'd forgotten to get Honey's crisps yesterday. In the shop. So, we brought some over for her. That's if she's not craving pickles this morning instead?' I wave the big sack of crisps. Patrick gives Dinny a look—not unkind, slightly puzzled.

'I know how fed up *I* get when Mum forgets my food when she goes shopping,' Eddie rescues me. At the sound of his voice, Harry looks up. Dinny shrugs one shoulder. He turns.

'Honey!' he yells at the ambulance.

'Oh! There's no need to disturb her . . .' I feel colour in my cheeks. Honey appears at one of the small windows. It frames her face. Pretty, petulant.

'What?' she shouts back, far louder than she needs to.

'Erica has something for you.' I squirm. Eddie edges closer to Harry, trying to see what he's working on. Honey appears, picking her way carefully down the steps. All in black today, hair arrestingly pale against it. She stands at a distance from me and watches me suspiciously.

'Well. Silly really. We got you these. Dinny said you fancied some, so . . .' I trail off, I dandle the bag. Slowly, Honey steps forward and takes them from me.

'How much do I owe you?' she asks, scowling.

'Oh, no, don't worry. I don't remember. Forget it.' I wave my hand. She shoots Dinny a flat look and he puts his hand in his pocket.

'Two quid cover it?' he asks me.

'There's really no need.'

'Take it. Please.' So I take it.

'Thanks,' Honey mutters, and goes back inside.

'Don't mind Honey,' Patrick grins. 'She was born in a bad mood, and then it got worse in puberty, and now that she's expecting . . . well, forget it!'

'Fuck you, Pat!' Honey shouts, out of sight. He grins even wider.

Eddie has got closer and closer to Harry. He is peering at the man's hands, and probably blocking his light.

'Don't get in the way, will you, Ed?' I say, smiling cautiously.

'What is it?' Eddie asks Harry, who doesn't reply, but looks at him and smiles.

'That's Harry,' Dinny tells Ed. 'He doesn't really like to talk.'

'Oh. Well, it looks like a torch. Is it broken? Can I see?' Eddie presses. Harry opens his hands wide, displays the tiny mechanical parts.

'So, will you be down for our little solstice party this evening, Erica?' Patrick asks.

'Oh, well, I don't know,' I say. I look at Dinny and he looks back, steadily, as if working out a problem.

'Of course you are! The more the merrier, right, Nathan? We're lighting a bonfire, having a bit of a barbecue. Bring some booze and you're most welcome, neighbour,' Patrick says.

'Well, maybe then.' I smile.

'Your dreadlocks are wicked,' Eddie tells Harry. 'You look a bit like *Predator*. Have you seen that film?' He has his fingers in the mess of torch parts, picking bits out, putting them in order. Harry looks faintly astonished.

'I've got to run. I'll catch you later.' Patrick nods at Dinny and me. He leaves the camp with a springing step, hands thrust into the pockets of a battered wax coat.

I look at the muddy toes of my boots, then at Eddie, who is piecing the torch back together before Harry's incredulous eyes.

'Ed seems a good lad,' Dinny says then, and I nod.

'He's the best. He's a great help.' There's a long silence.

'When I spoke to Beth . . . she seemed, I don't know,' Dinny says, hesitant.

'She seemed what?'

'Not like she used to be. Almost like there was nobody home?'

'She suffers from depression,' I say, hurriedly. 'She's still the same Beth. Only she's . . . she got more fragile.' I have to explain, even though I feel treacherous. He nods, frowns. 'I think it started here. I think it started when Henry disappeared,' I blurt out. This is not what Beth has told me, but I do think it's true. She told me it started one stormy day, driving home at dusk. The clouds were heavy, but on the western horizon as she drove towards it, they broke into slivers, and stripes of bright pale sky showed behind them. One of those wet mackerel skies. She said she suddenly couldn't tell what was the horizon and what was the sky. Hills or clouds. Earth or air. It was so bewildering that she almost drifted into the oncoming traffic, and she felt seasick all evening, as if the ground were moving beneath her feet. After that, she told me, she wasn't sure what was real any more, what was safe. That's when she thinks it started. But I remember her the evening Henry vanished. Her silence, and the uneaten beans on her plate.

'I would hate to think that what happened then has made her ill all this time,' Dinny says quietly. He knows what happened. He *knows*.

'Oh?' I say. If only he would go on, say more. *Tell me*. But he doesn't.

'It wasn't . . . well. I'm sorry to hear that she's not happy.'

'I thought coming back here would help, but . . . I'm worried it might be making her worse. You know, bringing it all back. It could go either way, I think. But it's good that Eddie's here. He takes her mind off things. Without him I think she'd even forget it was Christmas.'

'Do you think Beth will come to the party tonight?'

'Truthfully, no. I'll ask her, if you like?' I say.

Dinny nods, his face falling. 'Ask her. Bring Eddie too. He and Harry seem to be getting on well. He's great with kids—they're less complicated for him.'

'If you asked her, I'm sure she'd come. If you came up to the house, that is,' I venture. Dinny shoots me a brief, wry smile.

'Me and that house don't really get along. You ask her, and perhaps I'll see you both later.' I nod, bury my hands in the back pockets of my jeans.

'Are you coming, Ed? I'm going back to the house.' Eddie and Harry look up from their work. Two sets of clear blue eyes.

'Can't I stay and finish this, Rick?' I glance at

Dinny. He shrugs again, nods.

'I'll keep an eye out,' he says.

*   *   *

We smuggled Dinny into the house once, when Meredith had gone into Devizes for a dental appointment. Henry was at the house of a boy in the village with whom he had taken up. A boy whose house had a *proper* swimming pool.

'Come *on*!' I hissed at Dinny. 'Don't be such a baby!' I was desperate to show him the big rooms, the huge stairs, the enormous cellars. Not to impress him, not to show off. Just to see his eyes widen. To be able to show *him* something for a change, to be the one in charge. Beth hunkered down at the back of the three of us, smiling tensely. There was nobody about except the housekeeper—who never paid us much attention—but still we crouched to scuttle in. Behind the last sheltering bush, I was close enough to feel Dinny's knee pressing into my hip; smell the dry, woody smell of his skin.

Dinny was reluctant. He had been told enough times, heard enough stories from his grandpa, Flag, and his parents; had even had fleeting encounters with Meredith. He knew he wasn't welcome there, and that he shouldn't want to look. But he was curious, I could tell. As a child will be when a place is forbidden. I had never seen him that unsure; I'd never seen him hesitate, and then choose to carry on. We went from room to room, and I gave a running commentary: 'This is the drawing room, only nobody ever does any drawing in it, not that I've seen. This is the way to the cellar. Come and see! It's the size of another whole house! This is Beth's room. She gets the bigger room because she's older but from my room you can see right into the trees and I saw an owl, once.' On and on I went. The Labradors followed us, grinning and wagging excitedly.

But the more I went on, and the more we showed him, the more rooms we dragged him into, the quieter and quieter Dinny got. His words dried up, eyes that were wide fell flat again. Eventually even I noticed.

'Don't you like it?'

A shrug, a tip of the eyebrows. And then the sound of the car on the driveway. Freezing, panicking, hearts lurching. Trying to hear: were they coming in the front, or the back? A calculated risk and I chose wrong. We ran out onto the terrace as they appeared at the side of the house. Meredith, my father, and worst of all Henry, back from his visit. He grinned. After a hung moment I grabbed Dinny's arm, yanked it, and we tore across the lawn. The greatest act of insurrection I think I ever performed and it was to save Dinny. To save him from hearing what Meredith would say to him. She was shocked into silence, just for a second. Standing tall and thin in a crisp linen suit, duck-egg blue; hair set, immaculate. Her mouth was a hard red line of pigment, and then we were away and it cracked open.

'Erica Calcott, you come back here this *instant*! How dare you bring that *filth* into my house? How *dare* you! I *insist* that you come back here immediately! And you, you thieving gypsy! You'll scuttle off like vermin, will you? Like the vermin that you are!' I like to think my father said something. I like to hope Dinny didn't hear, but of course deep down I know that he did. Running away like a thief. Like a trespasser. I thought I was being brave, I thought I was being a hero for him. But he was angry with me for days. For making him go into the house, and then for making him run away.

*   *   *

I'm up in Meredith's room. This is the biggest bedroom, of course, with an ugly four-poster bed, heavy with carvings. The base is high and the mattress deep. How will the next owners move this bed? It's huge. Only by taking an axe to it, I think. To be replaced with something contemporary and probably beige. I fling myself across it, over the stiff brocaded bedspread, and count how long it takes me to stop bouncing. Who made this bed? The housekeeper, I suppose. The morning that Meredith collapsed on her way into the village. Gradually I become still and realise that I am bouncing on my dead grandmother's bed. The very sheets she slept in the night before she died.

In here more than anywhere the ghostly remains of her seem to linger. As is only natural, I suppose. Part of me wishes that I'd come to see her as an adult. That I'd pinned her down, made her tell me where all that bad feeling came from. Far too late now. Her dressing table is a huge thing—deep, wide; several drawers in columns on either side, a wide drawer in the middle that opens into my lap; a triptych mirror set on a box of yet more drawers. The top is satin smooth, a patina wrought by centuries of soft female fingers. I think Mum should have jewellery as well as photos. Meredith made no bones about telling us she'd sold off her best pieces, like the best of the estate's land, to pay for repairs to the roof. She told my parents this accusingly, as if they ought to have put their hands in their pockets, looked under the sofa cushions and produced thirty thousand pounds. But there has to be something left for my thieving hands to find.

Lipsticks and eyeshadows and blushers in the top right-hand drawer. Small dunes of loose make-up powder, shimmering underneath all the metal tubes and plastic compacts. Belts in the next, coiled like snakes. Handkerchiefs, hair clips, chiffon scarves. This drawer smells powerfully of Meredith, of her perfume, and the slightly doggy notes of the Labradors. In the bottom right drawer are boxes. I take them out, put them up where I can see them. Most are full of jewellery—dress pieces by the looks of it. One box, the biggest, shiny and dark, is full of papers and photographs.

With a prickle of excitement, I sift through the contents. Letters from Clifford and Mary; holiday postcards from my mum and dad; odd bank statements, secreted away into this secretive box for who knows what reason. I read odd snatches of each, feeling the illicit thrill of prying. Some photographs too, which I put to one side; and then I find the newspaper clippings. About Henry, of course. Local papers started the coverage. *Lady Calcott's Grandson Missing. Search for Local Boy Intensifies. Clothes found in Westridge woods did not belong to missing boy.* Then the nationals joined in. Abduction fears, speculation, a mysterious hobo spotted walking the A361 with a bundle that could have been a child. Boy matching the description seen lying in a car in Devizes. *Police very concerned.* I can't take my eyes from it. As if a hobo could have carried Henry any distance at all. Big-boned, solid Henry. We never saw any of this, Beth and I. Of course we didn't. Nobody reads the paper when they're eight years old, and we weren't allowed to watch the news at the best of times.

It looks like she bought several papers, different ones every day. Did she cut these out at the time, or later, years afterwards, as a way to keep hope alive, to keep *him* alive? I had no idea it was such a big story. I hadn't connected, until right now, the reporters milling at the gates with any kind of national infamy. Of course, I realise now why they were there, the reporters; why the story ran and ran, getting fewer and fewer column inches as the months went on, until it disappeared altogether. Children shouldn't just vanish without trace. That's the worst fear, worse even than finding the body, perhaps. Having no answers, having no idea. Poor Meredith. She was his grandmother, after all. She was meant to be looking after him.

I am staring, staring hard at a grainy, enlarged photo of Henry. A school photo, neat and tidy in a blazer and stripy house tie. Hair combed; toothy, decorous smile. That photo on posters in the shop window, on telegraph poles, on newspaper pages, in doctors' waiting rooms and supermarkets and garages and pubs. No websites back then, but I remember seeing this photo all over the village. The one in the shop window was in colour. It quickly faded in the sunshine, but it was bright when I first saw it. *Can I go to the shop? No! You're to stay indoors!* I couldn't understand why. Mum went with me in the end, and held my hand, and politely asked the reporters to let us through, to not follow us. A couple of them did anyway, took some pointless shots of us emerging from the shop with orange ice lollies. One tiny cutting from late August, 1987. A full year later. The regretful last line: *Despite an extensive police investigation, no trace of the missing boy has yet been found*.

There's an ache in my ribs and I realise I've been holding my breath. As if in anticipation; as if the story could have had any other ending. I notice the rain falling faster, louder. Eddie is out in the woods. He'll be soaked. It seems so unreal, reading about Henry in the press, reading about that summer. Unreal, and at the same time all the more real. All the more terrible. It did happen, and I was there. I put the clippings back in the box, careful not to crease them. I will keep these, I think; in the very same box, so coffin-like, that Meredith put them in twenty-three years ago.

I pick up the pile of photographs and flick through them, shaking off the shadow of the newspaper clippings. Random family portraits and holiday shots for the most part—the sort of thing Mum was after. A small black and white photo of Meredith and Charles on their wedding day—my grandfather Charles, that is, who was killed in World War II. Charles wasn't in the armed forces, but he went up to London on business one week and a stray V2 found its way to the club where he was having lunch. The best shots of their wedding day are on the piano in the drawing room, in heavy silver frames, but in this little shot Meredith is bent at an odd angle, twisting to look back over her shoulder, away from Charles, as if the hem of her dress has caught on something. They are emerging from the church, coming out of the dark into the light. In profile Meredith's face is young, painfully anxious. Her hair is very fair, eyes huge in her face. How did such a lovely girl, such a nervous young bride, ever become Meredith? The Meredith I remember, cold and hard as the marble shelves in the pantry.

Only one other photo arrests me. It's very old, battered around the edges; the image surfaces from a sea of fox marks and fade. A young woman, perhaps in her early twenties, in a high-necked dress, hair pinned severely back; and on her lap a child in a lace dress, not more than six months old. A dark-haired baby, its face slightly smeared, ghostly, as if it wriggled just as the exposure was taken. The woman is Caroline. I recognise her from other pictures around the house, although in none of them does she look as young as this. I turn it over, read the faint stamp on the back: *Gilbert Beaufort & Son, New York City*; and hand written, in ink that has almost vanished, *1904*.

But Caroline did not marry Henry Calcott, my great-grandfather, until 1905. Mary was seized by a genealogy fad a few years back—traced the Calcott family lineage that she was so proud to have married into and sent us all a copy in our Christmas card that year. They married in 1905, and they lost a daughter before Meredith was born in 1911. I frown, turn the picture to the light and try to find any more clues within it. Caroline stares calmly back at me, her hand curled protectively around her baby. Where did this child go? How did it fall from our family tree? I slip the photo into my back pocket, begin to pick through the jewellery, hardly seeing it. A brooch pin catches my fingertip, and I sit there a while, tasting my blood.

*   *   *

After dinner Eddie escapes from the table to watch TV. Beth and I sit among the dirty plates and bowls. She has eaten a little. Not enough, but a little. When she senses Eddie watching her, she tries harder. I steal one last potato from the bowl and lean back, feel something stiff in my back pocket.

'What's that?' Beth asks, as I pull out the photo of our great-grandmother. She hasn't spoken to me much since I asked her about Henry, and now her voice is slightly stiff. But I know an olive branch when I see one.

'I found it up in Meredith's room—it's Caroline,' I tell her, passing it over.

Beth studies the young face, the pale eyes. 'Gosh, yes, so it is. I remember those eyes—even when she was ancient, they stayed that bright silver colour. Do you remember?'

'No, not really.'

'Well, you were pretty small.'

'I used to be so scared of her! She hardly seemed human to me.'

'Were you really? But she never bothered us. Never paid us much attention.'

'I know. She was just so . . . *old*!' I say, and Beth chuckles.

'That she was. From another era, well and truly.'

'What else do you remember about her?' I ask. Beth leans back from the table, pushes her plate away from her. Half of her slice of quiche is still on

154

her plate, untouched.

'I remember that look Meredith used to get on her face whenever she had to feed her, or dress her. That look of such careful neutrality. I always remember thinking she must have been having terrible thoughts, such terrible thoughts to have been so careful not to let them show on her face.'

'But what about Caroline? Do you remember anything she said, anything she did?'

'Well, let me think. I remember the time she went mad at the summer party—when was it? I can't remember. Not long before she died. Do you remember it? With the fireworks and all the lanterns strung along the driveway to light the way up to the house?'

'God! I'd totally forgotten about that . . . I remember the fireworks, of course, and the food. But now you remind me I do remember Meredith wheeling Caroline inside, because she'd been shouting something about crows . . . what was it about? Can you remember?' I ask. Beth shakes her head.

'It wasn't crows,' she says. And as she tells me, the scene slides into focus in my mind, as if it had always been there, waiting for Beth to point it out to me.

*   *   *

The Storton Manor summer party was an annual affair, usually held on the first Saturday in July. Sometimes we were there in time for it, sometimes not, depending on the school calendar. We always hoped to be—it was the one occasion when we wanted to take part in something of Meredith's, because the lights and the people and the music and the dresses turned the manor into another place, another world. That year, Beth spent hours doing my hair for me. I'd been crying because my party dress had got too small for me, something we hadn't discovered until I put it on earlier in the evening. It was too tight under the arms and the smocking pinched my skin. But there was no alternative so I had to wear it, and to cheer me up Beth braided turquoise ribbons into my hair, fifteen or twenty in total, which came together in a plume of curled ends at the back of my head.

'Last one—sit still! There. You look like a bird of paradise, Erica!' she smiled, as she knotted the last one. I tipped my head this way and that, liked the brush of the ribbons against the back of my neck.

Flaming torches marched up the driveway, reeking of paraffin and guttering in the night air. They made a sound like flags flying. There was a string quartet on the sun terrace near where long tables had been set up, draped with white cloths and loaded with ranks of shining glassware. Silver ice buckets on long legs held chilled bottles of champagne, and the waiters raised their eyebrows at me when I dipped my fingers in, filching ice cubes to suck. The food was probably wonderful, but I remember snatching a caviare bliny, cramming it into my mouth and then spitting it into the nearest flowerbed. Adult conversation that we didn't understand volleyed over our heads; gossip and hearsay bandied back and forth, oblivious of we little spies, infiltrating the crowd.

Most of our extended family, people I never see any more, attended, as well as everyone who was anyone in county society. A photographer from *Wiltshire Life* circulated, snapping the more attractive women, the more titled men. Horsey women with flat hair and big teeth, who wore garishly expensive evening gowns in shades of pink, peacock and emerald. They dug out their diamonds for the occasion—rocks glittering against freckled English skins. The whole garden was flooded with the smell of their perfumes, and later, when the dancing started, that of fresh sweat. The men wore black tie. My dad fidgeted with his collar, his cummerbund, not used to the stiff edges, the layers of fabric. Insects swirled around the lanterns like sparks from a fire. The lawns rang with voices and laughter, a steady roar that grew with the number of empty bottles. Only the fireworks silenced it, and we children stared, rapt, as the purple night sky exploded into light.

A whole crew of staff was brought in to cater the party. Wine waiters; cooks who took over the kitchen; waitresses to ferry the trays of hot canapés they produced; calm, implacable butlers who lingered indoors, politely directing people to the downstairs bathrooms and discouraging the curious from peering into the family rooms. It was one of these anonymous workers that Caroline attacked, inexplicably. She had been positioned in her chair on the veranda, near enough to the terrace to hear the music, but still within the shelter of the house. People drifted over to pay their respects, bending forward awkwardly so as not to tower over her, but they drifted away again as soon as it was polite to do so. Some of them Caroline acknowledged with a faraway nod of her head. Some she just ignored. And then a waitress went over with a smile, offered her something from a tray.

She was dark, I remember that. Very young, maybe only in her teens. Beth and I had noticed her earlier in the evening because we envied her hair. Her skin was a deep olive and she had the most luxurious black hair, hanging in a thick plait over her shoulder. It was as deep and glossy as ink. She had a neat rounded body, and a neat rounded face with dark brown eyes and apples high in her cheeks. She might have been Spanish, or Greek perhaps. Beth and I were nearby because we'd been following her. We thought her incredibly lovely. But when Caroline looked up and focused on the girl her eyes grew huge and her mouth dropped open—a damp, lipless hole in her face. I was close enough to see that she was shaking, and to see a frown of alarm pass over the waitress's face.

'Magpie?' Caroline whispered, a ragged breath forming the word so loosely I thought I'd heard it wrong. But she said it again, more firmly. 'Magpie, is that you?' The waitress shook her head and smiled, but Caroline threw up her hands with a hoarse cry. Meredith looked over at her mother, drawing down her brows.

'Are you all right, Mother?' she asked, but Caroline ignored her, continuing to stare at the dark-haired waitress with a look of pure terror on her face.

'It can't be you! You're dead! I know you are . . . I *saw* it . . .' she wailed.

'It's OK,' the girl said, backing away from the old woman. Beth and I watched, fascinated, as tears began to slide down Caroline's cheeks.

'Don't hurt me . . . please don't,' she croaked.

'What's going on here?' Meredith demanded, appearing next to her mother, glaring at the hapless waitress, who could only shake her head, at a loss. 'Mother, be quiet. What's the matter with you?'

'No! Magpie . . . how can it be? I was sure I didn't . . . I didn't mean for it . . .' she begged, putting trembling fingers over her mouth. Her face was aghast, haunted. The waitress moved away, apologising, smiling an uncomfortable smile. 'Magpie . . . wait, Magpie!'

'That's quite enough! There's nobody here called Magpie! For goodness' sake, Mother, pull yourself together,' Meredith admonished her, sharply. 'We have guests,' she said pointedly, leaning forwards to speak right into Caroline's ear. But Caroline just kept staring after the black-haired girl, frantically searching the crowd for her.

'Magpie! Magpie!' she shouted, still weeping. She grasped Meredith's hand, fixed her daughter with wide, desperate eyes. 'She's come back! Don't let her hurt me!'

'Right. That's enough. Clifford—come and help me.' Meredith beckoned sharply to her son and between them they turned Caroline's chair and manoeuvred her in through the tall glass doors. Caroline tried to fight them, kept craning her head to look for the girl, kept saying the name, over and over again. *Magpie, Magpie*. It was the first and only time I remember feeling sorry for her, because she sounded so frightened, and so very, very sad.

*   *   *

'Magpie, that was it. Funny name,' I say, as Beth stops speaking, undoes her own long plait and runs her fingers through her hair. 'I wonder who she thought that girl was?'

'Who knows? She was obviously pretty confused by then. She was over a hundred, remember.'

'Do you think Meredith knew? She was so brusque with her about it!'

'No. I don't know,' Beth shrugs. 'Meredith was always brusque.'

'She was horrible that night.' I get up, clatter the kettle onto the hotplate for coffee.

'You should go and have a root around in the attic if it's old pictures and papers you're after,' Beth says, suddenly keen.

'Oh?'

'That old trunk up there—when we came here for Caroline's funeral I remember Meredith putting everything she could find of hers up in that old red leather trunk. It was almost as if she wanted everything of Caroline's out of her sight.'

'I don't remember that. Where was I?'

'You stayed in Reading with Nick and Sue next door. Dad said you were too young to go to a funeral.'

'I'll go and have a look up there later, then,' I say. 'You should come up, too.'

'No, no, I've never been that bothered about family history. You might find something interesting, though,' she smiles. I notice how keen she is for me to investigate this distant past rather than our more recent one. How keen she is to distract me.

LONGING

1902–1903

As spring became summer, Caroline grew more used to the presence of Joe and Magpie and the other Ponca women, who were Joe's mother White Cloud and widowed sister, Annie. She did not call upon them again, but Corin warned her that it was traditional for Indian womenfolk to drop in on one another, and to exchange gifts, and she received several such visits before the Ponca seemed to lose interest. Caroline dreaded seeing the trio approach the house, and she sat awkwardly through their visits, crippled by nerves, unsure of how to speak to them, or what to give in return for their gifts of honey, mittens and an elegantly carved wooden ladle. In the end she usually gave them money, which White Cloud accepted with a closed expression on her face. Caroline made them tea and longed for them to leave, but when their visits ceased she could not help but feel that she had failed in some way. And she watched Joe from the window as he went about the ranch, her eyes ever curious for the alien oddity of his features, his black mane of hair. He wore a long knife in a tooled leather sheath on his hip, and each time she saw it a cold shiver scurried down her spine.

She did not get used to the heat, which increased with each passing day. By noon the sun was a flat, white disc that seemed to press like a giant hand on her head whenever she stepped outside, pushing her down, making her heavy and half-blind. When the wind blew it seemed as hot as the blast from an oven. Accustomed all her life to rising at ten in the morning, Caroline now took to getting up with Corin, at first light, in order to have some time to exist, some time to live before the heat became unbearable. At that hour the sky in the east was violet and azure, pricked by faint, glimmering stars that winked out of existence as the day broadened. Corin drove her back to Woodward to order fabric for curtains, and rugs, and a large mirror to hang above the mantel, and he paid for all of these things with a slightly bemused expression. Caroline chafed with impatience in the intervening weeks it took for the goods to come by train from Kansas City, and she clapped her hands with excitement when they arrived. Gradually, she dragged the furniture in the house into a better arrangement, and she swept and swept to keep the sand out on windy days, until her hands blistered and she gave up in frustration, stopping up whatever gaps she could find around the windows and doors with rags.

It was even harder for her to get used to the work required, on a daily basis, just to keep the household up and running. She knew that as Corin's wife she should make his coffee and breakfast in the morning before he set out onto the ranch, but by the time she had put up her hair and washed her face and laced herself into her corsets, he had provided for himself and gone out to work.

'Why do you take such time with your hair, love? There's nobody here that's going to think badly of you if you just pin it back in a simple fashion,' Corin pointed out gently, scooping her hair from her damp neck and running his thumb across the fine strands.

'*I* would think badly of it,' Caroline replied. 'A lady can't go around with her hair unbound. It's just not decent.' But she took what she thought to be his meaning and began to rise even earlier in order to make herself presentable and still have time to cook breakfast.

When the cistern was dry, water had to be drawn from the well at the top of a rise to the north of the house; a well Corin was quick to point out was nothing short of a miracle, since most of the county's groundwater was tainted with gypsum that rotted the guts and tasted foul.

'Not even the finest house in Woodward has a supply of water this close and this sweet. They're still hauling it in from the south by wagon!' he told her proudly.

It took a long time to boil water on the stove and, since timber was so scarce, more often than not the cow chips Caroline had encountered in Hutch's camp fire were the only fuel. Upon finding out what these were—chunks of dried-out cattle manure—Caroline promptly refused to collect them, and could only be induced to use them by poking them into the stove with iron tongs. Not far away from the ranch was a shallow stream that the ranchers referred to as Toad Creek, along the banks of which grew a thin line of straggly cottonwoods, sand plums and walnut trees, giving the ranch a welcome dash of foliage.

'Why can't we just cut timber from the creek?' Caroline asked, wrinkling her nose as Hutch, a little disgruntled at the task, delivered a basket of cow chips to the door.

'Well, ma'am, we could. But only for a couple of months and then we'd be back to the chips and without any trees to pretty up the view,' Hutch told her, drily.

And each morning there was the water to bring in, the stove to sweep out and re-lay, breakfast to make and then pots to clean, laundry to wash— Caroline was used to dirty clothes being taken away and then returned to her two days later, clean, pressed and neatly folded; she was astonished to discover how much work went into those intervening two days—and then the endless battle with the sand in the house and on the porch. She had also to tend to her wilting, stunted vegetable garden. Corin had presented her with the seeds proudly, having traded them with a neighbour. Watermelons and marrows, peas and beans. He also bought her two tiny cherry trees, which she watered with great care and attention, fretting when the wind buffeted them. They struggled in the red soil, and did not flourish no matter how she cosseted them. Then there was lunch to prepare, clothes to be mended and then dinner. Caroline was not a good cook. She scorched the eggs and forgot to salt the beef. Vegetables went soft, meat went tough and stringy. Her beans had hard, gritty centres. Her coffee was weak, and her bread refused to rise, emerging from the oven solid and chewy. Each time she apologised, Corin reassured her.

'You've not been brought up to do it, that's all. You'll get the hang of it,' he smiled, manfully swallowing down whatever she put in front of him. Every time her hands got grimy she washed them at once, hating the feel of dirt on her skin, the dark crescent of earth and smuts beneath each nail. She scrubbed her hands so many times in a day that the skin grew red and angry and began to crack, and she sat mourning their lost softness, cradling them in her lap at the end of the day.

Hot baths could only be had by laboriously filling a large copper drum and lighting the fire beneath it, and then filling the tin tub by the bucketful, behind a wooden screen that Caroline had ordered for the express purpose of private bathing. Corin chafed at such wanton use of precious water, but at the end of her day's labour, with her movements hampered by her corsets, Caroline's body ached from fingertips to toes. She could feel each knobbly protrusion of her spine as it uncurled against the back of the tub, feel a tender crease between every single rib. Her hands, as she wrung out her washing cloth, trembled with fatigue. In the yellow glow of the kerosene lamps, she examined her broken nails and the tan colour of her arms where she had taken to pushing up her sleeves in the heat. She rubbed her thumb over her calluses now, massaging rose-scented vanishing cream into them to soften them, as lonely coyote song filled the darkness outside.

She did not complain of the work, not even to herself. Whenever she caught herself flagging, she pictured Bathilda, smiling in mocking triumph; or she thought of Corin, so full of admiration, calling her brave and beautiful, and how she would hate to prove him wrong. But on the occasions that her spirits did begin to sink, Corin seemed to sense it. He brushed the sand from her hair at the end of the day, singing softly as he pulled the bristles through in long, smooth strokes; or telling her tall stories to make her laugh: about the super-smart cow that drank beer and had learnt to count, or the impatient settler who'd painted himself all over with the wet red mud of Woodward County to pass himself off as Indian and settle on their lands. Or, as she lay in the tub and rubbed her calluses, he would appear around the bath screen and work his fingers into the tight muscles of her neck and shoulders until she was all but drowsing in his hands; then he would gather her up and carry her, dripping wet, to the bed. In the consuming, blinding joy of his lovemaking, she forgot all other aches.

One night they lay side by side on the bed, catching their breath after their exertions. Propping himself up on his elbow, Corin wiped the commingled sweat from Caroline's chest and slid his hand down to her stomach. She smiled and shifted under the heavy weight of it, the hot press of his skin.

'Boy or girl to start with?' he asked.

'Which would you rather?' she replied.

'I asked first!' he smiled.

Caroline sighed happily. 'I truly don't mind. Maybe a girl . . . a little girl with your brown eyes and hair the colour of honey.'

'And then a boy?' Corin suggested.

'Of course! You'd rather a boy first?'

'Not necessarily . . . although it would be good to get him up and running, get me some more help around the ranch . . .' he mused.

'Poor baby! Not even born yet and you've got him out riding the fences!' Caroline cried.

Grinning, Corin put his lips to her belly and kissed her damp skin. '*Psst!* Hey, you in there—

come out a boy and I'll buy you a pony!' he whispered.

Caroline laughed, putting her hands around Corin's head to cradle it, no longer noticing their roughness.

It was two months before a neighbour dropped by to visit. Caroline heard a shout at the front of the house, as she was glumly examining a sunken honey cake that she'd just taken from the oven.

'Hullo, Masseys!' the shout came again and, startled, Caroline realised it was a woman's voice. She smoothed back her hair, brushed flour from her apron, and opened the front door, stepping onto the porch with regal grace. Then she gaped. The woman, if such she was, was not only dressed as a man—in slacks, leather chaps and a flannel shirt tucked into a wide leather belt—but she was sitting *astride* a rangy bay horse, slouching as comfortably in the saddle as if she had been born there. 'You're home! I was beginning to think I was hollering at an empty house,' the woman declared, swinging her leg over the horse's back and dropping abruptly to the ground. 'I'm Evangeline Fosset. Pleased to meet you, and do call me Angie since everybody else does,' she continued, approaching with a smile. A long ponytail of orange hair swung behind her, and although her face was as tanned as Corin's it was also strong and handsome. Her blue eyes shone.

'I'm Caroline. Caroline Massey.'

'Figured you were.' The keen blue eyes swept over her. 'Well, Hutch told me you were a beauty, and Lord knows that man never lies,' she said. Caroline smiled, uncertainly, and said nothing. 'I'm your neighbour, by the way. My husband

Jacob and I have a farm about seven miles that way.' Angie pointed to the south-east.

'Oh! Well . . . um . . . won't you come inside?' Caroline faltered.

She cut little squares from the outside edge of her honey cake, where it was indeed more or less like a cake, and served them on a large plate, with tea and water. Angie took a long draught.

'Oh! How I envy you that sweet well of yours! To have water not tasting of gyp or the cistern is something wonderful, I can tell you,' she exclaimed, draining the glass. 'Did Corin tell you how they found it? The well, that is?'

'No, he hasn't . . .'

'Well, they'd tried digging about a hundred different holes and found nothing but gyp, gyp, and some more stinking gypsum water. They were relying on the creek but that dries up half of the year, as you'll soon see. And they were being so darn careful with the supply that not one of the men on this ranch had washed himself for more than a month. I tell you, no word of a lie: I could smell them from my front step! Well, one day a funny old man came riding by on a beaten-up mule and said did Corin want him to find sweet water on his land? Ever one to give a person a chance, although he didn't see how the old fellow was going to achieve what he hadn't managed in months, Corin tells him by all means.' Angie paused for breath and popped a square of cake into her mouth. Caroline watched her, mesmerised. 'This old fellow takes out a narrow, forked branch of wood that's all worn smooth with years of touching, and off he goes, wandering here, there and everywhere, holding this twig in his fingertips. The midday sun starts pounding down and still he goes hither and thither, back and forth, until he gets to the top of the rise and bam! That twig of his twists in his grip and points straight down at the turf like an arrow. 'Here's your sweet water, sir,' the old fellow announces. And digging down, sure enough, there was the well. Can you believe that, now?' Angie finished her tale with a nod and a smile, and watched Caroline, expectantly.

'Well, I . . .' Caroline began, her voice sounding frail after Angie's bold narrative. 'If you say so, of course,' she finished, smiling slightly. Angie's face fell a little, but then she smiled again.

'So, how are you settling in? You getting used to ranch life?'

'Yes, I think so. It's rather different . . . to New York.'

'I'll bet it is! I'll bet!' Angie chuckled; a low, throaty sound.

'I've never seen a woman ride astride before,' Caroline added, feeling rude to mention it, but too astonished not to.

'Oh, it's the only way to travel around here, believe me! Once you've tried it, you'll never go back to fiddling around sideways. When I heard Corin was bringing a gal back from the city, I thought, that poor thing! She can't know what she's getting into! Not that I don't love this place. It's my home, although Lord knows Mother Nature can be a bitch around here at times, pardon my language—but really, she can.' Again, Angie looked at Caroline, and Caroline smiled nervously, at a loss. She poured her guest some more tea. The china cup, with its pattern of pink roses and blue ribbons that had seemed so charming in the catalogue, looked as fragile and childish as a toy in Angie's strong hand. 'The loneliness gets to some women. Not seeing anyone—well, any other women—for weeks at a time. Months, sometimes. It can get to a person, being in the house by yourself all day.'

'I've been . . . keeping very busy,' Caroline said hesitantly, startled by the woman's forwardness.

'As we all do, for sure,' Angie shrugged. 'Kids'll help, when they start coming. Nothing like a houseful of little ones to keep you distracted, I can tell you!' Caroline smiled, and blushed a little. She could hardly wait to have her first baby. She longed for a tiny child to cradle, for the softness of its skin, the wholeness of a new family. The permanence of roots put down.

'Corin wants to have five,' she said, smiling shyly.

'Five! My good Lord, you've got your work cut out for you, girl!' Angie exclaimed with a wide grin. 'But—you're young yet. Spread them out, that's my advice. That way the older ones'll be able to help you with the tiddlers. Well, when you fall, be sure to let me know. You'll want more help then, and advice from an old hand. Just remember where I am, and send word if you need anything.'

'That's really very kind of you,' Caroline said, secretly sure she would need no such help. She knew, in her heart, that while her cooking refused to improve and her body would not harden to the housework, it was in motherhood that her calling lay.

When Angie left, an hour or so later, she did not set off in the direction of her home, but towards the corrals where some of the men were at work. Caroline tended not to venture there herself, feeling too shy of the men and too unsure of the nature of their work, despite Corin's urgings that she learn the running of the ranch. What she had seen she had found brutal. Animals brought roughly to the ground, their horns sawn off, their heads pushed beneath stinking, stinging dip to kill parasites, the Massey Ranch emblem, *MR*, burned into their skins. She hated the way they rolled their eyes in terror, so white and vulnerable looking. But seeing Angie lead her horse calmly over to Hutch, who was overseeing the branding of new calves in the nearest corral, Caroline suddenly felt left out and left behind. She hurriedly removed her apron, grabbed her bonnet and walked quickly in the same direction.

Hutch had come over to the fence and was leaning upon it, continuing to watch the branding even as he talked to Angie. Wondering how to announce her presence, feeling high strung with nerves, Caroline heard her name spoken and stopped instead, stepping sideways so that the shadow of the bunkhouse engulfed her. The stink of burning hair and skin made her gag, and she put her hand over her mouth to stifle the sound.

'She's none too friendly, is she?' Angie said, folding her arms. Hutch shrugged one shoulder.

'She's trying her best, I reckon. Can't be easy, with her brought up so soft. I don't think she ever walked more than a quarter mile at a time before, and I hear from Corin that she surely never cooked before.'

'Shame he didn't set up nearer town—she could have taught class or something. Made better use of those fine manners than she will out here,' Angie said, shaking her head as if in disapproval. 'What do the boys make of her?'

'Hard to say, really. She doesn't come out of the house much; she doesn't ride out, sure as heck doesn't bring us lemonade on a hot day,' Hutch grinned. 'Feels the heat a bit strongly, I think.'

'What was Corin thinking, marrying such a green tenderfoot and leaving her out here by herself?'

'Well, I reckon he was thinking she was a fine-looking girl with a good head on her shoulders.'

'Hutchinson, one of these days I'll hear you speak a hard word about someone or something and I will fall clean off my horse. Good head on her shoulders in the city maybe, but out here? Why, she's even setting about the chores with corsets on so tight she can hardly breathe! Does that sound like good sense to you?' Angie exclaimed. Hutch said something that Caroline could not hear above the calves' frightened bellows, and then he turned towards Angie. Fearing she would be seen, Caroline skirted the side of the bunkhouse and walked swiftly back to the house, angry tears smarting her eyes.

Later, at dinner, Caroline watched her husband as he ate the bland food she had given him without complaint. He had come in late from rounding up two stray beeves, arriving at the table ravenous and having performed no toilette but to splash his hands and face with water from the trough. In the lamplight he looked rough, older than he was. His hair stuck out at wild angles and there was prairie sand along his hairline. After a day outside he seemed to soak up the sun and then glow all night long, she thought. The sun loved him. It did not love her. It scorched her pale skin, burnt freckles into her cheeks and made her nose peel most unattractively. She watched him and felt a surge of love that was at once wonderful and somehow desperate. He was her husband, and yet she felt as though she might lose him. She had not known that she was failing until she met Angie Fosset and heard her verdict on Corin's soft new wife. She swallowed her tears because she knew she would not be able to explain them to him.

'Evangeline Fosset came by here today,' she said, her voice a little constricted.

'Oh? That's wonderful! She's such a good neighbour, and always so friendly. Didn't you find her so?' he asked. Caroline sipped from her water glass to forestall her reply. 'If ever there was an example of how the West gives women freedoms that they've never had, and of how best a woman might make good on those freedoms, Angie is that example,' Corin went on.

'She didn't leave a calling card before visiting. I wasn't prepared for a guest,' Caroline said, hating the cold tone in her voice, but also hating to hear her husband praise another woman.

'No, well . . . when you've got to ride seven miles to say you're going to call on a person, seems like sense to just go ahead and call on them once you get there, I suppose.'

'I heard her talking about me to Hutch. She called me tenderfoot. What does it mean?'

'Tenderfoot?' Corin smiled briefly, but stopped when he saw his wife's tight expression, the glimmer in her eyes. 'Oh, now, sweetheart—I'm sure she didn't mean anything bad by it.

Tenderfoot just means you're not used to the West, that's all. To the outdoor kind of life.'

'Well, how can I be used to it? Is it my fault, where I was born? Is that any reason to talk about a person, and use names? I'm *trying* to get along with life out here!'

'I know you are! I know.' Corin took Caroline's hands and squeezed them. 'Don't fret about it. You're doing great—'

'No, I'm not! I can't cook! I can't keep up with all the work! The plants aren't growing . . . the house is full of sand!' she cried.

'You're exaggerating—'

'Hutch knows I can't cook, so you must have told him! I *heard* him say it!'

At this Corin paused, and a little colour came into his cheeks. 'I'm sorry, sweetheart. I shouldn't have said it and I'm sorry that I did. But, my love, if you need some help just tell me, and we'll find you some help!' he assured her, stroking her face where tears were wetting the skin.

'I need help,' she said, miserably; and as she admitted it she felt the weight of it lighten on her shoulders. Corin smiled.

'Then you shall have it,' he told her gently, and he murmured soft words to her until she smiled back at him and stopped her crying.

So Magpie was recruited to come into the house and share the housework, and although Caroline was not sure that she wanted the Ponca girl beside her all day long, Magpie came with a ready smile and an ease of doing things that came from being born to it. Happily, Caroline relinquished the cooking to her and watched as old bones and dried beans became thick, tasty soup; and bread dough rose willingly between damp cloths when left in the sun on the window sill; and handfuls of mysterious herbs picked from the prairie made sauces savoury and delicious. The washing took less than half the time it had previously taken, and came up cleaner; and Magpie did the heavier jobs, like fetching water and carrying the wet linens out to the line so that Caroline, for the first time since her arrival, found time in the day to sit and read, or to start some sewing. She never thought she would feel anything other than glad to have another person take on these tasks, but at the same time she envied the ease with which Magpie performed them. Magpie worked with good cheer, and she taught Caroline tactfully, never implying that she ought to know such things, and never making Caroline feel inadequate, so it was impossible to resent the girl.

But she did find it hard to concentrate with Magpie in the house. The girl drew the eye and she sang softly to herself as she worked—odd melodies like none Caroline had ever heard, as alien and eerie as the voices of the prairie wolves. And she moved softly, so softly that Caroline hardly heard her. She was sitting at her sewing one morning, stitching a tiny flower garland into the corner of a table runner, when she sensed a presence behind her and turned to find Magpie right by her shoulder, appraising the work.

'Very good, Mrs Massey,' she smiled, nodding approvingly. 'You stitch very well.'

'Oh . . . thank you, Magpie,' Caroline said breathlessly, startled by the girl's sudden appearance. The sun, catching the long braid of the Ponca girl's hair, showed no sign of red, or of brown. It was as black as a crow's wing. Caroline noticed the thickness of it, and its inky sheen, and thought it coarse. With her round face and wide cheekbones, Magpie almost resembled the Celestial women Caroline had occasionally seen in New York, although Magpie's skin was darker and redder. Caroline could not help shuddering slightly when their arms accidentally brushed. But she was fascinated by the girl, and caught herself watching her in whatever task she was performing. In the heat of the day, while sweat blistered Caroline's brow and itched beneath her clothes, Magpie seemed unaffected. The sun had no power to discomfort her, and Caroline envied her this, too.

One suffocatingly hot day, when Caroline thought she would run mad if she had no relief from it, she went into the bedroom, shut the door, stripped off her blouse and corset and threw them to the floor. She sat still and felt the relative cool of the air in the room touch her sticky, stifling skin and, slowly, the light-headedness that had dogged her all that morning began to diminish. It was so humid, the air so thick, the sky so blindingly, glaringly bright that Caroline seemed to feel her blood thickening, simmering in her veins. When she dressed again, she left the corset off. Nobody seemed to notice, and indeed there was little *to* notice. The heat and her own cooking had reduced her appetite and the work had taken its toll. Beneath the rigours of her underclothes, Caroline had grown very thin.

Later that week it rained. It rained as though the sky were blackly furious with the ground and aimed to injure it. It rained in torrents, not in drops but in solid rods of water that lanced down from the glowering clouds and stirred the topsoil into a soup that ran away towards Toad Creek. That modest creek became an angry cascade. The horses stood stoically, nose to tail, with water streaming from their manes. Out on the pasture, the cows lay down and narrowed their eyes. Corin was in Woodward with Hutch, having driven seven hundred head of cattle to the stock pens, and Caroline lay on the bed in the early evening and prayed as hard as she could that the North Canadian would not flood, would not stay long in spate, would not prevent Corin's return. She left the shutters open, listening to the rain hammer the roof above her, waiting, arms outflung, for the air creeping in through the window to feel cooler—for the water to wash the heat away.

There was a tentative knock at the door, and Magpie appeared.

'What's wrong?' Caroline asked abruptly, sitting up with a start.

'Nothing wrong, Mrs Massey. I have brought you something. Something to make you relieved,' the girl said. Caroline sighed, smoothing back her sweaty hair.

'Nothing can make me relieved,' she murmured.

'Come and try,' Magpie pressed. 'It's not good to lie down too much. You don't grow used to things that way,' she insisted, and Caroline dragged herself to her feet, following the Ponca girl to the kitchen. 'Watermelon. The first one of the summer! Try some.' Magpie passed Caroline a wide slice of the fruit: a bloody-coloured crescent moon that stickied her fingers.

'Thank you, Magpie, but I'm really not very hungry . . .'

'Try some,' Magpie repeated, more firmly. Caroline glanced at her, met her bright black eyes and saw only goodwill there. She took the fruit and nibbled at it. 'It's good, yes?'

'Yes,' Caroline admitted, taking bigger bites. The melon was neither sweet nor sharp. It tasted mild and earthy, softly easing the parched, torn feeling at the back of her throat.

'And drink this.' Magpie passed her a cup of water. 'Rainwater. Straight from the sky.'

'Well, there's no shortage of that today!' Caroline joked.

'This is water from the land, this is water from the sky,' Magpie explained, pointing to the fruit and the cup. 'To eat and drink these things, it makes you . . . it makes you balance with the land and the sky. Do you see? That way, you don't feel so much like you are punished. You will feel like you are a part of this land and sky.'

'That would be good. Not to feel punished,' Caroline smiled slightly.

'Eat more, drink more!' Magpie encouraged her, smiling too. They sat together at the kitchen table, with the rain hissing down outside and their chins slick with melon juice; and soon Caroline felt a blessed cool begin to spread outwards from inside her, sluicing the fevered burn from her skin.

*   *   *

There was a dun-coloured mare called Clara, who had short, slender legs, a compact body, ribs like a barrel, neck a little scrawny. She was in her twilight years and had foaled a half-dozen times for Corin; foals that had grown into fine saddle horses, with just one exception—a colt who was never right between the ears, and could not be broken, and who snapped the bones of several fine bronco busters before his heart finally gave out with the strain of his own fury.

'Clara hung her head all sorrowful the day it happened, even though that colt was over the other side of Woodward by then,' Hutch told Caroline, as she stroked the mare's bony face tentatively. The pungent reek of horse and the leather of the tack was strong in the morning sunshine. Caroline squinted up at the foreman from the shade of her bonnet. Hutch's eyes were bright slivers between the furrows of his brows and the crow's feet scoring his temples. These marks on his face were deep, though he was only a little older than Corin.

'You think she knew her baby had died? How sad!' Caroline said.

'I reckon she knew. Inferno, we called that colt. He was the colour of fire, and when you walked up to him he fixed you a look in the eye that made grown men tremble.'

'How horrible! How could an animal as gentle as Clara have such an evil offspring?'

'Many a murderer was born to a decent, God-fearing woman, and I guess the same applies for horses as for humans,' Hutch shrugged. 'Now, Clara here wouldn't hurt a fly. You could get up on her back, yell at the top of your voice and give her a mighty wallop with a stick and she wouldn't even hold that against you.'

'Well! I don't think I'm going to do any of those things!' Caroline laughed.

'Well, sure you are—the getting up on her back

part, that is,' Hutch smiled.

'Oh, no! I thought I was just learning how to put the saddle on today?' Caroline said, a note of alarm in her voice.

'That's right, and that's taken all of five minutes. And what's the point of a horse with a saddle on it if nobody gets up and sits in it?'

'Hutch, I . . . I don't know that I can . . .' she faltered.

'Only one way to find out,' he said, but gently, and he took her elbow to draw her closer to the horse's side. 'Come on now, Mrs Massey. There's no way the wife of a rancher can go around not knowing how to ride. And it's nothing to be scared of. It's as easy as sitting in a chair.'

'Chairs don't run around! Or kick!' Caroline argued.

'No, but they don't get you from point A to point B in half the time a wagon does, neither,' Hutch chuckled. His smile was crooked and warm, and when he held out his hand to her she found it impossible not to take it.

'I'm really not sure about this,' she said, nerves making her voice small.

'In about ten minutes' time, you're going to be wondering what all the fuss was about,' Hutch assured her.

Hutch cupped his hand around her shin and boosted her into the side saddle, where she perched, her face pale, expecting at any moment to be cast back into the sand. He showed her how to hook her right leg around the pommel to keep herself secure, and to take her weight in the left stirrup for balance.

'All right now. Comfy?' he asked.

'Not really,' she said, but she found the beginnings of a smile for him.

'Now, give her a little nudge with that heel, loose those reins and say, "Get up, Clara!"'

'Get up, Clara! Please,' Caroline said, with as much conviction as she could manage, and then gave a little shriek as the mare moved obediently forwards.

'OK, now you're riding!' Hutch exclaimed. 'Just relax, she's not going anywhere. Relax, Mrs Massey!' he called, walking beside her with one hand loosely on the rein. 'You're doing a great job,' he told her.

For half an hour or so Hutch escorted her around the empty corral. Clara walked steadily, stopping and starting and turning left and right without the least hint of bad attitude or boredom. Caroline listened to what she was told, and tried to remember it all, tried to feel the movement of the horse and make it her own, as Hutch instructed, but she could not shake the feeling that the animal had no choice but to resent her being there, and would at any given moment revert to the wild and throw her as far as she possibly could. Her back and legs were soon aching, and when she commented on this to Hutch, he gave the side saddle a disparaging look.

'Well, that's bound to happen when you do something for the first time. But, to be honest, Mrs Massey, you'd be a heck of a lot more comfortable riding astride than you are sat sideways like that . . .'

'Men ride astride. Ladies take the side saddle,' Caroline said firmly.

'You're the boss,' Hutch shrugged.

At that moment, Corin came cantering in off the pasture with two of the line-riders. Sunlight rippled from Strumpet's black coat, and sweat was running down the mare's forelegs. Caroline sat up straighter, rigid with embarrassment. The line-riders, whose names she still could not remember, tipped their hats to her, and slowed their horses, and she thought for a hideous moment that they were going to stop and watch the rest of her riding lesson. She gave them a small wave, and her cheeks flared scarlet. They rode as naturally as Magpie cooked and worked, slouching in the saddle as though their bodies had been designed for that very purpose. To her immense relief, they carried on towards the water troughs and only Corin pulled up at the corral fence.

'Well, now! Look at you! You look fantastic up there, sweetheart!' he beamed, pulling off his hat and rubbing his hot scalp.

'You want to go on over?' Hutch asked, and Caroline nodded. 'Well, go on then. You know how,' he urged her. Cautiously, Caroline turned the mare's head and persuaded her to walk over to the fence.

'That's fantastic, Caroline! I'm so happy to see you up on a horse at last!' Corin told her.

'I'll never be able to saddle her alone—it's so heavy!' Caroline smiled, anxiously.

'Well, that's as may be. But you can just ask any one of the boys and they'll help you with it. There's always somebody around, and they'd jump through hoops if a pretty girl like you asked them to!' Corin grinned.

'Can I get down now, Hutch?' she asked.

'I think we've done enough for one day,' Hutch

nodded, hitching up his jeans at the waist. 'Couple more goes like today and we'll change your name to Annie Oakley!' he smiled.

Feeling altogether less of a tenderfoot, Caroline listened as Hutch described the best way to dismount, but somehow her foot got snarled up in the stirrup, and her skirts tangled her knees, so she sprawled forwards on the descent, landing on her front in the corral sand with the air whooshing out of her lungs. Behind her, Clara gave a small snort of surprise.

'Damn! Are you all right, Caroline?' Corin swore, scrambling out of his own saddle.

'Well, that wasn't exactly how it was supposed to go,' Hutch remarked calmly, taking her arm and helping her to sit up. 'Hang on there, catch your breath,' he instructed, but Caroline had no intention of staying in the dirt, or so close to Clara's hooves, for any longer than she had to. She climbed shakily to her feet, coughing, her eyes streaming where grit had got into them. Her neck was jarred and one wrist badly over-bent where it had taken the weight of her fall. She was covered in dust from hair to hemline. She glared at Corin, furious with herself and crippled with embarrassment.

'Why, you look every bit as fierce as Inferno, when you fire up like that!' Hutch said, admiringly.

'And every bit as red, too,' Corin grinned.

'Don't . . . *laugh* at me!' Caroline bit the words off, frustration and anger burning her up inside. She turned on her heel and stalked away towards the house, shaking with the shock of the fall, her legs jellied by the riding. She was more disappointed than she could bear—to have failed again, to have made herself a laughing stock.

'Ah, hell, Caroline! Come back! I wasn't laughing at you!' She heard Corin call out behind her, but she squared her shoulders the best she could and kept walking.

*   *   *

Autumn arrived on the prairie with a string of vicious thunderstorms and pounding hailstones rent from blackened skies. Hutch came in from the range one evening and warmed himself by the stove as he reported the loss of three head of cattle, felled that day by a bolt of lightning that had struck the ground amidst the herd and thrown them into the air like confetti. Caroline paled at the tale, and Corin gave his foreman a censorious look that the poor man, his teeth chattering and his hands curled into scalded red claws, failed to notice. This glowering season was short, and soon the true winter began. Corin came in for dinner with his movements stiff and clumsy, and granules of sleet clinging to his eyebrows; but he always found a smile for his wife, declaring:

'There's one *hell* of a blue norther blowing out there!'

Caroline, who would once have been shocked by such language, no longer was. Still, she frowned slightly, out of habit, and pulled her shawl tightly around her against the wave of cold air that entered with her husband. She, who never thought she would miss the summer's heat, found herself longing for the sun.

They saw out the end of 1902 and welcomed in 1903 with a party at the Fosset's farm, to which all of the nearby ranchers, their families and riders had been invited. The night was still and dry, the air hanging like a chill blanket, and on the buggy ride over, Caroline's fingers, toes, her nose and the tips of her ears grew quite dead with cold. There was no moon, and the lantern on the buggy lit the prairie a scant few yards ahead. The dark all around was like a living thing, like solid flesh that watched. Caroline shivered, and huddled closer to Corin. Behind them, she could hear the hooves of the Massey riders following, keeping close as if they too felt pursued. When the Fosset place hove into view ahead, lights blazing out into the night, Caroline uttered a short, silent prayer of relief, and breathed a little easier.

There were fires burning about the yard, and meat smoking and spitting on the griddle, and a mass of people and horses all gathered into this oasis of light and life on the dead, dark plains. Corin's arm was shaken, his shoulder clapped, and they were soon engulfed by the friendly crowd of their neighbours. An accordion, a fiddle and a drum struck up in the barn, and the heat given off by dancing bodies warmed it, filled it with the animal smell of breath and sweat. Angie's children had made a painted banner out of a ragged old sheet, and it hung above the gate, reading *happy new yere!* and easing to and fro in the slow shifting air. Angie had two girls, aged twelve and eight, and a little boy aged four, who had his mother's red hair and the bluest eyes anyone had ever seen. Even as she danced and laughed and talked, Angie kept one eye on this perfect, happy little lad, and when she saw Caroline admiring him, she called him over.

'Kyle, this here is our good neighbour Caroline Massey. Now, what do you say to her?' she whispered to the boy, swinging him up onto her hip.

'Please' t' meetya, Missus Massey,' Kyle mumbled shyly, around the fingers he was chewing.

'Oh, well I'm pleased to meet you too, Kyle Fosset,' Caroline smiled, taking the hand that wasn't in his mouth and shaking it gently. Angie set him down and he darted away, ungainly on his short chubby legs. 'Oh, Angie! He's just the most *beautiful* child!' she exclaimed, and Angie beamed.

'Yeah, he's my little angel all right, and don't he just know it!'

'And the girls too . . . you must be so proud of . . .' Caroline said, but she could not keep her voice steady and had to stop.

'Hey there, now—stop that! This here is a celebration of the new year, and all the wonderful new things it's going to bring. You hear me?' Angie said, significantly. 'It's going to happen for you. You just have to be patient. You hear?' Caroline nodded, and wished she could feel as sure as Angie sounded.

'Mrs Massey? Will you dance with a rough rider like myself?' Hutch asked, appearing beside them.

'Of course!' Caroline smiled, hastily blotting her eyes with her fingertips. The band played one tune into the next without pause, and Hutch led her in a swaying dance that was almost a waltz, but not quite so. The room was a blur of smiling faces, some of them none too clean, and Caroline remembered the Montgomery's ball, still not yet a year gone but seeming to belong to another lifetime altogether. She had come such a long way, she told herself. It was no wonder that she did not yet find herself feeling at home.

'Is everything all right, Mrs Massey?' Hutch asked, seriously.

'Yes, of course! Why wouldn't it be?' she said, too brightly, her voice thin.

'No reason,' Hutch shrugged. He was wearing his best shirt, and she noticed that the top button was hanging by a thread. She made a mental note to add it to the pile of mending back at the ranch. 'Are you ready for another riding lesson, yet? You did great, that first time we tried it, but I never saw you go back for another try.'

'No, well . . . I'm not sure I'm the world's most naturally gifted horsewoman. And besides, now the weather's turned so cold I would surely freeze if I tried it!' she said.

'There are some people that take naturally to it, that's for sure, and others that don't. But I've seen those that once struggled get to grips with it in the end, with practice. But you have to be willing to get back on the horse, Mrs Massey. You do have to get back on the horse,' Hutch said, intensely, and she was no longer sure that he was talking about riding.

'I . . .' she started, but could not think what to say. She looked down at her feet and saw how dusty her shoes were, and found her eyes swimming with tears.

'You're going to be just fine,' Hutch said, his voice so low that she hardly heard him.

'Hutchinson, I'm cutting in! That's my wife you're cradling and she's by far the handsomest girl in the room,' Corin announced, taking Caroline's hands and spinning her into his embrace. His eyes were alight with happiness, cheeks flushed from sipping whisky and dancing, and he looked glorious, so glorious that Caroline laughed and threw her arms around his neck.

'Happy new year, my darling,' she whispered into his ear, letting her lips brush lightly against his neck, so that he held her tighter still.

*   *   *

In February snow fell deeply, lying in thick drifts and making the world too bright to look upon. Caroline stared at the featureless scene beyond the window in wonder, and stayed close to the stove as much as she could, her hands curled inside the fingerless mittens the Ponca had given her, which kept as much of her skin covered as possible whilst still allowing her to do the mending. Her chilled fingers fumbled the needle and dropped it often.

'Now you are glad to have them,' Magpie said, nodding at the thick mittens. 'When White Cloud gave them to you, I saw in your face you thought you would never need them!' she smiled.

'I should have paid her double,' Caroline agreed, at which Magpie frowned slightly.

'Will you tell a story, while I do this work?' Magpie requested. She was kneeling at the wash tub, rubbing the stains out of Corin's work wear on a ridged wooden washboard.

'What kind of story?'

'It doesn't matter. A story of your people,' Magpie shrugged. So Caroline, unsure who her people were, told her the story of Adam and Eve in the Garden of Eden, and of the treacherous serpent, the delicious apple, and the subsequent fall from grace. She put down her sewing as she reached the finale, describing their sudden shame at their nakedness, and the scramble to find something with which to cover themselves. Magpie chuckled, which made her cheeks even rounder and her eyes sparkle.

'This is a good story, Mrs Massey—a missionary man told this same story to my father once, and do you know what my father said?'

'What did he say?'

'He said this is typical of a white woman! An Indian woman would have picked up a stick and killed the snake and all would have been well in the garden!' she laughed. Caroline, stung for a moment by the implied criticism, soon found herself smiling, and then catching the girl's infectious laughter.

'That's probably about right,' she conceded, and they were still laughing when Corin came in, brushing the snow from his shoulders. He looked at Caroline, sitting by the stove with her sewing to one side, and at Magpie on her knees by the tub, and he frowned. 'Corin? What's wrong?' Caroline asked; but he shook his head and came over to the stove to warm himself.

Later, as they were eating supper, Corin spoke his mind.

'When I came home today, I . . . I didn't like what I saw, Caroline,' he said.

'What do you mean?' she asked, her heart high in her throat.

'You just sitting there, keeping warm, when Maggie was working so hard—'

'It wasn't like that! I was working at the mending! Ask Magpie . . . I just stopped to tell her the story of Adam and Eve . . .' Caroline trailed off, unhappily.

'I know you're used to having servants, Caroline, but Maggie is no servant. I meant for her to help you in the house, of course, but she does not have time to do *everything* here. She has her own home to tend to, and soon she won't be able to do as much. You need to help her more, love,' he finished gently. He broke a piece of bread from the loaf and crumbled it distractedly between his fingers.

'She does help me! I mean, I help her too—we share the work! What do you mean, soon she won't be able to do as much? Why won't she?'

'Sweetheart,' Corin looked up at her through his rough golden brows. 'Maggie's pregnant, Caroline. She and Joe are going to have a baby. Their first.' He looked away again, his face sombre, and in that expression Caroline read an accusation. Tears sprang to her eyes and she was choked with an emotion a little like ire, a little like grief, a little like guilt. An insufferable mixture of the three that burned in her gut and made a roaring noise in her ears. She clattered up from the table, ran to the bedroom and closed the door behind her.

* * *

In a light buggy, harnessed to a bay horse with a high, proud head carriage, the journey to Woodward could be made in a day, with a dawn start and a break to rest and water the horse at noon time. Most of the ranch hands and riders accompanied them on horseback, including Joe and Magpie. Caroline watched the Indian girl, who rode a wiry grey pony, and wondered how she could have failed to spot the telltale swell at her middle, the slight deference in her movements.

'Is it wise for Magpie to ride in her condition?' Caroline whispered to Corin, although there was little chance of being heard above the thudding of hooves, the wind and the creak and whirr of the buggy wheels.

'I said the very same thing to Joe,' Corin smiled. 'He just laughed at me.' He shrugged. 'I guess Ponca women are a bit tougher than white women.' A few tiny flecks of rain blew out of the sky. Caroline made no reply to Corin's remark, but she felt the sting of it. The implication she heard, whether he had intended it or not, was that she was weak and that she was failing here in the West, as a woman and as a wife.

They arrived in Woodward as dark was falling and took a room at the Central Hotel. Joe, Magpie and the ranch boys melted into the town: to the Equity, Midway, Shamrock and Cabinet saloons, to the brothel run by Dollie Kezer at the Dew Drop Inn, and to the houses of friends. Caroline's back ached from the long drive and she was tired, but she nevertheless urged Corin to lie with her, and she shut her eyes as she felt him spend himself within her, praying that whatever magic it was that made a child coalesce into being, it would happen this time—*this time*.

Caroline's spirits had soared with the prospect of coming into town for the spring gala day, and for dancing. Visits away from the ranch were precious scarce and they had not ventured forth for four long months since the Fosset's shindig on new year's eve. Woodward, which had seemed upon her arrival from New York to be a one-horse town indeed, now seemed a vibrant hub of life and activity. But there was something about this very fact, even, that saddened Caroline. The following day dawned fair and the streets thronged with people, cowboys and settlers alike. They formed two thick cords that ran for several blocks along the length of Main Street, undulating where a raised sidewalk ran in front of a shop. The air thronged with the smells and sounds of thousands of bodies and excited voices, the stink of horses and manure, and the parched wood and paint fragrance of the buildings. Store fronts were strung with colourful bunting and had their doors flung wide open to welcome the unprecedented opportunity for new custom that day.

The crowd was entertained with a roping and riding contest, a mock buffalo hunt, and shooting competitions. There were fancy lariat tricks and a display of bull-dogging that looked unduly violent to Caroline, who turned her face away as the steer's head was pulled around, its lip clamped as they both crashed to the ground. Joe far outperformed all other competitors in a knife-throwing competition, sending his blade again and again into the centre of a paper target pinned to hay bales to win a box of fine cigars and a brand new Bowie knife. The applause for his victory was muted compared to that lavished upon the white victors of other events, but Joe smiled his wry half-smile nonetheless and admired the new blade. They ate barbecue, fresh peaches, ice cream and honey cakes, and the ladies drank iced tea while the men took beer. Caroline, who had been without ice or refrigeration since leaving New

York, found the chilled drink in her mouth to be not far short of heavenly. They caught up with neighbours, and Corin swapped the current prices of wheat and beeves with fellow ranchers; and they ran into Angie and Jacob Fosset, Angie clad in a lurid lilac gown with too much colour on her face. When Corin complimented her, she laughed and exclaimed:

'Oh, I look like a show girl, I know I do; but we gals don't get to dress up often enough! And I need a little help to look festive, Lord knows—we can't all be pretty as paint like your wife here, Corin Massey!'

'Well,' Corin told her, with a generous tip of his hat, 'you look just fine to me, Angie Fosset.' While the men talked, Angie took Caroline to one side.

'Any news, honey?' she asked in a low tone, in answer to which Caroline could only grip her lower lip in her teeth and shake her head. 'Well, I've thought of some things you could try . . .' Angie told her.

In the evening the band played waltzes and polkas, as well as some square dances—large sheets of canvas were laid over the sand of Main Street to facilitate the dancing, since no hall in town could accommodate such a large number of pairs. Caroline danced with the grace of her upbringing, even though Corin's steps were marred by beer and there were wrinkles in the canvas to snag unwary feet. With buildings all around her, and people, Caroline felt better than she had in months as they marked a Mexican waltz amongst the jostling shoulders of Woodward's citizens. For a while, the smile she wore was not a brave one, or a dissembling one, but a genuine one.

But later, as she stood talking to a circle of Woodward wives, Caroline saw Corin across the street, bending down in front of Magpie and putting his hands on her midriff. He seemed to cradle the bulge in her abdomen gently, almost reverently, and whilst Magpie looked embarrassed she also looked pleased. Caroline caught her breath and blood flooded her cheeks. Corin was in his cups, she knew, but this behaviour was too much. Soon, though, it was not for this reason that her cheeks burned. Corin's face was turned away, his gaze was unfocused. Waiting, she realised; waiting for the child to move inside the Ponca girl. And as she witnessed this act of intimacy, she suddenly thought she saw something possessive in her husband's touch—something altogether too interested.

4

It's cold as we walk down towards the woods on the longest night of the year. All three of us. Eddie pestered Beth into coming, and in the end she seemed almost curious. There's a brisk, bitter breeze that finds its way inside our coats, so we walk quickly, on stiff limbs. In the clear dark our torch beams stagger haphazardly. The moon is bright and the flowing clouds make it seem to sail across the sky. A vixen shrieks as we get near the trees.

'What was that?' Eddie gasps.

'Werewolf,' I say, matter-of-fact.

'Ha, ha. Anyway, it's not a full moon.'

'All right, then, it was a fox. You're no fun any more, Edderino.' I am in high spirits. I feel unfettered, like my strings have been cut and I can float free. Bright, restless nights do this to me. There is something about a wind blowing in the dark. The way it brushes by, its nonchalance. It seems to say: *I could pick you up; I could carry you away, if I wanted to.* There is a promise to this evening.

We can hear music now, and raised voices, laughter; and now the glow of the bonfire shines at us between the trees. Beth hangs back. She folds her arms tightly across her chest. The firelight follows every anxious line of her face. If Eddie wasn't with us I think she would stay here, in the sheltering woods, darting from shadow to shade and watching. I pull a flat bottle of whisky from my coat pocket, fight to open it with gloved hands. The three of us, in a circle, our breath pouring up into the sky.

'Swig. Go on. It'll warm you up,' I tell her, and for once she doesn't argue. She takes a long pull.

'Can I have some?' asks Eddie.

'Not on your life,' Beth replies, as she wipes her chin and coughs. She sounds so real, so there, so like Beth that I grin and take her hands.

'Come on. I'll introduce you to Patrick. He's super nice.' I take a drink myself, feel the fire in my throat, and then we move.

There's a moment of nerves as we step into the firelight. The same as before, of being unsure of our welcome. But then Patrick finds us and introduces us to a myriad people, and I struggle to keep their names in my head. Sarah and Kip—long hair shining in the firelight, stripy knitted hats;

Denise—a tiny woman with a deeply lined face and ink-black hair; Smurf—a huge man, hands like shovels, a gentle smile; Penny and Louise—Penny the more butch of the pair, her head shaved, her eyes fierce. Their clothes and hair are bright. They look like butterflies against the winter ground. There's a sound system in the back of a pick-up and vehicles parked all the way up the lane. Children too, dodging in and out of the crowd. Eddie vanishes and I see him a little while later with Harry, threading thick wads of dead leaves onto long twigs and thrusting them into the fire.

'Who's that with Eddie?' Beth asks, a note of alarm in her voice.

'That's Harry. I've met him, don't worry. He's a little bit on the slow side, you could say. Dinny says he's always got on well with children. He seems totally harmless to me,' I tell her, speaking loudly, right into her ear. The fire has put a dew of sweat along our lips and brows.

'Oh,' Beth says, not quite convinced. I see Honey, moving across the clearing, preceded by her enormous bump. Her face is alive this evening, she's smiling, and she is lovely. I feel a small prickle of despair.

'That's Honey, there. The blonde,' I say to Beth, in defiance of myself. Watching expressions veer wildly across Honey's face, I am sure of it—I have taught girls older than her: she is too young to be having that baby. I feel something close to anger, but I can't tell who or what it's aimed at.

Then Dinny appears beside Beth, smiling his guarded smile. His hair is unbound and it hangs around his jaw, messy and black. He stands half turned towards the fire, half away, so the light cuts him in two, throws his face into sharp relief. It stops a breath in my chest, holds it until it burns.

'Glad you came down to join in, Beth, Erica,' he says, and as he smiles again I see the faint blurring of alcohol about him—a true warmth, for the first time since I saw him again.

'Yes, well, thank you very much for having us,' Beth replies, looking around at the party and nodding as if we are at some society do.

'You've got lucky with the weather tonight, anyway. It's been foul,' I say. Dinny gives me an amused look.

'I don't believe in foul weather—it's all just weather,' he says.

'No bad weather, only the wrong clothes?' I ask.

'Exactly! Have you tried my punch? It has a certain . . . punch. Don't take any naked flames near it, whatever you do,' he smiles.

'I tend to avoid punch,' I say. 'There was an incident with punch, I'm told. Although, they might be lying because I sure as hell don't remember anything about it.'

'Beth, then? Can I tempt you?' Beth nods, lets herself be led away. She still looks slightly dazed, almost bewildered to be here. Dinny's hand is on her elbow, guiding her. For a moment I am left alone as he pulls her away, and some emotion scuttles through me. A familiar old emotion, to be left behind by Beth and Dinny. I give myself a shake, find faces that I know and foist myself upon them.

I can feel the whisky heat in my blood and I know I should be careful. Eddie tears past me, grabs my sleeve and pulls me round.

'You haven't seen me! Don't tell them you've

seen me!' he gasps, breathless, grinning.

'Tell who?' I ask, but he's gone, and seconds later a small tangle of children, and Harry, scurry by in his wake. I take another long pull of whisky then pass the bottle to a pixie-faced girl with rings in her nose, who laughs and thanks me as she passes. The stars wheel over my head and the ground seems to vibrate. I can't remember when I was last drunk. Months and months ago. I had forgotten how good it can feel. And I see Beth standing next to Dinny, in a knot of people, and even though she is not speaking, she looks almost relaxed. She is part of them, not locked up inside herself, and I am happy to see it. I dance with Smurf, who spins me until I feel a little sick.

'Don't fall in love with her, Smurf. These Calcott girls don't stick around,' Dinny shouts to him as we pass by. I am too slow to ask him what he means. I get as close to the fire as I dare, use a poker to rake a jacket potato from the ashes at the edge, then burn my tongue on it. It has the tang of the earth. I greet Honey, and even though her reply is stilted I don't care. And I watch Dinny. It's not even conscious after a while. Wherever I am I seem to know where he is. As if the fire lights him a little brighter than it does everybody else. The night spins out around the camp, dark and alive; then I see flashing blue lights, coming along the lane towards us.

The police have to park and walk down to the camp. Two cars, disgorging four officers. Marching in with an air of diligence, they start checking for drugs, asking people to turn out their pockets. The music goes quiet, voices fall away. A hung moment in which the fire snaps and roars.

'Is there a Dinsdale here?' a young officer asks. A pugnacious gleam in his eye. He is short, square, very tidy.

'Several!' Patrick calls back at him.

'Can I see some identification to that effect please, sir?' the policeman asks stiffly. Dinny waves Patrick back, dips quickly into his van and presents the officer with his driving licence. 'Well, even so I'm required to ask you all to disperse, as this is an illegal gathering in a public place. I have reason to believe that things may escalate, constituting an illegal rave. There have been several complaints—'

'This isn't an illegal gathering in a public place. We have the right to camp here, as you well know. And we have the same right as the rest of the population to have a few friends around for a party,' Dinny says coldly.

'There have been complaints about the noise, Mr Dinsdale—'

'Complaints from who? It's only ten o'clock!'

'From people in the village, and at the manor house . . .'

'From the manor house? Really now?' Dinny asks, glancing over his shoulder at me. I go over, stand next to him. 'Have you been complaining, Erica?'

'Not me. And I'm pretty sure Beth and Eddie haven't either.'

'And who might you be, madam?' the officer asks me, somewhat dubiously.

'Erica Calcott, the owner of Storton Manor. And that's my sister Beth, and since we're the only people *living* at Storton Manor, I think we can safely say all residents there give this party their full endorsement. And who might *you* be?' The whisky makes me bold, but I am angry too.

'Sergeant Hoxteth, Ms . . . Lady . . . Calcott, and I . . .' I have flustered him. At the edge of my sight, I see Dinny's eyes light up.

'It's *Miss* Calcott. Are you any relation of Peter Hoxteth, the old bobby?' I interrupt.

'He's my uncle, not that I think that has any relevance to—'

'Yes, well. I remember your uncle. He had better manners.'

'There have been complaints, nevertheless, and I am authorised to break up this gathering. I don't wish for there to be any unpleasantness about it, however—'

'The Hartfords over at Ridge Farm have their summer ball every year, with twice this number of people and a live band with a massive amp. If I ring up and complain about *that*, will you go trooping in and break it up? Start searching for drugs?'

'I hardly think—'

'And anyway, this isn't a public place. This is my land. Which, I suppose, makes this *my* party. My *private* party. To which you boys are not, I fear, invited.'

'Miss Calcott, surely you can understand—'

'We'll turn the music down now, and off at midnight, which we were planning to do anyway. The kids need to get to bed,' Dinny interjects. 'But if you want to send us all packing without making some arrests, you'd better come up with a better reason than made-up complaints from the manor house. *Officer.*'

Hoxteth bridles, his shoulders are high and tense. 'It is our *duty* as police officers to investigate complaints—'

'Well, you've investigated. So piss off!' Honey chips in, waving her belly aggressively at the man. Dinny puts a restraining hand on her arm. Hoxteth's eyes flicker over Honey's youth, her beauty, the swell of her midriff. He flushes, knots forming at the corners of his jaw. He nods at his officers and they begin to file away.

'Music off. And everybody gone by midnight. We'll be back to check,' he says, raising a warning finger. Honey raises a finger of her own, but Hoxteth has turned away.

'Tosser,' Patrick mutters. 'Full of youthful zeal, that one,' he adds. Once the cars have pulled away, Dinny turns to me with a smile, an arched eyebrow.

'*Your* party, is it?' he asks, amused.

'Oh, come *on*. It did the trick,' I reply.

'That it did. I never had you down as the anti-establishment type,' he says wryly.

'Shows what you know. I even got arrested once—do I get some kudos for that?'

'Depends what you got arrested for.'

'I . . . I threw an egg at our MP,' I admit, reluctantly. 'Not very anarchic.'

'Not very,' he says, flashing me a grin. 'But it's a start.'

'That was wicked,' Eddie tells me, appearing at my side, breathless. I put my arm around his shoulders and squeeze him before he can escape.

*   *   *

Beth is cooking something for lunch that's filling the ground floor with garlic-scented steam. The windows cloud with it and rain cloaks the outside world so that the house feels like an island. Eddie's gone off into the woods with Harry, and strains of Sibelius's fifth come creeping up the stairs with the steam. Beth's favourite. I take it as a good sign that she has looked it out in Meredith's music collection, and is preparing food that she might even eat. I wonder what Dinny and Honey are doing. In such rain, on such a depressing day. No rooms to wander through, no rows and rows of books or music, no television. Their lifestyle is a matter of pure speculation for me. If it were me, I suppose I'd be in the village pub. For a second I consider seeking them out there, but my stomach gives a lurch of protest and I remember the hangover I'm nursing. Instead I head for the attic stairs.

I do remember Sergeant Hoxteth's uncle. We would see him in the village sometimes, when we went for sweets or ice cream from the shop. He had a ready smile. And he came to the house, on more than one occasion. Either because Meredith had called him, or because the Dinsdales had. They have the right to camp there, just as Dinny said. There's a legal deed or warrant or whatever, from the time of my great-grandfather, before he married Caroline. He and Private Dinsdale were in the army together, in Africa I think. The full story has been lost down the years, but when they came back Dinsdale wanted a place to park up, and Sir Henry Calcott gave it to him. And to all members of his family, in perpetuity. They have a copy of it, and our family lawyer holds a copy. It really got Meredith's goat.

We'd see Sergeant Hoxteth standing in the hallway, waiting uncomfortably for Meredith to appear with her Gorgon glare. The time she made one of the farmers park a massive baler across the top of the track to keep the travellers out. The time she learnt that not all those at the camp were Dinsdales and wanted the *hangers-on* evicted. The time she saw someone drawing water from one of the estate troughs and wanted to press charges. The time food kept vanishing from the larder, and small articles from around the house, and Meredith insisted that it was the Dinsdales until it turned out that the housekeeper had an elderly mother to support. The time one of the travellers' dogs got into the garden and she *put the wind up it* with a twelve-bore shotgun. People in the village thought that they were under attack. *They will spread diseases to my animals*, was Meredith's clipped explanation.

We used to come up here to the attic sometimes, to root around in the junk. It always looked like there should be something exciting to discover, but it didn't take long for us to tire of the packing crates, broken lamps, offcuts of carpet. The hot-water tank, gurgling and hissing like a sleeping dragon. On such a wet day it is dark up here, the far reaches of the space hung in shadow. The tiny dormer windows are few and far between and they are crusted up with water marks and algae. It is so quiet I can hear the soft breathing sounds of the house, the rain making a musical chuckle as it filters through the choked guttering. Unconsciously, I tiptoe.

The leather of the old red trunk is so dry and brittle that it feels sandy when I touch it, comes away as grit between my fingers. I strain my eyes to see inside, dragging it around to face the nearest window. It leaves the ghost of itself in the dust on the floor and I wonder when it was last moved. Inside are wads of papers; boxes; a small, dilapidated valise of some kind; a few mystery objects wrapped in yellowed newspaper pages; a leather writing case. It doesn't look much, if this is all of Caroline's personal things. Not much for a hundred years of life. But then, old houses like this come ready-made, I suppose. The lives within come and go, but most of the contents stay the same.

I search avidly through the papers. Invitations to various functions; a government leaflet about what to do in an air raid; Caroline's telegram from the queen on the occasion of her one hundredth birthday; some prescriptions written out in a doctor's hand so typically wild that I can't make out the words. I unwrap a few of the paper parcels. There's a gold face-powder compact and matching lipstick; an exquisite tortoiseshell fan, so fragile I hardly dare touch it; a silver dressing table set, inlaid with mother of pearl, the brushes silky soft, the mirror cracked across its face; a curious bone ring, satin smooth, with a silver bell hanging from it that tinkles, startling me in the stillness. I wonder what sets these objects apart, what made them wholly Caroline's, what stopped Meredith selling them off like she did with so many of the other precious things. After a while, I notice it. They are all engraved, marked as hers. *CC*, drawn with a flourish into the metal. I turn the bone ring over in my fingers, looking for the same mark. The script, when I find it on the rim of the tarnished silver bell, is small and almost worn away, and it makes me pause. *For A Fine Son*, it reads.

I re-wrap these treasures and put them back in the trunk. I am not sure what will become of them. Technically, they belong to Beth and me now, but they don't really, of course. Any more than they belonged to Meredith, which was why she stowed them away up here. The valise, which has a wide, hinged-opening top, is empty. It once had a pink silk lining, now just in tatters. I take out the writing case instead, which is so full that the laces struggle to tie around the bulge of it. Inside are her letters, many of them still in their envelopes. Compact, white envelopes, much smaller than are commonly used these days. I flick through, realise that most of them have been addressed in the same hand—a small, slanting script in black ink. Just slightly too cramped to be called elegant. I open one carefully and skip straight to the end. Most of these letters are from Meredith and have a Surrey postmark.

My heart gives a strange little twist. I turn back to the first page of the one I am holding, and read.

April 28th 1931.

Dear Mother,

I hope this letter finds you well, and less troubled by your rheumatism than of late? You will be pleased to hear that I am settling in well here, and am gradually becoming accustomed to running my own household—even though I do of course miss you, and Storton. Charles is rather relaxed about the arrangements—his only stipulation is that breakfast be served at eight and dinner at nine! An easy man to please, and I have had the freedom to find my own way of doing things. The house is so much smaller than Storton, you would doubtless be amused by how many and varied the instructions have been that I've needed to give the staff in order to bring things along! I fear they have grown rather too used to having a gentleman alone in the house, and one unlikely to pay much mind to the rotation of linen, the freshening of flowers or the airing of guest bedrooms. It does seem rather unusual to be alone in the house all day whilst Charles is at his offices. There is a singular quiet in the afternoons here—I often look to my left to remark upon something to you, only to find the room empty! I suppose I ought to make the most of the peace and quiet before it is carried away by the patter of little feet . . . I find myself entirely pulled between two emotions: the thrill of anticipating the birth of your first grandchild, and utter dread of the same event! I remind myself daily that women have been giving birth successfully for a great many years, and that I am certain there can be nothing another woman might do that I might not. Were you afraid, when you were first expecting? I do hope you will come and visit, Mother—I should dearly love to have your advice. The house is smaller than you are used to, as I have said, but it is nevertheless quite comfortable. I have fitted out the largest guest bedroom with new drapes and bed linen—the existing ones were quite worn out—so it is every bit ready for your arrival. The garden is a riot of daffodils, which I know you like, and the countryside hereabouts is really very charming for a gentle walk. Write and let me know if you will come, and when you might like to. In anticipation of our happy event, Charles has sworn me off driving the motorcar, but I can arrange for our man Hepworth to collect you from the station at any time—it is a short drive, not at all arduous. Do come.

With much affection,
Meredith.

In 1931 Meredith would have been just twenty years old. Twenty years old, married and expecting a baby that she must have lost, because my mother was not born for some time after that. I read the letter again, try to re-imagine Caroline as a mother somebody loved, as somebody Meredith clearly missed. The letter makes me sad, and I have to read it again to work out why. It is such a *lonely* letter. From far below, I hear Beth calling me for lunch. I slip the letter back into the case and tuck it beneath my arm before going down to her.

*   *   *

The rain doesn't stop until Tuesday afternoon, and I am itching to get outside. I envy Eddie, who comes back as it gets dark, hair in damp curls and mud up to the knees of his jeans. At what age do you start to notice the cold and the wet and the mud? About the same time you stop moving everywhere at a run, I suppose. In the nursery the gap where the linen press stood yawns at me from the wall. An imprint of dust and cobwebs and unfaded paint. I cross to the piles of cloth I evicted from it, start to go through them, putting cot sheets, lacy sleep-sacks, tiny pillow cases and an exuberant christening gown to one side. A pile of muslin squares that I find tucked away, and a small feather eiderdown as well. I have no idea if any of it will be any use to Honey and her baby, when it comes. Will she even have a cot? But it is good, heavy linen, smooth to the touch. Luxurious. She might like that idea, perhaps: swathing the child in expensive bedding, even if the ambulance will be a more basic nursery. I catch sight of those pillowcases again, with the yellow stitched flowers. I make a mental note to look the flowers up, identify them, in case that will tell me why they tug at my subconscious so.

'Where are you going with that lot?' Beth asks, as I lug it down the stairs.

'I'm taking it over to Honey. It's all baby stuff—I thought she could use it.' Beth frowns. 'What's wrong?' I ask.

'Erica, why are you trying to . . .'

'What?'

'You know. I don't think you should be trying so hard to be friends with them again, that's all.'

'Why not? Anyway, I'm not trying that hard. They are our neighbours though. You seemed happy enough to chat to Dinny at the party the other night.'

'Well, you made me go, you and Eddie. It would have been rude not to talk to him. But I . . . I don't think we have much in common any more. In fact I'm not sure we ever knew him as well as we thought we did. And I don't see what purpose it serves, trying to pretend everything is how it was before.'

'Of course we knew him! What's that supposed to mean? And why shouldn't things be how they were before, Beth?' I ask. She seals her lips, looks away from me. 'If something happened between the two of you that I don't know about . . .'

'Nothing happened that you don't know about!'

'Well, I'm not so sure,' I say. 'Besides, just because you don't want to be friends with him any more, doesn't mean I shouldn't be,' I mutter, dragging the bag to the door and pulling on my coat.

'Erica, wait!' Beth comes across the hall to me. I turn, search her face for clues. Troubled blue eyes, closely guarded. 'We *can't* go back to the way things were. Too much has happened. Too much time has passed! It's far better to just . . . move on. Leave the past alone,' she says, her eyes sliding away from mine. I think of Dinny's hand, its gentle, proprietorial grip on her elbow.

'It sounds to me,' I say, steadily, 'that you don't want him any more, but you don't want me to have him either.'

'*Have* him? What is that supposed to mean?' she says sharply. I feel colour flare in my cheeks and I say nothing. Beth draws in a deep, uneven breath. 'It's hard enough being back here as it is, Erica, without you acting like an eight-year-old again. Can't you just stay away, for once? We're supposed to be spending time here *together*. Now Eddie is off with that Harry all day long, and you'd rather chase after Dinny than . . . I don't have to stay, you know. I could take Eddie and go back to Esher for Christmas . . .'

'Well, that's a great idea, Beth. Just the kind of unpredictable behaviour that Maxwell is always looking out for!' I regret this as soon as I say it. Beth recoils from me. 'I'm sorry,' I say quickly.

'How can you say things like that to me?' she asks softly, her eyes growing bright, blurred. She turns and walks away.

Outside, I take a deep breath, listen to the muted calls of the rooks, the gentle dripping and unfurling of soaked foliage. A living sound, a living smell in the middle of winter. I've never really noticed it before. I drop the bag of linens, suddenly unsure of myself, and sit down on a rusting metal bench at the edge of the lawn; feel the dead cold of it bite through my jeans. Perhaps I will take it down later. I can hear voices coming from the stream beyond the eastern edge of the garden. I make my way over, through the little gate at the side of the lawn and down across the scrubby slope. After the rain the ground is heavy with water. It squeezes up around my feet as I walk.

Eddie and Harry are in the stream, the water swirling perilously close to the tops of their wellies. All the rain of late has made the water fast, and even faster in the centre, channelled deep because Eddie and Harry have built a dam of flints and sticks reaching out from each bank. Harry's trousers are wet all the way up to his hips, and I know how cold the water must be.

'Rick! Check it out! We almost got it right the way across a moment ago, but then part of it collapsed,' Eddie calls, excited, as I reach them. 'But before it did the water got really high! That's when we got soaked, actually . . .'

'I can see that. Boys, you must be freezing!' I smile at Harry, who smiles back and points at a rock by my feet. I bend down and pass it to him gingerly, slipping on the muddy bank, and he adds it to the dam.

'Thanks,' Eddie says absently, unconsciously speaking for his friend. 'It's not that cold once you get used to it,' he shrugs.

'Really?'

'No, not really—my feet are bloody freezing!' he grins.

'Language,' I say, automatically and without conviction. 'It's a good dam, I have to admit,' I continue, standing in the mud with hands on hips. 'What are you going to do if you manage to finish it? It'll make a huge lake.'

'That's the idea!'

'I see. God, Eddie, you are *covered* in mud!' It's all up the sleeves of his jumper, where he has pushed them up with muddy hands; all up the legs of his cords where he's wiped his hands. There's a smear across his forehead, sticking his hair into clumps. 'How have you managed to get so filthy? Look—Harry's managed to stay clean!'

'He's further from the ground than I am!' Eddie protests.

'True enough,' I concede.

Grabbing a fistful of Harry's coat to steady himself, Eddie makes his way towards me, feet rocking over the stony stream bed.

'Is it lunch time yet? I'm starving,' he declares, losing his balance and bending forwards to steady himself, hands in the freezing mud.

'Yes, almost. Come back and get cleaned up— you can always finish this later. Here.' I hold out my hand and Eddie grabs it, taking a huge stride out of the stream, heaving on my arm. 'No—don't pull, Eddie, I'll slip!' I cry, but too late. My legs scoot from under me and I sit down abruptly, with an audible splash.

'Sorry!' Eddie gasps. Behind him Harry grins, makes an odd huffing noise, and I realise he is laughing.

'Oh, you think that's funny, do you?' I ask, slithering back to my feet, wet mud seeping into my knickers. I pull my trousers up, leaving vast muddy smears across them in doing so. Eddie wobbles again, takes a sloshing step forwards that kicks a wave of water over the tops of my boots. *'Eddie!'*

'Sorry!' he says again, but this time he can't keep from smiling, and Harry laughs harder.

'You little buggers! It's freezing! Here,' I find my muddiest finger, wipe it on Eddie's nose. 'Have some more!'

'Wow, thanks Rick! And here . . . here's some for you! Happy Christmas!' Eddie scoops some mud into his hand, chucks it at me. It lands messily on the front of my sweater, which is pale grey. I gasp, peer down at it. Eddie freezes, as if suddenly afraid he's gone too far. I scrape the worst of it off, weigh it in my palm.

'You. Are. *Dead!*' I say, lunging at him. With a yelp of laughter, Eddie darts past me, up the bank and into the scrub.

It takes me some distance to catch up with him and I have to discard the mud and swear a truce before he'll let me near him. I put my arm around him, more to warm my own throbbing fingers than anything else. Behind us, Harry had been following but he stops, stares up into a hawthorn tree where two robins are cursing one another.

'Is he coming?' I ask. Eddie shrugs.

'He's always stopping to watch birds and stuff like that. I'll see you later, Harry!' he shouts, giving him a wave. We ought to go in through the scullery, but it's locked and we have no choice but to use the front door. We discard our boots outside—a hollow gesture, since our socks are every bit as wet and muddy. Beth puts her head around the kitchen doorway.

'What on *earth* have you been doing?' she gasps. 'Your clothes!' Eddie looks a little contrite, glances at me for support.

'Um, being eight years old again?' I venture, painting my face with innocence. Beth gives me a hard look, but she cannot hold it. The ghost of a smile twitches her mouth.

'Perhaps you might like to get changed, the pair of you, before we have lunch?' she says.

*   *   *

I phone my mum in the afternoon, to check that all is well, and ask what time they plan to arrive.

'How is it going there? How's Beth?' Mum asks, in a casual tone that I recognise. The casual tone she uses to ask important things. I pause, listen for sounds of my sister close by.

'She's OK, I think. A little bit up and down, I suppose.'

'Has she said anything? Anything about the house?'

'No—what kind of thing?'

'Oh, nothing in particular. I'm looking forward to seeing you both—and Eddie of course. Is he having fun there?'

'Are you kidding? He loves it! We hardly see him—he's out playing in the woods all day. Mum—could you do me a favour?'

'Yes, of course, what is it?'

'Could you possibly dig out your copy of that family tree Mary drew up? And bring it along?'

'Yes, I think so. If I can find it. What do you want it for?'

'I just want to check something. Did you ever hear of Caroline having a baby before she was married to Lord Calcott?'

'No, I never did. I would doubt it very much—she was very young when she married him. What on earth makes you ask that?'

'It's just this photo I found—I'll show you when you get here.'

'Well, all right then. But you know any questions about family history really ought to be directed at Mary. She did all that research the other year, after all . . .'

'Yes, I suppose so. Well, I'd better crack on here—I'll see you very soon.'

I can't call my Aunt Mary—Henry's mother. I can't speak to her on the phone. I get a feeling that I can hardly bear, as if the air in my lungs is hardening. At Meredith's funeral, I hid. To my shame. I actually hid from her behind a vast spray of lilies.

For bedtime reading, I prop Caroline's writing case on my knees and read a few more of Meredith's letters. Some of the earlier ones date from her time away at college and speak of a fierce deportment tutor, dormitory politics, shopping trips into town. Then the lonely letters from Surrey begin. I flick through a few more of them and then, tucked into one of the pockets of the case, I find an envelope addressed in quite a different hand. The paper inside is like dried leaves, and I touch it lightly, unfold it with consummate care. Just one page, with one paragraph of script. Far larger lettering than Meredith's, written with emphatic pen pressure, as if in some urgency. The date given is the fifteenth of March, 1905.

Caroline

I received your letter this morning and with no slight concern. Your recent marriage and delicate condition are matters to be much celebrated, and no one could be more satisfied than I to see you settled and joined to a man such as Lord Calcott, who is well positioned to give you everything you require for a happy life. To put your current position in unnecessary jeopardy would be foolhardy in the extreme. Whatever it is that you feel you must confess, may I strongly urge you that all matters arising from your previous existence in America should by every means possible <u>remain in America</u>.No purpose can be served by revisiting such matters now. Be grateful for the new start you have been given, for the happy circumstance of your fortuitous marriage, and let that be the last word upon it between us. Should you bring embarrassment or infamy of any kind upon yourself or our family, I should have no other choice but to sever all ties with you, however it would grieve me.
   Your Aunt,
   B.

The scoring beneath the phrase *remain in America* has all but torn the paper. A heavy, violent strike.

In the quiet after I read these ringing words, I see all the secrets within this house lying in drifts as deep as the dust and shadows in the corners of the room.

*   *   *

On Christmas Eve our parents arrive, and their familiar car pulling into the driveway seems a small miracle of some kind. Proof of an outside world, proof that this house, Beth and I, are part of it. I meant to keep Eddie in this morning—I suggested to Beth that we should—but he is up before us and gone. An empty bowl in the kitchen sink, cornflakes drying hard, and half a glass of Ribena on the table.

'We've lost your grandson, I fear,' I say, as I kiss Dad and take bags from the back of the car. Perhaps not the cleverest thing I could say. Mum hesitates.

'What's happened to Eddie?' she asks.

'He's got a friend—Harry. He camps here, just like . . . Well. They're always off in the woods. We hardly see him these days,' Beth says, and we can hear that it bothers her. Just a little.

'Camping? You don't mean . . . ?'

'Dinny's here. And his cousin, Patrick, and some others,' I say casually. But I can't help smiling.

'Dinny? You're *kidding*?' Mum says.

'Well, well!' Dad adds.

'Hmm, well, now you know how we used to feel, I suppose,' Mum says to Beth, kissing her on the cheek as she goes indoors. Beth and I share a look. This hadn't ever occurred to us.

Beth looks like our mother. She always has, but

it's getting more pronounced the older she gets. They both have Meredith's willowy figure, the delicate bones of her face, long artistic hands. Meredith cut her hair short and set it, but Mum has always left hers natural, and Beth's is long, unchecked. And they have an air about them, which I lack. Grace, I suppose it is. I take more after our father. Shorter, broader, clumsier too. Dad and I stub our toes. We catch our sleeves on door handles, knock our wine glasses over, bruise ourselves on coffee table edges, chair legs, worktops. I have a huge affection for this trait, since it comes from him.

We drink coffee and admire the Christmas tree that came yesterday and now towers up into the stairwell. All the decorations we bought weren't quite enough. They look a little lost on such vast branches. But the lights twinkle and the resinous smell of it reaches every corner of the house, a constant reminder of the season.

'Bit extravagant, isn't it, love?' Dad asks Beth, who tips her eyebrows, dismissively.

'The house needed cheering up. For Eddie,' she says.

'Ah well, yes, fair enough,' Dad concedes. He's wearing a red jumper; grey hair standing up in tufts just like Eddie's does, and the hot coffee flushing his cheeks pink. He looks jovial, kind—just as he is.

There's a thump on the door, which I open to find Eddie and Harry on the step, out of breath, as ever, and damp.

'Hi, Rick! I came to say hello to Grandma and Grandpa. And I told Harry he could come and see the tree. That's OK, isn't it?'

'Of course it's OK, but kick those boots off before you take another step!'

Eddie is hugged, kissed, questioned. Dad proffers a hand to Harry for him to shake, but Harry just looks at it, bemused. He drifts over to the tree instead, crouches down to gaze up into it, as if trying to see it at its biggest, its most imposing. Dad shoots me a quizzical look and I mouth, *I'll tell you later*. We decide to keep Eddie, since lunch is not far off, and send Harry home with a box of Beth's mince pies, which he dips into even as he shambles off across the lawn.

'He seems a funny old thing,' Mum says mildly.

'He's wicked. He knows all the best places to go in the woods—where to find mushrooms and badgers' nests,' Eddie defends his friend.

'Badgers have setts, not nests, Eddie; and I hope you haven't been playing with fungi—that's really very dangerous!' Mum says. I see Eddie bridle.

'Harry knows which ones you can eat,' he mutters, defensively.

'I'm sure he does. It's fine, Mum,' I say, to quieten her. 'Old people don't know that wicked means good,' I whisper to Eddie. He rolls his eyes, escapes up the stairs to get changed.

'It's good for him, to have such an outdoor friend. He spends so much time cooped up at school,' Beth says firmly.

Mum raises a hand. 'I meant no criticism! Lord knows you two spent enough time out in the woods with Dinny when you came to stay here.'

'You didn't mind, though, did you?' Beth asks anxiously. She is all the more sensitive now to the slights of children against their parents. Mum and Dad exchange a glance, and Dad gives Mum a fond smile.

'No, not really, I suppose,' Mum says. 'It might have been nice if you'd wanted to spend a bit more time with us . . .' In the shocked pause after she says this, Beth and I exchange a guilty look and Mum laughs. 'It's fine, girls! It was the beginnings of my empty nest syndrome, that's all.'

'I don't know what I'll do when Eddie goes off to university. It's bad enough now that he boards all week,' Beth murmurs, folding her arms.

'You'll miss him like mad, you'll spoil him rotten when he comes down, and you'll find a new hobby—just like all mothers do, darling,' Mum tells her, putting an arm around her bony shoulders.

'It's a long way off yet, anyway,' I remind her. 'He's only eleven, after all.'

'Yes, but five seconds ago he was a tiny baby!' Beth says.

'They grow up fast,' Dad nods. 'And be happy about it, Beth! After six years of having a teenage boy around the house, I expect you'll be thrilled to have him go off to study!'

'And just think of all the fun stages you've got before then—the arguments about curfews, and driving lessons, and first girlfriends staying over. Finding porno mags under his bed . . . peering into his dazed eyes in the morning and wondering what drugs he took the night before . . .'

'Erica! Really!' Mum admonishes me, as Beth's eyes grow wide with horror.

'Sorry.' I smile.

'Rick, I think you've been teaching too long,' Dad chuckles. Beth raises her eyebrows at me.

'Smug aunt syndrome—that's your problem.

You get to watch me go through all of this and laugh into your sleeve as I get it all wrong and tear out my hair,' she says accusingly.

'Come on, Beth. I'm joking. You've never put a foot wrong as a mother,' I tell her, rushing on before a pause can form, before we all remember the huge wrong stride she took, not too long ago. 'Come and have some mince pies—Beth's outdone herself with them.'

Later on, I show Mum the photographs I've found for her. She identifies the people I didn't recognise—more distant relatives, people now dead, faded away, leaving only their faces on paper and traces of their blood in our veins. I show her the one of Caroline, taken in New York with the baby cradled in her left arm. Mum frowns as she scrutinises it.

'Well, that's definitely Caroline—such pale eyes! She was striking, wasn't she?'

'But what was she doing in New York? And whose baby is it, if she only married Lord Calcott in 1904? Do you think they had one before they got married?'

'What do you mean, what was she doing in New York? She was *from* New York!'

'Caroline? She was American? How can nobody have told me that before?'

'Well, how can you not have realised? With that accent of hers . . .'

'Mum, I was five years old. How would I have noticed her accent? And she was ancient by then. She hardly spoke at all.'

'True, I suppose,' Mum nods.

'Well, that explains why she was in New York in 1904. So, who's the baby?' I press. Mum takes a deep breath, inflates her cheeks.

'No idea,' she says. 'There's no way she could have had a child with Henry before they wed, even if that wouldn't have caused a huge scandal. She only met him late in 1904, when she came over to London. They married in 1905, soon after they met.'

'Well, was she married before? Did she bring the baby over with her?'

'No, I don't think so. You really would be better off asking Mary. As far as I know, Caroline came over from New York, a rich heiress at the age of around twenty-one or twenty-two, married a titled man at quite some speed, and that was that.'

I nod, oddly disappointed.

'Perhaps it was a friend's baby. Perhaps she was its godmother. Who knows?' Mum says.

'Could have been,' I agree. I take the picture back, study it closely. My eyes seek out Caroline's left hand, her ring finger, but it's hidden in the folds of the ghostly child's dress. 'Do you mind if I keep this one? Just for a while?' I ask.

'Of course not, love.'

'I've . . . been reading some of her letters. Caroline's letters,' I am strangely reluctant to confess this. Like reading somebody's diary, even after they're dead. 'Have you got that family tree? There was a letter from an Aunt B.'

'Here you are. Caroline's side of things is a bit sketchy, I'm afraid. I think Mary was more interested in the Calcott line—and all of Caroline's family records would have been in America, of course.' There is nothing, in fact, on Caroline's side, except the names of her parents. No aunts or uncles, a very small twig to one side before

221

Caroline joined the main tree in 1905. Caroline Fitzpatrick, as she was then.

I study her name for some time, waiting, although I'm not sure what for.

'In this letter, her aunt—Aunt B—says that whatever happened in America should stay in America, and she shouldn't do anything to mess up her marriage to Lord Calcott. Do you know anything about that?' I ask. Mum shakes her head.

'No. Nothing at all, I fear.'

'What if she did have a baby before she came over here and got married?'

'Well, for one thing she wouldn't have managed to get married if she had! Well brought up girls did not just have babies out of wedlock back then. It would have been unthinkable.'

'But what if she did get married to someone else before Lord Calcott? I found something up in the loft—in the trunk where Meredith put all of Caroline's stuff—and it says *To a Fine Son* on it,' I say.

Mum raises her eyebrows a little, considers. 'It was probably Clifford's. What kind of something?'

'I don't know—it's some kind of bell. I'll fetch it down later and show you.'

We have drifted into the drawing room. Mum picks up each photo from the piano and studies it at length, her face hung between expressions. She runs her thumb over the glass of Charles and Meredith's wedding portrait. A futile little caress.

'Do you miss her?' I ask. Normally a stupid question when somebody's mother dies. But Meredith was different.

'Of course. Yes, I do. It would be hard not to miss somebody who knew how to fill a room quite the way my mother did.' Mum smiles, puts the photo down, wipes her fingermarks away with the soft cuff of her cardigan.

'Why was she like that? I mean, why was she so . . . *angry*?'

'Caroline was cruel to her,' Mum shrugs. 'Not physically, or even verbally . . . perhaps not even deliberately; but who can say what damage is done when a child grows up unloved?'

'I can't imagine. I can't imagine how a mother could fail to love her child. But, *how* was she cruel to her?'

'Just in a thousand and one little ways,' Mum sighs, thinks for a moment. 'For example, Caroline never brought her a present. Not once. Not on birthdays or at Christmas, even when Meredith was small. Not on her wedding day, not when I was born. Nothing at all. Can you imagine how something like that might . . . chip away at you?'

'But if she'd never had a present, perhaps she didn't know to expect one?'

'Every child knows about birthday presents, Erica—you've only to read a storybook to learn about them. And the staff used to get her little things when she was small—Mother told me how much they meant to her. A rabbit—I remember her mentioning that. One year, the housekeeper gave her a pet rabbit.'

'That's . . . really sad,' I say. 'Didn't Caroline believe in presents?'

'I just don't think she was aware of the date, most of the time. I honestly don't think she knew when Meredith's birthday was. It was as though she hadn't given birth to her at all.'

'But if Caroline was so awful, why was Meredith

so devoted to her? Why did she move back here with you and Clifford when your father died?'

'Well, difficult or not, Caroline was her mother. Meredith loved her, and she was always trying to . . . prove herself to her.' Mum shrugs sadly, opens the piano lid and presses the top note. It floats out, fills the room, in perfect tune. 'We were never allowed to play this piano. Not until we'd reached a certain standard. We had that battered old upright in the nursery to practise on instead. Clifford never did get good enough, but I did. Just before I went away to university.'

'There are lots of letters from Meredith in Caroline's things. They all sound rather sad, as if she was always more or less by herself—even when she was married.'

'Well,' Mum sighs. 'I don't remember my father, so I don't know how things were before he died. She loved him, very much I think. Perhaps too much. Caroline once said to me that losing love like that left a hole you could never fill. I remember it clearly because she so rarely spoke to me. Or to Clifford—she hardly seemed to notice us children at all. I'd been watching Mum out in the garden, and I jumped when she spoke because I hadn't heard her sneak up behind me.'

'She could still walk, then?'

'Of course she could! She wasn't always ancient.'

'But why didn't Caroline love Meredith? I don't understand.'

'Neither do I, dear. Your great-grandmother was a very strange woman. Very distant. Sometimes I would go and sit next to her and try to talk to her, but I soon realised she wasn't listening to a word I said. She would just stare right through you, with those grey eyes of hers. No wonder Meredith married so soon—she must have been thrilled to find somebody who would listen to her!'

'It's amazing how normal you are. What a great mother you are.'

'Thank you, Erica. Your father helped, of course. My knight in shining armour! If I'd moved back here after my degree, if I'd stayed here long enough to resent them both . . . who knows?'

'Perhaps not everyone is cut out for parenthood. I can't imagine Meredith was the cuddliest . . .'

'No, but she was a good mother, for the most part. Strict, of course. But she wasn't as . . . sharp when we were small, as she was after we'd been living back here for a few years. As Caroline grew frail, she needed a lot of looking after. I think Mother resented that. She did her best for us, but I don't think she got over losing my father, or the disappointment of having life begin and end here—she and Caroline, cooped up in this old house. But we turned out OK, didn't we? Clifford and I?' she asks me, her face shaped with sudden sadness. I cross the room, hug her.

'More than OK.'

'I've come to collect some kisses!' Dad announces, finding us, brandishing mistletoe and a grin.

* * *

After dinner we put all our presents under the tree. Eddie looks like a miniature gent in his navy blue monogrammed dressing gown, stripy pyjamas and red felt slippers. He checks the gift tags and positions each parcel carefully, according to some private scheme. We drink brandy, listen to carols. Outside the rain is lashing at the house in waves. It sounds like handfuls of gravel, thrown against the windowpanes. It makes me shiver.

Sometime around midnight the rain stops, the clouds roll away, and a bright moon bedazzles the night sky. It lights the green paper vines climbing the walls in my room, the single wardrobe, the arched window looking east over the driveway. There's a rookery in the naked chestnut tree outside, the nests like clots in the twiggy branches. I can't get to sleep. My brain scrambles to life each time I start to drift, sending up a starburst of faces and names and memories to confound me. Brandy does this to me sometimes. I have to unpick each thought from the knotted mess, work it loose from my mind and let it float away. I keep the memories of Dinny, though; I don't let them go. New ones I've made, to add to the well-worn, sunshine ones. Now I know how he looks in winter light, in rain. I know how he looks in firelight. I know how alcohol takes him; I know how he makes a living, how he lives. I know how that wide, lazy childhood smile has grown up, changed, become a quick flash of teeth in the darkness of his face. I know he resents us, Beth and me. And soon, perhaps, I might begin to understand why.

*   *   *

Christmas morning passes in a rushed, comforting haze of food preparation, champagne and piles of torn shiny paper. Dad helps Eddie unpack his new games console, and they experiment with it on the inadequate television in the study while we women occupy the kitchen. The turkey barely fits into the Rayburn. We have to poke its legs in, and the tips of them blacken where they touch the sides.

'Never mind. Everyone prefers breast, anyway,' Mum says to Beth, who waves a nervous hand through the tendrils of smoke rising from the oven. It will take hours to roast and, pleading a slight headache, Beth retires to lie down. She shoots us a mute, angry glance as she goes. She knows we will talk about her now. I don't know if she sleeps at such times or if she just lies there, reading wisdom in the cracks in the ceiling, watching spiders enmesh the light shade. I hope she sleeps.

Mum and I slide ourselves onto the kitchen benches, link hands across the table, our conversation hanging awkwardly around the urge to talk about Beth. I break the silence.

'I found a load of newspaper clippings in with the photos in one of Meredith's drawers. About Henry,' I add, unnecessarily. Mum sighs, withdraws her hands from mine.

'Poor Henry,' she says, and strokes her fingers over her forehead, brushing back an imaginary hair.

'I know. I've been thinking about him a lot. About what happened—'

'What do you mean, about what happened?' Mum asks sharply. I look up from the thumbnail I was picking.

'Just, that he vanished. His disappearance,' I say. 'Oh.'

'Why? What do you think happened to him?'

'I don't know! Of course I don't know. I thought, for a while that . . . that perhaps you girls knew more than you were saying . . .'

'You think we had something to do with it?'

'No, of course not! I thought that, maybe, you were protecting somebody.'

'You mean Dinny.' Something flares inside me.

'Yes, all right then, Dinny. He had a temper, your young hero. But, Erica, Henry vanished! He was taken, I'm sure of it. Somebody took him, carried him off and that was the end of it. If anything had happened to him here on the estate, anything at all, then the police would have found some evidence of it. He was taken away, and that's all there is to it,' she finishes, calm again. 'It was a terrible, terrible thing, but nobody is to blame except the person who took him. There are just a few very dangerous people out there, and Henry was unlucky enough to meet one of them.'

'I suppose he was,' I say. None of this rings true to me. None of it convinces me. Eddie by the pond, throwing a stone; and that watery ache in my knees.

'Let's not talk about it today, shall we?'

'OK, then.'

'How has Beth been?'

'Not great. A bit better now. We went to a party at the camp the other night, and she chatted to Dinny a bit; and she seemed to pick up a little. And now that you and Dad are here too . . .'

'You went to a *party* with *Dinny*?' Mum sounds incredulous.

'Yes. So what?'

'Well,' she shrugs, 'it just seems so odd, after all these years. Taking up with him again . . .'

'We're not *taking up with him*. But we are neighbours now. For the time being, anyway. He's . . . well. He's not really much different, and neither am I, so . . .' For a terrifying moment, I think I will blush.

'He was so in love with Beth, you know. Back when they were twelve,' Mum says, staring into the past and smiling. 'They say you never forget your first love.'

I down the last of my champagne, get up to fetch the bottle. The heat of my blush remains, moves up to my nose, threatens to become tears. 'Come on. These spuds won't peel themselves!' I smile, proffering a paring knife at her.

'How long will Beth rest for?'

'A hour, perhaps. Long enough to dodge the potato peeling, that's for certain.'

*   *   *

My eyes strain against the gathering dark. It's not yet five o'clock but my feet are indistinct. They snag on tufts and twigs and roots that I can't see. I've come to fetch Eddie. I make a pass of the camp but all is quiet. I am still not sure who each vehicle belongs to, and they look so tight, so closed up against the world that I am too afraid to go knocking on doors, asking for Harry. I cut into the woods but the darkness is even deeper here. I should have brought a torch. Night is coming fast; the light feels exhausted.

'Eddie!' I call, but it's a pathetic sound. I can see the strict formations of the search teams, going through these woods twenty-three years ago. Five days after he vanished, but still they kept trying. Their faces grim; the dogs pulling at their leads. The crackle and click of CB radios. *Henry!* Their shouts were loud and clear but stilted even so, as if self-conscious, as if knowing the name was hurled in vain, would only reach their own ears. The weather was foul that weekend—it was the August bank holiday, after all. The tail end of Hurricane Charley, lashing Britain with wind and rain. *'Eddie!'* I try again, as loudly as I can. The quiet, when my clumsy feet go still, is astounding.

I come out of the woods beyond the dew pond. The barrow is a vague growth on the horizon. I skirt the edge of the field, along the fence, back towards the house, and slowly I see figures coming into being by the water. Two large, one small. I heave a lungful of air, feel a chill slide down my back. I had not known how afraid I was. Harry, Eddie, Dinny. They could be the three protagonists of a boy's own story, and here they are, at the dew pond. Skimming stones in the near dark on Christmas Day.

'Who's that?' Eddie says, when they notice me. His voice sounds high, childish.

'It's me, you muppet,' I say, mocking my own fear at his expense.

'Oh, hi, Rick,' he says. Harry gives an odd hoot—the first real sound I have heard him make. He runs around the water's edge to me—big clumsy strides. I hold my breath, wait for him to slip, stumble in, but he doesn't. He presents me with a small stone, flat, almost triangular. I can just about see his smile.

'He wants you to have a go,' Dinny says. I walk carefully around to them. I turn the stone over in my hand. It is warm, smooth.

'I came to get Eddie. It's time he was in—it's pitch black out here,' I say to Dinny. I feel prickly, endangered. The water is nothing but a blackness at our feet.

'You just need to give your eyes time to adjust, that's all,' Dinny tells me, as the others go back to their stones, the flat black water, the counting of white blooms in the gloaming.

'Still, we should go back. My parents are here . . .'

'Oh? Tell them hello from me.'

'Yes, I will.' I stand next to him, close enough for our sleeves to touch. I don't care if I am crowding him. I need something near enough to catch, something to anchor me. I can hear him breathing, hear the shape he makes in the echoes from the pond.

'Aren't you going to skim that stone?' He sounds wryly amused by the idea.

'I can hardly see the water.'

'So? You know it's there.' He looks sideways at me. Just a silhouette, and I want to put my hands on his face, to feel if he's smiling.

'Well, here goes.' I creep to the edge, find a firm footing. I crouch, swing my arm, and when I let go of the stone I follow it, towards the surface, towards the obsidian water. *One, two, three* . . . I count the splashes and then I stumble, my vision skids vertiginously, my feet slide over the edge of the bank and I gasp. What a place, I have sent that innocent stone to—what darkness.

'Three! Rubbish! Harry got a seven a little while ago!' Eddie calls to me. I feel Dinny's hands under my arms, the reassuring weight of him pulling me to my feet. Panic fluttering in my chest.

'Not a great night for swimming, I think,' Dinny murmurs. I shake my head, glad he can't see my face, the tears in my eyes.

'Come on, Eddie, we're going in,' I say. A ragged

edge to my voice.

'But I've just . . .'

'Now, Eddie!' He sighs, solemnly presents Harry with the rest of his stones. They make a warm, cheerful noise as they change palms. I walk away from the edge, back towards the house.

'Erica,' Dinny calls to me. I turn, and he hesitates. 'Happy Christmas,' he says. I can tell this is not what he had intended to say, and even though I wonder, I don't feel strong enough to ask right now.

'Happy Christmas, Dinny,' I reply.

LOSING

1903–1904

The summer swelled and Magpie's body ripened in time with it, seeming to expand by the day as her baby grew. She moved with an odd grace, as purposefully as ever but never suddenly, neatly angling her new width around the furniture and through the narrow door of the dugout she shared with Joe. Caroline watched her. She watched, and she wondered, her heart full of suspicions that she went from discrediting to confirming to herself twenty times a day. And more than anything, she was jealous. She felt sick and weak and full of something dark and bitter each time she saw the growing inches of the Indian girl's body. And if anything could have driven her from the house and out into the summer sun, it was this.

The wooden house just could not keep out the heat as the thick brownstone walls of New York had done. And, Caroline reflected, when it was hot in New York, it was never as hot as this, and she had never before had to be active in such temperatures. But Magpie's composure and Hutch's exhortation to her at new year were at work upon Caroline's mind; so one day, which dawned slightly overcast and a little cooler than usual, she decided to get out of the house. She packed a basket with a newly ripe melon, some biscuits and a bottle of tonic water, tied the ribbon of her sun bonnet in a bow beneath her chin, and set off for the nearest neighbouring farm, which belonged to an Irish family called Moore. It was six miles to the north-west and Caroline, who had no idea what it felt like to walk six miles, had nonetheless overheard Corin say that a man might easily walk four miles in an hour. Setting off early, she thought, she would be there in time to take coffee and maybe a bite of lunch, and then back again in plenty of time to help cook dinner. She told Magpie where she was going, and squared her shoulders when the Ponca girl gave her a level, incredulous stare and blinked slowly, like an owl.

She walked for an hour, at first admiring the flowers on the horse-mint and wild verbena and gathering a posy to present to the Moores, but soon found the basket a dead weight on her arm, bruising her skin. She was slick with sweat in spite of the clouds, and felt it prickling her scalp underneath her hat. Her skirts were fouled up and wadded together with sandburs and thistle barbs, and they swung ponderously around her legs, tripping her. The sandy ground, which undulated gently, pulled at her feet and was more strenuous to walk across than she'd thought. She battled slowly up a long rise, certain that from the crest of it she would see the neighbouring farm. She could not. Breathing hard, she saw the landscape roll away into the distance, as far as the eye could see. Putting the basket down, she turned in a slow circle, staring into the unbroken horizon. A hot wind blew, making waves in the long grass that looked, in the distance, like a green and gold ocean. The wind carried the scent of dry earth and sagebrush and it moaned a low note in her ears.

'There's nothing here,' Caroline murmured to herself. Something rose up in her then, something like panic, or anger. 'There's *nothing here*!' she shouted, as loudly as she could. Her throat felt raw and dry. The wind snatched her words away, and gave her no answer. She sank onto the prairie and lay back to rest. An endless sky above her, and endless land all around. If she did not rise again, she thought, if she stayed where she was, only wild dogs and buzzards would ever find her. It was an irresistible thought, a terrifying one.

Walking back at last, having never reached the Moore's place, Caroline nearly missed the ranch. She had veered to the north by a mile or more and only happened by chance to see smoke rising from the chuck hut to her right, where a silent Louisiana Negro called Rook would be cooking dinner for the ranch hands. Turning south, Caroline's legs wobbled with exhaustion. Her mouth was parched and her face, after a day in the harsh light and hot wind, was tight and stinging. Behind her she could feel the vastness of the prairie spreading out, watching, and beyond the ranch the grasslands stretched away to every point on the compass. The corrals, fences, wheat and sorghum fields her husband had mapped onto the land were pitifully small. The ranch was an island, a tiny atoll of civilisation in an endless patchy sea, and when she finally reached the house, gasping for breath and scattering wilted flowers behind her, she shut the door and burst into tears.

*   *   *

That night Caroline lay awake, in spite of her exhaustion. The clouds cleared as night fell, and the moon rose luminously full. It was not this that kept her awake, but the knowledge, the new understanding of how vast and empty the land she now lived upon truly was. She felt swallowed up by it; tiny, invisible. She wanted to grow, to expand, to take up more space somehow. She wanted to be significant. The air inside the bedroom was smothering, thick with the lassitude of summer. Beside her, Corin snored softly, his face pressed into the pillow, arms flung out to his sides. The moon caught the contours of the muscles in his arms and shoulders, and the sharp line where the tan of his neck became the pale of his back. Caroline rose, took a spare blanket and went outside.

She spread the blanket amongst the fecund orbs of the watermelons and lay down upon it. Something scuttled away into the foliage close to her face, and she shuddered. There were no other sounds, though her ears strained to pick up any movement from the bunkhouse, any sign of an approaching ranch hand. Then she pulled her nightdress up until it covered only her breasts, leaving the lower portion of her body bare to the night sky. Her hipbones stood proud, casting shadows of their own in the silvery light. Her heart beat fast in her chest, and she did not shut her eyes. Stars scattered the sky. She began to count them, lost her place and started again, and again; losing all idea of how long she had lain there and where on earth she was. Then the door banged behind her and she heard uneven steps, and Corin grabbed her beneath her arms and pulled her into his lap.

'What is it? What's wrong?' Caroline gasped. Painted in greys and blacks, Corin's face was pinched with fear and his eyes were wide. Seeing her awake and well Corin let her go, exhaling heavily, and put his face into his hands.

'What are you doing out here?' he mumbled. 'Are you all right?'

'I'm . . . fine. I just . . . it was so hot in the bedroom . . .' Caroline hurriedly pulled her nightdress down.

'But it's just as hot out here! What are you doing—why were you naked?' he demanded. Alarmed, Caroline saw that he was shaking. She bit her lip and looked away.

'Moonbathing,' she said.

'What?'

'I was moonbathing . . . Angie told me it might help,' Caroline said quietly. She had sneered inwardly at such superstition when their neighbour first mentioned it, but now it seemed she would try anything.

'Help with what? Love, you're not making sense!'

'Help a woman to get pregnant. To lie with the moon shining on her body,' Caroline said, shamefacedly.

'And you believed her?'

'No, not really. Not really. It's just . . . *why* aren't I pregnant yet, Corin? It's been over a year!' she cried. 'I don't understand.'

'I don't understand it either,' Corin sighed. 'But I'm sure these things happen when they're good and ready, that's all. A year is not that long! You're young and . . . it's been a big upheaval for you, moving out here to be with me. It *will* happen love, please try not to worry.' He tipped her chin up with his fingertips. 'Come back inside now.'

'Corin . . . why were you so afraid just now?' Caroline asked, as she rose stiffly to her feet.

'What? When?'

'Just now, when you found me out here. You looked so alarmed! Why? What did you think had happened?'

'There was a woman, on the other side of Woodward a couple of years ago . . . never mind. I just thought something might have happened to you. But you're fine, and it's nothing to worry about . . .' Corin reassured her.

'Tell me, please,' she pressed, sensing his reluctance. 'What happened to the woman?'

'Well, apparently she felt the heat badly, like you do too, and she was also pining for her home back in France, and she took to sleeping out in the yard to keep cool, but one night . . . one night she . . .' His fingers grasped the night air, searching for a way to tell her without telling her.

'She what?'

'She cut her own throat,' he said, in a rush. 'Three children waiting for her indoors and all.' Caroline swallowed convulsively, her own throat closing at the thought of such violence.

'And you thought I'd . . . done that to myself?' she breathed.

'No! No, love, no. I was just worried for you, that's all.' He ushered her back into the bedroom and said he would wait up until she slept, but soon his soft snores began again, and still Caroline's eyes stayed fixed upon the ceiling.

She wondered. She wondered where Corin went all day. It had never occurred to her to think about this before. He always gave an account of his day over the supper table, but how could she know that he was telling it true? How could she know how long it took to round up strays, to pursue rustlers, to brand the new steers, to set the stallion Apache to a brood mare, to mend fences, to plough or sow or reap the wheat fields, or cut hay, or do any of it? And Corin could, of course, send Joe anywhere if he wanted him out of the way. And Magpie had often already left, by an hour or so, before Corin came in for the evening. There were times, plenty of times, when she had no idea where either of them might be. And the way he had touched Magpie, that time—the way he had put his hands on her at the Woodward gala. These were Caroline's thoughts as she lay awake, and as she sat in the ringing silence at the end of each day, waiting for Corin's return. When Caroline saw her husband, her fears vanished. When she was alone, they flourished like weeds. Her solace was Magpie's plainness, as she saw it. The coarseness of her hair, the fat on her figure, the alien planes of her face. She noted these things and called to mind Corin's praise of her own beauty.

But one hard August day when a high, spiteful sun was bleaching the grassland, even this solace was taken from Caroline. Magpie was at the kitchen window, standing sideways so that she could lean her hip against the bench as she peeled carrots with a short, sharp blade. She was singing, as usual, her expression soft and her hands busy. Caroline watched her through the doorway from the main room, from behind a book she was supposedly reading, and a falter in the quiet song made her blink. Magpie stopped peeling, her gaze falling out of focus and one hand going to her distended belly. A tiny smile twitched her lips and then the song and the work continued. The baby had shifted, Caroline realised. It was awake, alive inside the girl. It was listening to its mother singing. Swallowing, Caroline put her hand to her own stomach. It was more than flat, it was concave; there was no welcoming fold of flesh, no fulsome vitality. She could feel her ribs and her hipbones, wooden and sharp. How dry and hard and dead her body seemed, compared to Magpie's. Like the dead husks, the chaff that the men beat out of the wheat. She looked at the girl again, and then her throat went tight and for a second she couldn't breathe. The sun streaming in through the window caught the gloss of Magpie's thick, black hair; the wide, bowed curve of her top lip; the high slant of her cheeks and eyes; the warm glow of her skin. Magpie was beautiful.

Before dawn the next day, as Corin stirred and began to wake, Caroline went on soft feet to the kitchen. She poured him a cup of cold tea and cut two thick slices of bread from yesterday's loaf, which she spread with honey. She presented him with these offerings as he sat up, blinking in the charcoal glow of near-day.

'Breakfast in bed. I always used to have breakfast in bed on Saturdays,' she told him, smiling.

'Well, thank you. How grand I feel!' Corin cupped her face in the palm of his hand, and took a long draught of the tea. Caroline propped the pillows up against the wall behind him.

'Sit back for a moment, love. You don't have to rush out just yet,' she urged him.

'Putting off a chore never got it finished faster,' he sighed, ruefully.

'Just five more minutes,' she begged. 'Try some of the bread. I spread it with that honey Joe collected for us.'

'That man is a marvel with bees,' Corin nodded. 'I've never seen anything like it. Just walks right up to the nest and puts in his arm, and never once takes a sting.'

'Some Indian magic, perhaps?'

'Either that or he's just got the toughest hide of any man alive,' Corin mused. Caroline thought of this—of Joe with his unforgiving black eyes and skin like the bark of a tree. She shuddered slightly, wondering how Magpie could bear to bed herself with him.

'Corin?'

'Yes?'

'You know, it's been more than a year now since we were wed and, well . . . we never have been back to go swimming again, like on our honeymoon.'

'I know. I know it, Caroline. It's so hard to find the time,' Corin said, leaning his head back against the wall, his face still languid with sleep.

'Can we go? Soon? I just . . . I want to spend the day with you. The whole day . . . we hardly ever do that! Not with all the work you have to do.'

'Well, I don't know, Caroline. There's just so much to do at this time of year! We've got the stupidest bunch of beeves as I've ever had on the ranch and they've been busting through the fences every chance they get, wandering off and getting themselves stuck in the creek and caught up in wire and I don't know what else. Maybe in a week. In a week or two . . . how about that?'

'You promised me we would,' she said quietly.

'And we will. We will,' he insisted.

Soon afterwards he rose, pulled himself into his clothes, stroked one hand gently over Caroline's hair and kissed the top of her head before going through to the kitchen to make coffee. Caroline sat and listened to the rattle of the coffee beans, the clang of the kettle hitting the stove, and she felt a peculiar weariness wash over her. For a moment, she did not think she had the strength to rise, to see another day through to its end. Every bone in her body seemed leaden. But she drew in a long breath, and she stood, and began to dress herself slowly.

*   *   *

At the end of September, Joe appeared at the house one wet afternoon, his hat in his hands, eyes half shut against the steady downpour and an air of impenetrable calm about him. Caroline smiled, but she could not help but draw back from him, and she saw a hardening in his eye when she did this.

'Magpie's time is come. She asks for you to go there,' Joe said.

'To go where? Why?' Caroline said, not understanding.

'To go to her. To help the baby,' Joe explained, in his guttural accent. His tone was as neutral as his expression, but something told Caroline that he did not necessarily approve of his wife's request. She hesitated, and felt her pulse quicken. She would have to go inside the dugout. However used to having Magpie around the house Caroline had become, she could not help thinking of that low, half-submerged dwelling as some kind of animal's den.

'I see,' she said quietly. 'I see.'

'In this way, she honours you,' Joe told her solemnly. 'Such work is only for family.'

After a hung pause, pinned by Joe's inscrutable gaze, Caroline went back inside. She squashed her hat onto her hair, took off her apron and felt panic rising like bubbles in her throat. She had no knowledge of birth, no idea what she should do to help. She was not sure that she wanted to help at all.

Outside, Joe showed the first and only sign of impatience Caroline had ever seen any of the Ponca show. He repositioned his hat in his hands and looked over his shoulder towards where his wife lay in labour. Seeing this, Caroline felt a stab of guilt and she hurried out, turning her face to the ground as they went so that she would not see the terrifying spread of land around them. Ever since her abortive walk to the Moore's farm, she had felt a dizzying horror of the gaping landscape of Woodward County. The expanse of it seemed to pull her thoughts apart, building an unbearable pressure behind her eyes. She felt the urge to run, to throw herself back indoors before she disintegrated into the mighty sky. Their footsteps splashed and Caroline's hem was soon soaked with water, stained ruddy from the soil.

Three steps led down into the dugout, and they dropped into a soft, warm darkness lit by a kerosene lamp that battled against the gloom outside and in. There was a strong smell, made up of smoke from the stove, animal hides, and herbs that Caroline could not identify. The blood thumped at her temples as she felt all eyes turn to her—Magpie's, White Cloud's, and those of Joe's sister, Annie. Joe himself stayed outside and disappeared into the rain. Magpie's face was slick with sweat, her eyes wide and fearful. The other women's expressions were cautious; not unfriendly, but reserved.

'Joe . . . said I should come. He said you had . . . had . . . asked for me to come?' Caroline stammered. Magpie nodded and smiled slightly before her body convulsed, and she ground her teeth together, an expression that made her look savage. 'What should I do? I don't know what I should do!' Caroline quailed. White Cloud said something rapid in the Ponca language and handed Caroline a small wooden pail, filled with rainwater, and a clean cloth. The old woman motioned dipping the cloth into the water, and then pressed her hand against her forehead, gesturing to Magpie. Caroline nodded and knelt beside the labouring girl, wiping her drenched face with the cool water, afraid, as she performed this intimate duty, that the girl would somehow see into her troubled heart.

In the semi-dark, White Cloud began to sing a soft monotonous song that lulled them all; lulled Caroline so that she had no idea how much time was passing, whether hours or minutes or days. The words were blurred and dry, and the song sounded to Caroline's ears like the long, drawn-out rush of the warm prairie wind, lonely and reverent. As regularly as waves on the shore, Magpie heaved against the pain inside her, screwing up her eyes and baring her teeth. She looked as feral as a cat, but she did not cry out. On and on these waves came, as the darkness deepened outside; and on and on White Cloud sang, mixing up a pungent drink that she gave to Magpie gradually, a spoonful at a time. Then, with a low sound in her throat like a strangled growl, Magpie's baby arrived into Annie's waiting hands, and White Cloud broke off her song with a sharp cry of joy, her wizened face breaking into a wide grin, and then into laughter. Caroline smiled with relief, but as Annie passed the wriggling, whimpering baby boy to its mother, she felt a splinter pierce her heart and lodge there. Tears sprang to her eyes and she looked away to hide them, seeing, in a dark corner of the dugout, a pair of spurs on leather thongs. A pair Corin had been looking for and had asked if she had seen about the place. She stared at them, and the splinter wormed its way ever deeper.

*　　　*　　　*

Two months later, the baby was chubby and delightful. He was named, in the Ponca tongue, *first born son*; but called by his parents and so everybody else, William. He rode around the ranch in a sling on Magpie's back, gazing out at the world with an expression of mild astonishment in his round eyes. And he slept there in a crumpled little heap, dribbling down his chin, not stirring as Magpie returned to work in the main house, her body not at all fatigued by the child. The cold, like the heat, seemed to have little effect on the girl's spirits. She appeared at the house swathed in her thick, brightly patterned blanket, her cheeks burnished dark red by the wind and her eyes as bright as jet beads.

And although it hurt her to hold William,

Caroline often asked to do so. Like exploring a wound, or pressing a bruise. She cradled him in the crook of her arm and rocked him gently. He was a good-natured baby and did not cry for strangers. He had an array of fledgling facial expressions that melted her heart and eased the splinter from it. A tiny frown of puzzlement at the noises she made; the sagging of his mouth and eyes as sleep took hold; wide-eyed wonder when she showed him her peacock-feather fan. But the pain of handing him back to his proud mother was a little stronger each time, the hurt a little worse; and the only thing harder than this was watching Corin play with the baby, when he came in from working. His brown hands looked impossibly large around the tiny child's body, and he grinned foolishly when he managed, by tickling and mugging, to make William smile. Each time he succeeded in this endeavour he glanced at his wife, to share it with her, but Caroline found it hard to find the smile she knew he wanted. Seeing him love this child, this child that was not hers, was almost more than she could bear.

There was to be no christening for William, which surprised Caroline, even though it made sense. She fretted briefly about the danger to the child's soul, but Magpie only laughed when she tentatively suggested that it wouldn't hurt him to go through the ceremony, just in case.

'Our ancestors are watching him, Mrs Massey. You don't have to worry,' she smiled.

Awkwardly, Caroline dropped the subject. But she suggested that they hold a welcoming lunch for him instead, and Magpie agreed to this. Caroline sent out some invitations, but only Angie Fosset was willing to celebrate the birth of an Indian baby, and she turned up on her tall horse with the saddlebags full of cast-off baby smocks and napkins.

'I'm stopping at three, so I've no need of these any more,' she told Magpie. Caroline had sent Hutch into Woodward the week before to collect the gifts she had ordered for William from Corin and herself. Magpie accepted each present with increasing embarrassment, and the atmosphere over the party grew awkward.

'Mrs Massey . . . this is too much,' Magpie told her, her eyes troubled. Annie and White Cloud exchanged a look that Caroline could not read.

'Oh, my goodness, what lovely things!' Angie exclaimed.

'Well,' Caroline smiled, feeling suddenly exposed. 'A lovely little boy should have lovely things,' she said, but felt that they could all see into her heart—that these were gifts she had wanted to give her own baby, not Magpie's. She turned to William in his carrier to hide her dismay, stroking one finger down his crumpled, sleeping face. But this was worse. Her cheeks flared red and her breath caught in her chest. 'Who'd like some cake?' she asked tightly; getting up and fleeing into the kitchen.

*   *   *

Caroline's second winter on the prairie was harder than the first. The four walls of the house became her gaol, trapping her with Magpie and William— two constant reminders of how she failed, day after day. For if Magpie's return to work, her cheery demeanour and the ease with which she coped proved anything to Caroline, it was that she would never belong on the prairie like the Ponca girl did. She would never get on as well, never thrive, never settle, never put down roots here, but remain blown about the surface like tumble weed. She found it harder and harder to talk to Magpie, to sing and tell stories as they'd used to. The words stuck in her throat and she feared that even genuine expressions of admiration for Magpie, for William, would come out tainted with the grief she felt, and would sound insincere.

When Hutch came to the house for coffee he would push her gently to speak her mind, to come out riding again, to do anything but stay cooped up inside the house. Caroline assured him, absently, that she was fine, and all was well; and the foreman had no choice but to drift away again, a thoughtful look in his eye. When the confinement got unbearable, and Caroline did gather her courage and venture outside, the wind hit her skin like knives, and the sky rained terror down upon her and, once chilled, it took hours for her to get warm again, however close to the stove she huddled. As she broke the ice on the water cistern one morning and felt the splashes on her hands burning coldly, she remembered the warm water of the pool where they had swum on their honeymoon; and she gazed down into the dark depths of the tank, rooted to the spot by sadness.

At night, Caroline and Corin often lay awake as the wind howled around the house, too loud to ignore. Beneath the blankets one such night, he drew lazy patterns on her shoulder that both soothed and aroused her. The smell of him was so dear to her, strong and rank and animal after a day's work under heavy clothes. She clung to him like a drowning person clinging to a float, keeping her eyes tightly shut, feeling as though the house, at any moment, might give in to the onslaught and be torn away with them inside it. The house was a fiction, she thought; a flimsy carapace between them and the empty fury outside; and it might vanish in a heartbeat. As long as Corin was there, she told herself. As long as he was there with her she didn't care. He seemed to sense her fears and he spoke to calm them, the way she had heard him speak to nervous horses. His voice was low and she fought to hear it above the din—words rolling in a steady rhythm, like water trickling, half awake and half asleep.

'I guess we should spare a thought for White Cloud and Annie, although I know the Ponca are born to this life and they are stronger than we are, still I would not want to have nothing but hides between me and the wind on a night like this. Hutch has told me of the Great Die-Up, in the winter of eighty-seven, which was before I had come out west, and we two, you and I, were still in New York City, unbeknownst to one another. Every bad winter we have, every time I mention the cold he just shakes his head and says it's nothing, not compared to the Great Die-Up. Whole herds of cattle froze where they stood. Riders died out on the ranges and they weren't found until the spring, when the snow melted back and left them sitting high and dry, with their knees drawn up to their chests in the last pose they ever struck, just trying to keep warm. The beeves were all skinny and weak because the summer before that winter had been a droughty one and there was precious little grass or feed to be had. And they just died in their *droves*. And the cows lost their calves before they were due to birth them, because there was hardly enough to fill one mouth, let alone two; and Hutch himself lost three toes—two on his right foot and one on his left. He'd been out riding in a blizzard so thick he strained to see his horse's ears, trying to keep the cattle moving so they didn't just huddle up and freeze into one great heap of dead meat, and when he climbed off his horse at the end of the day he couldn't feel his legs, let alone his feet. He told me he didn't get his boots off until three days later, and by that time his feet were big and black and the blood had just frozen right there in his veins. And it's true, too; I've seen the gaps where those toes of his should be. There were snowstorms the likes of which had never been seen, nor have been since; from Mexico to Canada and everywhere in between, and I remember—don't you remember having no beef one year, when you were little? Perhaps you were too young, but I remember there being no beef in New York. Cook tried everything she could to get some each week but there was none to be had. Not with nigh on every poor beast on the ranges lying under a snowdrift. So this storm, this wind—well, like Hutch says, it's nothing, my darling. This is the prairie being sweet to us, Caroline. And we're warm, aren't we? And we're safe, too. How could we not be when we have each other?' He spoke like this, on and on through the ragged night, as hailstones hit the roof like lead shot; and Caroline drowsed on the edge of sleep, drinking in the steady words and feeling a cold ache in her feet for

Hutch's lost toes, a cold ache in her heart for cowboys hugging their knees to their chests, out in the sweet prairie wind.

*   *   *

By the spring of 1904 there seemed to be infants everywhere. Several of the mares had gangling foals running at their heels, the yard hens bobbed on a sea of fluffy chicks, William's howls could at times be heard in every far corner of the ranch, and a small wire-haired terrier belonging to Rook, the Negro cook, gave birth to a litter of blunt-nosed puppies following a chance encounter with a Woodward mongrel of uncertain provenance. The weather was turning warm again, the days longer. No more ice in the cistern, no more hailstorms and blue north winds. The young wheat and sorghum was pale green, and there was a brave scattering of blossom on Caroline's spindly cherry trees. But, try as she might, Caroline could not be rid of the weight of her dashed expectations, or her fear of the open land that her husband loved so much.

They sat outside on the porch one fair Sunday afternoon, after a travelling preacher had called by to read a service for all the ranch's inhabitants, and, because of the contentment she read in Corin's face, rocking gently in his chair, Caroline felt a hundred miles from him.

'What are you reading?' he asked her eventually, startling her because she had thought him asleep beneath his copy of *The Woodward Bulletin*. She smiled and raised the book so he could see the cover. 'What, *The Virginian* again? Don't you get tired of reading it?'

'A little. But it's one of my favourites, and until you take me to town to buy some others . . .' she shrugged.

'All right, all right. We'll go next week, how about that? Once Bluebell's foaled. You could always go by yourself, if you didn't want to wait for me? No harm would come to you—'

'You don't know that! I prefer to wait for you,' Caroline cut him off. Just the thought of striking out for Woodward alone was enough to turn her stomach.

'All right, then.' Corin retreated back beneath his paper. 'Read some of that one to me then. Let's find out what's so special about it.' Caroline looked at the page she had been reading. Nothing was that special about it, she thought. Nothing but that the heroine, a civilised lady of the East, had made such a life for herself, had found such happiness in the wilderness; had been able to see beauty that Caroline could not, and to understand her man as Caroline could not. Caroline scoured the pages as if the secret to this was hidden there somewhere, as if she might be taught how to settle in the West, how to love it, how to thrive. But the passage she had been reading described Molly Wood deciding to leave—the dark spell before that girl's sunshine happy ending, and Caroline hesitated before reading it out, sitting tall as she had been taught and holding the book high in front of her so her voice would not be hampered by a crooked neck.

'*This was the momentous result of that visit which the Virginian had paid her. He had told her that he was coming for his hour soon. From that hour she had decided to escape. She was running away from her own heart. She did not dare to trust herself face to face again with her potent, indomitable lover . . .'*

'My, what drama,' Corin murmured sleepily when Caroline finished, and she closed the book, running her hands over the cover which had become dog-eared and creased with rereading.

'Corin?' Caroline asked hesitantly, a while later when the sun was getting fat in the western sky. 'Are you awake?'

'Mmm . . .' came the drowsy reply.

'I come into my money soon, Corin. I know I told you before, but I . . . I didn't tell you how much money it is. It's . . . a lot of money. We could go anywhere you wanted . . . you won't have to work so hard any more . . .'

'Go somewhere? Why would we go anywhere?' he asked.

Caroline bit her lip. 'It's just . . . so isolated here—so far from town! We could . . . we could buy a house in Woodward, perhaps. I could spend some of the week there . . . Or we could move everything closer, move the whole ranch closer! I could . . . join the Coterie Club, perhaps . . .'

'What are you saying, Caroline? Of course I can't move the ranch closer to town! Cattle need open grasslands, and the land nearer town is all given over to homesteaders now.'

'But you won't need to raise cattle any more, don't you see? We'll have money—plenty of money!' she cried. Corin sat up and folded the newspaper. He looked at his wife and she recoiled from the pained expression on his face.

'If money was what I was interested in, I'd have stayed in New York. Sweetheart! This life is everything I've dreamed of since my father took me to Chicago when I was a boy and I saw Buffalo Bill Cody's 'Wild West and Congress of Rough Riders of the World' at the Columbian Exposition . . . That was when I decided to come out here with him, when he came looking for fresh suppliers. I watched those ropers and riders, and I knew that *this* was what I wanted to do with my life! Ranching isn't just a job for me . . . it's our life, and this is our home, and I can't think I'll ever want to move or live anywhere else. Is that what you want? Do you want to live somewhere else? Somewhere away from me, perhaps?' His voice caught when he asked this question and she looked up quickly, shocked to see tears waiting in the corners of his eyes.

'No! Of course not! *Never* away from you, Corin, it's just . . .'

'What is it?'

'Nothing. I just thought . . . perhaps I might be happier, to have a little more company. More refined society than I have here, perhaps. And . . . perhaps if I was happier, we might start a family at last.'

At this Corin looked away across the corrals and he seemed to consider for a long time. Caroline, thinking the discussion over, sank back into her chair and shut her eyes, sad to her core and exhausted by this attempt to voice her fears.

'We can build. We could use some of the money to double the size of the house, if you like, and get a maidservant, perhaps. A housekeeper to take over from Magpie now that she has William to look after . . . An electricity generator, maybe. And plumbing! A proper bathroom for you, with running water indoors . . . How about that? Would

254

that fix this?' Corin asked. He sounded so hurt, so desperate.

'Yes, perhaps. A bathroom would be lovely. Let's see when the money comes,' she said.

'And I'll take you to town very soon. We can stay the night, maybe even a couple of nights, if you like? Buy you as many books and magazines as we can carry back; and I need to go to Joe Stone's for some new spurs. I've been idiot enough to break my spare pair and I've still not yet laid hands on the original ones . . .'

'They're at Joe and Magpie's place. In the dugout,' Caroline told him tonelessly.

'What? How do you know?'

'I saw them in there, when I was helping with the birth.' Hating herself, Caroline watched him closely. For signs of guilt or embarrassment, or a telltale blush. Instead Corin smacked a palm to his forehead.

'Lord, of course! I loaned them to Joe, months and months ago! Way out towards the panhandle that day we chased those thieves down—his snapped and since Strumpet was behaving and that gelding of his was being a brute, I gave him my spurs. I never thought to ask for them back at the end of that long ride—I was that ready to fall down and sleep! Why didn't you say, if you saw them, love?'

'Well, I . . .' Caroline faltered, and shrugged. 'I . . . just forgot, that's all. The baby came and that was something of a distraction . . .' Corin sprang to his feet.

'You clever girl to remember them now! I'll go over and fetch them right away, before we both forget again,' he smiled, and strode away from the house. Caroline watched him go and then she put her face into her hands for all the times since William's birth that she'd pictured the spurs, lying there in Magpie's home; all the times she'd imagined the haste and the urgency with which they might have been discarded there, flung aside by passionate hands in the desire to reach that hidden, adulterous nest of blankets.

*　　　*　　　*

After her suggestion that they move to town, and as the second anniversary of their marriage approached, Caroline caught her husband watching her more closely—for signs of malaise, perhaps, or melancholia. He must have noticed, then, that she was increasingly quiet and visibly enervated, but there was little he could do about it. Caroline smiled when he asked after her, and assured him that she was quite well. She did not say that when she opened the door she felt as though she might fall out, might tumble into the gaping emptiness of the prairie without man-made structures to anchor her. She did not say that gazing into the distance made her heart wince and then bump against her ribs so loudly she was sure Magpie could hear it. She did not say that the sky was just too dizzyingly huge for her to look at. Only cradling William seemed to soothe her. She marvelled at his increasing strength as he struggled to reach for things, to grasp and chew her fingers. The movement of his small body against hers seemed to fill a dark and gaping hole inside her, and Magpie smiled to see the tender expression on her face. But Caroline always had to give the baby back to his mother, and each time she did the hole inside her returned.

The plants in the garden wilted and were choked beneath encroaching weeds. Unharvested vegetables split and rotted in the sun. Magpie agreed to take over the tending of the garden, but she too watched Caroline with a slight, appraising frown. She forced Caroline to oversee the pulling up of the spent winter plants and the rearrangement of the garden for summer crops.

'You must tell me what to plant, Mrs Massey. You must tell me where to plant,' the girl insisted, although they both knew that Magpie was by far the wiser in such matters. Caroline demurred, but the raven-haired Ponca girl, with calm insistence, would brook no argument. As Magpie dug and hoed, Caroline remained always in the shadow of the house, her hands behind her, resting on the rough wood of the wall as if for support. Magpie jumped back with a gasp when she uncovered a rattlesnake in the shelter of the dying leaves, but then she killed it deftly with her hoe and tossed the limp coils to one side. 'Think, now, if the white lady had done it this way in the Garden of Eda!' she called to Caroline, laughing. But the violence made Caroline sick to her stomach.

'Eden,' she whispered. 'It was the Garden of Eden.' She went back inside without another word, her fingers never leaving the side of the house.

One evening, Caroline saw Corin stop Magpie as the girl, with William slung across her back, headed for the dugout where she would prepare another dinner, and keep another household. She stood at the window and held her breath as Corin jogged over to Magpie, put a hand lightly on her

257

arm to stop her. Caroline strained her ears as if she might hear what her husband asked, for even from inside the house she could see questions written all over his face. Magpie answered him in her usual contained way. No gestures, no telltale facial expressions—or at least none that Caroline could read. When Corin released the girl and started towards the house, Caroline turned away and busied herself plating up the meal Magpie had made for them. Roasted corn chowder, with thick slices of roast beef and warm bread.

Corin was troubled by whatever Magpie had told him, that much was clear. Caroline felt a stab of resentment towards the girl, but she smiled as she put food on the table, willing him reassured, willing him unconcerned about her, because she did not know what she would say to him, if he were to ask if she was happy. What he said, as they settled down to eat, was:

'I do think, sweetheart, that you should learn to ride and come out with me sometime to see more of the land we live on. There's nothing that lifts my heart more than a fast ride over the prairie, with the wind to buoy you up and the swiftness of a good horse . . .' But he broke off because Caroline was shaking her head.

'I just can't, Corin! Please don't ask me . . . . I tried! The horses frighten me. And they know it— Hutch says that they can sense the way people feel, and it makes them act badly . . .'

'But you were afraid of Joe and Maggie, until I introduced you to them. You're not still afraid of them now, are you?'

'Well, no . . .' she reluctantly agreed. Magpie she no longer feared, of course, but on the rare occasions that Joe came up to the house to speak to Corin, or to deliver supplies fetched in from Woodward, a knot of tension still clenched in the pit of her stomach. His face looked fierce to her, no matter what Corin said. His features spoke of violence and savagery.

'Well, it would be just the same with the horses. That mare you rode—Clara. Why, she's as gentle as a lamb! And that side saddle I bought you is just sitting in the shed, gathering cobwebs . . . The season's changing now, the weather's better . . . If you would only come out with me and see the beauty of God's virgin country here . . .'

'I just can't! Please, don't try to force me! I am far happier staying here . . .'

'Are you, though?' he asked. Caroline stirred her soup around with her spoon and said nothing. 'Maggie tells me . . .' He trailed off.

'What? What has she said about me?'

'That you don't want to go outside. That you stay indoors, and you're too quiet, and she has much more work to do. Caroline . . . I . . .'

'What?' she asked again, dreading to hear what he would say.

'I just want you to be happy,' he said miserably. He watched her with his eyes wide and she saw nothing within them but truth and love, and hated herself anew for ever thinking he could have betrayed her, could have passed over her infertile body to make a son elsewhere.

'I . . .' she began, but could not think what to say. 'I want to be happy too,' she whispered.

'Then tell me, please. Tell me what I can do to make you happy!' he implored. Caroline said nothing. What could she say? He had done everything a man could do to give her a child, but she could not manage it. He had loved her, and married her, and given her a new life, and she could not ask again for him to give that life up. 'We'll go swimming again. We'll have our honeymoon again. This Sunday—we'll go. Hang the ranch, hang the work—just you and me, my love. And we'll make a baby this time, I just know it. What do you say?' he urged. Caroline shook her head and felt a tremor shake the core of her. It was too late, she realised. Too late for their second honeymoon swim. She could never go back to that pool, not now. It was too far, the way too open; it was too much for her now, too frightening. But what remained? What else could she suggest?

'Only . . . only promise me you'll never leave me,' she said, at last. Corin put his arms around her and held her tightly with quiet, helpless desperation.

'I will *never* leave you,' he whispered.

*   *   *

The first hot night of June, Caroline woke in the darkness with sweat cooling between her breasts, pooling in the hollow of her stomach and slicking her hair to her forehead. She had been dreaming of waking up alone, out on the grasslands, as if she had fallen asleep that day she set out for the Moore's place and not woken since. No house, no ranch, no people, no Corin. She lay still and listened to the blood rushing in her ears, listened to her own breathing as it slowed, grew quieter. Goosebumps rose along her arms. She looked beside her at the comforting outline of Corin, edged in grey light from around the shutters. The coyote song that always haunted the night echoed outside, reaching out unhindered for mile after boundless, borderless mile. Caroline closed her eyes and tried to shut out the sound. It shook her very soul to hear it, waking from such a dream, from such a nightmare. It told her, over and over, of the wilderness outside the walls; of the empty, pitiless land.

Suddenly then, Caroline faced what she had long known but refused to acknowledge. This was where she lived. Here was her husband, here was her life, and this was it. No change, no move; Corin had told her so. And no children. It was two years since she and Corin had been wed and the failure to conceive a child certainly did not stem from a want of trying. She would watch Magpie and Joe raise a brood, she thought; and never have a child of her own. It would be unbearable. If Magpie were to conceive again, she would not be able to have her in the house all day. So, this empty house then, when Corin was away buying or selling beeves, delivering a thoroughbred saddle horse to its new owner, or arguing the price of wheat in Woodward. This empty house in this empty land, for the rest of her life. *I will lose my mind*, Caroline realised, seeing this fact clearly, like plainly printed words scrolling in front of her eyes. *I will lose my mind*. She sat up with a cry and beat her hands against her ears to block out the howling and the resounding silence behind it.

'What is it? What's happening! Are you ill?' Corin slurred, stirred from his sleep. 'What is it, my darling? Did you have a nightmare? Please, tell me!' he begged, grasping her hands to stop the blows she was raining onto them both.

'I just . . . I just . . .' she gasped, choking and shaking her head.

'What? Tell me!'

'I just . . . can't sleep with those god*damned* coyotes shrieking all night long! Don't they *ever* let up? All night! Every night! They're driving me out of my goddamned *mind*, I tell you!' she shouted, eyes wild with rage and fear. Corin took this in and then he smiled.

'Do you know, that's the first time I've ever heard you swear?' he said, releasing her, brushing her dishevelled hair from her face. 'And I have to say, you did a mighty fine job of it!' he grinned. Caroline stopped crying. She looked at the shadow of his smile in the darkness and an odd calm befell her—the numbness of exhausted sleep as it stole in and overcame her in seconds.

The next morning, Corin went out briefly before breakfast and then returned, smiling at his wife with a twinkle in his eye. Caroline's eyes were puffy and they itched. In silence, she went about making breakfast, but she burnt the coffee beans in the roasting pan and the resulting drink was bitter and gritty. She warmed some bean pottage from the night before and made a batch of flat biscuits to go with it, all of which Corin wolfed down with great relish. Before long there was a shout from outside. Caroline opened the door to find Hutch and Joe outside, mounted on their dun-coloured horses with rifles jutting up from the saddles and pistols at their hips. Joe held Strumpet's reins and the black mare was also saddled and ready to ride.

'I didn't think you were riding out today? I thought you were mending fences?' Caroline asked her husband, her voice a small thing after the furies in the night.

'Well,' Corin said, swallowing the last of his coffee with only the faintest grimace and walking out of the house. 'This is a little extra trip I've decided to take, on the spur of the moment.'

'Where are you going?'

'We're going . . .' Corin swung into the saddle, 'to hunt some coyotes,' he grinned. 'You're quite right, Caroline—there are too many of them living close to the ranch. We've been losing some hens; you've been losing some sleep. And it's a fine day for a bit of sport!' he exclaimed, wheeling Strumpet in a tight circle. The mare got onto her toes and snorted in anticipation.

'Oh, Corin!' Caroline said, touched by his efforts for her. The men tipped their hats to her, and with a whoop and a drumming of hooves they were away, leaving nothing but tracks in the sand.

By lunchtime the sky had closed over, filling with thick clouds that rolled steadily out of the north-west. In the kitchen, Caroline sat at the table with Magpie, shelling peas whilst William slept quietly by his mother's feet. Every now and then he stirred and whimpered as if dreaming, and while this made Magpie smile, it made Caroline's heart ache as if with cold. How much longer, she wondered, before this chill became irrevocable and her heart would be lost to her just like three of Hutch's toes had been lost to him? Magpie seemed to sense her sadness. At length the Ponca girl spoke.

'White Cloud is a very wise woman,' she said. In the stillness of the house the crisp pop of the green pods and the rattle of peas falling into the pail were loud. Caroline waited for Magpie to say more, unsure of how to reply to this statement. 'She can make many medicines,' Magpie went on at last. Caroline glanced up and Magpie met her gaze with steady, black eyes.

'Oh?' Caroline said, with as much polite interest as she could muster.

'In the days before, when she lived among our own people, in the lands far to the north of here, many Ponca would go to her for advice. Many *women* would go to her,' Magpie said, with heavy emphasis. Caroline felt warmth prickle her cheeks, and she got up to light a lamp against the dull afternoon. The yellow glow shone on glossy braids and brown skin. Caroline felt like a wraith of some kind, as if Magpie were real and she herself were not quite so. Not quite whole, not quite flesh. The lamp did not light her in the same way.

'Do you think . . . White Cloud would help me?' she asked, in barely more than a whisper. Magpie looked at her with great sympathy then, and Caroline looked down, studying the peas as they blurred in front of her.

'I can ask her. If you would like me to ask her?' Magpie said softly. Caroline could not speak, but she nodded.

Later, Caroline stood and watched from the window as the first drops of rain began to fall. It was not a violent rainstorm, just a steady soaking that fell straight down from the sky. Not a breath of wind was blowing. Caroline listened to the percussion of it on the roof, the gurgle of it in the guttering as it sluiced down into the cistern. It took a while for her to work out what was making her uneasy. The rain had come on slowly, out of the north-west, the same direction in which the men had ridden away. They would have seen this rain closing in, drawing a grey veil over the horizon. It would have found them long before it found the ranch, and yet they had not returned. There would be no hunting in rain like this, and it was late. Magpie had put a rabbit stew in the stove and had left, over an hour ago. The table was set, the stew was ready. Caroline had scrubbed her nails to get the stain of the pea pods out from underneath them. She stood at the window and her unease grew with each drop of rain that fell.

When at last she thought she saw riders coming, the end-of-day light was weak and made them hard to discern. Two hats only, she could see. Two riders only, and not a third. Her heart beat in her chest—not fast, but hard. A steady, slow, tight clenching that was almost painful. Two hats only; and, as they drew nearer, definitely only two horses. And as they drew nearer still, she saw two horses with dun coats and no black one.

For I was reared
In the great city, pent 'mid cloisters dim,
And saw nought lovely but the sky and stars.

Samuel Taylor Coleridge, *Frost at Midnight*

5

On Boxing Day I wake up to hear voices in the kitchen, the clatter of the kettle on the Rayburn, the tap running, water clunking through the pipes in the wall by my bed. It sounds so like the mornings of my childhood here that I lie still for a moment, with the dizzying feeling that I have gone back in time. I expect I am the last one up, as I always used to be. Still full and heavy with yesterday's rich food, I go up to the attic in my dressing gown, unwrap the bone ring from Caroline's trunk and take it downstairs with me. On the stairs hangs the smell of coffee and grilled bacon; and against all logic my stomach rumbles.

The four of them are at the table, which is properly laid with plates and cutlery, coffee mugs and a huge cafetière, a platter of bacon and eggs, toast tucked neatly into a rack. Such quirks of the generation gap make me so fond. I would never think of setting the breakfast table, putting toast in a rack instead of on my plate. The four people I care most about in the world, sitting together at a laden table. I lean on the door jamb for a second and wish that it could always be this way. Warm steam in the air; the dishwasher grinding through its noisy cycle.

'Ah! You've decided to grace us with your presence,' Dad beams, pouring me a coffee.

'Cut me some slack, Dad, it's only nine o'clock,' I yawn, sauntering to the table, sliding onto a bench.

'I've been out already, to fetch in loads more

wood,' Eddie boasts, smothering some toast with chocolate spread.

'Show off,' I accuse him.

'Ed, would you like some toast with your Nutella?' Beth asks him pointedly. Eddie grins at her, takes a huge bite that leaves a chocolate smile on his cheeks.

'Sleep OK?' I ask my parents. They took the same guest room they always did before. So many rooms to choose from, and we all of us have filed into our habitual ones like well-behaved children.

'Very well, thank you, Erica.'

'Here, Mum—this is that bell I was telling you about, that I found up in Caroline's things.' I hand it to her. 'The handle looks like it's bone, or something.'

Mum turns it over in her hands, glances up at me incredulously. 'It's not a bell, you dope, it's a baby's teething ring. A very lovely one, too. This is ivory, not bone . . . and the silver bell acts as a rattle. Added interest.'

'A teething ring? Really?'

'A very old-fashioned one, yes; but that's certainly what it is.'

'I saw something like that on *The Antiques Roadshow* not that long ago,' Dad adds.

'Ivory and silver—it must have been for a pretty rich kid,' Eddie observes, around a mouthful of toast.

'Was it Clifford's? Do you remember it?' I ask. Mum frowns slightly.

'No, I have to say I don't. But I may have forgotten. Or . . .' she reaches behind her, takes the family tree from the sideboard. 'Look at the gap between Caroline getting married, and Meredith

270

being born—seven years! That's rather unusual. There's my great aunt, Evangeline—she died before her first birthday, poor thing.' She points to the name preceding Meredith's, the pitifully short dates in brackets beneath. 'Two babies in seven years is not very many. Perhaps she had a son that died, before she had Meredith, and this ring belonged to that poor little chap.'

'Maybe. But wouldn't he be on the family tree, even if he'd died?'

'Well, not necessarily. Not if he was born prematurely, or was stillborn,' Mum muses. 'I know that Meredith lost a child before I was born. These things can run in families.'

'Perhaps we could talk about something else at the breakfast table?' Beth says quietly. Mum and I button our lips guiltily. Beth miscarried a child, very early on, before Eddie was born. It was little more than a slip of life, but its sudden absence was like a tiny, bright light going out.

'What are we going to do today, then?' Dad asks, helping himself to more scrambled eggs. 'I, for one, feel the need to stretch my legs a bit— walk off some of yesterday's excess.'

'To make room for today's excess, David?' Mum remarks, peering at his plate.

'Quite so!' he agrees cheerfully.

It is brighter today, but grey clouds nose purposefully across the sky and the wind is brisk, penetrating. We take a route through the village, westwards past the little stone church that nestles into a green slope studded with the gravestones of generations of Barrow Storton's dead. In the far corner is the Calcott plot, and in unspoken unity we drift over to it. It is about two metres wide, and as long. A cold bed of marble chippings for our family to sleep in. Henry, Lord Calcott, is in there, and Caroline, with the little daughter she lost before Meredith. Evangeline. And now Meredith has joined them. So recently that the remnants of the funeral flowers are still here in a small, brass pot, and the cuts of her name on the stone are sharp and fresh. I can't help thinking she would rather have had her own place, or lie next to her husband Charles, than spend eternity cooped up with Caroline, but it is too late now. I shudder, make a silent pledge that I will never lie in this claustrophobic family grave.

'I suppose if Caroline had had a son, he'd be buried here, wouldn't he?' I ask, breaking the silence. Beth sighs sharply and walks away, over to where Eddie is climbing the gabled lychgate.

'I suppose so. Probably. But, who knows? If he was very tiny, perhaps they'd have given him an infant's grave instead,' Mum replies.

'What would that look like?'

'Just like a grave with a smaller stone, usually with an angel on it somewhere—or a cherub,' she says. Dad looks at me sidelong.

'I have to say, you're taking a pretty keen interest in this all of a sudden,' he says.

'No, I just . . . you know. I never could stand an unsolved mystery,' I shrug.

'Then I fear you were born into the wrong family.'

'Hey, Eddie!' I call to him. 'Look for small gravestones with angels on them, and the name Calcott!' Eddie rips me a smart salute, begins to trot up and down the rows of stones. Beth folds her arms and glares at me.

'Can we please stop looking for dead babies!' she shouts, the wind pulling at her voice.

'Give me five minutes!' I call back.

'Perhaps we should get on, Erica?' Mum says diffidently.

'Five minutes,' I say again.

I run my eyes along the ranks of stones, in the opposite direction to which Eddie has gone, but they all seem to be of regular size.

'Sometimes there's a special area for the infant graves . . .' Mum sets her gaze to the far corner of the churchyard. 'Try over there—do you see? Under that beech tree.' I walk quickly to where the wind is seething through the naked beech, sounding like the sea. There are perhaps fifteen or twenty graves here. On the older graves are little cherubs, their features blurred with lichen, chubby arms wrapped forlornly around the stones. There are a couple of newer stones too, carved with teddy bears instead; less celestial guardians which seem somehow out of place. But then that's the point, I suppose. An infant has no place in a churchyard. Lives that had no chance to start, losses that must have torn their parents' souls. All those broken hearts are buried here too, alongside the tiny bodies that broke them. It's a melancholy sight and I scan the names and dates hurriedly, walk away from the sad little party with a shiver.

I have never before found graveyards eerie, or particularly depressing. I like the expressions of love on the stones, the quiet declarations of people having existed, of having mattered. Who knows what secret feelings lie behind the carved lists of offspring, siblings and surviving spouses—or if the memories they had were truly loving. But there is the hope, always, that each transient life meant something to those left behind; cast a vapour trail of influence and emotion to fade gradually across the years.

'Anything?' I ask Eddie.

'Nope. There's an angel over there, but the lady was seventy-three and called Iris Bateman.'

'Can we go, now?' Beth says impatiently. 'If you're that desperate to know if she had a son, go and look it up in the births, marriages and deaths register. It's all online now.'

'Perhaps she *was* married before, in America,' Mum says, taking my arm in a conciliatory manner. 'Perhaps the baby in the photograph died there, before she came over.'

To the north of the village is a web of farm tracks and bridleways, dodging through the drab winter fields. We take a circular route, at a brisk pace, falling into pairs to pass along the narrow pathways. Eddie drops back to walk beside me. He is leaving later on today. I look at his sharp face, his scruffy hair, and feel a pull of affection. It gives me such an odd, desperate feeling for a second that I pause to consider how Beth must be feeling. As if reading my mind, Eddie speaks.

'Is Mum going to be OK?' A carefully neutral tone he is too young to have developed.

'Yes, of course,' I tell him, with as much certainty as I can find.

'It's just . . . when Dad came to pick me up last time, before Christmas, she seemed . . . really unhappy about it. She's getting thin again. And, like, today, just now, she was really snappy with you . . .'

'Sisters always snap at each other, Eddie. That's

nothing out of the ordinary!' I find a fake laugh and Eddie gives me an accusing look. I drop the bravado. 'Sorry,' I say. 'Look, it's just . . . it's hard for your mum, being back at the manor house. Has she told you about your great-grandma's will? That we can only keep the house if we both come and live in it?' He nods. 'Well, that's why we've come to stay. To see if we would like to come and live here.'

'Why does she hate it so much? Because your cousin was kidnapped—and she misses him?'

'Possibly . . . possibly it's to do with Henry. And the fact that, well, this place is in our past now, and sometimes it can feel wrong to try and live in the past. To be honest, I don't think we'll come to live here, but I'm going to try to make your mum stay for a bit longer at least; even if she doesn't really want to.'

'But why?'

'Well . . .' I struggle for a way to explain. 'Do you remember that time your finger swelled up to the size of a sausage and it was so sore you wouldn't let us look at it properly, but it wouldn't heal up so finally we did look and you had a splinter of metal in it?'

'Yeah, I remember. It looked like it was going to explode,' he grimaces.

'Once we got the splinter out it healed, right?' Eddie nods. 'Well, I think your mum won't . . . heal because she has a splinter. Not of metal, and not in her finger, but she's got a kind of splinter inside her and that's why she can't get better. I'm going to get the splinter out. I'm going to . . . find out what it is and get rid of it.' I hope I sound calm, confident in this purpose; when what I feel is desperate. If I believed in God, I would be striking all kinds of fervent bargains right now. *Make Beth well. Make her happy.*

'How? Why do you have to be here to do it?'

'Because . . . I think this is where she got the splinter in the first place,' I say.

Eddie considers this in silence for a while, his face marked by worried lines I hate to see. 'I hope you do. I hope you can find out what it is,' he says, eventually. 'You will find out, won't you? And she will get better?'

'I promise you, Ed,' I say. And now I must not fail. I *cannot* let us come away from here without a resolution of some kind. The weight of my promise settles onto me like chains.

*   *   *

Our parents leave soon after lunch, and by teatime Maxwell has come for Eddie as well. Maxwell is grouchy, blotches of overindulgence on his cheeks. He looks mealy-mouthed. I load carrier bags of presents into the boot, Beth watching me blackly as if I am colluding in the theft of her son.

'See you, Edderino,' I say.

'Bye then, *Auntie* Rick,' he says, and climbs into the back. He is calm, resigned. He goes from one place of welcome to the next; he is practical, does not fret. He lets himself be ferried, and pretends not to notice Beth's anguish. There's the smallest hint of cruelty in this, as if he means to say, you made this situation, you set it up this way.

'Did you tell Harry you were going today?' I ask, leaning into the car.

'Yes, but you might have to tell him again, if you see him around. I'm not sure how much attention he was paying.'

'OK. Call your mum later on, won't you?' I keep my voice low.

' 'Course,' he mutters, looking at his hands.

The brake lights of the car gleam red as they pull out of the drive. It's raining again. Beth and I stand and wave like idiots until the car is out of sight. Our hands drop, in near-perfect unison. Neither one of us wants to turn back to the house now this event is past. Christmas. The preparation of the house, the feeding and entertaining of Eddie, of our parents. Now what? No deadline, no timetable. Nothing to guide us but ourselves. I glance at Beth, see tiny drops of water beading the stray hairs around her face. I can't even ask what she wants for lunch, can't even impose this small future on us. The house is bursting with leftovers, ready to be grazed.

'Eddie's so great, Beth. You've done so well there,' I say, needing to break the silence. But there's a chilly, sad edge to Beth's eyes.

'I'm not sure how much of it comes from me,' she says.

'All the best bits,' I say, taking her hand, squeezing it. She shakes her head. We turn and go inside again, alone.

When she is this quiet, when she is this pale and still, like a carving, I think of her in the hospital. At least I didn't find her. I've only got Eddie's descriptions, making pictures in my head. She was in her bedroom, lying on her side, bent at the waist as if she had been sitting up and then tipped over. He couldn't see her face, he told me. Her hair had fallen right over it. He says he doesn't know how long he stood there before going over to her,

277

because he was too afraid of moving her hair, of seeing what was underneath. His mother, or his dead mother. He needn't have touched her at all, of course. He could have just called an ambulance. But he was a child, a little boy. He wanted to make it right himself. He wanted to touch her and find her sleeping, nothing more. What courage he must have found. To do it—to push back her hair. I am so proud of him it hurts.

She had taken a lot of sleeping pills and then tried to cut her wrists—with the short-bladed paring knife that I had seen her use more than once, slicing banana onto Eddie's cereal—but the conclusion drawn was that she had hesitated. She had hesitated—perhaps because the first cut, deep enough to look bad but not deep enough to do any real damage, had hurt more than she expected. And while she hesitated the pills sank into her bloodstream and she passed out. She had cut her wrist the wrong way. Horizontally, across the vessels and tendons, instead of parallel to them as any serious suicide, these days, knows is best. The doctors called it a cry for help rather than a genuine attempt, but I knew different. I clattered into the hospital, waited while they pumped her stomach. Opposite me in the corridor was a window, blinds drawn. My reflection stared back at me. In the greenish light I looked dead. Lank hair, face drooping. I fed money into a machine; it expelled watery hot chocolate for Eddie. Then Maxwell came and took him away.

When she woke up I went in to see her, and I had no idea until I got to her that I was angry. *So* angry with her. Angrier than I have ever been.

'What were you doing? What about Eddie?'

These were my first words. Snapping like a trap.

A nurse with hair the colour of sharp sand scowled at me, said, 'Elizabeth needs her rest,' in an admonishing tone, as if she knew her better than I. There was a bruise on Beth's chin, purple hollows around her eyes, in her cheeks. *What about me?* I wanted to add. Hurt, that she would want to leave me. The same feeling as when she ran off with Dinny, snowballing down the years. She didn't answer me. She started to cry and my heart cracked, let the anger run out. I picked up a matted length of her hair and began chasing out the knots with my fingertips.

*   *   *

It's been a long time since I spoke to my Aunt Mary, let alone telephoned her. I am still reluctant to, but I have got a ball rolling now. I have started to learn things, started to uncover secrets. If I keep going, sooner or later I will get to the ones I am looking for. I shift uncomfortably in the chair as I wait to hear Mary's voice. She was always mousy, quiet; so mild and meek that half the time we didn't even notice her. A pink-skinned woman with pale hair and eyes. Neat blouses, tucked into neat skirts. It was a shock to hear her scream; to hear her shout and cry and curse in the aftermath of Henry's disappearance. Then when that stopped she was even quieter than before, as if she'd used up all the noise she possessed in that one burst. Her voice is fluting and quiet, as precarious as wet tissue paper.

'Mary Calcott speaking?' So timorous, as if she's really not sure.

'Hello, Aunt Mary, it's Erica.'

'Erica? Oh hello, dear. Happy Christmas. Well, I suppose it's a bit late for that now. Happy New Year.' There is little conviction behind these words. I wonder if she hates us, for surviving when Henry did not. For being around to remind her of it.

'And to you. I hope you're well? You didn't come down with Clifford, to collect those bits and bobs you wanted from the house?'

'No, no. Well, I'm sure you understand that Storton Manor is . . . not an easy place for me. It's not a place I like to think of often, or return to,' she tells me, delicately. I can't warm to her. To put losing her son in such limp terms, as if it was an embarrassing incident, best forgotten. I know how unfair I am being. I know she's not a whole person any more.

'Of course.' I struggle to find more small talk, fail. 'Well, the reason I was calling, and I hope you won't mind me asking, is that I wanted to pick your brains a little about the family research you did, the year before last.'

'Oh, yes?'

'I've found a photo of Caroline, you see, dated 1904, and it was taken in New York . . .'

'Well, that certainly sounds right. She came to London in late 1904. It's hard to be absolutely sure of the date.'

'Yes. The thing is she has a child with her, in the picture. A baby that looks about six months old or so. I just wondered if you had any idea who the baby might have been?'

'A child? Well. I can't think. That can't be right.'

'Was she married before, in the States? Only,

the way she's holding the baby . . . it just looks like a family portrait to me. She looks so proud . . . It looks to me like it's her baby, you see.'

'Oh, no, Erica. That can't be right at all. Let me just get the file down. One moment.' I hear rustling, a cupboard door creaking. 'No, I've got a copy of her marriage certificate to Sir Henry Calcott here, and it clearly says, in the 'condition' column, that she was a spinster. A spinster at twenty-one! Hardly seems an appropriate label, does it?'

'Could she have . . . got a divorce, or something?' I ask, dubiously.

'Goodness me, no. It was very rare in that day and age, and certainly not without it being well talked about. Or mentioned on the occasion of her subsequent marriage. The child must belong to somebody else.'

'Oh. Well, thank you . . .'

'Of course, Caroline was always rather reticent about her early years in America. All anybody could discover was that she had grown up without any close family and had come to England to make a fresh start when she came into her money. She married Henry Calcott very soon after meeting him, which, I have always thought, perhaps shows how lonely she was, poor girl.' Twice now, she has said his name.

'Yes, it does sound that way. Well, thanks for looking it up for me, anyway.'

'You're welcome, Erica. I wonder whether I might ask you to send me the photograph? To add to my presentation files? Early pictures of Caroline and her generation are so very scarce.'

'Oh, well actually, my mother has already asked

me to give her any pictures I find. But I'm sure she'd be happy to send you copies of them . . .'

'Of course. Well, I shall ask Laura when I next see her.'

There's a pause and I can't quite bring myself to say goodbye, to admit that this piece of information was all I was after, and that I do not want to talk to her. There is so much to say, so much not to say.

'So . . . how was Christmas?' I ask. I hear her draw in a breath, steeling herself.

'It was fine, thank you.' She pauses again. 'I still buy Henry a present every year, you know. Clifford thinks I am quite mad, of course, but he has never really understood. What it's like for a mother to lose a child. I can't just put it aside and move on, as he has managed to do.'

'What did you get him?' Before I can stop myself.

'A book about the RAF. Some new football boots, and some DVDs,' she says, her voice growing, as if she is pleased about choosing these gifts. Gifts she will never give. I can't think what to say. I would be strangely fascinated to know whether she buys child-sized football boots, or has hazarded a guess at his adult shoe size. 'Do you ever think about your cousin, Erica? Do you still think about Henry?' she asks, rushing the words.

'Of course. Of course I do. Especially now we're . . . back here again.'

'Good. Good. I'm glad,' she says, and I wonder what she means. I wonder if she senses guilt, hanging around Beth and me like a bad smell.

'So there's been no news? Of him—of Henry?' Ridiculous thing for me to ask, twenty-three years after he vanished. But what conclusion can I draw, from the gifts she still buys him, but that she expects someday to have him back?

'No,' she says flatly. A single word; she makes no effort to elaborate.

'Eddie's been here with us for Christmas,' I tell her.

'Who?'

'Edward—Beth's son?'

'Oh yes, of course.'

'He's eleven now, the same age as . . . Well, he had a fine old time, anyway, carousing around out in the woods, getting filthy.'

'Clifford wanted to have another, you know. After we lost Henry. There might still have been time.'

'Oh,' I say.

'But I told him I couldn't. What did he think— that we could just replace him, like a lost watch?' She makes an odd, strangled sound that I think is meant to be a laugh.

'No. No, of course not,' I say. There is another long pause, another long breath from Mary.

'I know you never got on. You girls and Henry. I know that you didn't like him,' she says, suddenly tense, offended.

'We did like him!' I lie. 'It's just . . . well, we liked Dinny too. And we kind of had to choose sides . . .'

'Did it ever occur to you that Henry used to . . . act up, sometimes, because you always left him out of your games and ran off to play with Dinny?' she says.

'No. I . . . never thought he wanted to play with us. He never seemed like he wanted to,' I mumble.

'Well, I think he did. I think it hurt his feelings that you couldn't wait to get away,' she tells me, resolutely. I try to picture my cousin this way—try to shape the way he treated us, treated Dinny, in these terms. But I can't—it won't fit. That's not the way it was, not the way *he* was. A flare of indignation warms me, but of course I can say nothing and the silence buzzes down the line. 'Well, Erica, I really must go,' she says at last, in one long exhalation. 'It was . . . nice to talk to you. Goodbye.'

She hangs up the phone before I can respond. She does not do this crossly, or abruptly. Absently, rather, as if something else has caught her attention. She's had lots of fads and projects in the years since Henry died. Tapestry, watercolours, horoscopes, brass rubbing, Anglo Saxon poetry. The family genealogy was the longest running, the one she really followed through. I wonder if she did it because she got to say his name, over and over again, when Clifford would not allow her to speak of their son. *Henry Calcott, Henry Calcott, Henry Calcott*. Learning everything she could about his ancestors, the source of each component part of him, as if she could rebuild him.

He's dead. This I know. He was not carried off. It wasn't him, lying in the back of a car in a Devizes car park. It wasn't him, being carried by a mysterious hobo on the A361. I know it because I can feel it, I can feel the memory of his death. I can feel it at the dew pond, even if I can't see it. The way I could hear the shape of Dinny in the darkness on Christmas Day. We were there, Henry was there; and Henry died. I have the shape of it. I just need to colour it in. Because I've stalled. I'm blocked. I can't go in any direction until I can fill this hole in my head, until I can work Beth's splinter free. Every other thought must detour around these missing things, and that will not do. Not any longer. And if I must start in 1904 and work my way towards it, then that is what I will do.

Through the kitchen window I see Harry, lingering by the trees at the far end of the garden. It's still raining, harder now. His hands are thrust into the pockets of his patchwork coat and he is hunched, damp, forlorn looking. Without thinking, I pull leftovers from the fridge and larder and start to carve fleshy slices from the cold turkey with its burnt leg stumps. I slather mayonnaise onto two bits of white bread, cram in turkey, and stuffing the consistency of chipboard. Then I take it down to him, wrapped in foil, my coat draped over my head. He doesn't smile at me. He shifts from foot to foot, in an apparent agony of indecision. Rain drips from the ends of his dreadlocks. I catch the scent of his unwashed body. A soft, animal smell, strangely endearing.

'Here, Harry. I made this for your lunch. It's a turkey sandwich,' I say, handing it to him. He takes it. I don't know why I expect him to speak, when I know he won't. It's such a fundamentally human thing, I suppose. To communicate with noise. 'Eddie's gone back to his dad's house now, Harry. Do you understand what I'm saying? He's not here any more,' I tell him, as kindly as I can. If I knew when Eddie was coming back, I would add this information. I don't. I don't know if we'll be here. I don't know anything. 'His father came today and took him home with him,' I explain. Harry glances at the sandwich. A tiny metallic tune, as rain hits the foil. 'Well, at least eat this,' I say gently, patting his hand on the sandwich. 'It'll keep you going.'

*   *   *

Beth finds me in the study. I am curled up in a leather bucket chair. I stood on the desk to get this book of wild flowers down from the top shelf. It brought a shower of dead flies with it, a smell of past lives. Now it's open, heavy across my knees, at a double-page spread of yellow marsh flags. Ragged, buttery irises. Nonchalantly drooped petals on tall stems, like pennants on a still day. I recognised them as soon as I saw them. Marsh flags.

'The rain's stopped. Do you fancy a quick walk?' Beth asks. She has plaited her hair, put on clean jeans and a jumper the colour of raspberries.

'Absolutely,' I say, all astonishment. 'Yes, let's.'

'What were you reading?'

'Oh, just about wild flowers. There were three old pillowcases up in the press. They had yellow flowers embroidered on them, and I wanted to know what they were.'

'What were they?'

'Marsh flags. Does that ring any bells with you?'

'No. Should it? What kind of bell?'

'Probably a misplaced bell. I'll just get some wellies on.'

We don't walk very far, since the sky is like charcoal on the horizon. Just down into the village and then up to the barrow. I am sure I see one of the girls from the solstice party through the window of the pub. Sitting by the fire, accepting a fresh pint from a man whose back is turned to me.

There's a welcoming drench of wood smoke and beer and voices from the doorway, but we carry on past. Lots of villagers out and about today. Walking off the cake and puddings. They all greet us, although I am sure we are not recognised. A few faces tug at me. They slot into my memories somewhere, but too seamlessly for me to pick them out. A stout woman rides past on her horse, silver tinsel woven into its tail.

We cross the tawny grassland up to the barrow, scare up two dozen glossy rooks that had been strutting purposefully. The wind whisks them away, and from a distance they look like ragged shot-holes in the sky. Beth links her arm through mine, walks with a swinging step.

'You seem happy today?' I ask her, carefully.

'I am. I've come to a decision.'

'Oh? What kind of decision?' We've reached the barrow. Beth lets go of my arm, conquers the mound in three long strides and turns to gaze over my head into the distance.

'I'm going. I'm not staying,' she says, throwing her arms wide, girlish, dramatic. She takes a huge breath, lets it out with emphasis.

'What do you mean? Going where?'

'Going home, of course. Later today. I've packed!' she laughs, as if she is wild, reckless. 'I'm taking *that* road,' she says, squinting and pointing to the line of tall poplars that march along the lane out of the village.

'You can't!' The thought of being alone in the house fills me with a dread I can't define. I would rather dive to the bottom of the pond, let it suck me down. I feel something like panic sputtering in my stomach.

'Of course I can. Why stay? What are we even *doing* here? I can't even remember why we came. Can you?'

'We came to . . . we came to sort things out. To . . . decide what we wanted to do!' I grope for words.

'Come on, Erica. Neither of us wants to live here.' She drops her arms as she says this, looks at me suddenly. 'You don't, do you? You don't want to live here? You don't want to stay?'

'I don't know yet!'

'But . . . you can't want to. It's *Meredith's* house. Everything about it says *Meredith*. And then there's . . . the other thing.'

'Henry?' I say. She nods, just once. Short and sharp. 'It's *our* house, Beth. Yours and mine now.'

'Oh my God, you want to stay. You do, don't you?' She is utterly incredulous.

'I don't know! I don't know. Not for ever, perhaps. For a while, maybe. I don't know. But please don't go, Beth! Not yet. I'm . . . I'm not done. I can't go yet and I can't stay here on my own. Please. Stay a bit longer.' On top of the barrow Beth sags. I have stabbed her, let out all the air. We are quiet for a while. The wind rolls over the ridge, trembles the grasses. I see Beth shiver. She looks impossibly lonely up there.

At length she comes down to me, her eyes lowered.

'I'm sorry,' I say.

'What do you mean, you're not done yet?' Her voice is flat now, lifeless.

'I need to . . . find out what happened. I need to remember.' A half-truth. I can't tell her about her splinter. I can't let her know what I am working towards. She would snatch herself away, not let me

288

touch; just like Eddie with his swollen finger.

'Remember what?'

I stare at her. She must know what I'm talking about.

'About *Henry*, Beth. I need to remember what happened to Henry.' She glares at me now, eyes reflecting the grey sky. She searches my face, and I wait.

'You remember what happened. Don't lie. You were old enough.'

'But I don't. I really don't,' I say. 'Please tell me.' Beth looks away, past the rooftops and chimney trails of the village below and into the east, as if projecting herself there.

'No. I won't tell you,' she says. 'I won't tell anyone. Not *ever*.'

'Please, Beth! I have to know!'

'No! And if . . . if you love me, you'll stop asking.'

'Does Dinny know?'

'Yes, of *course* Dinny knows. Why don't you ask him?' She flicks her eyes at me. There's a chilly touch of resentment there. For an instant, then it's gone. 'But you know, too. And if you really don't remember then . . . then maybe that's a good thing.' She walks away from me, along the ridge towards the house.

She stops at the dew pond. This is the first time she's been back to it, that I know of, and it halts her so abruptly that I almost run into her. The wind skids over its surface, turns it matt and ugly. I expect to see her crying, but her eyes are dry and hard. The sad lines on her face, etched deeper than ever. She stares down into it.

'I was so scared, the first time you swam here,'

she murmurs, so quietly I can hardly hear. 'I thought you wouldn't be able to get out. Like the hedgehog in the pond at home, that time. Do you remember? It had swum around and around until it was too exhausted to swim any more, and then it just drowned. All those videos we were shown at school—never to swim in quarries or rivers. I thought water without chlorine in it had some dreadful, lurking power that waited and watched and ate little kids.'

'I remember you yelling at me like a harpy.'

'I was scared for you,' she says, shrugging minutely. 'Now you spend all your time being scared for me. Except today. *Why* do I have to stay? You must see that . . . it's bad for me, being here?'

'No, I . . . I think it could be good for you,' I force myself to say.

'What do you mean?' she asks me, darkly. My heart beats faster.

'I mean what I say. You can't keep running from this, Beth! Please! If you would just talk about it—'

'No! I've told you—over and over. Not to you and not to anybody!'

'Why not to me? I'm your *sister*, Beth, nothing you could tell me would make me love you any less! Nothing,' I say firmly.

'That's what you think, is it? That there's something despicable in me that I'm trying to hide?' she whispers.

'No, Beth, that's what I *don't* think! You're not listening to me! But you *are* hiding something—you can't deny it. I have no secrets from you!'

'Everybody has secrets, Erica,' she snaps. It's true, and I look away.

'All I want is for us to be able to leave this place behind . . .'

'Good! That's what I want, too! So let's do it—let's leave.'

'Leaving it isn't the same as leaving it *behind*, Beth! Look at you—since we've been back here it's been like sharing the house with a ghost! You're . . . miserable and you seem determined to stay that way!' I shout.

'What are you *talking* about?' Beth shouts back at me, spreading her hands in fury. '*You're* the one determined to keep me here—you're the one determined to make me miserable! I only came here at all because you pressured me into it!'

'I'm determined to get rid of whatever it is that's keeping you down, Beth. And it's here—I know it is. It's here at this house—don't walk away from me!' I grab her arm, stop her. Beth is breathing hard, will not look me in the eye. Her face is pale.

'If you don't let me go, I might not ever forgive you. I don't know what I will do,' she says, her voice trembling. Startled, I drop my hand from her arm but I don't think this is what she means. I am afraid of what she will do. My resolve wavers, but I fight to hold on to it.

'Please, Beth. Please stay here with me. At least until the new year. Let's just . . . figure this out. Whatever it is.'

'Figure it out?' she echoes me, bitterly. 'It's not a riddle, Erica.'

'I know that. But life can't go on the way it has been. This is our *chance*, Beth—our chance to put things right.'

'Some things can't be undone, Erica. The sooner you accept that the better,' she whispers.

Tears are bright in her eyes, but when she looks up at me they are full of anger. 'It can't be put right!' she snaps, and storms away from me. I pause before I follow her, find that I am shaking.

*   *   *

For the rest of the day we play hide and seek. This house always was perfect for it. The rain comes in sideways, draughts creep down the chimneys. I bring Harry inside and make him a cup of sweet tea. He sits at the kitchen table sucking it from his teaspoon like a child. He drips water onto the floor, fills the room with the smell of wet wool. But I can't find Beth to give her a cup of tea. I can't find her to ask what she wants for dinner, if she wants to go out anywhere, if she wants to rent a film from the garage on the road to Devizes. I feel it is my job, now, to fill her time. Time I am forcing her to spend here. But she melts into the house like a cat, and I stomp from room to room in vain.

Henry once left her hiding for hours. Left her alone, trapped, panicked. He made me part of it, again. I was small. I must have been—Caroline was still alive. Earlier that day she'd been wheeled outside to the terrace. She had one of those grand old wicker wheelchairs. No grey NHS metal and plastic for her. It creaked as it rolled along, fine spokes glinting, but Henry said it was Caroline that creaked, because she was so old and mummified. I knew it was nonsense but even so, each time I heard it, I would think of papery skin tearing; of hair that would crumble to dust if you touched it; of a tongue gone stiff and woody in a shrivelled mouth. We were never made to kiss her, if we didn't want to. Mum saw to that, and thank goodness.

By then she was mostly bedridden, but it was a fine day and we were all there—Clifford and Mary, my parents. She was wheeled to the table, presented with her lunch on a tray that slotted into the frame of the chair. The housekeeper brought out the soup in a white china tureen shaped like a giant cauliflower, and there were potatoes and salad and ham on the table. I was told off for dipping my fingers into the melted butter at the bottom of the potato bowl. Meredith helped Caroline to eat, sometimes feeding her the way you feed a baby. Meredith frowned as she did it; pinched her lips tightly together. Caroline's hair was thin. I could see her scalp through it and it *did* look papery. The conversation went on around her, and I kept my eyes carefully on my plate. Only once did she speak up and, though her voice was louder than I expected, the words crept out ponderously.

'Is that man Dinsdale still alive?' She dropped her fork as she spoke, as if holding it and speaking were too many things to do at once. It clattered loudly, down onto the paving slabs.

'No, Mother. He's not,' Meredith answered, and I burned with the knowledge that there were in fact many Dinsdales, alive and well not two hundred metres from where we sat. I knew better than to speak at the table. Caroline made a small sound, high and wavering, which could have been anything. Satisfaction, perhaps. 'I believe his son is, however,' Meredith added.

'Can't you get *rid* of him, child?' Caroline asked, and I was as puzzled to hear Meredith called *child* as I was outraged at the question. Across the table, Henry smirked, kicked me in the shin.

'No more than you could,' Meredith countered.

'Travellers,' Caroline mumbled. 'They were meant to go. They were meant to move on,' she said.

'They go. And then they come back again,' Meredith muttered. 'And sadly there is very little I can do about it.' At this Caroline went still. An unnatural pause, as if she was going to say something else. Everybody at the table waited, but she did not speak again. Meredith folded her napkin crisply onto her lap, began to serve herself with salad. But the frown stayed, knitted between her brows, and when I looked at Caroline she was staring out across the lawn, eyes boring into the far trees as though she could see straight through them. Her head wobbled on her neck, and from time to time her hands would twitch involuntarily, but that far, pale gaze never wavered.

After that lunch we children were sent to have an afternoon nap—because I was small and cross, Henry had been rude at lunch, and that left Beth with nobody to play with. Henry instigated the game. He hid first, and we found him at length in the attic room, behind the same crumbling, burgundy leather trunk I have so recently rediscovered. We stirred up motes of dust that flashed and swirled in the light from the eaves, circling slowly. I found a peacock butterfly, wrapped in spider webs and as mummified as I feared Caroline to be. I clamoured for it to be my turn to hide, but Beth had found Henry first, so it was her turn. Henry and I knelt at the bottom of the stairs, shut our eyes, counted.

I don't think I could count to a hundred at that age. I was relying on Henry, and he normally counted *one, two, miss a few, ninety-nine, a hundred*; so after what seemed a long time, listening to the housekeeper clattering dishes in the kitchen, I opened one eye to check on him. He wasn't there. I looked up and saw him coming down the stairs. He smiled nastily at me, and I cast my eyes around. I did this instinctively, whenever I found myself alone with that look on Henry's face. In case help was at hand. My heart quick in my chest.

'Is it time to find Beth yet?' I whispered at last.

'No. Not yet. I'll tell you when,' he said. 'Come on, then, come with me.' He used his fake-nice voice, a high pitch that he also used to trick the Labradors. He offered me his hand and I took it unwillingly. We went into the study; he put the TV on.

'Is it time now?' I asked again. Something was wrong. I made for the door but he put out his leg, blocked me.

'Not yet! I told you—you can't go and look until I say it's time.'

I waited. I was miserable. I didn't watch what was on the TV. I looked at Henry, at the door, back again. What's time, when you're five years old? I have no idea how long I was made to wait. It must have been over an hour, and it felt like an eternity. When the door creaked open, I ran to it. My father came in, asked where Beth was. He studied my anxious face and asked again. Henry shrugged. Dad and I went all over the house, calling. On the top floor corridor we heard her—banging, and faint sounds of distress. The final set of stairs, up to the attic, had a cupboard underneath, an iron key in the lock. Dad turned it, lifted the latch and Beth tumbled out, her face pale and streaked with dirt and tears.

'What on earth?' Dad said, gathering her up. She was breathing so hard that her own sobs half choked her, and her eyes stared out in a way that frightened me. It was as if she had closed herself off from me, from the world. Fear had made her hide inside her own head. The cupboard was cramped and cobwebby, and the light switch was on the outside. Henry had turned it off and turned the key in the lock while I kept my eyes closed and assumed he was counting. Left her alone in the dark with the spiders and no room to turn around. I knew all this, I told my dad, and he demanded the truth from Henry. Beth stood behind him, unnaturally quiet. There were pale patches of dust on her knees, grazes on the heels of her hands; something had caught a lock of her hair, pulled it out of her Alice band in a sagging loop.

'It was nothing to do with *me*. I've been down here all the time. We got bored of looking for her,' Henry shrugged, swinging his legs to and fro with excitement although he managed to keep his face straight. Beth had stopped crying. She was looking at Henry with a bright hatred that shocked me.

* * *

It's mid-afternoon and I am upstairs, wedged onto the window sill in my bedroom. My breath has steamed up the glass, obscured the view, but I am reading so it doesn't matter. More of Meredith's letters to Caroline. I am surprised that Meredith kept them all—that she stowed them away with Caroline's things, as a record of their troubled relationship. Letters belong to the recipient, I know, but it would have been easy, and understandable, for her to destroy them after her mother died. But perhaps she wanted them for exactly what they recorded. The fact that she tried to have another life, even if she failed.

Dear Mother,

Thank you for the card you sent. I can only say that I am as well as can be expected. I have my hands very full with Laura, who has recently started walking and has consequently taken to running rings around me—it is nigh on impossible to keep her out of mischief. Her particular passion this week is for mud and worms. I have an excellent nanny, a local girl called Doreen, who has a calming influence on the child—and on me, I must say. Nothing seems to fluster her, and in these troubled days, that is a virtue indeed. I have given your invitation to return to live with you at Storton Manor a great deal of thought, but for the time being I intend to remain in my own home. I have the support of my neighbours, who have proved themselves most sympathetic in my hour of need. Many of the local women have sons and husbands away fighting, and each time the much dreaded telegram arrives a contingent is dispatched to make sure that there is food in the house, and the children clothed, and the wife or mother still breathing. I dare say you would not approve of the social classes mingling in this way, but I was greatly moved to receive just such a visit myself when word of Charles' death got about. I went to London last Friday, to collect what belongings of his remained at his club and offices. You would not believe the scenes of devastation I witnessed there. It was enough to chill the very heart of me. So I will stay for as long as I can manage to do so, because, though it pains me greatly to commit such a thing to paper, I have not yet forgiven you, Mother. For not coming to Charles' funeral. Your objections to him as a husband were never as great, and your dislike of travelling never so strong, that either should have prevented you from attending, and insulting him in this way. The snub did not go unnoticed amongst our acquaintances. And what of me? Do you not realise that I should have liked to have you there, that I needed your support on such a day? Surely there are limits to the stoicism a new widow should have to display? That is all I will say for the time being. I must grow accustomed to life without my husband, and I must take care of myself, little Laura and my unborn child. For now I do not think you or any one can ask anything more of me.

Meredith.

As I finish reading I am interrupted by the clang of the doorbell. I climb down from the sill, wincing, the blood rushing into my stiff legs. I make my way to the top of the stairs, pause when I hear Beth open the door, and Dinny's voice. My first impulse is to carry on, rush down the stairs to see him, to ease things for them. But my feet don't respond. I stay still, my hand on the banister, listening.

'How are you, Beth?' Dinny asks, and the question carries more weight than it normally would. More significance.

'I'm very well, thank you,' Beth answers, something odd in her tone that I can't identify.

'Only . . . Erica said that you—'

'Erica said that I what?' she says sharply.

'That you weren't happy to be back. That you wanted to leave.' I can't hear Beth's reply to this. If she makes one. 'Can I come in?' he says, almost nervously.

'No. I . . . I think you'd better not. I'm . . . busy right now,' Beth lies, and I feel her tension, making my shoulders ache.

'Oh. Well, I really just came up to say thanks to Erica for the baby things she took down to Honey. Honey even smiled when I got back—it was amazing.' I smile as I hear this, but I don't know if Beth will understand how rare Honey's smiles seem to be.

'Oh, well . . . I'll pass that on. Or shall I call her down?' Beth asks stiffly.

'No, no. No need,' Dinny says, and my smile fades. There's a pause. I feel a draught from the open door, whispering up the stairs to me. 'Listen, Beth, I'd like to talk to you about . . . what happened. There are some things I think you don't understand—'

'No!' Beth interrupts him, her voice higher now, alarmed. 'I don't want to talk about it. There's nothing to talk about. It's in the past.'

'Is it, though?' he asks softly, and I hold my breath, waiting for Beth's answer.

'Yes! What do you mean? Of course it is.'

'I mean, some things are hard to leave behind. Hard to forget about. Hard for me to forget about, anyway.'

'You just have to try hard,' she says bleakly. 'Try harder.'

I can hear the movement of feet, on the flagstones. I can picture Beth twisting, trying to escape.

'It's not that simple, though, is it, Beth?' he says, his voice stronger now. 'We used to be . . . we used to be able to talk about anything, you and I.'

'That was a very long time ago,' she says.

'You know, you don't get to call *all* the shots, Beth. You can't just pretend nothing happened, you can't wash your hands of it—of me.'

'I *don't want to talk about it.*' She emphasises each word, hardens them with feeling.

'You may not have a choice. There are things you need to hear,' Dinny says, every bit as firmly.

'Please,' Beth says. Her voice has shrunk, it is meek and afraid. 'Please don't.'

There's a long, empty pause. I daren't breathe.

'It's good to see you again, Beth,' Dinny says at length, and again this is not the flippant remark it usually is. 'I was starting to think I never would. See you again, that is.'

'We shouldn't be here. I wouldn't be, if it weren't for . . .'

'And you'll go again soon, will you?'

'Yes. Soon. After New Year.'

'Never a backward glance?' he asks, a bitter edge to the words.

'No,' Beth says, but the word does not sounds as firm as it should. The cold air makes me shiver and

I am shot through with desperation again, to know what it is that they know, to remember it.

'I'll go, then.' Dinny sounds defeated. 'Thank Erica for me. I hope . . . I hope I'll see you again, Beth. Before you disappear.' I do not hear Beth's reply, only the door shutting and a sudden loud sigh, as if a thousand pent-up words rush out of her at once and echo around the hallway.

I stay on the stairs for a short while, listen as Beth goes into the study. I hear the whoosh of a chair as she sits down abruptly, then nothing more. It would be easier, I think, to squeeze truths from the stones of these walls than to squeeze them from my sister. In frustration, I return to the attic, flip open the lid of the red trunk with none of my usual care, and run my fingers through Caroline's possessions once more. There has to be something more, something I have missed. Something to tell me who the baby in the photo was and what happened to him. Something to tell me why she hated the Dinsdales so much that there was no room left inside her to love her own child. But once I have taken everything out, I am none the wiser. I stop, sit back on my heels, notice that my hands are shaking. And as I pick up a paper parcel, reach in to put it back, something catches my eye. A tear in the lining paper at the bottom of the trunk; a tear that has left a loose flap. And, half hidden beneath the paper, an envelope. I reach for it, see that the handwriting is not Meredith's, and as I read the letter inside my pulse quickens.

Scrambling to my feet, I rush down to the study. The fire is devouring a huge pile of wood, pouring out heat.

'Beth—I've found something! Up in Caroline's

things,' I tell her. She looks up at me, her face drawn. She has not forgiven me yet, for the things I said at the dew pond.

'What is it?' she asks flatly.

'It's a letter to Caroline—it had got lost. I found it in the lining of her trunk, and it's very old—from before she came to England. Listen to this!' The envelope is another very small one; the paper inside it so old that the ink has faded to a weak brown colour. The pages are spotted and torn, as if much handled; read and reread over a spread of long years. When I open it out, the sheets tear along the folds a little. I touch it as gently as I can. In places, I can hardly make out what it says, but there is enough here, enough to prove a theory.

'*April 22nd, 1902,*' I read. '*My Darling Caroline—I received your letter and was much dismayed to hear that you had not received mine—nor the one before it, it would seem! Please rest assured that I have been writing—that I do write, almost every night. There is so much work to be done here, to ready it for your arrival, that I am ending each day fairly well beat, but nevertheless I think of you every night, I swear it to you. We have been greatly hampered by spring storms here—the day before yesterday hailstones the size of my fist came down in a shower that could have killed a man! This wild land needs a gentle female hand to tame it, love. And I know that I will not be troubled by any such tempests once you are here at my side.*

'*Please do not fret about your Aunt's departure—here you will have all the home and family that you will ever need! I know it troubles you to part on bad terms with her, but surely . . .* I can't make out what it says next. In fact, most of this paragraph . . .' I squint at it. '*I have seen to it that . . . It pains me to*

. . . Be patient for just a little while longer, my darling, and before you know it we will be together. I have found a place beside the house where I am going to make you a garden. I remember you told me once how much you would love to have a garden. Well, you shall have one of your very own, and you can grow in it whatever you wish to. The soil here is a little sandy, but many things will flourish in it. And we will flourish here, I know it. My heart reminds me of your absence every day, and I thank God that we will soon be reunited.

'There's a huge chunk here that I can't make out at all—it looks like it got wet or something, at some point,' I interrupt myself, scanning down the rest of the page. 'Then he finishes: *I long to see you again, and it gladdens my heart to know that you will soon be setting out to journey here to me. Be at ease, darling—very soon we will begin the rest of our lives. Yours always, C.* How about that, then?'

'So, she was married!' Beth exclaims.

'It would seem so . . . nothing actually says that they were but I can't think of another reason, back then, that he would write a letter like that—about starting their lives together and her having a new family and all the rest of it.'

'Where was she travelling to? What does the postmark say?' I study the envelope.

'I can't make it out. It's totally worn away.'

'Shame. What if she was meant to travel out to marry him and something happened before she got there?'

'But then what about the baby?'

'True. So she lost a husband and a baby before she even came over here. And she was how old at that point?'

'Twenty-one, I think. She'd just come into her money.'

'How amazing—that none of it was on her marriage certificate, or was known until now! I wonder how it was forgotten?' Beth muses.

I shrug. 'Who knows. If she divorced him, maybe she wanted it kept quiet? Mary said that Caroline never wanted to talk about her early years— perhaps she had something to hide. And remember that letter from Aunt B I showed you— that mentioned things that happened in America staying in America. She was definitely worried about a scandal of some kind. If her husband had died, it would have just said widow on her marriage certificate to Lord Henry. She must have left him. And if her baby died, that might explain why she was always so frosty, so impenetrable.' At this Beth falls quiet.

She has not mentioned Dinny's visit to the house. She has not passed on his thanks to me, and I can't find out if this is deliberate, or an oversight, without letting on that I was listening. But it is niggling me. I itch to hear what it is he wants to say to her.

'What's wrong?' I ask.

'Erica, why are you so keen to know all this? To know everything?' She looks across at me from the shadow of her hair, her long eyelashes. The fire behind her gives her an orange gleam.

'Don't you find it interesting? I want to know why . . . why our family hates the Dinsdales. Hated the Dinsdales,' I correct myself. 'I want to know how Meredith got as cruel as she did—as bitter and twisted as she did. And the answer seems to be that she inherited it from Caroline. And I just want to know *why* . . .'

'And you think you've found out?'

'Why they hated the Dinsdales? No. I have no clue about that. It couldn't just have been class prejudice—it had to be more than that. It *was* more than that. It was *personal*. And anyway, in her letters it sounds like Meredith wasn't that bothered when class barriers started to come down during the war. But at least I think I know why Caroline was so cold. Why, as Mum said, she never loved Meredith.'

'Because she lost a child?'

'Lost a whole life, by the sounds of it. You remember that time, at that summer ball, when Caroline thought she recognised the waitress?'

'Yes?'

'I wonder who she thought it was. I wonder why she was so upset by her.'

Again Beth doesn't answer, blocks herself from me in that way I can't stand. 'And I can't get those blasted marsh flags out of my head! I'm sure I remember something about them . . .' But Beth isn't listening to me any more.

'Losing a child . . . I can't imagine how that must feel. A child that has had the chance to grow, to become a real person. When your love for it has had years to deepen. I just can't imagine.'

'Neither can I.'

'No, but you can't even begin to, Erica, because you don't know what it feels like—you don't know how strong that love is,' she tells me intensely.

'There's lots I don't know,' I aver, hurt. In the silence, the fire pops, shifts as it burns down.

'We never missed Henry,' she murmurs, sinking back into the shadow of the armchair so that I cannot see her face clearly. 'We saw the search for him and the way it nearly pulled the family apart. In a way, we saw the consequences of . . . what happened. But we never *missed* him. We were only ever on the edges of it . . . of the mess. The pain it caused . . .'

'It was hard to miss him, Beth. He was vile.'

'He was vile, but he was just a little boy. Just a little boy, Erica. He was so young! I don't know . . . I don't know how Mary survived it,' she says, her throat tightening around the words. I don't think Mary did survive it, not entirely. For a hideous moment I picture Beth being like Mary. Beth, twenty years from now, every bit as empty and deadened as Mary. For surely that is how it will go, if I do not manage to heal her. If I have got it wrong—if I have made it worse, bringing her here. I do not trust myself to speak. In my hands the letter to Caroline is as light as air; so insubstantial, the words of this lost man barely touching the pages, his voice whispering down the years, fading into the past. I touch my fingers to the *C* with which he signed himself, send out a silent thought to him, back through time, as if he might somehow hear it, and take comfort.

* * *

It's late now and Beth went to bed hours ago. Only two days since Christmas Day, since I last saw Dinny, and yet there's a kind of quiet desperation gathering beneath my ribs. If Beth won't tell me what happened then Dinny has to. He has to. Which means I have to ask him; and I know, I *know* he does not want to be asked. Pitch black outside but I haven't bothered to draw the curtains. I like sitting in full view of the night. There's some stupid film on the television, but the sound is turned down and I have been staring at the fire as it dies, and thinking, thinking. Nobody else to hear this wild weather but me, but it's comforting to know she is up there. The house gives me an empty feeling. Without her it would be unbearable. Now and then a drop of rain makes it down to the embers, hisses as it lands. A shred of what was wrapping paper, now a grey ghost of itself, is stuck to the grate. It bends this way and that in the vacillating updraft, as the wind curls into the chimney pots. I am hypnotised by it.

What would have happened, if Henry hadn't vanished? Perhaps Meredith wouldn't have grown ever more unpleasant, as she did. Mum might not have fallen out with her as she did, finally driven to the end of her patience, the end of her forgiveness. Clifford and Mary would have kept on coming, would not have been passed over for the house when the time came. I know it irks Clifford terribly, to be missing out on the house. A king without a castle. He kept on visiting but it wasn't enough. Mary's refusal to come near the place peeved Meredith sufficiently. *Does she want to be a Calcott or doesn't she, Clifford? Such cowardice!* Henry would be the Honourable Henry Calcott, just waiting for Clifford to die before he could slip on the *Lord*. Beth and I would have spent more summers here. Perhaps we would have grown up with Dinny. Beth and Dinny, together; awkward, tentative, passionate teenagers. I shut my eyes, banish the thought.

There's a knock behind my shoulder, and a face

at the black glass that makes me gasp. It's Dinny, and I stare stupidly, as if he's walked right out of my thoughts. The rain has slicked his hair to his forehead and his collar is turned up against the cold. I open the window and the wind snatches it, almost pulls it out of my hand.

'I'm sorry to . . . sorry it's so late, Erica. I saw the light was on. I need help.' There is rainwater on his lips, and I can taste it. He is breathing hard, looks scattered.

'What's wrong? What's happened?'

'Honey's gone into labour and . . . something's wrong. Erica, something's going wrong and all the vans are bogged in after all this pissing rain . . . We need to get to hospital. Can you take us? Please? It'll be quicker than waiting for an ambulance to find the place . . .'

'Of course I will! But if I drive down to you my car will just get stuck too . . .'

'No, no—just go to the top of the green lane, can you? I'll carry her up to you.'

'OK. OK. Are you sure you can carry her?'

'Just go, please—we need to hurry!'

Dinny vanishes from the window, back into the dark. I scrabble for my car keys, my coat, pause only for a second to think I should tell Beth. But she is probably asleep and I can't wait to explain it to her. I shove my mobile into my pocket and run for the car. The rain streams over the windscreen in an unbroken wave. In the short sprint from the house my shoulders are soaked. I am breathing hard, too hard. My hands shake as I try to find the ignition and I have to stop, make myself calmer. The driveway is potted with puddles and I splash out onto the road, wipers flailing.

There's no sign of them as I pull in at the top of the green lane. My headlights flare on the hedgerow, flood away towards the camp. I trot down the track, slipping. The ground is slimy. Grass pulls away beneath my feet, dissolves to nothing. I hear the wind plaguing the trees in the darkness. They crash like an invisible ocean. I stop at the far reach of the car's headlights and stare into the blackness. Rain comes in through the seams of my shoes. Then I see them, making slow progress, and as I lurch towards them Dinny slips and falls onto one knee, fighting to keep his balance with the bulk of the pregnant girl teetering in his arms. Honey grips his shoulders, fear turning her hands into claws.

'Can you walk?' I ask Honey, as I reach them. She nods, grimacing. 'Dinny, let go! Let her get to her feet!'

He tilts to the side, lowers Honey's feet to the ground then levers her up. She is upright for a second before she doubles over, cries out.

Fuck!' she howls. I take her other hand and her nails bite into me. Drenched hair shrouds her face. 'This can't be right . . . it can't be right,' she moans.

'Her waters broke discoloured,' Dinny tells me.

'I don't know what that means!' I cry.

'It means trouble. The baby's in trouble,' he says. 'It means we need to move!' But Honey is still doubled up and now she is sobbing. In pain or fear, I can't tell.

'It's going to be OK,' I tell her. 'Listen—really, it's going to be OK. Are you sure you can walk? The car's not much further.' Honey nods, her eyes tight shut. She is breathing like bellows. My heart is racing but I feel calm now. I have a purpose.

We reach the car and manoeuvre Honey into the back seat. I have mud up to my knees. Honey is soaked to the skin, pale and shivering.

'I'll drive. You help Honey,' Dinny says, moving towards the driver's door.

'No! She needs you, Dinny! And it's my car. And the steering is a little snappy in the wet. It'll be safer if I drive,' I shout.

'One of you fucking well drive!' Honey shouts. I push past Dinny, take the driver's seat, and he climbs into the back. We skid off the verge, slalom down the lane, make for the main road.

I take us to Devizes at a reckless pace, as fast as I dare, squinting into the tunnelling rain. But when I corner Honey is thrown about in the back seat and so I slow down, unsure of what is best. She cries quietly between contractions, as if to herself, and Dinny seems dumbstruck.

'Not far now, Honey! You're going to be fine, please don't be scared! They'll whip that baby out faster than you can say *epidural*,' I shout, glancing at her in the mirror. I hope I am not lying to her.

'It's not far?' she gasps, eyes on my reflection, pleading.

'Five minutes, I promise. And they'll take good care of you and the baby. It's going to be fine. Right, Dinny?' He jumps as if I've startled him. His knuckles around Honey's hands are white.

'Right. Yes, right. You're going to be fine, sweetheart. Just hang in there.'

'Have you thought of any names?' I ask. I want to distract her. From her fear, from the cold, wet night, from the pain shining her face with sweat.

'Er . . . I think, um, I think . . . Callum, if it's a boy . . .' she pants, and pauses, her face curling up as a contraction ripples across her midriff.

'And for a girl?' I press.

'Girl . . . for a girl . . . Haydee . . .' she groans, tries to sit up taller. 'I need to push!'

'Not yet! Not yet! We're nearly there!' I press the accelerator flat as the orange glow of town grows in front of us.

I pull up right in front of the hospital and Dinny is out of the car before it stops. He comes back with help, and a wheelchair.

'Here we go, Honey.' I turn around to her, take her hand. 'You'll be fine now.' She squeezes my hand, tears rolling down her face, and there is no trace of her attitude, her fire, the disdainful tilt of her chin. She looks little more than a child. The rain batters the roof of the car for one quiet moment, then the back door is pulled open, and they take her out, and she shouts at them, and swears, and we pile into the building, blinking in the harsh light. I follow them as far as I can, along three clattering corridors, through several doors, until I am lost. At the last set of doors somebody stops Dinny and me. A hand on my upper arm, kind but implacable.

'Partners only from here, I'm afraid. You can wait back down the hall—there's a waiting room there,' the man tells me, pointing back the way we have come.

'You're Honey's partner?' he asks Dinny.

'Yes—no. I'm her brother. She's got no partner,' he says.

'Right. Come on then.' They disappear through the doors, leave them swinging in their wake. The doors make a sweeping sound and a thump, as they pass each other, once, twice, three times. My breathing slows with them, and then they fall still. Dinny is her brother.

The clock on the wall is just like the one that used to hang in my classroom at school. Round, white plastic with a yellowing fade, the thin red second hand ticking around with a tremble. It says ten to one as I sink into a green plastic chair, and I watch as it creeps round and round, wondering how it hadn't occurred to me that Dinny might have a sister. He didn't have one when we were little, so I assumed he still didn't have one. They look nothing alike. I think back, rake through all my memories, try to remember ever seeing them touch each other, or speak to each other as if they were a couple. They never did, of course. A feeling appears in me, to know he is not hers, it is not his baby. I feel a tentative hope.

Half past three and I am still the only person in this square waiting room. People go along the corridor occasionally, their shoes squeaking on the floor tiles. My legs are heavy from sitting too long. I am drifting into a kind of daze. I see Dinny's camp in my mind's eye, on a summer day—early summer, with spent tree blossoms raining down on a light breeze, and sunshine glancing from the metal grilles of the parked vans. Grandpa Flag dozing in his chair—the wind lifting the coarse ends of his graphite hair, but otherwise he would sit so still. He never said that much to us, but I always thought of him as kind, safe. He would slump, as if fast asleep, but then suddenly laugh at something that was said or done. A loud guffaw, booming from his chest. Always a battered hat, pulled low over his face; and in its shadow, dark eyes gleamed. Leathery cheeks, deeply scored. A lifetime outdoors had tanned him the colour of hazelnuts. The colour of Dinny's arms in the summertime. They made him move, again and again. The police, in the days after it happened. Grandpa Flag watched them with his calm, penetrating gaze. They made everybody move their vans, time and time again, with a roar of engines and plumes of diesel smoke. One trailer, belonging to a man called Bernie, needed a tow to move it. Mickey and the other men put their shoulders to it, shifted it, did as they were told even though Bernie's trailer was high enough from the ground to make looking underneath it easy. I asked Mum what they were looking for. *Fresh earth*, she told me shortly, and I didn't understand.

A figure passing the door rouses me—Dinny, walking slowly. I run clumsily into the corridor.

'Dinny—what's happened? Is everything OK?'

'Erica? What are you still doing here?' He looks dazed, battered and amazed to see me there.

'Well, I . . . I was waiting to hear. And I thought you'd want a ride back.'

'I thought you'd have gone—you needn't have waited all this time! I can take the bus back . . .'

'It's half past three.'

'Or a taxi then,' he amends, stubbornly.

'Dinny—will you tell me how Honey is? And the baby?'

'Fine, she's fine,' he smiles. 'The kid was upside down but she managed to do it, eventually. It's a girl and she's doing well.' His voice is rough, he sounds exhausted.

'That's great! Congratulations, Uncle Dinny,' I say.

'Thanks,' he grins, a touch bashfully.

'So, how long do they have to stay in?'

'A couple of days. Honey lost a fair amount of blood and the baby's a little jaundiced. They're both fast asleep now.'

'You look shattered. Do you want a ride home?' I offer. Dinny rubs his eyes with his forefinger and thumb.

'Yes, please,' he nods.

The weather has not let up. I drive at a more cautious pace. The countryside is so black, empty. I feel as though we're carving a tunnel through it, the only two people in the world. I am light-headed with fatigue but too tired for sleep. I have to concentrate hard on driving safely. I open my window a little; cold air hits me, flecks of rainwater. The roar of it fills the car, cloaks the weight of the silence between us.

'You never said Honey was your sister. I didn't realise,' I say, not quite lightly.

'Who did you think she was?'

'Well . . . I thought she was . . . I don't know . . .'

'You thought she was my girlfriend?' he asks incredulously, then laughs out loud. 'Erica—she's fifteen years old!'

'Well, I didn't know that!' I say defensively. 'What was I supposed to think? You didn't have a sister the last time I saw you.'

'No, I didn't. She was born well after you left. A late bonus, my mother called her.' He smiles slightly. 'Now she's not so sure.'

'What do you mean?'

'Well, you've met her. Honey doesn't have the easiest temperament.'

'So what happened? How come she's been staying with you?'

'The baby. When she got pregnant Mum wanted her to get rid of it. She thought it would ruin her life, having a baby so young. Honey refused. So Mum said fine, have it adopted, and again she wouldn't. They had a massive row and then Keith weighed in as well. So Honey flounced out and was told not to come back.' He sighs. 'They're just angry with each other, that's all.'

'Keith's your mum's new husband?'

'They're not married, but yes, to all intents and purposes. He's OK. A bit strait-laced.'

'I can't really imagine your mother with somebody strait-laced.'

'No, well, neither can Honey.'

'But Honey must be used to a more . . . conventional sort of life, mustn't she?'

'She travelled with us until she was seven, when Dad died. I guess it got into her blood. She's never really settled into the mainstream.'

'But now, with the baby . . . surely she can't stay with you for ever?'

'No, she can't,' he says firmly, and I glance across at him. He looks careworn, and the silence settles back into the car.

'What happened to the father?' I ask cautiously.

'What happened to him? Nothing, yet. That may change if I ever get my hands on him,' Dinny says grimly.

'Ah. He's not been a knight in shining armour about it all, then?'

'He's a twenty-year-old townie idiot who told Honey she couldn't get pregnant on her first time.'

'That old chestnut.' I wince. 'And twenty years old? He must have known he was lying . . .'

'Like I say, if I ever catch up with him . . . Honey

won't tell me his full name, or where he lives,' Dinny says, blackly.

I cast him a wry glance, smile slightly. 'I wonder why,' I murmur. 'Still, it must be a great way to raise a child—living the way you do. Travelling around, wherever you feel like. No mortgages, no nine-to-five, no juggling with childcare . . . The great outdoors, no keeping up with the Joneses . . .' I venture.

'It's fine for the likes of me, but for a fifteen-year-old with a fatherless kid? She hasn't even finished school yet,' he sighs. 'No. She needs to go back home.'

I park in front of the house. The study light I left on blooms out, lighting the stark tree trunks nearest the house.

'Thanks, Erica. Thank you for driving us. You were really great with Honey, back there—you've been great,' Dinny says, reaching for the door handle.

'Why don't you come in? Just to warm up. There's brandy, and you could have a shower, if you want. You're covered in mud,' I tell him. He looks at me, tips his head in that quizzical way.

'You're offering me a *shower*?' he smiles.

'Or whatever. I could dig out a clean T-shirt for you,' I flounder.

'I don't think that's a good idea, Erica.'

'Oh, for goodness' sake, Dinny! It's just a house. And you're welcome in it, now. You're not going to *catch* convention, just by using the plumbing.'

'I'm not sure how welcome I am. I came up to talk to Beth. She wouldn't let me in,' he says quietly.

'I know,' I say, before I can stop myself. He

shoots me a questioning glance. 'I was listening. At the top of the stairs,' I say apologetically.

Dinny rolls his eyes. 'Same old Erica.'

'So are you coming in now?' I smile. Dinny looks at me for a long moment, until I start to feel pinned; then he looks out at the hostile night.

'All right. Thanks,' he nods.

I lead Dinny through to the study. The fire has gone out but it's still very warm. I go to draw the curtains.

'God, it's black out there! In London you have to shut out the light, here you have to shut out the dark,' I say. The wind throws a dead leaf against the glass, holds it there. 'Still think there's no such thing as bad weather?' I ask him wryly.

'Yes, but I'll admit that I'm *definitely* wearing the wrong clothes for it tonight,' Dinny concedes.

'Sit. I'll get brandy,' I tell him. I creep to the drawing room, fetch the decanter and two crystal tumblers, make as little noise as I can. I shut the door softly. 'Beth's asleep,' I tell him, filling the glasses.

'The house looks just the same as I remember it,' Dinny says, taking a swig of amber spirit, grimacing slightly.

'Meredith was never one for unnecessary change,' I shrug.

'The Calcotts are part of the old guard. Why would she want anything changed?'

'*Were* old guard. You can hardly say that of Beth and me—I'm an impoverished schoolteacher, for God's sake, and Beth's a single working parent.'

Dinny smiles a quick, ironic smile at this. 'That must have really pissed the old bird off.'

'Thanks. We like to think so.' I smile. 'Do you

want another?' I ask as he drains his glass. He shakes his head, then leans back in his chair, stretches his arms over his head, arches his back, catlike. I watch him, feeling heat in my stomach, the blood pounding in my ears.

'I might take you up on that shower, though. I'll admit it's been a while since I had access to facilities like these.'

'Sure.' I nod, casually. 'This way.'

The room the furthest away from Beth's is Meredith's and its en suite has the best shower—the large glass cubicle is opaque with limescale, but it has one of those huge shower roses that pours out a wide cascade of hot water. I find new soap, a clean towel, and I turn on a bedside lamp because the main light is too bright and if Beth is awake she might see it as a strip under her door, might come and investigate. Dinny stands in the middle of the room and turns, taking in the huge bed, the heavy drapes, the elegant antique furniture. The carpet over the uneven boards is a threadbare sage green. That familiar faint smell of dust and mothballs and dog.

'This is her room, isn't it? Lady Calcott's?' Dinny asks. In the low light his eyes are black, unreadable.

'It has the best shower,' I say nonchalantly.

'It feels a bit . . . wrong, to be in here.'

'I think she owes you a shower, at least,' I say gently. Dinny says nothing, starts to unbutton his shirt while I hurry from the room.

Creeping softly away along the corridor I hear the shower come on, the pipes gurgling and popping in the walls, and I shut my eyes, hoping Beth won't wake up. But even as I think it she

318

appears, looking at me around the side of her door at the far end of the corridor. Her hair hangs down at either side of her face, bare feet white and vulnerable.

'Erica? Is that you?' Her voice is taut with alarm.

'Yes—everything's fine,' I say quietly. I don't want Dinny to hear that she is awake.

'What are you doing up? What time is it?' she yawns.

'It's very early. Go back to bed, love.' Beth rubs her face. Her eyes are wide, confused, newly awake.

'Erica? Who's in the shower?' she asks.

'Dinny.' I look at my feet in my grubby socks, shifting guiltily.

'What? What's going on?'

'It's no big deal. Honey had her baby tonight—I had to drive them to Devizes and we got soaked and muddy and . . . when we got back I said he could have a shower here, if he wanted,' I tell her, all in one breath.

'You've been to *Devizes*? Why didn't you tell me?'

'You were asleep! And I had to go in a rush— Honey didn't feel right and . . . and it was all in a bit of a hurry, that's all.' I crush one of my feet beneath the other. I am reluctant to meet her eye. I flash her a grin. 'Imagine how Meredith would have gone off—to know a *Dinsdale* was in her shower!' I whisper, but Beth does not smile.

'Dinny is in the shower and you're waiting outside the room like . . . like I don't know what,' she says.

'I'm not waiting outside the room! I was just

going to grab him a clean T-shirt . . .'

'Erica, what are you doing?' she asks me, seriously.

'Nothing! I'm not doing anything,' I say, but even though it's true it doesn't sound it. 'Are you going to tell me that I shouldn't have invited him in?'

'Maybe you shouldn't have,' she says shortly.

'Why not?'

'It's . . . he's . . . virtually a stranger, Erica! You can't just go inviting in random people in the middle of the night!'

'Not random people. Dinny,' I say firmly. I hold her gaze, see that I have won this argument. She can't explain her objection, not without explaining other things. She says nothing more, turns slowly and shuts the door.

I hurry to my room, pull one of the over-sized T-shirts I wear for pyjamas out of my case and drop it outside Meredith's door. Steam leaks out from under it, and the mineral smell of hot water. I hasten away down the stairs, retreat into the study, knock back the last of my brandy.

I emerge when I hear Dinny jogging down the stairs. The hallway is sunk in shadows. He pauses when he sees me.

'Erica! You made me jump,' he says, sounding tired, putting one hand up to his hair, raking it roughly with his fingers. Water drips from the ends of it, soaking the shoulders of my Rolling Stones T-shirt.

'So much for the dry clothes,' I say.

'Dry-er, anyway,' he smiles. 'I'll be wet again as soon as I go outside, but thanks all the same. That, I have to admit, is a great shower.'

I can't seem to answer him; I can't seem to breathe right. I feel as if I've forgotten how, as if breathing in no longer follows breathing out, as if I have lost the logic of it. He reaches the bottom of the stairs, is by my side, and I feel as if I am standing too close to him. But he does not move and neither do I. He tips his head, gives me a bemused look. The same look from decades ago, when I told him I saw trolls in the hollow on the downs, and I am suddenly beset by memories of him: teaching me to duck dive, watching my countless failed attempts; showing me how to suck the nectar from the white flowers of the dead-nettles, plucking one and offering it to me. Gradually his expression changes, grows more serious. I could dissolve under his scrutiny, but I can't seem to turn as I should, or move away. I watch a drop of water trickle down his arm; watch the faint scattering of goose pimples in its path. My hand moves without my bidding.

I touch the place where the droplet stops, trace my fingers along his forearm, wiping away its cold trail. The shape of the muscles over the bones. The warmth of his blood beneath the skin. My skin feels raw where it touches him, but I leave my hand on his arm; I am grounded, I cannot move. For a second he is still too, as still as I am, as if I have frozen us both with this uninvited touch. The vast hall, ceiling scattered with echoes, seems to shrink in around me. Then he moves away; just slightly, but enough.

'I should go,' he says quietly. 'Thanks for . . . all your help this evening—really.' He sounds puzzled.

'No . . . no problem. Any time,' I say, blinking, startled.

'I'll see you around.' He smiles awkwardly, lets himself out into the bleak early morning.

LAMENT

1904

Caroline found herself outside, found herself soaked and shivering, without even realising she had moved. Water ran into her eyes and through her hair and down the back of her cotton dress, and as the two horses trotted into the yard she splashed over to them from the house, caught the rank stink of hot, wet horse in her nostrils. She recognised Hutch and Joe, their hats pulled low over their faces, and as she drew breath to ask she saw the third rider, hanging bonelessly across the front of Hutch's saddle; bare-headed, the rain streaming from bronze hair gone slick and dark.

'Corin?' she whispered, putting her hand out to shake him slightly. She could not see his face, could not make him look up at her. 'Where's his hat? He'll get a chill!' she shouted at Hutch. She didn't know her own voice; it was too high, too brittle.

'Mrs Massey, come now, step aside. We have to get him inside the house. Quickly now!' Hutch told her sternly, trying to steer the horse around her.

'Where's Strumpet? What happened to Corin—what's wrong with him? Tell me!' she asked, frantic now. She knotted her fingers around the horse's reins, pulled its head around, stopped it walking past with its precious cargo. Hutch said something terse, and Joe swung down from his horse, taking Caroline's hands and freeing the reins. Joe shouted something, his voice loud and deep. Caroline paid no heed. More men arrived, to take the horses, to gather Corin up. Caroline stumbled behind them to the bottom step of the house; she fell, and could not rise again. She could not remember how to walk, how to make her legs bend or her feet rise or fall. Strong hands lifted her and even though they bore her in the direction she wanted to go, she fought them savagely, as if she could resist what was happening, and make it not so.

They laid Corin down on the bed. Caroline dried his hair carefully with a linen towel, peeled his wet shirt from his torso and pulled his sodden boots from his feet, splattering rainwater onto the floor. She fetched clean blankets and covered him thickly. His hands were like ice and she held them in her own, feeling the familiar calluses, trying to rub some warmth into them when she had none to give. She brought a bowl of the rabbit stew, steaming and fragrant, and set it by the bed.

'Won't you have some? It will warm you,' she murmured to him.

'He was riding hard after a big dog coyote. It was the last one we were going after, since we'd seen the rain coming in. Strumpet—she always was the quickest. Fast on her feet too—and that's not the same thing. She was nimble, that mare. Quick thinking. I never saw a horse and rider move so well together as Corin and that mare . . .' Hutch spoke in a low monotone; his eyes fixed on Corin and his hands working in circles, wringing and twisting and wringing again. Caroline hardly heard a word he said. 'But then, with no warning she just went over. High in the air, heels right up over her head. Whatever she stepped in, and I think it was some sinking sand, she never saw it coming or she'd have avoided it for sure. Corin was thrown down hard and . . . and then Strumpet came down on top of him. It was so fast! Like God reached down and turned that poor horse over with a flick of his finger. Her two legs were broke in front. Joe shot her. He shot her and we had to leave her out there for the damned coyotes. That brave horse!' He broke off, tears coursing down his cheeks.

Caroline blinked. 'Well,' she said eventually, slowly, like a drunken person. 'You'll have to go and fetch her back. Corin won't have any horse but her.' Hutch looked at her in confusion. 'Is the doctor here yet?' she asked, turning back to the bed. A dark water stain was ruining the silk squares of the quilt, seeping out around Corin. Patches of angry colour bloomed beneath the skin of his chest and arms, like an ugly blush. His right shoulder sat at a wrong angle and his head lolled to the left, always to the left. Caroline slipped her hands beneath the blankets to see if he was warming up, but his flesh was cold and solid and wrong somehow. She lay her head close to his and refused to listen to the quiet, terrified corner of her mind that knew he was dead.

*   *   *

They buried Corin on his own land, at the top of a green rise some hundred and fifty feet from the house and a good distance from the sweet-water well. The parson came out from Woodward and tried to persuade Caroline that it would be more seemly for the burial to be in the churchyard in town, but since Caroline was too numb to answer him Hutch had the final say, and he insisted that

Corin had wanted to be buried on the prairie. Angie Fosset and Magpie were responsible for Caroline's attendance that day, and for lacing her into a borrowed black dress that was too big and hung from her thin frame in folds. They also found her a veiled hat with two long, black ostrich feathers that swept out behind her.

'Have you written to his people, Caroline?' Angie asked, pulling a brush through Caroline's matted hair. 'Sweetheart, have you written to his mama?' But Caroline did not answer her. She had no will left to draw breath, to form words. Angie shot Magpie a dark look, and took the Ponca girl aside for a whispered consultation that Caroline did not attempt to overhear. They led her up the rise to stand by the graveside as the parson read the sermon to a crowd of ranchers, neighbours and a good portion of the population of Woodward. The sky was tarnished. A warm wind shook the wreath of white roses on the coffin and carried a few sprinkled raindrops onto the congregation.

When the proper prayers were said and done, Hutch walked a few steps to stand at the head of the coffin. The mourners waited, eyes turned respectfully downwards, and when Hutch did not speak they waited some more, glancing up at him from time to time. Even Caroline, eventually, raised her shrouded eyes to see what was happening. Then, at last, Hutch pulled in a long breath and spoke in a deep voice, soft and steady.

'The minister here has made a pretty speech, and I know he meant for it to be a comfort. And it may well be a comfort to some, to think of Corin Massey gone ahead of us into the kingdom of heaven. I daresay that, in time, I might be able to draw some comfort from that same thought. I hope he likes it there. I hope there are fine horses, and wide green spaces for him to ride. I hope the sky there is the colour of a spring dawn over the prairie. But today . . .' he paused, his voice cracking. 'Today I hope that God will forgive me if I object to him taking Corin from us so soon. Just for today, I think we can feel hard done by that our great friend has gone. For we will miss him sorely. I will miss him sorely. More than I can say. He was the best of us, and a fairer or a kinder man you could not hope to meet.' Hutch swallowed, two tears sliding down his cheeks. He wiped them away roughly with the back of his hand, then, clearing his throat, he began to sing:

'Where the dewdrops fall and the butterfly rests,
The wild rose blooms on the prairie's crest,
Where the coyotes howl and the wind sports free,
They laid him there on the lone prairie.'

His song was as mournful as the empty wind and it blew right through Caroline. She felt as insubstantial as air, as intangible as the clouds above. Her eyes returned to the pale wooden casket. Nothing about it spoke of Corin, nothing about it reminded her of him. It was as if he had been wiped from the earth, she thought, and it seemed an impossible thing to have happened. She had no photographs, no portraits of him. Already his scent was fading from his pillow, from his clothes. Hutch, Joe, Jacob Fosset and three other men stepped either side of the coffin, gathered the ropes into their weathered hands and took the strain. The parson spoke again but Caroline turned and stumbled away down the hill, the folds of the borrowed dress trailing her like a dark echo of her wedding gown. She could not bear to see the weight on those ropes, the tension in those hands. She could not bear to picture what was weighing that coffin down; and the blackness of the open grave awaiting it appalled her.

'Don't you leave her alone for a second. Not for a second, Maggie. She was lonely enough when Corin was alive, God help her,' Angie whispered to Magpie as she got ready to depart after the funeral. Caroline was standing right next to them, but Angie guessed that she did not care. Angie turned to her, put firm hands on her shoulders. 'I'll be back on Tuesday, Caroline,' she said, sadly, but as she opened the door Caroline found her voice at last.

'Don't go!' she croaked. She could not bear to be left, could not bear the emptiness. The spaces inside the house were as terrifying as those outside it now. 'Please . . . don't go, Angie,' she said. Angie turned, her face twisted up with pity.

'Oh, Caroline!' she sighed, embracing her neighbour. 'My heart is breaking for you, it truly is,' she said, and Caroline wept, her body sagging helplessly against Angie's.

'I . . . I can't bear it . . . *I can't bear it!*' she cried, and her anguish seemed fit to pull her slowly to pieces. Magpie dropped her face into her hands and bowed her head in sorrow.

But Angie had to leave at some point—she had a family of her own to look after. Magpie was around as much as she could be. She slept on a folded blanket in the main room, with William beside her. His cries in the night woke Caroline in a panic because they were so loud and unfamiliar. She thought coyotes were inside the house, or that Corin was back and crying in pain. But once fully awake a persistent, dull lassitude returned to her. One night she peeked at Magpie through a crack in the door and watched the dark-skinned girl nurse the baby by candlelight, singing so softly that the sound might have been the breeze, or the blood moving in Caroline's own ears. She felt the darkness at her back like a threat, like a ghoul she was too afraid to turn and see. The darkness of the empty bedroom, as empty now as everything else. The ache of missing Corin, as she lay in that dark bed, was like a knife lodged in her heart, slowly twisting. So she stayed at the crack in the door for a long time, clinging to the candlelight like a moth; and eventually Magpie stopped singing and changed her posture subtly, just enough to show that she felt herself watched.

The heat of high summer was hardly worth fighting now. Caroline did as she was told, and ate as long as Magpie sat with her and forced her to. In the evening, Magpie spoke softly of unimportant things as she undressed Caroline and brushed out her hair, just as the maid Sara had once done. Caroline shut her eyes and thought back to that time, to the dark spell after her parents had died and how she had thought that she would never again feel as lost and sad as she did then. But this was worse; it was much, much worse.

'Do you remember the time my father took us to the circus, Sara?' she murmured, with the ghost of a smile.

'Who is Sara?' Magpie asked sharply. 'I am Magpie, your friend, Mrs Massey.'

Caroline opened her eyes and caught the Ponca girl's gaze in the mirror.

'Yes, of course,' she said tonelessly, to hide the fact that for a moment she'd had no idea who or where she was.

As she went about the chores, Magpie took to putting William into Caroline's lap. She did this particularly when Caroline had not spoken for several hours, or was not responding to questions, her face fixed and unchanging. The child, by then ten months old, soon began to wriggle and climb about her person, and she would be forced to take hold of him, steady him, and focus her attention on him.

'Sing to him, Mrs Massey. Tell him the story of the Garden of Eda,' Magpie urged; and although Caroline could not find any stories or songs in her heart, she did find traces of a smile for the baby, and her hands woke up enough to tickle him, to hold and reposition him. She did not wince when her hair was pulled. William regarded her with his curious, velvet dark eyes and grinned wetly from time to time; and from time to time Caroline gathered him up and held him close, her eyes shut tight, as if drawing strength from his tiny body. Magpie hovered nearby when she did this, ready to take the child back when the embrace grew too much and made him cry.

Throughout the summer, Caroline spent long hours sitting out on the porch, tapping the runner of Corin's rocking chair with her toe and then shutting her eyes, listening to the sound it made as it creaked to and fro, to and fro. She tried not to think. She tried to not wonder how things might have been if she had not blamed the coyotes for her fears in the night. She tried not to wonder how things might have been if she had not had that nightmare, if she had not been afraid of the wild, if she had been a stronger person; a better, more adaptable person. A braver one. Any other kind of person than the kind that sent a husband out to die chasing wild dogs. She wept without realising it, and went about with her face encrusted with salt. And she had no child of his to keep and raise and speak to with quiet sorrow of how bronze and gold and glorious its father had been. Not even this trace of him was left to comfort her. She stared into the wide, far horizon and let herself be afraid of it. All day she sat, and was afraid. It was the only way she knew to punish herself, and she felt that abject misery was no worse than she deserved.

Some weeks later, Hutch came into the house with a respectful knock. Had Caroline not been so remote, so inward facing since Corin's death, she would have noticed the man's suffering, and that he avoided her, shouldering the blame for Corin's accident upon himself. He was thinner because he could not bring himself to eat. The accident had cut him too deeply. The lines on his face seemed deeper, although he could not yet be thirty-five. Guilt weighed heavy upon him and grief was ageing him, stamping its mark on him, just as it was on Caroline, but she did not have it in her to offer comfort. Not even to Hutch. She made coffee for him and noticed, solemnly and without satisfaction, that she had finally brewed a good strong cup, not weak, not bitter, not burnt. She pictured Corin sipping it, pictured the smile that would have spread over his face, the way he would have complimented her on it—slipping an arm around her waist, planting a kiss on her face. *Sweetheart, that's the best coffee I ever tasted!* Even her smallest triumphs had made him proud. Thoughts like this made her sway. Thoughts like this knocked her legs out from under her.

'Mrs Massey, you know I hate to bother you, but there are things that require your attention,' Hutch said, taking a cup from her. With a slight wave of her hand, Caroline invited him to sit, but although Hutch turned to look at the proffered chair, he remained standing.

'What things?' she asked.

'Well, with Mr Massey . . . gone, you're the owner of this ranch now. I know that may sound alarming, but it needn't be. I don't want you to worry about a thing. I'll stay here and run it for you. I know the workings of it more than well enough, and I've been here long enough to call this my home. Your husband trusted me with his business concerns, and I hope you can too. But there are things I can't do, and one of those things is pay the hands and riders their wages.'

'Pay them? But . . . I haven't got any money,' Caroline frowned.

'Not here, perhaps. Corin always drew the wages every couple of months from his bank in Woodward, and I can't see that there'll be any trouble in you doing the same.'

'You . . . want me to go to Woodward? I can't,' she refused, as completely as if he'd asked her to go to the moon.

'I'll drive you. We can stay one night only if that's what you want; or you can go visiting some of the ladies while we're there. I think . . .' Hutch paused, turning the cup around in his hands. 'I think you need to go to Woodward, ma'am. I think you need to see some people. I think you need to get some air into your lungs. And if we don't pay them, those boys'll go elsewhere. They're good and loyal, but they've had no money for two months now, and that's just not right. And I can't run the ranch without them.' Finally, he sipped the coffee, and his look of surprise at its rich flavour did not go unnoticed. Caroline imagined the trip to Woodward, and a great weariness came over her. She rocked back on her heels and fought to keep her balance, grasping the back of a chair for support.

'All right then, if it's the only way. Corin . . . Corin would have wanted the ranch to carry on.'

'That he would, Mrs Massey,' Hutch agreed. He paused, and lowered his head sadly. 'Your husband was a good man and no mistake. The best I ever knew. And this place was his pride and joy, so I reckon we owe it to him to keep it running, to make it bigger and better than ever,' he said, looking up to hear Caroline echo the sentiment, but she was gazing out of the window and hardly heard him. 'This is damn good coffee, pardon my language, Mrs Massey,' Hutch told her, draining the cup. Caroline glanced at him and gave a small nod of agreement.

*   *   *

She forgot her parasol and felt the sun burning her skin as soon as they set out for Woodward. With her eyes screwed up against the light, she thought of the lines that would take root in her face, and found that she didn't care. The wind was blowing, hot and dry, and a pall of dust sat around Woodward. Sharp grains got into Caroline's unblinking eyes, so that as they travelled down Main Street her face streamed with tears. She rubbed at it roughly, pushing hard with her fingers, feeling the odd solidity of her eyeballs behind the lids.

'Stop now. Stop it,' Hutch told her softly. He wet his handkerchief with water from his flask and held her hands still in one of his while he wiped the sand from her face. 'There,' he said quietly. 'That's better. I reckon your poor eyes have shed enough tears of late to last a lifetime.' The hand holding hers relaxed its grip, but did not relinquish them completely, and, tenderly, he brushed a final grain of sand from her cheek with his thumb.

'Is this the place?' she asked dully. They had pulled up outside Gerlach's Bank, a large building with a grand, handsome sign.

'This is it. Do you want me to come in with you?'

'No.' She shook her head. 'I'll be fine. Thank you.'

Inside the building it was quiet and cool, and Caroline's boots sounded loudly on the wooden floor as she entered. She approached the neat young clerk and saw him recoil from the disarray of her face and clothes and hair. A long-case clock ticked ponderously against the wall, a sound Caroline hadn't heard since leaving New York. She looked at the gleaming clock, very similar to one that had stood in Bathilda's hallway, and it seemed an object from another world.

'May I help you, madam?' he asked.

'I would like to make a withdrawal,' she said,

realising that she had no idea how this would be achieved, having never made such a request before.

'Do you have an account with Gerlach's, madam?' the clerk asked, making this prospect seem unlikely. Caroline looked at the precise trim of his moustache, and his immaculate suit and collar. His expression was haughty, she thought, for a boy who worked in a bank. She drew herself up and fixed him with a steady gaze.

'I believe my husband has kept an account here for many years. I am Mrs Corin Massey.' At this an older man appeared behind the young clerk and smiled kindly at her.

'Mrs Massey, do come and sit down. My name is Thomas Berringer. I've been expecting you. Everything has been put in order and you may of course have access to your late husband's account. May I bring you a glass of water?' Mr Berringer ushered her into a seat and waved a hand at the clerk for the water to be brought.

When it came to how much money should be withdrawn, Caroline realised that she had no idea. No idea how much a rider or a ranch hand should be paid, how much was owing, or even how many young men there were to be paid. She withdrew half of the available funds, and although Mr Berringer looked surprised, he filled out the necessary forms and passed them to her to sign without comment. The date he had written at the top gave Caroline a small jolt.

'It's my birthday,' she said dully. 'I'm twenty-one today.'

'Well, now.' Mr Berringer smiled, looking slightly uncomfortable. 'Many happy returns of the day, Mrs Massey.'

The resulting packet of bank notes was thick and heavy. Caroline weighed it in her hand, unsure of where to stow it. Seeing her predicament, Mr Berringer again beckoned to the clerk, and a cloth bag was found to conceal the money from prying eyes. Outside, Caroline stood on the raised sidewalk and gazed at all the people and horses and buggies. She had once felt so at home amidst people. Now she felt at home nowhere, she realised. Now was her chance to visit the town's stores, to buy books or foodstuffs or clothes, but she could not think of anything she wanted. Seeing a haberdashery, she bought a soft, white crocheted blanket for William, and an open carrycot made of close-woven straw.

'It'll be cooler in this heat than that leather papoose carrier he has currently,' she explained to Hutch.

'That's mighty kind of you, Caroline. I'm sure Maggie will be very pleased,' Hutch nodded, stowing the gifts beneath the seat of the buggy. A long while later, too late for her to comment, Caroline realised that Hutch, for the first time, had called her by her Christian name.

They stayed just one night, in the same hotel where they had stayed the night of the gala. Caroline asked for the same room, but it was occupied. She had wanted to be in a place where Corin had been, like a pilgrim visiting a shrine. As if the place would remember Corin, as if his essence would still be felt there. She watched from the window for a long time as the sun went down, painting the town in lavish shades of pink and gold. She watched the people who passed, and listened to snatches of their conversation, bubbles of their laughter, and she tried to remember what it had been like to be one of them. As dark was falling she saw Hutch go out, with his hair combed flat and a clean shirt on. He sauntered away along Main Street, and Caroline watched until she lost sight of him amidst the jumble of people.

The men were paid, and the wad of banknotes thinned by barely a third. Caroline returned the remainder to the cloth bag and put it into her vanity case. Her hand brushed something soft and she drew it out. It was her blue velvet jewellery fold, with her mother's emeralds and some other fine pieces inside. She unrolled it and looked at the bright stones, thinking of the last time she had worn them, the night she had first met Corin. When had she thought she would wear them out here? They looked ridiculous in the simple bedroom. Like glossy hothouse blooms in a field of wheat. She held them up against her skin and looked in the mirror. How different she looked now! So gaunt, so tanned; her nose a swathe of freckles, her hair dull and untidy. She looked like a lady's maid trying on her mistress's jewels, and she realised that she might never wear them again. They had no place on the prairie. She rolled them away and put them back in the case. Then, without thinking, she packed away some other things too— some clean undergarments and blouses; a nightdress with long sleeves too warm for the summer; some hair combs and face powder. She closed the lid and fastened the clasps tightly, wondering where on earth she thought she could go.

Late in August the ranch grew quiet. Hutch, Joe and several of the other men had gone out onto the grass with near a thousand head of cattle, for the final weeks of fattening up before the animals would be loaded onto trains and shipped north, to the meat markets of the eastern states. Many of those men who remained on the ranch were laid low with an illness that passed quickly from person to person, consigning them to their beds with a debilitating fever and tremors. Sitting on the porch early one morning, thinking of nothing and feeling nothing inside, Caroline saw Annie, Joe's sister, ride out of the ranch on Magpie's grey pony. She headed east, urging the pony into a brisk canter. The Ponca woman's face, as she passed, was set into deep lines of disquiet. Caroline watched until she was out of sight; then she thought for a while and realised that she had not seen Magpie since the previous afternoon. She stood and walked slowly across the yard.

The dugout was hot and rancid. Magpie lay still on the bed and William mumbled and grizzled to himself in the straw carrycot Caroline had bought for him. There was an unmistakable smell of ammonia and faeces coming from the baby, and a rank, metallic smell behind it which instinctively made Caroline afraid. With her heart beating fast, she knelt beside Magpie and shook her gently. The girl's face was deep red and dry. When she opened her eyes they had an odd, dull gleam and Caroline drew back slightly, frightened.

'Magpie, are you sick? Where has Annie gone?' she asked hurriedly.

'I am sick. White Cloud too. Her medicines have not cured us,' Magpie whispered. There was a wooden cup by the bed and Caroline picked it up. There was some concoction within, which smelt sharp and vinegary. She held it up to Magpie but the girl turned her head away weakly. 'No more of that stuff. No more of it,' she whispered.

'If you have a fever, you have to drink something,' Caroline said. 'I'll get some water. You have to get up, Magpie. William's dirty . . .'

'I cannot get up. I cannot change him,' Magpie replied, sounding so unhappy that Caroline faltered. 'You must do it. Please.'

'But I don't know how!' Caroline said. 'Magpie, why didn't you send word to me that you were sick?' she asked. Magpie gazed at her, and she read the answer there. Because none of them had thought she would be any help. Tears welled in her eyes. 'I'll clean him. I'll fetch you water,' she said, wiping her face. The smell of the sick girl and her soiled baby was nauseating, and a rush of dizziness assailed her. But she moved with a purpose, grabbing a pail and heading over to the cistern. 'Where's White Cloud? Where's Annie gone?' she asked again, from the doorway.

'White Cloud is sick too. She is in the teepee, resting. Annie has gone east, to our peoples' lands on the Arkansas River . . . she goes to fetch medicine . . .'

'The *Arkansas River*? That's nigh on two hundred miles! It will take her days and days!' Caroline cried.

Magpie just looked at her, her face slack with exhaustion and despair. 'Please, clean William,' she said again.

Caroline fetched a pail of water and a ladle. It took all of her strength to lift Magpie's head and shoulders so that the girl could drink, but Magpie could only manage tiny sips and found it hard to swallow.

'Please drink some more,' Caroline begged, but Magpie did not reply, lying back on her fetid bedding, her eyes closing. Searching the dugout, Caroline found clean napkins and a towel. She took William out of the carrycot and went outside with him. The filth she found when she undressed the baby made her gag, and she threw the rags onto the coals of the dying cook fire. The water was cold and William began to cry as she dunked him into the pail, swilling the congealed mess from his backside. His cries were weak though, his voice a little hoarse, and he seemed to tire himself out with it, falling into a kind of doze as Caroline finished bathing him and positioned a new napkin between his legs as best she could. Sitting on the ground, she lay him along her thighs and was stroking his arms, entranced, when she realised how warm he was and how flushed his cheeks had grown. She put her fingers to her own forehead to check, and the difference was unmistakable. Hurriedly, she gathered him up and went back into the dugout.

'Magpie . . . William's very hot. I think he has a fever too,' she said, bringing the baby to the bedside for Magpie to see. The Ponca girl's eyes filled with tears.

'I don't know how to help him. Please . . . he will get sick too. You must take him . . . take him to the house! Clean him, feed him. Please!' she said weakly.

'I have cleaned him, see? He will be fine . . . you'll both be fine, Magpie,' Caroline declared.

'White Cloud . . .' Magpie murmured indistinctly. Caroline lay William back in his cot and went over to the teepee. She hesitated outside, afraid to go any further. She thought of White Cloud's iron gaze, her alien voice raised in song.

'White Cloud? May I come in?' she called tentatively, but there came no reply. Breathing fast, Caroline lifted the tent flap and went inside. White Cloud lay crumpled on the ground like so many old rags. Her grey hair was slick with sweat, matted to her scalp. With her bright eyes closed she was just an elderly lady, small and weak, and Caroline felt ashamed for fearing her. 'White Cloud?' she whispered, kneeling beside her and shaking her as she had done Magpie. But White Cloud did not stir. She would not wake. Her skin radiated heat and her breathing was fast and shallow. Caroline had no idea what to do. She went back outside and then faltered, standing alone with her hands shaking, surrounded by people who suddenly had need of her help.

At Magpie's insistence, Caroline took William back to the house with her. He was fast asleep, his fist wedged into his mouth. She put him in the coolest, shadiest spot she could find and began to explore the kitchen cupboards, looking for food she could take over to Magpie. Steeling herself, she went over to the bunkhouses and found three of the beds occupied. The stricken riders murmured in helpless embarrassment when she entered, assuring her that they were quite well even though they were too weak to rise. Caroline fetched pails of water and made each of them drink, before leaving a further cup of water beside each man's bed. She had been hoping to find somebody able to ride to town and fetch the doctor, but there was no way any of those remaining could do so. The thought made panic close her throat. She went back to the house and began to make a soup from dried beans and the carcass of a chicken Magpie had roasted two days before. She also fetched a pumpkin up from the root cellar and cooked it up into a mash for William.

In the night William woke her up with thin cries of distress and she rose, holding him to stop his crying with comforting words and kisses. She laid him back down as he went back to sleep, then sat on the edge of the bed and cried quietly to herself, because it was all she had ever wanted to have a baby sleeping next to the bed, and to comfort it and love it. But this child was not hers, and Corin was not lying beside her, and this tiny taste of what should have happened, of how things should have been, was so bitter and sweet.

By morning, there was no denying that William had caught the fever as well. He slept too much, he was hot, and was groggy and limp when he woke. Caroline went over to the bunkhouses with the soup she had made, and then to the dugout to Magpie, pausing outside the teepee. She knew she should go in and try to wake White Cloud again, try to make her drink some water. But fear gripped her, a new and horrible fear born of instinct rather than conscious thought. It made the hair stand up on the back of her neck as she forced herself to lift the tent flap. White Cloud had not moved. She did not move. Not at all. Not even her chest, with the rise and fall of breathing. Caroline dropped the tent flap and backed away hurriedly, horror squeezing her insides, shaking her from head to foot. Breathing fast, she went down into the dugout.

Magpie was weaker, and harder to wake. The whites of her eyes looked grey, and her skin was even hotter. Caroline washed her face with a wet cloth, and ladled more water through her cracked lips.

'How is William? Is he sick?' Magpie whispered.

'He . . .' Caroline faltered, unwilling to speak the truth. 'He has a fever. He is quiet, this morning,' she said gravely. Fear lit a dull light in Magpie's eyes.

'And White Cloud?' she asked. Caroline looked away, busying her hands with the cloth, the water pail, the ladle.

'She is sleeping,' she said shortly. When she looked up Magpie was watching her, and she could not hold the girl's gaze.

'I don't know what to do. I don't know how to help myself or White Cloud,' Magpie whispered, despairingly. 'We must hope for Annie to come back soon, and to bring medicine.'

'That will take far too long!' Caroline said desperately. 'Somebody will have to go! You can't wait for Annie!' She stood up, pacing the dugout. 'I'll go,' she said in the end. 'I'm well enough. I'll go, and . . . I'll take William with me. The doctor can see to him straight away and then come back with me and look after you and everybody else. It's the best way.'

'You will take William with you . . . ?'

'It's the best way. You can't look after him,

Magpie! I can do it. I'll take the buggy and that way the doctor will see him this evening. Tonight, Magpie! He could have medicines *tonight*! Please. This *is* the best way.' Now that she had decided, she was desperate to start. She thought of White Cloud—her denuded, too-still form. 'It might be too late, otherwise,' she added. Magpie's eyes widened with fear, and she blinked tears away.

'Please, take care of him. Please come back quickly,' the girl implored.

'I will! I'll send the doctor to you at once. It will be fine, Magpie—truly it will,' Caroline said, the speeding of her heart making her voice tremble. She took Magpie's hand and squeezed it hard.

She loaded her vanity case, the carrycot and a bag of William's things into the buggy and drove it as quickly as she dared, steering the horse between thickets of brush as she had watched Hutch and Corin do. The North Canadian was low between its banks and cool droplets of water spun up from the wheels as they took the ford, stirring up the sweet, dank, mineral smell of the river bottom. Pausing to rest herself and the horse, Caroline lifted William into her arms. He was still hot and cried fitfully each time he woke, but now he was sleeping, and his face had settled into a calm slump that so reminded Caroline of how Corin's face had looked when he'd slept in his chair that she caught her breath. Thinking again, even for a second, that this might be Corin's child stole the air from her lungs. She sat down in the sand with William in her lap, and she studied him, running a finger from his hairline to his toes. Long toes, spaced widely apart, just like Corin's. His hair was dark, but his skin was lighter than either Magpie's or Joe's. His eyes, although brown, had a greenish ring around the iris that lightened them. In the furrow of the tiny brow, and the pout of his lips above a tucked-in chin, Caroline thought she saw traces of her husband. She cradled the child to her chest and she wept. She wept for Corin's betrayal, and for the loss of him, and for the perfect, agonising feeling of holding his baby to her.

*   *   *

The doctor took one look at Caroline's frantic face and the child in her arms and ushered her inside. He took William and examined him closely, quizzing Caroline about the symptoms the adults at the ranch were showing and how long the illness had been rife. He listened to the baby's heart and breathing, and felt the heat glowing in the soft skin.

'I think he will be well. His fever is not too high as yet, and his heart is strong, so please, try not to worry too much. Are you staying in town tonight? Good. Keep him cool. The main thing is to bring his fever down as soon as possible. Cold wet cloths, changed regularly. Give him three drops of this on his tongue, with a teaspoon of water afterwards, every four hours. It's an antipyretic—it will help break the fever. And if he will eat or drink, try to let him do so. I believe he will recover quickly. Don't look so afraid! You brought him to me in time. But I must leave for the ranch, for if it goes unchecked this sickness could prove more serious. You will follow on tomorrow, so I can check the child again?' Caroline nodded. 'Good. Rest, for both of you. And cold cloths for your child. Are there any others at the ranch as young as this, or any of great age?' The doctor asked as he ushered her from the room. *Your child.*

'There are no other children. White Cloud . . . she is advanced in years, although I cannot say how old she is,' she whispered. 'But I think . . . I think she has died already,' she said, her throat constricting. The doctor shot her an incredulous glance.

'I must leave at once and travel through the night—I can hope to be there by sunrise. A fellow doctor can be found at this address—if William takes a turn for the worse, call upon him.' He handed Caroline a card, nodded briskly, and stalked from the room.

Caroline did not sleep. She fetched a basin of cold water from the hotel kitchens and laid damp cloths gently onto William's skin, as instructed. She was loath to take her eyes from him, studying each line of his face, each hair on his head. She checked the clock obsessively, giving him his dose when four hours had passed. He woke up from time to time and studied her in return, grasping her finger in a strong grip that reassured her. By morning she was light-headed with fatigue, but William's colour was better, and his skin was cooler. He ate some rice pudding that the landlady had made for him, studying the women with a calm appraisal that made them smile. Caroline wrapped him in the crocheted blanket, laid him in the carrycot, put a pacifier into his chubby hands and gazed at him. He could be hers—the doctor had immediately thought so. He could be the child of a respectable white woman—nothing about his person marked him out as a Ponca. Indeed, he could have been hers, she thought. He should have been hers.

Caroline was reluctant to go back to the ranch. She should have left hours before, with the sunrise, but the thought of starting back made her so tired inside that she averted her eyes from the black buggy, parked outside in the yard, and from the corral where the buggy horse had spent the night, chewing hay and scratching its sweaty head against the fence. The doctor would see to the sick, and when Caroline returned she would have to give William back. She thought of White Cloud's body, lying untended in the teepee. She thought of Magpie, helpless and sick. She thought of life, stretching on for year after empty year, and all of them without Corin. But when she looked at William she smiled and felt something swelling up inside her. Something that pushed the other thoughts aside and made it bearable to go on. She could not go back. It was a prospect as black and terrifying as the grave Hutch had cut into the grassland to take Corin's coffin. *She could not go back.*

Across town, plumes of steam rose from the railway track. Caroline walked in that direction, her case in one hand, the carrycot in the other. The weight of these two items made her unsteady on her feet, but she moved purposefully, her mind now empty of thought, because her thoughts were too dark. The platform was wreathed in steam and the hot metal smell that had accompanied her to Woodward in the first place. But this immense, black locomotive was facing the other way. Northwards, to Dodge City, Kansas City and beyond. Back the way she had come, away from the prairie that had torn out her heart.

'Look, William, look at the train!' she exclaimed, holding the baby up for his first sight of such a thing. William eyed it distrustfully, putting out a hand to grasp at a wisp of steam as it scrolled by. Then the guard's whistle startled them both and the train exhaled a vast, ponderous cough of steam, its wheels easing into motion. A latecomer ran onto the platform, wrenched open a carriage door and leapt aboard, just as the train began to inch slowly along the platform.

'Come along, ma'am! Quickly now, or you'll miss it!' the man smiled, holding out his hand to her. Caroline hesitated. Then she took the man's hand.

6

Meredith's laughter was the rarest of things. Even at the summer ball, or at the dinner parties she sometimes hosted—where children were not allowed and we would creep from our beds to eavesdrop—I hardly ever heard it. She would just smile, and sometimes make a single, satisfied sound in the back of her throat when something pleased her. Like most little girls, laughter came as easily to me as breathing. I remember thinking it must be something that got used up as you got older, as if laughter was like a mass of coloured ribbons, bundled up inside you, and once it had all spooled out, that was it.

But I did hear it once, and I was stunned. Not just by the sound—high and loud, with a rusty edge like an old hinge—but by what had caused it. An overcast day, not long before Henry disappeared, with a quiet breeze blowing. We were in Mickey and Mo's motor home, listening to the radio and playing rummy with Dinny, who had a slight temperature and had been told to stay indoors, much to his disgust. I tried to tempt him out, up into the tree house to play there instead, but he did what Mo told him. He was more obedient than Beth and I. The camp was quiet, most of the adults out working. Outside, sheets were drying on a line strung between the vehicles. They drifted in and out of view through the window, moving with a regular swell and fall. I could see them, in the corner of my eye, as I shifted my thighs against the vinyl bench and silently urged Beth to discard a four or a Jack. So I saw it first—the change in the view from the window. The sudden oddness of the sheets, the colour, the way the sky above them thickened.

The sheets were on fire. I gaped at them, stunned by this unexpected thing. Pale yellow and blue flames tore across them in odd patterns, scribbling lines of charred black, pouring smoke up in clouds, reducing the fabric to dark shreds that tore away like cobwebs. There was a shout from outside and Dinny got up, leaned past me to look out of the window.

'Look!' I gasped uselessly.

'Erica! Why didn't you say!' Beth admonished me as Dinny ran out and we followed. Outside, two women who had been laid up with the same bug as Dinny were yanking the sheets from the line, stamping at them frantically. The plastic-coated line itself had melted and fallen into pieces, scattering the burning remains of the sheets on the ground, which was perhaps for the best. On the side of the motor home, an ugly, brownish smear showed how close the flames had got.

'How the *bloody hell* did that happen?' one of the women swore, catching her breath as the last flames went out. Hands on hips, surveying the smouldering remnants.

'If we hadn't been here . . . Mo only hung those just before she went off—they can't even have been all the way dry yet!' the other exclaimed, fixing us kids with a serious eye.

'We were inside playing cards! Swear to God!' Dinny said emphatically. Beth and I nodded in frantic support. The smoke got into my nose, made me sneeze. The first woman crouched, picked up a shred of fabric with her fingertips, sniffed at it.

'Paraffin,' she said grimly.

Beth and I left then, running as soon as we were out of sight. We skirted the stables, looked in the coach house, found Henry in the woodshed. He had a flat plastic bottle of something, with a squeezy red nozzle on it. I thought of the patterns the flames had made, almost as though they'd been following lines. He put the bottle back on a high shelf, turned to face us, smiling.

'What?' He shrugged.

'You could have set the vans on fire. You could have killed somebody,' Beth said quietly, watching him with such a grave and serious look that I was even more upset, even more afraid.

'I don't know what you're talking about,' Henry said loftily. The stink of paraffin clung to him, was on his hands.

'It *was* you!' I declared.

'Prove it.' He shrugged again, smiling now.

'I'm telling. You could have killed somebody,' Beth repeated, and now Henry stopped smiling.

'You're not supposed to go to the camp. You won't tell,' he sneered. Beth turned on her heel, stalked away towards the house. I followed, and so did Henry, and soon it became a race, and we thundered into the hall, shouting for Meredith, out of breath.

We thought that it was too serious not to tell. We thought that, even though Henry was her favourite, she would have to reprimand him for this. Making dogs sick was one thing, but Beth was right. The fire could have killed somebody. Even for Henry, it was too much.

'Henry set fire to the Dinsdales' washing!' Beth got her words out first, gasping them as Meredith looked up from the letter she was writing, sitting at the davenport in the drawing room.

'What is all this racket?' Meredith asked.

'We were at the camp, and I know we're not supposed to go, but we were only playing cards, and Henry set fire to the sheets that were hanging out on the line! He did it with paraffin from the shed! And the motor home nearly caught on fire, and somebody might have been killed!' Beth said, all at once but enunciating clearly.

Meredith took off her glasses, folded them calmly. 'Is this true?' she asked Henry.

'No! *I* haven't been near their filthy campsite,' he said.

'Liar!' I shouted.

'Erica!' Meredith silenced me, the word like a whip crack.

'So how did this fire start, if indeed there has been a fire?'

'Of course there's been a fire! Why would I say—' Beth protested.

'Well, Elizabeth, you also said you weren't going to associate with the tinkers, as I have repeatedly requested, so how am I to know when you are lying and when you are not?' Meredith asked, evenly. Beth clamped her lips together, her eyes fierce. 'Well, Henry? Do you know how the fire might have started?'

'No! Except—well . . . these two seem to get on with the gyppos like a house on fire. Perhaps that's what did it,' he said, looking up at her carefully, almost smiling, gauging her reaction. Meredith studied him for a moment, and then she laughed. That rare, loud sound that startled us all, even Henry. Two bright spots of pleasure bloomed in his cheeks.

*　　　*　　　*

In spite of the fact that Caroline never, apparently, went to visit her in Surrey, in spite of her no-show at Charles' funeral, Meredith did come back to live here with her. Perhaps life got too hard, with no husband and two children. Perhaps Caroline needed looking after, and Meredith loved her in spite of everything. And she was to be the next Lady Calcott, after all; perhaps she thought it was her duty to return to the family seat. I'll never know, of course, because the letters stop upon her return. I think of the care and attention she showed Caroline when she was ancient—feeding her, dressing her, reading to her. What if she did all that and still got no love back for her pains? What if she'd hoped for some deathbed confession that never came—that her mother had always loved her, that she had been a good daughter? What if she'd had dreams of marrying again, of starting over? Perhaps she expected Caroline to die soon after she returned, and had ideas about bringing the house back to life, of tempting a new husband with it, of having more children to fill it? But like the queen, Caroline lived on and on; and the heir grew old, waiting to ascend. I think it must have been something like that—some crushed hopes, some vast disappointment. To make Meredith turn out the way she did. To make her treat our mother so harshly, when our mother refused to make the same sacrifices.

These are my thoughts on Monday morning, as I dress in warm cords and slide the teething ring into my pocket. The bell makes a cheerful little giggling sound. I go to the study, look in the desk drawers for a pen and a pad of paper and stuff them into my bag. Outside is another of those crystal-clear days, painfully bright. I try to feel the optimism I felt the last time the sky was this blue, and we went to Avebury, and Eddie was here to make us glad. I leave Beth on the phone to Maxwell, bargaining for the return of her son. She sits by the kitchen window in a shaft of incandescent light that blanches out her expression.

The sun is low in the sky, inescapable. It stabs at me through the windscreen, lances up from the wet road so that I must drive through a blinding wall of light. I turn gingerly out of the village onto the main road and see a familiar figure walking along the frosty white verge. Light clothes, as ever; hands thrust into his pockets the only concession to the biting cold. Something leaps up inside me. I pull over, wind down the window and call to him. Dinny shades his face with one hand, hiding his eyes, leaving only his jaw visible—that flat line of his mouth that can look so serious.

'Where are you headed?' I ask. The cold stabs at my chest, makes my eyes water.

'To the bus stop,' Dinny replies.

'Well, I gathered that. Where then? I'm going into Devizes—do you want a lift?' Dinny walks over to the car, drops his hand from his face. With the sun this strong, I can see that his eyes are brown, not black. The warm colour of conkers; touches of tortoiseshell in his hair.

'Thanks. That'd be great,' he nods.

'Shopping?' I ask, as I pull away from the verge, the engine sluggish with frost.

'I thought I'd get something for the baby. And I need a few supplies. What about you?'

'I'm going to the library—they'll have internet access there, won't they?'

'I don't know—never been in, myself,' he admits, a touch sheepishly.

'For shame,' I tease.

'There's more than enough drama in the newspapers, without reading made-up dramas as well,' he smiles. 'Checking your email?'

'Well, yes, but I'm also going to look something up in the births, marriages and deaths index. I've been tracking down a Calcott family secret.'

'Oh?'

'I found a picture of my great-grandma, Caroline—do you remember her?'

'Not really. I think I saw her from afar a couple of times.'

'She was American. She came over to marry

Lord Calcott late in 1904, but I've found this picture of her in 1904, in America, with a baby.' I fumble blindly in my bag and pass it to him. 'Nobody seems to know what happened to that baby—there's no record of her marrying before, but I've also found a letter that suggests otherwise.'

'Well, the baby probably died there, before she came over.' He shrugs slightly.

'Probably,' I concede. 'But I just want to check—just in case he's mentioned in the records. If he is . . . if I can prove that Caroline lost a child—another child, since we know she lost a daughter here in Barrow Storton—it might help explain why she was the way she was.'

Dinny says nothing to this. He studies the photo, frowning slightly.

'Perhaps,' he murmurs, after a while.

'I've been trying to find out, you see, why the Calcotts—the earlier Calcotts—had such a bee in their bonnets about you Dinsdales. Caroline and Meredith, I mean. I've been trying to find out why they behaved the way they did towards your family,' I say, suddenly keen to have his support in this quest.

'A bee in their bonnets?' he echoes quietly. 'That's a gentle euphemism.'

'I know,' I say apologetically. I change the subject. 'So, how's Honey doing?' We chat about his sister for a while, until I try to park in Devizes and am met by swarms of people, row upon row of parked cars.

'What on earth is all this?' I exclaim.

'Sale mania,' Dinny sighs. 'Try Sheep Street.'

Eventually, I creep the car into a space, bumping the one next to me when I open the door.

Skeins of exhaust twist up into the sky and the town hums with voices, the ring of purposeful footsteps. It all seems too loud, and I feel as though the quiet at Storton Manor has snuck into me, somehow. It's performed a stealth coup; and now I notice its absence like something vital gone.

'Do you want a lift back as well?' I offer.

'How long will you be?'

'I'm not sure. An hour and a half? Maybe a bit longer?'

'OK—thanks. I'll meet you back here?'

'How about in that café on the High Street—the one with the blue awning? It'll be warmer if one of us has to wait,' I suggest. Dinny nods, twists his hand in salute and strides away between the packed cars.

The library is on Sheep Street, so I don't have far to walk. The fan above the doors pours out a stifling wave of warmth and I stop the second I am through, struggle out of my coat and scarf in the cloying heat. It's almost empty inside, with a few people perusing the shelves and a severe-looking woman at the desk who is busy with something and does not look up at me. Seated at a computer, I search for deaths in 1903, 1904 and 1905, to cast a wide net, and the names Calcott and Fitzpatrick, in London and in Wiltshire. I skim these results for the deaths of children under the age of two. My pad of paper remains blank on the desk beside me. After an hour, I scrawl on it: *He's not here*.

I stare at the last list of names on the screen, until my eyes slide through the pixels, focus on a point in the middle distance. The baby probably died in America. That, and whatever happened to make Caroline leave the man who signed himself

C, might even be what made her come over to England in the first place, and could certainly have contributed to her distance, her frigidity. So why can't I let it go at that? What is it that is pulling at a far corner of my mind, begging me to grasp it? Something else—another thing—that I know and have forgotten. I wonder how many of these things are lurking in my head, waiting for me to chase them out. I pull the teething ring from my pocket, run my fingers around the smooth, immaculate ivory. Inside the bell, on the rim, is the hallmark. A tiny lion cartouche, an anchor, a gothic letter G, and something I struggle to make out. I turn it to the light, hold it close to my face. A flame? A tree—a skinny tree like a cypress? A hammer? The light bounces from it. It's a hammer head. Vertical, as if viewed from the side when striking something.

I turn back to the computer, search for *American silver marks G.* Several online encyclopedias and silver-collecting guides appear. Searching entries under the letter G, it takes no time at all to find the stamp on the bell. Gorham. Founded in Rhode Island in 1831. An influential silver maker—made various tea sets for the White House, and the Davis Cup for tennis, but their primary trade was in teaspoons, thimbles and other small gift items. I find the vertical hammer head in the list of Gorham's date marks—1902. This then I have managed to prove—whoever the baby in the photo is, and whoever his father was, and whatever became of him, this silver and ivory teething ring belonged to him. He was the fine son it was offered to. Not Clifford, not any other child Caroline lost once she had come over to England. I close my hand around it, feel my skin warm the metal; the stifled movement of the clapper inside, like a tiny, tremulous heartbeat.

It is slow work, making my way to the High Street, through knots of purposeful browsers. Shop windows ablaze with lurid banners promising unmissable bargains, ludicrous discounts; music and heat blaring out; people with four, five, six fat carrier bags, sprouting from the ends of their arms. I am barrelled this way and that and the café, when I reach it, is full to the brim. I feel a wash of irritation, until I see Dinny already at one of the small tables in the steamed-up window. The reek of coffee grounds is strong and delicious in here. I edge my way through the crowded tables.

'Hi—sorry, have you been waiting long?' I smile, draping my coat over the empty seat opposite him.

'No, not long. I got lucky with this table—a couple of old dears were just getting up as I came in.'

'Do you want another coffee? Something to eat?'

'Thanks. Another coffee would be good.' He clasps his hands on the sticky table top and looks so odd suddenly that I stare, can't work out what I am seeing. Then I realise—this is one of only a scant handful of times I have seen Dinny indoors. Actually sitting at a table, in no hurry to be outside again, doing something as mundane as having coffee in a café. 'What's up?' he asks me.

'Nothing,' I shake my head. 'I'll be right back.'

I buy two big mugs of creamy coffee, and an almond croissant for me.

'Didn't you have breakfast today?' Dinny asks, as I sit.

'Yes, I did,' I shrug, tearing off a corner, dunking

it. 'But it is Christmas,' I add, and Dinny smiles, tips one eyebrow in concession. The sunlight through the window gives him a bright halo; he is almost too dazzling to look at.

'Did you find what you were looking for?'

'Yes and no. There's no record of the baby dying this side of the Atlantic, so I suppose he must have died on the other side of it, like you suggested.'

'Or . . .' Dinny shrugs.

'Or what?'

'Or, the baby didn't die at all.'

'So where is he?'

'I don't know—it's your project. I'm just pointing out one reason why there might be no record of his death.'

'True. But on her marriage certificate, it says spinster. It couldn't have said that if she'd come over with another man's baby,' I counter. Dinny shrugs again. I pass him the teething ring. 'I checked the mark on this, though. It's a—'

'Teething ring?' Dinny says.

'Which apparently everybody knows but me.' I roll my eyes. 'It's an American mark—and it was made in 1902.'

'But didn't you already know the baby was born in America? What does that prove?'

'Well, if nothing else, I think it proves that Caroline was his mother. When I showed Mum the photograph she suggested Caroline could have been its godmother, or it could have been a friend's baby, or something. But for her to have kept his teething ring this whole time—she has to have been his mother, don't you think?'

'I suppose so, yes.' Dinny nods, hands me back the ivory ring.

I gulp the hot coffee, feel it bring blood into my cheeks. Dinny casts his eyes back out to the thronging street, seems deep in thought.

'So, how does it feel to be the ladies of the manor? Are you starting to get used to it yet?' he asks suddenly, still looking out of the window, away from me.

'Hardly. I don't think we'll ever feel that the place is ours. Not really. And as for staying on to live . . . well. Aside from anything else, the upkeep costs alone would stop us.'

'What about all the Calcott riches village rumour has it you've inherited?'

'Just rumour, I'm afraid. The family wealth has been in decline since the war—and I mean the *first* war. Meredith was always complaining to my parents that they didn't help enough—with the upkeep of the place. That's why she had to sell off so much of the land, the best paintings, the silver . . . the list goes on. There was some money left, when she died, but it'll be spent once the death duties are paid.'

'What about the title?'

'Well, that's gone to Clifford, Henry's father.' As I say his name I raise my eyes, lock with Dinny's for a fleeting moment. 'My great-grandfather, who was also a Henry, changed the letters patent by act of parliament, because he had no sons. He fixed it so that the barony could pass to Meredith, and then revert to male offspring. Her heirs-male of the body, or whatever they call it.'

'So that's why Meredith stayed Calcott, even though she married? And why your mother is a Calcott too? But how come you and Beth are Calcotts, then?'

'Because Meredith bullied my parents into it. Poor Dad—didn't stand a chance. She said the Calcott name was too important to cast off. Apparently, Allen just doesn't have the same clout.'

'Odd, that she left the house to you girls if the title was going to your uncle, and she was so keen to keep the family line going and all the rest of it,' he muses, swirling his coffee around the bottom of the mug.

'Meredith *was* odd. She had no say in where the title went, but she could do what she liked with the house. Perhaps she thought we represented the best chance of keeping the family going.'

'So, after Clifford, it will be . . . ?'

'Extinct. No more title. Theoretically, Clifford could go to court again, and have it pass to Eddie, but there's no way in the world Beth would allow it.'

'No?'

'She wants nothing more to do with it. Or the house, really. Which kind of makes my decision for me, too—we would both have to live here if we wanted to keep it.' Dinny is silent for a while. I can feel the shape of Beth's reluctance, the reason for it, trying to coalesce in the air between us.

'Not really surprising,' Dinny murmurs at last.

'Isn't it?' I ask, leaning forward. But Dinny shrugs, leans back from the table.

'Why are you here, then? If you know you aren't going to stay?'

'I thought it would be good. Good for Beth. For both of us really. To come back for a while and . . .' I wave one hand, struggle for words. 'Revisit. You know.'

'Why would it be good for her? It doesn't seem to me like she even wants to think about it, let alone revisit it. Your childhood here, I mean.'

'Dinny . . .' I pause. 'When you came up to the house to see her, what did you mean when you said there were things she needed to know? Things you wanted to tell her?'

'You really were eavesdropping, weren't you?' he says, his tone ambiguous. I try to show contrition.

'What things, Dinny? Something about Henry?' I press, my heart thumping.

Dinny looks at me with lowered brows.

'I think I owe it to her . . . no, not owe. That's the wrong word. I think she ought to know some things about when we were young. I don't know what she thinks, but . . . some things might not have been what they seemed,' he says quietly.

'What things?' I lean forward, make him meet my eye. He hesitates, stays silent. 'Beth keeps telling me you can't turn back the clock, and we can't go back to the way things were,' I flick my eyes up at him, 'but I just want to tell you that . . . that you can trust me, Dinny.'

'Trust you to do what, Erica?' he asks, and his voice has an edge of sadness.

'To do whatever. I'm on your side. Whatever happens, or happened,' I say. I know I am not making myself clear. I don't know how to. Dinny pinches the bridge of his nose, screws his eyes shut for a second. When he opens them again I am shocked to see tears there, not quite ready to fall.

'You don't know what you're saying,' he says quietly.

'What do you mean?'

Again he pauses, lost in thought.

'You all done in town, then?' he says, ready to leave.

*   *   *

When I check my phone, there are three missed calls from my flatmate, Annabel. The name seems to come from another time, another world entirely. I wonder absently if there is some problem with the rent, or the radiator in my room that keeps leaking, staining the carpet. But these questions seem so very distant, irrelevant. And then I realise: that is not my life any more. It was the life I was living, and at some point, without me even realising it, I stopped living it. And I don't have very long to work out where that leaves me. I go up to my room to read letters, to think. I listen to the quiet, which resounds after the bustle of town. The muted yelping of the rooks outside. No musical bird song to charm the ear, no church bells pealing, no children laughing. Just the deep quiet that so upset me at first. I let it sink back into me. How amazing, that this could ever feel like home.

*   *   *

On Tuesday I drive to West Hatch, squinting into the lazy sun. It's not a big village. I drive around it twice until I see what I'm looking for. In front of a compact brick bungalow, a piece of sixties-built convention, there's a battered old motor home taking up the whole of the driveway. It was new once, cream coloured with a wide coffee-brown stripe running along each side. Now it's green with algae, bald of tyre. But I know it at once. I have been inside it, sat on a padded, sticky plastic bench and gulped down savage home-made lemonade. I am almost choked up at the sight of it now. Mickey Mouse's house. I picture Mo as she was, round and slightly wry, leaning on the door jamb drying her hands on a blue cloth as Dinny and Beth and I turned our backs to her. Mickey with his elaborate moustache, in overalls always streaked with engine oil, black grime in the creases of his hands.

*   *   *

At the door I find my nerves fluttering. Excited rather than scared. The bell makes a soft, electronic *ping . . . pong.* I never thought Mo would answer to such a bell, but answer she does. She looks smaller, older, slightly denuded, but I recognise her at once. More lines on her face, and her hair a solid, unlikely chestnut colour, but the same shrewd eyes. She looks at me with a steady, measuring gaze and I'm glad I'm not trying to sell her anything.

'Yes?'

'Um, I've come to see Honey? And the baby. It's Erica. Erica Calcott.' I smile slightly, watch her recognise the name and search my face for the features she knew.

'Erica! By Christ, I would never have known you! You look so different!'

'Twenty-three years might do that to a girl.' I smile.

'Well, come in, come in, we're all in the front room.' She ushers me inside, gestures to a doorway on the left and suddenly I'm nervous about going in. I wonder who *we all* are.

'Thanks,' I say, hovering in the hall, hands clammy on the plastic flower wrapper.

'Go on in, go on,' she says, and I have no choice. 'I hear you nearly met little Haydee already, on the way to the hospital!'

'Nearly!' I reply. I find myself the only one standing in a room full of seated people. It's stiflingly hot. The view from the window wobbles slightly in the radiator haze and I feel my face flush crimson. I glance around, smile like an idiot. Dinny looks up sharply from one end of the sofa, and he smiles when he sees me.

Honey sits next to him, an empty carrycot at her feet and a bundle in her arms. There's another young girl I don't recognise, with shocking-pink hair and a crystal in her lip. Mo introduces her as Lydia, a friend of Honey's, and an older man, thin and beady, is Mo's partner Keith. There's nowhere for me to sit so I dither awkwardly in the small room, and Honey struggles to sit up straighter.

'Oh, no—don't get up!' I say, proffering the flowers and chocolates, then shunting them onto the table through a clutter of empty coffee mugs and a plate of rich tea biscuits.

'I wasn't. I'm passing her to you,' Honey says, flicking her kohled eyelids and carefully manoeuvring the baby towards me.

'Oh, no. No. You look comfortable.'

'Don't be chicken-shit. Take her,' Honey insists, half smiling. 'How did you find us?' she asks.

'I went down to the camp first—bumped into Patrick. He told me you were home.' I glance at Dinny, I can't help it. He is watching me intently, but I can't guess his expression. I drop my bag and take Haydee from her mother. A small pink face, still creased and angry, below a shock of dark hair finer than cobwebs. She doesn't stir as I perch on the arm of the sofa, or as I kiss her forehead and smell the baby smell of brand-new skin and milky spit. I am suddenly curious to know how it would feel if this baby were mine. To be in on those secrets—the strength behind Beth's gaze when she watches her son; the way he raises her up, makes her whole, just by being in the room. These little creatures that have such power over us. The beginnings of a need in me that I hadn't known was there.

'She's *tiny*,' I say, breathlessly, and Honey rolls her eyes.

'I know. All that heaving and all this flab for a five pound midget!' she says, but she can't hide how pleased she is, how proud. This initiation over, the atmosphere in the room seems to ease.

'She's beautiful, Honey. Well done you! Is she a screamer?'

'No, not so far. She's been pretty chilled out.' Honey leans towards me, can't stay even arm's length from the child for long. Up close I see the dark shadows under her eyes, skin so pale that blue veins show through it, winding across her temples. She looks tired, but thrilled.

'She'll get the hang of the yelling, don't you worry,' Mo says ruefully, and Honey flashes her a mildly rebellious look.

'I'll put another brew on,' Keith says, levering himself from his chair and collecting empty mugs onto a tin tray. 'You'll take a cup, Erica?'

'Oh, yes please. Thanks.' I can feel eyes on me and I look to my right. Dinny watches me, still.

Those dark eyes of his, black as a seal's again now; unblinking. I hold his gaze for two heartbeats and then he looks away, stands up abruptly. I suddenly wonder if he minds me gatecrashing his family like this.

'I have to get going,' he says.

'What? Why?' Honey asks.

'Just . . . things to do.' He bends down, kisses his sister on the top of her head, then he hesitates, and turns to me. 'We're all heading to the pub tomorrow night, if you and Beth want to come?' he asks.

'Oh, thanks. Yes—I'll ask Beth,' I say.

'Raise me a glass,' Honey grumbles. 'New Year's Eve and I'll be at home and in bed by nine.'

'Oh, you'll soon get used to missing out on all sorts of occasions, don't you worry,' Mo tells her brightly, and Honey's face falls in dismay.

'I'll be back later. Bye, Mum,' Dinny smiles, briefly presses his hand to the side of Mo's face and then stalks from the room.

'What have you done to him, then?' Honey asks me, and she smiles but she's guarded.

'What do you mean?' I reply, startled.

'He jumped like a rabbit when you walked in,' she observes; but her attention is back on Haydee, and I pass the baby back to her.

Keith returns with a fresh tray of steaming mugs, and the lights on the Christmas tree in the corner wink on and off; slow, then fast, then slow again. Mo asks me about the house, about Meredith and Beth and Eddie.

'Nathan tells me young Eddie was out playing with our Harry, when he was here,' she says.

'Yes, they got on brilliantly. Eddie's such a great

kid. He never judges,' I say.

'Well, Beth was always such a good girl. It's no wonder really,' Mo nods. She blows on her tea, her top lip creasing like Grandpa Flag's did. It gives me a shock to notice this resemblance, this sign of how much time has passed. Mo, becoming an old woman.

'Yes. She's . . . a wonderful mum,' I say.

'God! It makes me feel ancient, to see you all grown up, Erica; and Beth too . . . with her own child, no less!' Mo sighs.

'Well, you are a grandma now, after all.' I smile.

'Yes. Not something we were quite ready for, but I am a grandma now,' she says, giving Honey a wry glance.

'Oh come *on*, Mum. We've had this conversation about a *hundred* times already,' Honey says, exasperated. Mo waves a conciliatory hand at her, then passes it wearily over her eyes.

'God, haven't we though?' she mutters; but then she smiles. We sit quietly for a moment, as Haydee murmurs in her sleep.

'Mo, I wanted to ask you about something—if you don't mind?'

'Fire away,' she says, but she laces her fingers in her lap, as if bracing herself, and there is tension around her eyes.

'Well, I was wondering if you'd tell me again why Grandpa Flag was called Flag? I know someone told me before, when we were little—but I can't remember it properly now . . .' At this she relaxes, unknots her hands.

'Oh! Well, that's an easy enough one to tell. His proper name was Peter, of course, but the story goes, as it was told to me, that he was a foundling.

Did you know that? Mickey's grandparents found him in the woods one day, in a patch of marsh flags—those yellow flowers, you know them? It was something like that, anyway. He'd been ditched by some young lass who'd got herself in trouble, no doubt'—a mutinous scowl from Honey, at this—'so they picked him up and took him in to raise as their own, and called him Peter; but more often than not Mickey's grandma just called him 'her baby of the flags', or some such fancy, and the name just stuck.'

'I remember. In a patch of marsh flags . . .' I say, and everything else about the story I remember being told before, except this part. With a tingle of recognition, I realise that this detail is not exactly right. 'Do you know when that was? What year?'

'Lord, no! Sorry. In the early years of the last century, it would have been; but I couldn't say any surer than that. Poor little mite. Can you imagine, leaving a baby out like that? No knowing if anyone would find it or if it would just lie there and suffer to the end. Terrible thing to do.' Mo slurps her tea. 'Mind you, in those days once you had a kid no one would touch you, I suppose. Not for work or for marrying or nothing else.' She shakes her head. 'Rotten bastards.'

'Do you know where they found him? Where in the country, I mean?'

'Well, here, of course. In Barrow Storton. He was a local baby, whose ever he was.'

I take this in, and I almost tell them what I think, but I don't. It seems suddenly too big, the incredible, disturbing, seasick idea that I have; and the way it chimes with something Dinny said to me in the café yesterday.

'Why do you ask?' Mo says.

'Oh, just curious. I've been looking into the history of the Calcotts, and what have you, since I've been back. Shuffling through what I remember, trying to fill in the gaps,' I shrug. Mo nods.

'It's always the way. We wait until the people who could answer our questions are dead and gone, and only then do we realise we had questions to ask them,' she says, somewhat sadly.

'Oh, I'm not sure Meredith would have answered any questions of mine, anyway,' I say wryly. 'I was never her favourite.'

'Well, if it's the history of the house you're after, you should go and talk to old George Hathaway, over at Corner Cottage,' Keith tells me, leaning his sinewy elbows on his bony knees.

'Oh? Who's George Hathaway?' I ask.

'Just a pleasant old boy. He ran the garage on the Devizes road most of his life. Retired now, of course. But his mother was a maid at the big house, back in the day.'

'How far back?' I ask eagerly.

'Oh,' Keith flaps a gnarled red hand over his shoulder, 'right back. You know, they used to go into service at an early age, back then. I think she was only a girl when she started there. Before the First World War, it would have been.' I breathe deeply, excitement tickling the palms of my hands. 'You know which one Corner Cottage is? On the way out of the village, towards Pewsey, where the lane bends sharp to the left? It's the little thatched place with the green gates just there.'

'Yes, I know it. Thank you.' I smile. I leave them shortly afterwards, as Honey starts to drowse on the sofa and Mo takes the baby from her, puts her down in the carrycot.

'Come again, won't you? Bring Beth—it'd be nice to see you both,' Mo says, and I nod as the cold outside makes my nose ache.

*   *   *

I go straight to Corner Cottage, which sits by itself on the outskirts of Barrow Storton; walls that were once white now streaked and grey. The render is cracking in places, the thatch is dark and sagging. The gate is closed, but I let myself in, cross the weed-choked driveway. I knock three times, hard; the heavy knocker so cold it burns my fingers.

'Yes, my love?' An old man, short and spry, smiles at me, keeps the chain on the door.

'Um, hello. Sorry to bother you—are you George Hathaway?' I say, hurriedly marshalling my thoughts.

'That's me, my love. Can I help you?'

'My name's Erica Calcott, and I was wondering if—'

'*Calcott*, you say? From the manor house?' George interrupts.

'Yes, that's right. I was just—'

'Just a tick!' The door shuts in my face, opens a second later without the chain. 'Never in all my years did I expect a *Calcott* to arrive at my door. What a turn up! Come in, come in; don't dawdle on the step!'

'Thank you.' I step inside. The interior of the cottage is clean, tidy, warm. Pleasantly surprising, compared to the exterior.

'Come on through. I'll put the kettle on and you

can tell me whatever it is that brings you here.' George bustles ahead of me along a narrow corridor. 'Coffee suit you?' The kitchen is low and crowded. The usual build up of paraphernalia—biscuit tins, spatulas, rusting sieves and onion skins; but other things besides. Things that speak of the absence of a woman about the house. A black and greasy engine part on the table. A set of spanners on top of the fridge. George moves with a speed and deftness that belies his years. Neat curls of white hair around a thin face; eyes a startling pale green, the colour of a driftwood fire.

'I've only just got back myself, last night—you're lucky to find me home. Been at my daughter's for Christmas, over in Yeovil. Lovely to see her, and the grandkids of course, but just as lovely to be home again, isn't that right, Jim?' He addresses a small, fat, wire-haired mongrel, which waddles from its basket to investigate my legs. It has the penetrating aroma of elderly dogs everywhere, but I scratch behind one of its ears, all the same. Pungent grease gathers under my nails. 'Here you go. Sit down, my love.' He passes me a mug of instant and I cup my hands around it gratefully, slide onto a chair at the enamel-topped table. 'You've moved into the big house, now, have you?'

'Oh, not really, no. We've been here for Christmas—my sister and I. But I don't think we'll be staying on permanently,' I explain. George's face falls.

'Now that's a shame! Not selling up, I hope? Shame for the place to fall out of the family, when it's been in it so many years.'

'I know. I know it is. Only, my grandmother was rather specific about the terms of her will, and . . .

well, let's just say it might be very hard for us to keep to them,' I say.

'Ah, well, say no more. None of my business. Families is families, and they all have their ins and outs, Lord knows, even the grand ones!'

'Perhaps especially the grand ones.' I smile.

'My mother worked for your family you know,' George tells me, pride in his voice.

'I know. That was why I've come to see you, actually. The Dinsdales put me on to you—'

'Mo Dinsdale?'

'That's right.'

'Lovely lady, Mo. Bright as a button. Normally, it's the menfolk that brings a car in for work—I used to run the garage, you know, on the Devizes road. But when that big wagon of theirs needed fixing it was always Mo that came in with it, and she watched me like a hawk! Needn't have—I knew better than to try to pull the wool over her eyes. Lovely lady,' George chuckles.

'I was wondering if your mother ever used to talk about the time she spent working at the manor?' I ask, sipping my coffee, letting it scald my throat.

'If she ever talked about it? Well, she never *stopped* talking about it, my love—not when I was a lad.'

'Oh? Did she work there a long time, do you know? Do you know when she started there?' I am keen, I lean towards George. Beneath the table, Jim sits on my foot, plump and warm. George grins at me.

'It was the length of time she worked there that was the cause of all the natter!' he says. 'She was let go, you see. Only eight or nine months after she started. It was a bit of a source of shame, in our family.'

'Oh.' I can't hide my disappointment, because I doubt that she can have learnt much in so short a time. 'Do you know why? What happened?'

'Lady Calcott fingered her for stealing. Mother denied it with every breath she had, but there you go. The gentry didn't need proof back then. Off she went packing, with no character reference or nothing. Stroke of luck that the butcher here—my dad—was in love with her from the second he set eyes on her—she married him soon afterwards, so she wasn't without means for very long.'

'Which Lady Calcott was it? Do you know the year your mother was there?'

'Lady Caroline, she was. 1905, as I remember Mother telling me.' George rubs his chin, squints into the past. 'Must have been,' he concludes. 'She married my old man in the autumn of '05.'

'Caroline was my great-grandmother. Would you like to see a picture of her?' I smile. I have it with me, in my bag. The New York portrait. George's eyes widen with delight.

'Why, yes, look at that! She looks much the same as I remember her! Nice to know the old grey cells haven't packed all the way up just yet.'

'You knew her?' I am surprised at this.

'Not *knew* her, so much—the likes of her didn't come around to tea with the likes of us. But when I was a lad we used to see her, from time to time. She opened the church fête a couple of times, you know; and then there was the big bash we had for the coronation in fifty-three. They opened up the manor gardens, put some bunting around and the like. About the only time I remember them doing something so community-minded. The whole village poured in to have a gander, since, even for a bunch of toffs, and if you'll pardon my saying, miss, the Calcotts have always been tighter than a gnat's chuff. None of us was ever invited in for any other reason.'

'Please, call me Erica,' I tell him. 'So, did your mother say anything else about her time working for Caroline? Like why she was accused of theft, if she said she didn't do it?' At this, George looks a little sheepish.

'It's a bit of a wild story, that one. Mother was always very straight, very honest. But most people had trouble believing what she claimed, so after a long old while she finally stopped talking about it. But I do remember, from when I was a lad, that she reckoned she knew something she wasn't supposed to. Found something out she wasn't supposed to—'

'What was it?' The air expands in my chest, makes it hard to breathe.

'I'll tell you, if you give me half a chance!' George reprimands me with a smile. 'She said there was a *baby* vanished from the house. She didn't know whose baby it was—it just appeared one day, which was one of the things that made people doubt her. Babies don't just appear, after all, do they? Some gal had to have carried him and birthed him. But she swore it—that there was a baby in the house, and that it vanished again, just as quick as it arrived. And about the same time, one was found out in the woods and the tinkers— Mo's people—took it all round the village, asking who it belonged to. Nobody put their hand up, so they raised the child. But my mother could not let it lie—she swore blind to anybody that'd listen that that baby was in the manor house one day, and that Lady Calcott took him out and left him. So, of course Lady C wanted her gone. Accused her of stealing some trinket, and that was that. She was out of there so fast she never had time to get her coat on. Make of that what you will. Some in the village said my mother cooked this baby story up, to get her own back, you understand? To bring some heat on the Calcotts who'd left her without a job to go to. And maybe, maybe there's some truth in that. She was so very young when all this went on, my mother. No more than fifteen or so. Perhaps she was too young for such a responsible position. But I can't credit her just lying about something like that. Nor stealing, for that matter. She was straight as a die, my old mum.' George stops, stares into the past, and I realise I am holding my breath. My heart bumps painfully, makes my fingers shake a little. I tap one nail on the blurred baby in the New York picture.

'That's the baby. That's the baby that appeared at the manor. The baby that Caroline dropped out in the woods. Your mother wasn't lying,' I tell him. George goggles at me and I feel the blessed relief of closure, of solving a puzzle, however distant from me it may be.

I tell him what I know, what I have gathered from her letters, from this photo, the teething ring, and the missing marsh flag pillowcase. And the age old animosity towards the Dinsdales. I talk until my mouth is dry and I have to swig cold coffee to wet it. And when I am done I feel bone weary but glad. It feels like finding something precious I thought I'd lost; like filling in a huge hole in my past—in our past. Mine, Beth's, Dinny's. He is my cousin. Not two families at war, but one family. At length, George speaks.

'Well, I'm staggered. Proof, after all these years! My mother—if she can hear you from wherever she is, believe me, my love, she's doing a little victory dance right now! And you're sure about all this, are you?'

'Yes, I'm sure. It probably wouldn't stand up in a court of law, or anything, but I'm as sure as I can be. That baby came with her from America, and somehow she kept him hidden while she married Lord Calcott. But then he wound up here at the manor, somehow, and she had to get rid of him. That's the part I'm most in the dark about—where he'd been in the meantime, and if she was married before and had a baby, why keep it hidden? But it's too much of a coincidence. The baby that vanished and the one that was found *have* to be one and the same.'

'It is a pity that all those people who called my mother a liar aren't around to find out better.'

'What was your mother's name?' I ask, on a whim.

'Cassandra. Evans, as she would have been back then. Hold on, I'll show you a photo.' George moves over to the dresser, opens a drawer and rifles through it. The picture he gives me is of Cassandra Evans on her wedding day. Cassandra Hathaway, as she had recently become. A small, delicate-looking girl with a determined glint in her eye and a broad smile. Smooth skin, dark hair caught up in coils, a garland of flowers pinned to it. Her dress is simple, shift-shaped with a panel of lace in the bodice and touches of net at the collar.

This girl saw Grandpa Flag while he was still Caroline's *fine son*. She might have known what it was that Caroline longed to confess to her Aunt B. I stare into the grainy dark spots of her eyes, trying to see that knowledge there.

*   *   *

I leave Corner Cottage a short while later, promising to go back and visit. 'A new entente cordiale between Calcotts and Hathaways!' George announced, quite delighted, as I left. I hadn't the heart to say I might never be back; to the village, the manor, any of it. Unexpected, the way this thought makes me feel, when for twenty years or more I have lived away quite happily. I feel at the edge of a terrible sadness, a deep pool of it that I could fall into, never climb out of; just as Beth feared I would at the dew pond. And yet I haven't even unpacked, back at the manor. My clothes are still in my case. They are in disarray, like me. I've lurched out of my established trajectory and now I am freewheeling, uncertain of where to go next.

I think about blood as I drive back to the manor. About those little traces, the little tendencies all our ancestors have left in us. My propensity to clown in awkward situations; my mother's ability to draw; Beth's grace; Dinny's straight brows and jet eyes. A blizzard of tiny traces, whirling at the core of each of us. I think about my blood and Beth's. About Dinny's, about Grandpa Flag's. And Henry's of course. Henry, the last scion of the Calcott line. He showed us Dinny's blood once, up at the barrow. I think even Henry was a little shocked by it, just for a second. Shocked and then pleased, of course. Jubilant. It was the summer he disappeared, but it was early in the holidays. It might have been the first time they'd seen each other that year, but I don't know for sure.

I'd seen boys fight before, of course. At school, in the far corner of the playground where the side of the games hall shielded the combatants from the watchful eyes of the break monitor. *The corner.* That's what it was called. Whispered from ear to ear during lessons—the next assignation, the next death match. *Gary and Neil in the corner at lunchtime!* The scandal always thrilled me, although the fights never lasted long. Coat pulling; somebody spun around, thrown to the ground. Hair yanked, perhaps; a kicked shin, bruised knees. Then the monitor would notice the crowd, or one boy would start to cry. The victor won the right to escape, the loser had to stay and protest that nothing had happened.

But with Dinny and Henry it was different. We'd gone up to the barrow to test-fly the model aeroplanes we'd spent all morning making from brown paper and ice-lolly sticks. We needed a good launch site, was the verdict—proper thermal updraughts, Dinny said. Meredith was stirring trouble in the village, as ever. She'd forbidden the estate's tenant farmers to give work to any kind of itinerant worker, which left the farmers without the help they needed and could afford, and the Dinsdales without the summer jobs that they relied upon finding here. That was her aim, of course— although I'm not sure of that now. She must have known she'd have to back down eventually. I think she just did it to remind them. Remind them that she was there, and that she hated them. There were all sorts of arguments at the house, and we'd overheard a lot of them. And so had Henry, of course. He followed us up to the barrow with this as his ammunition.

'Shouldn't *you* be out begging? Your whole family will have to go out begging soon, I expect; or thieving of course.' Sneering at Dinny; no preamble. 'There's no way you'll be able to *buy* any food. Not if you stay around here.'

'Shut up, Henry! Go away!' Beth ordered, but he curled his lip at her.

'*You* shut up! You can't tell me what to do! And I'm going to tell Grandma you've been playing with the dirty gyppos!'

'Tell her! See if I care!' Beth cried. She was rigid, as taut and straight as a javelin.

'You *should* care—if you're friends with him then you might as well become a gyppo too. You already smell like one. You're stupid enough to be one too, I suppose . . .' He was breathing hard from running up the hill to us; spite made his neck mottle. Dinny glared at him with such fury that I launched my paper plane in anxious desperation.

'Look! Look—look how far it's going!' I cried, jumping up and down. But none of them looked.

'What's the matter with you? Haven't you learnt to talk yet? Are you too stupid?' Henry taunted Dinny. Dinny stared at him, knotted his jaw, said nothing. His silence was a challenge, and Henry didn't back down. 'I saw your mother just now, actually. She was looking in our dustbin for your supper!' Dinny flew at him. So fast that I wasn't aware he'd moved until he cannoned into Henry and they both went staggering down the hill.

'Don't!' Beth shouted, but I don't know which of them she was talking to. I stood stock-still, rooted with shock. This was no playground scuffle, there was no coat pulling. They looked like they wanted to kill each other. I saw bared teeth, fists, young muscles straining.

Then Henry landed one lucky punch. Truly blind luck, because Dinny was clawing at his face so his eyes were shut. Henry flailed his arms, raining blows, and got lucky. His fist cracked Dinny's nose and knocked him down. Dinny sat for a second, astonished, and then a rush of bright blood poured from his nose and began to drip from his chin. Beth and I were mute with horror. That Henry had won. That Dinny was bleeding so much. I had never seen blood like that. So red, so quick. Not like the dull smears on the butcher's block when I went shopping with Mum. Dinny cupped his hand under his chin and caught the blood as if he wanted to keep it. It must have hurt. Tears welled in his eyes, slipped mutinously down his cheeks to join the blood. Henry, when he realised what he'd achieved, stood over Dinny and grinned. I remember his nostrils flaring whitely in triumph, how haughty he looked. He walked away with a swaggering step. Dinny watched him, and I watched Dinny. His eyes blazed, and for a long moment Beth and I were too afraid to go near him.

*   *   *

New Year's Eve is a Wednesday and it really just feels like a Wednesday. None of the old excitement. It was always excitement tinged with dread anyway, I can tell myself now. The buzz and riot of the fireworks over the Thames, the grim knowledge of how long it would take to get clear of the crowds afterwards. Now it's just a Wednesday, but with an encroaching deadline of another kind. Beth said she would stay until the new year. That's what I begged from her—just until the new year. Tomorrow. There's only one thing that I can think of that might make her stay longer, and that's if she won the argument with Maxwell. If Eddie is coming again before school starts, then she might stay.

I am excited about something, of course. Excited about the announcement I plan to make this evening. It's wild outside. I turn the radio up to drown out the moaning wind, harrying the corners of the house. It took a long time to convince Beth to come to the pub—I had to lie, say it might be the last time she sees Dinny before we leave. The wrenching sound of the wind might be all it would take to dissuade her.

'Hair up or down?' I ask Beth as she comes into the bathroom, holding my hair up in a twist to show her, then dropping it, shaking it out. She considers me, tips her head to one side.

'Down. We're only going to the pub, after all,' she says. I rake my fingers through my hair.

'Yeah, I'm only going to put jeans on,' I nod. She stands behind me, bends to put her chin on my shoulder, peers at her own reflection. Can she see? That the bones of her face are so stark, compared to mine? That her skin looks too thin, too pale?

'I know it's New Year's Eve. But I just . . . I just don't really feel like going out. We don't *know* these people . . .' she says, moving away again.

'I'm starting to—you would, if you came out

more. Please, Beth. You can't just stay in on your own. Not tonight.'

'Why are you so obsessed with spending time with him, anyway? What good will it do? We don't *know* him any more. We live utterly different lives! And soon we'll have left and we'll probably never see him again anyway.' She paces the floor behind me, agitated.

'I'm not obsessed,' I murmur, drawing silver powder across my eyelids and examining the effect in the mirror. I can feel her looking at me. 'It's *Dinny*,' I shrug. 'He's about *the* most important person from our childhood. Look,' I turn to her, make her look at me. 'Let's just not even think about any of that this evening, OK? Let's just go out, drink the new year in and have a good time. OK?' I give her a little shake. She takes a deep breath, holds it for a moment.

'OK! You're right. Sorry,' she relents. She sounds relieved, and smiles a little.

'That's better. Now, go and pour us some whisky. *Lots* of whisky,' I command.

*   *   *

'Here you go,' she says, as I come down to the kitchen.

'This should get us a bit more in the party spirit.' I smile and take a glass from her. We clink, and drink. Beth's smile looks a little forced, but she is trying. 'How was Maxwell? Is Eddie coming back to stay?'

'What, here? No,' she says. 'I want him to come and stay with me at home for the last weekend of the holiday. Max says they're going to his parents

. . . I don't know,' she sighs. 'I always feel like the one who has to fight to get the better slots in the timetable.'

'Well, we did have him for Christmas . . .' Disappointment bites me. Nothing will keep her here now. Something scrambles inside me, twists, tries to find a way to hold on to her, to hold on to our time here. I am not finished. I am jittery with need.

'A few days out of a four week holiday! It's hardly fair.'

'A few pretty important days, though,' I argue, my voice high. I have lost track of the conversation. I should be urging her to fight harder, to get Eddie back—back here to his friend Harry. Beth sips her whisky. I watch the cartilage in her neck move as she swallows.

'I know. I just . . . I miss him so much, Rick. I don't really see what the point of me is, when I don't have him to look after,' she says forlornly.

'The point of you is to be his mother, whether he's in the room or not. And to be my big sister. And, more importantly right now, your purpose is to drink whisky with me, because I don't intend to be the only one starting the new year with a headache,' I say.

'Bottoms up, then,' Beth says gravely, tipping the entire contents of her glass down her throat, spluttering and laughing as it burns her nose.

'Now, that's more like it!' I laugh.

It's bitter outside. The air bites right through our clothes, and the glow of the alcohol; makes our eyes stream, our lips crack. We walk quickly with gritted teeth, hunched and inelegant. It's clear; the sky is inky, torn across by the unrelenting wind.

There are lights on all through the village, warding off the lonely night, and the heat and humanity of the White Horse crashes out like a wave when I pull the door open. It's cheek by jowl. We breathe in the breath of others, swim through it; the heavy, happy stink of alcohol and bodies. Voices so loud, so close. I am sure the silence at the heart of Beth will be battered into submission. I thread us a path to the bar, searching the crowd for Patrick or Dinny, or anybody else I recognise. It's Harry's dreadlocks that I spot, in the snug room at the back of the pub. I buy two whisky and waters, tip my head and smile at Beth to follow me.

'Hi!' I shout, arriving next to the table. I recognise faces from the solstice party, faces I have seen coming and going around the camp. Denise, Sarah and Kip. Dinny and Patrick, of course. Patrick grins at me, and Dinny smiles, his eyes widening with surprise as they alight on Beth. A second later I wonder if it was Beth he was smiling at, not me, but I can't be sure.

'It's the ladies of the manor! Come join us, ladies!' Patrick calls, waving a magnanimous arm over the group. His cheeks are pink, eyes bright. Harry pats my arm and on impulse I bend to him, kiss his cheek, feel the brush of his whiskers. Dinny stares. There's a shuffling, a bunching together along the horseshoe-shaped bench, and room is made for Beth and me at either end.

'I've never actually been in here before,' I shout. 'We weren't old enough the last time we came to stay!'

'That's a crime! Well, this is your local now, so let's get you acquainted with it. Cheers!' Patrick clatters our glasses together. Cold liquid see-saws out, catches the back of Dinny's hand.

'Sorry,' I say, and he shrugs.

'No problem.' He sucks the whisky from his skin, grimacing. 'I don't know how you can drink that poison.'

'After the fourth or fifth nip you get used to it,' I reply jovially. 'So, how are you getting used to being an uncle?'

'I'm not! I still can't believe she's had a baby— five seconds ago she was a baby herself, you know?' Dinny tips his head wryly.

'Make the most of her when she's tiny,' Beth tells him, her words struggling to rise above of the mash of voices. 'They grow so quickly! You won't believe how quickly,' she tries again, louder now.

'Well, I do have the best of both worlds, I suppose. I get to have fun with the kid and then give her back when she stinks or starts howling,' Dinny smiles.

'That's always been my favourite part of being an aunt,' I say, smiling at Beth. And so just like that we chat. We sit and talk like neighbours, like nearly friends. I try not to think about it, how miraculous it is; I don't want to break the spell.

'How's your family research going?' Dinny asks me a while later when my body is warm, my face slightly numb. I peer at him.

'You mean *our* family history?' I ask.

'Do I? What do you mean?'

'Well, what I've found out, basically, is that we're cousins,' I say, smiling widely. Beth frowns at me, Dinny gives that quizzical look of his.

'Rick, what are you talking about?' Beth asks.

'Quite distant—half cousins, twice removed, or thereabouts. Seriously!' I add, when I am met with scepticism all round.

'Let's hear it, then,' says Patrick, folding his arms.

'Right. We know that Caroline had a baby boy before she married Lord Calcott in 1904. There's a photograph, and she kept hold of the kid's teething ring for the rest of her life—'

'A baby boy who more than likely never came over the water with her, or she would have had trouble remarrying as a spinster, which she apparently did not,' Beth interjects.

'Just hear me out. Then there's a pillowcase missing from one of the antique sets in the house—a pillowcase with yellow marsh flags stitched onto it. Now, Dinny, your grandpa himself told me the story of how he got his name, and your mum reminded me the other day, when I was over there. But I think some of the finer details have got scrambled over the years—Mo said Flag was found in a patch of marsh flags and got the name that way, here, in the Barrow Storton woods which slope and are pretty well drained and aren't really good ground for marsh flags to grow in. I'm *sure* I remember Grandpa Flag telling me himself that he was found in a blanket with yellow flowers on it. It has to be the pillowcase—it has to be!' I insist, as Patrick scoffs and Dinny looks even more sceptical. 'And today, I met George Hathaway—'

'The bloke who used to run the garage on the main road?' Patrick asks.

'That's him. His mother worked at the manor house when Caroline first arrived there. She was sacked—ostensibly for stealing, but she insisted, George says, that she was sent away because she knew there had been a baby in the house—right at the time the Dinsdales found Flag. There was a baby in the house and then it vanished. Your grandpa was my great-grandmother's son. I'm sure of it,' I finish, jabbing a tipsy finger at Dinny. He studies me, rubs his chin, considers this.

'That's . . .' Beth gropes for the word. 'Ridiculous!' she finishes.

'Why is it?' I demand. 'It would explain Caroline's hostility to the Dinsdales—she dumps the kid, wants rid of him, and they pick him up and raise him right on her doorstep. Every time they came back here, they brought that baby with them. It must have driven her mad. That was why she hated them so much.'

'Answer this, then,' Dinny says. 'She brings the baby over with her. She has him with her while she remarries—for some reason her previous marriage is not recorded, but there's no way she'd have wound up marrying a lord if the baby was illegitimate. So, she keeps the baby until she gets here, to Barrow Storton, and then she dumps it in the woods. My question would be why? Why did she do that?'

'Because . . .' I trail off, study my drink. 'I don't know,' I admit. I think hard. 'Was your grandpa disabled in any way?'

'Fit as a fiddle, sharp as a tack,' Dinny shakes his head.

'Maybe Lord Calcott wouldn't let her keep another man's son?'

'Then he would have just not married her, surely, if he minded that much?'

'Isn't it possible,' Patrick begins, 'and indeed rather more plausible, that Caroline's baby died in the States, one of the *servants* at the manor got herself in trouble—perhaps Hathaway's mum—took a pillowcase from the house in a moment of desperation, and got rid of her illegitimate baby? It would hardly be surprising if she lied about it, or got fired for it,' he suggests cheerfully.

'He has a point,' Beth tells me. I shake my head.

'No. I *know* it was the baby in the picture. It has to be,' I insist.

'And as for her attitude towards me and mine,' Patrick goes on with a shrug, 'she was just a product of her time. God knows we come up against enough prejudice these days, let alone a hundred years ago! Vagrancy used to be an actual crime, you know.'

'All right, all right!' I cry. 'I still think I'm right. What do you say, Dinny?'

'I'm not sure. And I'm not sure I want to be a Calcott. They haven't been very kind to the people I love, over the years,' he says, and his gaze is so direct that I have to look away.

'Well, drink up, cousin,' Patrick says. Conciliatory, but not convinced. The subject is changed, my parade rained upon.

'It was a good theory, though,' Beth says, chucking me with her elbow.

*　　　*　　　*

By midnight my ears are buzzing and when I turn my head the world blurs past, takes a while to settle back into the right order. I lean against Harry, who sits up straight and has drunk so much cola that he climbs over me go to the toilet every twenty minutes or so. There is talk all around me and I am part of it, I am included. I am happy, drunk, blinkered. At midnight the barman turns the radio up loud and we listen to Big Ben, waiting with our breath paused in the gap before the first toll of the new year. The pub erupts and I think of London, of hearing those bells all the way from there, of my old life carrying on without me. I find I don't want it back. Patrick and Beth and several others kiss me and then I turn to Dinny, proffer my cheek, and he plants a kiss there that I can still feel long after it's gone, wonder if it will leave an indelible mark.

Not long afterwards Beth pulls my arm, says that she's going. The crowd is thinning out, leaving the drunker people behind, of which I am one. I want to stay. I want to keep this party going, maintain the false impression that I belong with these people. Beth shakes her head and speaks into my ear.

'I'm tired. I think you should come too, so we can see each other safely back. You've had quite a bit to drink.'

'I'm fine!' I protest, too loudly, proving her point.

Beth gets up, smiles her goodbyes, starts to pull on her coat and hands me mine.

'We're off,' she says, smiling in general but not meeting Dinny's eye.

'Yep. Party's pretty much over,' Patrick yawns. His bright eyes have turned pink.

'You can all come back to ours, if you want. Plenty of booze there,' I offer expansively. Beth shoots me a worried glance, but nobody takes me up—pleading lateness, drunkenness, impending headaches. I pull on my coat. I am clumsy, can't find the arms. I knock the table as I climb out from behind it, rattling the glasses. As we turn to go Dinny catches Beth's arm, pulls her down to him and speaks into her ear.

'Good night, cousin Erica!' he calls as I weave away.

'I'm right!' I insist, tumbling out of the pub.

'Erica! Wait for me!' Beth shouts into the wind as she emerges from the pub behind me. But I can't seem to slow down. There's a fire in my blood and it's working my body, and I have no control. 'Wait for me, will you!' She jogs to my side. 'That was actually quite fun,' she says.

'Told you,' I say, loud above the buffeting air. I can't quite name what I'm feeling. A huge impatience, the boundless frustration of knowing nothing for sure.

'What were you and Dinny whispering about back there?' I ask.

'He, uh . . .' She looks taken aback. 'He just said to . . . see you safely to bed, that's all.'

'That's all?'

'Yes, that's all! Erica, don't start—you're drunk.'

'I'm not that drunk! You two always did have your secrets and not much has changed. Why won't either of you tell me what happened back then?'

'I . . . I've told you—I don't want to talk about it and neither should you. Have you asked Dinny, then?' She sounds alarmed, almost frightened. I think back, muzzily, realise that I haven't. Not outright.

'What did he really say just now?'

'I just *told* you what he said! My God, Erica . . . are you *jealous*? Still—after all this time?' I stop walking, turn to look at her in the last scatterings of light from the village. It never occurred to me

391

that she knew. That they knew, that they noticed me clamouring for attention. Somehow, it's worse that they did.

'I'm not jealous,' I mutter, wishing it were true. We walk on, stumble up the driveway in silence. As we get to the house I realise that I am uneasy. Some warning bell is trying to ring, beneath my drunken haze. It's Beth's silence, I think. The quality of it, its breadth and depth.

Beth opens the front door but I step back from the darkness inside. In the graphite glow of the moon, it looks like a grave mouth. Beth steps in, flicks on a blinding yellow light, and I turn away.

'Come on—you're letting all the heat out,' she says at last.

I shake my head. 'I'm going for a walk.'

'Don't be ridiculous. It's half past one in the morning and it's freezing. Come inside.'

'No. I'll . . . stay in the gardens. I need to clear my head,' I tell her flatly, backing away. She is an outline in the doorway, faceless and black.

'I'll wait for you to come in, then. Don't be long.'

'Don't wait. Go to bed. I won't be long.'

'Erica!' she calls, as I turn away. 'You're . . . you're not going to let it drop, are you? You're not going to leave it alone.' Real fear in her voice now. It sounds as brittle as glass. I am frightened too, by this change in her, by her sudden vulnerability, the way she braces herself in the door frame as though she might fly apart. But I steel myself.

'No. I'm not,' I say, and I walk away from her.

I won't let this evening end until I have something, until I have resolved something. Until I have remembered something. I stride across the choppy lawn, my legs running away with me, joints swinging, elastic. Under the trees, the dark is solid. I look up at the sky, put my hands in front of me to feel the way, continue. I know where I am going.

The dew pond is just more blackness at my feet. The stone-and-mud smell of the water rises to greet me. Above me the sky hangs motionless, and it seems unreal that the stars should not move, should not be swept away in the wind. Their stillness makes me dizzy. Here I sit in the dead of winter, in the dead of night, a woman with a head full of whisky trying to go back, trying to be a child full of fantasies under a hot summer sky. I stare at the water, I take myself there. My breathing slows and I notice the cold for the first time, the press of the ground through my jeans. I hug my knees into my chest. *Have you pissed yourself, Erica?* Henry laughing, Henry smiling that nasty smile of his. Henry bending down, looking around. What was he doing? What was he looking for? What was I doing? I went back into the water. I'm sure I did. It was a diversion—I was trying to break the tension. I turned and took a run up, and made as big a splash as I could, scrabbling under the surface because my knickers threatened to desert me. And when I came up . . . when I dashed the water from my eyes . . . had Henry found what he was looking for?

Before I know what I am doing, I am in. I have put myself there. I take a run up, I make as big a splash as I can; and then reality comes pouring all around me and my skin catches fire at the cold of the water. The pain is incredible. I have no idea which way is up, no idea where to go, what to do. I have no control over my body, which flails and contorts itself. The air has vanished from my lungs, they have collapsed, my ribs are crushed. I will die, I think. I am sinking like a stone. I will reach the bottom at last, just like I always strove to. The water has no surface, there is no sky any more. And I see Henry. My heart seems to stop. I see Henry. I see him, looking down at me from the bank, eyes wide and incredulous. I see him teetering, and I see blood running down into his eyes. So much blood. I see him start to fall. Then I am in the air again and it is a blessing—so warm, so full of life after the knife strike of the water. A gasp rushes air into my lungs; I cry out in pain.

I can see the bank. It tips and blurs in my view as my body threatens to sink again. I try to make my arms work, to kick my legs. Nothing will move as it is supposed to. My heart beats wildly now, too fast, too big in my chest. It's trying to escape from me, from this leeching chill. I can't get air to stay in my lungs. It whistles out as the water squeezes me. I am flayed alive; I am burning. One hand hits the bank and I can't feel it on my skin, only the resistance of it. I claw at it, force my fingers into the mud, try to make my other hand reach it, try to pull myself out. I struggle. I am a rat in a barrel, a hedgehog in a pond. I am whimpering.

Then hands grab me, under my arms, pulling me further out until my knees are grounded. One more pull and I am out, water streaming from my clothes and hair and mouth. I cough and start to cry, so happy to be out, hurting so much.

'What the *fucking hell* are you *doing*?' It's Dinny. His voice echoes oddly in my ears and I can't look up at him yet, can't move my heavy head on my wooden neck. 'Are you trying to kill yourself, for fuck's sake?' He is rough, furious.

'I'm . . . not sure,' I croak, and concentrate on coughing again. Behind his head the stars judder and wheel.

'Get up!' he commands. He sounds so angry, and the last of my will leaves me. I give up. Lying down on the ground, I turn my head away from him. I can't feel my body, can't feel my heart.

'Just leave me alone,' I say. I think I say. I'm not sure if I have formed words, or just exhaled. He turns me over, stands behind my head and pulls me up by my armpits.

'Come on. You need to warm up before you can lie down and have a rest.'

'I am warm. I'm boiling hot,' I say, but tremors are starting to come, from my feet to my fingertips, convulsing every muscle. My head pounds.

'Come on, walk now. It's not far.'

A short time later I become aware of myself, of the peeled feeling of my skin, the ache in my ribs and arms and skull. My fingers and toes are throbbing, agonising. I am sitting in wet underwear in Dinny's van. Wrapped in a blanket. There's hot tea beside me. Dinny pours in sugar by the heaped spoonful, instructs me to drink it. I sip it, burn my tongue. I'm shaking still, but less now. The inside of the ambulance is warmer than I'd imagined. The embers in the stove light our faces. Narrow bunks along one side, cupboards and shelves and a worktop along the other. A space for billycans. A kettle on the stove top, pans hanging on hooks.

'How come you were at the dew pond?' I ask. My voice has an unhealthy rattle to it.

'I wasn't. I was going home when I heard the bloody great splash you made. You're just lucky the wind's blowing in from the east or I wouldn't have heard it. I wouldn't have come. Do you know what could have happened if I hadn't? Even if you'd managed to get out and then lain on the bank for half an hour . . . do you understand?'

'Yes.' I am contrite, embarrassed. There is no trace of the whisky in me now. My swim has washed it all away.

'So what were you doing?' He sits opposite me on a folding stool, rests one ankle on the opposite knee, crosses his arms. All barriers. I shrug.

'I was trying to remember. That day. The day Henry died.' *Died*, I say. Not *disappeared*. I wait to see if Dinny will correct me. He doesn't.

'Why would you want to remember?'

'Because I *don't*, Dinny. I don't remember it. And I have to. I need to.' He doesn't answer for a long time. He sits and he considers me with hooded eyes.

'Why? Why do you have to? If you really don't remember, then—'

'Don't tell me I'm better off! That's what Beth says and it's not true! I am not better off. There's a bit missing . . . I can't stop thinking about it . . .'

'Try.'

'I know he's dead. I know we killed him.' As I speak I shudder again, scattering drops of tea onto my legs.

'*We* killed him?' Dinny glares at me suddenly, his eyes alight. 'No. *We* didn't kill him.'

'What does that mean? What *happened*, Dinny? Where did he go?'

The question hangs between us for a long moment. I think he will tell me. I think he will. The silence stretches.

'These are not my secrets to tell,' Dinny says, his face troubled.

'I just want things to be as they were,' I say quietly. 'Not things—people. I want Beth to grow up the way she should have grown up, if it hadn't happened. It all starts there, I know it does. And I want for us to be friends, like we were . . .'

'We could have been, perhaps.' His voice is flat. I look up for an explanation. 'You just stopped coming!' he exclaims, eyes widening. 'How do you think that felt, after everything I—'

'After everything you what?'

'After all the time we'd spent, all the growing up . . . You just stopped coming.'

'We were kids! Our parents stopped bringing us . . . there wasn't much we could do about it . . .'

'They brought you here the summer after. And the one after that. I saw you, even if you didn't see me. But you never came down to the camp. My family were turned *inside out* by the police, looking for that boy. Everybody treated us like criminals! I bet they didn't turn the manor upside down, did they? I bet they didn't keep looking in the herb garden for a grave.' I stare at him. I can't think what to say. I try to remember the police searching the house, but I can't. 'At first I thought you'd been forbidden to come down here. But you'd always been forbidden before and that had never stopped you. Then I thought perhaps you were scared, perhaps you didn't want to talk about what had happened. Then I finally hit on it. You just didn't care.'

'That's not true! We were just children, Dinny! What happened was . . . too big. We didn't know *what* to do with it—'

397

'*You* were just a child, Erica. Beth and I were twelve. That's old enough. Old enough to know where your loyalties lie. Would it have killed you to come? Just once? To write down your address, to write a letter?'

'I don't know,' I say. 'I don't know what happened. I . . . watched Beth for all my cues. Even now I can't tell if I knew what we'd done, what had happened. I don't know when it went out of my head. I can hardly remember anything I thought or did in those summers afterwards. And then we stopped coming.'

'Well, no wonder. If you were both acting so vacant, your mother must have thought it was damaging you.'

'It *was* damaging us, Dinny.'

'Well, there you go. What happened, happened. There's no changing it now, even if you want to.'

'I *do* want to,' I murmur. 'I want Beth back. I want *you* back.'

'You're lonely, Erica. I was too, for a long time. Nobody to talk to about it all. I guess we have to take what's due to us.'

'Whose secrets are they, Dinny, if they're not yours or mine?'

'I never said they weren't yours.'

'Mine and Beth's?' He stares at me, says nothing. I can feel tears in my eyes, feel them start to run, impossibly hot.

'But I don't *know*!' I say quietly.

'Yes. You do.' Dinny leans towards me. In the low light I can see every dark eyelash, outlined by the orange glow from the stove. 'It's time you went home to bed, I think,' he says.

'I don't want to go.' But he is on his feet. I wipe

my face, notice that my hands are red and angry, mud under the nails.

'You can keep the blanket for now. Give it back to me whenever.' He rolls my wet clothes into a bundle, hands them to me. 'I'll walk you back.'

'Dinny!' I stand up, stagger slightly. In the small space we are centimetres apart but that is too far. He stops, turns to face me. I can't think of any words to say. I clasp the blanket close to me and lean towards him, tilt my head so my forehead can touch his cheek. I take one step closer, shut my eyes, put one hand on his shoulder, curling my thumb into the hard jut of his collarbone. I stay that way for three heartbeats, until I feel his arms circle me. I lift my chin, feel his lips brush mine, and I lean into his kiss, clumsy with desire. His arms tighten around me, chase my breath away. I would halt the world, if I could; stop it spinning, make it so I could stay here for ever, in this dark space with Dinny's mouth against mine.

He walks me back to the manor's ponderous front door and as I shut it behind me, I hear a sound that makes me pause. Water running. The sound of it echoes faintly down the stairs; and in the walls, the corresponding wrenching of the pipes.

'Beth?' I call out, my teeth chattering. I struggle out of my soaked boots, make my way to the kitchen, where the light is on. Beth is not there. 'Beth! Are you still up?' I shout, flinching from the glare of the lights, my head thumping. The water running still, drenching my thoughts with nauseating unease. I fight to focus my eyes, because there is something not right in here, in the kitchen. Something that makes the blood beat in my temples, dries my throat. The knife block, knocked roughly over and lying on its side on the worktop, and several of the knives pulled out, discarded beside it. For the second time on this black night, I cannot breathe. I turn, race to the stairs on legs that won't move fast enough.

LASTING

1904–1905

The stationmaster at Dodge City was most sympathetic. He listened patiently to Caroline's tale of her lost ticket and allowed her to pay there and then for her whole journey, from Woodward to New York. She spent the long days of the train ride watching out of the window, at grey storm skies and blistering white skies and china-blue skies so pretty they hurt her head. She thought of nothing, but tested the kernel of grief inside herself from time to time, to see if it would diminish with distance when it hadn't with time. William, still recovering from his fever, slept a great deal, whimpering fretfully when he awoke. But he knew Caroline and allowed her to soothe him. She sacrificed lunch at the Harvey hotel in Kansas City to shop instead for clean napkins, blankets and a bottle for the baby, hurrying back to the train with her heart fluttering anxiously, in case it left without her. The train was the only home she had at that moment. It was her only plan, the only thing she knew.

'Oh, he is just *beautiful*! What's his name?' a woman exclaimed one evening, pausing on her way through the carriage to bend over the carrycot and clasp her hands together over her heart.

'William,' Caroline told her, swallowing; her throat suddenly, painfully, dry.

'That's a handsome name, too. Such dark hair!'

'Oh, yes, he takes after his father in that

respect,' Caroline smiled. She could not keep the sorrow from her voice as she spoke, though, and the woman glanced at her quickly, saw her red-rimmed eyes and the paleness of her face.

'Just you and William now, is it?' the woman asked kindly. Caroline nodded, amazed by how easily the lie came to her.

'I'm taking him to live with my family,' she said, smiling a wan smile. The woman nodded in sympathy.

'My name's Mary Russell. I'm sitting in the third car and if you need anything—even if it's just company—you come and find my husband Leslie and me. Agreed?'

'Agreed. Thank you.' Caroline smiled again as Mary moved away, wishing that she could accept the offer, wishing that she could seek out some company. But that could only be in another world, where Corin was not dead and they were just visiting his family in New York, perhaps, and with a baby that Caroline had carried in her womb, not just in her arms. She returned to her quiet study of the landscape, and William returned to sleep.

New York was impossibly loud and huge. The buildings seemed to lean over from their vast heights, casting deep, murky shadows, and the noise was like a tidal wave, crashing and foaming into every corner of every street. Heavy with fatigue, and with her mind wound tight with nerves, Caroline hailed a hansom cab and climbed aboard. Her clothes were travel-stained and smelt stale.

'Where to, madam?' the driver asked. Caroline blinked, and her face grew hot. She had no idea where to go. There were girls whose addresses she knew, whom she would once have called her friends, but she could not think of calling on them after more than two years without a word, with a black-eyed baby and her face dirty with smuts from the train. She thought briefly of Corin's family, but William squirmed in her arms and she blinked back tears. There was no way she could have carried and borne them a grandson without Corin having written to them about it. And she did not want to be anywhere she might be found. This knowledge came like a sluice of cold water. She *could* not go anywhere somebody might look to find her.

'A . . . um, a hotel. The Westchester, thank you,' she answered at length, naming a place where she had once had lunch with Bathilda. The driver flicked the reins and the horse started forwards, narrowly missing a motorcar that drew to a halt to let them go ahead, tooting its horn impatiently.

Bathilda. Caroline had not thought of her, had deliberately not thought of her in months and months. She knew what her aunt would have made of her fears, and of the wreck that life had become out in Woodward County. Now Caroline shut her eyes and at once she could see Bathilda's knowing look, her scathing expression. She could imagine Bathilda hearing of Caroline's plight and responding with a weighty, sanctimonious *Well* . . . She would not have gone to her, even if the woman had remained in New York, Caroline told herself defiantly. She would not have gone to Bathilda even now, now that she knew nobody and had no idea where to go, or what to do. She suppressed the treacherous longing she felt just to see a familiar face, even if it was not a friendly one. For whose faces would remain friendly to her now? She thought of Magpie, waiting in the dugout—but only for a second. The thought was too terrible. She thought of Hutch, of what emotions his face would register when he rode back in from the ranges, found White Cloud dead, maybe others too, and she and William gone without a word. Her insides seemed to burn her, seemed to writhe around themselves, and pain snapped behind her eyes. With a small cry she buried her face in her hands and concentrated hard on staying upright on the cab's padded bench.

At the Westchester she paid for a respectable room, and enquired after a nursemaid for William, explaining that her own maid had been taken seriously ill and been forced to return to her family's care. One was found without delay, a pug-faced girl with bright ginger hair, called Luella, who looked nothing but terrified when Caroline handed William to her. William took one look at the strange girl's frightened eyes and garish hair and began to wail. Holding the child awkwardly, Luella backed out of the room. Caroline went into the bathroom and, realising in a way she never had before just how miraculous indoor plumbing was, she ran herself a hot bath, sank into it and tried to quiet her mind, which rang with unanswered questions and thoughts and fears, and threatened at any moment to tip her into panic.

In the end she did not stay more than a week in the city where she had been born and raised. It no longer felt any more like home than the ranch house, or Woodward, or the railway car that had brought her back. The oily fumes of the motorcars that had proliferated in her absence stuck in the back of her throat, and the throng of people made her feel every bit as invisible as she had felt out on the prairie. The buildings were too close, too solid, like the cliff walls of some labyrinth from which escape was impossible. *There's nowhere I belong*, Caroline thought, as she walked William in his new perambulator down streets she had never seen before, had never heard of before, hoping in this way to reduce the risk of anybody recognising her. She paused on a corner and looked up, high above, to where a crane was swinging a steel girder that looked like a toothpick into the waiting arms of a gang of workmen. The men stood at the edge of this unfinished tower with nothing to keep them but their balance. Caroline felt a sympathetic clench in her stomach for the danger they were in, for the nearness of the fall. But she soon walked on again, recognising the feeling as one she had herself, one she'd had for a long time. The creeping knowledge of life's precariousness, of the transience of it.

Passing a photographic studio, with a handsome gilt sign that read *Gilbert Beaufort & Son,* Caroline paused. Inside the cluttered, stuffy shop she recoiled from the vinegar stench of the developing chemicals. Not quite finding a smile for the camera, she commissioned several portraits of herself and William, arranging to have them delivered to the Westchester when they were ready.

Her fingers shook as she opened the package. She had hoped to create something permanent, to prove to herself, in some way, that she existed; and that even though she was widowed, she had Corin's child, the child that was rightly hers, to show for her marriage. She was part of a family. She would have some record of herself and of her life, which she was so unsure of that she sometimes wondered if she might still be lying out on the prairie somewhere, dreaming everything that had happened since. But in nearly every picture William had moved, blurring the image of himself so that his face was tantalisingly obscured; and in nearly every picture Caroline, to her own eyes, stared out from the paper every bit as ghostly and insubstantial looking as she felt. One photo alone had captured an intangible trace of what she'd hoped to see—in one shot she looked like a mother, proud and calm and possessive. She slid this picture into her case and threw the rest into the grate.

On the fourth day she saw Joe. She was walking with William in search of a park or a garden, a green space of some kind to feel a breeze and, she hoped, to calm the child. Fully recovered from his illness and returned to his strength, William was loud and unsettled. He cried in the night and snatched his arms away when Caroline tried to comfort him, squirming in her embrace as she rocked him and tried to sing to him as Magpie had done. But she could no more capture the Ponca girl's odd melodies than she could howl like a coyote, and her efforts were drowned out by William's shouts. Thinking it was the open prairie he missed, Caroline walked him most of the day, growing increasingly aware of how different the noises and smells and sights must be for the child, and how heavy the unclean air must feel in his tiny lungs. This was not his home, any more than it was hers, she realised; but unlike herself, William did have a home. She should take him back. The thought stung her like a slap to the face. Even if he was Corin's, even if he should have been hers, he belonged in Woodward County. She stood rooted to the spot, knocked senseless by this realisation, whilst pedestrians flowed around her like a river. But how could she? How could she explain—how could she be forgiven? She could see the pain, the accusation in Hutch's eyes, the anger and fear in Magpie's. All the times they had helped her, all the times they had encouraged her. And this was how she had repaid their belief in her—she was an outrage, a despicable failure. It was not possible. She could not face them. There *was* no going back.

And then she saw Joe, coming around the corner towards her, his face set into a grimace of hard fury, his black hair flying behind him as he strode towards her, knife ready in his hand to kill her. Caroline went cold from her head to her toes and stood petrified as the man walked past her, the black hair in fact a scarf, the knife a piece of rolled up paper, the face not Joe's at all but belonging to a swarthy, Mexican-looking man who was late for something and hurrying. Shaking uncontrollably, Caroline sank onto a nearby bench, the din of the city receding as a strange, muffled thumping invaded her head. Black speckles swirled like flies at the edges of her vision, and when she shut her eyes to be rid of them they turned brilliant white and danced on undeterred. In the distance, a passenger liner sounded its whistle as it slid gracefully into the docks. The deep blast echoed all around and brought Caroline back to herself, and to William's cries. Swallowing, she stroked his cheek, made some broken, soothing sounds, and then she stood up, turning to cast her eyes southwards towards the docks, the ship, and the sea. Five hours later she was aboard a steamer, bound for Southampton.

*   *   *

Joe was indeed in New York, but not on that very day. He and Hutch arrived two days after Caroline's ship had departed, where they made their way directly to the home of Mrs Massey, Corin's twice-bereaved mother, ignoring the stares that their country clothes and Joe's Indian blood elicited. No trace of Caroline or William had been found since she had been seen taking breakfast at the hotel, the morning after she'd left Woodward. The manager of Gerlach's Bank confirmed that there had been no transactions on the Massey account since the recent wages withdrawal. Word was sent out with every passing traveller, and to every outlying rancher, to report any sighting or signs of her; and although the ticket office clerk at the station swore that no fair-haired women carrying babies had bought a ticket for any train from him that day, or indeed that week, Hutch followed a hunch of his and took Joe and himself to New York, making fruitless enquiries at each station after a Mrs Massey.

Mrs Massey Senior had not, of course, seen or heard anything of her daughter-in-law, and was most distressed to hear that she and a young child had vanished. She was able to supply the men with Caroline's maiden name and former address, but their enquiries in the city after Miss Fitzpatrick were every bit as fruitless. They retraced their

408

steps, trying the name Fitzpatrick instead of Massey, and then had little choice but to return to the ranch, to where Magpie had fallen into a trance, at times tearing at her hair and making long cuts down her arms with a blade that sent rivulets of bright blood to drip from her fingertips. Joe let his wife mourn in this way; he was impassive, the rage had burned from him, and his own heart was empty without his son. Between them, the men raised the money to pay a Pinkerton man for one month, but this was just enough time for the detective to follow the same path that Joe and Hutch had, and he finished the term unable even to say whether Caroline and William had been abducted or had run away. Hutch lay awake night after night, mystified and suspicious at once; scared for Caroline and for the ranch, which, having no owner, no longer had a future either.

*   *   *

Dreading her arrival more with each mile that passed, Caroline took the train from Southampton to London, and upon arriving found a hotel she could afford once the shrinking packet of dollars from Gerlach's Bank had been converted into pounds sterling. William was heavy in her arms and his cries made her ears wince, as if withdrawing inside her skull to protect themselves. During the long days of the sea crossing she had felt sick, distracted by a pounding at her temples that made it hard to think. William had cried for hours at a time, seemingly without pause, and although Caroline told herself that he must be feeling the same sickness as she, the same pain in his head, she could not shake the belief that he somehow knew he was being carried further and further from home, and that his cries were of rage at her for doing it. She saw an accusation in his face each time she looked at him. She stopped trying to quiet him, to sing to him or to hold him, leaving him instead to cry in the carrycot that he was rapidly outgrowing, so that she herself could remain in bed, curled against the cabin wall in misery.

Now, in an unfamiliar city, so tired she could barely think and with the ground still rolling beneath her feet, Caroline hefted the child higher in her arms and propped him against the smooth marble counter in the hotel lobby.

'I need a nursemaid,' she announced, with a note of panic in her voice. 'My own has been laid low with some fever.' The man behind the counter, tall and thin with immaculate hair and clothing, inclined his head condescendingly at her, twitching one eyebrow at her accent. She knew she was creased and careworn, and that William smelt bad, but these facts only served to make her crosser with the hotelier.

'Very well, madam. I shall make enquiries,' he told her smoothly. Caroline nodded, and toiled up the stairs to her room. She bathed William in the porcelain bowl of the washstand, trying not to ruin the towels with the filth smearing his bottom and legs. He stopped crying as she washed him, and made small, happy noises, slapping his feet in the water. Clearing her raw throat, Caroline hummed a lullaby until he began to drowse. Her ears rang with the quiet left by his absent cries, and she held him tightly to her, still humming, forgetting everything else but the warmth of him, the trusting weight of him, as he slept. There was no more water to wash herself with, and she put William to sleep on the bed as she fruitlessly paced the corridors of the hotel in search of a maid to remove the foul water, and to ask about the possibility of a hot bath.

Later a woman came to the room, announcing herself with a quiet knock. She was plump and florid with pale, frizzy hair and grimy smears on her dress, but her eyes spoke of warmth and intelligence as she introduced herself as Mrs Cox, and they lit up when they fell upon William.

'Is this the little chap in need of a nursemaid?' she asked. Caroline nodded and waved her forward to gather him up from the bed.

'Whereabouts in the hotel do you stay? In case I have need of you or the child?' Caroline asked.

'Oh, I'm not attached to the hotel, ma'am, although I have often been called upon to look after the young children of guests when they find themselves in unusual situations, like you, ma'am . . . I live with my own children and my husband not far from here in Roe Street. Mr Strachen downstairs will always know where to find me, if you need him to. How long will you be needing me to watch him, ma'am?'

'I . . . I don't know. I'm not sure yet. A couple of days, perhaps? A little longer . . . I'm not sure.' Caroline hesitated. Mrs Cox's face fell, but when Caroline paid in advance she smiled again, and was jouncing a startled-looking William merrily on her hip when she left with him not long afterwards. Caroline's heart gave a sickening little lurch as William disappeared from view, but then a vast and numbing weariness pulled at her. She lay down on the bed in her dirty clothes and, with her stomach rumbling, fell instantly asleep.

The next day, wearing the cleanest, least creased clothes she could find in her bag, Caroline gave the slip of paper upon which Bathilda had written a Knightsbridge address to a cab driver and let him transport her there with all the quiet resolution of a person going with dignity to the scaffold. The house she arrived at was four storeys high and built of pale, grey stone clamped into a strict row of identical such houses with handsome, red front doors. Caroline reached for the doorbell. Her arm felt as heavy and stiff as the iron railings, and by the time her finger was near to its target it was trembling with the effort. But she rang it, and gave her name to the elderly housekeeper, who admitted her to a gloomy entrance hall.

'Please, wait here,' the housekeeper intoned, and moved away along the corridor at no great speed. Caroline stood as still as stone. She looked inside her head and found no thoughts at all. Nothing but an echoing space, hollowed out like a cracked and discarded nutshell. *Oh, Corin!* His name rushed into that space like a thunderclap. Reeling slightly, Caroline shook her head, and the emptiness returned.

Bathilda was fatter, and the hair at her temples was a brighter white, but other than that the two years since they had last met had wrought few changes upon her. She was occupying a brocaded couch with a cup of tea in her hand, and she stared at her niece in astonishment for several seconds.

'Good gracious, Caroline! I should never have known you if you weren't announced!' she exclaimed at last, raising her eyebrows and adopting her old familiar *froideur*.

'Aunt Bathilda,' Caroline said in a quiet voice, quite tonelessly.

'Your hair is quite wild. And you're so tanned! It's disastrous. It does not suit you at all.'

Caroline accepted this criticism without blinking, saying nothing while Bathilda sipped her tea. She was aware of her heart beating, hard and slow, just like when they had brought Corin home from the coyote hunt. This was another kind of death, but a death all the same.

'Well, to what do I owe this honour? Where is that cow-herding husband of yours? Has he not joined you on this foreign expedition?'

'Corin is dead.' It was the first time she had said the words. The first time she had had to. Tears scalded her eyes. Bathilda absorbed this news for a moment and then she relented.

'Come and sit down, child. I'll send for some more tea,' she commanded, in a softer tone of voice.

Bathilda soon took control of Caroline and seemed happy enough to do so now that the younger woman was meek and broken, and no longer defiant. Caroline went back to the hotel to collect her things that afternoon, and moved into a spare bedroom at the pale grey town house with the smart red door. She was introduced to the owner of the house, Bathilda's cousin by marriage, Mrs Dalgleish, who was thin and dry and wore a censorious look above a lipless mouth.

'Where is Sara?' Caroline asked hopefully.

Bathilda merely grunted. 'The foolish girl has wed herself to a grocer. She left last year,' she said.

Caroline's heart sank a little more. 'Did she love

him?' she asked wistfully. 'Was she happy?'

'I really don't know. Now, to the matter in hand,' her aunt swept on.

Bathilda took Caroline to the bank and arranged for her money to be transferred from her parents' New York bank into an English account. She took Caroline shopping, accepting the story that all of her old clothes had been ruined on the ranch. They visited a hairdressing salon, where the rough ends and stray wisps of Caroline's hair were trimmed and tamed and curled neatly against her head. She applied to a chemist for Sulpholine Lotion, which was wiped, stinging, over Caroline's face and hands to bleach the tan from her skin. Fingernails were shaped and buffed, calluses worked from the skin with pumice stone. And, for the first time in over a year, Caroline's tiny form was tied tightly into corsets once again.

'You are too thin,' Bathilda said, scrutinising the end product of this beautification. 'Was there no food, out in the wilderness?' Caroline was considering the answer to this when Bathilda continued. 'Well, you are almost fit for society. You will have to remarry, of course. Two widows in this household are more than enough already. I know of just the gentleman, and he is in town now, to see the newest girls. A Baron, if you please—land-rich but cash-poor, and in need of an heir. He would make you a *lady* . . . from farmer's wife to nobility in the space of a couple of months! What a resolution that would be!' Bathilda exclaimed, reaching out for Caroline's shoulders and pulling them back a little straighter. 'But, although he is not as young as once he was, he's known to prefer fresh young things . . . not the world-weary widows of backwater cattlemen. It will be best if we do not mention to anyone your unfortunate first marriage. Can you do that? There's no evidence to the contrary? Nothing you haven't told me?' she asked, fixing Caroline with stern blue eyes.

Caroline took a deep breath. Words clamoured to be spoken, and her pulse raced. But she knew that if she confessed to having brought a child with her, this new life Bathilda was building for her would fly apart like a mirage and she would instead have to remain in this agonising present, with no chance of a more bearable future. She would have to remain with Bathilda, or alone, for ever. Neither could she stand. Caroline knew the answer she was expected to give, and she gave it. Biting down on her tongue to silence it, she shook her head. But when she raised her left hand and worked the wedding ring free, it left a perfect white band on her skin. She kept the ring in a closed fist and later slipped it into the satin lining of her vanity case, next to the photograph of herself and William.

The white band soon faded, kept hidden under satin and kid gloves until it was wholly invisible. Caroline met Lord Calcott at a reception that Bathilda took her to the following week, and she remained obedient and demure and nearly silent as he spoke and they danced and he looked at her with a heat in his eyes that left her cold inside. He was lightly built, not tall, perhaps forty-five years old, and he walked with a slight limp. His hair and moustache were speckled with grey amidst the dark, and his fingernails were neatly manicured. His hands left damp patches on her silk gowns when he held her waist to waltz. They met twice more, at a ball and a dinner party, in rooms stuffily heated against the late autumn chill. As they danced he asked her about her family, and her favourite pastimes, and how she liked London, and the English cuisine. Later he spoke to Bathilda and enquired after Caroline's temperament, her lack of conversation, and her income. After one such evening she accepted his proposal of marriage with a nod of her head and a smile as fleeting as winter sun. He drove her back to Knightsbridge in a smart black carriage pulled by a team of four, and his goodnight kiss roamed from her cheek to her mouth, his hands shaking with rising lust.

'Darling girl,' he whispered hoarsely, pushing up her skirts and kneeling between her legs to shove his way inside her, so abruptly that she gasped in shock. *Do you see?* She hurled the anguished thought out, silently, to wherever Corin had gone: *Do you see what has happened because you left me?*

*   *   *

Caroline spent Christmas of 1904 with Bathilda and Mrs Dalgleish, and she arranged to marry Henry Calcott late in February the following year. This time her engagement was properly announced, and a picture of the happy couple, taken at a celebratory ball, was published in *The Tatler*. As the wedding approached Caroline began to suffer from a consuming lassitude, the taste of copper in her throat, and a sickness in the mornings that made her long for the strong, cowboy coffee that Bathilda and her cousin considered too vulgar to keep in the house. Bathilda kept a stern eye on these developments. 'It seems the wedding won't come a day too soon,'

416

she commented one morning, as Caroline lay in bed, too dizzy and weak to rise. When the nature of her condition dawned upon her, Caroline was stunned.

'But . . . but I . . .' was all she managed to reply to her aunt, who raised an eyebrow and ordered beef tea for her, which she could not look at without gagging. Caroline remained still for several hours, and thought and thought, and tried not to see the clear implications of her pregnancy. For she was every bit as thin as she had been in Oklahoma Territory, if not thinner; and every bit as unhappy, indeed if not more so. The only thing that had changed was the man with which she lay.

*   *   *

Storton Manor seemed unlovely to Caroline. It was grand, but graceless; the windows too stern to be beautiful, the stone too grey to be welcoming. The driveway had been colonised by leggy dandelions and couch grass, the paint was peeling from the front door and the chimney stack was missing several pots. Her money was much needed, Caroline realised. The staff lined up crisply to meet her, as if determined to outshine the shabbiness of the house. Housekeeper, butler, cook, parlourmaid, chambermaid, scullery maid, groom. Caroline descended the carriage steps and swallowed back a threatened storm of weeping as she pictured the scruffy ranch hands who had lined up for her presentation to her first marital home. *And you left them*, she accused herself. *You just left them all without a word.* She smiled and nodded for each as Henry introduced them, and they in turn bobbed a curtsy to her, or made a short bow, muttering *Lady Calcott* in lowered voices. She took hold of her real name, *Caroline Massey*, and squeezed it tightly to her heart.

Later, walking around the broad sweep of the grounds, Caroline began to feel a little better; the snowstorm pieces of herself began to settle, just softly, into a kind of order. The air of the English countryside had a sweetness, a kind of soft greenness to it, even at the far end of winter. No clamour of city streets, horses, carts, or people; no empty prairie wind, or coyotes crying, or mile after unbroken mile of horizon. She was neither too hot, nor too cold. She could see the rooftops and smoke plumes of the village through the naked trees around the house, and it soothed her to know that within a moment's walk there were lives being lived. A swathe of bright daffodils lit up the far end of the lawn, and Caroline walked slowly through them, her hem brushing them flat and then springing them free again. She meditated on the emptiness of her mind, on the hollow feeling she couldn't shake, but she allowed herself to think, just for a moment, that she was safe and could bear it all.

*   *   *

Henry Calcott was a lusty man, so Caroline suffered his conjugal attentions every night in the first few weeks of their wedded life. She was passive and turned her face away from him, amazed at how different love-making felt when undertaken with a person for whom she felt nothing. Her mind and senses completely free of passion, Caroline noticed the wet sounds enjoined by the meeting of their bodies; the fleshy, slightly fetid smell; the way her husband fought for breath, and the way his eyes crossed as he neared his climax. She tried to keep her face neutral and not let her distaste show.

Workmen appeared at Storton Manor and began to tidy the grounds and make repairs to the house, both inside and out.

'Will you be all right, if I go up to town? The men shan't bother you?' Henry asked Caroline at breakfast, three weeks after her arrival at the manor.

'Of course they won't bother me,' she replied calmly.

'You are more than welcome to come to town with me . . .'

'No, no, you go. I prefer to remain here and get better acquainted with . . . with the house, and . . .'

'Very well, very well. I'll only be a week, I should think. Just a few matters of business to attend to,' Henry smiled, returning to the morning's papers. Caroline turned to look out of the window at the overcast day. *Matters of business*, she repeated to herself. At one London ball, a thin-faced girl with platinum hair had whispered to her that Henry Calcott loved a game of poker, even though he almost always lost. Caroline did not mind as long as his habit took him to London every few weeks, and left her well alone.

The second day after his departure was a day of steady rain that hung a wet curtain around the house. The view from the window was of greys and browns and muted greens, a sludgy smear of countryside blurring through the glass. Caroline

419

sat close to the fire in the drawing room, reading an overblown romance by a woman called Elinor Glyn. Her eyes skimmed the text and her thoughts were on the child inside her: why she could not tell how she felt about it; when she should tell Henry; and why she had not done so already. This last answer at least she knew—because it was unbearably bitter, to have to give Henry Calcott the news she had yearned, fruitlessly, to give Corin. The parlourmaid, a timid girl called Estelle, interrupted her reverie with a quiet knock.

'Begging your pardon, my lady, but there's a woman here to see you,' Estelle announced in her wispy voice.

'A woman? What woman?'

'She wouldn't state her business, my lady, but she gave her name as Mrs Cox. Should I show her in?'

Caroline sat mesmerised with shock. There was a long pause, in which the sound of approaching feet could be heard.

'No!' Caroline managed at last, standing up abruptly but too late, as Mrs Cox pushed past Estelle and stood before Caroline with rainwater dripping from her hem onto the Persian rug. She fixed Caroline with a fiery eye and a determined set to her jaw. 'That will be all, thank you, Estelle,' Caroline whispered.

Mrs Cox looked immense but as she unbuttoned her raincoat the reason for this became clear. William was asleep, safely warm and dry beneath the coat, in a sling the woman had fashioned from a length of cotton canvas.

'I don't know what you mean by it!' Mrs Cox exclaimed at last, when it became clear that

Caroline was lost for words. 'Leaving the child with me all these many weeks . . . I don't know what you can mean by it!'

'I . . .' But Caroline had no answer to give. Her careful neutrality, her passive acceptance of her fate, had written William out of the script. She had distanced herself from all thoughts of him, all responsibility. Seeing him again, waking up now as light and fresh air reached him, gave her a feeling like a blow to the stomach, a hard spike of love that was riddled with guilt and fear. 'How did you find me?' was all she could think to ask.

'It wasn't that hard, not with news of your wedding published in all the papers. I waited a bit longer, thinking you'd wanted the child kept safe and quiet while you got wed, but then I saw you weren't going to come for him at all! You weren't, were you? And him such a good, healthy boy . . . I don't know what you mean by it!' Mrs Cox repeated, her voice growing thick. She took a handkerchief from her pocket and dabbed at her eyes. 'And now I've had the expense of bringing him here on the train, and the trouble of walking him here through all this rain without him catching his death . . .'

'I can pay you. For the train, and . . . for the time you've had him. I can pay you more than that, even—here!' Caroline rushed to the dresser, withdrawing a purse of coins and holding it out to the woman. 'Will you keep him?' she asked suddenly, fear making her voice shake. Mrs Cox stared at her.

'*Keep him?* What can you mean? I'm not running a baby farm, I'll have you know! You're his mother—a child belongs with its mother. And look

421

at the life he'll have here!' She gestured at the grand surroundings. 'I've enough mouths to feed and enough bodies to find beds for without taking on another one!' The woman seemed distraught. Caroline could only stand and stare in desperation as Mrs Cox began to work at the knot holding the sling around her shoulders. 'Here. I've brought him back to you now. Fit and well. All his things are in this bag—all but the carrier, for which he has grown too big, and I could not carry it as well as him to come down here. I . . . I hope you'll love him, ma'am. He's a good boy and he deserves to have a mother's love . . .' She seated William on the red silk cushion of a winged armchair. He held his arms up to her and smiled. 'No, lovey, you're staying with your real mam now,' she told him, her eyes again filling with tears. Now that it came to leaving him, Mrs Cox hesitated. She looked from William to Caroline and back again, and then her face creased in anguish and she knotted her hands in the folds of her skirts. 'Take good care of your boy, Lady Calcott,' she said, and hurried away. William sat quietly for a minute, his eyes darting around the room from one unfamiliar object to another. Then he began to cry.

Frantic to hide him, Caroline scooped William up and went quickly via the back stairs to her bedroom. She put him down on the bed and stepped back, clasping her hands to the sides of her head, trying to still her thoughts, and her heart, which was clattering far too fast in her chest. Her breathing came in short, panicked snatches. Quickly, she found a pacifier in William's bag of things and gave it to him to distract him. He stopped crying and grasped at the familiar, tinkling object, making small conversational noises to himself. Gradually, Caroline calmed down. He had grown so much! But then, he was a year and a half old now. His skin was darker and his hair was thicker. His face was beginning to show the high, slanting cheeks and straight brows of the Ponca. How could she ever have thought he was Corin's child? William was Indian, through and through; it would have been obvious even if she had not come to realise that her failure to give Corin a child had more to do with Corin than with herself. Which meant that she had stolen Joe and Magpie's baby. The enormity of this heinous crime hit Caroline like a poleaxe, and she sank to the floor, cramming a fist into her mouth to stifle uncontrollable sobs that surged up from her stomach and near strangled her. And she could not undo this terrible thing. There was no redress she could offer to Magpie—kind, gentle Magpie, who had been nothing but loyal and friendly, who was missing her child thousands of miles from where he now lay. Thousands of miles that neither she nor William would ever traverse again. It was another world, another lifetime. In bringing him here she had crossed a one-way boundary. In that moment, Caroline did not know how she was going to live with what she had done. She sat slumped on the carpet, and she wished to die.

Half an hour later, the maids and the housekeeper, Mrs Priddy, saw Lady Calcott struggling across the waterlogged lawn, carrying something heavy in what looked like a cloth bag. They called after her, and wondered whether to accompany her and make sure she was well, but if Lady Calcott heard them she showed no signs of pausing. She vanished with her burden into the trees at the furthest edge of the gardens, and when she appeared again, pale and shivering, at the mudroom door, she was without it.

'What a day for a walk, my lady!' Mrs Priddy exclaimed, as they found clean towels for her and unlaced her muddy boots. In truth it was a mild day, beneath those soggy English clouds, and certainly not cold enough to have brought on the storms of shuddering that wracked their new mistress's frail body. 'Let's get you up to your room. Cass will bring you some hot tea, won't you, Cass?' Mrs Priddy addressed the chambermaid, a girl of fifteen who goggled at Caroline with round, green eyes. If any of the staff thought anything more of Mrs Cox's short visit, Caroline's walk in the rain or the pillowcase missing from the bed, they knew better than to say anything about it. All except Cass Evans, that was, who whispered things late at night to Estelle, up in the small room on the top floor that they shared.

*　　　*　　　*

Caroline kept to her bed for several days. She lay in a state of dread and sorrow, which deepened when she slid her hand beneath her pillow and found William's pacifier there. The one she had given him, to quieten him as he lay on the bed; the one she and Corin had presented to him as a welcoming gift. She ran her fingers around the silken ivory, cradled the silver bell gently in her hand. She ought to get rid of it, she knew. She ought not to have anything in her possession that could link her to the child, to any child. But she

424

could not. As if some essence of William, of Magpie, of life and love, remained caught up in that one precious talisman, she clasped it tightly in her fists and held it close to her heart. And when Lord Calcott returned from London with an empty wallet, she finally delivered the news of her delicate condition with an expressionless face and a calm demeanour.

*   *   *

The tinker family did not move on, as Caroline had assumed they would; as she had prayed they would. Instead, a few days later, they brought William to the door, to ask politely if anybody in the household had any idea to whom the child belonged, since their enquiries in the village had proved fruitless. Caroline saw them coming along the driveway from her position at the drawing room window. Her heart squeezed fearfully in her chest—just as it had when Corin had first told her she had Indian neighbours—and she jumped up to flee before realising that there was nowhere to go. She waited as the butler opened the front door, heard muffled words spoken, then the approach of footsteps and a subtle knock.

'Yes?' she called, her voice wavering.

'I'm sorry to disturb you, my lady, but Mr Dinsdale and his wife say they have found a child in the woods and they wonder if we have any idea to whom it might belong or what they ought to do with it?' The butler, Mr March, sounded puzzled, as if the etiquette surrounding lost babies was new to him. Feeling like she was going to be sick, Caroline turned on the man.

'What can that *possibly* have to do with me?' she demanded coldly.

'Yes, my lady,' Mr March intoned, every bit as coldly, making the slightest of bows as he withdrew. So the Dinsdales went away again, still carrying William and casting looks back at the house over their shoulders, as if bewildered by their dismissal. Caroline watched them go with increasing unease and a rush of blood to her head that dizzied her, and she traced this feeling to the way Mr March had referred to them—*Mr Dinsdale and his wife.* As if he knew them.

'Dinsdale? Ah, you've met our young campers, have you?' Henry exclaimed when Caroline asked him about the tinkers. She put down her knife and fork, her throat too tight to swallow. 'Harmless folk. Now, I know it may seem a little out of the ordinary, but I've given them permission to stay on that stretch of land—'

'What? Why would you do that?' Caroline gasped.

'Robbie Dinsdale saved my life in Africa, my dear—at Spion Kop, some years ago. Were it not for him, I would not be here today!' Henry announced dramatically, putting a huge forkful of potatoes *dauphinoise* into his mouth. A drop of hot cream ran down his chin, and Caroline looked away.

'But . . . they are *gypsies*. Thieves and . . . and probably worse! We *cannot* have them as our neighbours!'

'Now, my dear, I *will* not have that, I'm afraid. Private Dinsdale stayed with me in our pitiful trench when I was shot, and defended my prone body against a dozen Boer snipers until the Twin

Peaks were taken and the buggers pulled back!' Henry waved his knife emphatically. 'He was wounded himself, and half dead with thirst, but by my side he stayed, when he could have run. All that was left of the rest of my men was a bloody mess like a scene from hell. The war changed him, though . . . He was eventually discharged on medical grounds, although they never did settle on what was wrong with the chap. Lost a few of his marbles out there, I would say. One day he just stopped talking, stopped eating, and wouldn't get up from his bunk no matter who ordered him to. I had to step in with a good word for the fellow. He's much improved now, but he was never quite able to fit back in to his civilian life. He was apprentice farrier in the village here, but that soon finished. He couldn't pay the rent and was thrown out of his cottage, so he took to the road. I told him he could stay here as long as he made no trouble, and he never has done. So here they stay.' Henry wiped potato from his moustache with a crisp, white napkin. Caroline studied her plate, fidgeting nervously.

'He took to the road, you say? So they move around the country, they're not often here?' Her voice was little more than a whisper.

'They're here a lot of the time. It's close to both their families, and Dinsdale can get work here and there where his name's known; mending metalwork and the like. So I fear you will have to get used to them, my dear. They need not trouble you—indeed, if you avoid that area of the grounds, you need not encounter them at all,' Henry concluded, and Caroline knew that the matter was closed. She shut her eyes, but she could feel them.

She could sense that they were there—or rather that William was there, not two hundred yards from where she now sat at dinner. If he remained always there to remind her, she knew it would prey upon her, and slowly devour her. She prayed that they would give the child up, or move on, taking the object of her guilt and anguish with them.

*　　　*　　　*

When her baby was born, Caroline wept. A little girl, so tiny and perfect that she did not seem real, but wrought of magic instead. The soaring, consuming love that Caroline felt for her daughter only served to show her just how great the ill which she had done to Magpie truly was. The mere *thought* of being separated from this child of hers was painful enough. So Caroline wept, with love and with self-loathing, and nothing that was said could console her. Henry patted her head, at a loss, and did a poor job of hiding his disappointment that he had a daughter, not a son. Estelle and Mrs Priddy told Caroline, over and over, what a beauty the girl was, and how very well she had done, which brought fresh tears that they ascribed to exhaustion. At night she was beset by dreams of Magpie, her heart in flames, eyes fever-bright, failing, fading, dying of grief; and when she awoke the taint of her crime made her head throb as though it would burst. The baby was dressed in white lace gowns and named Evangeline. For four months Caroline loved her to distraction, and then the tiny girl died, one night in her crib, for no reason that any one of three doctors could ascertain. She flickered out of existence like a snuffed candle, and Caroline was shattered. What little will to go on she had kept since losing Corin now ran out of her like blood from a wound, and there was nothing left that could staunch it.

On a Tuesday, months later, Caroline went down to the kitchen and found Mrs Priddy and Cass Evans preparing a basket of vegetables from the garden with which to pay Robbie Dinsdale. He was out of sight in the scullery, sharpening the kitchen knives with a stone treadle wheel, sending sparks flying and filling the air with the piercing whine of stressed metal. Caroline would not have sought out the source of the racket if she hadn't seen guilt in Mrs Priddy's eyes; if the woman hadn't stopped what she was doing so suddenly, with such a start, when her mistress appeared in the room. Cass pressed anxious fingers to her mouth. They all knew how Lady Calcott felt about the Dinsdales, although they did not know why. Caroline strode through to the scullery and interrupted Dinsdale, who looked up at her with soft, amber eyes. Slowly, the wheel ground to a halt. Dinsdale was wearing rough clothing, and his hair was long and greasy, tied at the back of his head with string. His face was quite lovely, as fresh and innocent as a boy's, but somehow this only made it worse. Caroline's grief had turned her heart to stone. She knew herself to be punished, forced by fate to suffer the same anguish that she had inflicted upon Magpie, but so great was her pain that she did not accept it—she *could* not. She fought it, and bright anger coursed through her veins

'Get *out*!' she shouted, her voice vibrant with rage. 'Get *out* of this house!' Dinsdale started up from his stool like a jack-in-the-box and fled. Caroline turned on the housekeeper and the chamber maid. 'What is the meaning of this? I thought I had made my feelings about that man perfectly clear!'

'Mr Dinsdale has always done the knives for us, my lady . . . I didn't think any harm could come—' Mrs Priddy tried to explain.

'I don't care about that! I don't want him in the house—or anywhere near it! And what's this?' she demanded, gesturing to the basket of vegetables. 'Are you stealing from the gardens as well?'

At this Mrs Priddy swelled, and she pinched her brows together. 'I've worked here for more than thirty years, my lady, and never once been accused of any such thing! The excess from the kitchen garden has long been used to pay local men for their labour—'

'Well, not any more! Not that man, anyway. Do I make myself clear?' Caroline snapped. She fought to contain her voice. It was wavering, reeling; it threatened to rise to a shriek.

'They 'as extra mouths to feed!' Cass Evans piped up.

'Hush, child!' Mrs Priddy hissed.

'What?' Caroline said. She stared at the green-eyed girl in incredulous fear. *'What?'* she repeated, but Cass shook her head minutely and did not speak again.

Only Lord Calcott's intervention kept Mrs Priddy in her job in the wake of this misdemeanour. He did not understand his wife's objection to Dinsdale, and he did not try to. He merely silenced her and then took himself to London to avoid her vitriolic mood. The staff began to give Caroline a wide berth, fearing her unpredictable rages, her spells of sudden weeping. Late one night, after retiring, Caroline rose and went down to the kitchens in search of liver salts to calm her stomach. She went on soft feet, her slippers making almost no sound, and paused outside the scullery, hearing the girls still clearing up the dinner plates, and chatting to the stable boy, Davey Hook.

'Well, why else do you think she's took against them so fierce?' Cass's village accent was instantly recognisable.

' 'Cause she's a nob—they're all like that! Noses up in the air,' Davey said.

'I think she's half lost her reason since little Evangeline died, poor mite,' Estelle spoke up.

'I'm telling you, I heard it. There weren't no mistaking it—I *heard* it. That woman who came in from the station had something hidden under her coat, and then I heard a baby crying up in the mistress's chamber—I did! And then all of a sudden Robbie Dinsdale finds a lad out in the woods—and we *saw* her go over there, carrying something with her. We saw her.'

'But you never saw what it was she carried, did you?'

'But what else could it have been?'

'Why, anything at all, Cass Evans!' Estelle exclaimed. 'Why ever would the mistress take a child out and leave it in the woods?'

'You said yourself she's lost her reason!' Cass retorted.

'Only since she lost the little 'un, I said.'

'Maybe it's hers. Maybe that's her baby—another man's baby! And she had to keep it hid from the master—how about that, then?' Cass challenged them.

'It's you 'as gone soft in the head, Cass Evans, not her upstairs! Toffs don't go about dropping babies like farmers' daughters!' Davey laughed. 'Besides, you've seen that bairn the Dinsdales have got—swarthy as a blackamoor, he is! He's not her boy, he couldn't be. Not with her so pale. That there's a gypsy child, through and through. Some other lot probably cast it off, too many mouths to feed, and that's the beginning and end of it,' the boy said.

'You mustn't say such things about her ladyship, Cass,' Estelle warned her, softly. 'It'll fetch you nothing but trouble.'

'But I know what I heard. And I know what I saw, and it ain't right!' Cass stamped her foot. Outside the room, Caroline's chest was burning. A pent-up breath escaped her in a rush, not quiet enough, and the conversation within halted abruptly.

'*Shhh!*' Estelle hissed. Footsteps approached the door. Caroline turned on her toes and fled back to the stairs as silently as she could.

Henry Calcott was not at home when Cass Evans was dismissed. Caroline dealt with Mrs Priddy, Cass having been sent to her room to pack her meagre possessions.

'The girl's family is well known to me, my lady. I am certain she is not the thieving kind.' The housekeeper's face was clouded with concern.

'Nevertheless, I came in to find her rifling through my jewellery box. And now a silver pin is missing,' Caroline replied, marvelling at the dispassion in her voice when inside she was wrought with panic.

'What kind of pin, my lady? Perhaps it has been mislaid and is around the house somewhere?'

'No, it has not been mislaid. I want the girl removed from the house, Mrs Priddy; and that is all I have to say on the matter,' Caroline snapped. Mrs Priddy watched her, helplessly, with eyes so sharp that Caroline could not hold her gaze for long. She turned back to the mirror above the mantelpiece and saw no trace of fear, or guilt, or nerves in her own face. Her features were pale, immobile. Like stone.

'May I give her a good reference, at least, my lady? To give her a start elsewhere? She's a good girl, she works hard—'

'She steals, Mrs Priddy. If you write a reference, you must include that information within it,' Caroline said quietly. Behind her, she saw Mrs Priddy's expression change to incredulity. 'That will be all, Mrs Priddy.'

'Very well, my lady.' The older woman spoke coldly, and walked stiffly away. When the door closed behind her, Caroline sagged, holding the mantel for support. Her stomach churned, and she tasted bile. But she swallowed it down and steadied herself. Cass left via the kitchen door, with tears and highly vocal outrage, an hour or so later. Caroline watched from the upstairs hall window, and when Cass turned to look back at her former home she met Caroline's guarded gaze with a glare of such fury that it would have scorched a more feeling person.

Lord Calcott merely grunted when the new girl, who was fat and plain, opened the bedroom curtains one morning.

'What happened to that other lass? The brown-haired one?' he asked, idly.

'I had to let her go,' Caroline replied flatly. He said no more on the topic, since it was hardly an inconvenience to himself. Indeed, he was in residence less and less, and spent scant enough time with his wife for a second child to be conceived—the pregnancy was a long time coming. Caroline feared that nothing would ever again feel as wonderful as holding Evangeline for the first time, but the changing of her body brought with it an anticipation of love that was irresistible, and she succumbed to it, turning in on herself, humming softly to the unborn baby, feeling it wedged tightly beneath her ribs, a kernel of warmth and life in the dead husk of her being. But the boy, for boy it was, was born months too soon and had no chance of life. The doctor was all for taking it away with the bloodied sheets, but Caroline demanded to see her child. She studied the tiny, unformed face in wonderment—that she could still feel loss, that her eyes had tears left to shed. But it was the last of the love she possessed poured into that one gaze, that one long look she took at the dead baby's face. The very last touch of warmth inside her, she passed to him; and then the doctor did indeed take him out with the bloody sheets and all was lost.

Caroline's recovery was slow, and never complete. By the time she was well enough to receive visits from friends, and Bathilda, they found her slow and dull, her conversation near non-existent, her movements sluggish and her beauty much diminished. There were hollows at her eyes and cheeks, her hands were as bony as bird claws and there were touches of grey at her temples even though she was not yet near thirty. She seemed ghostly, as if part of her had left for another plane. People shook their heads sadly and thought twice before adding the Calcotts to any invitation list. Left alone, Caroline walked a great deal. Around and around the gardens, as if looking for something. One day she went through the woods, to the clearing where the Dinsdales still camped. They had learnt to give the house a wide berth, and never came again to swap labour for food. Caroline, therefore, had no excuse to argue for their removal, and to be thwarted this way made her ever more bitter towards them.

She waited in the trees, staring at their brightly painted wagon and the patchwork pony tethered nearby. Their home looked so jaunty, pitched there on the green summer grass; so practical, so wholesome. Caroline was reminded of White Cloud's teepee, and this, like any thought of the ranch, made her vision swim and her mind close up in misery. Just then the Dinsdales returned from the village. Mrs Dinsdale, whose blonde hair hung in angelic ringlets, had a babe in arms, and holding onto Mr Dinsdale's hand was a sturdy boy of about three years, dark coloured and round. His steps were sure but they made slow progress, pausing every few steps for the boy to crouch down and examine something on the ground with an endless curiosity. Caroline's breath caught in her throat. William so resembled Magpie that it was near unbearable to look at him.

She watched them for some time. Mrs Dinsdale put her baby down to sleep inside the wagon, then sat on the steps and called to William, who came running to her with his arms aloft to be carried.

She did not call him William, of course. It was some other name that she used, that Caroline could not entirely hear, but that sounded like *Flag*. Watching them, Caroline was so torn apart with sorrow and envy that she did not know how to contain it. But she was so angry too, that this family of drifters should flourish when her own had been snatched from her, twofold. She stared at William and she hated him. She hated them all. *No more*, she thought, *I can take no more*. The price she had been made to pay was far too high, and though some part of her thought that this injustice must, somehow, be redressed, she knew that it could not be. She sat down in the shadows and cried quietly for Corin, who could not help her.

Therefore all seasons shall be sweet to thee,
Whether the summer clothe the general earth
With greenness, or the redbreast sit and sing
Betwixt the tufts of snow on the bare branch
Of mossy apple-tree, while the nigh thatch
Smokes in the sun-thaw; whether the eve-drops fall
Heard only in the trances of the blast,
Or if the secret ministry of frost
Shall hang them up in silent icicles,
Quietly shining to the quiet Moon.

Samuel Taylor Coleridge, *Frost at Midnight*

The stairs take the last of my energy, so when I reach the bathroom door I am gulping, fighting for breath. The light is on inside, tendrils of steam creeping under the door. And the tap still running. With my hand on the door I freeze, shut my eyes for a second. I am so afraid; so afraid of what I might see. I think of Eddie, pushing back Beth's hair when he came home after school and found her. How I need his courage right now.

'Beth?' I call, too meekly. No reply. Swallowing, I give two tiny knocks then throw open the door.

Beth is in the bath, her hair floating around her, water perilously close to the rim, escaping into the over flow. Her eyes are shut and for an instant I think I have lost her. She is Ophelia, she will ebb away from me, float off into serene oblivion. But then she opens her eyes, turns her face to me, and I am so relieved I nearly fall. I stumble in, sit abruptly on the chair where her clothes are folded.

'Rick? What's going on? Where are your clothes?' she asks me, pushing the tap closed with her big toe. I dropped them and Dinny's blanket in the hallway, before I ran. I am wearing wet, muddy underwear, nothing more.

'I thought . . . I thought . . .' But I don't want to tell her what I thought. It seems a betrayal, to think that she would do that to herself again.

'What?' she asks, her voice flattening out, growing taut.

'Nothing,' I mumble. The light stabs at my eyes, makes me flinch. 'Why are you in the bath at this time of night?'

'I said I'd wait for you to get back,' she replies. 'And I was cold. Where have you been?' she asks, sitting up now, wet hair smoothing itself to her breasts. She bends her knees, wraps shining arms around them. I can see every rib, every bump of her spine, marching down into the water.

'I was with Dinny. I . . . fell into the dew pond.'

'You did *what*? What was Dinny doing there?'

'He heard me fall in. He helped me out.'

'You just fell in?' she asks incredulously.

'Yes! Too much whisky, I suppose.'

'And did you just . . . fall out of your clothes? Or did he help you with those as well?' she asks tartly. I give her a steady look. I am angry now—that she scared me so. That I scared myself so.

'Who's jealous now?' I ask, just as tart.

'I'm not—' she begins, then puts her chin on her knees, looks away from me. 'It's *weird*, OK, Erica? You chasing after Dinny is weird.'

'Why is it weird? Because he was yours first?'

'Yes!' she cries; and I stare, amazed by this admission. 'Just don't get involved with him, all right? It feels incestuous! It's just . . . wrong!' She struggles to explain herself, stretching her hands wide. 'I can't stand it.'

'It's not wrong. You just don't *like* the idea, that's all. But you needn't worry. I think he's still in love with you,' I say quietly, feeling my own heart sink inside me.

I wait to see her expression change, but it doesn't.

'We should go, Erica. Can't you see? We should leave here and not come back. It would be by far the best thing. We could go tomorrow.' Her voice gains conviction, she fixes me with desperate eyes. 'Never mind sorting out all Meredith's things—that's not why we came here, not really. The house clearance guys can do it! Please? Let's just go?'

'I know why I came here, Beth.' I am tired of not talking about it, tired of tiptoeing around it. 'I wanted us both to come because I thought I could make you better. Because I want to find out what it is that torments you, Beth. I want to bring it to the surface. I want to shine a light on it, and . . . show you that it's not so bad. Nothing is as bad in the light of day, Beth! Isn't that what you tell Eddie when he has nightmares?'

'Some things *are*, Erica! Some things are as bad!' she cries, the words torn from her, terrified. 'I want to *leave*. I'm leaving, tomorrow.'

'No. You're *not*. Not until we've confronted this. Whatever it is. Not until we've faced up to it!'

'You don't know what you're talking about!' she shouts harshly. She stands abruptly, sends water cascading onto the bathroom floor, reaches for her dressing gown and shrugs it on violently. 'You can't stop me if I want to go.'

'I won't drive you to the station.'

'I'll take a taxi!' she hisses.

'On New Year's Day? Out here in the sticks? Good luck.'

'God*damn it*, Rick! Why are you doing this?' she swears, anger snapping in her eyes, clipping her words. They echo from the tiled walls, attack me twice.

'I . . . I promised Eddie. That I'd make you better.'

'What?' she whispers.

I think carefully, before I speak again. I think

about what I saw, as the dew pond closed over my head.

'Tell me what Henry was looking for at the side of the dew pond,' I demand softly.

'What? When?'

'At the side of the dew pond that day. The day he disappeared, and I'd been swimming in the pond. He was looking for something on the ground.' I hear Beth's sharp intake of breath. Her lips have gone pale.

'I thought you said you didn't remember?' she says.

'It's coming back to me. A little. Not all of it. I remember jumping back into the pond, and I remember looking up at Henry, and he had been looking for something on the ground. And then I remember . . .' I swallow, 'I remember him bleeding. His head bleeding.'

'Shut up! *Shut up!* I don't want to talk about it!' Beth shouts again, puts her hands over her ears, shakes her head madly. I watch, astonished, until she stops, stands snatching at the air, chest heaving. I take her arm carefully and she winces.

'Just tell me what he was looking for.'

'Stones, of course,' she says, quietly, defeated. 'He was looking for stones to throw.' She pulls away from me then, slips from the bathroom into the dark of the corridor.

*　　*　　*

No sleep for me. I try counting my breaths, counting my heartbeat; but when I do this my heart speeds up, as if startled by such scrutiny. It rushes along, makes my head ache. I shut my eyes so tightly that coloured shapes bloom in the dark and flounce across the ceiling when I open my eyes again. There's a bright moon tonight, and as I skim sleep, as the hours spin past, I see it sail heedlessly from one pane of the window to the next.

I feel dreadful when I get up: heavy and tired. My throat is sore; there's an ache behind my eyes that won't go. It was a hard frost last night—Dinny was right about what might have happened if I'd lain about on the ground, drunk and befuddled. Now there's a dense mist, so pale and luminous that I can't tell where it ends and the sky begins. The thing is, we ran. That day. Beth and I ran. I remember scrambling out of the pond as fast as I could, bruising my feet on flints. I remember Beth's fingers closing tightly on my arm like little bird claws, and we ran. Back to the house, back to lie low, to hide and stay quiet until the trouble started. Or rather, until the trouble was noticed. We didn't go back, I am sure of it. The last time I saw Henry he was by the side of the dew pond; he was teetering. Did he fall? Was that why I got out, so desperately fast? Was that why I told them all he was in the pond—why I insisted upon it? But he wasn't, and there was only one other person there. There is only one person who can have moved Henry, who can have taken him somewhere else, because I know he didn't take himself. He was taken somewhere so secret and so hidden that twenty-three years of searching couldn't uncover him. But I am close now.

It could be this memory that I've fought so hard to regain that's hurting my head. I don't have to concentrate to recall it now. It capers in my mind's eye of its own accord, again and again. Henry

443

bleeding, Henry falling. It worries me that I didn't want breakfast. I looked at the food and I remembered Henry and there was no question of eating anything. No question of putting anything into my mouth, of enjoyment or satisfaction. Is this how Beth has felt, for twenty-three years? The thought turns me cold. It's like knowing there's something behind you, following you. That neck-prickling feeling, a constant distraction. Something as dark and permanent as your shadow.

The doorbell startles me. Dinny is there, wearing a heavy canvas coat for once, his hands thrust deeply into the pockets. In spite of it all my cheeks glow and I feel a wave of something ill-defined. Relief, or perhaps dread.

'Dinny! Hello—come in,' I greet him.

'Hi, Erica, I just wanted to check you were all right. After last night,' Dinny says, stepping over the threshold but staying on the doormat.

'Come in—I can't shut the door with you standing there.'

'My boots are muddy,'

'That's the least of our problems, believe me.' I wave my hand.

'So, how are you? I wondered if . . . if you'd swallowed any of that pond water, it might have made you sick,' he says. An awkwardness about him that wasn't there before, a diffidence that touches me.

'I'm fine, really. I mean, I feel like death, and I'm sure I look like death, but other than that, I'm OK.' I smile nervously.

'You could have killed yourself,' he tells me gravely.

'I know. I know. I'm sorry. That wasn't my

intention, believe me. And thank you for rescuing me—I really owe you one,' I say. At this he looks at me sharply, his eyes probing my face. But then he softens, puts out his hand and brushes cold knuckles lightly down my cheek. I catch my breath, shiver slightly.

'Idiot,' he says softly.

'Thanks,' I say.

There's a thump from upstairs. I picture a full suitcase, pulled off a bed. Dinny drops his hand quickly, puts it back in his pocket.

'Is that Beth?' he asks.

'Beth or the ghost of Calcotts past. I expect she's packing. She doesn't even want to stay for one more day.' I give a helpless little shrug.

'So you're leaving?'

'I . . . I don't know. I don't want to. Not yet. Maybe not at all.' I glance at him. I really don't think I could stay in this house by myself.

'No more Dinsdales or Calcotts at Storton Manor. It's the end of an era,' Dinny says, but he does not sound regretful.

'Are you moving on?' I ask. My heart gives a little leap of protest.

'Sooner or later. This is a rotten place to camp in the winter. I was only really here because of Honey—'

'I thought you said you saw Meredith's obituary?'

'Well, yes, and that. I thought there was a good chance you and Beth might be around.' For a moment we say nothing. I am still too unsure of him to test this tide that's towing us apart. Perhaps Dinny feels the same way.

'I'd like to say goodbye to Beth before you

disappear,' he says quietly. I nod. Of course he does. 'I didn't get the chance, the last time you went,' he adds pointedly.

'She's upstairs. We had a fight. I don't know if she'll come down,' I tell him. I study his hands. Square shaped, smeared with grime. Black crescents under the nails. I think of the mud by the dew pond, him hauling me out. I think of the way he held me, just for a while, while the embers sank low and my body shook. I think of his kiss. How I want to keep him here.

'What did you fight about?'

'What do you think?' I ask bitterly. 'She won't tell me what happened. But she *has* to face up to it, Dinny—she has to! It's what's making her ill, I know it!' Dinny sighs sharply, shifts his weight onto the balls of his feet, as if he would run. He rubs a hand over his forehead, exasperated. 'You never did get to tell her the things you wanted to, Dinny. But . . . you can tell me instead,' I say.

'Erica—'

'I want to know!'

'What if knowing changes everything? What if, for once, your sister and I are right and you're better off not remembering?' Fierce eyes lock on mine.

'I *want* it to change everything! Change what, anyway? She's my sister. I love her and I'll love her no matter what she does. Or did,' I declare adamantly.

'I'm not just talking about Beth,' he says.

'Who, then? What then? Just tell me!'

'Don't shout at me, Erica, I can hear you. I'm talking about . . . you and me.' His voice grows softer. I am silent for two heartbeats. They come quickly, but seem to take for ever.

'What do you mean?'

'I mean . . . whatever this is . . . whatever it might have been, it would all change.' He looks away from me, folds his arms. 'Do you understand?' he asks. I bite my lower lip, feel my eyes stinging. But then I see Beth, in the bath, as she was last night; whole in body, but slipping away. I swallow the hot little flame that Dinny has just lit inside me.

'Yes. But I have to know,' I whisper. My nose is running. I scrub it with the back of my hand. I wait for him to speak, but he doesn't. His eyes dart from the floor to the door to the stairs and back again, focusing on nothing. Knots in his jaw, tying themselves tighter. 'Just tell me, Dinny! Beth and I ran off. I don't know what happened, but I know we ran off and left you and Henry at the pond. And that was the last anybody saw of him and I want you to *tell me*!' My voice sounds odd, too high.

'Beth should—' he begins.

'Beth won't. Oh, maybe she will, one day. Or maybe she'll try to kill herself again, and this time she'll manage it! I have to get this *out* of her!' I cry. Dinny stares at me, shocked.

'She tried to *kill* herself?' he breathes. 'Because of this?'

'Yes! Because she's depressed. Not just *unhappy*—ill, Dinny. And I want to know what caused it. If you don't tell me then you're just helping keep her like she is—haunted. Just tell me what you did with his body! Tell me where he is!' I plead. My blood is soaring like a tidal wave, roaring in my ears.

'Erica!' Beth's shout echoes across the hallway.

Dinny and I jump, like guilty children. *'Don't!'* she cries, running down the stairs to us. Her eyes are wide, face marked with fright.

'Beth, I wasn't going to tell her—' Dinny starts to say, holding up a hand to placate her.

'What? Why not—because *Beth* has told you not to?' I snap at him.

'Don't tell anybody! *Ever!*' Beth says. I hardly recognise her voice. I grasp at her hands, try to make her look at me, but her eyes are fixed on Dinny's and something passes between them that I can't bear.

'Beth! Please—Beth, look at me! Look at what trying to keep this secret has done to you! Please, Beth. It's time to get rid of it. Whatever it is, let it go. Please. For Eddie's sake! He needs you to be happy—'

'Don't bring Eddie into this!' she snaps at me, her eyes awash with tears.

'Why not? It's *his* life that this is affecting too, you know! He's your responsibility. You owe it to him to be strong, Beth—'

'What would *you* know about it, Erica? What would you know about responsibility? You haven't even got a permanent job! You change flats every six months! You've been living like a student since you left home—you've never even had a pet so don't tell me about *my* responsibilities!' Beth shouts, and I recoil, stung.

'You're my responsibility,' I say quietly.

'No. I'm not,' Beth replies, holding my gaze.

'Beth,' Dinny says. 'I've been trying to talk to you since you got back here and I know you don't want to hear what I have to say, but it's important, and . . . I think Erica has a right to hear it too—'

'She was *there,* Dinny! If she doesn't remember then she doesn't need to. Now can we please leave it alone? Dinny, I . . . I think you should go.'

'No, he shouldn't! Why should he go? I asked him in. In fact,' I cross to the door, stand with my back to it, 'nobody's going until I have had the truth from one or both of you. I mean it. The truth. It's long overdue,' I say. My heart trips, hurls itself against my ribs.

'Like you could stop me,' Dinny mutters.

'Erica, stop asking!' Beth cries. 'Just . . . *stop asking!'*

'Beth, maybe it would be better to just tell her. She's not going to tell anybody. It's just the three of us. I think . . . I think she has a right to know,' Dinny says, his voice soft. Beth stares at him, her face so pale.

'No,' she whispers.

'*Christ!* I don't know why you even came back here!' he shouts, throwing up his arms in exasperation.

'Dinny, tell me. It's the only way to help her,' I say firmly. Beth's gaze flickers from me to Dinny and back again.

'No!' she hisses.

'Please. Tell me where Henry is,' I urge him.

'Stop it!' Beth commands me. She is shaking uncontrollably. Dinny grinds his teeth together, looks over his shoulder, looks back at me. His eyes are ablaze. He seems torn over something, undecided. I hold my breath and my head spins in protest.

'Fine!' he barks, grabbing my arm. 'If you think this is only way to help her. But if you're wrong, and when everything is different, don't say I didn't warn you!' He is suddenly angry, furious with us. His fingers bruise me; he tows me away from the door and wrenches it open.

'No! Dinny—*no!*' Beth shouts after us, as he pulls me outside.

'*Ow*—stop it! What are you doing? Where are we going?' On instinct I fight him, try to dig my heels in, but he is far stronger than me.

'You want to know what happened to Henry? I'll show you!' Dinny spits the words out. Fear grips my insides. I am so close to finding Henry, so close that it terrifies me. Dinny terrifies me. Such strength in him, in his grip; such an implacable look on his face.

'Dinny, *please* . . .' I gasp, but he ignores me.

'Erica! *No!*' I hear Beth's ragged shout chasing us but she does not follow. I look back over my shoulder, see her framed in the doorway, mouth distorted, hands grasping the jamb for support.

Dinny marches me across the lawn, out of the garden through the trees, and I think we are going to the dew pond. Suddenly I know, for absolute sure, that I do not want to go there. Dread makes my knees weak; I renew my struggle to get free.

'Come on!' he snaps, pulling me harder. He could wrench my arm clean away from my body. But we are not going to the dew pond. He is heading west now. We are going to the camp. I follow him like a reluctant shadow, weaving and stumbling behind him. My heart pummels inside me. Dinny pulls open the door of the nearest van, not bothering to knock. Harry looks up, startled; smiles when he recognises us. Dinny propels me up the steps into the van, which smells of crisps and dog and damp clothing.

'What the hell is this?' My voice is shaking, I can't get my breath, I am ready to shatter.

'You wanted to know where Henry was.' Dinny raises his arm, points at Harry. 'There's Henry.'

I stare. My head empties, the plug is pulled. I'm not sure how long I stare, but when I speak my throat is dry.

'What?' The word is a feeble little thing, a faint shape around the last scrap of air in my chest. The floor is tipping underneath my feet; the earth has rolled off its axis, is wheeling away with me, dizzy and helpless. Dinny lowers his arm, shuts his eyes and puts a hand over them, wearily.

'That's Henry,' he repeats; and again I hear the words.

'But . . . how *can* it be? Henry's dead! How can this be Henry? Not *Henry*. Not him.'

'He's not dead. He didn't die.' Dinny drops his hand and the fire has gone out of him. He watches me but I can't move. I can't think. Harry smiles, uncertainly. 'Try not to shout. It upsets him,' Dinny says quietly. I can't shout. I can't anything. I can't breathe. Pressure is building inside my head. I worry that it will explode. I put my hands to my temples, try to hold my skull together. 'Come on— let's go. Let's go outside and talk,' Dinny murmurs, taking my arm more gently now. I snatch it away and lean towards Harry. I am so scared as I look at him. Scared enough for my knees to sag—there's a hollow thump as they hit the floor. Scared enough for a shocking nausea to sweep through me. I am chilled to the roots of my hair, and burning all over. I push stray dreadlocks back from Harry's face, peer into his eyes. I try to see it. Try to recognise him, but I can't. I won't.

'You're wrong. You're lying!'

'I'm neither. Come on, we can't talk about this here.' Dinny pulls me to my feet and takes me outside again.

For the second time in twelve hours I sit in Dinny's van, shivering, stunned, stupid. He makes coffee on the stove in a battered steel pot, the liquid spitting and smelling delicious. Sipping from the cup he gives me scalds my mouth, and I feel it revive me.

'I . . . I can't believe it. I don't understand,' I say quietly. Outside a door bangs. Popeye and Blot woof gently behind their teeth; more a greeting than a warning. Dinny has one ankle propped up on the other knee, his familiar pose. He looks both hard and nervous. He sighs.

'What don't you understand?' He says this quietly, in the spirit of genuine enquiry.

'Well, where has he *been* all these years? How come he was never found? They searched *everywhere* for him!'

'Nobody ever searches *everywhere*.' Dinny shakes his head. 'He's been here, with us. With my family, or with friends of my family. There's more than one traveller camp in the south of England. Mum and Dad had plenty of friends to leave him with, friends who looked after him, until it had blown over. As soon as I was old enough to keep an eye on him myself, I did.'

'But . . . I saw him bleeding. I saw him fall into the pond . . .'

'And then you two ran away. I fished him out and I fetched my dad. He wasn't breathing, but Dad managed to get it going again. The cut on his head wasn't as bad as it looked . . . head wounds just bleed a lot.' He looks at his boot, twists the frayed end of a lace between his finger and thumb.

'And then? Didn't you take him to the hospital? Why didn't you come and find somebody at the manor?' I ask. Twenty-three years of my life are rewriting themselves behind my eyes, unravelling like wool. I can hardly focus, hardly think. Dinny doesn't answer for a long time. He grips his chin in his hand, knuckles white. His eyes burn into me.

'I . . . wouldn't say what had happened. I wouldn't tell them how he'd got hurt . . . or by who. So Dad . . . Dad thought it was me. He thought Henry and me had got into a fight or something. He was trying to protect me.'

'But, you could have told them it was an accident—'

'Come off it, Erica. Everyone's always looking to be proved right about us—all my life, people have looked to be proved right. That we thieve, that we're criminals—that we're scum. The social would have leapt at the chance to take me away from Mum and Dad. A spell in juvy, then a *proper* home, with a *proper* family . . .'

'You don't know that . . .'

'Yes. Yes, I do. It's you who doesn't know, Erica.'

'Why is he . . . the way he is?'

'Not from the knock on the head, that's for sure. Dad took him to an old friend, Joanna, who used to be a nurse in Marlborough. This was that same afternoon, before anyone even knew he was missing. She put a couple of stitches in his head, said he might have a concussion but it was nothing to worry about. We were going to wait for him to wake up, make sure he was OK, then drop him within walking distance of the village and disappear. That was the plan. Joanna looked after him for the first few days. He was out of it for two days straight and . . . then he woke up.'

'You could have brought him back then. You could have left him somewhere he'd be found, like you said. Why didn't you?'

'By then the search was enormous. We were being watched. We couldn't move without some keen copper noting it down. Henry would have told them we'd had him—when he was found, of course. But we thought we'd have a head start to vanish. By the time we realised there was no way we could bring him back without being seen, it was too late. And he wasn't right, when he woke up. Anybody could tell that. Dad took me to see him, since I knew him best, out of all of us. *Just tell me what you think*, Dad said. I didn't know what he was getting at until I saw Henry and spoke to him. Sitting up in Joanna's spare bed, holding a glass of orange squash like he didn't know what to do with it. I'd rather have been anywhere else in the world than in that room with him.' Dinny pushes his fingers through his hair, grips his scalp. 'I tried talking to him, like Dad said I should. But he wasn't the same. He was wide awake, but . . . distant. Dazed.'

'But why? You said his head wasn't hit that hard?'

'It wasn't. It was the time he spent not breathing. The time before Dad got to him and got air back into his lungs.' Dinny sounds so tired now, leaden. There's a sparkle of pity, at the core of me, but I can't let it fill me yet. Too many other things to feel.

I've finished my coffee before I speak again. I hadn't noticed the silence. Dinny is watching me, tapping his ankle with one agitated thumb, waiting. Waiting for my reaction, I suppose. A defensive gleam in his eye.

'It didn't blow over, you know. Not for his parents. Not for our family . . .'

'Do you think it blew over for me? For *my* family? I've had to see him nearly every day since then, wondering if it would have been different if I'd tried to revive him myself, that bit sooner . . . If we *had* taken him to hospital.'

'But you've never told. You've kept him—'

'Not *kept* him. Looked after him . . .'

'You've kept him and let his family—let his *parents* think he was dead! You've let Beth and I think he was dead.'

'No, I had no idea what you and Beth were thinking! How would I know? You *ran*, remember? You ran and washed your hands of it! You never even came to ask me about it! You left him with me and I . . . we . . . did what we thought was best.'

This I cannot dispute.

'I was eight years old!'

'Well, I was twelve—still just a kid, and I had to let my parents think I'd nearly killed another boy. That I'd *brain-damaged* another boy. At least, that's what I thought I had to do. That's what I thought was right. By the time I realised you two were never coming back, it was too late to change anything. How much fun do you think that was?'

I feel the blood run out of my face when he says this. *I had to let them think* . . . A memory fights its way through the clash in my head. Henry bending down, surveying the ground, gathering four, five stones. Water in my eyes and in one ear, which boomed and wobbled, mangling their voices; Henry, taunting, throwing names at Dinny; Beth's shrill commands: *Stop it! Go away! Henry, don't!* Henry said, *Pikey! Filth! Dirty gyppo! Thieving dog! Tramp!* With each word he threw a stone, whipping it from the shoulder with that throw boys are taught at school, but girls never are. A throw that would have sent a cricket ball back from the boundary, and a good aim. I remember Dinny crying out as one hit him, grabbing his shoulder, wincing. *I remember what happened.* And I picture Beth, in the doorway just now; her shout following us, and the terror on her face. *No!*

'I have to go,' I whisper, stumbling to my feet.

'Erica, wait—'

'No! I have to go!'

I feel sick. There's too much inside me, something has to come out. I rush back to the house, tripping over my feet. In the cold downstairs toilet, where the frigid toilet seat makes your thighs ache, I collapse, throw up. But with my throat burning and the stink of it all around me, I somehow feel better. I feel justly punished. I feel as if some kind of retribution is beginning. Now I know what has tortured Beth all these years. Now I know why she has punished herself so, why she has sought such retribution. Splashing my face in the basin, I gasp for breath, try to find the strength to rise. I am cold with fear—I think I know what retribution she might seek from herself.

'Beth!' I call, coughing at the ragged feeling in my throat. 'Beth, where are you—I have to tell you something!' On trembling legs, I run in and out of all the downstairs rooms, my heart skittering, making me dizzy. *'Beth!'* My voice is rising, almost a scream. I pound up the stairs, run to the bathroom first then along the corridor to Beth's room. The door is shut and I throw myself against it. Inside, the curtains are closed, the room in darkness. And what I fear the most, what I dreaded to see is there in front of me. It fills my vision, hollows me out. *'No!'* I rush into the shadowed room. My sister, curled on the floor, her face turned away from me. Long-bladed scissors gripped in her fragile hand, and a dark pool around her. 'Beth, no,' I whisper, with no more air in my lungs, no blood in my veins. I fall to my knees, gather her up; she is so light, insubstantial. For a second I am struck dumb by the pain, and then she turns her face to me, and her eyes are open, focused on mine, and I laugh out loud with relief.

'Erica?' Her voice is tiny.

'Oh, Beth! What have you done?' I smooth her hair back from her face and then I realise. She has hacked it off, all of it. The dark pool on the floor is the severed length of her hair. Without it she looks like a little girl; so vulnerable. 'Your hair!' I cry, and then I laugh again and kiss her face. She has not cut herself, is not bleeding.

'I couldn't do it. I wanted to but . . . Eddie . . .'

'You *didn't* want to do it! You *don't* want to do it! I know you don't, not really,' I tell her. I pull her further into my arms, rock her gently.

'I did! I did want to!' she weeps angrily, and I think she would pull away from me if she had the strength. *'Why* did you make him tell you? *Why* wouldn't you *listen* to me?'

'Because it had to happen. It did. But listen to

me—Beth, are you listening? This is important.' I glance up, catch my reflection in the dressing table mirror. I look grey, spectral. But I can see it in my own eyes—the truth, waiting to spill out. I take a deep breath. 'Beth, Henry's not dead. *Harry* is Henry! It's true! Dinny told me the whole story . . . he didn't die. They took him off to some friend of theirs for first aid and then they moved him around different camps for years and years. That's why none of the searches ever found him.'

'What?' she whispers. She watches me like she would a snake, waiting for the next strike.

'Harry—the Harry your son just spent the Christmas holiday playing with—Harry is *our cousin Henry*.' Oh, I want to release her; I want to mend her! In the silence I hear her breathing. The fluttering of air, pushed from her body.

'That's not true,' she whispers.

'It's true, Beth. It's true. I believe it. Dinny wouldn't tell anyone what had happened, so Mickey thought *Dinny* had done it, and they didn't want him to be taken away . . .'

'No, no, *no!* None of that is right! I killed him! I *killed* him, Rick.' Her voice rises to a wail, wanes to a sliver. 'I killed him.' She says it more calmly now, as if almost relieved to let the words out.

'No, you didn't,' I insist.

'But . . . I threw that stone . . . it was too big! I should never have thrown it! Even Henry wouldn't have thrown one that big. But I was so angry! I was *so* angry I just wanted to make him *stop*! It went so high,' she whispers.

I can see it now. Finally, finally. Like it was there all along. Girls aren't taught to throw properly. She flung her whole body behind it, let go of it too soon, sent it too high. We lost sight of it against the incandescent summer sky. Henry was already laughing at her, laughing at the ineptness of the throw. He was already laughing when it came back down, when it hit his head with a sound that was so wrong. Loud, and wrong. We all knew the wrongness of that sound at once, even though we'd never heard it before. The sound of flesh breaking, of a blow to the bone. It was that sound that made me sick just now. As if I were hearing it again for the first time, and only now rejecting it. And then all that blood, and his glazed look, and my scramble from the water, and our flight. I have it now. At last.

'I didn't kill him?' Beth whispers at last, eyes boring into my face, mining me for the truth.

I shake my head, smile at her.

'No. You didn't kill him.'

I see relief seep into her face, slowly, so slowly; like she hardly dares believe it. I hold her tightly, feel her start to cry.

*　　　　*　　　　*

Later, I go back to the camp. In the early afternoon, with the sun burning through the mist. As the first glimpses of sky appear—gauzy, dazzling shreds—I feel something in me pouring out, pouring up. I'm left with a neutral feeling that could become anything. It could become joy. Perhaps. I sit next to Harry on the steps of his van. I ask him what he's doing and although he doesn't speak, he shows me, opening his hands. A tiny penknife in one hand, a half-cylinder shard of tree bark in the other, and patterns scratched into it,

459

geometric shapes bumping and overlapping. He is miraculous to me now. I try to take his arm but he shuffles, doesn't want me to. I don't force it. Miraculous. That Henry could grow into this gentle soul. Was he damaged or, rather, was something knocked out of him by Beth's blow? The spite? The childish arrogance, the aggression? All the base things, all of Meredith's legacy, all the hate she taught him. He is a cleanly wiped slate.

I let him keep working, but I tie his dreadlocks into a chaotic knot behind his head so I can see his face. I sit, and he works, and I watch his face. And slowly, familiar things surface. Some of his features settle back into the shapes I knew. Just here and there, just traces. The Calcott nose we all have, narrow at the bridge. The blue-grey shade of his irises. He doesn't seem to mind me watching. He doesn't seem to notice.

'He recognised you, I think,' Dinny says quietly, coming to stand in front of us. His arms hang loosely at his sides, hands in fists, as if he's ready for something. Ready to react. 'That first time you saw him in the woods and he stopped you passing by. I think he recognised you, you see.' I look up at Dinny, but I can't speak to him. Not yet. Tendons standing out on his forearms, ridges under the skin, tense with the clench of his hands. He was right. Everything has changed. Across the clearing, Patrick emerges from his van and gives me a solemn nod.

I go up to fetch Beth as the light is failing. She has been lying down for hours. Assimilating. I tell her who is downstairs and she agrees to see him. All the solemnity and the dread of one going to the gallows. Her bluntly cropped hair lies at odd angles, and her face is immobile, unnaturally still. Some force of will it must be costing her, to keep it that still. In the kitchen the lights are on. Dinny and Henry, sitting opposite each other at the table, playing snap and drinking tea as if the world has not just tensed itself up and thrown off everything our lives were based upon, like a dog shaking off muddy water. Dinny glances up as we come in, but Beth only looks at Henry. She sits down, at a safe distance, and stares. I watch and wait. Henry shuffles the cards clumsily, dropping a few onto the table that he slides back into the deck, one by one.

'Does he know me?' Beth whispers; her voice so thin, so precarious. Something about to break. I sit beside her, put my hands out to catch her.

Dinny shrugs slightly. 'There's really no way of knowing. He seems . . . comfortable around you. Around both of you. It usually takes him a while to warm up to strangers, so . . .'

'I thought I'd killed him. All this time, I thought I'd killed him . . .'

'You did,' Dinny says flatly. Her mouth opens in shock. 'You knocked him out and left him face down in the water—'

'Dinny! Don't—' I try to stop him.

'If I hadn't pulled him out, he *would* be dead. So just remember that before you start judging what *I've* done, what my family's done . . .'

'Nobody's judging anybody! We were just kids . . . we had no idea what to do. And yes, it was lucky you thought so fast, Dinny,' I say.

'I'd hardly call it lucky.'

'Well, whatever you want to call it then.'

Dinny draws in another breath, eyes narrowing at me, but Beth starts to cry. Not soft, self-pitying tears. Ragged, ugly sobs, torn out from the heart of her. Her mouth is a deep red hole. Low wails, rising from a darkness inside that's almost palpable, horrible to hear. I sit back down, put my arms around her as if I can hold her together. Dinny goes to the window, leans his forehead against the glass as if he wants nothing more than to be gone from this place. I press my cheek against Beth's back, feeling shudders pass up through her and into me. Henry sorts the cards into their suits in neat piles on the table. I can't begin to decipher what I feel about Dinny, about this secret he's been keeping. Henry, squirrelled away in England's labyrinth of lay-bys and green lanes; in vans and motor homes and caravans and lorries; a simple side-step but a world away from the door-to-door search for him in the neat and tidy villages. It's too big. I can't see it clearly.

We part some time later, to deliver our respective charges to bed. Dinny goes into the night with Henry; I walk up the stairs with Beth. She cried for a long time and now she's quiet. I think her mind is rewriting itself, like mine had to, and that she needs time. I hope that is all she needs. Her face looks raw. Not just red, not just rubbed. Raw like it is new-made, like it has yet to be shaped, yet to be marked by life. A childlike delicacy. I hope I see something wiped from it, some of her caginess, some of the shadow and fear. Too soon to tell. I pull the blankets up to her chin like a mother would, and she smiles a half-mocking smile.

'Erica,' she says, and sighs a little. 'How long have you been in love with Dinny?'

'What?' I shrug one shoulder to dismiss her,

realise too late that it's a gesture of his that I've picked up.

'Don't deny it. It's written all over you.'

'You need to sleep. It's been a rough day.'

'How long?' she presses, catching my hand as I move away. I look at her. In this light her eyes are unreadable. I can't lie, but I can't answer.

'I don't know,' I say shortly. 'I don't know that I am in love with him.' I walk to the door, stiffly, feeling betrayed by every line of my body, every tiny move I make.

'Erica!'

'What?'

'I . . . was pleased, when you said you didn't remember what had happened. I didn't want you to remember. You were so young . . .'

'Not *that* young.'

'Young enough. None of it was your fault, I hope you know that. Of course you know. I didn't want you to remember, because I was so ashamed. Not of throwing a stone back at him, but of running. Of leaving him there, and never telling Mum and Dad. I don't know why. I don't know why I did that! I've never known!'

'It wasn't—'

'It was a thing to be decided on the instant. That's what I've come to think, as I've got older. A decision made in an instant and once it's made you can't go back on it. Do you face up to a mistake, even one so terrible, or do you run away from it? I ran. I failed.'

'You didn't fail, Beth.'

'Yes, I did. You only ever did what *I* did. I was the leader, the eldest. If I'd spoken up straight away he could have lived.'

'He did live!'

'He could have lived *normally*! Not been so damaged . . .'

'Beth, there's no point to this. He lived. It can't be undone now. Please stop torturing yourself. You were a child.'

'When I think of Mary, and Clifford . . .' Tears blur her eyes again, spill over. I can think of nothing to say to this. Clifford and Mary. Their lives were ruined more completely than ours. The thought of them settles like lead around my heart.

*   *   *

I am awake in the clinging darkness before sunrise, and creep quietly to the kitchen. That odd state, exhausted and electrified at once. I make coffee, drink it strong and too hot. The cold of the floor numbs my feet through my socks. The little clock on the microwave tells me it's half past seven. Silence in the house but for the creak of the heating as it fights its losing battle. I fetch yesterday's paper, stare at it blankly and fail to do the crossword. The caffeine bustles my brain awake, but it doesn't help me think. How can we not tell Henry's parents that he's alive? How can we not? We can't not. But they will want to know what happened. Even placid Mary, so broken, will want to know what happened. And Clifford will want *justice*. Justice as he would see it. He will want charges brought against the Dinsdales for kidnapping, for withholding medical treatment. He will probably want charges brought against Beth and me, although these would be harder to bring. Grievous bodily harm, perhaps. Perverting the

464

course of justice. I have no idea what charges apply to children. But I can see him clearly, with the three of us in his teeth, shaking and shaking. So how can we tell them?

Outside the sky lightens slowly. Beth appears, fully dressed, at ten o'clock. She stands in the doorway with her bag on her shoulder.

'How are you doing?' I ask her.

'I'm . . . OK. I've got to go. Maxwell's dropping Eddie off after lunch tomorrow and nothing's ready, and . . . and I need to get to a hairdresser before he arrives. I've got him until he goes back to school on Wednesday.'

'Oh, right. I thought . . . I thought we were going to talk about it? About Henry?' I ask.

She shakes her head. 'I'm just not ready to talk about it yet. Not yet. I feel better, though.'

'Good, good. I'm glad, Beth. Really, I am. I want nothing more than for you to be able to put all this behind you.'

'That's what I want too.' She sounds lighter, almost bright; smiles in readiness to depart, grips her bag convincingly.

'Only . . . I don't know what we should do about Clifford and Mary. What we should do about telling them . . .' I say. Her face falls. She is on the same train of thought as me, I think, only I am some hours ahead of her. She licks her lips, quickly, nervously.

'Right now I have to go. But honestly, Rick, I don't think I should have any say in what happens next. I don't have the right. I don't want the right. I've done enough to him. To them. I don't think any idea of mine would be a good one.' Little shadows chase across her face again.

'Don't worry about it, Beth. I'll sort it out.' So sure of this, I sound. She smiles at me, diaphanous and wonderful as new butterfly wings; comes over and hugs me.

'Thank you, Erica. I owe you so much,' she says.

'You don't owe me anything.' I shake my head. 'You're my sister.'

She squeezes me with all the strength in her willow-switch body.

It starts to sleet from a flat grey sky as we get into the car, and I have just started the engine when Dinny appears from beneath the trees, knocks on the window.

'I was hoping I'd catch you. I guessed you'd be off this morning,' he says to Beth. Just the faintest hint of a rebuke, but enough to put a line between her brows.

'Beth has to catch the next train,' I say. He flicks his eyes to me and nods.

'Look, Beth, I just wanted to say . . . I just . . . when I said last night that you'd killed him, I didn't mean that . . . that you'd done it deliberately or anything,' he says. 'I used to ask my parents why Henry was such a bastard. Why he was such a bully, such a vicious little git . . . They told me over and over again that when children behave that way it's because they aren't happy. For whatever reason they're full of fear and anger and they take it out on other people. I didn't believe them then, of course. I thought it was just because he was an evil sod, but I believe it now. It's true, of course. Henry wasn't happy then, and, well, he is happy now. He's the happiest, most peaceful soul I know. I just . . . I just thought you should think about that.' Dinny swallows, tips his chin at us and steps back from the car.

'Thank you,' Beth says. She can't quite look him in the eye, but she's trying. 'Thank you, for what you did. For never telling anybody.'

'I'd never have done anything to hurt you, Beth,' he says softly. My knuckles on the steering wheel are white. Beth nods, her eyes downcast. 'Will you ever come back this way?' he asks.

'Perhaps. I think so. Sometime in the future,' she replies.

'Then I'll see you around, Beth,' Dinny says, with a sad smile.

'Goodbye, Dinny,' she says quietly. He smacks the roof of the car with the flat of his hand and I pull away obediently. In the rear-view mirror I see him standing there, hands in his pockets, dark eyes in a dark face. He stays until we have driven out of sight.

*   *   *

Saturday the third of January today. Most people will be back at work on Monday. I will call the Calcott family lawyer, a Mr Dawlish of Marlborough, and tell him he can put Storton Manor on the market. I have decisions to make, now that I can go forward again. There's nothing missing any more, no cracks, no excuses to stall. I am quiet as I move around the house. I don't want the radio on, or the TV for company. I don't hum, I try not to bang; I put my feet down softly. I want to hear the clear bell-tone of the truths I know ringing in my head. I could leave it all—leave the huge tree and all the holly I painted gold. They could stay, gathering dust and cobwebs until the auctioneer has been and gone with all the good stuff, and the house clearance men have been for the rest. Relics of this odd, limbo Christmas of ours. But I can't bear the thought of it. That shreds of our lives should be left like Meredith's apple core in the drawing room bin. Discarded and repugnant.

Industry is good. It keeps my thoughts from overwhelming me. Three things only I will keep: Caroline's writing case and the letters within it, the New York portrait and Flag's teething ring. The rest can go. I strip the tree of baubles and beads and clear the last of the Christmas leftovers from the fridge and the larder, scattering the lawn with anything the birds or foxes might fancy. I find pliers in a scullery drawer, climb the stairs to where the Christmas tree is fixed to the banisters, and cut the wire. 'Timber!' I cry, to the empty hallway. The tree sags slowly to one side, then flops to the floor like an elderly dog. A delicate, muffled crunch tells me I didn't find every bauble. Dry needles cascade from the branches, carpet the flagstones. With a sigh, I fetch a dustpan and brush and set to chasing them around the floor. I can't help conjuring a life for myself with Dinny, picturing staying with him. Sleeping on a narrow bunk in the back of his ambulance; cooking breakfast on the tiny stove; perhaps working in each new town. Short contracts, sick-leave cover. Tutoring. As if anybody would hire a supply teacher with no fixed address. Lying close each night, hearing his heartbeat, woken by his touch.

There's a knock, and Dinny's voice startles me from my reverie.

'Is this a bad time?' His head appears around

the front door.

'No, it's perfect timing, actually. You can help me drag this tree out.' I smile, climbing to my feet and wincing. 'I've been on my knees for too long. And not for any of the best reasons,' I tell him.

'Oh? And what are the best reasons?' Dinny asks, with an arch smile that warms me.

'Why, prayer, of course,' I tell him, all sincerity, and he chuckles. He hands me an envelope.

'Here. A card from Honey. For your help the other night, and for the flowers.' He takes an elastic band from his pocket, holding it in his teeth while he gathers up his hair, pulls it back from his face.

'Oh, she didn't have to do that.'

'Well, after you'd left Mum's the other day she realised that she hadn't actually *said* thank you. And now that the hormones are settling down, I think she appreciates how vile she's been for the past few weeks.'

'She had good reason, I suppose. Not an easy time for her.'

'She didn't make it easy. But it all seems to be working out now.'

'Here—grab a branch.' I open both sides of the front door wide and we grasp the tree by its lowest branches, tow it across the floor. It bleeds a green wake behind it.

'Perhaps you shouldn't have swept up until after we'd moved the tree?' Dinny observes.

'Could be,' I agree. We abandon the tree on the driveway, brush the needles from our hands. Everything is dripping wet out here, weighed down with water. Dark streaks on the trees, like a fever sweat. The rooks clamour from across the garden.

Their disembodied voices hit the house, come back again as metallic echoes; I think I can feel them watching us with their hard little eyes like metal beads. My heart is the quickest thing for miles around. My thoughts the least quiet. I look at Dinny, suddenly shy. I can't give a name to what's between us, can't quite feel the shape of it. 'Come for dinner tonight,' I say.

'OK. Thanks,' he replies.

*   *   *

I've made a meal with the last of anything edible from the larder, the fridge, the freezer. This is the last time. I will throw the rest away. Ancient tins of custard powder; dog biscuits; jars of treacle with rusted-on lids; sachets of ready-mix béchamel. The house will go from lived-in to empty, from home to property. Any time now. I said he could bring Harry, if he wanted. It seemed only right. I feel I ought to have some part in looking after him, in supporting him. But Dinny sensed this, and he frowned, and when he arrives at seven he's alone. A tawny owl shrieks in the trees behind him, heralds him. A still night, cold and dank as a riverbank pebble.

'Beth seemed a bit better when she left,' I say, opening a bottle of wine and pouring two large glasses. 'Thank you for saying . . . what you said. About Henry being happy.'

'It's true,' Dinny says, taking a sip that wets his lower lip, traces it with crimson.

All along, he has known. All this time, all these years. He can't know, then, how I feel now— looking down and seeing I wasn't walking on solid ground after all.

'What is this, anyway?' he asks me, turning the food over with his fork.

'Chicken Provençal. And those are cheese dumplings. Mixed bean salad and tinned spinach. Why? Is there a problem?'

'No, no problem,' he smiles, and gamely begins to eat. I take a forkful of dumpling. It has the texture of plasticine.

'It's horrible. Sorry. I never was much of a cook,' I say.

'The chicken's not bad,' Dinny says diplomatically. We are so unused to this. To sitting and eating together. Small talk. The idea of us together, in this new world order. The silence hangs.

'My mum told me that you were in love with Beth back then. Is that why you would never say what had really happened? To protect Beth?'

Dinny chews slowly, swallows.

'We were *twelve*, Erica. But I didn't want to tell on her, no.'

'Do you still love her?' I don't want to know, but I have to.

'She's not the same person now.' He looks down, frowns.

'And me? Am I the same?'

'Pretty much,' Dinny smiles. 'As tenacious as ever.'

'I don't mean to be,' I say. 'I just want to do the right thing. I just want . . . I want everything to be all right.'

'You always did. But life's not that simple.'

'No.'

'Are you going back to London?'

'I don't think so. No, I'm not. I'm not sure where I'm going.' I look at him when I say this and I can't keep the question from my eyes. He looks at me, steadily but without an answer.

'Clifford will make trouble,' I say at length. 'If we tell them. I know he will. But I'm not sure if I could live with myself, knowing what I know and letting him and Mary think Henry's dead,' I say.

'They wouldn't know him now, Erica,' Dinny says seriously. 'He's not their son any more.'

'Of course he's their son! What else is he?'

'He's been with me for so long now. I've grown up with him. I've seen myself change . . . but Harry just stayed the same. Like he was frozen in time the day that rock hit him. If anything, he's my brother. He's part of *my* family now.'

'We're all one family, remember? In more ways than one, it seems. They could help you look after him . . . or I could. Help support him . . . financially, or . . . He's their *son*, Dinny. And he didn't die!'

'But he did. Their son did. Harry is not Henry. They'd take him away from everything he knows.'

'They have a right to know about him.' I shake my head, I cannot let this lie.

'So, what—you're picturing Harry living with them, cooped up in a conventional life, or in some kind of institution, where they can visit him whenever they like and he'd be plonked in front of the TV the rest of the time?'

'It wouldn't be like that!'

'How do you know?'

'I just . . . I can't even imagine what it must have been like for them, all this time.' We are quiet for a long time. 'I'm not going to decide anything

472

without you,' I tell him.

'I've told you what I think,' Dinny says. 'It would do them no good to see him now. And we don't need any help.'

He shakes his head and looks sad. I cannot bear this thought, that I am making Dinny sad. I put my hand across the table, mesh my fingers into his.

'What you did for us—for Beth—taking the blame like that . . . it's huge, Dinny. That was a huge thing that you did,' I say quietly. 'Thank you.'

*   *   *

'Will you stay?' I ask him, late in the evening. He doesn't answer, but he stands up, waits for me to lead. I won't take him into Meredith's room. I choose a guest room on the top floor, in the attics of the house, where the sheets are chilly with the long absence of warm bodies and the floorboards creak as we cross them. The silence makes us quiet, and the night outside the bare window sketches us in silvery greys as we undress. My skin rises where he touches me, the tiny hairs on me reaching out. He is so dark in this monochrome light, his face a depth of shadow I can't fathom. I kiss his mouth, bruise my lips against his, drink him in. I want there to be no space between us, no part of my body not touching his. I want to wind myself around him like ivy, like a rope, binding us together. He has no tattoos, no piercings, no scars. He is whole, perfect. The palms of his hands are rough on my back. He coils one through my hair, tips my head back.

I close my eyes and watch with my body—each sure move of his hands, the warm brush of his breath, his weight over me. I pull his elbows out from under him. I want him to cover me, to crush me. Nothing guarded about him now, no hesitation, no thinking. A frown of a different kind as he puts his hands under my hips, lifts me, fits me to his body, pushes hard. I want to ink my mind with this, always keep him in this room with me; keep the taste of him on my tongue, make the beat between each second last, unending. Salt sweat on his top lip, ragged words mumbled into my hair. I want nothing else.

'I could stay with you,' I say afterwards. My eyes are shut, trusting. 'I could stay and help you with Harry. I can get work anywhere. You shouldn't have to support him alone. I could help. I could stay with you.'

'And travel all the time, and live like we do?'

'Well, why not? I'm homeless now, after all.'

'You're a long way from being homeless. You don't know what you're saying.' His fingers are curled around my shoulder, and they smell of me. I lean myself against him. His skin is hot and dry beneath my cheek.

'I do know. I don't want to go back to London, and I can't stay here. I'm at your disposal,' I say, and the absurdity of this statement makes me chuckle. But Dinny does not laugh. There's a growing tension in his frame that makes me uneasy. 'I don't mean . . . I'm not trying to foist myself on you, or anything,' I add hurriedly. No grip of mine could hold him, if he wanted to go. He sighs, turns his head to press a kiss onto my hair.

'It wouldn't be so bad having you foisted on me, Pup,' he smiles. 'Let's sleep on it. We can sort it out tomorrow.' He says it so softly, so quietly that I decipher the words from the rumble in his chest beneath my ear. Deep and resolute. I am awake long enough to hear his breathing deepen, slow down, grow even. Then I sleep.

When I wake up I'm alone. The sky is flat, matt white, and a fine drizzle sifts down through the trees. A rook perches on a bare branch outside the window, feathers fluffed against the weather. Suddenly, I long for summer. For warmth, and dry ground, and a mile-wide sky. I run my hand across the side of the bed where Dinny was when I fell asleep. The sheets aren't warm. There's no indent in the pillow, no echo of his head. I could have imagined him here with me, but I didn't. I didn't. I won't race down there. I won't be alarmed. I make myself get dressed, eat breakfast cereal with the last of the milk. Today I will either have to shop or leave. I wonder which it will be.

I slip across the sodden lawn, wellies slick with water, papered with dead leaves. I feel clear-headed today, purposeful. It's misplaced, perhaps, when I have not yet made the decisions that need making, but perhaps I am finally ready to make them, perhaps that's what this feeling is. I've got a box of things for Harry. I found them in some drawers in the cellar, had earmarked them for the bin when I realised he might like them. A broken Sony radio, some old torches and batteries and bulbs and small metal objects of unknown provenance. They rattle against the cardboard under my arm. My back aches from the strain of Dinny's weight, pushing against my pelvis. I shiver, cradle this physical memory close to me.

I stand for quite some time in the centre of the camp clearing, while the rain begins to soften the box I carry. No vans here now, no dogs, no columns of smoke. It is deserted and I am left behind—alone in an empty clearing churned muddy by feet and wheels; and me, churned muddy by him. By the getting of him, and now the losing. My long-lost cousin, my childhood hero. My Dinny. Perfect calm, and stillness. No breath of a breeze today. I can hear a car, speeding along the lane from the village, tyres crackling in the standing rainwater. I have no phone number for him, no email address, no clue in which direction he has gone. I turn in a slow circle, in case there is something behind me, something that waited for me, or someone.

LEGACY

1911–

Caroline's last child was born in 1911, long after the occupants of Storton Manor had given up hope of there being a Calcott heir. There had been other pregnancies, two of them, both a long time in the conceiving, but Caroline's body had rejected the children and they had been lost before they even really began. The little girl was born in August. It was a long, hot summer the likes of which no one could remember, and Caroline sweltered, shuffling into the garden to lie swollen and prone in the shade, drowsing. The heat was such that sometimes, as she hovered on the edges of sleep, she imagined herself back in Woodward County, sitting on the porch and gazing out at the yard, waiting for Corin to ride home; so that when she was approached by a servant or her husband, she stared at them in no little confusion for a while, before remembering who they were and where she was.

The gardens were scorched and brown. A village boy, Tommy Westenfell, drowned in the dew pond. His feet got tangled in weeds at the bottom and he was found hours later by his distraught father; pale, still, and sleepy-eyed. Mrs Priddy took a bad turn walking back from the butcher with a whole leg of lamb and was consigned to her bed for three days, her skin mottled and puce. Estelle and Liz, Cass's plump replacement, worked hard to cover for her, with perspiration soaking their uniforms.

The smell everywhere was of parched earth, sweat and hot, dry air. The stone flags of the terrace burnt Caroline's feet through the soles of her slippers. Henry Calcott, who was by then uncomfortable around his own wife, remained at home long enough to see the child safely born, and then quit Wiltshire to stay with friends by the sea in Bournemouth.

The labour was long and arduous, and Caroline was delirious by the end. The doctor forced fluids into her through a tube pushed down her throat, and she gazed at him from the bed with uncomprehending terror. Liz and Estelle kept the baby those first few days, taking turns to lay cold cloths onto their mistress's skin to cool her. Caroline recovered, at length, but when they brought the child to her, her gaze swept over it impassively, and then she turned her face away and would not nurse it. A wet nurse was found in the village and Caroline, who wanted to be sure that the girl would live before she dared to love her, found, as months and then years passed, that she had left it too late. The little girl did not seem to belong to her, and she could not love her. The child was two years old before she was given a name. Estelle, Liz and the wet nurse had been calling her Augusta all that time, but one day Caroline looked dispassionately into her cradle and announced that she would be named Meredith, after her grandmother.

*   *   *

Meredith was a lonely child. She had no siblings to play with and was forbidden to play with any of the

478

village children that she saw roaming the fields and lanes around the manor house. The household was in decline by then, and the village of Barrow Storton was a sad, quiet place with most of the young men gone off to fight and die on the continent. Henry Calcott kept mainly to town, where his gambling consumed so much money that several of the staff, including Liz and the scullery maid, were laid off, leaving Mrs Priddy to keep the house as best she could with only Estelle to help her. Mrs Priddy was kind to Meredith, letting her eat the leftover pastry scraps and keep a pet rabbit in a pen outside the kitchen door, where she fed it carrot tops and ragged outer lettuce leaves. A tutor came, five mornings a week, to teach Meredith her letters, music, needlework and deportment. Meredith hated the lessons and the tutor both; and escaped into the garden as soon as she could.

But Meredith longed for her mother. Caroline was an otherworldly creature by then, who sat for hours in a white gown, either at a window or out on the lawn, staring into the distance and seeing who knew what. When Meredith tried to hug her, she tolerated it for a moment and then disentangled the child's arms with a mild smile, telling her vaguely to run along and play. Mrs Priddy admonished her not to tire her mother out, and Meredith took this instruction to heart, fearing that she was somehow responsible for her mother's persistent lethargy. So she kept away, thinking that if she did her mother would not be so tired, and would get up and smile and love her more. She played alone, watching pigeons on the rooftops courting and bowing to one another. She watched the frog spawn in the ornamental pond slowly grow tails and hatch into tadpoles. She watched the kitchen cats as they chased down hapless mice and then devoured them with swift, perfunctory crunches. And she watched the Dinsdales in the clearing through the woods. She watched them whenever she could, but she was too shy to ever let them see her.

The Dinsdales had three children: a tiny baby who went around in a sling on his mother's back, a little girl with yellow hair like her mother's, who was a few years older than Meredith herself, and a boy, a dark, strange-looking boy whose age Meredith was unable to guess at, who went everywhere with his father and played with his little sister, grinning as he teased her. Their mother was pretty and she smiled all the time, laughing at their antics and hugging them. Their father was more serious, as Meredith understood fathers should be, but he smiled often too, and put his arm around the boy, or lifted the little girl high into the air to sit astride his shoulders. Meredith could not imagine her own father ever doing such a thing with her—the very thought made her uneasy. So Meredith watched this family, fascinated, and even though they were happy and bright she came away from her clandestine visits feeling tearful and dark, unaware that she watched them because she envied them and was filled with yearning for her own mother to hug her that way.

One day she made a mistake. Her mother was on the lawn in her wicker chair, an untouched jug of lemonade on the table beside her with thirsty flies settling unafraid on the beaded lace cover. Meredith emerged from the woods and was startled to see her there, immediately brushing down her skirts and tucking her hair behind her ears. Her mother did not look up as she approached, but managed a wan smile once her daughter was standing right in front of her.

'Well, child, and where have you been today?' her mother asked her in a voice that was soft and dry and seemed to come from far away. Meredith went right up to her and tentatively took hold of her hand.

'I was in the woods. Exploring,' she said. 'Shall I pour you some lemonade?'

'And what did you find in the woods?' her mother asked, ignoring the offer of lemonade.

'I saw the Dinsdales—' Meredith said, and then put her hand over her mouth. Mrs Priddy had warned her never to mention the Dinsdales to her mother, although she had no idea why not.

'You did what?' her mother snapped. 'You know that's not allowed! I hope you have not been talking to those people?'

'No, Mama,' Meredith said quietly. Her mother settled back into her chair, pressing her mouth into a bloodless line. Meredith steeled herself. 'But, Mama, *why* can I not play with them?' Her heart beat fast at her own temerity.

'Because they are filth! Gypsy, tinker villains! They are thieves and liars and they are not welcome here—and you are *not* to go near them! Not *ever*! Do you understand?' Her mother leant forward in her chair like a whip cracking, and grasped Meredith's wrist so that it hurt. Meredith nodded fearfully.

'Yes, Mama,' she whispered.

They are not welcome here. Meredith took these words to heart. When she watched them next her envy became jealousy, and instead of wanting to play with them, and share their happy existence, she began to wish instead that they did not *have* their happy existence. She watched them every day, and every day she grew crosser with them, and sadder inside, so that it came to seem to her that it was the Dinsdales who were *making* her sad. Her and her mother both. If she could make them go away, she thought, her mother would be pleased. Surely, she would *have* to be pleased.

On a hot summer's day in 1918, Meredith heard the Dinsdale children playing at the dew pond. She edged closer, through the dappled light beneath the trees, then stood behind the smooth trunk of a beech and watched them jumping in and out of the water. It looked like tremendous fun, although Meredith had never been swimming so she could not know for sure. She wished she could try, though. Her skin was itchy with the heat, and the thought of all that clear, cold water washing over it was so tempting it made her weak. The Dinsdales were splashing up arcs of crystalline droplets, and Meredith noticed how dry her mouth felt. The boy's skin was so much darker than his sister's. It was a kind of nut colour, and his raggedy hair was inky black. He teased the girl and dunked her under the water, but Meredith saw that he secretly watched her and made sure she was still laughing before he dunked her again.

She leant out for a better view, and then froze to the spot. The Dinsdales had seen her. First the boy, who had climbed out and was standing on the bank, water streaming from the hems of his short breeches, then the girl, who paddled in a circle to see what her brother was looking at.

'Hello,' the boy said to her, so casual and friendly, when Meredith felt like her heart might explode in her chest. 'Who are you?'

Meredith was amazed that he didn't know, when she herself felt that she knew *them* so well. It outraged her that they did not know who she was. She stood, stock still and breathless, not knowing whether to stay or to run.

'Meredith,' she whispered, after a long, uneasy silence.

'I'm Maria!' the girl called from the water, her arms windmilling madly beneath the surface.

'And I'm Flag. Do you want to come in for a swim? It's quite safe,' the boy told her. He put his hands on his hips and examined her, head tipped to one side. His wet skin shone over the curves of his arms and legs, and liquid light from the water danced in his eyes. Meredith felt almost too shy to answer him. She thought him beautiful, and was not sure what to say.

'What kind of name is *Flag*?' she asked, haughtily, in spite of herself.

'My name,' he shrugged. 'Do you live at the big house, then?'

'Yes,' she replied, her words still reluctant to come.

'Well,' Flag continued, after a pause, 'do you want to swim with us or not?'

Meredith felt her face burn and she tipped her chin down to hide. She was not allowed to swim. She never had been—but the temptation was so strong and, she reasoned, who would ever find out?

'I . . . I don't know how to swim,' she was forced to admit.

'Paddle then. I'll fetch you out if you fall in,' Flag shrugged. Meredith had never heard the word *paddle* before, but she thought she understood. Fingers trembling with the illicit thrill of disobedience, she sat down on the cracked earth and pulled off her boots, then crept carefully to the water's edge. It wasn't *really* disobeying, she told herself. Nobody had ever said anything to her about not paddling.

She slithered the last few inches down the steep bank and gasped nervously as her feet stumbled into the water.

'It's so cold!' she squeaked, hastily scrambling backwards. Maria giggled.

'It's only cold when you first jump in. Then it's perfect!' she said.

Meredith edged forwards again and let the water rise to her ankles. The bite of it made her bones ache and scattered silvery shivers all over her. With a yell, Flag took a short run up and leapt into the middle of the pool, bending his knees and wrapping his arms around them. The splash caused a wave to engulf Maria and soak the bottom six inches of Meredith's dress.

'Now look what you've done!' she cried, afraid that Mrs Priddy or her mother would see and she would be found out.

'Flag! Don't,' Maria told him gaily as he surfaced, spluttering.

'It'll soon dry out,' Flag told her carelessly. His hair was plastered to his neck, as slick as otter fur. Meredith climbed out crossly, sat down on the bank and studied her feet, which had gone from pink to bright white after their wetting.

'Flag—say you're sorry!' Maria commanded.

'Sorry for getting your dress wet, Meredith,' Flag said, rolling his eyes at his sister. But Meredith didn't reply. She sat and watched them swim for a while longer, but her sullen presence seemed to spoil their fun and they soon climbed out and pulled on the rest of their clothes.

'Do you want to come and have tea?' Maria asked her, her smile a little less ready than before. Flag stood half turned to go. Water ran from his hair and wet his shirt, slicking it to his skin. Meredith wanted to look at him but her eyes slid away infuriatingly when she tried.

She shook her head. 'I'm not allowed,' she said.

'Come on then, Maria,' Flag said, a touch impatiently.

'Goodbye, then,' Maria shrugged, and gave Meredith a little wave.

It took nearly two hours for the thick cotton of her dress to dry out completely, and during that time Meredith kept to the outer edges of the garden where only the gardener might see her. He was ancient and didn't pay much attention to anything except his marrows. She thought about her paddle, and about Maria inviting her to tea, and about Flag's wet hair shining, and each of these things gave her a fizzing feeling quite at odds with the resentment she had felt before. It made her skip a little and smile excitedly. She imagined how it might be to go to tea, to see the inside of the covered wagon that she had watched so many times from the trees, to meet their blonde and affectionate mother, who put her arms around them and smiled all the time. *How do you do, Mrs Dinsdale?* She practised the phrase under her breath in the safe, silent confines of the greenhouse. But there could be no arguing that this would be a huge disobedience. And that talking to Flag and Maria had been one as well, even if she could argue her way around the paddling. Just thinking about what would happen if Mama found out about it brought her spirits low again, and when she was called in for tea she made sure that she was quiet and dull and gave nothing away.

For days, Meredith was consumed with thoughts and daydreams about the Dinsdales. She had so rarely encountered other children—only visiting cousins, or the children of other guests who stayed only fleetingly so she never really got to know them. She knew she was supposed to despise the tinkers, and she knew all the things her mother had told her about them, and she still longed more than anything to please her mother and to make her happy, but the idea of having friends was irresistible. A week later, she was playing in the barred shadow of the tall iron gates when she saw Flag and Maria walking along the lane towards the village. They would not see her unless she called out and for a second she was paralysed, torn between longing to speak to them again and knowing that she shouldn't—least of all from the gate, which was visible from the house if anybody happened to be at one of the east-facing windows. In desperation she came up with a compromise of sorts and burst loudly into song—the first thing that came to mind, a song she had heard Estelle singing as she pegged the laundry out to dry.

'I'd like to see the Kaiser, with a lily in his hand!' she bellowed, tunelessly, hopping from one bar of shadow to the next. Flag and Maria turned and,

seeing her, came over to the gates.

'Hello again,' Maria greeted her. 'What are you doing?'

'Nothing,' Meredith replied, her heart yammering behind her ribs. 'What are you doing?'

'Going on to the village to buy bread and Bovril for tea. Do you want to come too? If we can get a broken loaf, there'll be a ha'penny left to buy sweets,' Maria smiled.

'Not necessarily,' Flag qualified. 'If there's enough left over we're to buy butter, remember?'

'Oh, but there's never enough for butter as well!' Maria dismissed her brother.

'You have to go to the shops yourselves?' Meredith asked, puzzled.

'Of course, silly! Who else would go?' Maria laughed.

'Suppose *you've* got servants to run around buying *your* tea, haven't you?' Flag asked, a touch derisively.

Meredith bit her lip, an awkward blush heating her face. She hardly ever went into the village. A handful of times she had accompanied Mrs Priddy or Estelle on some errand, but only when her father was away, and her mother laid low and guaranteed not to hear of it.

'Do you want to come, then?'

'I'm not allowed,' Meredith said unhappily. Her cheeks burned even more, and Flag tilted his head at her, a mischievous glint coming into his eye.

'Seems to be a fair bit you're not allowed to do,' he remarked.

'Hush! It's not *her* fault!' Maria admonished him.

'Come on—I dare you. Or maybe you're just

scared?' he asked, arching an eyebrow.

Meredith glared at him defiantly. 'I am not! Only . . .' She hesitated. She *was* scared, it was true. Scared of being found out, scared of her mother's lightning-fast temper. But it would be so easy to slip away and back again without being noticed. Only the worst luck would mean she was discovered in this outrageous behaviour.

'Cowardy, cowardy custard!' Flag sang softly.

'Don't listen to *him*,' Maria advised her. 'Boys are *stupid*.' But Meredith was listening, and she did want to impress this black-eyed boy, and she did want to be friends with his sister, and she did want to be as free as they were, to come and go, and to buy sweets in the village and bread for tea. The gates of Storton Manor seemed to rear up above her head, ever higher and starker. Jangling with nerves, she reached for the latch, pulled open a narrow gap and slipped out into the lane.

Flag strode on ahead, leaving Maria and Meredith to walk side by side, picking wild flowers from the hedgerows and firing questions to and fro—what was it like living in a caravan, what was it like living in a mansion, how many servants were there and what were their names and why didn't Meredith go to school, and what was school like and what did they do there? In the village they stopped at the door to the farrier's shed to watch as he pressed a hot iron shoe onto the foot of a farm horse, whose hooves were the size of dinner plates. Clouds of acrid smoke billowed past them, but the horse did not blink an eye.

'Doesn't it hurt him?' Meredith asked.

' 'Course not. No more than it hurts you to have your hair cut,' Flag shrugged.

'Get on with ye, casting shadows o'er the work,' said the farrier, who was old and grizzled and stern of eye, so they carried on towards the grocer's. They bought a broken loaf and a jar of Bovril, and even though there was only enough left for two small sugar mice, the lady behind the counter smiled at Meredith and gave them a third.

'Not often we see you in the village, Miss Meredith,' the lady said, and Meredith caught her breath. How did the woman know who she was? And would she tell Mrs Priddy? Her face went pale and panicked tears came hotly into her eyes. 'Now, now. Don't look so aghast! Your secret's safe with me,' the woman said.

'Thank you, Mrs Carter!' Maria called brightly, and they went outside to devour their sweets.

'Why aren't you allowed to go into the village? No harm could come to you,' Flag asked as they stopped by the pond to watch the ducks circling idly. They sat down on the grass and Meredith nibbled at her sugar mouse, determined to make it last. She so rarely had sweets.

'Mama says it's not seemly,' Meredith replied.

'What's seemly?' Maria asked, licking her fingers with relish. Meredith shrugged.

'It means she's too good to go mixing with the hoi polloi. The likes of us,' Flag said, sounding amused. The girls thought about this for a while, in meditative silence.

'So . . . what would happen if your ma found out you was along here with us, then?' Maria asked at length.

'I would be . . . told off,' Meredith said uncertainly. In fact, she had no real idea. She had been told off for even watching the Dinsdales. Now she had sneaked out of the gardens and come into the village with them, and talked to them lots, and been seen in the grocer's by a woman who knew her name, and it had all been wonderful. Painfully, she swallowed the last of her sugar mouse, which had lost all its sweetness. 'I should go back,' she said nervously, scrambling to her feet. As if sensing the change in mood, the Dinsdales got up without argument and they began to walk back along the lane.

At the gates, Meredith slithered back through the gap as quickly as she could and pulled the gate closed, not daring to look up at the house in case somebody was watching. Her blood was racing and only once the gate was shut did she feel a little safer. She held on to the bars for support while she got her breath back.

'You're an odd one and no mistake,' Flag said, with a bemused smile.

'Come and have some tea with us tomorrow,' Maria invited her. 'Ma said you can—I asked her already.'

'Thank you. But . . . I don't know,' Meredith said. She was feeling exhausted by her adventure and could hardly think of anything except getting away from the gates without being seen talking to them. The Dinsdales wandered off and Meredith put her face to the bars to watch them go, pressing the cold metal into her skin. Flag pulled a leggy stem of goose grass from the hedge and stuck it to the back of Maria's blouse, and the blonde girl twisted and craned her neck, trying to reach it. As they passed out of sight Meredith turned and saw her mother standing in the upstairs hall window, watching her. Behind the glass, her face was ghastly pale and her eyes far too wide. She looked like a spectre, frozen for ever in torment.

Meredith's heart seemed to stop, and at once she thought desperately about running away to the furthest part of the garden. But that would only make matters worse, she realised in a moment of cold clarity. She suddenly needed to pee and thought for a hideous second that she would wet herself. On trembling legs she made her slow progress into the house, up the stairs and along the corridor to where her mother was waiting.

'How dare you?' Caroline whispered. Meredith looked at her feet. Her silence seemed to enrage her mother further. *'How dare you!'* she shouted, so loudly and harshly that Meredith jumped, and began to cry. 'Answer me—where have you been with them? What were you doing?' Mrs Priddy appeared from a room down the hall and hurried along to stand behind Meredith protectively.

'My lady? Is something the matter?' the housekeeper asked, diffidently.

Caroline ignored her. She bent forwards, seized Meredith's shoulders and shook her roughly.

'Answer me! How *dare* you disobey me, girl!' she spat, her gaunt face made brutal by rage. Meredith sobbed harder, tears of pure fear running down her cheeks. Straightening up, Caroline took a short breath that flared her nostrils whitely. She measured her daughter briefly, then slapped her sharply across the face.

'My lady! That's enough!' Mrs Priddy gasped. Meredith fell into shocked silence, her eyes fixed on the front of her mother's skirts and not daring to move from there. Caroline grasped her arm again and towed her viciously to her room, pushing her inside so abruptly that Meredith stumbled.

'You will stay in there and not come out until you have learnt your lesson,' Caroline said coldly. Meredith wiped her nose and felt her face throbbing where her mother had hit her. 'You're a wicked child. No mother could ever love you,' Caroline said; and the last thing Meredith saw before the door closed was Mrs Priddy's stunned expression.

For a week, Meredith was kept locked in her room. The staff were given orders that she was to have nothing but bread and water, but once Caroline had retired, Estelle and Mrs Priddy took her biscuits and scones and ham sandwiches. They brushed her hair for her, told her funny stories, and put arnica cream on her lip where the slap had made it swell, but Meredith remained silent and closed off, so that they exchanged worried looks above her head. *No mother could ever love her.* Meredith dwelt on this statement for a long time and refused to believe it. She would *make* her mother love her, she resolved. She would prove that she was not wicked, she would strive to be good and obedient and decorous in all things, and would win her mother's heart that way. And she would shun the tinkers. Because of them, her mother could not love her. *They are not welcome here.* She lay listlessly on her bed and felt her old anger at the Dinsdales, her old resentment, well up into a stifling pall that cast a dark shadow over her heart.

EPILOGUE

Spring is finally looking like it might win. We're through the muddy daffodils stage, past the week where soft tree blossoms were stripped by wind and rain and left to rot at the roadside in pink and brown drifts. Now there are tiny cracks in the earth of my sparse lawn, and fledgling sparrows line up along the fence, wide yellow mouths and fluffy feathers. I might get a cat, if it weren't for these absurd little birds, sitting shoulder to shoulder like beads on a string. I check their progress daily. The last tenant here parked his motorbikes on the lawn, and piled up the debris of his DIY, so there isn't much grass, but it will grow now, I think. The sun finally has some warmth. I sit out in it, tilt my face to it like a daisy, and I can feel the summer coming at last.

It was a relief, in the end, to have all my decisions made for me. Made by Dinny. What could I tell Clifford and Mary? That Henry was alive but damaged, and although I had seen him many times over Christmas and not told them, I now had no idea where he was? And why would I even try to stay at the manor, with all of them gone? Beth, Dinny, Harry. Henry. But I didn't go far. That was a decision I had already made, I think. There was no question of me going back to London—it would have been like walking backwards. And on the edge of Barrow Storton was this cottage to rent. Not pretty, not quaint, but fine. A 1950s two-up, two-down at the end of a short row of identical cottages. Two bedrooms, so

Beth and Eddie can come and stay, and a great view from my bedroom at the front. It's on the opposite side of the village to the manor. I can see right across the valley, with the village at its bottom, and one corner of the manor is visible through distant trees. Less and less of it now that the trees are swelling into leaf. Then the downs roll away, bounding up to the barrow on the horizon.

It makes me very serene, living here. I feel like I belong. I have no sense of there being anything else I should be doing, or working towards, or changing. I am not even waiting, not really. I make a special point of not waiting. I teach in Devizes, I walk a lot. I call in on George Hathaway for cups of tea and biscuits. Sometimes I miss the people I used to see in London—not specific people as such, but having so many faces around me. The illusion of company. But here I tend to notice the faces I do see all the more. People aren't part of a crowd like they were. I've made friends with my neighbours, Susan and Paul, and sometimes babysit for them for free because their little girls wear patched trousers far too short for them and don't go to ballet or judo or have riding lessons. There's no trampoline in their back yard. Susan's expression moved from suspicion to incredulous joy when I offered. The girls are good-natured and they do as they're told, most of the time. I take them on nature walks up on the downs or along the riverbank; we make cornflake cakes and hot chocolate while Susan and Paul go to the pub, the cinema, the shops, their bed.

Honey knows I'm here, and so does Mo. I went back to see Haydee and told them where I was and they've both been to visit since. I polished the tarnish from the silver bell on Flag's teething ring, brought it to a high shine and tucked it into Haydee's cot. She grabbed it with one fat hand, crammed it immediately into her mouth. *It was your great-grandpa's*, I whispered to her. I wrote down my address, told Honey to keep it in case anybody asked for it. She gave me a straight look, solemn, then arched one eyebrow. But she didn't say anything. She's back at school now and Mo comes around with Haydee in her pram. She walks from West Hatch, says the fresh air and movement is the only thing that makes the baby sleep. I revive her with tea at this, the furthest point of her journey. Mo walks with a waddle, her back aches, and when she gets to me she is usually hot, pulling at her T-shirt to unstick it from her breasts. But she loves Haydee. As I make tea she twitches the blanket over the child and can't keep herself from smiling.

I have the photo of Caroline with her baby in a frame on the window sill. I never did get around to giving it to Mum. I am still proud to have uncovered the child's identity, to have found the source of the rift between my family and Dinny's. Mum was astonished when I told her the story. I can't prove it all, definitively; but I know it to be true. I've decided to like the fact that I can't find out completely; that I can't fill in all the blanks— why Caroline hid her earlier marriage, why she hid her child. Where Flag was before he appeared at the manor and then fell into the Dinsdale's loving arms. Some things are lost in the past—surely that's why the past is so mysterious, why it fascinates us. Nothing much will be lost any more—too much is recorded, noted, stored in a file on a computer somewhere. It would be easy, not to be fascinated these days. It's harder to keep a secret, but they can be kept. Harry is living proof that they can be kept. I find I don't mind secrets half so much when they are mine to keep, when I am not excluded.

The manor house was sold at auction for a figure that gave me a sinking feeling inside, just for half an hour, imagining where I could have gone and what I could have done with such wealth. Clifford came to the auction but I hid from him, at the back of the conference room in a Marlborough hotel, as the figures bounced to and fro, got bigger and bigger. I could sense his anguish just by looking at the back of his head, rigid on stiff shoulders. I felt sorry for him. I think perhaps he'd hoped nobody else would come, nobody else would want to buy it; that he could snap it up for the price of a semi in Hertfordshire and tell everyone for ever that it was his birthright. But plenty of people did come, and a developer bought it. It's being converted into luxury flats, just like Maxwell suggested, because this is considered commutable now—from Pewsey to London and back every day. I can't imagine how it will look inside when it's done. What will my little back bedroom be? A kitchen with black granite worktops? A fully tiled wet room? I can't imagine it, and I'm half tempted to go and see the show flat when it's ready. Only half tempted though. I don't think I will. I don't want my memories of it muddied.

I think about Caroline and Meredith a lot. I think about what Dinny said—that people who bully and hate, people who are cold and aggressive are not happy people. They behave that way because they are unhappy. It is hard to find sympathy for Meredith when I have such memories of her, but now that she is dead I can manage it, when I try. Hers was a life of disappointment—her one bid to free herself from a loveless home over so soon after it began. It might have been harder still to feel sympathy for Caroline when I never really knew her, when she chose to abandon one child and then raised another without love. It would be easy to conclude that she just could not love. Wasn't able to. That she was too cold to be truly human, that she was born flawed. But then I found the last letter she wrote before she died; and I know better.

It lay undiscovered for weeks in the writing case, after I left the manor. Because she never sent it, of course, never even tore it from the writing pad. It was there, all along, beneath the cover, the line guide still in place underneath it. Her spidery writing tumbles across the page as if unravelling. 1983 is the date. No day or month specified, so perhaps that was the best she could do. She was over a hundred by then, and weakening. She knew that she was dying. Perhaps that was why she wrote this letter. Perhaps that was why she forgot, for a while, that she could never send it, that it would be read by nobody until me, more than a quarter of a century later.

My Dearest Corin,

It has been so long since I lost you that I cannot count the years. I am old now—old enough to be waiting to die myself. But then, I

*have been waiting to die ever since we were
parted, my love. It is strange that the long years
I have spent here in England seem, sometimes,
to have passed by in a blur. I cannot recall what
I can have possibly done to fill so much time—I
really do not remember. But I do remember
every second I spent with you, my love. Every
precious second that I was your wife, and we
were together. Oh, why did you die? Why did
you ride out that day? I have been over it so
many times. I see you mounting up, and I try to
change the memory. I convince myself that I
ran after you, told you not to go, not to leave
me. Then you would not have fallen, and you
would not have died, and I would not have had
to spend these long dark years without you.
Sometimes I so convince myself that I did run
after you, that I did stop you, that when I realise
you are gone it comes almost as a shock. It
hurts me dreadfully, but I do it over and over
again. I did a terrible thing, Corin. An
unforgivable thing. I ran away from it but I
could not undo it, and it has followed me
through all the years since. My only consolation
has been that I never forgave myself, and that
surely this life I have endured has been
punishment enough? But no, there could never
be punishment enough for what I did. I pray
that you do not know of it, for if you did, you
would not love me any more and I simply could
not bear that. I pray that there is no God, and
no heaven or hell, so that you cannot have been
looking down, cannot have seen what crimes I
committed. And I can never join you in heaven,
if that is where you are. Surely, my soul belongs*

in hell when I die. But how could you not go to heaven, my love? You were an angel already, even on earth. Being with you was the one time in my whole life that I was happy, that I was glad to be alive, and everything since then has been ashes and dust to me. How long you have lain under that empty prairie? It is aeons since I saw you. The whole world could have been born and died again in the vast age since we touched. I wish I could see you one more time, before I die. Part of me believes that there would be some justice in this—that if the world was a fair place, I would be allowed just a second of your embrace, to make up for losing you. No matter what I did in the madness of grief, no matter how I compounded my mistake or how much worse I have made it—have made myself—ever since. I would gladly give myself up to an eternity of torment just to see you one more time. But it cannot be. I will die, and be forgot, just as you died. But I never forgot you, my Corin, my husband. Whatever else I did, I never forgot you, and I loved you always.

Caroline.

I read and re-read this letter in the weeks after I found it. Until I knew it by rote, and each word broke my heart a little. Such a vast depth of regret and sorrow that it could cloud a sunny day. When I feel it take hold of me, when I feel I have absorbed too much of it, I remember Beth. Her crime will not follow her any more. She will not compound it, or let the regret tear at her for ever. The chain has been broken, and I helped to break it. I remember that, and I let it cheer me, fill me up with hope. I will never know what Caroline did. Why she took her baby and ran to England, why she then abandoned him. One thing I do notice, though, from my many readings of this letter: she does not mention her son. If the child was hers, and Corin his father, why doesn't she mention him? Why doesn't she tell her Corin about his son? Try to explain why she abandoned him? This may well be the crime she hopes he never saw, but surely that must have come before her flight from America? And this abandonment seems inexplicable, really unbelievable, when matched to the love she professes for the child's father. I remember the dark young girl at the summer party—the girl whom Caroline called Magpie. Her hair, as black as Dinny's. I will never know for sure, but this omission from the letter hints at a crime indeed, and makes me doubt the claim of kinship I made to Dinny.

Beth came to stay a couple of weeks ago. She wishes, I think, that I'd settled in a different village, but she's getting used to the idea. She doesn't shy away from this place any more.

'Doesn't it bother you, seeing the house over there?' she asked. Expressions fly across her face these days. They rise and jostle like balloons. Something tethered her features before and now it's gone. And I may well settle somewhere else, sometime; soon, or eventually. I'm not waiting, but I need to be where he can find me. Just until the next time he does. And he's got reasons to come back here, after all. More to pull him here than just me, and my desire for him. A mother, a sister, a niece. I think Honey would tell me, if he'd been back.

My happiness at seeing Beth improve bubbles up whenever I set eyes on her. No miracle cure, of course, but she's better. She can split the blame for what happened with Dinny now; she no longer has to think that she and she alone dealt fate to Henry Calcott. The truth of it, the right and wrong, is more diffuse now. She didn't take a life, she just changed one. There's even a fragment of leeway, just a hint of grey as to whether the change was for the better or worse. So no miracle cure, but she talks to me about it now—she'll talk about what happened, and because she's turned around and looked at it, it's not dogging her steps like it used to. I can see the improvement and so can Eddie, although he hasn't asked me about it. I don't think he cares what's changed, he's just pleased that it has.

It takes a while to see somebody differently when for years you've seen them in a particular way, or not seen them at all. I still saw Harry, when Dinny told me to see Henry. And I still saw Dinny as I had always seen him, always loved him. I tell myself that he needs time to see me differently, to see me as I am now and not see a child, or a nuisance, or Beth's little sister, or whatever else it is he sees. Perhaps the time is not now; but it will come, I believe. There was a legal wrangle over the plot of land where the Dinsdales are allowed to camp. The developer didn't want a load of travellers parking up in the communal gardens of his new flats. In the end that piece of ground, along with the rest of the woods and pasture, was sold to the farmer whose land adjoins it, and he has known the Dinsdales for years. So it's still there, waiting for them. Waiting for him. A beautiful place to camp in the summer, green and sheltered, and unmolested now.

I'm hoping for a hot summer. Weather to bake the bones and excuse this languid life I've adopted. Weather to give Honey freckles, and to make ice-lollies from lemon squash with Susan and Paul's girls, and to darken Dinny's skin. Weather to sneak to the dew pond, to paddle, to swim, to chase its ghosts away. And today a small parcel came in the post for me. Inside, crumbling, was a piece of tree bark with patterns scratched into it. Nothing I could distinguish in the designs, except the name at the bottom—*HARRY*—in crooked, angular, almost unreadable letters. A declaration, I take it to be, of who he is now, of who he wants to be. And an unspoken message from Dinny, who wrapped it up and posted it. That he knows where I am, and that he thinks of me. For now, I find I am quite happy with that.

ACKNOWLEDGEMENTS

My love and thanks to Alison and Charlotte Webb for their reading, critiquing and endless enthusiasm over the years; and to John Webb for never suggesting that I get a proper job!

Thanks to the members of WordWatchers in Newbury for all their support, comments and cake.

Finally, my thanks also to Edward Smith and the members of youwriteon.com for getting the book read, reviewed and noticed; and to Sara and Natalie at Orion for taking it the rest of the way.

WAIT FOR ME!

Memoirs of the Youngest
Mitford Sister

Deborah Devonshire

WINDSOR
PARAGON

First published 2010
by John Murray (Publishers)
This Large Print edition published 2011
by AudioGO Ltd
by arrangement with
John Murray (Publishers)

Hardcover ISBN: 978 1 445 85621 6
Softcover   ISBN: 978 1 445 85622 3

British Library Cataloguing in Publication Data available

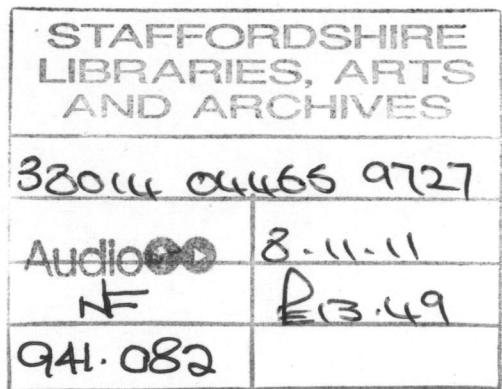
Printed and bound in Great Britain by
MPG Books Group Limited

To
Charlotte Mosley, my editor
Helen Marchant, my secretary
and my old friends Richard Garnett
and Tristram Holland
who gave me the confidence to keep trying

Contents

Illustrations

With the 'guns' at Bolton Abbey, DD and Harold
Macmillan mounted, early 1960s
Shooting at Chatsworth, 1960
With Stoker at the Game Fair, Chatsworth, 1966

Section Four
Lagos, 1962
With Dr Nnamdi Azikiwe and Elizabeth
Cavendish, Chatsworth, 1961
Visit of the Shah of Persia to Chatsworth
Invitation to the Inauguration of President John F.
Kennedy
Greeting Robert Kennedy on his visit to
Chatsworth, 1964
Pushing over a pile of pennies at a charity event in
Whitwell, Derbyshire
Serving behind the counter at the Orangery Shop,
Chatsworth
With Sophy at the Countryside March, 1997
Celebrating our Golden Wedding at Chatsworth
Tercentenary of the dukedom, Chatsworth, 1994
With the Prince of Wales, 2000
With Sybil Cholmondeley at Houghton
Diana, Pamela and DD at Chatsworth
With my granddaughter Stella Tennant
With Jean-Pierre Béraud at his fortieth birthday
party, 10 August 1996
At Andrew's and my eightieth birthday party,
Chatsworth, 2000
Feeding the hens
With my great-grandchildren, 2009
Aged ninety at the Old Vicarage, 2010

Note on Family Names

My family used nicknames usually as terms of affection, but sometimes the opposite. To spare the reader the irritation of ever-changing names, I have generally used those we were given at our christening. This seems strange to me because I never did so in real life but I hope it will make things plainer for my readers.

For the record, my parents were *Muv* and *Farve*—obvious enough. Muv had a string of other names including *Aunt Sydney*, because that is what our cousins called her, and *Lady Redesdale*, which strangers called her. Farve was *Morgan* to Jessica and Unity, for no particular reason. Nanny was *Blor* or *m'Hinket*; she did not like either but did not try to stop us. Because of her black hair, Muv and Farve called Nancy *Koko* after the Lord High Executioner in *The Mikado*. Pam and Diana called her *Naunce* and to me she was the *Ancient Dame of France*, the *French Lady Writer* or just *Lady*. Pam was *Woman* to us all, with variations thereof. Tom was *Tuddemy* to Unity and Jessica ('Tom' in Boudledidge, their private language) and this was taken up by the rest of us. Diana was *Dayna* to Muv and Farve, *Deerling* to Nancy, and *Honks* to me. I still have to think who I am talking about when she is 'Diana'. Unity was *Bobo*, but *Birdie* or *Bird* to me. Jessica called her *Boud* ('Bobo' in Boudledidge). Jessica was *Little D* to Muv, *Steaake* to Pam and *Hen* or *Henderson* to me, but she was *Decca* universally—and remains so in this book. I have always been *Debo* to most, but *Hen* to Jessica,

Swiny to Unity, and *Nine*, *Miss* and lots more to Nancy. I was *Stubby* to Muv and Farve, after my short fat legs which could not keep up (hence the title of this book). Our names changed with the wind but the ones none of us ever spoke were Nancy, Pamela, Thomas, Diana, Unity, Jessica and Deborah.

I always had nicknames for my husband, Andrew, which changed over time. For many years it was *Claud*, because when he was Lord Hartington he got letters addressed to 'Claud Hartington'. My mother-in-law was *Moucher* to one and all (after the character in *David Copperfield*)—I never heard anyone call her Mary. My elder daughter, Emma, is *Marlborough* or *Marl* because of her Girl Guide uniform, which was smothered in badges like the much-decorated Mary, Duchess of Marlborough. My younger daughter, Sophy, is *Moffa*—goodness knows why. The only one of my children's nicknames I have used throughout the book is *Stoker*, which for some reason he has never managed to throw off. He now signs himself 'Stoker Devonshire'. I call him *Sto*.

1

We Are Seven

Blank. There is no entry in my mother's engagement book for 31 March 1920, the day I was born. The next few days are also blank. The first entry in April, in large letters, is 'KITCHEN CHIMNEY SWEPT'. My parents' dearest wish was for a big family of boys; a sixth girl was not worth recording. 'Nancy, Pam, Tom, Diana, Bobo, Decca, *me*', intoned in a peculiar voice, was my answer to anyone who asked where I came in the family.

The sisters were at home and Tom was at boarding school for this deeply disappointing event, more like a funeral than a birth. Years later Mabel, our parlourmaid, told me, 'I knew what it was by your father's face.' When the telegram arrived Nancy announced to the others, 'We Are Seven', and wrote to Muv at our London house, 49 Victoria Road, Kensington, where she was lying-in, 'How disgusting of the poor darling to go and be a girl.' Life went on as though nothing had happened and all agreed that no one, except Nanny, looked at me till I was three months old and then were not especially pleased by what they saw.

Grandfather Redesdale's huge house and estate in Gloucestershire, Batsford Park near Moreton-in-Marsh, was inherited by my father in 1916. It was too expensive to keep up and was sold in 1919. My father looked for somewhere more modest near Swinbrook, a small village where he owned land, fifteen miles from Batsford. There was no house there suitable for a family of six children and a seventh on the way, so he bought Asthall Manor in the neighbouring village. I was born soon after the move and my earliest recollections are of the ancient house and its immediate surroundings. Asthall is a typical Cotswold manor, hard by the church, with a garden that descends to the River Windrush. It was loved by my sisters and Tom, and the seven years spent there were probably the happiest for parents and children, the proceeds of the sale of Batsford giving the family a feeling of security that was never repeated.

There was, and is, something profoundly satisfying in the scale of Asthall village. It was a perfect entity where every element was in proportion to the rest: the manor, the vicarage, the school and pub; the farmhouses with their conveniently placed cowsheds and barns; the cottages, whose occupants supplied the labour for the centuries-old jobs that still existed when we were children; and the pigsties, chicken runs and gardens that belonged to the cottages. Before cars and commuters, you lived close to where you worked and the shops came to you in horse-drawn vans. This was the calm background of a self-contained agricultural parish, regulated by the seasons, in an exceptionally beautiful part of England.

My father planted woods to hold game, as well as a short beech avenue leading up to the house, and his dark purple lilacs outside the garden wall are still growing there after nearly a hundred years. The house itself needed much restoration. My mother's flair for decoration and her talent for home-making ensured that the French furniture and pictures from Batsford were shown at their best. My father installed water-powered electric light—just the sort of contraption he adored; drawing heavily on his umpteenth cigarette, he would lean over the engineer, itching to do the job better himself. He made sure he had a child-proof door to his study by putting the handle high up out of reach. Sometimes we heard the voice of Galli-Curci singing Farve's favourite aria, coming loudly from the outsize horn of his gramophone—a twin of the one in advertisements for His Master's Voice. In another mood he might put on 'The Diver' ('He is now on the surface, he's gasping for breath, so pale that he wants but the stillness of death'), sung by Signor Foli in a terrifying and unnaturally low bass voice.

With foresight, or perhaps by luck, Farve converted the barn a few yards from the house into one large room with four bedrooms above and added a covered passage, 'the cloisters', to connect the two buildings. Tom and the older sisters lived in the barn, untroubled by grown-ups or babies, and made the most of their freedom. My father, who was famous for having read only one book, *White Fang*, which he enjoyed so much he vowed never to read another, entrusted Tom, aged ten, with the task of choosing which books to keep from the Batsford library. Nancy and Diana later said that if they had any education, it was due to the unrestricted access they had had to Grandfather's books at Asthall. Later, a grand piano arrived for Tom who showed great musical promise. Music and reading were his passions.

The First World War was not long over and life for the survivors was limping back to normal. There was little to record in our family in the first few years of my life. Nancy went to Hatherop Castle, a finishing school near by, and was taken to Paris with a group of friends where she first saw the architecture and works of art that inspired in her a lifelong love of that city. She wrote enthusiastic letters to our mother about the shops, the food and the days spent at the Louvre. Pam busied herself with her ponies, pigs and dogs. Tom was at Lockers Park prep school in Hemel Hempstead. His orderly mind was already preparing for a career in the Law and he paid Nancy to argue with him all day during the holidays. Diana was an unwilling Girl Guide and played the organ in church, putting into practice her theory that 'Tea for Two', if played slowly enough, did very well as a voluntary.

The years at Asthall passed in a haze of contentment from my point of view. I was aware of The Others but they were so old and seemed to Decca (Jessica, my daily companion) and me to be of another world. It was not until later that I got to know them. Unity, next up in age from Decca and not yet in the schoolroom, made her huge presence felt but, although always kind to me, she was not an intimate. Our life in the nursery consisted of the daily round, the common task, secure and regular as clockwork.

At the age of five we started lessons with Muv, who followed the admirable Parents' National Education Union (PNEU) system with its emphasis on learning through direct contact with nature and good books, and its disapproval of marks, prizes, rewards and exams. She taught us reading, writing and sums, and read us tales from the famous children's history book, *Our Island Story*. She was a natural teacher and never made anything seem too difficult. At the age of eight, I moved on to the schoolroom and a governess (trained at the PNEU's Ambleside College) and never enjoyed lessons again.

Our nursery windows overlooked the churchyard with its graves of wool merchants long since dead, the beautiful tombs topped with fleeces carved in stone. We were fascinated by funerals, which we were not meant to watch but of course did. Decca and I once fell into a newly dug grave, to the delight of Nancy who pronounced fearful bad luck on us for ever. At that age, I was sure Farve would be buried by the path leading to our garden and even today I expect to see his big toe sticking up through the turf, which is what he warned me would happen if I misbehaved.

Beyond the churchyard to the left were stables, kennels and a garage. Early on at Asthall my father had a horrible accident in the stable yard: he was getting on to a young horse when it reared and fell backwards on to him, breaking his pelvis. The injury did not heal properly and, unable to throw his leg over a saddle, he never rode again. To the right of the churchyard was the vicarage. We adored the vicar's wife and long after we had left Asthall, Pam and I used to ride over and trot briskly up the drive, shouting for ginger biscuits. Across the road was the kitchen garden with its glasshouses and glorious white peaches, reserved strictly for grown-ups. Unity and our cousin Chris Bailey committed the heinous crime of sneaking into the greenhouse and stealing some peaches. There was a stony silence throughout the house while they were reprimanded by my father, which made a big effect on the younger ones. Farve has gone down in history as a violent man, mainly because of Nancy's portrayal of him as the irascible Uncle Matthew in her novels. While he could indeed get angry, he was never physically violent and his bark was far worse than his bite. We would tease him, goad him as far as we dared, until he turned and roared at us.

As soon as I could walk I shadowed Farve, struggling to keep up. He used to pick me up, throw me on to his shoulder and carry me over winter ditches and summer stinging nettles; the comforting feel of his velveteen waistcoat is inseparable from my memories of him. I must have been a great nuisance, but we saw eye to eye about everything. He took me fishing in the magic moment of the year when the mayfly were hatching and let me carry his net. As time went by, he showed me how to slide it under the hooked trout—no talking, no jerking—and land it on the bank. The sound of a reel when a line is cast on a trout rod equals early summer to me and the smell of newly cut grass, cow parsley, thrushes and 'All the birds of Oxfordshire and Gloucestershire' (Edward Thomas's Adlestrop is not far from Asthall) take me back to our stretch of the Windrush. No health, no safety, no handrail on the single planks that were our bridges as we crossed and recrossed over the river. It was paradise and I knew it. The river water had its own smell that rose from the easily stirred-up mud, and many years later when swimming among the weeds and mud in a pond high above Chatsworth, in the company of moorhens and mallard, nostalgia for the river at Asthall was almost too much and I was six again.

My father loved the river, described in the estate agent's brochure when Asthall was sold as 'of the most attractive character to a fisherman, including rapids, gentle swims and pool', but he was plagued by the idea of the coarse fish that competed with the trout. Like Uncle Matthew, he called on the services of a chubb fuddler who came and scattered magic seed on the water till hundreds of chubb rose to the surface, 'flapping, swooning, fainting, choking, thoroughly and undoubtedly fuddled'. Nancy's account of this annual event is one of the funniest passages in any of her books.

Farve made a pool in the river, even adding a diving board for the brave, where we learned to swim, held up by water-wings and wearing rubber bathing caps that cruelly pulled our hair. His own bathing costume was made of thin, harsh, dark-blue serge bound with braid. For the sake of modesty it had a skirt—'my crrino-leeene' he called it in an exaggerated French accent. Unexpectedly, Farve and his brothers spoke perfect French, thanks to their tutor Monsieur Cuvelier, who lived at Batsford and taught them when they were boys. The old tutor came to stay at Asthall during the holidays and his presence always put Farve in the sunniest of moods; according to Diana, 'He and our uncles became boys again before our astonished eyes.' Walking back to the house after bathing, Farve used to pick up sticks and stones with his toes to amuse us.

'Look what my prehensile extremities can do,' he said, but however hard we tried our toes could not be as clever or useful.

In the name of culture, my sisters started the Outing Club. Farve's brother, Uncle Tommy, drove the older children in his car, an envied open-tourer that had a roof like the hood of a pram—with as many finger-pinching hinges—and windows of yellowing celluloid that cracked easily and were striped with sticking plaster. Unity, Decca and I went in Farve's car. I was the Club Bore as we had to keep stopping for me to get out and be sick; all I remember of these outings is the grass by the roadside. We visited Kenilworth Castle and Stratford-upon-Avon in pursuit of history and literature. Another uncle, my mother's brother George Bowles, accompanied us in the role of visiting professor and told us about the past glories of which Farve and Uncle Tommy were blissfully ignorant. I was too young to go on the outing to Stratford that passed into family lore, when Farve, pressed by Muv, took the older children to see *Romeo and Juliet*. Uncle Matthew's reaction in *The Pursuit of Love* is unmistakably that of Farve: 'He cried copiously and went into a furious rage because it ended badly. "All the fault of that damned padre," he kept saying on the way home, still wiping his eyes. "That blasted fella, what's 'is name, Romeo, might have known a blasted papist would mess up the whole thing. Silly old fool of a nurse too, I bet she was an R.C., dismal old bitch."'

When I was four, my parents, Decca and I drove to Scotland in stages to stay with a friend of my father. An obvious stopping place on the way was

Redesdale Cottage in Northumberland where Farve's mother lived. Grandmother Redesdale was fat, pink-cheeked and smiling, with wispy white hair tucked into a small black cap. She was always dressed in black, unlike widows of today, and was a wonderful storyteller. She kept a Berkshire pig instead of a dog, the double of Beatrix Potter's Pig-Wig, which she took to church on a lead. No one thought it a bit odd—affection for animals was taken for granted—and she had a similar affection for my father whom she called 'Poor Dowdie', with an indulgent smile.

Christmas parties at Asthall were homemade and on Christmas Night we wore fancy dress—nothing grand, we picked up whatever was to hand. My father's only concession was to put on a red wig, but he never appears in the photographs as he was always behind the camera. Pam dressed as Lady Rowena from *Ivanhoe* and wore the same outfit every year: a long, floppy, low-necked gown, embellished with a row of orange-red beads. The beads are on my dressing table now and remind me of her every time I see them. Nancy was a dab hand at disguise and her costume was always the best. She loved making a bit of trouble and went missing one year when the family photograph was about to be taken. We shouted and looked for her everywhere. Eventually there was a knock at the back door and a filthy, cold, wet tramp appeared. It was Nancy. When Asthall was for sale, it was the sister of Mrs Hardcastle, wife of the prospective buyer, who became Nancy's inspiration. Mrs Hardcastle's sister was no beauty: she had a thick black moustache and wore a cloche hat and mothy fur slung around her neck. Nancy used to appear quite often in this dreary disguise and once took in Mabel, who showed her into the drawing room.

My mother gave a Christmas tea party every year for the village schoolchildren between the ages of five and fourteen. Lists of names and ages were kept from one year to the next and each child was given a toy and a garment by Father Christmas, who was played by the vicar. He arrived to an atmosphere of tremendous excitement: the big drawing room was darkened except for a few candles, handbells were rung and in he came through the window carrying his sack on his back. 'I come from the land of ice and snow,' he intoned in a deep voice to the dumbstruck children. The magic never failed. After an enormous tea, the children trooped out clutching their parcels and an orange, a treat in itself in those days.

My father did not wish for a social life. Muv would have enjoyed one but seldom suggested anything he would not want—she was aware of the hazards. Lunch guests were rare, but a memorable exception was the Duchess of Marlborough, the American Gladys Marie Deacon, second wife of the Ninth Duke, who came over from Blenheim. She produced a paper handkerchief, the first any of us had seen, blew her nose and stuck it into a yew hedge. My father was outraged. At lunch she asked him if he had read Elinor Glyn's *Three Weeks* (everyone was talking about the writer and her work at the time). Farve glared at her. 'I haven't read a book for *three years*,' he barked. That was the end of that subject and of the Duchess of Marlborough. Years later, when Nancy invited some undergraduate friends from Oxford to lunch, my father waited for a pause in the conversation and said loudly to my mother at the other end of the table, 'Have these people no homes of their own?'

But Muv was amused by Nancy's friends. She once asked Henry Weymouth (later the Marquess of Bath, who opened a safari park at his Wiltshire family seat, Longleat) what his favourite way of spending the day was. 'Ratting,' he replied with conviction. There were even a few weekend parties where strangers were well diluted with aunts, uncles and cousins—relations were always first on the list. When Nancy was eighteen, Farve conceded that a dance must be given for her. Muv was unable to gather enough young men for the event and, according to Nancy, my father trawled the House of Lords and netted a few middle-aged fellows; they must have been surprised to be invited to a debutante dance. As the day drew near, Farve asked my mother what time the 'on-rushing *convives*' were expected. The poor fellow had to endure a repeat of this torture five more times as each daughter grew up.

My parents seldom had friends to stay. One exception was Violet Hammersley, who came on prolonged visits. 'Mrs Ham' was a near contemporary of Muv but seemed much older. She was born and had spent the first years of her life in Paris, where her father, Mr Freeman-Williams, was a diplomat. When he died, Mrs Freeman-Williams took her young family to live in London, where Muv remembered her as a friend of her own father. Mrs Ham was an unexpected friend of my mother: her circle was intellectual and artistic—from Somerset Maugham to Bloomsbury and beyond—while Muv was taken up with children and domestic affairs. According to Nancy she looked like El Greco's mistress and, with her dark hair and sallow complexion, would certainly have made an ideal model for the painter. She always wore black and was draped in shawls from head to foot. We called her 'the Widow' or 'Wid', not to her face, but when it occasionally slipped out she put on the expression of resignation usually reserved for Nancy's teases.

By the time I knew her her late husband's bank, Cox & Co., had failed and Mrs Ham's means were much reduced. Gone was the house on the river at Bourne End and with it the Venetian gondola and gondolier. She had retired to a small Regency house in Totland Bay on the Isle of Wight, where her garden shed, known as 'The Mansion', had been converted into two guest bedrooms. It was dreadfully damp but because it was Mrs Ham's we loved it. We never tired of asking her how she had lost her money. Her face would take on a tragic look and, with exaggerated pronunciation of every syllable, she said, 'and th*i*en the b*i*ank f*i*ailed', which was met with howls of laughter from us all. She was a strict pessimist: according to her the past was black, the future blacker. It was a triumph when my sisters persuaded her to dance her version of the cancan to the tune of 'Ta-ra-ra-boom-di-ay'. She lifted her layers of skirt, pointed her toe and was off. But just the once.

Mrs Ham was famously mean. One day, when told that some friends were coming to call on her, she asked me in a sepulchral voice, 'Does that involve sherry?' When she came to lunch with us in London, my father would stand waiting on the steps with half a crown in his hand to pay the taxi;

he knew she would fumble in her purse and say she had no change. Her arrival in our house was marked by the strong antiseptic smell of TCP that filled the bathroom and the passage. Farve teased Mrs Ham mercilessly. She thrived on the attention but was never quite sure when he was joking—that was his way with many people and the pair of them were a regular turn.

In spite of the difference in generations, Mrs Ham became an intimate friend of my sisters and mine because of her deep interest in our doings. My mother kept a distance from our passions; she looked on them with amusement but did not get involved. Mrs Ham, on the other hand, seemed fascinated by whatever we told her, however exaggerated and dotty—chiefly about love and romance, of course—and we confided in her as in an agony aunt. To sit on the sofa next to her, her face close to mine, to have her listening with intense concentration to me and me alone, was something I had never experienced and found irresistible. It was thrilling when she said, *'Child, are you in love?'* Naturally we always were and told her about it in lengthy detail. The idea of any grown-up being in the least bit interested amazed us; no wonder she was a welcome guest. I wrote hundreds of letters to her, as did we all, and we got lovely ones back, usually beginning, 'Horror Child', and admonishing us for not writing more frequently.

*   *   *

Many years after we left Asthall, I went back to see the house and found to my joy the old telephone, thin as a parasol handle, still on its cradle, the same plate rack above the sink in the pantry and the same lino still on the nursery floor. The feel of it underfoot and all that went with that room made me long for Nanny Blor, for the comfort of her lap, her hymn-singing and prayers at bedtime. Nanny's real name was Laura Dicks. Her father was a blacksmith and she came from Egham in Surrey. How she got the nicknames 'Blor' or 'm'Hinket' I do not remember. In 1910, when my mother interviewed her, she was thirty-nine and not robust, and it seemed doubtful whether she could push the pram up the hill from Victoria Road to the park, laden with heavy toddlers in the shape of Pam, aged three, Tom, nearly two, and four-month-old Diana. My parents havered and then Nanny saw Diana. 'Oh, what a lovely baby!' and that was it. She arrived to stay for more than forty years.

Like my mother, Nanny was always there, unchanging, steady, dependable—the ideal background for a child—and, like my mother, she was always scrupulously fair. If Nanny did have a favourite it was Decca, an irresistibly attractive child, curly-haired, affectionate and funny. But I was unaware of this and loved her with all my heart, as we all did. She was the antidote to Nancy and a very present help in time of trouble, 'the still small voice of calm'. She was neither tall nor short and you would not have picked her out in a crowd. Her clothes were those of her profession: grey coat and skirt, black hat and shoes and, in the summer, a quiet cotton dress with a white collar. On car drives, when I always felt sick, I used to cling to her gloved hand. The gloves were made of something called 'fabric', which must have covered a lot of possibilities. I never saw her lose her temper or even be really cross though she muttered at us sometimes. She must have been more sorely tried than any other Nanny, but we were always forgiven and treated to a bedtime hymn. Her favourites were 'The Ninety and Nine' ('There were ninety and nine that safely lay/In the shelter of the fold,' Nanny sang, 'But one away on the hills had strayed /Far off from the gates of gold'), 'Shall We Gather at the River?', 'Loving Shepherd of Thy Sheep' and 'Now the Day is Over'. She was deeply religious and must have suffered from not being able to attend her own Congregational church when we were at Asthall, or later Swinbrook, but she never said so.

She did not criticize us much, neither did she praise. 'No, darling, I shouldn't do that if I were you,' or 'Very nice, darling,' was as far as it went, her eyes on her needle or the iron, the regular tools of the nursery. Signs of arrogance, conceit or vanity she called 'parading about' and discouraged them with a little sniff and cough. 'It's all right, darling, no one's going to look at you,' became her standard saying when we complained that our dresses were not smart enough for a party. She carried this dictum a bit far when Diana, eighteen years old and staggeringly beautiful in her wedding dress, said, 'Oh Nanny, this hook and eye doesn't work. It looks awful.' 'It's all right, darling,' Nanny soothed, 'who's going to look at you?'

I read now about the necessity of self-esteem in children. We would have become impossibly pleased with ourselves had we been indulged with such a thing. As it was, our ups and downs were high and low enough, and Nanny sat on any ups. Her own childhood had been strict no doubt, but she never imposed her parents' rules on us. She accepted our governesses and their different ways without a murmur, as she did my mother's unusual, not to say eccentric, rules about food and medicine. When the time came for us to leave the nursery for the schoolroom, she never questioned the authority of the governesses, though I am sure she must have suffered at losing the little ones and sometimes suspected, rightly, that the governesses were not all they should be. As soon as we could after lessons, we rushed back to talk to her. She was the one we loved.

We seldom went shopping or had new clothes. When I was eight, Diana married and her sister-in-law, Grania Guinness, was the same age as me but taller. She had the most wonderful dresses from Wendy, the ultimate in children's clothes for style and beauty, and when a parcel arrived with a dress she had outgrown, my excitement was intense. Otherwise, Fair Isle jerseys and a 'smart' coat for church were about it. Skating was an exception and I was allowed one of those lovely short full skirts that make whatever you do on the ice look better.

Our underclothes were woollen vests and knickers and an extraordinary, but apparently necessary, concoction called a liberty bodice, which had no freedom about it so how it got its name I cannot imagine. It was tight and made of some harsh stuff, with here and there straps and buttons that did nothing. The nursery fireguard with an extra brass rail was Nanny's drying place; it answered perfectly and the faint smell of damp wool was part of childhood. Nanny did her best to make us self-reliant and tidy and to instil in us the other qualities she thought necessary. It was an uphill task. When I threw my underclothes into a heap on the floor, she said, 'Put them the right way, they're all inside out.' 'Well, m'Hinket,' I replied, 'tomorrow they won't be inside out.' 'Now, darling,' she said, 'what if you had an accident and were taken to hospital? Think what a shock the nurses would have if they saw your vest inside out.' Even when very young I thought nurses might have seen worse things, but I have not forgotten what she said.

One of the rare holidays we had as young children was going with Nanny to stay with her twin sister, whose husband kept a hardware shop in the main street of Hastings. They lived above the shop and we lodged with them. The smell of paraffin and polish, the brushes, brooms and besoms that hung from the ceiling, the freezing-cold grey sea with a ginger biscuit reward for going in—all were lovely in their way but as we could not take our ponies, goats, rats, mice, guinea pigs and dogs it seemed a waste of a fortnight to me. Nanny's own holiday was the worst moment of the year. Diana told me that, aged three, I refused to eat, in spite of our Churchill cousins' nanny coming to take Blor's place for those fourteen ghastly days. It was Diana herself who persuaded me to swallow the shovelled-in food.

We never considered Blor's own life. Like Mabel and Annie, the head housemaid, she was so much part of the family that she was not consulted about moves or anything else that might affect her. She just came with us. Long after her role in the nursery was over, she remained a vital part of the household, washing, ironing, sewing and darning; just her being there meant the world to me and my sisters. She accompanied Decca and me on our rare shopping trips to Oxford. We stopped for tea at the Cadena Café or, if we were feeling rich, at Fuller's which meant walnut cake with a perfect icing, the acme of a good tea.

Being the youngest of a family had its advantages. Rules were stretched a bit and I was my father's favourite—whether that was because I was the last or because I shared his interests I do not know. The disadvantage was being an object of The Others' derision, 'So *stupid*, you can't keep up, you're such a BORE.' They made a circle round me, pointing and chanting, 'Who's the least important person in this room? YOU.' But this was outweighed by the fun of being with the older ones, even though I could not keep up. We fought, of course, as well as baited and teased each other, but after tears came the laughter and I look back on my childhood as a happy time. I thought our upbringing was exactly like everyone else's. Perhaps it was not.

2

Farve and Muv

Nancy wrote about our childhood in her novels, which to her amazement, and ours, became best-sellers. People still ask me, 'Was your father really like Uncle Matthew?' In many ways he was. Nancy made him sound terrifying but there was nearly, though not always, a comic undercurrent not apparent to outsiders. I adored him. He was an original, with a total disregard of the banal or boring. He had a turn of phrase he made his own, delivered with a deadpan face and perfect timing. Strangers stared at him nonplussed but we knew just what he meant. 'That feller whacked merry hell out of the piano,' described an admired musician's performance. Ordinary words were memorable when they came from him and two favourites were 'mournful' and 'degraded': 'Take your degraded elbows off the table,' he ordered Diana, aged fourteen. He was easily irritated by a non-favourite and encouraged them to 'go to hell judging your own time'. An unloved was dismissed as 'some mournful woman' and whatever this anonymous female did was wrong. She (and other people's babies) might also be 'a meaningless piece of meat' and that was that. A 'putrid sort of feller' could never aspire to anything better. In our family Farve was all-powerful: we appealed to him when we thought something was unfair and he could overturn any order given by a governess or anyone else in authority over us. Even my mother did not question his word.

Like others of his kind, David Mitford did not care a hang what people thought of him, take him or leave him, and it never occurred to him to toe the line or trim. He was honest and looked honest: tall and upstanding, blue-eyed and extraordinarily handsome, he had thick white hair and moustache by the time I remember him. He was unmistakably an English countryman. His prized possessions were his rod and gun, locked away and untouched by anyone except himself, and his car. After the financial crash of 1929, the Daimler and beloved chauffeur had to go and were replaced with a Morris that Farve drove himself. He had been friends with William Morris, later Lord Nuffield, since the motor magnate's Oxford bicycle-shop days and we were brought up on the legend that Farve had been asked to invest in Morris's business but decided against it—one of several unlucky financial decisions on his part. The car was treated as if it were alive, safely put away in the garage at night and never expected to go long distances without a rest. Propping up the bonnet, Farve would check the oil, wiping the dipstick on a clean rag to ensure accuracy, and top up the radiator water religiously. The petrol tank was replenished from cans, except when we went to Oxford and an adored attendant at the Clarendon Yard Garage, another William, was given the job of filling up while he talked to my father about engines. Farve was a good driver and enjoyed driving, but the sight of a female in charge of a vehicle was sometimes too much for him. If a car came too close or made the smallest mistake with the rules of the road he shouted, 'Blasted woman driver', to which my mother was often able to say, with truth, 'Funny thing, she's dressed as a man.'

'My good clothes' were cosseted like his car and gun. Mabel the parlourmaid was in charge and he was always well dressed. In the country, his appearance was indistinguishable from that of a gamekeeper, an occupation that would have suited him down to the ground. He wore a brown velveteen waistcoat, alternating with moleskin; a gunmetal watch—no silver chain but a leather bootlace; gaiters with huge chunks of shoes that were made for him; and he carried a stout thumbstick that completed the illusion. As years went by, the gaiters gave way to trousers fashioned from an impenetrable material called Mount Everest cloth—'thorn proof, dear child'. In London he was conventionally dressed but for one garment: a black cloak inherited from his father (Farve would never have bought such a thing himself), which he wore when forced to go out in the evenings. In his mid-thirties he went to a dentist and asked him to take out all his teeth. The dentist refused, saying it was dangerous. 'All right then,' said Farve impatiently, 'I'll go to someone who will.' An hour or so later there was not a tooth left in his head. Thereafter 'my good dentures' chewed up Muv's excellent food.

Farve shopped only where he was known. His regular ports of call were the best, and certainly the most expensive: Solomon's, a fruit shop in Piccadilly opposite the Ritz; Fortnum and Mason, where he was friends with the tail-coated assistants; Berry Bros, where he bought wine for our occasional guests (he drank only water); and Locke's the hatter. All these were within a stone's throw of each other and on the way to his club, the Marlborough in Pall Mall. His favourite shop, however, was the Army and Navy Stores, which stocked all the stuff of Empire: folding chairs with canvas seats and backs, enamel bowls with buttoned waterproof lids, a chronometer for his desk (so he could see if anyone was a quarter of a minute late), string and labels of lasting quality, the latest in camp beds, rust-proof filing cabinets, gritty Lifebuoy soap that smelt strongly of carbolic (his idea of complete cleanliness), thick woollen underclothes (stocked no doubt for Arctic explorers) and the precious Primus stove for his early-morning tea.

He walked to this holy of holies in Victoria Street with a lurcher and Labrador at heel—no leads. He put the dogs to sit in the entrance and waited with them for the doors to open at 9 a.m. My mother asked him why he had to be there so early. 'If I am any later I am impeded by inconveniently shaped women,' was the reply. He often brought back a little present for us, always beautifully packed, which gave it an air of importance. My mother was not sure of his taste in anything decorative and he told me that when buying something for her, he always said to the shop assistant, 'A lady will be in to change these next week.' And so she was.

Punctuality was drilled into us. If one of us dawdled before an outing Farve went without the laggard. Pam, daydreaming, was once left behind on a longed-for afternoon at the zoo—a lesson learned the hard way and cited again and again as a purple warning. Nancy's portrayal of Uncle Matthew standing at the front door, watch in hand at 11.55 a.m., awaiting someone expected at midday, muttering to himself, 'In six minutes the damn feller will be late,' is Farve exactly. He also had a horror of anything sticky. I once asked him what his idea of hell was. 'Honey on my bowler hat,' was the answer. His all-seeing eyes spotted a spill anywhere down the long dining-room table. Honey, jam and marmalade were all high-risk, but the sight of Golden Syrup in its wonderful green and gold tin made him particularly nervous, and he insisted on it being ladled on to the suet pudding by a grown-up. This was a regular occurrence because suet pudding was a favourite with us all. Farve got up and hovered as Mabel went round the table and we were relieved when the last person had been served with no spillage. What a mercy that no modernizer at Tate & Lyle has tampered with the design of the Golden Syrup tin, with its picture of bees buzzing round a dead lion and the line from the Bible, 'Out of the strong came forth sweetness'. I have always been fascinated by it and only wondered much later how it came to be associated with a pudding made of beef fat.

Two things annoyed Farve in my mother's otherwise impeccably run house. If a housemaid was rash enough to remove the deepest ashes from the grate where a wood fire burned, she was in trouble. Farve was right: it is the ashes that hold the heat and ensure a quick start in the morning. He found a way of avoiding the second annoyance. After breakfast he refilled his coffee cup and took it to his study. He let it get cold and drank what he called his 'suckments' at intervals during the morning. A tidy, new-to-the-job maid took the cup back to the pantry, emptied and washed it. This enraged my father: 'Some monkey's orphan has taken my suckments.' Thereafter he locked the cup in his safe.

Farve was impatient, intolerant, impulsive, loyal, courageous, loving, fastidious, unread and possessed of great charm, all underwritten with courtly good manners—to most. Every now and then his short fuse made him lash out. He was profoundly irritated by some of the young men Nancy invited to the house and more than once lost his temper with her friend James Lees-Milne, the future author and diarist. On one occasion Jim leant down to pick something up and a comb fell out of his pocket: 'A man carrying a comb—well!' On another famous occasion, Jim advocated friendship with Germany and Farve turned him out of the house. Poor Jim went to his motorbike but it was raining hard and it would not start. In despair he found the back door and was rescued by Mabel who hustled him upstairs. As he was creeping out of the house the next morning he met Farve. 'Good morning,' said Farve. He had forgotten the whole episode and offered Jim our usual generous breakfast.

Farve either liked you or he did not, there was no middle way. My mother sometimes tried to reason with him, but reason was not part of his makeup and, unlike her, he had favourites. This was unfair but he never tried to hide or moderate his feelings, it was part of his honesty. There was often a 'Rat Week' when he would pick on one of us for sometimes imaginary offences. Decca, who was able to twist him round her little finger and take liberties with him that none of the rest of us would have dared, fell out of favour for a while for no apparent reason. Unity became more silent and unresponsive in her teens because Farve was always watching her for some trifling misdemeanour.

It had been the same with his own brothers and sisters. He never liked his younger sister Joan but was fond of the man she married, Denis Farrer. 'The very desiccated Old Dean', he called him affectionately. Denis was not a dean, it was just a play on his name, but it was a spot-on description of that thin, sharp-featured fellow in middle age. Farve was once talking to an acquaintance about the Farrers and said, 'The only trouble with the Old Dean is that he married a ghastly woman.' 'Oh?' said the acquaintance, 'I thought she was your sister?' 'Yes, she is. A poisonous creature.' It was no wonder that people were surprised by him. Aunt Dorothy, wife of his adored brother, Uncle Tommy, was a non-favourite. She was said to be 'frightfully rich' but we never saw any sign of this alleged wealth and she was 'careful', to put it mildly. My parents went to lunch with Uncle Tommy and Aunt Dorothy in their house at Westwell, near Burford. The fare was sheep's hearts. 'Still beating on the plate,' my father told us afterwards. He did not go again.

*   *   *

Farve was the second son in a family of nine—five boys and four girls, none of whom inherited Grandfather Redesdale's love of art and architecture or his passion for the Far East. The eldest son, Clement, was killed in action on the Western Front in 1915. Clem was a heroic figure to his siblings, and my father and his other brothers were brought up in his shadow. He was better at everything than any of them, an example to be emulated, and was his parents' great hope for the future. Clem acted as guardian to his first cousins, the six Ogilvy children, after their father, the Sixth Earl of Airlie, was killed leading a cavalry charge against the Boers at the Battle of Diamond Hill in 1900. Their mother, Mabell, widowed at thirty-four, devoted the rest of her life to her children, the Cortachy estate in Angus and Queen Mary (whom she served as Lady of the Bedchamber for forty-three years).

Clem married one of his wards, Helen Ogilvy, in 1909. Helen had startling blue eyes and black hair, a rare combination, but she went completely white at the age of twenty-three. Their first daughter, Rosemary, was born in 1911 and their second, Clementine, shortly after Clem's death. As Clem had no son, my father was next in line to inherit the Batsford and Swinbrook estates. Farve was very much a second son and his childhood had been blighted by unhappiness at school. He hated every moment of it and longed to be home, free from lessons and out of doors at all hours with the keepers. As a boy he had a terrible temper, which worried his parents and anyone in authority over him. Clem had gone to Eton but Grandfather decided that Farve should be sent to Radley. I believe Grandfather was afraid that one of Farve's outbursts of temper would have damaging repercussions for Clem's school career.

It was towards the end of his time at Radley that Farve first set eyes on Sydney Bowles. Grandfather Redesdale (before his peerage) was newly elected to Parliament and invited a fellow MP, Tommy Bowles, to speak at a meeting. As was his wont, Bowles brought his children with him. Sydney described her first sight of David as he stood with his back to the fire at Batsford, wearing an old brown velveteen coat: 'A wonderful figure of a young man . . . He looked splendid to me, and he was indeed very handsome. So when I was fourteen and he was seventeen, I fell in love with him.' No doubt Muv kept the picture of this beautiful young man in her mind but, as happens with teenage girls, it was superseded by other fancies.

After leaving Radley, Farve's dearest wish was to join the Army but he could manage only 19 marks out of 2,000 for Latin, or so he told us, and he failed the entrance exam. Whether or not this unlikely score was the reason, history does not relate, but fail he certainly did and he often used to say to us, 'What good would Latin have been to me in the Army?' Grandfather Redesdale had a friend with tea estates in Ceylon and Farve was sent out there to work as a planter. When he arrived he was shocked by the hard drinking of his colleagues and decided then and there to be a teetotaller, a decision he kept for the rest of his life. 'Sewer' was Farve's word for the worst of the bad, usually prefaced by 'damned', and it became part of the language of our family. In truth it was *suar*, Hindi for pig, 'the accursed one', picked up while he was in Ceylon; but it sounded better in English, especially when you pictured what he meant.

My father's escape from Ceylon was the Boer War. His first home leave in four years coincided with the outbreak of hostilities and he seized the chance of joining the Army at last. Clement was already serving in the 10th Hussars and in January 1900 my father enlisted as a private in the Oxfordshire Yeomanry, and later transferred to the Northumberland Fusiliers. He was in his element, popular with men and officers alike, and was immediately given a commission. In 1902 he fought at the Battle of Tweebosch under Lieutenant General Lord Methuen and was lucky to survive a chest wound that destroyed one lung. (This did not stop him from being a chain-smoker. 'Have a gasper,' he would say when greeting any man he met, opening his neatly packed gunmetal cigarette case. A woman smoker was, of course, taboo, his daughters included. Only Decca broke the rule when she grew up.) After being wounded, Farve lay for three days, near death, on an ox cart, trundling over rutted roads to the field hospital at Bloemfontein. He was invalided home for a long convalescence. His strong constitution pulled him through, but it was a close-run thing.

My parents met again some ten years after they had first set eyes on each other, and this time it was David who fell for Sydney. Whatever and whoever had come between them since their last meeting, there must have been an immediate rapport. Farve went to Tommy Bowles to ask permission to marry his daughter. 'How do you plan to support her?' asked Bowles. 'I've got £400 a year and *these*,' said Farve, holding up his hands. The engagement was announced and they were married on 6 February 1904. Their honeymoon was spent on board Bowles's schooner and nine months later Nancy was born. Farve wrote to his mother just before the birth, 'I am sure I only wish that everyone could be so happy, there would be little left in life to complain of. I don't deserve it, but I am grateful.' Grandfather Bowles gave my father a job in the office of *The Lady*, the magazine he had founded in 1885. A more unsuitable occupation for the country-loving would-be gamekeeper is hard to imagine.

When they were first married, my mother was shocked to realize that my father had read only one book. She persuaded him to listen to her reading aloud some classics, starting with Thomas Hardy. She chose *Tess of the d'Urbervilles* with its descriptions of farm and heath land, which she thought he would enjoy. When she got to the sad part, my father started crying. 'Oh, darling, don't cry, it's only a story.' 'WHAT,' said my father, his sorrow turning to rage, 'do you mean to say the damn feller made it up?' I was born after the days of *White Fang* and never saw my father open a book.

Farve stuck at the office of *The Lady* for ten years until the outbreak of the First World War. As a result of his one lung, he was regarded as permanently unfit for active service but this did not deter him, aged thirty-seven, from joining his old regiment. He was sent to France in September 1914 as an officer reinforcement to the 1st Battalion of the Northumberland Fusiliers. Soon afterwards, his health broke down and he was invalided home. Determined to return to the front, he again succeeded in getting passed fit and rejoined his regiment's 2nd Battalion in April 1915. He was appointed transports officer, in the belief that it would be less strenuous than the front line, but his arrival coincided with the opening of the Second Battle of Ypres. As Brigadier H. R. Sandilands wrote in Farve's obituary:

Night after night (and sometimes twice nightly) he had to take up supplies to the battalion through the town of Ypres, which was under constant heavy bombardment. His method was to quicken the pace on approaching the town, and then to lead his wagons at full gallop through Ypres until clear of the Menin Gate. The men worked in two shifts, but David Mitford declined the offer of any relief, and accompanied every convoy. Thanks to his leadership, the battalion, throughout the Battle of St Julien, was never without its supplies: and, miraculously, he succeeded in delivering these without the loss of a man.

The strain of these days proved too much and Farve was once more invalided to England, where for the remainder of the war he trained the Special Reserve.

*   *   *

Grandfather Redesdale died in 1916, a year after his beloved Clem was killed. His finances had been hard hit by the enormous cost of rebuilding and maintaining Batsford. The place had been run on the extravagant lines of Edwardian England, with palatial stables for carriage horses, riding horses and Grandfather's famous stud of Shires. My grandmother's little book that records menus of many courses opposite the names of her guests (to ensure no repetition from one visit to the next) was usual in such a household, but my grandfather was also a gardener and I have never seen, except in this little book, a description of the flowers on the dinner table.

When my father inherited Batsford, it was obvious to him that his old home would have to be sold. Soon after the end of the war, a buyer was found in Gilbert Wills, later Lord Dulverton, chairman of the tobacco company W. D. & H. O. Wills, makers of the Virginian cigarettes Farve always smoked. Gilbert and my father became lifelong friends. Farve seldom stayed in other people's houses but made an exception for Gilbert and joined him in Scotland to shoot grouse on a moor rented from Lord Cawdor. (After the Second World War, Nancy was asked by the film director Alexander Korda to work on a script. She was proud of this coup and told my father about it. 'What?' he said, incredulous. 'I never knew old Jack Cawdor was interested in films.') Farve did not care for Gilbert's wife, Victoria, and, to irritate her, took his own apples and Keiller's Dundee marmalade—'my anti-scorbutics'—whenever he went to stay. When we asked him why he did it, he said he did not want to get scurvy and could not 'rely on her housekeeping'.

Our own household added up to too many women; a wife, six daughters and a governess at every meal must have made Farve long for male company. This he found at the Marlborough Club and in the House of Lords. I am glad for his sake (and for theirs) that peeresses in their own right did not arrive in the House until after Farve died. Although he was a firm believer in the hereditary system, the idea of women making a nuisance of themselves in those hallowed surroundings would have 'fair turned him up', to put it in his own language. As for life peeresses, I can imagine his reaction to that 'army of unkempt females', all 'lower than the belly of a snake'. As it was he enjoyed his work, representing the needs of country people. He was thorough and served on several committees, chairing the one to do with drains. I expect it had a grander name but drains was its job. He brought a world of common sense, unknown to politicians today, to these deliberations. He came back from London with rich tales of his fellow peers, all told in his deadpan way, with the ancient titles of Black Rod and Sergeant-at-Arms trotted out as though they were next-door neighbours. According to him, Lord Someone-or-Other had 'passed a motion on the floor of the House . . . (long pause) . . . and left it on the paper for weeks'. To us, used to cleaning up dogs' messes on the floor of our house, this was screamingly funny.

In May 1934 Farve moved rejection of Lord Salisbury's Private Member's Bill to reform the House of Lords. Reform had been discussed for years and was to be mooted for another six decades before it was eventually passed. In his speech my father said, prophetically, that those who wished for reform did so because they were afraid that if a Socialist government came to power, it would want to abolish the House of Lords. If it found a reformed Upper Chamber, however, it might tolerate it. 'But would they?' asked my father. 'Let their lordships make no mistake, they would not. Such a government would tolerate precisely nothing that interfered in any way with their plans and arrangements, and they would abolish anything that did. They would find no greater difficulty in abolishing a Constitution made in 1934 than one of greater antiquity.' (All but ninety-two hereditary peers were turned out of the House of Lords in 1999 by Prime Minister Blair, who had no plan with which to replace them; a stranger to common sense, he preferred the grand gesture and the big spin.)

In the same speech—he was known as 'the peer of but a single speech'—Farve reiterated his faith in the hereditary principle. He believed that a man who had spent all his life in politics or public affairs was more likely to have a son capable of following in his footsteps than a man who had never paid attention to either, 'especially when that son had been brought up in the atmosphere of public work and in the knowledge that the day would come when he would have to bear his part in that work'. The idea of public service is so out of fashion now that to mention it is to court criticism, even ridicule. Jack Kennedy's words, 'Ask not what your country can do for you, ask what you can do for your country', have been turned on their head. Yet you only have to think for a moment to realize that there is much sense in what Farve believed.

When it came to business my father was easily tempted by romantic ideas of making a quick fortune. In 1912 he joined the gold rush to Canada but, unlucky as always, the ground he staked out was the only bit for miles around where there was no gold. He believed everyone to be as honest as he was and gullibility made him an easy target for charlatans. On a legendary occasion, one Andia (Marquis of) persuaded him to invest in a business that made tasteful cabinets for hiding wirelesses, which in those days were huge and hideous. It all ended in court with the 'Marquis' suing for slander. The case was dismissed and Andia unmasked. Randolph Churchill went to the court hearing with his sister Diana (their mother was Farve's first cousin). 'It's so unfair,' said Diana, 'Cousin David was *bound* to win because he looks like God the Father.'

*   *   *

I never knew my mother in her full beauty. She was

forty when I was born, sixteen years after Nancy. Like my father, she had blonde hair and blue eyes, and her fine, regular features were a softer version of his. Totally without vanity, she did not seem to care what she looked like in everyday life, but when dressed up for an occasion she outshone her contemporaries. She loved clothes but possessed few and must have worn the same ones for years. I remember individual coats, skirts and dresses and an occasional evening dress; they were always original and exactly right for her. She was selfless to a rare degree and lived for her husband, children and other dependants. She belonged to a generation of women who were brought up to accept their husband's decisions and to make the best of their circumstances. 'For better, for worse, for richer, for poorer,' were the widely accepted conditions of marriage then.

Muv has been written about in books and newspapers, not because she sought recognition but because of her daughters. She is usually portrayed as vague, undemonstrative and cold, but I do not recognize her from this description. Vague she may have seemed to strangers, but she noticed and always understood our worries, real or imagined, and carried out her role as mother, wife and housekeeper in a way that a vague woman could never have done. In the 1920s and 30s she was responsible for what now seems an enormous indoor staff, as well as her family. She must have been sorely tried by us and there was seldom a day when a meal went smoothly. She presided above the noise, pretending not to notice the quick exit, banged door and tears, or the uncontrolled laughter sparked off by the silliest remark. She would sometimes go into a kind of reverie, abstracting herself from the ceaseless banter but remaining still present, a much-needed influence for calm. Telling Muv something thrilling or frightening seldom evoked more than, 'Orrnnhh, Stubby, fancy'; or 'Did you really? I do hope not.' She had heard it all before, of course, from each sister in turn. She rarely gave advice and when she did it was to underline what Nanny said, 'Don't draw attention to yourself.' Muv tried to prevent what she called 'announcements' such as 'I'm just going to wash my hands,' 'I'm going upstairs,' or, a shade more worthy, 'Help, I've forgotten to feed the guinea pigs.' She said, oh-so-truly, 'All that is not of interest to anyone.' What none of us realized at the time was just how much she taught us by her own example—and I cannot imagine a better one. By the time we were old enough to be aware of this, it was too late to tell her.

I have never known anyone as fair as Muv. She had neither favourites nor victims. That alone must have been almost impossible with such a disparate lot of girls, with diverse personalities and interests. Whether her disappointment every time another girl was born had an effect on us, perhaps a psychiatrist could say; certainly I was never aware of it. Tom, being the only boy, was always the exception. Her insight into the characters of each of her daughters gave her an uncanny knowledge of what we were doing; she did not have to be told by a busybody friend, she knew by instinct. We (or certainly Unity, Decca and me—I was too young to know about the older ones) were aware of this and our feeling of guilt when overstepping the mark was a steadying influence. Long after it was all over Muv told me that each daughter had had two or three years of adolescent rebelliousness or just bad temper, which had made life difficult for everyone in the house. As there were six of us, she went through twelve years of this kind of tension and it is not surprising that she retreated into her own thoughts from time to time. Her deafness in old age increased the impression she gave of being miles away. Two naughty grandsons fighting each other almost to the death said with glee, 'Granny Muv doesn't mind, she's so lovely and deaf.'

My sisters complained that she was strict. Perhaps after trying to make five girls stick to the rules she got tired of saying no and I was allowed a little more rope—but only a little as the tramlines of approved behaviour were still in force. It was not till the 1939 war that circumstances swept these away. One surprising indulgence was that I was allowed to go out hunting alone from the age of twelve. A friend of mine, an only child who longed to do the same, told her mother about this. 'Oh, it's all right for Lady Redesdale,' said the mother, 'she's got five more girls so it doesn't matter if anything happens to Debo.' As ever, my mother's reasoning was wise: out hunting someone is always around to look after you, but my friend was still forbidden.

My mother liked figures. She remembered our London telephone number, Kensington 6476, by saying 'six for seven-and-six is one-and-three each'. Her household account books recorded every penny she spent: 'Utensils 15s 9d, Cleaning Materials 1s 2d, Vegetables 2s 10d'. In 1933 the under parlourmaid was paid £18 a year, Nanny £74 (up from £45 when she first arrived) and Mr and

Mrs Stobie, the cook and gardener, £116. We all knew that if Muv had been in charge of our family finances everything might have been different. As it was, she had to juggle with what she was given and somehow remain solvent; intuition took her in the right direction and she never overspent. She was the one who put down roots and became part of the place where she lived, and it was she who bore the brunt of my father's extravagances and unlucky investments. It must have been hard for her each time we moved but I never heard her say so. I wonder now how much Farve told her when another crisis was building up. As children, none of us was privy to such discussions—if indeed they took place. Money was not spoken about as it is now, when it is often the sole subject of conversation, with a bit of illness thrown in.

Muv told me that had she had to earn her living she would have been happy as the woman at the *caisse* in a Paris restaurant, usually a formidable female dressed in black who sat enclosed in a raised glass cage above the tables and collected the cash from the diners' bills. The nearest Muv got to her ambition was to be County Treasurer of the Oxfordshire Federation of Women's Institutes. When she was totting up at the end of the year, a few pence out caused her major anxiety and we knew to keep out of her way. She was determined that we should all be as good managers as she was, and she started us off with a few pence a week pocket money. We graduated at the age of twelve to what was grandly called 'an allowance', eleven shillings a month, out of which we had to buy stockings, gloves, sweets, presents and any other extras we wanted. The amount was increased annually, bringing more responsibility, until we were seventeen and £100 a year had to cover most of our travelling as well as a complete wardrobe. When you compare our allowance with the wages of my parents' indoor staff, the Great Unfairness of Life is brought home.

When I was about ten, Muv got us all together to test our future housekeeping skills for an as yet unknown husband. Under the headings 'rent, rates, wages, heating, cleaning materials, food, clothes, travelling, and other necessities', she instructed us to account for an income of £500 a year. We pored over our sheet of paper, trying our best to apportion the money. Nancy finished almost before the rest of us had started. We read out our proposals and when it came to her turn, she waved her paper and said, 'Flowers: £499. Everything else: £1.' Muv gave up.

*   *   *

Muv's own childhood was unconventional, to say the least. Her mother, Jessica Bowles, née Evans-Gordon, died in 1887 when expecting her fifth child. Sydney was just seven years old. The family consisted of two brothers, George and Geoffrey, and Sydney and her younger sister Dorothy, known as Weenie all her life. A governess, Miss Henrietta Shell (Tello), joined them soon after their mother's death.

Sydney's father, Thomas Gibson Bowles, was illegitimate—a fact of no consequence now but in the second half of the nineteenth century the sins of the father were visited on the children and his origins carried a slur. His was an unusual case in that he was brought up by his father, Thomas Milner Gibson, a Radical MP, and little is known about his mother, a Miss Susan Bowles. When he was three years old Tommy Bowles was taken to live at his father's house in Suffolk (Mrs Milner Gibson must have been a generous woman to include him in her own brood). No public school would accept an illegitimate boy, so from the age of twelve he was educated in France. After a brief stint as a junior clerk in the Succession Duty office at Somerset House, he became a freelance journalist and magazine publisher, and was elected to Parliament in 1892.

Tommy Bowles' brains, forceful character and originality of thought made him a man to be reckoned with and he was a strong influence on his children. The sea was his passion. He held a master mariner's certificate and spent as much time as possible on board ship. After the death of his wife, he sold Cleeve Lodge, the house near the Royal Albert Hall in Kensington where he and Jessica had lived since their marriage, and moved his family to the country. But he could not settle to life in England and in August 1888 set off in his schooner, the *Nereid*, to Egypt and the Holy Land, taking with him Miss Shell, his four children and a dog. My mother was eight and Weenie only three. The eight-month voyage made a deep impression on the children. A habit learned at sea stayed with Muv all her life: the fear of running out of fresh drinking-water meant she never filled a glass, even of tap water, more than one-third full.

The *Nereid* was nearly wrecked in a hurricane off the coast of Syria, Grandfather having left Alexandria against the advice of the port authorities. Muv's account of the storm and their eventual safe landing enthralled us as children. Many years later she told me that they set sail in such dangerous conditions because Grandfather had discovered that while he was away exploring Upper Egypt, Tello was having an affair with a young naval officer. Muv remembered the man coming on board the *Nereid* and singing, 'You Are the Queen of my Heart Tonight'. Grandfather, who was enamoured of Tello himself, was so angry he insisted on leaving immediately.

Tello went out of the children's lives for some years after they returned to England. Then one day my mother was walking down Sloane Street when she saw, to her joy, Tello accompanied by four little boys in sailor suits. It transpired that the eldest was the son of the naval officer in Alexandria, but the next three were sired by Grandfather and were my mother's half-brothers. He had forgiven Tello her peccadillo, set her up in a house in London and made her editor of *The Lady*, a position she held for many years. My mother always wondered why he had not married her but guessed it would have been because of the eldest boy. Tello and Muv took up their friendship where they had left off and after her marriage Muv often invited her old governess to stay at Asthall. Tello was an inspired storyteller and we delighted in her company.

Back from the voyage, Grandfather took his family to Wilbury House, in Wiltshire, belonging to Sir Henry Malet. Sir Henry was hard up and had welcomed Grandfather's offer to share the household expenses. My mother was not fond of the daughter of the house, Vera, with whom she had to do lessons, but the beautiful Palladian house made a lasting impression on her at an age when sensitive children notice the details of their surroundings. Muv never again lived in a fine eighteenth-century house like Wilbury, her ideal, but her ability to make her succession of houses attractive and original on little money was one of her outstanding talents. Her stamp was unmistakable and I thought the results perfection. Junk shops drew her like a magnet and in the streets behind Marylebone Station she found bargains in furniture, china and anything that took her fancy. She never employed a decorator or sought advice; she knew what she wanted and got it done. When she was first married and living in a small house in Graham Street, Pimlico, she was amazed when a fashionable older woman asked her, 'Is your drawing room green and white or white and green?' To her chagrin Muv had to admit that it was indeed white and green. This must have been the nearest she ever came to following a trend.

Grandfather was MP for King's Lynn from 1892 to 1906 and when the House was sitting the family lived at No. 25 Lowndes Square. When Muv was fourteen, her father gave her the job of running his household, which she performed to his entire satisfaction. Not only did he have a beautiful daughter but a dependable housekeeper too. Grandfather had other lady friends besides Tello, including Lady Sykes, whom my mother particularly disliked and whose visits she dreaded. She described her as 'drinking and painting her face too much'—both were habits Muv abhorred.

The widowed father did not wish to cope with

dressing his two daughters so he decided they should wear thick serge sailor suits, day and evening, winter and summer, at home or away. Not till Muv was eighteen did a woman friend of Grandfather's tell him that it was time for her to be dressed more conventionally. One evening he was the guest of honour at a dinner given in Hammersmith Town Hall by the mayor. He was ready to leave, dressed in tails and a white waistcoat, but could not find Sydney who was to accompany him. So he called Weenie, who was in the garden with the dogs. Still in her grubbiest sailor suit, with no time to wash or tidy, she grabbed her cap and was whisked off. The elegant ladies in gloves, gowns and jewels must have been surprised to see her being led into dinner on the arm of the mayor and placed on his right at the top table. Muv and Weenie were used to their father's eccentric behaviour. He never gave them birthday or Christmas presents and when they complained that their friends all got something, he rounded on them saying that he housed, fed, watered, clothed and educated them and that was enough.

When they were in London, Sydney rode every day with her father in Rotten Row. She rode side-saddle, as all women did at the time, and for a few weeks every year when she was a child, the pommel of her saddle was fixed on the off (right) side, to ensure that her left hip grew in alignment with her right. The daily ride in Rotten Row provided not only exercise but also the opportunity to meet friends, part of the social life that Muv enjoyed. But the real fun for the two sisters was skating at the Prince's Club, the ice rink in Montpelier Square. Muv fell for the skating instructor,

Henning Grenander, a Swedish champion figure-skater, who was the equivalent of today's ski-guides, so adored by their clients. Waltzing with him seemed to Muv the height of romance.

In August, Grandfather sometimes took his family—along with some of his unusual habits—to a rented house on Deeside. He believed in Turkish baths and set one up in an empty dog kennel which was heated to the desired temperature with hot bricks. He sweated in the kennel and emerged sometime later to be drenched with buckets of cold water thrown from the roof by the butler. Muv's abiding love of Scotland dated from these visits. She had holiday romances there, including one with a young suitor called Eustace Heaven. My sisters and I thought this the most wonderful name when she told us about him, half-laughing, years later.

When Sydney was a debutante the first dance she went to, curiously enough, was given by the Duke and Duchess of Devonshire at their London house in Piccadilly. She was chaperoned by her father and they were early arrivals. I remember her telling me of Louise Duchess's painted face and fixed smile, and how the Duke stood behind her, half asleep as usual. What Sydney did not know was that the Duke woke up the next morning and saw thick fog outside. He turned over in bed, muttering that there was no point getting up—not realizing that the window was covered by the tent left over from the night before.

When Weenie was eighteen, Grandfather unwillingly agreed that a dance must be given for her. The guest list became too large for Lowndes Square, so Weenie brought in builders to break through the wall into the next house, whose owners were conveniently away. After Sydney married, Weenie, aged eighteen and equally as capable as Sydney, took over her tasks and faced the same difficulties with the drunken menservants in the household. There was a troublesome chef who was given notice several times but refused to leave. In order to get rid of him, Grandfather decided to shut the house and go to China, taking Weenie with him. On the day of departure the trunks were packed and stowed in the 'growler' that was to take them to the station to catch the boat train. Grandfather came down the steps and said, 'It's raining, my dear Piggy. We won't go.'

Weenie soon became engaged to Percy Bailey but knew nothing of what was in store. Grandfather was told that someone must explain the facts of life to her before she married. When these were disclosed, she exclaimed, 'Surely no *gentleman* would ever do a thing like that!' On her wedding day, she arrived at the church with Grandfather and his last words to her before walking up the aisle were, 'Piggy, I shall never know what I owe the Aylesbury Dairy now.' He had no more daughters to look after his household bills.

Grandfather died in 1922 so I never knew him but he was a strong influence on Muv in many ways, including diet. He had noticed that among the children living in London the Jewish ones were the healthiest, and decided to bring up his own family according to the dietary laws of the Old Testament. Muv adopted these rules and we were fed accordingly. The language in which the Lord spoke to Moses is as threatening as a thunderstorm. We did not feel deprived of 'eagle, ossifrage and osprey', which are an 'abomination' and therefore banned from the table, but swine being 'cloven-footed' but not chewers of the cud meant no bacon, and the rule against eating anything without fins and scales but that lived in the water meant no shellfish. I did not taste lobster until I was eighteen.

In spite of her unusual views, Muv's cooks always produced good food. She was influenced by Grandfather's foreign chefs and her table combined the best of French and English styles. She was no cook herself and when she and my father lived in a shack in Canada while prospecting for gold, she told us that she had bought a chicken, put it in the oven and was horrified on carving it to discover the crop and gizzard still full of corn which floated into the gravy. She was unexpectedly indulgent about our own food fancies, which many parents would have forbidden. Unity was addicted to mashed potatoes in her early teens and ate them to the exclusion of almost everything else. Bread sauce was my favourite, eaten with a spoon. My other craving was for Bovril, which Muv believed to be full of hated preservatives. She refused to buy it, but let me have it and charged it against my pocket money.

Muv flirted with Christian Science but could not take Mrs Baker Eddy. Her simpler creed was that, if left alone, the Good Body would cure itself without Mrs Eddy's help. She mistrusted the medical profession and used to say, 'Doctors are so nice but if only they could get away from their training.' Perhaps as children we were lucky that ninety per cent of the time, the Good Body did the job. When there was a crisis, Muv did get in a doctor but she preferred more unorthodox treatment. I once had a fierce attack of indigestion and a masseur, a follower of the Swedish osteopath Dr Kellgren, was called in. He gave me a rough pummelling all over and after a while I turned bright yellow. 'That's good,' he said, 'that's the bile coming out,' and I felt better. Muv was criticized by other parents who were sceptical of massage and disapproved of the infrequency of the doctor's visits, but their children envied us because, like sausages, Syrup of Figs and castor oil were banned. Muv paid no attention to whether or not we went to the lavatory; she knew that the Good Body would see to it in the end.

In 1931 tuberculin testing for cows became mandatory. Three of Muv's herd of Guernseys reacted positive to the test. This annoyed her and she refused to get rid of them, telling the cowman, 'What? Get rid of those beautiful animals. Certainly not! The children can have the milk', and have it we did. She believed that wholegrain, stone-ground wheat—nothing added and nothing taken away—was 'the bread of life'. She was critical of Lord Rank, 'the wicked miller', and regarded his ghost-white loaves (the cheapest kind of bread bought by the greatest number of people) and pale brown Hovis a confidence trick because the germ of the wheat had been removed, thereby lowering the bread's nutritional value. All such processed food was described as 'murdered food' by Muv's brother, Uncle Geoffrey, whose maxim was 'Don't keep it, eat it'. (He lived on bread, chocolate and the occasional herring.) All tinned food was considered close to poison; sardines were the exception and my father also bought something called 'glass tongue', which was visible through the jar. When refrigerators came into fashion, Muv said in a faraway voice, 'I don't really like refrigerators; they make the food so cold.'

3

Sisters and Tom

Until she married in 1933, my favourite sister after Decca was Nancy. She called me Linda, sometimes adding 'May' when it suited for a rhyme ('Linda May drives the clouds away/What would life be without Linda May? Grey'). She made me laugh and cry about equally but what I remember now is the laughter. She was so funny, lively and imaginative that, in spite of the tears, I could not resist her company. The sixteen years between us made her almost another generation, but whenever she was at home I spent hours sitting on the end of her bed listening to gossip and secrets about the people she had met while staying with friends. The confidences were safe with me as I had no one to repeat them to: Muv and Nanny would not have listened and Decca was not interested. They were a window on a glamorous life, embellished no doubt, and they made me long to meet the butterfly people she described, a world away from the nursery and schoolroom.

Nancy was a conundrum if ever there was one. She was everything and its opposite: loyal–disloyal, generous–mean, kind–unkind, steadfast–treacherous, hardworking –lazy, tolerant–intolerant. No wonder her biographers have found it difficult to steer through this maze of contradictions to arrive at the person she was. In life she exaggerated until the truth was hard to dig out but she often hit the nail on the head in her books. Sophia, a character in her novel, *Pigeon Pie*, who had a talent for 'embroidering on her own experiences', and who rushed from hyperbole to hyperbole, ending on a wild climax of improbability with the words 'it's absolutely true,' could be a portrait of Nancy. The one constant, however, was the pure pleasure Nancy's company gave; the way she lifted spirits when she came into a room, her talent for turning serious into ridiculous and for seeing people and situations as no one else did. She sparkled, not only her eyes but all of her, and was the star of any gathering. Her elegance was inborn, her figure unchanging, never too fat or too thin, and long before she had money to spend on herself, her clothes were always just right. Her swinging walk took her for miles in town and country and few could keep up with her.

She was not happy in youth, being well and truly unemployed for those years, with nothing to live on except the small allowance from our parents. Marriage was the career that we all aspired to—we were not trained to do a paid job. We learned how to keep house by example, but even that was with a future husband and family in mind. No work equalled no money. Any unskilled job, working in a hat shop, for instance, was frowned upon as 'taking money from someone who really needed it'. Nancy did not marry until she was nearly thirty and until then led an aimless existence, staying with friends for long periods but coming home in between to wherever we were living at the time. 'Sat about' are words which recur in my own diary as I grew up, and I well remember what we called 'aching voids of boredom'. It was a teenage disease, like being rude to our parents—especially to Muv who came in for criticism from all of us. It was not surprising that there was discontent on all sides. In *The Pursuit of Love* Nancy describes the agonizingly slow passing of the hours and days: 'What's the time?' asks Linda. 'Guess,' says Fanny. '"A quarter to six?" "Better than that." "Six?" "Not quite so good." "Five to?" "Yes."'

Nancy's fertile mind found an outlet in teasing—not difficult in my case as the slightest hint of pathos was guaranteed to bring tears, but none of us was spared; being laughed at was part of the rough and tumble of life in a large family. One day there was a headline in the paper: 'SLOWLY CRUSHED TO DEATH IN A LIFT. MAN'S LONG AGONY IN THE LIFT SHAFT'. Nancy only had to say SLOWLY and Decca and I dissolved into tears. It became too much for the grown-ups and was banned, so Nancy tapped it out with her hand or foot, watching our faces to see the effect. When my bedtime was at seven, she started looking hopefully at the clock at a quarter to. When the blessed moment came at last and it was time for me to go, she shooed me out saying, 'As soon as you've gone I shall do the Joy Dance.' Sure enough, when I got upstairs I heard loud stomping and clapping of hands coming from down below.

'No one will want to marry *you*,' she used to say. 'WHY?' I wailed. To be told by a grown-up sister that there was no chance of happiness as a wife and mother, when marriage was the only prospect, was a crushing blow. 'Why? Well, not only have you got a deformed thumb, there is the *gland* . . .' Perhaps because we drank milk from the cows that had reacted to the tuberculin test, I did indeed have a lump in my neck, which is still there. Nancy explained that it hubbled and bubbled when I was asleep and that no man could stand it. She sang:

> The hounds and the horses
> Galloping over the land
> All stopped to hear
> The hubbling, bubbling of the gland.

And added a second verse:

> The lords and the ladies
> Dancing to the band
> All stopped to hear
> The hubbling, bubbling of the gland.

I was convinced there was no hope for my future.

When Muv was expecting Nancy, Farve's letters make it clear how certain she was that her first child was to be a boy. She referred to the unborn as 'him', named him Paul and knitted and sewed blue garments. After a punishing fourteen hours in labour, the nine-and-a-half-pound baby was not blue-eyed, fair-haired Paul but dark-haired, green-eyed Nancy. The birth was far from the fairytale experience that Muv had looked forward to and was followed by weeks of extremely painful breast-feeding. We were all born at home. The doctors' rule in those days was that after giving birth, a mother should stay in bed for three weeks, flat on her back for the first two; the 'patient' was then allowed up for a few hours each day, extended as time went by until a normal daily routine was restored. Muv found this regime frustrating but kept to it. The pendulum has now swung too far in the opposite direction and she would have deplored the way mothers and their newborn infants are turned out of hospital after a few hours.

My father's sister Frances, Aunt Pussy, was five years older than my mother. She was the most beautiful of my father's sisters and was full of memorable sayings, such as 'I love this coat. It looks so cheap and was so expensive.' Aunt Pussy had no children of her own when Nancy was born and no experience of what is now called 'childcare'. But she had theories on how children should be brought up: they must never be crossed, corrected or criticized and must be allowed to develop in an atmosphere of heavenly peace. Muv was impressed by Aunt Pussy's notions about bringing up children and put them into practice with Nancy—at least until Pam was born. When Aunt Pussy eventually married and was expecting a baby, she spent hours in museums gazing at portraits of children by Greuze, hoping her baby would resemble them. Alas, her only child, Clementine (Pussette), was the opposite of one of Greuze's exquisite children and was mentally retarded.

Nancy always told me that she was perfectly happy till she was three when Pam arrived, although how she remembered is open to question. The birth of a new baby and the attention it receives can be hard on an older sibling and this was perhaps the origin of Nancy's jealousy, which later focused on Diana whose beauty and brains were unsettling to her eldest sister. The jealousy was hidden but to those of us who knew her it was very much there.

*   *   *

Pamela was as different from Nancy as you could imagine. She was called Woman, with a few variations, by all of us for the simple reason that she was so womanly. She had huge cornflower-blue eyes and naturally stripy blonde hair of the kind envied by many girls and achieved with difficulty by expensive hairdressers. She was slightly lame, after an attack of polio at the age of three left her right leg weaker and shorter than her left. She was nursed at home and made an almost complete recovery. Later on she adored riding, but because her grip on the saddle was too weak to manage jumps she was never able to go hunting.

Pam had much in common with Muv, her interests fixed firmly on the kitchen and garden rather than some fanciful library or the political leaders chosen by her siblings. There was no risk of extreme views or controversial talk; she was just herself, a comforting, sensible presence with no sharp edges. She was not quick-witted and could not keep pace with words and nuances, which made her a sitting target for Nancy whose teasing verged on bullying. But Pam's good nature saw her through a persecuted childhood and she laughed about it later on. She was never out of favour with Farve and because she never deviated from the steady path of a country person she was the favourite of our aunts and uncles.

Dogs played an important part in Pam's life; she invested them with human characteristics and organized her existence around their needs, to an extent unusual even in an Englishwoman. Food was of paramount importance and she was a stickler for well-chosen menus. A friend of my mother once turned up unexpectedly for lunch. As bad luck would have it, Muv must have taken her eye off the ball early that morning when meals for the day were being planned. To Pam's dismay, rice appeared twice: savoury in a risotto and creamy in a rice pudding. 'Stublow,' she told me, wide-eyed with horror, 'it was ghoul, *two* rices at *one* meal'—a kitchen gaffe remembered for the rest of our lives and any disaster was called 'two rices', in Pam's voice. At a smart dinner party in Paris she once surprised the guests by explaining a cut of pork to her neighbour, emphasizing her point by standing up, slapping her thigh and saying, 'Il faut le couper *là*'—you have to cut it *there*.

During the General Strike of 1926 Pam came into her own. A canteen for volunteer lorry drivers was set up in a big barn by the main road to Oxford, always called the Top Road (it is a smart restaurant now but it is still the canteen to me). So off went the sisters with heaps of sandwiches and an oil stove to brew the tea. Pam did the early shift. She had got everything ready, but no one came. Disappointed, she lay on the road pressing her ear to the tarmac, hoping to hear the sound of rumbling wheels. Silence. After a while a dirty old tramp wandered in and demanded tea. Pam, half afraid, brought him a cup. He sidled up to her and said with a leer, 'Give us a kiss, Miss.' Pam was terrified, and tripped and twisted her ankle as she fled. Once again, the tramp was Nancy.

*   *   *

I hardly knew Tom. He was eleven when I was born and already more than halfway through prep school. He was a serious, thoughtful child, adored by parents and sisters and, although aware of his unique position in the family as the only boy in a troop of girls, he somehow remained unspoilt. He had a carved head of regular features and, like my father, the steady, confident gaze of an honest man. It is not enough to say that he was good-looking—which is how all his contemporaries described him, he had the kind of personality that drew attention and made you look at him even when he was silent. Unlike Nancy, whose face changed with every passing thought, Tom's expression was impassive. He did not join in our silliness but was amused by it and when he laughed, sometimes unwillingly, at our idiotic jokes, a one-sided smile, which we called 'blithering', appeared. To make him blither was a small triumph and worth the try. He once got that curious complaint called Bell's palsy and the muscles on one side of his face froze and for a while the smile did too. A sister took a photograph and it records his bizarre, lop-sided smile.

Tom had the gift of making one want to please him, which was perhaps the secret of his success with women, and he left a trail of disappointed lovers who did not quite come up to his standards. His bugbear was depression, an affliction from which my sisters and I did not suffer. He sometimes came home unexpectedly and hardly spoke for days but sat, at times reading at times not, oblivious to his surroundings and to Decca and me jabbering away in Honnish, our private language. The depression lifted as mysteriously as it came and off he went to whatever he was supposed to be doing. He was the peacemaker of the family and managed to remain friends with everyone throughout all the political upheavals. He was the most steadfast and attractive person in the background of our lives and we all deferred to him, including Muv and Farve.

Tom's letters to Muv from prep school chiefly concerned food. The hungry last years of the 1914–18 war must have been hard on growing boys and 'sossages' and fried bacon are often mentioned, perhaps as a tease because they were outlawed at home. Tom made lifelong friends at school with Basil Blackwood, later the Marquess of Dufferin and Ava, and Jim Lees-Milne. Nanny told me of my introduction to Jim. At three months old I was taken with parents and sisters to a school cricket match in which Tom and Jim were playing. Jim lobbed a ball into my pram, which got him a brisk telling off from Nanny—the closeness of the near-fatal blow no doubt exaggerated. (I do not suppose Muv noticed.)

From prep school Tom won a scholarship to Eton and could have gone there for nothing, as a 'Tug' in Eton language, but because Farve could afford the fees it was decided that he should go as an 'Oppidan Scholar', leaving the place for a needier boy. Tom thrived at Eton, where his friends Jim and Basil were also pupils. His musical talent flourished and his tutor allowed him to have a piano in his room—an unusual concession, but he realized it was a part of Tom's being.

*   *   *

Diana left home to get married when I was nine. I saw little of her until after the war and did not really get to know and love her till then. Her beauty was the first thing that struck you; she was beautiful when she was born in 1910 and remained beautiful until her death. Without make-up or artifice, and often in clothes that she wore till they were threadbare, she was always the best-looking woman at any gathering. She was a great reader with a huge appetite for literature and was the intellectual equal of Tom, to whom she was closest in age and interests. Like Decca and Unity, once Diana had decided on a course of action there was no deviating or turning back and, like them, she was drawn to extreme politics. It was more surprising in her case as almost everything else about her was open-minded and tolerant.

Her immediate understanding of human frailty and her extraordinary sensitivity made Diana doubly attractive, and later on it was interesting to see how people who were prejudiced against her because of her politics melted on meeting her. Her rigid views on race were partly influenced by Grandfather Redesdale, an advocate of Teutonic supremacy, and were hardened by the experience of war and her unyielding nature. I do not share her views but my love for her overcame this side of her character, the greater part of which was pure and selfless. She was always the one to volunteer for some boring family chore and went out of her way to be kind to anyone in difficulty. As she grew old, she became almost saint-like in her goodness.

*   *   *

Unity was always the odd one out. She arrived in this world in August 1914 to the sound of troops marching to war and departed it thirty-four years later in tragic circumstances. Larger than life in every way, she could have been the model for a ship's figurehead or Boadicea, with her huge navy-blue eyes, perfectly straight nose and fair hair worn in two long plaits. Perhaps because of her teenage diet of mashed potatoes, her teeth were her only bad feature. (In those days cosmetic dentistry was in its infancy and you took what nature gave you.) As a child she was a dreamer, obstinate, fearless of authority, disobedient, affectionate and easily hurt, with a precocious talent for drawing and design. When she was about eight she made an unforgettable picture of a man walking in a field wearing a turban and little else. He had a bag hanging around his middle and was broadcasting seed as though it were peas and beans. The title of the drawing was 'Abraham and his Seed Forever'.

Unity was devoted to Decca, a closeness that withstood their political differences. They communicated in Boudledidge, a private language invented by Decca that no one in the family understood except me, but I would never have dared speak it—it was their language, not mine, and I would have been pulled up sharply had I tried. I was satisfied with Honnish, which had a background of the local Gloucestershire accent, elongated and shortened according to the importance of the words. If someone upset Unity at meals, she slid slowly and noiselessly to the floor and remained under the table while the chat went on above, surfacing only when she thought the episode was forgotten. My parents never drew attention to it. She understood the power of silence and carried it to such a degree that it was sometimes what the Army describes so well as 'dumb insolence'. One of the lessons in the PNEU programme was 'narration', when pupils had to recount a passage that the teacher had read out. Muv asked Unity to do this simple task but for some reason she dug in her heels and refused. 'Come on, darling, you must remember something,' said Muv. Unity shook her head. 'Not one word?' Muv insisted. 'Very well then,' said Unity, staring furiously ahead, *'the'*.

*   *   *

Decca was my boon companion all through childhood. She was bold, original, imaginative, generous, vulnerable, lazy, clumsy and comical in the extreme. We shared everything and life without her was unimaginable. We talked all day in Honnish, and when we slept in the same room we chatted for half the night as well—what about, heaven knows, but no secrets were hid. We had each other when the grown-ups and older sisters were difficult or when the Great Unfairness of Life seemed too much to bear.

Having opposite interests, we did not compete: Decca was a reader, an observer rather than a doer, and clever, with a talent for words that eventually made her famous. She was not interested in sports or games of any kind, she disliked the out-of-doors and was oblivious to the seasons. (When loyally accompanying her second husband, Robert Treuhaft, on a hiking holiday in an American national park, she intoned, 'Nature, nature, how I hate yer,' as she stumbled along a rocky path.) A feeling for interior decoration—so strong in my mother and inherited to the last degree of perfection by Nancy and Diana—was left out of her. Nor did she seem to care about her appearance: clothes were merely coverings to keep her warm; colours and shapes were thrown together hugger-mugger and made you wonder at her choice. Her mind and energies were engaged elsewhere, mainly with people and politics. Her unswerving loyalty to those she loved and biting criticism of the many she did not, were shades of my father—perhaps the only trait they had in common. When you were with her, all else faded in the face of her strong personality and you forgot everything except her company.

Decca had two pet animals and a bird, adored and transformed by her into human characters and, like Pam with her dogs, they were invested with considerable importance. The bird was a ring dove, complete with a beautiful wicker cage, which she had bought with long-saved pocket money. The dove became tame and flew above her head as she bicycled down the long hill to Swinbrook village, looking like the picture of the Holy Ghost in our children's illustrated Bible. It was an object of envy to me, who had neither bird nor bicycle. Her black spaniel, Tray, was a later shadow and was named after the dog that gained the upper hand over Cruel Frederick in *Struwwelpeter*, Heinrich Hoffmann's cautionary tales. Their terrifying pictures were a constant reminder of what could happen if we overstepped the mark. The Great Agrippa, so tall he almost reached the sky, was my father to the life in his dressing gown when he had just got out of 'my good clothes'. Little Suck-a-Thumb, blood pouring from the boy's amputated thumbs, and the smoking remains of Harriet, the result of her disobedience with matches, all hit the targeted conscience.

Decca's other creature was Miranda, an orphan ewe lamb she had brought up on the bottle. Miranda soon grew into a clumsier, pushier version of Tray and went everywhere with her loving owner, shoving people and furniture out of the way with a butt from her bony forehead. After the annual shearing, her fleece was sent to the Witney Blanket Company where the wool was transformed into a blanket with 'Miranda' woven in red into the border. The sheep and the annual blanket were an important part of nursery life. Miranda became the symbol of all the virtues, backed up by no less an authority than the Bible, which regularly harps on the necessity of separating the sheep from the goats (sheep being the superior of the two). Whenever a passage referring to this ancient state of affairs was quoted in church, Decca got excited and made the faces and sounds she kept for Miranda. If the parson noticed he must have wondered what had possessed one of the younger members of his congregation.

I sometimes wondered what it would be like to be an only child, but the stimulation of being one of a crowd, all older than me, was an education in itself. I could never keep up but I learned to hold my own.

4

Swinbrook House

Asthall manor was host to a poltergeist, one of those nuisances that accompany teenage girls. It crashed and banged in the attics and, according to legend, pulled off the cook's bedclothes. My sisters thought it was one of the reasons why Farve decided to sell the house in 1926. He loved building and having a project on the go and set about enlarging a farmhouse above Swinbrook village. I have never seen a photograph of the original house and do not know if Muv was consulted before Farve got to work on it. Judging by what emerged, I imagine not.

While the house was being finished we went to Paris and stayed in a cheap hotel. Farve took his car. He got into trouble with a policeman, who stood blowing his whistle and waving his windmill arms at this driver on the wrong side of the road. Farve wound down his window and shouted, '*Sorry, no Frrrench*,' in an exaggerated French accent (to make it easier for the policeman to understand). There was a bidet in our hotel bathroom and Nanny, Decca and I, who had never seen such a thing, hurried out to buy goldfish assuming that was what it was for.

After a few months we came home to Swinbrook

for the first time. Farve was delighted with his new house. My mother had done her best to make the interior as attractive as possible, given the newness of the shell. Neither of my parents were gardeners, surprisingly in the case of my mother as people who are good at decorating are often good at gardening. She particularly disliked white flowers, saying they were like bits of paper blowing about. My father's favourite flower was scarlet *Anemone fulgens*, a specialist's bloom not often seen in a garden. He treasured the two or three bulbs that succeeded out of the many he planted, and it was the end of the world if a rampaging dog or child were to step on one of these objects of untold value.

I loved the house from the start. The others did not. They had lost the Asthall barn and their freedom and had only the long drawing room to sit in, which they had to share with Muv. They were of an age to complain to whoever would listen and the cry, 'It *is* unfair', was often heard. Lesser complaints ruled the day: 'The knives and forks are so cold we can't eat with them' or 'Unity's got a rat and I've only got hens.' Our bedrooms and Nanny's were on the top floor and were painted white, each with a border of a different colour. Mine was green. The interior doors of the house were made of elm which, as every skoolboy knows, is prone to warping. Farve insisted that it was 'damn good wood', but Nancy said that even when it was locked, you could put your head round the visitors' bathroom door and see what was happening inside. The dining-room table was made of two long pieces of oak, sixteenth-century style (perhaps it was sixteenth-century; it is not the sort of thing children notice). The boards did not quite meet, making a little valley down the middle which we sowed with seeds and watered. It was the usual game of Tom Tiddler's Ground and, greatly daring, we would taunt Farve with this until he shouted at us to stop.

My mother stretched at meals. From her outspread arms her hands made circles in the air, first one way then the other, which she said was good for the digestion. She also yawned. I expect the governesses were surprised by this but they were surprised by many of her foibles. Farve drank water out of Grandfather Redesdale's magnificent goblet made from the melted-down gold medals won by his Shire horses. Farve did the carving. Mabel noticed short commons for the unloved and used to push the plate against his arm till he topped up the helping. She kept the remains of breakfast—forbidden sausages and ham—that came out of the dining room on shooting days, and we were into the pantry like lightning.

Mabel's domain was a refuge for us children. Like Nanny, she was usually unflustered but even she set about us when she had work to do and we annoyed her too much. 'GET OUT OF MY PANTRY,' was always followed by a kiss, her aquiline nose coming first, followed by kindly eyes. She and the under parlourmaid wore the same uniform: a dress of blue-and-white toile de Jouy in a traditional bird pattern, smart and clean-looking (my mother's idea, of course) with a white linen apron and white organdie cap threaded with black velvet ribbon.

Farve and Mabel understood each other perfectly. In most such households her position would have been held by a man, a butler, but because of my mother's bad experiences with drunken men in her father's pantry, she preferred a woman. After twelve years with us Mabel accepted a proposal of marriage from Mr Woolven, a regular visitor who was in charge of preparing the inventory of whichever of our houses was, for reasons of economy, being let. He was probably the only eligible man Mabel ever met. When she told my father the glad news he was furious. 'I would never have engaged you if I'd known you would leave at once,' he stormed. Yet they remained friends and Mabel always came back in an emergency. I thought her home address the most romantic imaginable: 'Mabel Windsor, Peacock Cottage, Queen Camel'.

*   *   *

Swinbrook village and its inhabitants seemed eternal. Winnie Crook, whose initials gave us children such pleasure, ran the post office. She served tuppence-worth of acid drops in a twist of paper, weighed on the same brass scales as the letters. Our other delights were Fry's peppermint cream, which broke off into conveniently sized bits, and good old Cadbury's tuppenny bars. I do not know if she sold anything more expensive but these were what we could afford. There was the village idiot who chased Nancy and no one thought anything of it, Mrs Price, who lived up a bank and was nearly a hundred years old, and at the Mill Cottage, Mrs Phelps, whom Farve mistook for a heifer calf when she was bent over weeding her garden.

The formidable Mrs Bunce was in charge of the Swan Inn and kept strict order; anyone out of step had to beware of the consequences and we never heard of any late-night fracas, even on a Saturday. She wore a black dress fastened at the neck with a cameo brooch and a sacking apron over her substantial front to keep off the meal that she mixed and fed to her turkey poults. The turkeys lived in a paddock opposite the pub and Mrs Bunce's stately figure could be seen slowly crossing the road—a car was a rare sight in those days and there was no need to hurry. There was sawdust on the stone floor of the pub and a charming curved settle in the parlour. The box tree that grows by the door had already reached its full height and I would love to know when it and the ancient wisteria next to it were planted.

The blacksmith, a huge man and a Methodist preacher, was a great figure in the village. His forge was as good as Vulcan's own to me (with Venus nowhere to be seen) and he let me pump the giant bellows. He was one of those men with whom animals are calm and the horses stood peacefully to be shod, resting their foot on his leather apron. I loved the hiss and smell of the smoke billowing from the smouldering hoof when the red-hot shoe was fitted. It left a mark where the hoof had to be trimmed and out would come an enormous file and the ragged edges fell away. What a skill it was and taken for granted by us.

There was also my father's gamekeeper with his broody hens and pheasant chicks, and his gruesome larder of magpies, jays, stoats and weasels, nailed to the branch of a tree. The Gibbet Oak (where men, not birds, were hanged) still stands by Widley, the wood where I found my first butterfly orchid. Farve put a stoutly built railway van in the main ride of Hensgrove Wood to serve as a shelter in the worst weather and for the keeper to store his multifarious kit. I was taken to see it the other day and it still stands, nearly a hundred years later, just as I remembered it.

We went to church of course, at St Mary's, Swinbrook. Muv and Farve sat on the short pew at the back and we directly in front of them. The effigies of the Fettiplace family on the north wall near the altar fascinated us: six life-sized stone men lying on their sides, heads supported by their hands, elbows resting on stone pillows. John Piper described them in the *Shell Guide to Oxfordshire* as 'intelligent, wicked-looking former lords of the village, lying on slabs like proud sturgeon'. This powerful family's claim to fame is that they disappeared some two hundred years ago, as did their house, although traces of the garden terraces are still visible in a field. We all believed this story but many years later a mention of the family in one of my books sparked a letter from a Fettiplace, to whom I wrote to apologize for saying she did not exist.

My parents made several contributions to the church, replacing the Victorian tiled floor with stone flags and installing oak pews. Farve had promised to give the pews should he ever have an unexpected windfall. This unlikely event came about in 1924 when he placed an ante-post bet at huge odds on Master Robert in the Grand National and the horse won. It belonged to our cousin Joe Airlie and there was a great celebration. My father had originally wanted a horse's head carved on the end of each pew to record how the munificent gift had been paid for, but the Bishop refused. Farve thought this hypocritical of the Prince of the Church as he knew perfectly well where the money had come from. Muv gave four brass chandeliers including a small pair with double-headed eagles at the apex that stand out to good effect against so much stone.

The weekly repeated prayers were not crystal-clear to a seven-year-old. What did 'dissembleth', 'cloke,' 'unfeignedly' and 'abhor' mean? And what on earth was the Virgin's womb? 'His servant David' was Farve—though it was difficult to imagine him as anyone's servant unless it was Lieutenant General Lord Methuen's; 'We have erred and strayed from thy ways like lost sheep' brought on Decca's grimaces reserved for Miranda; 'And thou, child,' was Mrs Ham speaking. It was a language that seeped into my subconscious and I cannot bear to hear the new version. Prayers seemed interminable and held up the longed-for freedom when I could be out of doors again. Fidgeting about, I licked the pew beneath my face (the taste of the polish is with me now). I thought everybody did this, but apparently not. Years later I buttonholed a few friends and they vehemently denied such a disgusting habit. I then asked my old friend, the writer Patrick Leigh Fermor, 'Did you lick the pews?' 'Yes, of course,' he said without hesitation, his understanding and memory of childhood undimmed.

Farve took the collection and tortured us by stopping twice in front of Aunt Iris, his penniless sister, nudging her the second time round. She used to frown and slap his hand which started us on the peculiar agony of church giggles. Decorating the church for Easter was our job. I never got further than primroses regimented along the window sills in potted-meat jars. If Easter was late, I included a few cowslips (picking these offerings for Our Maker is illegal now). None of us was much good at decorating but at least we tried. We regularly signed the visitors' book 'Greta Garbo' and 'Maurice Chevalier'. We must have been an almighty nuisance to those in charge.

*   *   *

The poultry farm at Swinbrook was Muv's one chance of running a profitable business. The man who looked after it was called, unbelievably, Mr Lay. The hen's food smelt delicious: warm mash in the mornings made of sharps, middlings and household scraps; wheat and maize in the afternoons. I too kept hens for commercial reasons and sold the eggs to Muv to bolster my pocket money. In Honnish, 'hon' meant 'hen' and had nothing to do with 'Honourable', as some ignoramuses later thought. (As the children of a baron 'The Hon.' was affixed to our names.) The Honnish Hons were Decca and me; the Horrible Counter Hons were Nancy, Tom and Diana. The Hons' meeting place was the linen cupboard, private and warm. We spent hours sitting on the slatted shelves writing our rules, enlarging Honnish vocabulary and eating Cadbury's cooking chocolate from its blue wrapper, wheedled out of Mrs Stobie in the kitchen. Mrs Stobie was a wonderful cook but, like so many of her profession, prone to moods. We knew by the loudness of the banging of pots and pans how she was feeling and kept out of her way when the decibels rose.

Decca and I were by then in the schoolroom where more serious lessons had succeeded my mother's grounding in reading, writing and sums. I am sorry to say there was not just one governess but a succession of them, and my sisters had already been through a fair few by the time we came on the scene. We were perfectly foul to them and made their lives intolerable, so naturally they left. But awful as we were, some of them were pretty peculiar too and I do not know how they thought they could teach. The usual subjects were a dead loss but one of the governesses, Miss Dell, encouraged us in the difficult art of shoplifting—stealing really. My mother found out (the shopkeepers did not, thank goodness) and Miss Dell disappeared.

Decca and I spent a lot of time answering advertisements and sending off for free samples, anything from shampoo and deodorant to milk powder for babies. Decca let her imagination rip when describing the maladies that affected her non-existent babies and the hopes she held out for the various patented foods and remedies. This made the arrival of the postman, Mr Beckinsale, the highlight of an otherwise dull day. Mr Beck, his waterproof canvas bag slung over one arm, pushed his heavy bicycle up the hill to Swinbrook House. He went straight to the pantry to drink tea and talk to Mabel, while Decca and I hovered until Mabel sorted the post and a little parcel addressed to '*Mrs* Jessica Mitford' appeared (the idea of an unmarried mother was unthinkable). This meant milk powder.

Decca also wrote to the agony aunts of women's magazines with wildly improbable tales, or asking for advice on imagined predicaments. To her delight these were sometimes published. 'Dear Mag, I have a little plum-coloured silk dress which has gone under the arms, the rest of this garment is fine and I am reluctant to throw it away. Please advise. Worried, Swinbrook House, Burford, Oxon.' I often wondered if the recipients of these requests ever guessed that they were from an under-employed eleven-year-old, practising the style which was one day to make her fortune.

*   *   *

The first big change in our everyday lives came in September 1929 when Unity went to boarding school. It had been her dream to join our Mitford and Farrer cousins at St Margaret's, Bushey, a church school in Hertfordshire. As she was so naughty with the governesses (she used to pick up poor Miss Dell, who was rather small, and put her on the sideboard) my parents gave in. She loved the school but her difficult characteristics came to the fore and she was what Nanny would have called 'her own worst enemy', longing to be part of school life but incapable of accepting its rules. To Unity's surprise and sorrow, she was sacked after just over a year. The reason, so she said, was that when reciting 'A garden is a lovesome thing, God wot' she added the word 'rot', but I imagine she also caused general unrest in her class and that the other girls looked on her rebelliousness with some awe. Decca and I were thrilled at the idea of her being expelled but my mother always said, 'No, children, she was asked to leave', as though it was quite different.

Unity going away to school brought rumblings of discontent from Decca, who was just twelve and longed to go to boarding school herself. She became moody and critical, no longer the comical, charming little girl she had been. She kicked against anything conventional and eventually took up the politics of malcontents. Although I had her to myself in term time, I was no good as a confidante as I could not understand, nor had I sympathy for, her longing to escape from home. I was pleased with life and the idea of boarding school was anathema. She opened a 'Running Away' bank account with her pocket money and the Christmas envelopes from aunts and uncles. It was treated as a joke by the rest of us, but to her it was deadly serious.

My older sisters never stopped saying how much they disliked Swinbrook—Nancy called it 'Swinebrook' or 'The Buildings'—and this must have been depressing for Farve. Perhaps because I was completely happy there, he was especially indulgent to me when a new entertainment to enliven Sunday afternoons opened in Oxford: the grand ice-skating rink in the Botley Road. Farve and his younger brother, Uncle Jack, were keen on the Austrian instructresses, known as the Ice Maidens, and they were part of the attraction.

Muv and Farve were already proficient skaters; waltzing and elementary figure skating came easily to them, as they did to me. The afternoons on the ice were sheer joy. I had learnt to skate on a family holiday in Pontresina in 1930. We went over to the

Suvretta House Hotel in St Moritz and I found an unlikely partner in the Conservative statesman Sir Samuel Hoare. We skated together and even gave a little show one afternoon. Back at the Oxford rink, I improved quickly and 'they' (I suppose the 1930s versions of talent spotters) asked Muv if I could be trained for the national junior team. She refused, realizing no doubt that it would be a full-time job. I did not know of this till much later and was sorry not to have had the chance of excelling at something at last.

Our old groom Hooper was my best friend during the Swinbrook years and for a long time afterwards. He had worked for Grandfather Redesdale at Batsford before the war and came back to the family immediately after the Armistice. Farve was aware that he suffered from shellshock after his terrible experiences in the trenches, and that his temper could explode without warning. When Unity's lack of interest in her horse irritated Hooper or when she made some clumsy gesture that frightened it, he would shout, 'I'll take yer in that wood and do for yer!' But he never did. In spite of these outbursts, Muv and Farve trusted him. Ponies and hunting were my passions and it was thanks to Hooper that I was able to enjoy them. As soon as I could escape from lessons I was in the stables watching and learning the daily routine. Hooper was the first of several professionals, whose lives were devoted to country and sport, with whom I felt entirely at home and whose companionship I valued.

One of Hooper's jobs was to drive our horse-drawn float laden with egg boxes twice a week from my mother's chicken farm to the station at

Shipton-under-Wychwood to catch the London train. I went with him and was sometimes allowed to drive. The eggs were packed in wooden boxes that held several trays lined with woolly brown felt, which was all very well until an egg broke. The boxes were padlocked and were treated with respect by the porters, who would have the empties ready for us to take home on the return journey. They had huge labels attached, one addressed to 'Lady Jean Bertie' and the other to 'The Marlborough Club'. I never met Lady Jean Bertie and, of course, never went to the Marlborough Club, but those names are engraved on my memory.

One of these journeys took place on 11 November 1927, nine years after the end of the First World War when memories of that terrible conflict were still vivid. Everyone observed the two-minute silence on Armistice Day. Hooper took out his watch and exactly at 11 a.m. brought the cart to a halt, removed his cap and got down to hold the horse's head. No sooner had he done so than the old mare swayed and fell dead. I suppose she had a heart attack. She had been brought out of the Army at the end of the war, having seen service in France. Her death during the silence made a terrific impression on all us children and Hooper wept for her.

Sunday afternoons meant skating and Saturdays meant hunting. Nothing in this world can touch the latter for excitement: the huntsman's horn, the shiver of the horse that presages something thrilling, the whimper of the first hound to find a fox and the crashing noise when the whole pack joins in—it has been described *ad infinitum*, but nothing comes up to the real thing. My father refused to pay more than £35 for a pony but I was lucky to get one of the best for that. Doughnut was everything to me. We had no horse box so I rode to meets, anything up to eight miles away. Coming home on the Stow–Burford road in horizontal sleet (there was nowhere to shelter) I was sometimes joined by Tony Hardcastle, son of the man who had bought Asthall from my father. When the weather was at its worst and we were soaked through and freezing, he would say that he would come back and haunt the road when he was dead. Driving to Swinbrook now, I look for him as we pass the Merrymouth Inn, but he eludes me.

I was always in love with one or other of the followers of the Heythrop. When I was nine Dermot Daley, who wore a swallow-tailed pink coat out hunting, was the particular attraction and I came home full of tales about him. Nancy tortured me by saying that she had heard that he was head over heels in love with M., a dreary girl who lived near Swinbrook. Nancy was too clever for words and knew exactly how to pick on what I would mind most.

*   *   *

It was at about this time that Nancy fell in love for the first time. Her affair with Hamish St Clair Erskine was never going to lead to marriage but it simmered on—half-heartedly on his side, wholeheartedly on hers—for several years. My parents could not bear him, especially Farve who realized that he was homosexual. Hamish was also a Roman Catholic, had no proper job and was soon banned from the house. Nancy's friends included many who were decidedly effeminate and they were usually disliked by Farve. Among them was Mark Ogilvie Grant. Teetering down to breakfast one morning at the dreaded hour of 8 a.m., he was greeted by my father who made a grand gesture of taking the lid off a sizzling dish, 'Brains for breakfast, Mark, PIG'S THINKERS.' (Familiarity eventually made Farve quite fond of Mark.)

There were several other young men, however, whom Farve could not help liking in spite of his prejudice, and he excused their lack of interest in field sports with, 'Well, I suppose he is a *literary cove.*' Peter Watson, a gentle, innocuous fellow, was one of these. The only telephone at Swinbrook was in Farve's business room and it was his property, not to be used lightly for a chat with a friend and certainly not without Farve's formal consent. If he thought a daughter was taking too long over some arrangement, he cut her short with, 'Put the telephone down, you're paralysing the line.' Peter Watson rang up one day and asked to speak to Nancy. Farve answered the telephone and, without moving the mouthpiece, shouted into the hall, 'Nancy, that hog Watson wants to speak to you.' Poor Peter was Hog from then on.

On another occasion Nancy's friend Mary Milnes-Gaskell came to lunch with her nails painted a dashing blood-red (the first time I had seen newly fashionable nail varnish). My father looked at her. 'I am so sorry,' he said, deadly serious. 'Why?' she asked. 'I am so sorry to see you have been in a bus accident.' As I got older and we moved to smaller houses, I was quite pleased that we did not have room for guests because you never knew what my father would say to make them feel uncomfortable.

By the time she was sixteen Diana longed to be grown up and leave home. She was sent to learn French in Paris where she met the painter Paul César Helleu, a friend of Grandfather Bowles, who had made several portraits of my mother and became an immediate admirer of Diana, the first of many to sit at her feet. Two years later, in 1929, Diana married Bryan Guinness, heir to a brewing fortune. Decca and I missed being bridesmaids because we had whooping cough, but after their marriage we often went to stay with them at beautiful Biddesden House, near Andover. Diana immediately made friends with her neighbours: Robert Byron, a contemporary of Bryan at Oxford, came over from Savernake Forest, Lytton Strachey and Dora Carrington at Ham Spray adored her, as did John Betjeman, Henry and Pansy Lamb, Augustus John's daughter Poppet and her younger sister, Vivian, whom I admired as a rider. All these writers, painters and poets were figures of fascination to Decca and me. One of them, Harold Acton, did something that horrified me. He took a log out into the snow, pretended it was a baby and murdered it. So realistic was his performance that the scene haunted me for years.

The enigmatic Carrington fascinated all who knew her and I too fell under her spell. She gave me some fan-tail pigeons which I treasured. I was interested in botany at the time, with the help of Bentham and Hooker's books on plant classification. One of the volumes described wild flowers in scientific language far beyond my ken, but a thinner one had four line-drawings to a page with every known native variety of flower, tree, grass, fern and sedge in the British Isles. I coloured these in as and when I found them, recording the date and place. Carrington was quite taken with this and I looked on it as a bond between us. She wrote to Lytton saying I had won her by my 'high spirits and charm'. It was certainly mutual and I was sad when, unable to face life after Lytton died, she borrowed a gun from Bryan, ostensibly to hunt rabbits in the garden at Ham Spray, and shot herself. Her death was a terrible loss for Diana who had become very fond of her.

Tom left Eton in 1927 and decided to study music and see something of Europe rather than go to an English university. He travelled to Italy and Spain, and to Austria, where a series of lucky chances took him to Schloss Bernstein in the Burgenland. The castle had been in Hungary until the end of the First World War when it became part of Austria. It was owned by a Hungarian, János Almásy, who became a friend of Tom and had him to stay for several months as a paying guest.

On his return to England in 1929, Tom settled in London to read for the Bar. His friends included the future politicians Nigel Birch, Jack Donaldson and Viscount Hinchingbrooke, Garrett Moore, who, as Lord Drogheda, became chairman of the Royal Opera House, Robert Byron, the writer, and the film producer John Sutro, as well as Jim Lees-Milne and Basil Dufferin—an urbane and talented collection of contemporaries whom Muv called 'the Fat Fairs', as good a description of them as any (with the exception of Garrett Moore who was neither fat nor fair). They started the Worst Play

Club and when the actors saw Tom and his friends sitting in the front row of the stalls, they knew how the young and clever rated their production. Alfred Beit, who was the son of the financier and art collector Sir Otto Beit and who later married our cousin Clementine Mitford, sometimes joined the group. The Club went to Bayreuth and Vienna for opera and concerts (to enjoy, not denigrate) and were amused by Alfred's meanness over small sums of money—'Will you buy the newspaper? I don't want to break into another sixpence'—as he was far better off than most of them.

In summer 1929 Tom took part in an art hoax at Diana and Bryan's London house in Buckingham Street. Two hundred people were invited to meet the self-taught 'artist', Bruno Hat, who came from somewhere in Germany. Brian Howard, the poet, and the artist John Banting produced a series of works on cork bathmats framed with rope— pictures of extraordinary ugliness, forerunners of the kind of thing we are asked to admire today. Evelyn Waugh wrote an introduction to the catalogue, 'An Approach to Hat', and the party was a great success. Guests inspected the paintings, murmuring their appreciation of the avant-garde. Lytton Strachey bought a picture to please Diana. Bruno Hat was in poor health but managed to make an appearance. Pushed in a wheelchair and muffled in scarves, he wore a black moustache and tinted glasses. After uttering a few words of an unknown dialect in guttural growls he was unmasked as Tom, who stepped out of the chair, threw off his coat, moustache and specs, delighted with the success of the joke. (In 2009 one of Bruno Hat's pictures was sold at auction for £18,000—I wish we had kept an outhouse full of them.)

One of Tom's friends was the MP and art collector Philip Sassoon, a highly civilized charmer and host, who in August 1930 asked Tom to stay with him at Port Lympne, his house in Kent. Philip provided an unusual entertainment for his guests: seven small aircraft, one piloted by Philip himself, the rest by professional pilots. Tom recorded the outing in a letter to Muv:

The party consists of Cousin Clementine and Winston, Sir Samuel Hoare & wife, Cousin Venetia [Montagu] and Aircraftsman Shaw [T. E. Lawrence].

I am a little disappointed with Shaw. He looks just like any other private in the air-force, is very short and has in his five years of service become quite hardened. He is not a bit like the Sargent portrait of him in his book. Last night I sat next him at dinner and he had Winston on the other side. Winston admires him enormously. He said at one moment 'If the people make me Prime Minister, I will make you Viceroy of India.' Lawrence politely refused and said he was quite happy in the air-force. When asked what he would do when in five years time he has to leave, he said simply 'Go on the dole I suppose.'

It is curious that he should enjoy such a life, with no responsibilities, after being almost king in Arabia. Some say it is inverted vanity: he would have accepted a kingship, but as he didn't get it, he preferred to bury himself and hide away.

This morning we flew over to see Colonel

Guinness at Clymping, about 80 miles away. We had 7 machines and flew in perfect formation over Brighton and other resorts— very low to frighten the crowd. Lawrence was thrilled at flying: he said the air ministry had stopped him flying a year ago. Winston drove his machine a little way. I hadn't realized that he had done a lot of piloting before the war.

We flew in arrow-head formation

Philip
Winston   Sam Hoare
Me   Lawrence
Venetia   Bryan Thynne
(Each with a pilot)

and landed in the field next door to Diana's cottage . . . It took about an hour getting there, and 3/4 hour back, as we didn't return in formation.

It was amusing flying *very* low on the edge of the sea and jumping the piers at Brighton and Littlehampton—to the astonishment of the people there.

Tom's fellow guests and their aerial expedition sound like something out of a Hollywood production. Few other letters from Tom to my parents have survived and none about politics, which is a pity as I would have loved to have known his thoughts.

Pam never lacked admirers and in 1928 became engaged to Oliver 'Togo' Watney, a neighbour at Swinbrook. My father detested Togo's mother whom he called 'the Witch of Cornbury' (the

Watneys' marvellous house near Charlbury). A London wedding was planned. The dining room was filled with presents—in those days the merest acquaintance sent something—and an oyster-coloured silk trousseau had been ordered. But as the day grew closer it became obvious that Togo would not go through with it. To Pam's disappointment, he broke off the engagement and the piles of presents had to be packed up and returned. My mother, who realized that Togo would not have made Pam happy, was relieved—better to make the break before than after the marriage.

In order to give Pam a complete change of scene, my parents, who were planning to sail for Canada on one of their gold-prospecting trips, decided to take her with them. It was long before ocean liners provided gyms and swimming pools for exercise, and Pam and my parents marched round and round the deck of the big ship, greeting their fellow passengers. 'I would like to introduce you to my cook,' my father said, indicating Pam. They walked on and in due course bumped into the same people. 'I would like to introduce you to my housemaid,' and so on, down the domestic hierarchy each time they met, to the bemusement of their fellow passengers. Pam blossomed at The Shack, the wooden cabin built by my father on land he had staked out. With no domestic help and my parents all to herself for the first time, Pam's innate talents, which were just waiting to be appreciated, came to the fore. On practical matters she always knew best (which was sometimes irritating, especially to Decca and me when we were still of an age to be bossed about).

When they returned, Diana realized that Pam would be at a loose end at Swinbrook and suggested to Bryan that she take charge of the farm at Biddesden. It was a time of agricultural depression and no farms were profitable, but Bryan could afford to run his as a hobby rather than a business. Although she had no formal training, Pam understood intuitively the work involved and did her best to keep expenditure down. She bought replacement stock for the herd of Guernsey dairy cows at local markets. Once in a while she made a bad purchase. We were all treated to her description of how thrilled she had been with a well-bred bargain and her dismay when she got her home and discovered *'the brute was bagless'*—her exaggerated voice rising to a scream. It became a family saying for any failure, and, like many family sayings, found its way into one of Nancy's novels, this time *Wigs on the Green*.

Pam lived in a farm cottage at Biddesden and was independent for the first time. Her car was as important to her as her dogs. She dug deep and bought a rare Italian breed called an OM ('For comfort, Stublow, she's a Rolls') and set off to explore Europe with friends. Her memory for food was remarkable. 'In Austria we had a most wonderful first course. It wasn't a soufflé and it wasn't an omelette, in a dish about that high,' she said, indicating two or three inches with her fingers, 'Oh Stublow, it was SO delicious.' While farming at Biddesden she met John Betjeman, one of Diana's legion of friends. He fell for her and wrote a poem, 'The Mitford Girls', which ended, 'Gentle Pamela/Most rural of them all'. Pam thought John comical in the grubby trousers he bought at a WI jumble sale for a shilling but, although fond of him, she had no thoughts of marriage.

5

Rutland Gate and Old Mill Cottage

When Asthall was sold, Farve bought the lease on a house in London: No. 26 Rutland Gate, Knightsbridge; a big house for a big family. It stood alone, with the graveyard of the Russian Orthodox church on one side and the entrance to No. 4 Rutland Gate Mews, which also belonged to my father, on the other. Opposite was Eresby House, belonging to Lord Ancaster, and from our nursery window I could see the Willoughby girls playing tennis on the two courts in their garden. Our house had nine indoor staff, who came with us from Swinbrook, a ballroom as well as a drawing room and enough bedrooms for all of us (though Decca and I shared). There was a wonderfully unhygienic communication system between each floor. You blew down a mouthpiece with an almighty puff that made the connecting device on another floor fly out with a whistle. With your ear pressed to this dual-purpose mouthpiece, you could hear the caller talking from the floor above or below.

The dining room, the scene of lunches and dinner parties for whichever of us was a debutante at the time, was decorated in the newly fashionable stipple—one of the rare occasions when my mother followed fashion. The drawing room, which had large, south-facing windows, was one of Muv's great successes. Pale grey and gilded, it was furnished with pieces of Grandfather Redesdale's French furniture that had survived the Batsford sale and these gave it an air of importance. Muv sat bolt upright at her *secrétaire à abattant* (a marvellous, plain and perfectly proportioned bit of furniture made by Charles Saunier) from 8.30 a.m. until she had finished her housekeeping chores and accounts. She was very fond of chocolate and in one of the drawers there were always boxes of Terry's langues de chat and chocolate pastilles in their round boxes.

Muv ordered food over the telephone from 'Wicked Old Harrod' (her name for expensive but reliable Harrods), which was delivered a couple of hours later in a silent, electrically driven van. More often she walked to the Brompton Road where she could find Mac Fisheries on a raised pavement with fish of all colours, shapes and sizes displayed in picturesque fashion on miniature icebergs. Muv was always on the lookout for herrings and used to say, 'It's not the price that makes the dish, the herring is the king of fish,' though I suspect the price did make her rather like herring.

Mrs Munro's was well established in Montpelier Street, near the auction house Bonhams, where rolls of good-taste chintz and trimmings were sold. Owles and Beaumont (Owls and Bowels to us, of course) was a decent draper a few doors from Harrods. Muv always started there because it was 'reasonable' but when she could not find what she wanted, she sighed and went back to 'Wicked Old'. Long after the war was over, my sisters and I used

Harrods Bank as a meeting place. Conveniently situated on the ground floor (which is now all marble and make-up), the Bank had green leather chairs and sofas. Our dogs joined the Kensington ladies' Pekes and Poms in the Harrods underground kennels, while we sat above them, chatting and watching the world go by. Sometimes Muv and Aunt Weenie met us there and the real customers stared when we made too much noise. The Bank hosted a carol service every Christmas, where God, Aunt Weenie, Muv and mammon met. I cannot imagine such a performance in Cosmetics now, where supercilious girls sell ultra-packaged face creams.

Tattersalls, the horse auctioneers behind Knightsbridge, was still just going when I was a child. The atmosphere of the place was cleverly evoked by the artist Robert Bevan, whose paintings bring back the clatter of hooves and the horse copers of his time. I wish I had a roomful of Bevans. A pony drew the Express Dairies' milk cart and knew at which houses to stop. It gave Pam's arm a sharp bite one day when she had some sugar for it. When a huge bruise appeared on the night of a dance she tied a satin bow round her arm. Coal and coke were delivered on a long wagon drawn by a Shire horse that wore a canvas nose bag containing oats and chaff—his 'bite'. There was plenty of time for the horse to eat while the men, dressed like Stanley Holloway in *My Fair Lady*, shovelled the fuel down the coal hole. There was a water trough in nearby Knightsbridge so all the Shire's needs were catered for.

The basement of Rutland Gate was the domain of the odd man, Mr Dyer, guardian of the boiler, who received and stacked the fuel to his (and Farve's) satisfaction. Mr Dyer slept by his boiler. I never saw him upstairs nor heard him complain of his subterranean existence. The basement was connected by a door to the garage in the Mews, which was for the cars and chauffeurs that had succeeded carriages, coachmen and grooms. Tom referred to it simply as 'the garage', as though that was all it was, but it had in fact several small, low rooms on the upper floor. My mother made the most of things, as she always did, and the little rooms were transformed by her colours, curtains and covers. During the Season, whenever the main house was let, we retreated to the Mews. Coming home from parties we had to pick our way in long evening dresses between the cars and pools of oil to reach the narrow stairs.

Decca was fascinated by the white slave trade which she had read about in some book. She saw white slavers everywhere and so, of course, did I—half-thrilled and half-repelled at the idea. She was certain that a perfectly innocent fellow living in Rutland Gate was a slaver. 'Why?' asked Muv. 'Well, when Debo and I are taking the dogs out in the morning he looks at us and says "Good morning". He's just waiting his chance to bundle us into a taxi and we'll wake up in South America.' The 'slaver', who carried a rolled umbrella and doffed his black homburg to us on his way to work, turned out to be Anthony Sewell, who later married a daughter of the architect Edwin Lutyens. He was a friend of Nancy, who no doubt told him what Decca thought.

*   *   *

86

The financial crash of 1929 changed our lives drastically. Farve was badly hit and was lucky to find tenants for his houses during those disastrous years. Swinbrook was let to Sir Charles Hambro and Rutland Gate to Mrs Warren Pearl, an American who annoyed my mother by painting everything, including the floors, green. We retreated to the Mews and to Old Mill Cottage in High Wycombe. The cottage had been in the background of our lives ever since I can remember. Grandfather Bowles leased it for my parents and their growing family in 1911 and when he died in 1922 Muv was able to buy it for £1,250. It proved a good investment, a place to go back to whenever money was short, and we came and went according to the state of Farve's finances.

A small, cheerful, rambling house, it was made up of two cottages, joined at right angles around an open yard; the third side was formed by Marsh Green Mill, which was let to Mr Mason, the miller. With its stables, outhouses and big mill pond, it formed a busy, harmonious whole. Our dining room looked out on to the yard where the lorries arrived with sacks of wheat and left with bags of flour. When we overstepped the mark at lunch—and we often did—Muv tried to change the subject by pretending to see the miller out of the window and saying in a languid voice, 'Mr Mason, there you are!' It never worked, but became part of our language.

In the dining room, once a kitchen, Decca and I found a new place for the Hons' meetings: the old brick bread-oven. The cottage had no walk-in linen cupboard like the one at Swinbrook, only useless shelves, so this oven hiding-place was ideal. There Decca and I and the third Hon, Margo Durman, my friend who lived across the road, sat in the dark, giggling and pondering our futures, totally happy away from the grown-ups. No one stopped Margo and me from playing in the loft or on the ladder-like stairs of the mill, whose banisters were as smooth as satin from the thin layer of flour that lay on every surface. No one bothered about the unprotected machinery whirring away and the hundredweight sacks ready to fall on us.

The mill pond was a world of frogs, dragonflies and myriad other summer insects. Across the road were beds of watercress, dark green and deliciously peppery, which grew on gravel in crystal-clear water that flowed from an artesian well. My mother gave the mill pond to the town of High Wycombe. It was what is now described as a 'feature' and she thought the town would like to have it as an adjunct to the Rye, a big open space that had been bequeathed by the Carrington family. She would be dismayed to know that the City Fathers of High Wycombe have thought fit to fill it in.

A large garden, with an orchard and fields beyond, completed the property. The famous Chiltern beeches covered the protecting hill, which was laced with public footpaths and bridleways. It was so different from Swinbrook, where the woods belonged to my father and we never met a soul. Here we often saw what we thought were sinister-looking men walking alone; we called them 'singletons', fully expecting to be murdered by them. A little way along the road was a sewage farm and a sawmill. We imagined that the loud sigh from the saws as they cut up the tree trunks came from the sewage farm—though how those lightweight rotating arms dripping water could have made such a giant sigh, we did not know.

Farve escaped his children and their animals by turning the garden shed into his study. Decca said that it was where his 'old eyes would close for ever', so it became the Closing Room. He thought it perfect—quiet, isolated and full of the ugly furniture that my mother had banned from her domain. The ponies came with us to High Wycombe and my father bought Hooper a house for £480 on a new housing estate just above our field. Hooper used to knock on the window of the Closing Room, push his 'book' under my father's nose, saying, 'Is your Lordship vacant?' My father settled the carefully itemized accounts—linseed hoof oil and the like. Soon after tea he would disappear into the only bathroom, which was in our part of the house, change into his Great Agrippa dressing gown and set off to the Closing Room to luxuriate with the weather forecast and the six o'clock news. At this hallowed moment of the day no one dared disturb him.

Farve had taught himself to crack a stock whip after seeing the American Rodeo at Wembley in 1924 and he practised his skill on the lawn at High Wycombe. The whip had a short, stout stock and a long, plaited cowhide thong which required great strength in the wrist to get it going. Farve stood winding it round and round above his head until it had gathered enough momentum and flew out at full length, making an almighty crack like a rifle shot. To be accurate took skill—it was like fly fishing with a very heavy line. Farve could slice a chosen twig off an apple tree from a distance and told us that experts could knock a cigarette out of the mouth of a brave volunteer.

Our governess at the time was Miss Pratt. She was not interested in education but loved playing cards, especially Racing Demon. We played from 9 a.m. till 11 a.m., had half an hour's break, then more Demon until lunchtime. We became expert at this testing game, which depends on speedy co-operation of hand and eye. My mother discovered what we were doing and Miss Pratt left. There was no time to engage another governess, so Decca and I (aged eleven and nine) were packed off to a day school in Beaconsfield. Every morning at assembly we sang the same hymn: 'For Those in Peril on the Sea'. I asked why. Answer: 'The Head's brother is in the Navy.' I could not imagine why it was so perilous to be in the Navy in peacetime.

Decca liked the school. She was clever and appealing; I was dense and cross, and hated every moment of the crowded world of lessons. I did not understand what the teachers wanted or why. It was made worse by the horrible lunch, to which we said 'No thank you'. My mother was informed and was sympathetic. She persuaded my father to see the headmistress and tell her that we would bring a banana instead. We could rely on Farve when it came to the crunch, and that lunch *was* the crunch. I wish I had been a fly on the wall at the interview between those two people who were both accustomed to getting their own way. My father won and it was bananas from then on.

Decca had acute appendicitis while we were at the Old Mill Cottage and the operation was performed on the nursery table. I was jealous of all the attention paid her and when the stitches came out, she put them up for sale and I bought one for sixpence. (In her memoirs, *Hons and Rebels*, she says she sold her appendix to me for £1, which was impossible as I did not have £1.) Another difficult time was when Muv, aged fifty-seven and not used to being unwell, got measles. She was dangerously ill but the only evidence was a sheet dipped in disinfectant every few hours and hung over her bedroom door. In spite of these precautions, I caught the disease (the only one in the house who did) and although not as ill as my mother, I remember having to spend Christmas in bed.

6

Back to Swinbrook

By April 1931, Farve's finances had improved enough for us to return to Swinbrook. For me this meant freedom to go riding again without meeting anyone, to fish on the Windrush and follow Farve on his rounds of the woods and farms. In the schoolroom, Decca and I had Miss Hussey, another product of the PNEU system and by far the best teacher we ever had. Each term we had to learn a hymn, a psalm and a poem, and at the end of term we recited our choices to Muv—and anyone else who would listen. It was normally easy to bamboozle a new governess; we simply turned the pages of the relevant book till we came up with the pieces we had learned the previous term (the hymn book fell open readily at 'Now the Day is Over') and off we went. My mother never noticed the repetition but when Miss Hussey arrived there was no fooling her and, to our annoyance, she made us learn new pieces. My poem was 'The Lament of the Irish Emigrant' by Selina Dufferin. The first lines, 'I'm sittin' on the stile, Mary/Where we sat side by side/On a bright May mornin' long ago/When first you were my bride', made me cry, but I learnt to look on it as a game and was able to go on—just. Decca chose Edgar Allan Poe's 'Annabel Lee', which she spouted at a tremendous rate, running all the words into one. There were so-called exams at the end of the summer term but I often managed to have flu at the appointed time. Luckily Muv was not interested in exams.

In 1932 our ordered life received a shock when after four years of marriage Diana left Bryan for Sir Oswald Mosley. Sir O had been a political figure since the age of twenty-one, first as a Conservative and then as a Labour MP. He had resigned in 1930 because of his disillusionment with Ramsay MacDonald's failure to deal with unemployment. Supremely confident that he himself had the answers to Britain's economic problems, he was about to launch the British Union of Fascists when he and Diana met.

Muv and Farve did not talk about Diana in front of us younger children; it was not the way then—any disagreeable subject was discussed privately. I was conscious of some pall of sorrow and anger affecting my parents, but was barely aware of the reason. Sir O was married with three young children and had no intention of leaving his wife. My parents were dismayed when Diana openly became his mistress and were shocked that Bryan was named the guilty party in her divorce. Bryan went through the motions of spending a night with a prostitute in a Brighton hotel, which in those days was how many divorces were arranged, but Muv and Farve considered it dishonest. Bryan was miserable about the separation—nothing could have been further from his wishes—but Diana was a forceful character and had decided on her future. My parents continued to see her and her two Guinness sons, Jonathan and Desmond, and she often came to Swinbrook, spending Christmas with us there in 1934. But Decca and I were not allowed to visit her at her house in Eaton Square because she was 'living in sin' (now so ordinary—you 'take a partner' as though going into business). It never occurred to us to question Muv and Farve's wishes and it is why I did not get to know Diana until after the war.

In April 1932 Tom qualified as a barrister and was called to the Bar. He began the slow process of getting briefs and making a name for himself in the chambers of Norman Birkett KC. He had many girlfriends. The first, Penelope (Pempie) Dudley Ward, was the prettiest, most lively and charming girl imaginable. They were both too young to think of marriage but remained friends until Tom's death. He moved on to more sophisticated women, most of whom were married and did not threaten his independence. They never came to Swinbrook, for obvious reasons, and Tom was discreet about his private life. Diana knew of his various friendships but she was not one to betray confidences.

Nancy was leading her unsettled life, staying away with willing hosts but still dependent on my parents for a home. She began writing, at first short articles for *The Lady*, which had been handed on by Grandfather Bowles to Uncle George. Her usual fee was £2 and sometimes £3, which caused much rejoicing. Articles for *Vogue* and *Harper's Bazaar* followed but they did not provide a regular income. Things were made more difficult by Farve's passionate dislike of any reference to us in the papers, so Nancy had to hide these whenever she had anything published. In 1931 her first novel, *Highland Fling*, was well received by the reading public and brought in a little more money. Decca and I were excited to see the finished book and thought the portrait of Farve as General Murgatroyd highly comical. There was a pile of the book at W. H. Smith in High Wycombe with a big notice announcing 'Local Authoress', which we also thought funny.

Nancy's rocky affair with Hamish Erskine dragged on, but after four years he grew tired of what was for him a charade and he broke it off by telling Nancy he was engaged to someone else. Nancy may have half expected it, but it was nevertheless a cruel blow. Diana understood her miserable existence and gave her a room at Eaton Square. Almost at once Nancy met Peter Rodd. It was a classic case of the rebound, but she believed herself to be truly in love. I wrote in my diary on 14 July 1933 that Nancy had sent me the most extraordinary letter, and that I could hardly believe it. In it she said that she was 'perhaps' going to be married to 'a very choice' person and wanted me to be the first to know. 'I love him a most terrific lot,' she wrote. 'If we can get some money we shall marry, and if we can't we shan't and that's why it's an important secret because if we don't it's a bore if everyone knows.' I am afraid I told Miss Hussey and Decca, but swore them to secrecy so that when Nancy announced the news they would pretend they knew nothing.

I liked Peter. He talked to me as he would to a grown-up, which was unusual—at thirteen you were still considered very much a child. The wedding was an excitement for Decca and me, particularly after missing Diana's. I thought carefully about what to wear and decided on a midnight-blue velvet dress. The stuff, as always, came from John Lewis, and Gladys, my mother's retired maid who ran up our clothes, did her best. The dress was to have a fur collar made from an unknown creature with jaws that snapped on to its tail to fasten it. It had been given to me by an aunt and I thought it most glamorous. I proudly showed it to Nancy a few days before the wedding. 'Oh,' she said, 'I see you've got a mouse's skin at last.' Down went self-esteem once more and furs were 'mouse's skins' thereafter.

Nancy and Peter went to live at Rose Cottage, Strand-on-the-Green, near Chiswick. It seemed an idyllic start but it was not long before the marriage began to falter. Nancy did her best to keep up appearances but Prod, as she called Peter, was no good at marriage—he lived from hand to mouth, never held down a job and disappeared for long periods. After the outbreak of war things got worse. He started bringing drunken pick-ups back from the pub who were prone to steal any money left around. Nancy was miserable.

After leaving St Margaret's, Unity briefly attended Queen's College in London. She enjoyed it but, once again, was asked to leave. Years later I met one of her school friends and asked why. 'Because she plucked her eyebrows,' was the reply. It is more likely that Unity's huge personality was too much for the staff. She 'came out' in 1932 and Decca described her in this her first year of grown-up life as 'a rather alarming debutante'. The round of dances took place and Unity went as was expected. Legend has it that she sometimes took her rat, but legends cannot be relied upon.

Her great new friend was Mary Ormsby Gore and they used to meet under the clock at Selfridges to go to the cinema. Unity was always punctual, Mary always late. Unity said she got flat feet from waiting but that it was worth it. She adored the cinema and often went to the Empire in Leicester Square as soon as it opened in the morning, and sometimes stayed to watch the whole programme through two or three times. She invited friends to spend the weekend at Swinbrook who were called the 'Saturday afternooners' by my mother, because by that time Unity was bored with them and poor Muv had to entertain them as best she could for the rest of their stay. One or two remained friends, among them the writer Micky Burn, a stalwart defender of the alarming debutante.

Unity first went to Germany in 1933 with Diana, who had been invited by Hitler's press chief, Putzi Hanfstaengl, with the promise that he would introduce her to the newly appointed Chancellor. Both Diana and Unity were enthralled by the wave of enthusiasm that was gripping Germany, but for

Unity National Socialism came as a call. In adolescence her difficult character had been waiting for just such an outlet and now that she had found one, she threw herself into it with religious fervour. She saw in Hitler the saviour of a country that had been humiliated by defeat, whose economy was in ruins and whose people were demoralized. Germany took up her whole being. With her blonde hair and blue eyes, Unity even embodied the Nazi ideal of womanhood and her classic face, till now always serious in photographs, was suddenly lit from within. Having discovered that Hitler often lunched or dined at the Osteria Bavaria, a small restaurant in Munich, she went there day after day in the hopes of seeing him. (She would be arrested as a stalker today.) In February 1935, Hitler eventually noticed her and sent someone across the room to invite her to his table. It sealed her fate.

Unity's life has been gone over by journalists and biographers, but they often miss the fact that she was not the only English girl to fall for National Socialism. Her uncompromising nature took her to further extremes than most but there were many other girls who, like her, were sent to Germany as part of their education and were swept up by the movement. Away from home for the first time and hungry for new experiences, they were almost without exception fascinated by what they saw and thrilled by the excitement that surrounded Hitler. At their impressionable age, the music and glamour were infectious. Among these girls was our cousin Clementine Mitford who struck up a close friendship with an SS officer (an episode in her life that was conveniently forgotten after her marriage to Alfred Beit).

Decca left home when she was sixteen to learn French in Paris with her best friend and cousin, Ann Farrer. I imagine Muv and Farve debated as to what to do with me now that I was the only one left in the schoolroom. Money was becoming a worry once again and it was less expensive for me to go as a weekly boarder to a school in Oxford than to have a governess. One of my great friends, Lilah McCalmont, was already at the school, which would have made everything easier. Unluckily she was ill at the start of the autumn term, so off I went alone. The school was in the Banbury Road where it occupied two gaunt Victorian houses—a couple of rabbit warrens with no escape. It was crowded with pupils who greeted each other like a Joyce Grenfell reunion, ignoring the new girl who had no idea of what to do or where to go. At the age of fourteen, I felt at home with animals but was nervous of people, and this building crammed with strangers was the worst kind of misery.

The house smelt strongly of lino, girls and fish. The smell flowed up the stairs and lodged under the ceiling of the attic room that I shared with Lilah's empty bed. I was miserable—no dog, no pony, no Nanny. Supper the first night was cod, encased in a thick blanket of black skin—horrible to look at and revolting to taste. The second night it was hot blackberries. Even now, over three-quarters of a century later, I can still smell those hateful suppers. I arrived at the school on a Wednesday and went home for the weekend on Friday. By that time I had fainted in geometry, failed to understand the point of netball and been sick several times. Muv kept me at home for a few days and I begged her not to send me back to that hell-hole. We came to a compromise: I would go back for the rest of the term (it was already paid for and it was too late to make other arrangements) but as a day girl.

So it was me instead of the eggs that arrived at Shipton Station every morning for the stopping train to Oxford, and came back at teatime—both journeys in the dark. I have never ceased to be thankful to Muv for allowing it. My aunts and most of her friends said it would be the ruin of me, 'So *spoilt*, that girl will be impossible.' But Muv stuck to the plan and I survived. At the end of that awful term, she understood that another experiment at another school would end in more tears, so Miss Frost, a nice, steady governess, came to teach me. Celia Hay, the daughter of friends of Muv, joined me and we did lessons together.

*   *   *

In 1935 Farve's money worries came to a head. Swinbrook House and its estate were extravagances he could not afford, and in April the house was let to Duncan and Pamela Mackinnon. Three years later it was sold to them, together with all the land. I minded more than I can say. I have seen it happen elsewhere, when children are uprooted from the place they love just when they are at their most vulnerable, when all their antennae are out and they have become almost physically attached to a house and its surroundings: the loss of all that is familiar is a kind of amputation. As one who becomes hopelessly addicted to sticks and stones, gateways with their ruts and puddles, anthills, thrushes, freshwater springs, kingcups, dog roses and may (soon to be hips and haws), wood anemones under oaks, silent woods in August, milk-white walnuts in autumn, the smell of new creosote on chicken houses, saddle soap and horse manure—having to abandon all these made leaving Swinbrook, 'the land of lost content', hard to bear.

The prospect of the upheaval no doubt occupied my parents for months beforehand. This time there could be no compromise: it was hard cash—or the lack of it—which decided the sale. Unhappy myself, it never occurred to me how much Farve must have minded the finality of losing the last link with his father's Oxfordshire legacy. Unity understood and wrote to him in May 1935, 'Poor old Forge, I AM sorry you have had to leave Swinbrook . . . I'm sorry for myself too because although I didn't like living there, it was lovely to come back to. But I do think it's dreadful for you.'

After leaving Swinbrook, we moved between London and High Wycombe. I went to the Monkey Club, a 'finishing school' off Sloane Street, for a few months. It was not a domestic-science kind of place: we attended lectures on politics, history, art and the other subjects thought necessary to be tucked away in our bird brains for future reference. I met Georgina (Gina) Wernher, who became a friend for life through shared interests, including a passion for hunting; and the beautiful Ayesha of Cooch Behar, who later married the Maharaja of Jaipur and pursued a political career in her own country, surviving a spell in prison in the 1970s. I planned to marry all the Maharajas in

India and, failing that, the President of Turkey with the irresistible name of Mustafa Kemal Atatürk.

Lessons over at last, I lived for pleasure. I refused to go to Paris to learn French, horrified at the idea of missing a season's hunting, and never did learn the language. The only time I minded this uncivilized gap was when I was invited to a grand dinner in Paris years later and sat next to Georges Pompidou. He could not (or would not) speak English. We smiled at each other and crumbled bread for what seemed an endless evening. Our host, Nancy's friend Gaston Palewski, sat opposite and was highly amused—I think he may have done it as a joke.

I spent the winter of 1936–7 with Aunt Weenie and Uncle Percy Bailey in their tiny cottage at Maugersbury by Stow-on-the-Wold, and hunted twice a week with the Heythrop. Hooper and my horse lodged in Stow. He rode down in the morning, stopped outside my bedroom window— which was the same height as he was on the horse—and we discussed plans. It was out hunting that I first met Derek Jackson and became fascinated by this strange being who rode unruly thoroughbreds with short leathers, like the jockey he aspired to be. The older, steadier followers of the hounds were deeply suspicious of him. Derek owned some steeplechasers, trained by Bay Powell, which he often rode himself and I persuaded Pam to take me to Windsor races where I knew Derek would be riding. They fell in love and were married in December 1936. I was mortified, having decided that in a few years I would marry Derek myself.

While Pam and Derek were on honeymoon his

identical twin, Vivian, was killed in a sleigh accident in St Moritz. Derek never recovered from this tragedy. Not only did the brothers look alike and talk alike, they both loved riding, had a total disregard of what others thought of them and followed the same scientific speciality— spectroscopy. I only once saw them together. 'I agree with Derek,' 'I agree with Vivian,' I heard them repeat, with a quack and a grunt for emphasis, in hoarse and breathless voices that seemed to emerge—all passages to the nose closed—from deeper throats than anyone else's.

Pam's marriage brought happiness to begin with, though being married to Derek was never an easy proposition. He was vital, generous, courageous, bisexual, unfaithful, unpredictable, rich—and therefore able to indulge every whim—and he was also rude and loved to shock. He must have been an embarrassing companion at times and Pam was witness to many scenes. They were at Paddington Station one day to catch a train to Oxford and found all the doors into the first-class carriages locked—the kind of incompetence that drove Derek into a rage. They had to walk along the platform and through a third-class carriage to find their seats. Derek waited till the train had got up steam then pulled the communication cord. The brakes went on and the express train ground to a halt. The guard entered their carriage but before he had time to speak, Derek held up his right hand, his pale suede glove blackened by the dirty chain. He told the guard that it was a disgrace to the GWR and that the glove must be taken and cleaned immediately. On another occasion he was riding in a race at Sandown Park and, not unusually for him, committed an infringement of some rule. He was had up before the stewards who fined him £20. Derek handed the chief steward a £100 note and told him to keep the change.

Derek worked at the Clarendon Laboratory in Oxford under Professor Lindemann and lectured at Oxford University. He and Pam lived at Rignell, an undistinguished twentieth-century house built of the almost orange stone that is quarried on the borders of Oxfordshire and Warwickshire. The furniture came from Heal's and Derek's fine collection of Impressionist paintings decorated the walls. Pam added her own touches and persuaded him to buy a hauntingly romantic picture by Corot of a pool in a wood, the shimmering green of the trees reflecting mysteriously in the water. She also reigned in the garden and on the farm. Her naturally calm nature could alter in a flash if anyone was thoughtless with the animals. In the great frost of 1940, when the farmhands had been called up, a couple of lads were left in charge of the cattle and horses. Pam found the tank that supplied water to the heifers frozen solid. 'Oh,' shrugged the boy looking after the cattle, 'they're all right, they'll lick the ice.' 'How do *you* know?' Pam exploded, *'you've* never been an in-calf heifer.'

I will never be sure whether Pam's professed dislike of children sprang from her unhappiness at being childless. We never spoke of it, but it was obvious that Derek did not want children. When she became pregnant, he took her to the north of Norway and drove for miles over bumpy roads with the inevitable result of a miscarriage. Her dogs, which Derek also adored, took the place of children. Trudy, the first of her long-haired dachshunds, was a special favourite and Pam's highest praise for anything, human or animal, was, 'just like the little dog herself'.

*   *   *

In April 1936 Muv took Unity, Decca and me on a Hellenic cruise aboard the SS *Letitia*. The purpose was Education. An impressive list of lecturers was advertised, including Sir Mortimer Wheeler, director of the London Museum at the time, and all was set for an uplifting fortnight round Greece with stops in Turkey and Asia Minor. We thought a cruise was for fun and romance and we treated it accordingly. On the first night Muv called us to her cabin. 'Now, children,' she said, 'we must all stick together.' What a hope. Decca fastened on to an unsuspecting fellow called Lord Rathcreedan, half-hero, half-butt. I expect he was suitably embarrassed by her attentions but equally intrigued. Unity discovered a political adversary in the Duchess of Atholl, a small dark woman known as the Red Duchess because of her support for the Spanish Republicans. She looked as if she had never enjoyed herself or laughed in her life. Towards the end of the fortnight, for the entertainment of the passengers, she and Unity had a political set-to on the platform used by the lecturers.

There was one man we took against. He had a beard, wavy fair hair and wore a hairnet on trips ashore. 'He looks like a chicken,' Decca said, and so the Chicken Man he was.

Heaven, I'm in heaven
And my heart beats so that I can hardly speak
And I seem to find the happiness I seek
When I'm out with the Chicken Man
Dancing beak to cheek

Decca sang, looking straight at him, getting as close as she dared.

I want my wings about you
The things about you
Will carry me through to heaven ...

We named one of the distinguished academics who we wished were not on board 'the Lecherous Lecturer', for no reason other than we liked the alliteration. (In *Love in a Cold Climate* Nancy turned him into Boy Dougdale, who did have a taste for young girls.) We were always playing with words. 'In a way', was 'in an Appian way' to me and Decca. It did not mean anything, it just seemed to suit.

I found a handsome man on board called Adrian Stokes, 'incredibly old, over thirty', I wrote in my diary. He looked like a blond eagle and I fell for him. He was a painter, art critic and ballet-lover, and when I got back to London he took me to Covent Garden to see the Ballets Russes. We saw Léonide Massine and the three 'baby ballerinas', Tamara Toumanova, Irina Baronova and Tatiana Riabouchinska, and Alexandra Danilova in *Symphonie Fantastique, Shéhérazade* and *L'Après-midi d'un Faune* and, my favourite of all, *La Boutique Fantasque*. At sixteen, I was not allowed to go out alone with a man so Nanny Blor came as chaperone. Goodness knows what Adrian (or Nanny) made of this, but it was the rule, take it or leave it, and luckily for me Adrian took it. Fixed in my memory is the 10 p.m. delivery of letters at Rutland Gate. I was always hoping for one from Adrian and used to sit in the hall ten minutes before the post was due. When, absolutely to time, a loving letter fell on the mat, squashed between Hansard and various circulars addressed to my parents, it was unbelievably exciting.

One of the *Letitia*'s last ports of call was Constantinople, to see the Blue Mosque and other necessities. The highlight was a visit to Topkapi Palace where two pathetic eunuchs were on show to the tourists. The idea was to get them to talk in their squeaky voices. When we got back to the ship, Muv summoned us to her cabin. 'Now, children,' she said very slowly, 'you are NOT to mention those eunuchs at dinner.' We dined every night at the Purser's table and the poor fellow must have had enough of us.

My father had taught me to drive a car when I was nine. We went into the big, flat field at Swinbrook called the Prairie and I was put through the paces of gears, accelerator, brake and clutch. The movement called 'double declutching' was easily mastered when there was no traffic and only endless grass to drive over. My father was extraordinarily patient (he was not, however, entrusted with teaching my mother to drive—one of my sisters had to do that) and the result of his tutorials was that I passed my test on my seventeenth birthday. The examiner seemed to be on my side. We drove down a lane and he asked, 'What does that sign mean?' 'Sorry,' I said, 'I don't know.' 'Do you think it's a humpback bridge?' 'Oh, *yes*,' I said, 'a humpback bridge,' which indeed it was. I have a feeling examiners would not be so helpful now.

High on the list of places I loved going to was Cliveden, the Astors' palace overlooking the River Thames. The younger sons of the house, Michael and Jakie, were two of the funniest, most attractive fellows I knew. I whizzed over from High Wycombe in the new freedom of my third-hand Austin Seven, a ramshackle object that looked a bit odd parked next to the Royces in the forecourt at Cliveden. But it got me there and that is surely the point of a car. The huge house, the very height of luxury, was arranged for the comfort and pleasure of its guests: flowers such as I had never seen— young apples trees covered in blossom, and jardinières full of pelargoniums arranged in blocks of colour; a vast red velvet sofa in front of the hall fire, big enough for several people to sleep in; the white- and gold panelled dining room, imported lock, stock and barrel from Madame de Pompadour's dining room at the Château d'Asnières. Adding to the continual excitement was the uncertainty of whom I might sit next to and what on earth I would talk to them about. Mr Lee was the king of butlers and the superb food was handed round at speed. At a crowded Sunday lunch, Lord Astor's valet, Mr Bushell, helped at table. He was unable to resist a grumble and when handing the soufflé to Jakie, I heard him say in a loud whisper, 'Life's a bugger, Mr Jakie.'

Nancy Astor was the star. Small, upright and sharp as a needle, she was a born entertainer— often at someone else's expense. She would fix her ice-blue eyes on her victim and stop them dead in their tracks. A dreary educationalist from the Midwest was droning on and on until she cut him off with, 'That's very interestin'' (a Virginian, she dropped her g's) 'but I'm not interested.' She was the first woman to take her seat in the House of Commons and was heckled one day by another Member. 'Why don't you think before you speak?' he jeered. 'How do I know what I think till I've heard what I've said?' came her quick reply.

She was always kind to me, perhaps because she saw me as no threat to any of her four sons. They had many serious girlfriends to whom she could be unfriendly, but I was never one of them and I loved her. Michael and Jakie pricked any pompous bubble coming from the mouths of the motley crew of politicians, writers, clergy and royal people who gathered at Cliveden. They both became MPs after the war, if rather unwilling ones. Michael had a safe seat in Surrey which he treated in cavalier fashion, disappearing for months at a time. His Chairman needed him on urgent business one day, but no one knew where he was. Eventually he turned up and got a ticking-off, to which he retorted, 'You must take me as you find me—if you can find me.' I was lucky to have been an extra in the theatrical performance that was Cliveden in those days.

The rules of the game of staying in other people's houses were incomprehensible to those who had not experienced them. They were brought home to me when I spent a glorious winter week with Gina Wernher at Thorpe Lubenham in Leicestershire. Her mother, Lady Zia, was a great-granddaughter of Tsar Nicholas I and her father, Sir Harold Wernher, was Master of the Fernie

Hounds. I was lent two superb horses, a revelation of what tip-top hunters could be. To lend a horse is always risky and I was flattered to be trusted with these two beauties. The niceties of behaviour meant that you simply proffered grateful thanks for this generosity, but should you need a stamp (cost 11/2d) you must pay for it. You may not use the telephone or send a telegram, unless you had broken your neck or some other disaster (in which case you must pay for the call). You may not leave your car right by the front door, nor should you lock it or take the key as this would be a slur on the honesty of the household. As a female, the downstairs lavatory was strictly out of bounds.

Nearly all my contemporaries smoked, which was not only acceptable, it was usual. I did not as Farve forbade it. Food fads did not exist or were certainly not discussed. The idea of answering a dinner invitation with a note of what you could or could not eat would have been preposterous and did not happen. Punctuality was essential and you must not keep the grown-ups waiting. You must try to talk to your dinner neighbours and not sit hunched, silent and hidden under a canopy of long hair (like the girls of the next generation). The status of an unmarried girl was low but as soon as she married, even if only eighteen, she qualified as a chaperone. All very odd, but that is how it was in 1937.

At Castle Howard there were no grown-ups. The parents of Christian, Mark, George, Christopher and Katie Howard had died by the time I first went there. (My mother told me that their father, Geoffrey Howard, had a glass eye and used to surprise people by tapping it with a fork at meals.)

The freedom of being able to say and do what you liked was rare in those days of convention. At Castle Howard the rules were there for breaking and we had riotous fun in that glorious house with no one to tell us to stop. Mark, two years older than me and my great friend in the family, was handsome in spite of a broken nose, clever, and with an infectious enthusiasm that made him popular wherever he went. His rambunctious family was full of wild Stanley blood, and Liberal politics and religion were subjects of fierce argument under Vanbrugh's roof. There were Bonham-Carters and Toynbees galore, intellectuals and politicians in the making, all arguing, with Christian, aged twenty, the eldest of the group, shouting to be heard above the din, and spitting in her hurry to get out her words. She became a Lay Canon and was active in bringing about the ordination of women—no doubt she would have been the first female Archbishop had she lived fifty years later.

*   *   *

Decca did the Season in 1935. She said she 'rather guiltily' enjoyed it, but it was obvious that she was longing to get away from home and begin a life of her own with people who shared her strengthening left-wing convictions. Perhaps she was jealous of Unity, who by this time had made friends with the German leaders, and her success may have driven Decca further into the opposite camp. Muv saw it all and understood Decca's unhappiness. She cast around for something to engage her attention and decided to take us both on a world cruise. It was an example of her concern for each of us when we most needed it—I am sure she did not want to go for herself but thought it would fill a gap for Decca. To make it even more fun, she suggested that Decca bring a friend, so Virginia Brett, a fellow debutante, was invited to come too.

In January 1937 Decca went to stay for a weekend with a cousin, Dorothy Allhusen, where she met another cousin, eighteen-year-old Esmond Romilly. He had run away from Wellington and had already seen action fighting for the International Brigade in the Spanish Civil War, and was planning to return. For Decca it was love at first sight; romance and ideals rolled into one. It was the perfect match at the perfect time—except that the world cruise was now nearly upon us. How could she go to Spain with Esmond and escape into her dream? Esmond devised a cunning plan. They forged a letter purporting to come from Mamaine Paget, a debutante friend of Decca, in which they pretended that Decca had been invited on a motoring tour of northern France with Mamaine and her twin sister. This tempting invitation was for two weeks, so Muv would be reassured that she would be back in good time for the cruise. Muv was completely taken in and, even though it was cutting it fine, she wanted Decca to enjoy herself. Perhaps we also looked forward to two weeks without her discontented presence in the house.

On 7 February Muv and Farve saw Decca off at Victoria Station to catch the boat train to Dieppe, where she was to join the Pagets. Or so they thought. After waving goodbye to her, my father never saw her again. The plan was for Decca to meet Esmond on the train and for them to make their way together to Paris to obtain a Spanish visa for Decca. When they arrived, however, they were told they would have to apply in London. In Dieppe, while waiting for the ferry to take them back to England, they discovered that the fictitious address that Decca had given Muv actually existed. There were letters waiting for them and Decca was able to answer a letter from Muv, sending her news of the imaginary sights she had seen in France.

While she was in London, Decca composed another letter to Muv telling her that she had run away with Esmond and asked Peter Nevile, a friend of Esmond, to deliver it to Rutland Gate when instructed. By this time Esmond had fallen in love with Decca and they decided to head for Spain, visa or no visa, and get married. In mid-February Decca wrote to Muv from Bayonne (hundreds of miles from where she was supposed to be) saying that she was staying with the twins longer than expected, but would be back by 20 February at the latest. Muv had a premonition that all was not as it should be. She rang a Paget aunt in London and learned that the twins were in Austria. Decca had vanished. My parents had no idea where she had been for the last fortnight or how to begin to find her. They were desperate.

Rutland Gate was like a morgue. No gramophone. No one laughed. We talked quietly when we did talk, going over the same old ground again and again. Where had she gone? And why? Was she alive? Someone sat permanently by the telephone. Farve contacted Scotland Yard and the Foreign Office. Decca was a missing person. On 23 February, after what seemed an eternity, Peter

Nevile arrived at Rutland Gate with Decca's letter. 'Worse than I thought,' said Farve when he read it. 'Married to Esmond Romilly.' Peter Nevile tried to persuade Farve to give him a story to sell to the newspapers (Decca and Esmond were short of money) but Farve was disgusted by the idea and sent Peter packing.

Muv wrote immediately to Decca at her last known address in Bayonne, begging her to come home. The web of deceit was as much a blow to my parents as her actual disappearance. In the hopes that it might help find her, Farve gave an interview to the *Daily Express* and a full-page article appeared headed, 'PEER'S DAUGHTER OF 17 ELOPES. SPAIN SEARCH'. It carried a picture of me instead of Decca. Tom advised us to have the paper up for libel, which we did, and the case was settled out of court. I was awarded damages of £1,000 on the grounds that the article had put me out of the marriage market for the rest of my life, but even this unexpected windfall meant little to me. I had lost my old Hen. I adapted Harry Roy's song 'Somebody Stole my Gal' to 'Somebody stole my Hen/Somebody stole my Hen/Somebody came and took her away/She didn't even say that she was leavin'.' Too true.

Decca and Esmond were traced to Bilbao. Peter Rodd came up with the idea of making Decca a ward in chancery so that she could be extradited legally and placed under court supervision, which indeed happened. Nancy and Peter went to France to try to persuade her to come home but without success. Soon after this, Muv made the journey to Bayonne where Esmond and Decca were now living. Decca told her that she was pregnant and when Muv got home she persuaded Farve and the judge that the marriage should go ahead.

I did not go to her wedding. There was a long-standing plan for me to visit Florence after the now-abandoned cruise, with Margaret Ogilvy, my much-loved cousin, to learn some Italian and see the sights. My parents said I should stick to the arrangement. Perhaps they were sparing me an emotional meeting with Decca after the nightmare of her elopement, perhaps they were afraid that the press might fasten on to me for a story. Her disappearance was devastating and severed the deep ties of childhood for ever. Although fears for her safety were now in the past, a mixture of misery and anger was still very much with me. Looking back, I realize that Decca could not have told me about Esmond and her plans as it would have put me in an impossible position, but at the time I could not see it. So I went to Florence. My diary tells of the famous galleries, museums and buildings, and of our visits to San Gimignano, Padua and Siena. If we had seen the Palio, the horse race round the Piazza del Campo in Siena, I might have taken some notice, but the memories I have of this slice of my education are of delicious bread and coffee and little else.

Decca and Esmond were married in Bayonne on 18 May 1937. Esmond's mother, Nellie Romilly, and Muv were present. Muv wrote to me that afternoon:

My Darling Stubby,
    There has not been a minute to write till now . . . this morning Decca came early & we had a great rush to get her ready in time for the

114

wedding at 12 o'clock. I took a silk dress from Harrods for her to be married in and we bought a hat and brown coat and brown shoes and gloves in about half-an-hour. She looked very nice in all her new clothes and Nellie had brought a suit for Esmond and he looked quite smart too & a red carnation in his buttonhole. There was quite a small crowd outside and of course the frightful newspaper men with cameras. The *Daily Express* man of course surpassed himself and said to me could he ask me when our consent was given to the wedding. I said yes he could ask but that I should not answer.

The one thing that really delighted little D[ecca] was the gramophone. She talked of it the whole time, how wonderful it would be to have it to play. It is a very nice one, it is supposed to be a 'club' from you and Bobo. It cost about £7 or a little less and there is a nice case for the records. I think they are leaving here tomorrow & going to Dieppe for a week or a fortnight. It will be very nice for them to have a change. They are evidently very happy together and I feel much happier about them . . .

All love darling,
Muv

The letter illustrates Muv's selflessness and the effort she made to give her blessing to 'Little D' and Esmond. She travelled to Bayonne (third class no doubt) laden not just with a dress for Decca, but with Unity's and my present of a gramophone and heavy records as well.

After the wedding Muv joined Margaret and me in Florence, and we went on from there to Venice. After a few days Margaret had to go back to Florence to finish the term. I was sad to see her go. Had she been allowed to stay with us, she would have had some unforgettable experiences instead of stumping round picture galleries with a well-meaning but dull Italian hostess who had done it thousands of times before.

Muv and I set off through Austria, taking the train to the Burgenland to stay at Kohfidisch with Countesses Jimmy (confusingly, a woman—Joanna) and Baby (Francesca) Erdödy. Tom had fallen under Baby's spell when he was living in Austria and they had been fond of each other for some time. The sisters collected us at the station in the local version of a shooting brake drawn by a pair of horses, and we drove along the tracks through endless woods to their house. It gave us a taste of the size of some of the great Central European estates—those that had managed to survive the fall of Austria-Hungary and the First World War. Jimmy said something surprising, but in such a matter-of-fact voice that it sounded as if it happened all over the place, 'My father was also the father of a number of the people who work here.' I suppose the *droit de seigneur* lasted in those parts of Europe longer than elsewhere and she took it absolutely for granted. I looked at the farm workers and stable staff with renewed interest.

After two nights with the Erdödys we went on to Schloss Bernstein, where Tom had spent contented months with the Almásys. I had never seen such beautiful country: from the terrace of the ancient castle we had a view across half of Europe and I understood why Tom was so enchanted by the place. The morning of our arrival, our host, János Almásy, was arrested for being a suspected Nazi sympathizer. He did not return until 10.30 p.m. that night and was told to report to the police the next morning, so I barely saw him.

From Bernstein, our lightning tour took us to Vienna for a night and on to Salzburg, where Unity met us in her little car and drove us to Munich. On the way we stopped at Königssee, where Unity telephoned to see if Hitler was in his house at Berchtesgaden. The answer came back that he was in Munich, which we reached the following day. I described our arrival in my diary:

7 June 1937
We went straight to Hitler's flat to see if he was there & as there were two soldiers outside we knew that he was, so we rushed to the Osteria Bavaria where they said that he had left 5 minutes before, so we rushed back to his flat & saw his cars all being prepared for him to go to Berchtesgaden. We left our car down a side street & Bobo & I rushed across the square to his house. One of the guards said 'Wait in the hall' so we went in & after a bit someone came down & said 'Hitler would like you to come up' so Bobo & I went up & she was shaking all over & the door of his room was opened & there he was standing there. He seemed very pleased to see Bobo & she introduced me & we all three went & sat on some chairs by the window. He isn't very like his photos, not nearly so hard looking. Soon Muv came up & tea was brought in & we all went to wash in his

bathroom & he had some brushes there with 'AH' on them. The flat was all in brown and white, really rather ugly & quite plain. He talked quite a lot about the Spanish war & the bombing of the *Deutschland*. He said we must all go to the Parteitag. We sat there for about 2 hours & then he got up & we all said goodbye & he shook hands twice with each of us. When we got down stairs there was quite a crowd waiting to see him go.

Neither Muv nor I could speak German, so Unity interpreted. There was no formality. Noticing that we were grubby and travel-stained when we arrived, Hitler showed us to the bathroom himself. He and Unity were at ease with each other and the tea party went on as it would have done with anyone anywhere in the world. Our host rang the bell on the tea table. No one came. He rang again, shook his head and gave up. No one else was present at tea and that a small domestic nuisance like a broken bell could happen even to a head of state made us feel at home. I wrote to Decca: 'We have had quite a nice time here & we've had tea with Hitler & seen all the other sights.' Looking back, what is surprising is that he postponed his departure for two hours so as to be able to sit and chat to Unity and, through her, to us.

7

Debutante

In March 1938 I was eighteen, the age to 'come out', which meant being a debutante. Those who took part in this curious and artificial way of life considered it as normal as the summer sporting calendar on which the London Season hung: Royal Ascot, the Epsom Derby, Lords and Henley. Dance bands, dressmakers, milliners, hairdressers, caterers, hotels, restaurants, florists, hire car firms and photographers all benefited from the trade whipped up by the frenzy of the Season.

It was a vintage year for beautiful girls. Two Sylvias (Lloyd Thomas and Muir); Ursula (Jane) Kenyon-Slaney, tall, blonde and willowy; June Capel, unbeatable for looks and charm; Gina Wernher, of unmistakable Russian descent, with high cheekbones and slanting eyes; Pat Douglas, striking, with veritable violet eyes; Sally Norton, whose perfect figure in Victor Stiebel was made for jealousy; Clarissa Churchill, with more than a whiff of Garbo in a dress by Maggy Rouff of Paris. Pamela Digby—whose famous career was to culminate in the American ambassadorship to Paris—was rather fat, fast and the butt of many teases; and there was Kathleen (Kick) Kennedy, sister of John F. Kennedy, not strictly a beauty but by far the most popular of all.

Joseph P. Kennedy had arrived as US Ambassador to the Court of St James's at the beginning of March and nothing like the Kennedy family had been seen before in the rarefied atmosphere of London diplomatic circles. For the next seventeen months they enlivened the scene. Vital, intelligent and outgoing, Kick was able to talk to anyone with ease and her shining niceness somehow ruled out any jealousy. Suitors appeared instantly but I noticed from the start that none of the other girls was annoyed by her success and I never heard a catty remark made behind her back. She was five weeks older than me and we soon made friends.

My other great friends were my cousins, Jean and Margaret Ogilvy, whose father, Joe Airlie, we all loved, though we were not so fond of their mother, Bridget. She was narrowly conventional to a ridiculous degree and her daughters had to be dressed just so before they were allowed out: shoes, stockings, gloves, hats, all had to be approved. When we were young Decca and I feared that if our parents were killed in an accident we might be left to Bridget in their wills, and what misery that would be (misery for Bridget too now I come to think of it).

The Ogilvy girls, Gina Wernher, Kick and I met for lunch at each other's houses time and again in the heady atmosphere of that summer. Gina lived at Someries House, which stood in its own big garden in Regent's Park. (It was demolished after the war and is now the site of the Royal College of Physicians, an unimaginable change in the landscape of pre-war London.) Our afternoon diversions included the Pathé newsreel cinema in Piccadilly, 'the eyes and ears of the world', a one-hour programme that included news, a Walt Disney film and an inferior imitation. If there was talk of war to come we did not believe it and continued to live for the present.

Royal Ascot in mid-June was the social highlight of the Season. I had first been in 1936 when I persuaded Muv to take me to see the Gold Cup. We went on to the Heath where you could go 'for nothing' and get close to the winning post. No reason to dress up, you just joined the crowd. Muv would have been far happier staying at home but did it to please me, which was typical of her. The race turned out to be the epic struggle between Lord Derby's mare Quashed and the American Triple Crown winner Omaha, belonging to the New York banker William Woodward, and Muv and I saw the final strides of this British triumph close to. It fired my interest in flat racing (I already followed National Hunt steeplechasing because of being so keen on Derek) and I still follow it with interest today. In 1937, Muv took me to Aintree by train for the day and we saw Royal Mail win the Grand National. It was a long day and I cannot believe she enjoyed it, but she knew I passionately wanted to go so booked some seats and off we went.

I went to Ascot again as a debutante, this time to the Royal Enclosure with friends. You wear a badge with your name pinned on your coat (I have often wished this happened at other social events when I am stumped as to who is who) and dress up in your best. I persuaded Madame Rita—who displayed her hats on sticks with padded tops in her cheerful showroom on the first floor of a house in Berkeley Square—to make a copy in spotted muslin of a 'fore and aft', the traditional tweed cap worn by deer stalkers, the ear flaps tied with a white satin ribbon on top of my head. It was ridiculous, but lots of Ascot hats are ridiculous. It was the racing I loved more than the social side, but both were all they were cracked up to be. We rattled down from London in one of the many special trains that took you to the racecourse. The sight of a crowd of overdressed women and top-hatted, tail-coated men assembled on one of our dirty old stations is somehow incongruous, like women in evening dress and men in black tie leaving for Glyndebourne in the middle of the afternoon.

I was as fascinated by the carriage horses in the King and Queen's procession—the famous Windsor Greys and Cleveland Bays—as I was by the thoroughbreds. There was something moving about the King and Queen's carriage appearing on the racecourse as a tiny dot a mile away and getting slowly bigger as it drew nearer; it was thrilling to see the skill of the postillions as they swung the carriage round to enter the paddock, judging to perfection the width of the entrance, and to hear the cheer of the crowd and the band playing the National Anthem. When the King had a winner, it was hats off all round and it was wonderful to see the tumultuous reception given to the horse and its owner. The feel of the crowd was much the same on the smart side of the course as it was on the Heath, an interest in horses bringing them together.

My allowance of £100 a year had to pay for the clothes I needed for the Season. My two or three evening dresses were run up by Gladys at £1 a time and the stuff came, as usual, from John Lewis. I never remember a failure and although I envied girls with dresses by Victor Stiebel, mine were always unique. A coat and skirt from Mr Nissen, tailor of Conduit Street—a major item but one that lasted—cost 81/2 guineas. We were never without Madame Rita's hats. Our hairdresser, Phyllis Earle in Dover Street (reached by a number 9 bus, getting off at the Ritz), charged 3/6 for a wash and set. My shoes, which came from Dolcis in Oxford Street, were cheap and decent to look at but painful after a few nights of round and round the dance floor. Muv gave me some of her elbow-length evening gloves made of doeskin, so gleaming white and smart they set off the dullest dress. They had to be cleaned each time they were worn and were posted to a firm in Scotland, so famous that 'Pullars of Perth' on the printed labels was enough of an address. The gloves were returned, pristine, in no time. I also had some white cotton pairs (which were looked down on) as reserves.

The shops in Brompton Road were reached through the Hole in the Wall at the bottom of Rutland Gate. Dangerously tempting were the two furriers who sold skins from the whole gamut of the animal kingdom, from rabbit to sable, including now-banned species such as baby seal, ocelot and leopard. Red fox was frowned upon by hunting people. Silver, blue and white Arctic fox were all right, but priced miles out of reach. Wool shops selling a kaleidoscope of coloured skeins from Sirdar and Paton & Baldwin were a feature of every London street; there were patterns and wool for rug-making and darning, and for knitting everything under the sun, including dogs' coats, which I knitted for my whippet Studley.

There were balls on Mondays, Tuesdays, Wednesdays and Thursdays, and often two on the same night. From time to time there was a Friday dance in the country (but not on a Saturday as it was not thought seemly to dance into Sunday morning). The hostess asked friends to give dinner parties before the ball and sent a list of prospective guests. At dinner, which was given in a private house or hotel restaurant, a debutante was seated between two young men who were expected to dance the first two dances with her on arrival at the ball since she might not know anyone early in the Season. Some obeyed this rule, but others often spied a more attractive friend and abandoned their dinner partners. Popular girls were booked up at once but the ladies' cloakroom was a refuge for those who had no partners. 'Can I borrow your powder?' 'Yes, but no crevice work please.' Chat about last night's dance, who was doing what, and the rest of the talk common to girls of our age in ladies' cloakrooms all over the world (seemingly idiotic now but very real then), filled the gap till the next dance when, with luck, a partner was booked. The dances were numbered so you somehow found who you were supposed to meet and took to the floor, stepping on each other's feet and exchanging banalities.

With no partners to seek them out, some of the debutantes hated every minute of this nightly routine, yet it was an admission of failure to go home before 1 a.m. At dances in the country you were given a programme with a tiny pencil attached by a silk thread, and a space to write the name of your partner next to the number of the dance. Men would say, 'May I see your programme?' All very well, but what if it was blank? I learned to put 'John', 'George', 'William', 'James'—none of whom existed but it looked better. Sometimes you got caught by an unwanted fellow, sometimes the one you wanted did his best to get away. It was a kind of game and a lesson in how to struggle through as best you can.

Meanwhile the unlucky chaperone—in my case Muv, who had already been through this charade five times with my sisters—changed into evening dress and, eyeing her turned-down bed with longing, telephoned for a taxi to take her to the ball. Mothers, aunts, or anyone who fitted the chaperone bill, sat on the caterers' gold chairs that surrounded the dance floor and waited until their charge had had enough. Occasionally Farve gave Muv a night off. He refused to take part in the festivities and never penetrated as far as the ballroom, but sat on one of those rickety hall chairs common to all big London houses, still in his evening cloak. One distraught hostess approached him and asked, 'Lord Redesdale, would you take the French Ambassadress into supper?' (a sumptuous meal that appeared between dinner and breakfast for the greedy or for those who had not yet dined). 'NO,' he said furiously, 'I'm waiting for Stubby.' The poor woman had no idea who Stubby was but wisely retreated and left him alone.

The sprinkling of older men who might take one of the patient mothers to supper were mostly unknown to Muv, so she often spent the late-night hours chatting to her neighbours. She watched the dancing and enjoyed seeing the wild gyrations of the Big Apple and the more staid Lambeth Walk. The bands—Joe Loss, Carroll Gibbons, Roy Fox,

Nat Gonella, Ambrose and sometimes even the great Harry Roy—were indefatigable. Tunes and lyrics by Cole Porter, Noël Coward and Irving Berlin, which have never been bettered, went through our heads night after night. Robert Cecil and Hugh Fraser were the two most energetic dancers: coats off, pouring with sweat, stumping and thumping with no real steps, just enjoying themselves madly. Muv said, 'If young men all go on like this there will be a war.'

At a ball given by Lady Louis Mountbatten for Sally Norton I danced with Jack Kennedy. 'Rather boring but nice,' I wrote in my diary. We danced again the next evening: 'I don't think he was enjoying the party much,' I recorded. Muv who, like everyone else, was intrigued by the Kennedys and full of admiration for Mrs Kennedy (who had easily outdone her in the childbearing line) observed the goings-on at one of these dances from her usual place with the other chaperones. She noticed Jack and, after watching him for a while, turned and said to a friend of mine (who later repeated it to me): 'Mark my words, I would not be surprised if that young man becomes President of the United States.' I do not know what made her say it, but she sometimes had that sort of premonition. I had none whatsoever and did not get to know Jack well until after he became President.

Gina Wernher was six months older than me and came out in 1937. Because we were friends I was allowed to go to her dance, even though it was a year before my official coming out. Her mother, Lady Zia, was related to many of the royal houses of Europe and these were represented in strength at the party. Our own recently crowned King and Queen were also there which lent glamour to the assembly. I dined with the Wernhers at Someries House, terrified of all the unknown bejewelled ladies, and found myself next to a girl who was obviously put out by the absence of the man who should have been sitting between us. She was Ann de Trafford, later the wife of a great friend, Derek Parker Bowles. We got through dinner somehow. Luckily Tom was at the dance and, realizing how nervous I was, rescued me when I needed him.

A change from dancing was the night when, among a crowd of other girls, I was presented at Court. This was the formal confirmation of having arrived—grown up at last. Before the days of television, the queue of hired cars lining up in the Mall to drop their passengers at Buckingham Palace was a free show for Londoners—like watching film stars arriving at a Leicester Square première. The cars could be stationary for some time, so the occupants were sitting ducks for any critical onlookers and their outspoken opinions. Gossip columnists sharpened their pencils, but for nothing worse than a description of the debutantes' clothes. The girls all wore white, with three white ostrich feathers in their hair and no jewellery. Their mothers, or whoever was presenting them (it was rumoured that two peeresses were paid to bring out debutantes by the mothers of girls who would not otherwise have been eligible), wore diamonds and every brooch they could lay their hands on.

I was presented in May. Muv and I waited in a room in the Palace for an hour and a half before making our entrée, while in the background 'The

Donkey's Serenade' (So I'll sing to a mule/If you're sure she won't think that I am just a fool/ Serenading a mule) played through amplifiers. When it came to our turn, I followed Muv, careful not to step on her train, and curtseyed first to the King and then to the Queen. I was not nervous because I knew exactly what I had to do and everything was so precisely organized, as it always is at Court. We made a quick getaway afterwards to have our photographs taken by Lenare.

One of my first big dances in 1938 was at Chandos House, given by Lady Kemsley for her daughter . The men armed the girls into dinner— already an old-fashioned custom then—and I was allotted to Lord Howland. The poor fellow was as shy as I was and we felt silly walking down the long passage, clamped unhappily together and with nothing to say. At that age Ian Howland (later the supremely comic Duke of Bedford who brought thousands to Woburn Abbey with his antics) was what we described as 'wet'. 'If all the dances are going to be like this,' I said to Muv, 'I'm not going.'

My own dance was held at Rutland Gate on 22 March, early in the Season; the bigger, smarter parties took place from May onwards. Three hundred guests were invited, including the familiar sprinkling of elderly uncles and aunts. Basics ran along the usual lines: gold chairs and a butler were hired for the evening, helpers were brought in to greet the guests and serve at table, and a bedroom near a bathroom became a ladies' cloakroom. (Nanny presided over the Ladies—goodness knows who looked after the Gents.) But the food at supper was not the usual Hunca Munca beef, ham or chicken-à-la-king that we saw every night.

Muv had a talent for making the commonplace original. Kedgeree (when the all-wild salmon was real and red) was the best dish imaginable and the guests fell on ours with delight. Instead of ice cream, rich mousses and pastries, she gave us black cherries and Devonshire cream. We ate off eighteenth-century Berlin porcelain decorated with European birds, butterflies and moths; even the steel knives and silver forks had painted china handles. The service had belonged to Warren Hastings and was bought by a Mitford ancestor at the sale to raise funds to pay for Hastings' trial. Heaven knows how much of this priceless china was smashed in the hurried washing-up after midnight. It is now wrapped in cotton wool at Chatsworth.

*   *   *

Two weeks after my party, I was invited to a dinner given by Lady Blanche Cobbold for her daughter Pamela before Lavinia Pearson's dance. I sat next to Andrew Cavendish. We were both just eighteen. Ignoring our neighbours, we never stopped talking throughout dinner. That was it for me—the rest of the Season passed in a haze of would-he-wouldn't-he be there; nothing and nobody else mattered. Meeting him was the beginning and end of everything I had dreamed of. A month later he left for Lyons 'to learn French' for a term (I never saw, or rather heard, any evidence of this in later life but it did not seem to matter). I missed him during his absence, but it was all the more exciting when he came back, and we managed to meet at parties time and again.

Three dances stand out in my memory that year. Mrs Kennedy gave a dinner-dance for Kick and her eldest sister Rosemary at the American Embassy in Prince's Gate on 2 June. My cousin Jean Ogilvy, who came out the year before we did, had taken on the pleasurable task of introducing Kick to her English contemporaries and to the unwritten rules and nuances of social life in this country. It was Jean who helped Kick arrange the seating at table and that was perhaps why I was lucky enough to find myself at Kick's table with Jean, Elisabeth Moncrieffe, Prince Frederick of Prussia, and, according to my diary, a 'very dull', nameless American. The three other men at the table—John Stanley, Robert Cecil and Eric Duncannon—were of a similar age, all heirs to large estates. Ambrose's famous band played and the cabaret was Harry Richman, brought over from America for the night. But it was the Kennedys themselves who lit up the evening.

Three weeks later the Speaker Fitzroy gave a dance for his granddaughters Anne and Mary at the Speaker's House. (No one made anything of it at the time but what a fuss there would be now if that historic house were used for such a frivolous purpose, and presumably free to Mr Speaker—a permissible perk that went unquestioned in those days.) The sun was well up over the Houses of Parliament when Muv and I left at 5 a.m. She had had a long wait that night. I remember the taxi-ride home because she was so angry with me. Dancing more than two dances with the same partner was strictly against the unwritten rules, but I was missing Andrew and had danced all night with Mark Howard. I expect Muv had had enough anyway without my bad behaviour. My diary for the next day says, 'Very dull day', and 'Duller still' the following. Perhaps this was a result of Muv's anger; it was rare for her to give us a ticking-off and it made a strong impression.

On 1 July I went to a ball at Bowood House in Wiltshire, for the coming of age of Charlie Lansdowne who, with his younger brother Ned Fitzmaurice, had become my great friends. After Andrew, I loved them best. The main house at Bowood, a large square Adam block, was still standing (it was pulled down after the war) and there was ample room for hundreds of guests. The garden with its eye-catching lake and cottage are set in the sort of idyllic eighteenth-century landscape that makes you gasp at the sheer beauty and Englishness of it. It was the most enjoyable evening I remember of all the glorious evenings we had that year. Andrew was back from Lyons and he and Tom Egerton stayed at the Swan Inn in Swinbrook. A girlfriend and I stayed next door at the Mill Cottage, which Farve rented after selling the Swinbrook estate. Tom and Andrew had met, aged thirteen, on their first day at Eton and remained lifelong friends. I too had grown to love Tom, and Andrew and I seldom planned anything that did not include him. Like Andrew, he was in the Coldstream Guards during the war and became famous in the regiment for rescuing the marmalade from the Officers' Mess at the Siege of Tobruk.

At the end of July, Andrew and I went to stay at Compton Place, his parents' house in Eastbourne, for Goodwood races. Also staying were Tom Egerton, Robert Cecil, my friends Irene (Rene)

Haig, Zara Mainwaring and Jakie Astor. Andrew's brother, Billy Hartington, had invited Kick. Rene must have been irritated by Kick joining the party because until then she had been Billy's favourite. In September we all went to Cortachy Castle, Jean Ogilvy's home, for the Perth races and the Highland balls. After the riotous fun at Compton Place, we had to be on our guard when we got to Cortachy under the critical eye of Bridget Airlie, Jean's mother. Hugh Fraser and Andrew got into trouble for running on to the Perth racecourse in front of the crowds and jumping the water jump.

Kick had by now become part of the scene and was as much with Billy as I was with Andrew. The rest of the Kennedy family were in the South of France that summer but Kick had struck out and was determined to spend those few days with Billy. Rose Kennedy, a forceful character of whom all her children were in awe, was not pleased and I wondered what reception Kick would get when she eventually joined her family. As far as Mrs Kennedy, a staunch Catholic, was concerned, it was out of the question for Kick to marry Billy because he was a practising Protestant. Kick went back to America when war was declared, but her heart was in England and in 1943 she returned, ostensibly to work for the American Red Cross, but really to join Billy; and despite the opposition from both families, they were soon engaged.

In August I got a stiff letter from Muv, who was in Germany with Unity, criticizing me for going to Castle Howard without telling her and spelling out what was expected of me when I stayed with Andrew. 'I hope if you went to Derbyshire that the Duchess invited you to visit and not only Andrew, as I *do not* wish you to visit about at the invitation of this boy or that.' By this time Andrew and I considered ourselves unofficially engaged but there were some hiccups. He became fond of Dinah Brand, a niece of Nancy Astor, and more or less deserted me for her. I minded terribly and had gone to Castle Howard to dry my eyes. He also liked the look of Maxine Birley, daughter of the painter Oswald Birley—a real beauty of whom I was deeply jealous. For a while Andrew and I did not meet, but then all obstacles seemed to dissolve and we took up as though we had never left off.

Like Farve, Andrew was very much a second son. His parents, Eddy and Mary (always known as 'Moucher') Devonshire, adored their elder son, Billy, the epitome of all that was good, clever and handsome. When they were in London, the Devonshires leased No. 2 Carlton Gardens from the Crown Estates (Devonshire House had been sold in the 1920s). These big London houses were built for entertaining, not for family life, and the grander the house, the less the younger members of the family and the household staff were considered. Andrew had no bedroom at Carlton Gardens and slept on a camp bed in his mother's sitting room. Edward, the butler, slept in a cupboard on the stairs.

In the autumn term of 1938 Andrew went up to Trinity College, Cambridge, where he enjoyed himself to the full. Unlike me and my girlfriends, he and his friends were conscious of the looming danger of a war and this added to their frenetic search for pleasure. They got into scrapes and baited the Proctors to within an inch of being sent down. They drank too much, danced all night and rode hopeless hirelings in point-to-points. There was a rule that undergraduates had to be back in College by 6 a.m. and there were many early morning accidents as they raced back from London to be in on time. Andrew had a lucky escape when the car he was sharing with two friends overturned, landed on top of him and damaged one of his kidneys beyond repair. He was in hospital for a month and told me that his time there conveniently coincided with end of first year exams, so he did not have to take them. He was greatly relieved as he was sure he would have failed. After one escapade, Bernard van Cutsem, later Andrew's racehorse trainer, was described on a newspaper hoarding of the *Cambridge News* as 'MILLIONAIRE JESUS PLAYBOY'. Anyone not conversant with the names of the Cambridge Colleges might have wondered at this headline.

Newmarket was near by and more time was spent at the races than at lectures. I do not think Andrew or any of his friends went in much for learning—it came a long way down their scale of priorities. There were exceptions, of course, and there was a sharp drawing-in of breath when George Jellicoe, one of the principal party-goers, got a First in modern history. Andrew planned to visit me at the Mill Cottage. As he did not drive, he came by rail, cross-country from Cambridge to Oxford, but missed three trains running. I drove the nineteen miles to Oxford Station and back to meet him off each one. Muv grew exasperated and said, 'I should give up seeing him if I were you, he's unreliable.' I went to see him at Cambridge just once and even I, philistine that I am, was stunned by the beauty of the place.

The spring and summer of 1939 brought more freedom for me, now an ex-debutante. I was invited to a few dances and was allowed to see Andrew unchaperoned. Our meeting place was often Keith Prowse in Bond Street, where we spent hours listening to 78 r.p.m. records in enclosed, so-called soundproof, booths. We lunched at Luigi's in Jermyn Street, the embodiment of new-found freedom, where a minute steak and all that went with it, including a bottle of wine, cost a guinea. (When war broke out Luigi was bundled off to Canada as an Enemy Alien—anyone less of an enemy I cannot imagine.) The place for evening entertainment was the Café de Paris. It was expensive and a rare treat. We were sometimes invited by friends, but often it was Andrew who paid. The cabaret never failed to be the best: Beatrice Lillie and Douglas Byng were the funniest; Frances Day, who sang 'It's De Lovely', the most glamorous; and the black band leader, Ken 'Snakehips' Johnson, was fascinating to look at. The last tune, signalling that it was time to go home, was always 'Goodnight Sweetheart'.

After war was declared, the Café de Paris went on as if nothing had happened—best dresses for women, uniforms for the men who had joined up and black tie for the others. In March 1941 when the bombing was at its height, the Café de Paris received a direct hit and many people were killed, including Snakehips, aged only twenty-six. An acquaintance of mine who passed by on foot later that night (the raid was so bad that even the taxis had gone home) said that he would not have believed the corpses and the mixture of blood and jewels had he not seen it with his own eyes.

The nightclub we loved best was the 400 in Leicester Square. Drink laws at the time were peculiar: members could buy a bottle of spirits, write their name and the date on it, and on their next visit the unfinished bottle would be waiting for them. Sometimes overseas service meant a long absence for a member, but the bottle was always there. A hazard at the 400 was that it was also a favourite of Andrew's father, who was apt to sit at a table near the narrow entrance with his friend Lady Dufferin. We had to pass close by, which was embarrassing for Andrew and Billy. In an attempt at anonymity, my future father-in-law labelled his bottles with the name of a fish beginning with 'H' (for his courtesy title 'Hartington'). Billy and Andrew discovered this and would ask Mr Rossi, the maître d'hôtel, 'Have you got a bottle belonging to Mr Hake or Herring or Halibut?'

This way of life cost Andrew far more than his allowance and he owed money to his tailor and bookmaker. After a day's racing at Brighton, he was chased by a Ladbroke's man the length of the train at Victoria Station. His long, nineteen-year-old legs enabled him to escape into the crowd, but the bills kept coming. One extravagance he did not fall for was a car of his own. He never liked the idea of driving and only did so under duress—and to the terror of his passengers. When he was in Italy during the war, he sometimes had to take the wheel but never afterwards. I became the driver when we married, except when he was on some official engagement and then the chauffeur drove.

On 6 July 1939 the last grand ball before the war was given at Holland House by Hon. Mrs Cubitt for her daughter Rosalind. The King and Queen were there and it was full of friends—so many that it was difficult to circulate in the succession of small rooms of the old Elizabethan house. It rained so hard that arriving guests had to queue for an hour and a quarter because only one car at a time could drop its passengers under the covered porch. The awful weather was somehow a portent of things to come; most of us realized that it was the last time we would see anything like it and in spite of being one of the best parties of the Season, it was also a kind of farewell.

8

War

In 1938, soon after the sale of Swinbrook, my father saw an advertisement for Inch Kenneth, a small island in the Inner Hebrides off the west coast of Mull. He went to look at it, fell under its spell and bought it. Perhaps the fact that it was so far away made the island all the more attractive. Muv went to see it for herself and her love of Scotland and the sea made her pleased with it. The house with its modern exterior—the latest addition was built in 1934—fits surprisingly well into the landscape. Sheltered to the north by a hill and fearsome cliffs, it faces south on to white sands and small coves. The ruins of the ancient chapel of St Kenneth, a follower of St Columba, are close by and there is a farmstead and walled kitchen garden. I veered between wanting to live there for the rest of my life and hating it. The weather was more important than in any place I have ever known: sublime when it was fine and the distant islands seemed to hover above the sea, infinitely depressing when the weather closed in and there was no escape until it was calm again.

I was on Inch Kenneth with Muv, Farve and Nancy on 3 September 1939, the day war was declared. The farm man, John McFadyen, was called up immediately. He came to the house in his uniform of the Argyll and Sutherland Highlanders to say goodbye and we were all in the kitchen in floods, including him. (He came back safely, I am happy to say.) I was left with three cows to milk. Two were of uncertain lineage but with a distinctly Shorthorn look, the third was a lovely little Jersey heifer, a first calver—on the skittish side. The cows' routine was sacrosanct: morning milking at about 7.30 a.m., then they were turned out to graze till 5 p.m. when the evening milking was due.

I do not know how many of my dear readers have milked a cow—not just tried their hand at it but been in total charge of this wonderful animal, who would be in considerable pain if left unmilked. The best part is burying your head into the warm and comforting flank; the worst is the flick of a tail over your eyes or hair, with a thin wet film of muck. Each cow is different. The older Shorthorns were relatively easy—their big floppy teats yielding the milk with a satisfying sizzle and spurt, hitting the bucket held tight between my knees. The little Jersey was my trouble. Her teats were short and embedded in her udder. The double squeeze which brings the milk was hard on my hands, using unaccustomed muscles. Had I been a pianist, the muscles might have been ready and waiting, but no such luck, and the sharp ache in my fingers and across the back of my hands became acute. I cut my nails as short as I dared to spare the flesh on the lower part of my palms, but even the satisfaction of an endless supply of fresh milk and enough cream to please the greediest seemed a high price to pay for the pain. The poor little Jersey was restless and I was in despair when a cow kick (a hind leg flashed forward—the opposite of a horse's kick) turned me and the bucket over. The three-legged milking stool was upside down with the rest. Being told not to cry over spilt milk is ridiculous; of course you cry when all that effort goes to waste.

As soon as war was declared, we feared for Unity. She had always said that in the event of war between England and Germany, her life would be over. True to her word she went to a public park in Munich, took out the small mother-of-pearl pistol she had bought for the purpose (she used to show it to us, telling us what she would do with it) and fired a bullet into her right temple. My parents were well aware of her threat and when they heard nothing from her they suffered the same awful anxiety as they had when Decca disappeared—not knowing whether she was alive or dead. Communications with Germany during the Phoney War were uncertain but eventually they heard from Teddy Almásy, János's brother, who wrote from neutral Hungary to say that Unity was ill in hospital but was being well looked after. The letter arrived on 2 October. There was no further news for six weeks. We were at Rutland Gate on Christmas Eve when the telephone rang. It was János, who was with Unity. He had taken her on an ambulance train from Munich to Berne, arranged by Hitler who kept in touch with her progress. 'When are you coming to fetch me?' Unity asked. To Muv she sounded her old self.

I was the only sister available to go with Muv on the long and possibly hazardous train journey through France to Switzerland. Although there had been little fighting so far, no one knew when a German attack might come. We set off together immediately after Christmas. The journey seemed as dark during the short days as it was during the long winter nights. Arriving in brilliantly lit Berne after blacked-out England and France lifted our spirits, as did the thought of seeing Unity again. It was a false dawn. Our first sight of her was a shock: her face was the same greyish-brown as her hair, which was matted and almost solid with dried blood—she had not been able to bear anyone touching her head since the day the bullet had smashed into her skull, nearly killing her. Even her huge eyes looked different: one glance showed that the light had gone out. She smiled and was pleased to see us but she was another person. Muv and I looked at the sad, thin creature that was left and tried not to let her see how horrified we were.

Unity had been unconscious for two months after shooting herself but had slowly regained the use of her limbs. The clinic pronounced her fit to travel and on New Year's Eve, accompanied by a nurse, we started back to Calais in an ambulance carriage attached to the train. Long halts at dark stations were followed by a few miles of jerky progress, accompanied by bangs and squeals of metal on metal. The whole process then began again. The jolts every time we stopped and started were painful and unsettling for the patient. The journey took so long that we missed the boat to Folkestone and had to endure two interminable nights in a hotel in Calais, where we were besieged by a hostile press.

Finally, on 3 January, Unity's stretcher was lifted on to the boat and off again at Folkestone, where Farve was waiting for us; then into an ambulance and at last we were on our way to the Old Mill Cottage in High Wycombe. But not for long. The engine started making strange noises and we drew to a halt. There was a long wait until another ambulance arrived to take us back to Folkestone. After all these alarms, it was too late to make the long drive to High Wycombe and we spent the night in a Folkestone hotel. Meanwhile the photographers, who had not been able to get close to us on the dock because it was a prohibited area, were snapping away and the reporters got their pictures and story when Unity was transferred from one ambulance to another. Farve was certain the breakdown had been fixed by the press. It was not till the following afternoon that we arrived home, after a journey that had taken four days instead of one.

Three weeks later, Unity was examined by Sir Hugh Cairns, Nuffield Professor of Surgery at the Radcliffe Infirmary in Oxford, who confirmed that the doctors in Germany were right not to have tried to remove the bullet which was lodged in her brain. Muv devoted herself to looking after Unity from the day we brought her home from

Switzerland and it gradually became clear to us all that she would never be the same again. Muv wanted to take her to Inch Kenneth but the island was a protected area and as Unity was regarded as a dangerous individual by the authorities, permission was refused. Little did they realize her condition. The press was still plaguing us, so Muv and Farve decided that the Mill Cottage in Swinbrook would be less accessible than High Wycombe, where the yard could not be closed off and the miller's lorries came and went.

We were at close quarters at Swinbrook. My bedroom measured seven by eight feet (against the law now but it seemed perfectly all right to me). Unity slept in the next room and there was just a flimsy door between us. Since her suicide attempt she had taken against me, as she had done with others. 'It's awful,' I wrote to Diana in October 1940, 'she *so* hates me that life here has become almost impossible. The sitting room is so small and two enormous tables in it belong exclusively to her and if one so much as puts some knitting down on one for a moment chaos reigns because she hies up & shrieks "bloody fool" very loud.'

She was unable to concentrate and jumped from one subject to another, using the wrong words and getting angry when we could not understand her. She sometimes spoke of the Führer, but as from a great distance; her grasp on reality was that of a child. To add to the misery, she was incontinent. Muv washed her sheets every day in the small kitchen sink and when they were hung out to dry they dominated the little garden. Mrs Stobie (now married to Philip Timms, my father's old foreman) came in to help. I overheard my mother interviewing an applicant for the job once when Mrs Stobie was ill. 'I do the rough,' I heard Muv say. That meant sawing the logs with what became known as a 'Queen Mary' (so called because the widowed queen spent the war at Badminton House where she delighted in cutting down the Duke of Beaufort's trees), chopping the wood for kindling, cleaning the grates in the morning and sweeping out the ashes.

The doctor advised Muv to encourage Unity to be independent and after a few months she was able to take the bus to Oxford on her own, sometimes asking her fellow passengers for money on the way. The highlight of her day was lunch at the British Restaurant, a kind of soup kitchen where the doubtful stew and potatoes cost one shilling. She sometimes queued up a second time, which you were not meant to do, but the good-natured customers and staff never reported her.

She would attach herself to various people for a time and then take up with someone else. Two people stand out for their patience: Mrs Wells, the parson's wife ('*Blissful* Mrs Wells', Unity called her), and Miss Bannerman who had an antique shop in Burford. These two good, unprejudiced women often kept her company. Unity still needed a cause, something to replace her love of Germany, and she turned to religion. Over the years she joined—or tried to join—the Roman Catholic Church, the Christian Scientists and everything in between. This led to terrible muddles with the local organizers of these different faiths and Muv had to sort them out. Had Eastern religions been as popular as they are today, I am sure Unity would have worked her way through those as well. I was entirely selfish and thought of nothing except being with Andrew and did precious little for either mother or sister.

Nearly all her contemporaries are dead so there are very few people who remember Unity as she was before she tried to kill herself. (One who does and who has fond memories of her is her old friend Micky Burn, now aged ninety-eight.) Those who are interested in her life can read thousands of words about her, written with the benefit of hindsight. All are hostile because of her friendship with Hitler. She has become a symbol of evil, her name synonymous with anti-Semitism. So why did we all love her? I have searched for the answer, tried to find a word to describe what it was about her, but cannot. Decca could not explain it either: the strongest possible political division separated her from Unity but nothing could extinguish their love for each other. We knew the bad side, we knew she had condoned Nazi cruelty and that she had taken a flat from a Jewish couple who had been evicted; yet in spite of her racist views, vehemently expressed, and her admiration for the most extreme of Hitler's lieutenants, there was something innocent about Unity, a guileless, childlike simplicity that made her vulnerable and in need of protection. Nancy and Pam in their own ways, Tom, undoubtedly, Diana to a much greater degree, Decca, amazingly, and I, certainly, could not help loving her. Our parents, of course, and cousins felt the same way. It was not that those who loved her forgave her her beliefs, they went on loving her in spite of them. None of this will impress her enemies but it goes some way to account for the feelings of those who knew her.

Perhaps it is too easy to say that she was inexplicable, but it is a fact.

*   *   *

Decca and Esmond returned to England three months before their baby daughter, Julia, was born on 20 December 1937. They lived in a house in Rotherhithe Street in south-east London which I visited two or three times. Esmond made no secret of his dislike of our family and Decca and I usually met on neutral ground. Esmond was not there when I went to see the baby, who was suspended in a cradle out of a window that overlooked the River Thames—a bit of Nanny's lore to do with fresh air, no doubt. Decca was guardedly welcoming. Unsurprisingly, the old intimacy had gone but we had a good chat.

Then came their tragedy: Julia caught measles, which turned into pneumonia, and she died, aged five months. Decca wrote an agonizing account of her baby's illness and death in her memoirs, but never spoke of her misery to me or any of the family; she buried her sorrow deep. To my shame, I was entirely taken up at the time with dances and friends—following 'the devices and desires' of my own heart. Decca resisted any attempt at sympathy on my part and, understandably, cut herself off from me and the frivolous life I was leading. The day after Julia's funeral, at which none of the family were welcome, the Romillys went to Corsica where they remained out of communication for three months.

Tom acted as a bridge between Decca and our parents and was the only member of the family to make friends with Esmond. A great arguer, he was fascinated by the theory of politics rather than their practical application and was able, unlike my sisters, to discuss politics dispassionately. He was present at Mosley's infamous Olympia meeting in 1934, where he was photographed giving the Fascist salute, but he also spent hours talking to Esmond. He was as interested to meet Hitler with Diana and Unity as he was to debate communism with Decca and Esmond's friends. As a result, he was claimed by both sides as 'one of us' and remained on good terms with everyone throughout all the political upheavals.

In early 1939 the Romillys left for America to start a new life. Esmond joined the Royal Canadian Air Force in July 1940 and this brought about the greatest sorrow of Decca's life. On 30 November 1941 Esmond's disabled plane came down in the North Sea and he was posted missing. The word 'missing' is particularly cruel, leaving as it does a ray of hope that the person will turn up safe and well, even in the most doomed circumstances. As days go by, it becomes increasingly unlikely and yet, and yet . . .

It was in Decca's nature to be optimistic and she clutched at every straw, hoping against hope that Esmond was a prisoner of war. In December, Winston Churchill (whose wife, Clementine, was Farve's first cousin) went to America to confer with President Roosevelt and asked Decca, who was living in Washington, to meet him at the White House. Churchill told her that he had looked carefully into the matter of the plane's disappearance and that there was no chance of Esmond being alive. Even then Decca could not believe it. As she left the White House, Winston gave her an envelope containing $500. She was enraged at this display of charity—as if she could not look after herself. She was certainly not going to accept money from Churchill and she gave it away to friends.

After Esmond's death, Muv wrote to Decca telling her how delighted we would all be to have her back and pleaded with her to come home. Decca's Air Force pension was derisory, but a prouder woman you could not find; she decided to stay in America, take a secretarial job and manage somehow. Esmond's death must have nearly destroyed her. I do not doubt that their marriage would have lasted: they were so exactly right for each other. Her saviour was Constancia, 'Dinky', her ten-month-old daughter—all that she had left of Esmond and the dizzy few years they had spent together.

*   *   *

Diana and Sir Oswald married in 1936, after the sudden death of his first wife, Cimmie, following an appendicitis operation that went wrong. In May 1940 Sir O was arrested under Defence Regulation 18B, a wartime ruling that empowered the government to detain anyone considered a threat to the country, and he was sent to Brixton Prison. He was not charged with any offence and so was not tried in a court of law. A month later Diana was also arrested under 18B and taken to Holloway, the women's prison. Max, her fourth son (and second by Mosley), was eleven weeks old and she was still breastfeeding him. She was given the chance to take the baby with her, but the bombing of London was expected at any moment and she decided to leave him with his brother, eighteen-month-old Alexander, in the capable hands of Nanny Higgs.

What happened to Diana and my brother-in-law is well documented. What is less well known is that the day after Diana was arrested Gladwyn Jebb, private secretary to Sir Alexander Cadogan at the Foreign Office and an acquaintance of Nancy, summoned Nancy to his office. He wanted to know whether she thought Diana's friendship with Hitler and other high-ranking members of the Nazi party made her a threat to the country, and asked her if she knew the purpose of Diana's visits to Germany. Nancy told Gladwyn that she thought Diana 'an extremely dangerous person'. What she based this statement on I do not know—Diana never spoke politics to Nancy—and why she agreed to be questioned about a subject of which she admitted she knew nothing I shall never understand. Diana had always been generous to Nancy and they loved each other's company, which makes Nancy's denunciation all the more inexplicable. But I do know that her underlying jealousy of Diana, which went back to childhood, was still very present. It had been exacerbated by Diana producing four healthy boys and Nancy being unable to have children following an ectopic pregnancy. Diana did not learn of Nancy's action until 1985, twelve years after Nancy's death. It must have been a fearful shock, however well she thought she knew Nancy, such duplicity being entirely foreign to her own nature.

Diana described her experiences in Holloway in

her memoirs, *A Life of Contrasts*, and there is little I can add. I visited her several times and saw enough to realize what an ordeal her imprisonment was. She was allowed one visitor for half an hour every fortnight. The precious thirty minutes was usually used by my mother, with or without Diana's children. There was always a wardress present at these meetings, one of whom became Diana's friend. The prison was overcrowded and there were many women to each lavatory. One of these had a red 'V' painted on the door and was usually empty, so Diana decided to use it. 'I shouldn't if I were you,' her friend the wardress warned her, 'it's for people with venereal disease.' Muv was so shocked by the filth of the visitors' lavatory that, in an uncharacteristic gesture, she wrote on the wall: 'This lavatory is a disgrace to HM Prisons'. Sir O also wrote an account of his imprisonment, but one detail he failed to mention is that the Lascar seamen held in the cells on the floor above him used to urinate out of the window and the wind blew the results down into his cell below.

Tom, who was with the 11th Battalion King's Royal Rifle Corps (surprising his old friends by the eagerness with which he embraced army life), visited Diana whenever he was on leave. One day in autumn 1941 he went to see both Sir O in Brixton and Diana in Holloway. He told Diana that he was dining that night with Churchill and asked if there was anything she would like him to say to the Prime Minister. 'Only the same as always,' she answered, 'that if we have to stay in prison couldn't we at least be together?' After dining at 10 Downing Street, Tom wrote to

Churchill on Diana's behalf, repeating her request. In December 1941, after eighteen long months apart, Diana and Sir O were re-united in Holloway, as were other husbands and wives held under Regulation 18B. Diana said that, unlikely as it may seem, one of the happiest days of her life was in prison: the day she and her husband were together again. The press made a great deal of this and it was picked up by the bus conductor on the north London route, who used to announce at the top of his voice, 'Holloway Jail. Lady Mosley's suite. All change here.' My mother gave him a stern look as she got off the bus to go through the huge prison gates.

Two years later, Sir O fell ill with phlebitis. The authorities were frightened that he might die in prison and in November 1943, after much discussion, the Home Secretary, Herbert Morrison, unwillingly agreed that the Mosleys should be released under house arrest. When this was announced, Nancy again performed her 'patriotic duty' and went to MI5 to volunteer that in her opinion Diana sincerely desired 'the downfall of England and democracy generally' and should not be released. This time Nancy's fantasy had gone too far; she had no evidence whatsoever for her claim and luckily the government took no notice. Diana was never to know of this second betrayal since the relevant government papers were not made public until four months after her death. To me, Nancy's behaviour is so incredible that I would not have believed it had I not read it in black and white in an official document.

*   *   *

Derek Jackson worked at Professor Lindemann's Oxford laboratory until the Fall of France. He then joined the RAF as a wireless operator/air gunner, making over sixty sorties with 604 Squadron. At thirty-four, he was older than most of his comrades and Lindemann did not want to let him go, but by force of character Derek succeeded in joining up. Pam followed him around the country and was there to look after him in rented houses whenever possible. From 1943 until the end of the war he played a vital role in helping to develop ways of interfering with enemy radar.

Derek behaved in the air force much as he had done on the racecourse, astonishing his pilot on one occasion by giving instructions in German. When the Mosleys were released from Holloway and had nowhere to live Derek invited them to Rignell, but after a few days the Home Office woke up to the fact that Derek was doing top secret scientific work and the Mosleys were told they had to leave. Derek was incensed and when aroused could be a formidable opponent. He grabbed the telephone and rang the Home Office, demanding to speak to Morrison who, as Derek knew, had been a conscientious objector in the First World War. To everyone's surprise Derek was put through and—as he enjoyed recalling later— he went into the attack: 'When *you* have got the DFC, the AFC and the OBE for valour, you can tell me what to do.' In spite of Derek's protestations, the Mosleys had to leave Rignell and went to a nearby inn, The Shaven Crown, where they spent Christmas 1943.

By 1940 the Free French had their headquarters

in London and it was there that Nancy met Gaston Palewski, General de Gaulle's chief of staff. He was the lover she had been waiting for all her life and she fell for him hook, line and sinker. Gaston, always called 'Colonel' by Nancy, was in some ways an English person's idea of a typical Frenchman: not only did he adore women, he showed it (which does not often happen in England). He was not handsome, but the speed of his clever talk soon made you forget his appearance. He had studied at Oxford and somehow knew reams of English poetry, nursery rhymes and quintessentially English jokes. He was as good a tease as Nancy and used to go on at her until she said, 'Oh Colonel, do shut up.' I got to know him in Paris after the war when staying with Nancy and became fond of him. He was one of those people you instantly felt you had known all your life.

Nancy spent much of the war working at Heywood Hill's bookshop in Mayfair. Heywood and his wife, Anne, had been her friends for years and he made a wise choice when he invited her to join the staff. No sooner did she appear in the Curzon Street shop than all her friends and acquaintances followed. In the bookshop, she was pinned down, available for chat anytime during business hours. Sometimes the laughter grew a bit much for serious book buyers and one customer said pointedly, 'May I be allowed to buy this volume please?' But the business Nancy brought was worth more than the odd lost sale. Household names from the writing fraternity, who also happened to be her friends, gathered at the shop and customers could see at close quarters what are now called 'celebrities'.

The wages were meagre, £3 10s a week, and Nancy was so short of money that she usually walked the two miles home to Blomfield Road to save the bus fare. On one flush day she was waiting in the queue at the bus stop in Park Lane after dark when a huge black American soldier came up and hugged her. 'Go away,' she screamed, 'I'm FORTY.' At one point she became a firewatcher and was asked to give lectures on fire-fighting. These soon came to an end. When she enquired why, she was told, 'Well, you see, it's your voice. We've had several complaints, someone even wrote in and said they wanted to put you on the fire.'

*   *   *

Enough has been written about the war for people who did not live through it to know that it brought tragedies and upheavals to everyone's lives. For each inhabitant of the British Isles there was a tale to tell. In our family, an unexpected sadness was my parents' decision to separate. The events leading up to the war—Decca's elopement and estrangement, Unity's attachment to Nazism, Diana's relationship with Sir O—had all poisoned life at home. Added to this was Muv and Farve's fundamental disagreement over Germany. At first, Farve had been impressed by Hitler but, as a born patriot, from the day war was declared he publicly renounced his former opinion and stood firmly behind the government. Muv refused to consider Hitler a threat and believed that it was a mistake to go to war. Neither of these strong characters would budge from their positions and it was painful in the extreme to see their unhappiness. Farve was permanently cross and for the first time I saw my mother truly angry.

Unity's suicide attempt was the last straw. Farve could not bear to see the day-in day-out hopelessness of her condition, which seemed to embody all the suffering brought on by the war. It became clear that he and Muv would be better apart so that the wireless news and propaganda would not provide daily fuel for their arguments. Muv never talked to me about the situation but I was, of course, acutely aware of it. Farve retreated to Inch Kenneth with Margaret Wright, who had been parlourmaid and later housekeeper at the Mews when 26 Rutland Gate was sold. Margaret was handsome and competent at her job but she was not used to the rough and tumble of family life. I felt her to be critical of my sisters and me— the opposite of Mabel—and she gave all her attention to Farve. She was one of those highly conventional women whose answer, in a prissy voice, you could guess before you had asked the question. She was such a boring companion that I often wondered how Farve could stand it, but he found her restful and undemanding. There was never any danger of a political argument and after a while she became indispensable to him.

These must have been terrible months for my poor mother. Added to her feelings about the war was the unhappiness of her marriage going awry, the ongoing worry of Unity's condition, Diana's imprisonment and Decca losing her soulmate in harrowing and uncertain circumstances. My own life was humdrum and almost carefree in comparison. According to Nancy, I was 'having a wild time with young cannon fodders at the Ritz', which was only partly true. Soon after the outbreak of war I worked in a canteen for servicemen at St Pancras Station and after Unity came home I did the same in Edinburgh to be with my Ogilvy cousins.

When war was declared, Andrew wanted to join the Coldstream Guards, in which his brother Billy was already serving as an officer, but there was a rush to join up and Andrew was told that he had to wait until there was a place for him. Frustrated, he returned to Cambridge. In December 1939, while he was marking time, he met Lady Digby (mother of my fellow debutante Pamela). 'What, Andrew? Still not in uniform?' she exclaimed. Andrew was incensed by this insult and never spoke to her again. I do not suppose she noticed, but she could not have said anything more wounding to a young man impatiently awaiting his call-up. This eventually came in June 1940.

When Andrew and I were in London we continued to drive around in my flimsy Austin Seven and when one nightclub got too hot with incendiary bombs falling close by, we moved to another. We took no notice of the bombing—it never occurred to us that we might be hit. In late 1940, on a visit to Andrew's parents' house in Derbyshire, we became officially engaged. My future mother-in-law said to Andrew, 'You have either got to marry that girl or stop asking her here.' So that is how it happened.

9

Marriage

Churchdale hall, where Andrew's parents had lived since 1923, sits like a broody hen spreading itself over the top of a hill above the village of Ashford-in-the-Water. It was a home if ever there was one, made so by the presence of Moucher, Andrew's mother, who in her self-effacing way was quite unconscious of the effect her goodness, beauty and ready understanding had on all around her. Andrew's sisters, Elizabeth and Anne Cavendish, respectively six and seven years younger than me and still in the schoolroom, soon became, and have remained, my great friends.

If my own father was thought eccentric, Eddy Devonshire ran him close. He wore paper collars, did not possess an overcoat and would stand, oblivious of the weather, in the freezing wind on Chesterfield Station in a threadbare London suit. He was a heavy smoker of ready-rolled Turkish cigarettes called Pasquale that he lit with a tinder cord, a curious bit of orange rope that looked like a dressing-gown cord. It smouldered away merrily even in a gale and was a useful lighter on outdoor occasions. It also smouldered away merrily in Eddy's coat pocket and made some decent holes, blackened around the edges; these became part of the suit, which he would never have dreamed of replacing. His ancient clothes sometimes let him down: he got both legs stuck in the ragged lining of one of the trouser legs of an old dinner suit and we waited a long time for him that night.

An expert fly-tier, Eddy was keen eyed and neat fingered, and told me he would have practised dentistry had his life been different. He made an odd sight, a white apron over his well-worn, blue velvet smoking-jacket, leaning across a table covered with all the ingredients for fly-tying. The smell of the glue was to become very familiar. He begged plumes from the hats of his women friends and, picking one up, would sigh with nostalgia and say things like, 'Ettie Desborough, Ascot, 1921.' Once the flies were ready, he lay in the bath imagining he was a salmon while Edward, the butler, pretending to be a fishing rod, jerked them over his submerged head. The ones the Duke judged most attractive were used on his stretch of the Blackwater in County Cork at the start of the salmon fishing season.

Eddy was not much good at small talk and often remained silent. Coming from a family that never drew breath, I found this silence intimidating, but our mutual interest in British wild flowers helped to break the ice. His copy of Bentham and Hooker is as good as a diary, with its neatly coloured-in line drawings of flowers and annotations of where and when he had found them. He returned from the funeral of his brother-in-law Evan Baillie, at Ballindarroch in the north of Scotland, delighted because he had stumbled on a *Trientalis europæa* in that remote glen.

Eddy was MP for Derbyshire West for fifteen years, until 1938 when his father, Victor, the Ninth Duke, died and Eddy moved to the House of Lords. He kept score of the number of votes cast in his constituency, one of the largest in the country, by planting crocuses at Churchdale in the parties' colours: blue for Conservative, yellow for Liberal, and he had to make do with white for Labour, there being no red crocuses. In the early years, Eddy was driven to meetings by his chauffeur, Lewis James, in a brownish-yellow 1914 Humber known as the Yellow Peril. (It is still roadworthy today.) Outside a rowdy meeting in a quarrying village one day, a man shouted insults about Eddy in front of Lewis. 'So what did you do?' asked Eddy as they drove away. 'I gave him one with my spanner,' said Lewis.

Keenly interested in the animal kingdom, Eddy was president of the Zoological Society of London from 1948 until his death. Herbrand, the Eleventh Duke of Bedford (whose best friend was a spider), was a member of the Society. On one occasion when Eddy was being driven home by Lewis James from the London Zoo, he heard a strange grunting, gabbling noise coming from the boot. 'James,' said Eddy, 'that is not a mechanical noise.' 'Geese, Your Grace. A present from the Duke of Bedford.' They drove on in silence.

*   *   *

Soon after Andrew and I became engaged, he went to Rutland Gate to talk to my father. A lucky thing happened, an incident when they both behaved out of character: Farve put his jumbo teacup, full to the brim, on the edge of a card table that sloped a little. It started to slide. Quick as a flash, Andrew grabbed it with both hands just before the fatal moment when the strong milky tea would have made a hateful puddle on the carpet—the sort of occurrence Farve abhorred. Andrew handed him the cup and was immediately accepted as part of the family. We decided to be married in London, at St Bartholomew the Great in Smithfield. We loved the ancient church and, perhaps subconsciously, craved the feeling of permanence it gave in the upside-down world of war and bombs when everything we knew was changing.

Miraculously, the church survived the Blitz and we were married there on 19 April 1941. My parents-in-law were kindness itself, letting us have the furniture we needed for the tiny mews house off Regent's Park where we lived while Andrew was stationed in London, making us presents of a car and a huge double bed, and giving me a pair of beautiful diamond and aquamarine clips. A sign of the formality of those far-off times was that they never asked me to call them by their Christian name: she was Duchess to me and he was Duke. It was the same for Andrew: Lord and Lady Redesdale never turned into David and Sydney. But these old rules did not interfere with friendship.

I was staying at the Mews with Muv and Farve two nights before our wedding when there was one of London's heaviest air raids of the war. For the first time I was frightened. Two houses at the bottom of the street were sliced in half by a direct hit, and a bed was left hanging precariously over the edge of a floor. All the buildings near by were damaged and every window in No. 26 was blown out. The ballroom, where the reception was to be held, was covered in broken glass and the curtains, which were torn to shreds, had to be put out with the rubbish. Muv bought rolls of grey and gold wallpaper, shaped them into pretend curtains and nailed them to the windows. Luckily the weather was mild as the house was open to the elements. The caterers brought a cake in a white cardboard casing (no icing because of sugar rationing) and when the time came to cut it, all they had to do was lift the cover. Muv somehow got hold of champagne. The wine merchant begged her not to take too much of his precious supply as no more could be had from France.

I was married from the Mews and a photograph shows the wedding group in front of the dustbins. We had no pages or bridesmaids (although Mrs Ham offered to be one, dressed in black, of course). Victor Stiebel made me a dream of a dress from eighty yards of white tulle. I never thought I should own such a thing, and had we been married six weeks later I could not have done: clothes rationing came in and my dress would have taken several years' worth of coupons. Farve gave me away in his Home Guard uniform. He had refused promotion from Private to Corporal because he did not want the responsibility, but his shoes were better polished than many of his comrades'. He was only sixty-three but looks old and sad in the photographs. After it was all over, Andrew and I drove to the government office where I had been summoned to register for war work, along with a crowd of other girls of my age.

We went to my parents-in-law's house Compton Place for our six precious days of honeymoon. It was a week of intensive air raids. All night long the German planes throbbed overhead on their way to London—a constant drone of engines bent on their mission to destroy. Eastbourne was a restricted area because of being on the coast and, with the enemy only a few miles away across the Channel, it may seem a strange place for Andrew's family to have gone in wartime, but we all loved it and I often stayed there when Andrew was away. It suited my father-in-law as the train from Eastbourne to London was quicker and surer for him than the long journey from St Pancras to Miller's Dale, the nearest station to Churchdale. Compton Place had an Elizabethan core, brought up to date in the early eighteenth century by Colen Campbell, no less, and its plasterwork and furniture were superb. The lawns and tennis court were left unmown during the war and masses of bee orchids, which had lain dormant since the First World War, came up through the chalky soil.

Our great friend John Wyndham, a contemporary of Andrew at Eton and Cambridge, lodged with us at our cottage off Regent's Park. His appalling eyesight ruled out military service and he was a civilian, working for Harold Macmillan who was then Parliamentary Secretary to the Ministry of Supply. Like Andrew, John owed money. The bailiffs soon discovered where he was living and two of them spent one day sitting on a wall by the entrance to our cottage. John arrived back from work and asked them what they were doing. They explained and with presence of mind John said, 'Yes, Mr Wyndham is very elusive. I am looking for him too,' and joined them on the wall.

Soon after our honeymoon Andrew was posted to the newly formed 5th Battalion Coldstream Guards, later part of the Guards Armoured Division. For two and a half years they were sent to different camps around the country and I joined

Andrew whenever I could. It was a period of intense activity and intense boredom for him. He said that the training in England was tougher in some ways than actually facing the enemy. On one bitterly cold night his battalion had to cross a swollen river in the north of England where several men lost their lives. On another occasion they were sprayed with blood from the local slaughterhouse; when the exercise was over they returned to camp, hungry and exhausted, to be given almost raw liver to eat. Such was the toughening-up programme. When the battalion was posted to Wiltshire we took a cottage in the main street of Warminster. Andrew went to the training camp by bus and on the way home he always brought a handful of wild flowers (to be identified in our Bentham and Hooker), including tall thistles which brushed the bosoms of the stout women sitting opposite. The battalion camped in the park of Siegfried Sassoon's house, Heytesbury, and Andrew was intrigued to see the writer, whom he greatly admired, wandering around his garden. He longed to talk to him but did not dare.

There was terrific excitement one summer's day when the Queen visited the troops on Salisbury Plain. Our friend Anthony Mildmay was the officer in charge and the men lined up to see Her Majesty drive by. They duly cheered and were bucked by her visit. Following her, sitting bolt upright in another stately Daimler, was the Queen's lady-in-waiting, Lady Nunburnholme, a cool, classic and correct English beauty. As the car drove by, Anthony was delighted to hear a soldier say loudly to his neighbour, 'Oo's the tart?'

We spent many evenings at Sturford Mead, on

the edge of the Longleat estate, with Daphne, the beautiful, lively wife of Nancy's old friend Henry Weymouth. Daphne's house was always full of a cross-section of the British Army, all of whom were in love with her. (Henry Weymouth was in the Royal Wiltshire Yeomanry and spent the entire war in the Middle East, without home leave.) It was at Daphne's that we first met Evelyn Waugh. The phenomenal amount of drink that the writer downed made him tricky company and, as I was still shocked by drunkenness, I kept my distance. One night he poured a bottle of Green Chartreuse over his head and, rubbing it into his hair, intoned, 'My hair is covered in gum, my hair is covered in gum,' as the sticky mess ran down his neck.

When sober, Evelyn's charm was winning, but you had to catch him early in the evening. He wanted to be friends and was full of compliments, but they turned to insults before you knew where you were. The cleverness came through but so did the criticisms; everything was wrong, including me. After the war he made up for his sharp remarks at Sturford by buying me a hat at Rose Bertin in Paris, which he tried on himself in the shop. It was made of white felt, with two white birds perched above its blue straw brim. A Paris hat was a thing of the past and was a welcome present if ever there was one. Good old Evie.

Another figure of Sturford days was Conrad Russell, a dairy farmer, cheese-maker and intimate of the Asquith gang at Mells. Blue eyed and silver haired, he was clever like all Russells. We made friends on the farming level—I could not compete with his brainy neighbours or his adored Diana Cooper. He realized that I was interested in the land and when he died left me his copy of Primrose McConnell's *Agricultural Note-Book*, which ranks high among my unstealable books.

One night when staying with Daphne we were awakened by the smell of burning. The house was on fire. We ran round the bedrooms, shouting to the sleeping guests to leave the house. Daphne's own door was locked; too much had been drunk that evening and it took what seemed an age to wake her. To add to the misery of that night, I put my bare foot in a huge dog's mess in the passage before we all got out—just in time. Panic produces strange reactions. In that house full of what are now described as 'decorative arts', all we managed to grab as we left were a few gramophone records. Poor Daphne lost many precious belongings and, to add insult to injury, was reported for infringing the blackout regulations. We were at Sturford Mead the night Henry came home. He was the handsomest man you ever saw and all seemed happy between him and Daphne. But the separation had been too long and their twenty-five years of marriage ended soon after his return.

Andrew's battalion was later posted to Norfolk, where I stayed in a pub at Hunstanton. We went botanizing in country that was new to both of us and, sitting on a straw stack, I fiddled with my wedding ring and dropped it. A gold ring in a pile of wheat straw is a goner so the ring is in that wheatfield still. Its replacement is a 'utility' one, gold in colour but probably of some baser metal. The loss of the wedding ring was made up for, however, by finding a corncockle—a rare flower in those days.

When I could not be with Andrew, his parents

were the kindest of hosts. My mother-in-law was universally loved. She was vague and always late, but she never interfered or criticized and I was well aware of what a wonderful woman she was. In 1940 an unwelcome guest arrived at Churchdale to disturb our routine: Sir Edward Marsh CVO, CB, CMG, scholar, translator and long-time private secretary to Winston Churchill. He had been knocked down in the blackout by a London taxi and was taken, badly shaken but with no bones broken, to nearby Pratt's Club (owned by my father-in-law) to be tidied up. The Duke took pity on him and invited him to Churchdale to recuperate. He arrived. Almost at once, Elizabeth, Anne and I were irritated by him and his boring tales of his old boss and the stage folk he knew. There he was at supper every night with only us for an audience—my parents-in-law were often in London. He insisted on listening to the nine o'clock news, which interrupted our records of Harry Roy and the like, but as soon as Alvar Liddell's soothing voice came over the wireless telling of the latest disaster, Eddie fell asleep. The little click when we turned off the wireless to go back to our favourite dance bands woke him with a start, and it was back to Alvar Liddell.

For exercise, Eddie tossed a pack of playing cards on the floor and picked them up one by one. I often wondered why he could not do something more useful—dig the garden for instance—but no, he was too special for that. After he had been with us for about a month, a van arrived at Churchdale with his cellar (many cases of Drambuie) and we realized that he was in for a long stay. He was so dug in, and I suppose thought himself part of the

165

family, that whenever the Devonshires moved from Compton Place to Churchdale and back, Eddie Marsh went too. He was head over heels in love with Ivor Novello (whose name he maddeningly pronounced 'I-*vor*') and was in a state of high excitement the day Novello came to tea at Compton Place, as Eddie's guest. Novello looked at my whippet, Studley, and said, his head to one side, 'What an enchanting bit of beige.' Studley was a serious dog, the hero of many hare-coursing days, and was not to be dismissed as 'a bit of beige'. That was the end of the composer of *The Dancing Years* as far as I was concerned. After fourteen and a half months, Eddie finally left. He would have stayed longer but Edward, the butler, and my sisters-in-law formed up to his hosts and said enough was enough. He arrived in November 1940 and left in January 1942. Talk about the man who came to dinner . . .

*   *   *

In November 1943 Andrew embarked for Italy with his battalion. Our daughter Emma was eight months old and we needed a house of our own. I moved into the Rookery, a dark, damp house in Ashford-in-the-Water (the Derbyshire River Wye flows through the garden) belonging to the Chatsworth estate. There were pigsties, stables and a paddock where I kept my driving pony. In the kitchen, a huge coal range took up one wall and smuts penetrated everywhere. The stove gave off such fierce heat, rapidly followed by the depressing sight of cold grey ashes, that our wartime rations were often inedible. Rationing and coupons ruled our lives. When I was in London for Andrew's last few days of leave before he left for Italy, he entrusted me with three hundred of the clothing coupons issued to soldiers to buy all the special kit they needed for going abroad. I was meant to be the reliable one, but I left the precious coupons in a taxi. It was a disaster because they could not be replaced, but Andrew never reproached me.

I lived at the Rookery with Emma, her nanny Diddy, three dogs, a pony and trap, a pig, a cow, and Violet, an evacuee with two small sons. I was blessed with Diddy—Ellen Stephens—who had arrived two months earlier, sent by Divine Providence. She was fifty-four, the minimum age at which any job other than 'war work' could be taken up, and it was our luck that her age coincided with our need. Babies thrived under her care: put a screaming infant into her arms and it immediately calmed down. Her influence went much further than the nursery and her intelligence, common sense, knowledge of the natural world and devotion to the children in her care gave them the best possible start in life. Diddy looked after Emma while I pretended to sort things at the Red Cross county clearing house in Bakewell. I was not much use to them as I was pregnant again and was sick over everything without warning.

I got about in an old milk float drawn by a splendid pedigree Hackney mare and sometimes drove up the steep hill past Sheldon to the limestone plateau of the Peak District. Along the broad grass verges, stretching for a mile or more, were piles of bombs, long and thin, short and fat, unguarded, waiting. They became part of the scenery and then disappeared one day as mysteriously as they had arrived. The mare trotted along the empty A6 to Bakewell in no time. I tied her to a post near Mr Thacker's butcher's shop, where he let me help him cut up the meat in the back room and get a few scraps for the dogs. Tongue was offal and therefore not rationed. 'Any chance of a tongue?' I would ask. 'You're thirty-sixth on the list,' was always the answer. I do not think I ever got to the top. (A woman next to me in the queue, listening to people talking about the end of rationing, said one day, 'Well, if they give it up, meat will be rationed by price and that would never do.' As the years have gone by I have often thought about what she said.) One day a wounded soldier repatriated from Italy brought home a lemon. Such a luxury had not been seen for a long time and it caused a minor sensation when he put it on the post office counter at Ashford-in-the-Water and charged tuppence a smell—proceeds to the Red Cross.

We paid rent to the Chatsworth estate to live at the Rookery. Our income was small at the time and I was appalled by the size of the estate bill for logs, our only form of heating apart from the ancient kitchen range. (My mother-in-law always said that the bill for logs was the land agent's way of trying to balance the forestry accounts.) In one of the snowy winters of the war, I fell ill while on a prolonged visit to Churchdale and Dr Sinclair Evans was called. His practice took him up rough tracks to remote farms and he always dressed in the same thick tweeds and gumboots for any bedside he was called to; with the sleeves of his woollen vest showing round his wrists, he was a reassuring sight in an emergency. Dr Evans was an excellent diagnostician and pronounced pneumonia, which in those days was treated with pills called M & B. In spite of the pills, I was delirious for a while and he told me afterwards that I shouted, 'I'm not in debt, I'm not in debt', obviously the result of the huge bills for firewood from Chatsworth Estates Co.

*   *   *

In January 1944, Henry Hunloke, MP for Derbyshire West, my father-in-law's old constituency, resigned his seat and a by-election was quickly called. Henry had been with his regiment in the Middle East since the outbreak of war and felt that he could no longer adequately represent the voters' interests. More significant, perhaps, he was married to Eddy Devonshire's sister Anne and was in the process of getting a divorce. Derbyshire West had been held almost exclusively by a member of the Cavendish family since the sixteenth century. Andrew's brother, Billy, yet another Cavendish nominee, was selected as the Conservative candidate and in February 1944 got leave from his regiment to fight the election. His selection turned out to be unwise as it made people feel the influence of Chatsworth was too strong: Conservatives were annoyed because the selection procedure had been so hasty and the opposition felt that they had not been given enough time to mount their campaign.

Billy and Andrew did not get on well and there was jealousy on both sides. As the second son, Andrew felt left out of things, and Billy suffered because Andrew was more attractive—not better looking, but quick, funny and popular with girls. It did not help matters that when Andrew was commissioned in 1940 the brothers sometimes found themselves near-neighbours when training. They were wary of stepping on each other's territory and the result was that I saw little of Billy in pre-war days. It was only in the run-up to the by-election that I got to know him and grew fond of him. He used to drop in for a drink on his way home to Churchdale and unwind after the punishing round of political meetings in village halls scattered over the constituency. Billy's opponent was Charles Frederick White Jr, a Socialist who had been active in local government for over thirty years. The fight was personal and grubby, and the meetings rowdy and sometimes rough. White's supporters taught children to chant:

> Charlie White's a gentleman
> Hartington's a fool
> Before he goes to politics
> He ought to go to school.

The country as a whole was fed up with rationing, discipline and the worsening conditions at home; and there seemed to be no light at the end of the tunnel. Nationalization of the coal industry was on everyone's lips and although mining was minimal in Derbyshire West, the constituency was surrounded by coal mines and heavy industry and the electorate was longing for change. As heir to one of the largest land holdings, and perhaps the greatest private collection of works of art in England, as well as several huge houses, Billy was a target for the anti-establishment brigade. He was beaten by 4,561 votes, receiving 41.5 per cent of the vote to White's 57.7 per cent. Billy's speech at the declaration of the poll was as memorable as his appearance: tall and fit from five years of army service, he was as handsome as a film star. 'It has been a hard fight,' he told his audience, 'and that is the way it goes. I am going out now to fight for you at the front. After all, unless we win the war there can be no home front. Better luck next time.' There were loud cheers, some of the women were in tears—perhaps they had a premonition of what was to come. One old lady standing next to me said, 'It's a shame to let him go, a great tall man like he is, he's such a target.'

The result of the by-election was a personal blow for Churchill, foreshadowing the defeat of Conservatism and Labour's landslide victory the following year. Derbyshire West had decided it wanted out with the old and in with the new, but the 'old' in this case was young and full of promise, while the 'new' was a grey man, lacking in distinction or appeal, with a bitter twist to his speeches. C. F. White sank without trace in the House of Commons. He hung on to his seat by only 156 votes in the 1945 General Election and decided, wisely, not to stand again in 1950.

Billy rejoined his regiment, now preparing for the invasion of France. Sadly, I could not go to his wedding to Kick on 6 May 1944 as I was still in bed after the birth of our son, Stoker. That Billy and Kick managed to marry at all was a tribute to their love for each other. It is difficult to realize the depth of antagonism that still existed in the 1940s between Protestants and Catholics. Billy came from a deeply religious Protestant background and Kick's Irish-Catholic parents felt just as strongly about their creed. At the eleventh hour, after a series of discussions with the head of the Roman Catholic Church in England and the Archbishop of Canterbury, the seemingly insurmountable obstacles were overcome and it was agreed that any sons of the union should be brought up in the Church of England and any daughters as Roman Catholics. My father-in-law had been haunted by the possibility that if his beloved Billy married a Roman Catholic any eventual heirs would be brought up in that faith, and the outcome satisfied him. Both he and Moucher became devoted to Kick, who was welcomed into the family by all. Rose Kennedy never accepted the decision and her relationship with her daughter suffered accordingly.

Billy and Kick had ecstatically happy moments together, snatching days and nights while preparations for D-Day were gathering speed. Six weeks after their wedding Billy left with his battalion for France and was part of the Allied advance that pushed towards Belgium at a fearful cost of British lives. They reached the border at the beginning of September, where they met stiff enemy resistance. Unbelievably, officers were allowed to wear pale-coloured corduroy trousers, a beret and to carry a swagger stick—an obvious target for a sniper. And so it was. On 9 September 1944 Billy, now a Major, was walking ahead of his company to lead an assault on the village of Heppen, when he was shot through the heart by a single bullet and died where he fell. His men were enraged. 'We took no prisoners that day,' one of them wrote to my father-in-law. Billy was buried at Leopoldsburg, one of nearly 800 Commonwealth dead in that cemetery.

Eddy and Moucher were devastated. Their hopes for the future died with their son. Kick, a widow at twenty-four, was in America for a memorial service for her elder brother, Joe Jr, who had been killed in action. She returned immediately to Compton Place, where Billy's parents, sisters and I tried to comfort each other. I wrote to Muv, 'As always when someone you know intimately has been killed, it seems quite impossible that you won't see him again. I am afraid of writing to Andrew. I don't know what to say or how to say it . . . They don't hold out any hope of getting Andrew home till after the war. I wish Winston was here as it's possible he might understand and send for him. I do so want to see him and he would make the whole difference to his mother and father.' To Diana I wrote that I was worried that Andrew might go right under for a time.

When the news of his brother's death reached him, Andrew was in the front line of some of the fiercest battles of the Italian campaign. The enemy were holding every inch of the ground and his company was in the thick of it. It was a miracle that he came out alive.

He wrote to me on 22 September:

My Own Darling,

In an odd sort of way I have always known that the happiness of our family life was too good to last and now the tragedy has happened. It seems odd that Billy, with everything to live for and so brilliantly capable of carrying out the life that he had to lead, should be taken just when that life was beginning, but I do not doubt for one moment that there is a reason. Wherever he has gone, he has gone in the good company of his and our friends.

My darling, you must be having a difficult and utterly miserable time. If only I could be there to be of some use—but it is the greatest comfort to me to know that you are there. I know what a difference it will make to Mummy and Daddy. The thought of their grief is terrible. That is the wicked part of death—the grief and sorrow it leaves behind.

Darling, it seems out of place among the misery of the moment and I only mention it on the chance it will give you all a bit of pleasure, I have been given an MC—most undeserved. It is nice to have it and I hope Mummy and Daddy will be pleased.

Darling, I suppose our life is going to be very different to what we had planned. But I know whatever life has in store, with you beside me life has no fears.

God bless you, my darling. Don't grieve for me.

It was so typical of Andrew just to throw in that he had received the Military Cross, as though it had been at a vicarage tea party. He was, in fact, decorated for 'the cheerfulness and leadership he displayed' when his Company had to dig in under heavy shelling near a village called Strada, south of Florence, and was trapped for thirty-six hours in scorching weather with nothing to eat and, worse, nothing to drink.

Andrew's time in Italy changed him. He saw many of his comrades dead or wounded and had a particularly horrifying experience when his mentor, Sergeant King, was killed. He had told the Sergeant to stay put while he went to look over a ridge to see if there was any sign of the enemy. When he got back the gallant Sergeant had been blown to bits by a mortar bomb. Andrew rarely spoke of this or any other of his experiences during the war, but they must, as they did for millions, have had a traumatic effect. The process of becoming an adult was concentrated into a few hard weeks.

After Billy's death, my parents-in-law continued their peregrinations between Churchdale and Eastbourne, but Eddy vowed never to set foot inside Chatsworth again. He had lost heart and could not bring himself to be interested in the future of a house which five years previously had been the scene of joyous celebrations for his adored son's twenty-first birthday.

*   *   *

For me 1944 was a momentous year. Two events of the greatest joy were the birth of Stoker and the news in October that Andrew was coming home. But the bad news came thick and fast. A few weeks before D-Day I was staying at Compton Place. Eastbourne was crowded with troops and my mother-in-law invited Ned Fitzmaurice, who was in the Irish Guards, Luke Lillingston, from the Leicestershire Yeomanry, and other young officers to tea. She told them to go to the kitchen garden and help themselves to strawberries. 'Awfully sorry,' said Luke, 'I've done that already.' He had scaled the high brick wall and gorged on a private feast. Two weeks later he was dead from wounds received in action. He left a lasting memory of a most attractive man with a reputation for being a fine horseman and an old-fashioned thruster out hunting.

That was the start. During the months of July and August my four greatest friends were killed. Mark Howard was the first to go, hit by shellfire on 2 July near a village called Marcelet, north-west of Caen. (Billy replaced him as Company commander.) Then Ned Fitzmaurice, aged just twenty-two, was killed on 11 August in a hail of machine-gun fire as he was leading his platoon. 'He was game to the last,' wrote a Lance Corporal in his regiment, 'no one could ever imagine him to possess the guts he had. I only wish a good many more could have had half of his, he is the gamest little lad I have ever seen. His first time in battle and Second-in-Command of the Company that morning.' Nine days later Ned's elder brother, Charlie, was blown up with his tank in Italy. He had been in the Middle East and Africa and away from his family and friends for years. He was posted as 'missing', giving false hope to his mother. His body was never found. On 12 August Dicky Cecil, aged twenty-two, a Sergeant Pilot in the RAF, died from injuries suffered in a motorbike accident in this country. The deaths of these four, so soon to be followed by Billy, left their family and friends numb.

Tom had gone through the North African campaign and thence to Italy, where in January

1944 he happened to meet Andrew. He found him sitting by the side of a road brewing tea with his Company. 'Tell Debo that he was very cheerful,' Tom wrote to Muv the next day. Tom gave Andrew some chocolate and a bottle of whisky, and they parted. Tom returned to England at the beginning of July 1944 and enrolled on a course at the Staff College in Camberley. His friendship with János and Teddy Almásy, and others in Germany, made him recoil at the idea of being part of the victorious army that would advance through Germany to finish the job. He asked to be transferred to the Devonshire Regiment, which was engaged against the Japanese in Burma. It must have been a wrench to leave his old comrades of the King's Royal Rifle Corps but it was his decision.

He arrived in Burma on 22 February 1945 and three weeks later was appointed Brigade Major. He knew not a soul in his new regiment, but the fact that they were face to face with the Japanese Army was good enough for him. Five weeks after his arrival he was hit by a burst of machine-gun fire from the enemy position. He was taken, still conscious, to the regimental aid post and operated on to remove a bullet that had penetrated his neck and lodged in his spine. He died six days later on 30 March and is buried near the Irrawaddy River, north-west of Mandalay.

Muv was at Inch Kenneth when the news came and Farve broke it to her in a telegram. 'I do not know how to tell you this,' he began. Tom's commanding officer sent a letter to my parents: 'It would be difficult to imagine a better regimental soldier,' he wrote.

He had courage, an iron sense of duty, an immense capacity for work, perfect manners and an unfailing interest in all the details of soldiering which can be so tedious and are yet so important for the efficiency and happiness of the battalion. Tom was not the easiest of men to get on with. He held strong views which he defended with skill and wit and he did not suffer fools gladly: but those to whom he gave his confidence and affection will have to travel far before they find a better or more loyal friend.

At the end of the war, a memorial to Tom was installed above my parents' pew in Swinbrook Church, and I am glad it is there for all to see. It is my lasting regret that I did not know my brother better.

After D-Day, Muv and Unity were given permission to go to Inch Kenneth, where I joined them in August 1944. It was misery. Farve, who had spent much of the war on the island, sat stony-faced at table while Margaret's trite remarks about what she had heard on the news dampened any attempts at conversation. It was hard to believe that Farve was the same man who, whenever one of us children made a critical remark about Muv, used to get up from his dining-room chair at Swinbrook and rush round to tell her that her hair was molten gold and that she was more beautiful than the day. (It used to make us laugh—she was well past middle age and was indifferent to her appearance.) Now he seemed to hate her. Instead of joining us after supper, he washed up with Margaret. There were no more jokes. Muv's piano was silent. It was no longer her house.

Unity's odd behaviour added to the strained atmosphere. She summoned Muv and me to the island's ruined chapel one day, wound a sheet round her waist as a cassock and pretended to be a clergyman taking the service. She forgot the words to the 'Te Deum' and 'Jubilate' and stumped back to the house, angry with herself and us for witnessing these shortcomings. It was all unbearably sad and the feeling of wretchedness was intensified by the isolation of the island; there was no one to talk to and nowhere to go—no cinema for Unity, no club for Farve, no antique shops for Muv. What should have been an idyllic place for a summer holiday was a kind of hell.

Recently a young journalist came to interview me about what I was doing the day war broke out. During the course of the interview, I recounted the deaths of my only brother, Andrew's only brother, a brother-in-law and my four best friends. 'So,' she said, 'did the war affect you in any way?'

10

Childbirths and Deaths

You might think having a baby is a natural function that happens when women wish it—and sometimes when they do not. But unforeseen hazards arise and things can change quickly from good to bad. When Andrew and I were first married, the false calm of the Phoney War was over and we did not know when he would be ordered abroad or whether either of us was likely to survive. We both wanted children and there was no question of postponement. We never imagined that everything might not go according to plan.

Almost immediately a baby was on the way and, like so many of our friends and contemporaries, we were happily anticipating the birth. Andrew's battalion was stationed in Hertfordshire at the time and we were living in a rented house at Shenley. I booked into Lady Carnarvon's nursing home, the Claridges of such places, which had been evacuated from London to Barnet, a few miles away. I went to a gynaecologist, Mr Gilliatt (later Sir William), generally accepted to be the leader in his profession, and all seemed to be going well. In November 1941, two and a half months before the baby was due, I fell ill with pain in my back and a high fever. (I was told later that *e-coli* was to blame.) Before the local doctor realized that something was wrong I went into labour and was hurried to the nursing home.

The baby was born after the well-named labour, which lasted several hours—an experience as every mother knows of extreme pain replaced by euphoria when the child is finally born, a new life starts and there is joy all round. But it was not like that. I heard the baby cry—animal instinct plays a big part during and after a birth and the cry of a newborn is the reward for the immense physical effort—and although I knew it was born too early, I had a wild hope that he (for it was a boy) would survive. The famous gynaecologist arrived when it was all over. He walked into the room, gave my stomach a rough push saying that was to get rid of the afterbirth, and added as he left, 'You don't expect the baby to live, do you?'

A few hours later, a nurse came to tell me that the baby had indeed died. I realized then what wonderful people nurses are; the worst jobs are always left to them, especially by grand doctors. Andrew arrived on compassionate leave and that was an immense comfort. It was a difficult time for him too as it had never occurred to him that such a thing could happen and that the outcome could be so sorrowful. The poor little baby was named Mark and buried in St Etheldreda, the parish church at Hatfield, just outside an entrance to the garden of Hatfield House where Andrew's Salisbury grandparents lived.

Despair slowly gives way to a sense of emptiness, grief for what might have been and feelings of self-reproach. Was it my fault? What did I do wrong? It was not easy to get back to day-to-day life. The loss of a premature baby was nothing in comparison to the sufferings caused by the war—the deprivations, the indiscriminate bombings and the daily deaths of young servicemen—but my own sense of failure, of being unable to achieve what most women can, remained. It was made worse when I heard of friends who had produced healthy babies with no difficulty. One of these friends, thinking to be kind, made me godmother to her child, not realizing how painful it would be.

Sixteen months later, on 26 March 1943, Emma was born, naturally and happily. Andrew's battalion was still in England and I spent the last six weeks before the birth with the Salisburys at Hatfield, to be near the nursing home in case of a second disaster. Their kindness has never been forgotten. Alice Salisbury, Andrew's grandmother, was a woman of irresistible charm—liberal, worldly-wise and funny. She used to stand in front of one of Hatfield's huge log fires and hitch up the back of her skirt to warm her behind. The house had become a hospital for wounded soldiers and the resident doctors often came to dinner. The fare was meagre by that stage of the war and was served on a Lazy Susan that revolved in the middle of the table. It whizzed so fast that you had to be quick to grab a bite to eat. I loved that visit and its successful ending.

Just over one year later, in April 1944, our son was born under rather different circumstances. Andrew had left for Italy, and I was staying at Churchdale with the Devonshires. Dr Evans arranged for 27 April to be his day off so as not to be interrupted. I was in the kitchen garden looking for something green to eat when he arrived armed with an injection to set me off. In what seemed no time at all it was over, the easiest birth of all my babies, and off went a message to Andrew, by now advancing on Rome. On 4 May Andrew wrote saying that he had received the news and what huge pleasure it gave him.

Sister O'Gorman, the Irish monthly nurse who had seen me through good times and bad, was with me for the confinement. (I suppose she had a Christian name, but 'Sister' was what we all, with great respect, called her.) As smart as paint when on duty in Lady Carnarvon's pink uniform, impatient when a patient was not really ill, Sister O'Gorman was a brilliant nurse and nothing could detract from that. But I was surprised when I opened a drawer after she had left to find dirty stockings mixed up with broken biscuits—an unexpected legacy from this loved woman. She was an extraordinary support during my strange experiences, genial and funny as only the Irish can be. Rather shame-faced I told her that when I was pregnant my craving had been for coal. Derby Brights were my particular favourites and I ate a good deal of them, breaking off the shiny bits and blackening my teeth in the process. 'Oh,' she said, 'that's nothing. My last patient ate Vim.'

Before Andrew left for Italy, we had decided on names. If a boy, he wanted 'Peregrine', to which I added 'Andrew' and 'Morny' after Mornington Cannon, a jockey I admired. Our family is famous for nicknames and, inevitably, when he was about four, the name 'Peregrine' became rather a mouthful and was replaced by all sorts of nicknames. The ugliest, I suppose, was 'Stoker', but it stuck. When Andrew came home in March 1945, his contented, easy-going son was eleven months old.

The following autumn I was pregnant for the fourth time. That is to say, I was pregnant for a while. In December, for no apparent reason, I had a miscarriage—no illness, no shock, no accident— and I lost a lot of blood before the doctor could get to me. Being fairly early on, I was sad, but it was not advanced enough to compare with the loss of the baby in 1941. Life went on without too much disruption. A couple of months later I could not do up my skirt and felt the stirrings of another baby. Incredulous, I went to Dr Evans. 'Yes,' he said, 'you must have miscarried a twin,' and explained that it could sometimes happen.

By this time, Andrew and I had moved from the Rookery to Edensor House in the small village within the park at Chatsworth. I went into labour six weeks early, for no particular reason that I know of but far enough on for the baby to be all right. Dr Evans came and so did the district nurse, an old friend. I heard them talking through the haze, the pains grew to be almost unbearable and there was the baby. 'A lovely boy,' they reassured me, wrapping him up and putting him in his cot. Sister O'Gorman had not yet arrived from London and they left me, saying they would be back in a few hours. Dr Evans and Nurse Parry returned when the baby was seven hours old and apparently healthy, to hear him give a great sigh and die. The shock of the loss of this baby must have gone deep with Dr Evans. As he was leaving the house he fainted dead away and poor Andrew arrived from a distant engagement to face not just the misery of the dead baby but Dr Evans lying unconscious in the hall. We named the child Victor and he was buried in the family plot at St Peter's, Edensor.

For this last confinement, Dr Evans had borrowed a contraption called a gas and air machine, used as an analgesic in childbirth. As the pains get more severe you clamp a mask on to your face with both hands and gulp the blessed gas as hard as you can. As you lose consciousness, your hands drop and with them the mask; then back to normal till it is repeated all over again. It is such a clever idea: you cannot overdo the gas and it helps at the worst moments. The Baslow practice did not own such a machine, which I thought I could remedy and did. Dr Evans brought the new device with him on an ordinary visit and we tried it out sitting on my bed, flopping over backwards as we each blacked out in turn. (I suppose today we would be had up for charges under all sorts of new laws.)

There was a third unhappy ending in 1953. Again premature, she too was alive and crying before quietly fading away. We gave her the name Mary and she is buried at Edensor alongside her brother Victor. Andrew had the harrowing duty of arranging the funerals, each with its tiny coffin. I was spared this because in those days, where possible, the mother was kept in bed for two or three weeks after giving birth. No one suggested that I should go to the services and I remained completely removed from them.

The cumulative effect of these failures made me wonder how it was that we had two perfectly healthy children, who were progressing just as children should. People sympathized at the losses and with the kindest intentions would say, 'Look at those two. How wonderful to have them.' It was indeed wonderful, but people who have not been through the searing experience cannot understand that you mourn the lost ones and that nothing can replace them. Nevertheless, had Emma and Stoker not survived I think the tragedies would have overwhelmed me.

When Sophy was born on 18 March 1957 and all was well, there was much rejoicing. For the first four months of pregnancy I stayed in or near my bed, constantly fearful of what now seemed the inevitable disaster. The reward for this slight inconvenience was inestimable and went a long way in restoring a sense of achievement. Sophy was born in a London hospital, where the doctor brought his spaniels to cheer his country patients. I was so apprehensive that I did not buy any new clothes for the baby, and the washed-out woolly things and old-fashioned gowns surprised the nurses in the smart maternity wing. As soon as Sophy was born I remember shouting, 'Is the baby all right?' Then, louder, 'IS THE BABY ALL RIGHT?' I could hardly believe it when they said that she was perfect. The fourteen-year gap between Emma and Sophy sometimes caused people to ask, 'Who was your first husband?'

As time went on, I appreciated more and more the incredible good fortune of having Emma, Stoker and Sophy, and the sadness for the other three faded. But writing about them now made me wonder whether the three who did not survive had been christened. Bleak notices of the burials of Mark, Victor and Mary appear in the Records Offices in Hertfordshire and Derbyshire, giving their ages as five hours, seven hours and four hours respectively (their short lives contrasting pathetically with all the old people on the lists). The vicar at Hatfield kindly made some enquiries and found a note about Mark's burial, but no record of a christening. Nor were there any records of a christening at St Peter's, Edensor. It is only recently that I discovered from Mrs Symonds, widow of the Reverend Tom Symonds, Vicar of Edensor 1954–71 (who had been told by Francis Thompson, the long-serving librarian at Chatsworth), that my mother-in-law baptized all three children in an emergency ceremony, recognized by the Church of England (and the Roman Catholic Church). I cannot imagine a better person to do it. I am glad I know the recorded facts of these births and deaths so their sorry chapter can now be closed.

11

Inheritance

In October 1944, six weeks after Billy was killed, I received a letter from Andrew telling me that he was coming home. I could hardly believe it. 'Oh dear, I am nearly off my head,' I wrote to Muv, 'I don't know whether I'm coming or going.' Andrew wrote that he would be back about the middle of December as he had to stay at a Reinforcement Depot for about a month and would then get a boat and come home. 'Oh can you imagine how wonderful it will be for me and for his mother and father,' I told Muv, 'I am nearly dying.'

Andrew eventually arrived home in March 1945. He had been withdrawn from his battalion and sent to a training camp near Naples at the request, as he later discovered, of Harold Macmillan, who at the time was Minister Resident with Cabinet status at Allied Force Headquarters in Algiers. Macmillan was married to Eddy Devonshire's sister Dorothy, and was known as 'Uncle Harold' in the family. In spite of the relief Andrew knew it must have brought his mother and father, he bitterly resented being taken away from the front. He never spoke to me about it, but I know that the order to go to the training camp was the hardest to obey in his five years of army service. In his memoirs, *Accidents of Fortune*, he wrote that when he rejoined his comrades who had fought on during three hard months, he was unable to look them in the eye.

With the horrors of the Italian campaign still fresh in his mind, it must have been difficult for Andrew to adjust to a calm life in the country where there was no petrol and the strictest food rationing yet. He had to decide his future. He was now heir to his father's estates but Eddy, aged fifty, was still in charge. Andrew's mind turned to politics, which had always been his overriding interest. He knew that he had no chance of being selected for a winnable seat so had to make a start with a safe Labour seat, which would serve as a good apprenticeship. He tried for two constituencies in the East End of London—Mile End and Shoreditch—but was turned down by both. The fact that he was the son of a duke and had been to Eton and Cambridge was enough to ensure he was not selected; his war record counted for nothing. He tried for North East Derbyshire but was again unsuccessful and was beginning to lose heart when Councillor Ernest Robinson, chairman of the few Conservatives in Chesterfield, persuaded the committee to hear Andrew put his case. To Andrew's joy, he was adopted and it was the beginning of our long association with that town and the many men and women of all political opinions with whom we made friends.

Andrew's father seldom gave him advice but when he did it was taken and used again and again. 'There is something you should ram home,' Eddy said to Andrew, 'and you cannot repeat it too often. No government has any money of its own, the only money it has to spend is what it gets from you and me in taxes.' You could see by the expression on the faces of some of Andrew's audience that they did not believe it (and some people probably still do not). I remember another piece of advice Eddy gave, delivered in his usual dry manner. 'Andy,' he said, 'mark my words, wherever there is trouble in the world there is a clergyman behind it.'

I have always voted Conservative and would never do otherwise. When we were young, Decca used to say in a sarcastic voice, 'There you go again. You're a Conservative policeman,' whenever I attempted to forestall a row with our parents. I was never tempted to follow any extreme cause, but I did get worked up in the 1945 General Election (and in subsequent elections), partly because of the personalities involved and partly because of my dislike of any Socialist government and their pretences. I was not interested in Communism or Fascism—I had had too much of them in my childhood.

Nationalization of the coal mines was the main topic in the run-up to the 1945 election, and feelings ran so high that the police were often present at meetings. We were spat at and our car was rolled till it nearly turned over. Audiences were rowdy and the heckling sometimes aggressive. On one occasion, a man at the back of the hall shouted to Andrew that he wanted to shake his hand. Andrew was so surprised at this friendly gesture that he jumped off the stage and ran down the aisle, where an accomplice shot out his leg and sent him crashing to the floor. He picked himself up, dismayed but unhurt, and returned to the platform with the audience laughing. I always thought that the way the Socialists presented nationalization to the coal miners was grossly unfair. The miners were led to believe that their lives would be transformed from one day to the next when the National Coal Board took over. In the event they found themselves back underground, the old hierarchy still in place. The only change, it seemed to me, was that there were more managers, while the men who mattered came to the surface as grimy as ever.

The election was a landslide victory for Labour, following the trend set in Derbyshire West the previous year. Andrew was beaten by over 12,000 votes, but he had whipped up such enthusiasm among his supporters that we had almost persuaded ourselves he could win. He stayed with Chesterfield after 1945 and spent a great deal of time in the constituency where he became well known. In the 1950 General Election, the boundaries of the constituency were changed to include the industrial district of Staveley and some of the worst housing in the neighbourhood. Labour won again with an even larger majority.

*   *   *

In March 1946 we moved to Edensor House, less than a mile from Chatsworth. My father-in-law thought Andrew should be nearer the big house and the estate office, and learn how things were run. Eddy had no intention of going to live at Chatsworth himself—Billy's death had seen to that. As far as I know, he kept his vow of never setting foot in the house again, with one exception: he gave away his daughter, Anne, at her wedding to Michael Tree in the chapel at Chatsworth in November 1949. But he did not sleep in the house and chose to stay with Andrew and me at Edensor, as he had always done since the end of the war whenever he came to Derbyshire on business.

Even before the tragedy of Billy's death, the house had never held happy memories for Eddy, and his childhood had been made miserable by continual criticisms from his mother, Granny Evie. He told me that every time he came home from boarding school his mother made him cry on the first day of the holidays. (Surprisingly, he later wrote affectionate letters to her, showing that his regard for his mother was ambivalent.) In 1925 his father, Victor Duke, had a stroke. He lived on for thirteen years but was very different to the benign person he had once been. He lost his temper with everyone and lay about him with his stick: station masters and footmen were his regular targets. When Victor became acutely ill, my old friend Dr Evans visited him daily and described the ordeal:

Every morning the routine was the same. I must enter the sick room and sit down quietly in a chair at one side of the fire, His Grace would be sitting on the other side reading *The Times*. Whatever happened I must not make a sound until he lowered the newspaper and peered over the top. His temper was known to be uncertain. I was told that sometimes his valet had to crawl under the breakfast table to lace up his boots. In this position His Grace found it impossible to belabour him with his walking stick.

Victor went on shooting after his stroke and was extremely dangerous, swinging round with his gun with no regard for his neighbours. Billy and

Andrew were placed either side of him, which naturally put Andrew off the sport as he was in mortal fear of his grandfather's gun. (Moucher even went so far as to buy the boys bullet-proof spectacles.) The only person at Chatsworth liked by the Duke was John Maclauchlan, the autocratic head keeper, who took him rabbit shooting, which Victor preferred to set-piece pheasant shoots. On one occasion, the Duke took a grandson, Peter Baillie, with him on this ploy. Peter, aged about six, created a legend in the family by turning a sackful of ferrets upside down on to the Duke's head and, surprisingly, did not get into trouble for this bold action.

No wonder Chatsworth was an unhappy place during those years. Granny Evie tried to carry on as if nothing had happened but the house and estate lacked a leader and it showed. Victor paid no attention to the head land agent and things gradually went downhill. Neither Eddy nor Moucher had the authority to run the many departments, including woods, farms, farm buildings and the hundreds of other houses and cottages on the estate. It was a relief to everybody when, in May 1938, Victor's life came to an end. Eddy and Moucher delayed moving into Chatsworth while essential plumbing work was carried out and camped there the following Christmas before setting off in the New Year for a long tour of Australia and South Africa. Eddy was Parliamentary Under Secretary for Dominion Affairs, a post he held until 1940. As soon as war was declared, he and Moucher packed up Chatsworth and went back to Churchdale.

After the war Eddy spent more and more time in

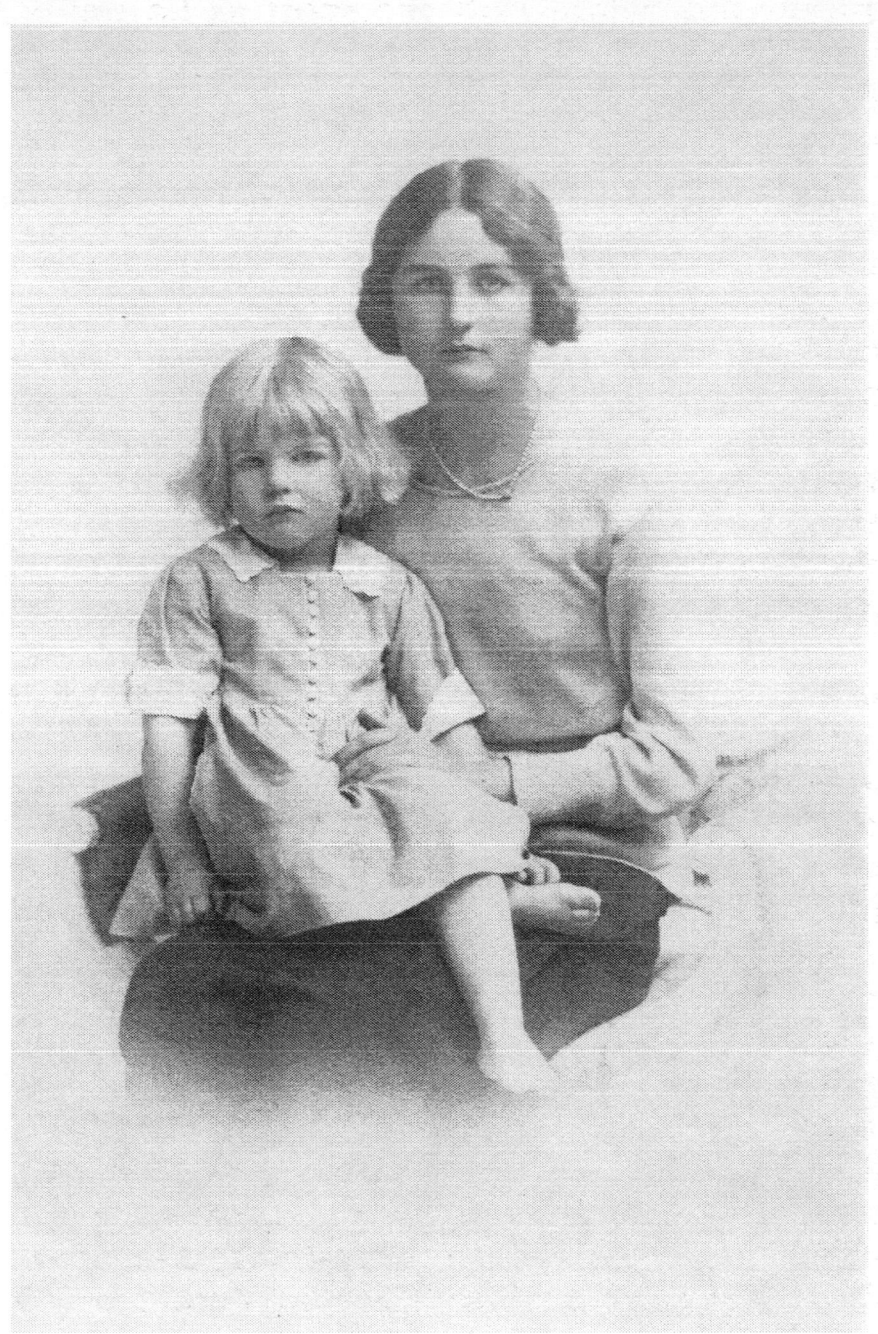

Aged three, with my eldest sister, Nancy

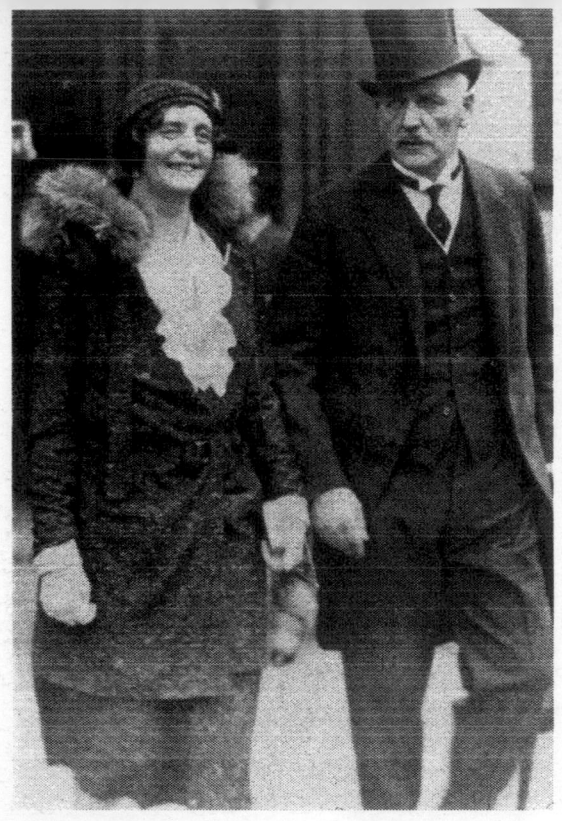

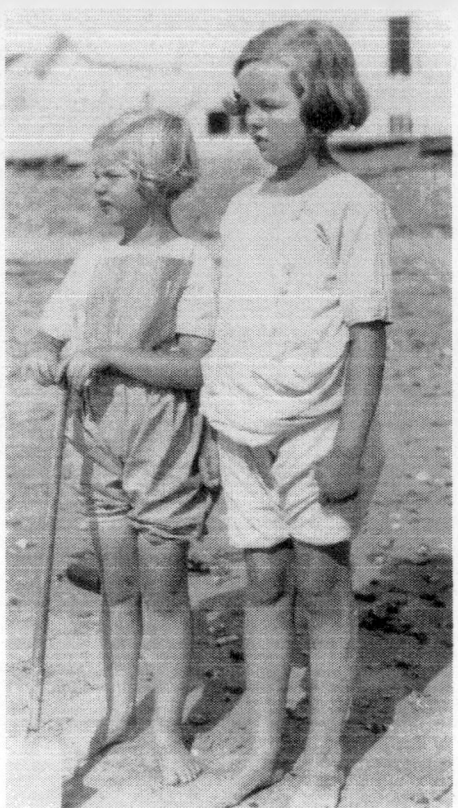

My mother and father (Muv and Farve)

With Decca (*right*) at Hastings

By the River Windrush at Asthall

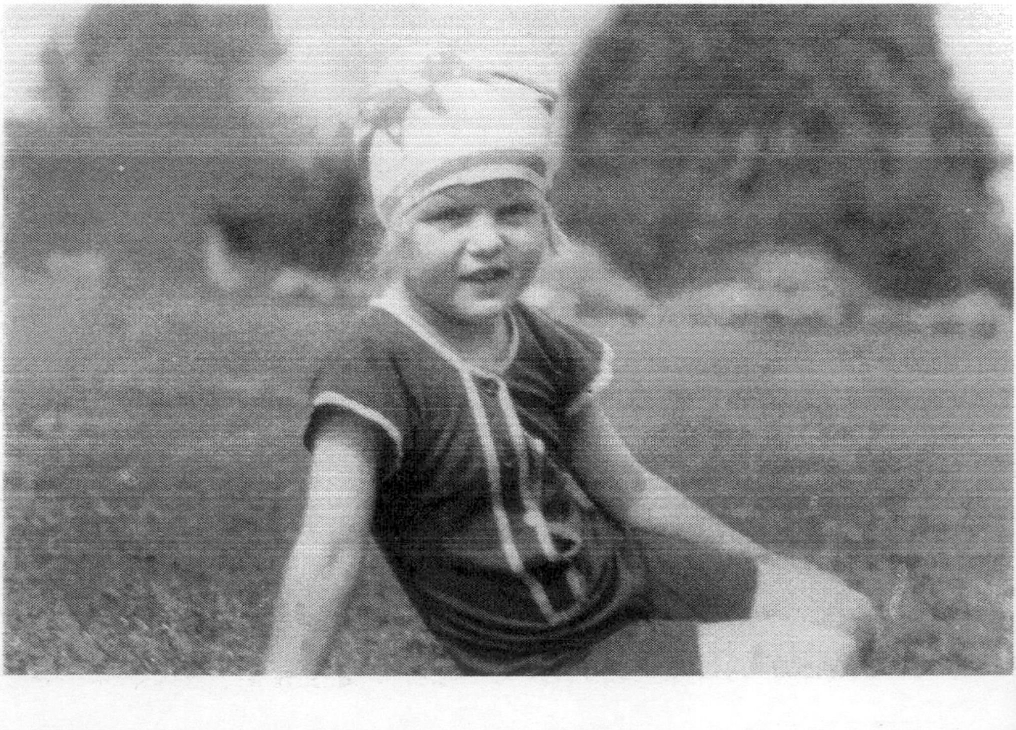

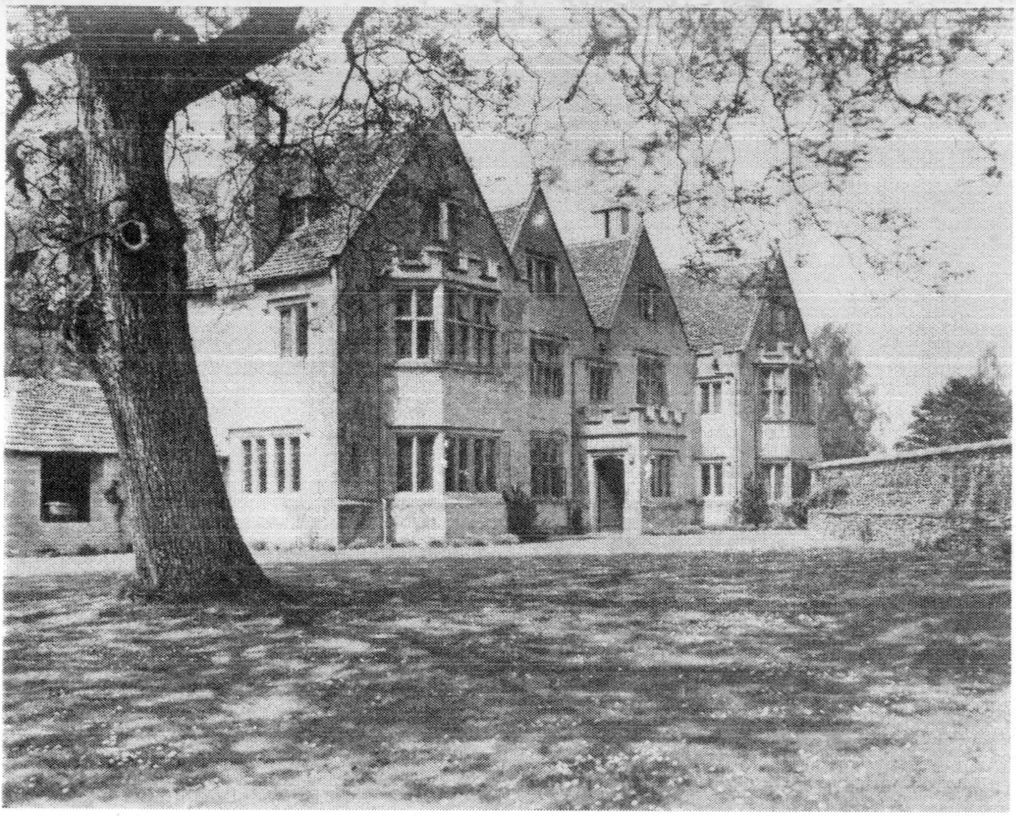

Asthall Manor

Muv and Farve with (*back row*) Nancy, Tom; (*middle row*) Diana, Pamela; (*front row*) Unity, Decca, DD. Asthall, 1926

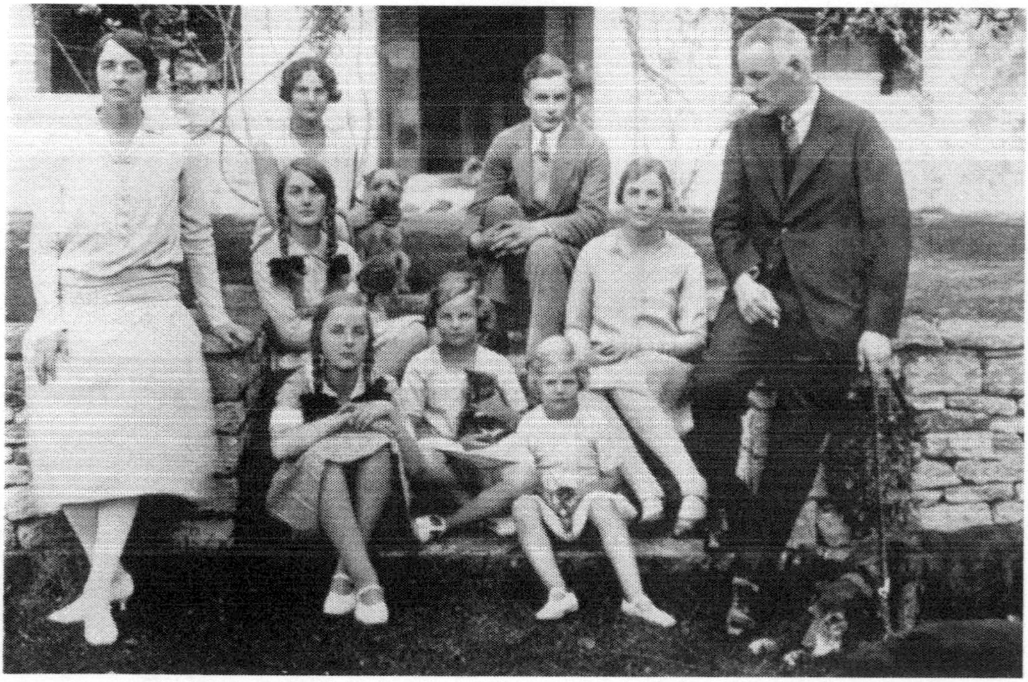

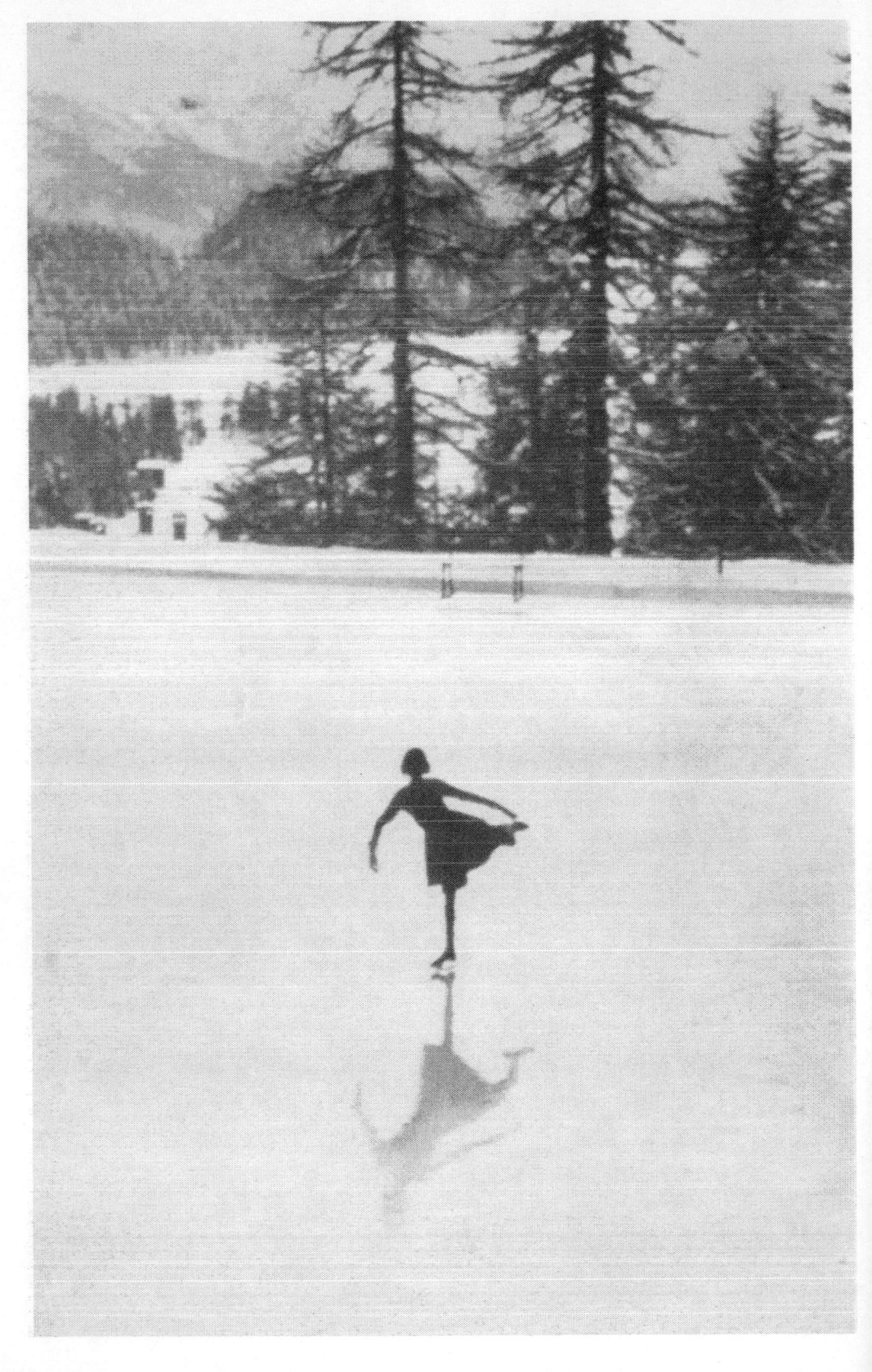

Left: Skating at the Suvretta House Hotel, St Moritz, 1930

Right: At Swinbrook with Nanny Blor

Below: Driving my donkey, Tonks, with Cecilia Hay (*left*), 1934

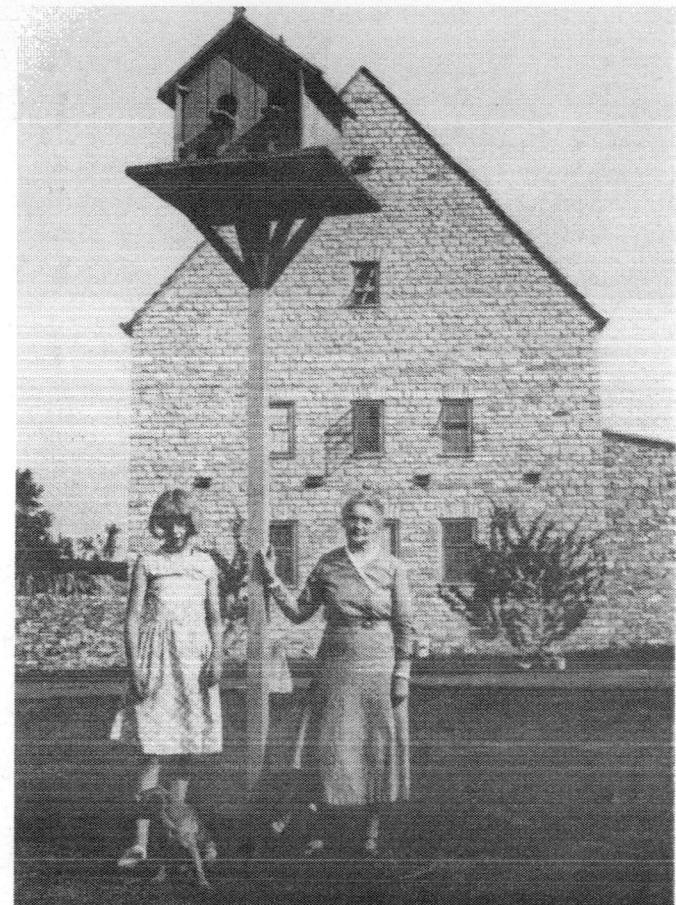

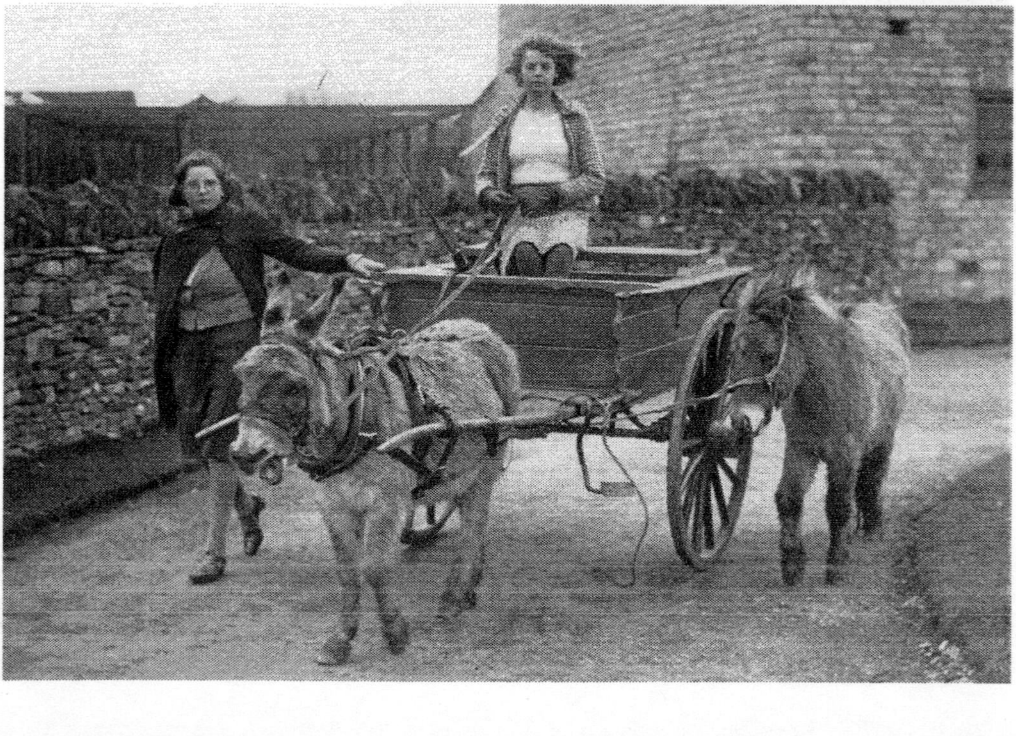

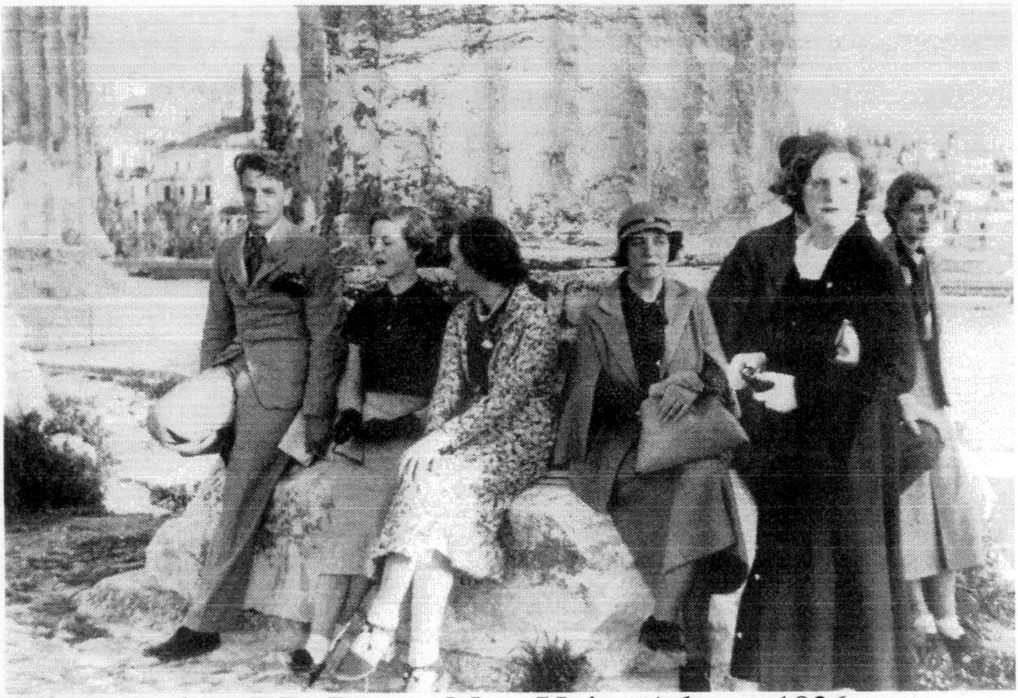

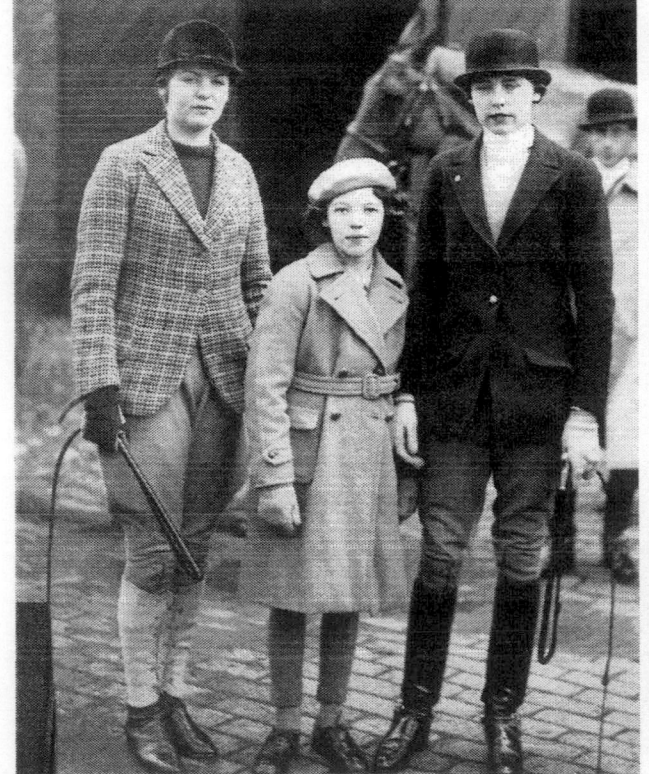
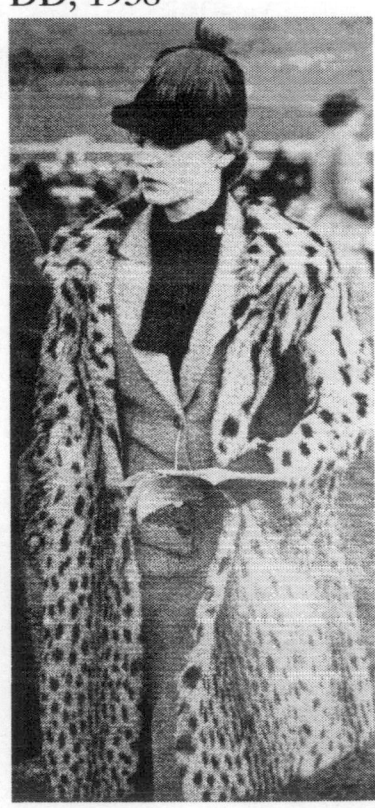

Adrian Stokes, DD, Decca, Muv, Unity. Athens, 1936

DD (*left*) with Myra and Gina Wernher.
Thorpe Lubenham, 1937

DD, 1938

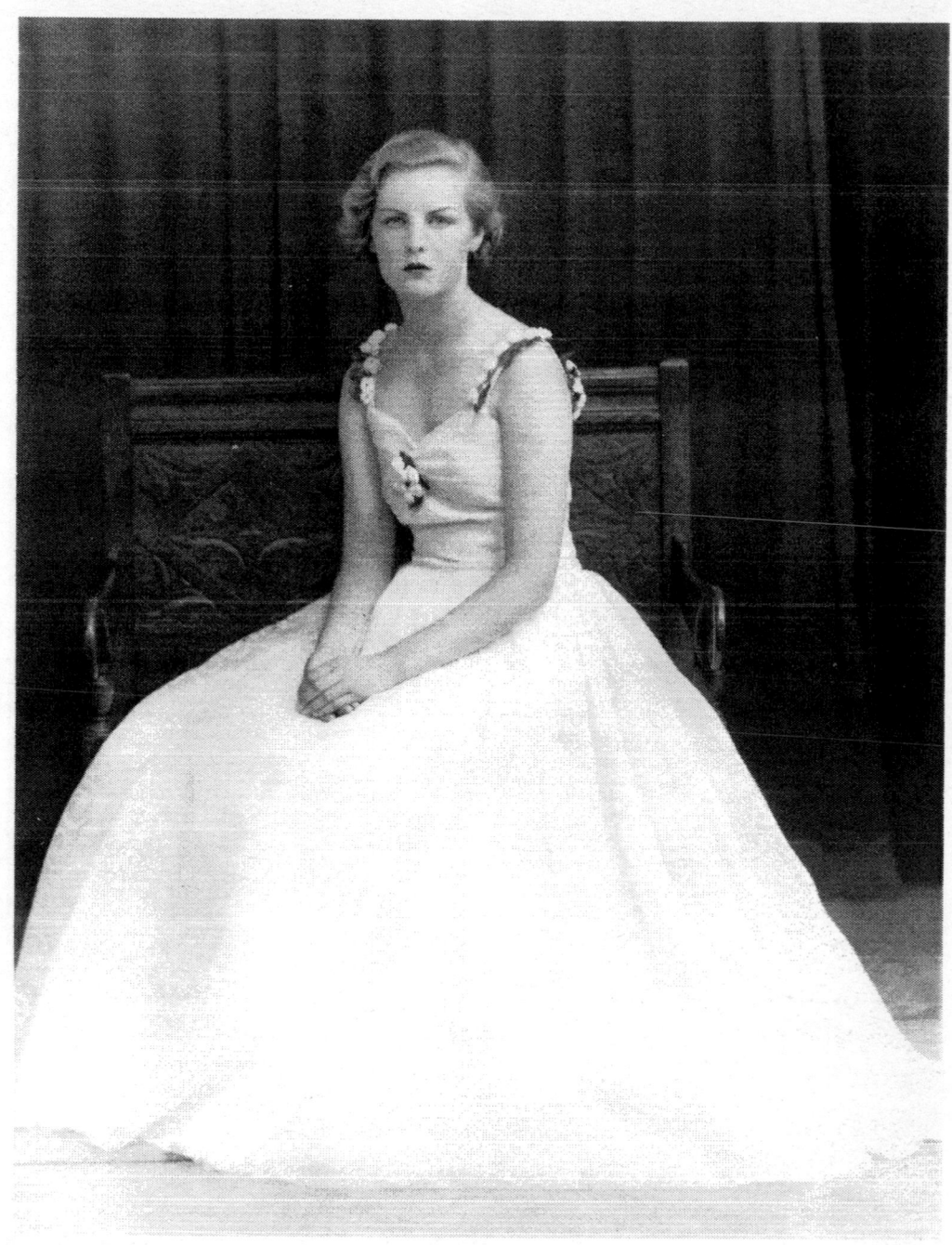

Debutante, 1938

Right: Muv's account book showing the cost of my coming-out party

Below: Muv at 26 Rutland Gate, London

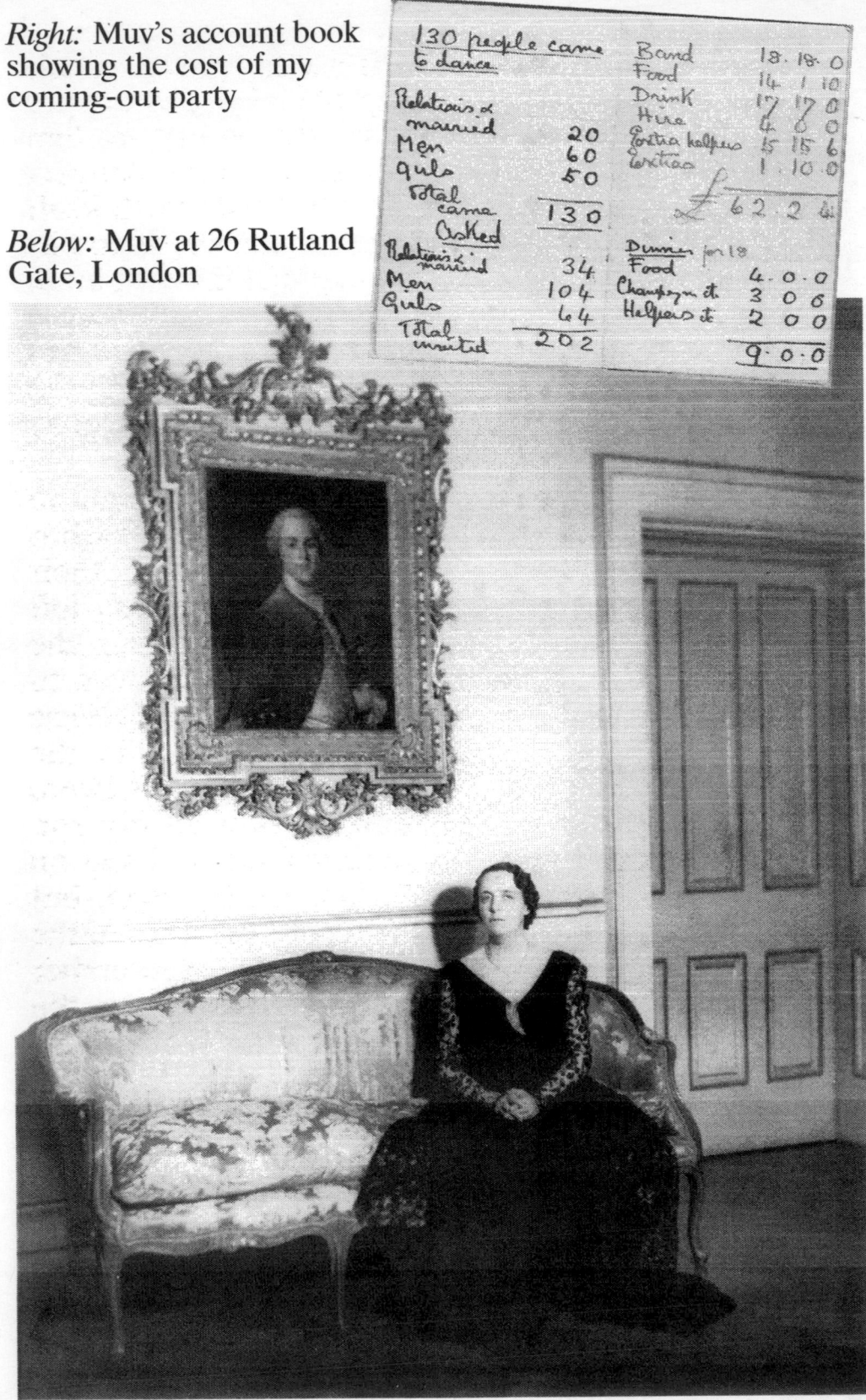

London and Compton Place. In 1947 Francis Thompson, the long-serving librarian and keeper of the collection at Chatsworth, wrote to him warning him in no uncertain terms of the dangers to the family's reputation and to Chatsworth itself if no action was taken to preserve the house and its collection. He advised the Duke that in his opinion Chatsworth should be opened to the public on a proper commercial footing. Eddy and Moucher had already started thinking about reopening the house on a small scale and Mr Thompson's letter must have given them a jolt.

During the war Chatsworth had been brought to life by the three hundred girls and staff of Penrhos College. In March 1946 they returned to their North Wales premises and Chatsworth was left empty. Andrew and I often walked along the footpath from Edensor and across the river to explore the cold, dank, echoing rooms. Basic maintenance was being carried out, and in the bitter winter of 1946–7 house carpenters were shovelling snow off the roof to forestall dry rot. Once a week the clocks were wound, so bang on the hour they struck and chimed in unison, but there was no one to hear them. The contents of the house had not been touched since September 1939, when they had been packed up to allow the Penrhos girls to start the autumn term in their new quarters. All manner of things, from the Memling Triptych to wastepaper baskets, were piled up in the library; Old Master drawings were stuffed into drawers and smaller objects had been stored in a walk-in safe.

My parents-in-law decided that the garden at Chatsworth should be kept up and the house 'maintained' and, for the first time, the money paid by visitors went to the upkeep of the house instead of to local hospitals. When work on reopening the house began, the old generation of carpenters, electricians, masons and plumbers were all nearing retirement age but they knew every inch of the place and its contents, and their help was invaluable. The women's side of things was less straightforward. No English women would do domestic work in such a place; they had had enough before the war of 'going into service', the memory of the long hours and the old discipline was too much and they took other jobs.

Moucher turned for help to two Hungarian sisters, Ilona and Elisabeth Solymossy, who had worked for Kick at her London house. To Moucher's relief the Solymossys not only liked the idea of coming to Chatsworth, they also recruited a polyglot collection of nine other Eastern Europeans. To walk down the back passage when they were on their way to lunch was like going into the Tower of Babel, and the smell of goulash (or its first cousin) pervaded all. I often wondered how my family and I would have got on had we been in their shoes, turned out of our homes for ever and left to fend for ourselves in a foreign country. This wonderful team, dressed like Miss Moppet with cotton handkerchiefs tied round their heads, dusted, sorted, scrubbed, polished and sewed throughout the winter of 1948–9. The shabby, grubby rooms were slowly made presentable and were ready when the house reopened at Easter 1949.

* * *

Eddy was drinking too much and risking his health for all to see, which created a worrying atmosphere at home. He was obsessed with chopping wood and had learned from the woodmen how to fell a tree and use the iron wedges that enabled the saw to cut without 'binding'. At Compton Place he would disappear for hours on end to an outhouse where he worked away, sawing and stacking piles of logs. He came in for dinner but went back to the outhouse immediately afterwards and did not return until after midnight, his old velvet suit impregnated with sawdust.

The physical effort, coupled with too much alcohol, was to prove a fatal combination. On 26 November 1950, while engaged in his favourite occupation, Eddy suffered a massive heart attack and just managed to reach the hall of the house before collapsing. He was fifty-five. (The death certificate was signed by the infamous Dr John Bodkin Adams, our GP at Eastbourne, who the following year was accused of murdering one of his patients; it was then discovered that more than 160 others in his care had died in suspicious circumstances. This suspected serial murderer had seemed very affable to me when he looked after Stoker and Emma while they had whooping cough during the war.)

Andrew was in Australia when his father died. Eddy had asked him to look for suitable places for investment, as he had already done in Kenya and Tanganyika. I was staying with Aunt Weenie at her cottage near Stow-on-the-Wold. Moucher and Andrew's sisters were at Compton Place, where I joined them to await Andrew's return from the

Antipodes. Even though Eddy had looked so ill lately, my mother-in-law was stunned and blamed herself for not doing more to stop him drinking.

The effect on his family of Eddy's death was, of course, immediate; the financial consequences, however, took years to unravel and absorbed almost all Andrew's attention for two decades. In 1926 Victor Duke had formed the Chatsworth Estates Company and at the time of his death the majority of the shares belonged to Eddy, his son and heir. Eddy made a similar arrangement in 1946 and handed over the bulk of his fortune to the Chatsworth Settlement Trust for the benefit of his descendants. Five years had to elapse before this became free of death duties, which under Mr Attlee's Labour government had soared to a dizzying eighty per cent. Eddy died fourteen weeks before the five years were up and Andrew was faced with raising millions of pounds to satisfy the Treasury's demands. Four-fifths of the value of the land and investments, and of works of art that had been collected by the family for over four hundred years, had to be found. It seemed strange to me that the family of a man who had given a lifetime of public service should have to pay such a vast fine on his death.

There was much heart searching, but as I knew little about the works of art at Chatsworth or the value of individual objects in the collection, I had nothing to do with the decisions. It was not my business and I did not see any of the reports of Andrew's meetings with Currey & Co., the family lawyers who played such a big part in subsequent transactions. But, as was his habit, Andrew often left letters from Currey lying about, thrown down wherever they landed after breakfast; I regarded these as fair game and sometimes had a sideways squint at them to try to glean what was happening. It was the first time I had heard money spoken of so freely (like illness it was not discussed in my youth); now, suddenly, the value of everything was being tossed around. Andrew conferred with his mother but Moucher was not exactly the right person to talk to as she was unaware of the value of anything. I once asked her the price of some object she liked the look of: '£40,' she said. 'No, £4. No, £400,' it was all the same to her. As a storehouse of sympathy, however, she was unbeatable.

Andrew took the decision to sell 12,000 acres of agricultural land in Dumfriesshire, 42,000 acres in Derbyshire, town property and woodlands in Sussex, and a house in London. Most of the glorious furniture and books from Compton Place were sold and the house was let to a language school. The kitchen garden (scene of the strawberry theft just before D-Day) was built on and a brutish 1950s edifice took the place of that beautiful, productive garden. Nine of Chatsworth's most important works of art went to the nation in lieu of duty and found their way to major institutions. The lion's share went to the British Museum in the form of Claude's *Liber Veritatis*, the Greek bronze head of Apollo, the Van Dyck Italian sketchbook (luckily Professor Michael Jaffé, who later worked on the catalogue of Dutch drawings at Chatsworth, found another at the back of a cupboard), the tenth-century Benedictional of St Aethelwold and over 140 early books, including fourteen works by Caxton's head printer, Wynkyn de Worde.

Holbein's life-size cartoon of Henry VII and Henry VIII went to the National Portrait Gallery; Rubens' *The Holy Family* to the Walker Gallery in Liverpool; the fifteenth-century Dutch hunting tapestries were allocated to the Victoria and Albert Museum; *The Donne Triptych* by Memling and *The Philosopher* by Rembrandt (which to Andrew's delight was later relabelled by scholars a 'studio production') went to the National Gallery. There was a purple warning to the followers of fashion in art (and they are many): when the contents of the Sculpture Gallery, including several Canovas, were valued, the total lumped together (it was evidently not thought worthwhile to list them separately) came to under £1,000. The scrap of paper it was written on looks a bit ridiculous sixty years later.

All this was still not enough to clear the debt. On 12 August 1954 Andrew was sitting in the train to London when he had the inspired idea to offer Hardwick Hall, the magnificent sixteenth-century house not far from Chatsworth built by Bess, progenitrix of the Cavendish family, to the Treasury in lieu of cash. Granny Evie, who was nearly ninety, was still living in the house at the time. She loved Hardwick very much, having always preferred it to Chatsworth, but to her credit she accepted the plan. Before the agreement was signed, Moucher kept reminding me of things I should take from the house. 'You must go and get the Minton dinner service which is in the cupboard behind the kitchen,' she said, and suggested a few other easily portable bits and pieces. I was pregnant with Sophy and could not trudge round the seemingly endless rooms to rescue some of the eighteenth- and nineteenth-century items of furniture that were not contemporary with the house. But I did save the pretty, blue-ribboned Minton dinner service and we used it at Chatsworth during all the years we lived there.

Protracted negotiations were finally completed and the house, together with 3,000 acres of surrounding farmland, was accepted by the government and handed over to the National Trust in 1959. The Trust has looked after it as we never could have done, and the family are eternally grateful both to Andrew for arranging the transfer of ownership and to the Trust for its fine stewardship.

The final payment of death duties was made on 17 May 1967, but interest had been accruing since 1950 and the full debt was not cleared until 1974.

12

Edensor House

We spent thirteen years at Edensor House, from 1946 to 1959. Emma and Stoker were three and two respectively when we moved in, and Sophy was born in 1957. While Andrew was busy sorting out the financial repercussions of my father-in-law's death, the day-to-day implications seeped more slowly into my life. Two occasions gave me a jolt and made me aware of what was to come. I was in the garden at Chatsworth one day and Bert Link, the head gardener, came up and asked me, 'What would you like us to do?' I realized then that the 105-acre garden was now part of my remit. And a few weeks after Eddy's death, Moucher handed me an old Elastoplast tin fastened with a rubber band. When I opened it I was amazed to see some family jewels, including row upon row of pearls. The pearls were such an inseparable part of my mother-in-law—I had seldom seen her without them, town or country, day or night—that I could not imagine wearing them and gave them straight back to her. But I kept the other pieces, including a star ruby brooch which I had made into a clasp for my own cultured pearls. This necklace, together with a high-collared shirt that appears in many portraits and photographs of me, became my uniform. After Andrew's death, I handed the family jewellery on to my daughter-in-law, Amanda. It was not mine, just as it had not been Moucher's: it belongs to Chatsworth, to be worn by the wife of the Duke of Devonshire.

I gradually began to take on more of the tasks of former duchesses of Devonshire, and found myself responsible for seven houses: Chatsworth, Hardwick Hall, Bolton Hall, Lismore Castle, Compton Place, a London house and Edensor. No wonder I put down 'Housewife' when filling in a form that demanded my occupation; I was wife to all of them. People sometimes ask what it is like being a duchess. The answer is that I honestly do not know because after it happened none of my intimates—either among the people who worked at Chatsworth or my friends far and wide—treated me any differently. I sometimes notice a change of gear, rather than attitude, when I am introduced to people but it does not last long—they soon see how unnecessary it is and behave normally.

Granny Evie had lived at Edensor House during the war and took to austerity with a will; the degree of cold she tolerated and her hateful food (nettles downward) were a lesson to us all, and she continued in the same vein when she moved to Hardwick. She indulged in various imaginary illnesses, finding something wrong with her womb caught from her dog, or catching tulip fire from the tulips. Dr Evans told me that she had a 'somewhat macabre' interest in medicine. 'To prevaricate was risky,' he said. On one of his visits, Granny told him that she was trying out a new cure for rheumatism and showed him a length of frayed electric light flex knotted around her waist. Dr Evans remained non-committal. 'I am not sure how I should wear it,' said Evie, untying the flex and putting it on the other way round. 'It does not matter, Your Grace,' said Dr Evans, deadpan, 'it's an alternating current.'

Granny Evie was not altogether easy to get on with, being critical of the younger members of her family, but she was fond of Emma and Stoker and was kind to me, I think because of Diddy, a paragon among nannies. When the children were about six and seven, they often went over to see Granny at Hardwick. Gardening and painting were on the agenda for these visits. One wet day Granny looked at the tapestry that hung on the curve of the magical stairs between the first and second floor of the house and thought it rather gloomy. She got out some poster paints and encouraged the children to do their best to cheer it up, and I do believe that if the tapestry has not been moved they could still find signs of their unusual graffiti.

From the age of ten, Emma went daily to St Elphin's School, five miles away in Darley Dale. St Elphin's was founded in the early nineteenth century for the daughters of clergy and there were a number of such girls during Emma's years. When John Betjeman went to talk to the school on Speech Day, he was delighted by an item on the programme: 'Tug of War between Clergy and Laity'. I had been appointed a Visitor (I never knew what it meant but it sounded good) and sat next to John on the platform. I glanced at his notes and saw, 'Oh you do look nice, ALL of you.' I was much encouraged to see that this famous poet needed prompting on big occasions like the rest of us.

Even though I never liked Edensor House—it faces north and east, has no view and was impossible to heat during fuel rationing—my memories of living there are full of laughter. Family and friends often came to stay, for no other reason than the fun of it. The house had only two spare rooms and when we had more people staying we used Moor View, a large cottage at the top of the village. Guests did not like having to turn out on cold winter nights and those chosen to go up the hill were known as the 'Suicide Squad'. But they kept coming back and many were to remain lifelong friends.

I inherited Jim Lees-Milne from Tom and Diana, and saw more of him as years went by. It is a pity that people reading about him now are told of his sexual proclivities and seem to overlook the work he did for the National Trust during and after the war. I loved Jim's company and I loved both him and his wife, Alvilde. His private life was his own.

Randal, Eighth Earl of Antrim, was also a regular. I did not know him well when he first arrived and called him 'Lord Antrim'. The name stuck and became a nickname, confusing those who heard it and knew that he was a friend. In 1966 he realized his ambition when he was made chairman of the National Trust; he brought the best of amateurism to that organization and a light-hearted feel that it has never regained.

Another regular was Kitty Mersey, the sister of my friends Charlie and Ned, killed in the war. Their father, the Sixth Marquess of Lansdowne, was a brother of Granny Evie so Kitty was Andrew's cousin. She and her husband, Edward Bigham, stayed with us for a night in summer 1947 and we made friends immediately. Kitty had the same irresistible sense of humour that had made her brothers such wonderful companions and it was good to find them again through her. She had suffered terribly over their deaths; they were by far her favourite human beings, and it was a bond between us. How she got her nickname 'Wife' is convoluted. There was a famous Lothario whom neither of us knew but whose wife was called Kitty. To make sure that people knew he was referring to his wife and not to one of his many mistresses, he would say, 'Kitty-my-wife', almost as one syllable. We took to doing the same with Kitty Mersey. This was soon shortened to 'my wife' or 'the wife', and it became a habit, like ridiculous nicknames often do, and was applied to any best friend of either sex.

Evelyn Waugh was a difficult guest and when he drank too much he was impossible. Everything was wrong: the wine, his bedroom, the outlook and, judging by his behaviour, the other guests too. Try as I might to remedy housekeeping shortcomings, I failed. Kitty was staying at the same time as Evelyn on one of her visits and when we went up to bed she came to talk to me in my bedroom. In no time Evelyn was in with a complaint. 'The curtains don't meet and I won't be able to sleep,' he grumbled. 'So sorry,' I said, 'but there is nothing I can do about it now.' Off he stumped but was soon back. 'If you turn the hall light off, I won't see my way to the bathroom.' 'All right,' I said, 'I'll leave it on.' A while later, another knock on the door, louder and more insistent this time. 'What is it now?' I said. 'I thought you ought to know,' Evelyn announced with a look of triumph on his face, 'that the pot in my bedside table is full.' I shall never know if it was true but doubted it as he did not bring the evidence with him. The next day he was going to stay with Osbert Sitwell at nearby Renishaw and I begged him not to tell of this appalling oversight. Two days later I received Evelyn's bread-and-butter letter, which ended, 'No one has shown any curiosity about the strange Trove of Edensor. They wot not of the pot.'

In spite of his uncertain ways, Evelyn remained a friend and a generous one. He sent us the limited edition of *Brideshead Revisited* in its floppy dark blue cover, which is in the library at Chatsworth, and he sent me his other works as they were published, inscribed in friendly terms. In *Love Among the Ruins* he wrote, 'For Darling Debo, the Beardless Duchess, with love from Evelyn' (the frontispiece depicts a goddess with a beard); he also sent me a copy of John Betjeman's *Continual Dew*, inscribed on the blue endpapers: 'A blue rose for Debo from Evelyn'. The best is his *Life of*

Ronald Knox. I was sitting with Kitty Mersey when it arrived. As soon as I saw the unprepossessing beige cover and title, I put it down with the rest of the day's post, thinking, 'I'll have to write and thank for that but I certainly won't read it.' Kitty, being a reader, picked it up and flipped through the pages. The inscription read, 'To Darling Debo with love from Evelyn. You will not find a word in this to offend your protestant sympathies.' There were no words—all the pages were blank. The perfect present for a non-reader. When *The Antiques Roadshow* came to Chatsworth, I proudly took *Ronald Knox* with its virgin white pages to the book expert, longing to know what price he would put on it. He was amused but would not risk a valuation and moved on to the next person in the queue.

Osbert Sitwell came to see me one day when I was ill in bed. Poor Osbert, the wretched Parkinson's disease had taken hold and his hand shook violently. He looked at it sadly and said, 'All this wasted energy, it ought to be working a mill.' He invited Andrew and me to the annual fête in the garden at Renishaw. Osbert was doing his duty by the stallholders, having a chat here and there, and he spotted a man in uniform. Thinking it was the leader of the band, he said, 'Thank you, my man. Your music was excellent.' He was talking to the local head of the St John Ambulance Brigade, but that little mistake passed him by. His sister, Dame Edith, did not come into the garden but swished about indoors wearing her usual ground-length skirt and huge rings on long, white fingers. On another occasion when we lunched at Renishaw, she wore a feather hat and long fur coat that she never unbuttoned. She told me that the chief things she remembered her mother saying were, 'We must remember to order enough quails for the dance,' and 'If only I could get your father put into a lunatic asylum.'

*　　　*　　　*

My sisters also came to stay at Edensor. Muv brought Unity for our first Christmas there. Our other guest was Adele Astaire, sister of Fred and the widow of Andrew's uncle Charles Cavendish. Farve said he could not come because he had no clothes, which was nonsense—Margaret was a more likely reason. Andrew insisted on having the Christmas-tree party for the village children either before Unity arrived or after she left because she embarrassed him so much with the vicar. I saw his point. She used to ask any man of the cloth she met why he had chosen that profession, whether he wished he had been made a bishop and if he enjoyed sleeping with his wife.

Eighteen months later Unity was on Inch Kenneth with Muv when she collapsed with a violent pain in her head and a high fever. They got her as far as the hospital in Oban, but she had meningitis and there was nothing the doctors could do. She died on 28 May 1948 and was buried in Swinbrook churchyard. Muv had devoted her life to Unity since we had brought her home in January 1940, and I know how much she worried about what would happen to Unity should she outlive her. This haunting fear may have made the parting easier.

Pam, the only one of my sisters who went on

telling me what to do when I was grown up, used to knock on our door in the morning and tell Andrew and me that it was time to get up. Once she had let her dachshund out no one could have gone on sleeping anyway—the din was loud enough to waken the dead. The dog had many nicknames, as did her litter of puppies. Walks with Pam and these loved ones were punctuated with stops while, holding a riding crop aloft as a threat (never carried out), she shouted, 'Come AT ONCE,' followed by a string of names and nicknames.

Nancy stayed with us when Stoker was about two and a half. 'Can you talk?' she asked him. 'Not yet,' he replied. She judged teenagers by their behaviour at bonfires: the slouching laggard who hardly picked up a stick to keep the blaze going was 'no good' (the sort my father would have dismissed as 'a meaningless piece of meat'). I have often thought this as good a way as any of assessing a sixteen-year-old, to be recommended to Human Resources. Trial by bonfire is now my rule.

Nancy wrote *The Pursuit of Love* in 1945 in the first flush of love for Gaston Palewski and it glows through the pages. The novel was an instant success and made her financially independent for the first time. We were all amused by it, including Farve, who laughed at the caricature of himself (although we knew that the entrenching tool really belonged to and was wielded by Sir Iain Colquhoun of Luss). Nancy put her family life into the book, including expressions that were part of our inter-sister shorthand. As a child, I had shortened the Whyte Melville quote that headed the cover of *Horse & Hound* ('I freely admit the best of my fun I owe it to Horse & Hound') to 'You must freely admit', which was shortened to 'Do admit', and used when trying to get Nancy's attention. It appears again and again in the novel, where I suppose I am Linda. Much as we enjoyed it I do not remember any of us thinking *The Pursuit of Love* would last, yet sixty-five years later it is still hugely popular and is considered a classic.

In 1946 Nancy moved to Paris to be near Gaston and remained in France, the country she adored, for the rest of her life. She had a theory that when you were travelling to the Continent the sun came out exactly halfway across the Channel and, going the other way, threatening clouds gathered as soon as you approached England. She found a ground-floor flat in a house on the Rue Monsieur in the Seventh Arrondissement, and often let me squeeze into the dressing room behind her bathroom. She had a large drawing room with an iron stove around which everything revolved in the winter. It gave out terrific heat but took a lot of looking after, having to be fed regularly with logs—like a horse with oats. Nancy knew its ways and stood over it with yet more logs to satisfy its voracious appetite. She loved the flat, which was a mixture of England and France, just as she was. There was an exquisite Sheraton roll-top writing table in the drawing room, more for show than work, an Aubusson carpet under an English sofa and a French chaise longue. The dining-room chairs were a wedding present from Diana.

When she was working, Nancy pulled the telephone out by its roots, stayed in her room and wrote in bed. Her housekeeper Marie, a comfort-maker if ever there was one, looked after her. Marie came from Norman farming stock and was shaped like a cottage loaf. She wore black shoes and stockings and had a shuffling walk that one thought must end in disaster when she was carrying a tray, but it never did. She was a natural cook and could make any potato taste delicious; her only shortcoming was that she could hardly bear to make English puddings and they were what Gaston loved. Nancy and Marie had long talks on the subject and, although Marie disparaged them, her efforts pleased Monsieur Palewski. She shopped at the local market and came home one day with a live hen which was to be the main dish for a lunch party the following day. The hen was shut in the oven for the night and in the morning there was an egg. She was reprieved and lived in the garden, faithfully laying for several years.

English friends visiting Paris were delighted to find Nancy there. Cecil Beaton was one of them. He and Nancy were always ready for a skirmish, scoring hits and spurring each other on to near-lethal digs. It was an entertainment for their friends that never failed to amuse. The jokes got nearer and nearer the knuckle till there was an explosion, then silence for a while until neither could resist starting up again. Soon after the opening of *My Fair Lady* in New York, where his costumes had brought gasps of wonder from the audience, Cecil came back to Europe, tired out by the pressures but thrilled by the acclaim. The papers had been full of it and everyone knew that it was just as much Cecil's triumph as Julie Andrews' and the composers' Lerner and Loewe. Cecil lunched with Nancy in the Rue Monsieur. She knew all about the success of the musical and of how Cecil had lived and worked with it day and night for weeks on end. A pause in their chatter and Nancy asked casually, 'When you were in New York, did you see *My Fair Lady*?' 'Yyyesss,' replied Cecil in his sheep-like bleat.

I never saw Nancy in fussy or ugly clothes. She bought few, but of the best, her perfect figure showing them off as their creators would have wished. She took me to see the clothes at Dior, Lanvin, Jean Dessès, Madame Grès, Balmain and Schiaparelli. Compared to the shops in England, they were fairyland during those early post-war years. A walk down the Faubourg St Honoré, which we called Main Street, was made impossibly tempting by the window displays and we longed for everything. Usually we looked and longed, but did not buy—like going to a gallery to admire the pictures. When we did fall for something there was huge excitement. I dug deep for a grand evening dress made of white organza covered with velvet appliquéd flowers, which went over a silk under-dress in Schiaparelli's famous shocking pink. Some years later Cecil asked to borrow it for an exhibition at the V&A. What he meant (but did not say) was that it would join the permanent collection, so it was goodbye to my best dress—which is still there.

Hubert de Givenchy had just started his own house and was a natural successor to the great Balenciaga, the acknowledged master of couture. When he opened a boutique on the ground floor of the house where he had his workshop, it became our first port of call. The *vendeuses*' interest in every detail of dress, coat or whatever it was they were selling, made them so much more appealing than their English counterparts, who gazed out of the window thinking of men, hunting, or whatever English women think of—anything except the dresses they were trying to sell. Hubert's staff would make the necessary alterations so that the finished garment fitted exactly, then one of them would go upstairs to see if 'Monsieur' was available. Hubert himself would come down to talk to us, wearing a white coat like a doctor, and tweaked the shoulders and hem before casting an approving eye. It was the height of pleasurable shopping. I still wear some of Hubert's clothes, made forty years ago and as good as ever.

In the 1950s my mother-in-law did voluntary work in the East End of London. She was a friend of Bunny Mellon, wife of the Anglophile philanthropist Paul Mellon. Bunny was curious to know more about Moucher's charity. She heard of the poverty among the women and how cheered they would be by some new clothes, so on her return to America she arranged for what looked like cardboard coffins to be sent to Moucher at Eaton Square. Out came wondrous garments by Balenciaga: brocade evening dresses, a black winter coat lavishly trimmed with black mink, and piles of less showy but beautifully made coats, skirts and cocktail dresses. Moucher said that my sisters and I could take our pick, which we did, replacing the Balenciagas with decent, unworn clothes of our own that satisfied my mother-in-law's charitable purposes.

The master couturier's clothes had come to a good home: they were well out of our reach to buy first-hand, but no one could have appreciated them more and we wore them time and again. Diana looked dangerously beautiful in the black coat with black mink facings. We met for lunch one day in London, at the Aperitif Restaurant in Jermyn Street, she a vision in The Coat. We sat down and looked round. I spied Paul Mellon and said, 'Oh, I must go and say hello.' Diana gave a scream and tried to make herself look small (impossible), terrified that he would recognize his wife's coat and snatch it off her back. She and Nancy shared a white satin evening dress they called 'Robeling', which was kept for the grandest occasions. Nancy also had one of those simple linen dresses that are immediately recognizable (by those accustomed to such luxuries) as the very height of haute couture. She wore it in Venice where a friend remarked on it. 'Oh well,' said Nancy, 'I always think one should have ONE good dress.' It was so like her not to admit to its origin.

In 1951, the Mosleys bought the Temple de la Gloire at Orsay, twenty miles from the centre of Paris. Built in 1801 as a folly, it was a small, classical building of faultless proportions, the perfect background for Diana. A lofty drawing room on the first floor opened on to a balcony, which was supported by two generous flights of stone stairs that led to the garden. The balcony overlooked a pond (referred to as a 'lake', but not exactly Windermere). I first went to the Temple on a misty evening; a travelling circus was encamped outside the gates and a camel was tethered to the railings, which added to the surreal atmosphere.

When the Mosleys bought the house it was surrounded by strawberry fields, but as time went by villas grew up around it. Every new house seemed to have dogs that barked, yapped and bayed in unison at certain times of the day. It was an unholy din, not unlike a pack of foxhounds that has suddenly picked up the scent of a fox. As a young man Sir O loved hunting and had the best of it with the Quorn at Melton Mowbray. He knew reams of sporting verse by heart and when the dogs set up their racket, I would say to him. 'Listen! *They've found!*' This provoked a torrent of word-perfect recitations of 'The Dream of an Old Meltonian' and 'The Good Grey Mare', which made me cry every time I heard them. Diana's laughter at his recital alternated with my tears. I loved my visits to the Temple: not only did I often have Diana to myself, but the atmosphere she created wherever she lived was the perfect antidote to any worries.

I met all sorts of people while staying with the Mosleys (some of them could not speak English, which served me right for preferring hunting to learning French when I was sixteen). When the Duke and Duchess of Windsor moved to an old mill at Gif-sur-Yvette, they became the Mosleys' neighbours. Andrew and I had first met them years before in the South of France when staying with our friends Loel and Isabel Guinness in Cannes. The Windsors lived at nearby Château de la Cro' and when they invited the Guinnesses to dinner, they included us in the invitation. The Duke was very attractive, with his shining blond hair and irresistible touch of pathos. He wore a kilt at dinner with all its extras, including laced-up pumps and a dirk in his stocking. A piper went round the dinner table playing his deafening music—more suited to the misty glens than the Côte d'Azur in the heat of July.

'Are you the Duchess of Devonsheer?' the Duke

asked me. I said I was. 'Aw, I didn't like her. She used to tell on me and it got back to my mother.' (Granny Evie passed on information, probably got from her son Charlie Cavendish, to Queen Mary about the Duke's visits to nightclubs when he was a young man.) I asked him if Granny Evie had been nasty when he met her face to face. 'Nasty? Smarmy as be damned,' he said. We got over this poor start and dinner was extremely enjoyable, the Duke speaking with nostalgia of England and the English, whom he called 'the British'.

The Windsors had a pack of pugs that had superseded their Cairn Terriers. 'Aren't they beguiling?' said the Duchess, using an adjective I had never before heard attached to any member of the canine race, let alone a pug. I could not like her, she seemed so brittle, her face bony, angular and painted, her body so dangerously thin she might snap in half. It was difficult to understand why the Duke adored her, but he certainly did and was in love with her until the day he died. He never took his eyes off her during dinner and shouted down the table, 'Wallis, Wallis, did you hear that?' when there was something he thought she might have missed.

I saw the Windsors again in August 1963, on a visit to the Mosleys, and wrote to Mrs Ham:

I'm in the plane going back from Paris to Manchester and the old homestead having had two days on the other side of the medal with the Mosleys. We dined with some Bismarcks and there were the Windsors. He was in a hilarious mood and made Diana and me laugh so hopelessly that we were nearly out of control. He said when Grandfather Redesdale used to go to Sandring-*ham* to advise on trees and gardens, 'us bunch of kids' used to get very excited as he always gave a pound to each. He told me he (the Duke) stopped quite often with Queen Mary at Marlborough House and that, although she was much more forthcoming when she was old, 'that woman was as hard as nails'.

He got me and Diana and Sir O together and said 'Now we are us four Britishers'. He told of romances at Melton 1,000 years ago. Altogether the charm, the pathos and the Cockney American accent finished me. She (the Duchess) kept pointing at me and Diana, saying 'Look at those brilliant Mitford brains. I'm not going to let them go on talking to the Dook unless I can hear what they're saying.' So she came over to listen to the pearls.

Years later I discovered a curious quirk of the Duchess. Our Chatsworth housekeeper, Dorothy Dean, who had been housemaid to the Windsors at Château de la Cro', was discreet and never gossiped about her old employers. But one day she did open up a little and told me that the Duchess would only employ blondes in the house: the footmen, the housemaids and even the people in the kitchen were all fair-haired. Why, I do not know. She herself was dark.

*   *   *

In February 1952 Decca invited me to stay in California. I had not set eyes on her for thirteen years, and then only briefly because of Esmond's hostility, but we had kept in touch by letter. In the intervening years she had married her second husband, Bob Treuhaft, and had had two sons, Nicky and Benjy. Dinky, her daughter with Esmond, was now eleven years old. I was nervous as to what I should find after so long. The flight to California was punctuated by many stops for refuelling and seemed endless, and when we eventually touched down at San Francisco, I felt weary and bemused. And there was Decca. A new person, trousered, American in appearance and accent—someone I did not recognize. It was the oddest sensation and filled me with a feeling of intense loneliness. What was I doing, thousands of miles from home, meeting a stranger who had once meant more to me than anyone in the world?

My engagement book for the week in California reads: 'Tuesday 12 February: dinner with Communists.' 'Wednesday 13 February: dinner with more Communists.' King George VI had died a week earlier and the left-wing extremists of California did not let this pass. The sarcasm that spewed from Decca's dinner guests was relentless and difficult to bear; none of them had ever been to England yet they launched into bitter criticism of everything I knew. Whatever I tried to say in defence of the King and our way of life was laughed out of court or greeted with a 'You would say that, wouldn't you' sort of look. One evening, the conversation turned to how to do away with the royal family. Manners were not their priority.

Decca and Bob were generous hosts and took me to Carmel, where we stayed in a hotel for a couple of nights. There I met 'brunch' for the first time and thought it perfect: all my favourite foods laid out. As we were leaving, I noticed that Decca had packed the towels. I asked her if she had done it by mistake. 'Oh, no,' she said, 'they are lovely and white and ours are horribly grey.' When I said, 'Hen, that's stealing', she replied, 'Oh, it's all right, hotels are insured for that sort of thing.' So my reputation for being the 'Conservative policeman' rose, as did my surprise at her thieving ways.

The visit was dispiriting. I knew Decca had tried hard to make me enjoy myself, introducing me to her friends and political colleagues, but it fell on stony ground because of their hostility and lack of understanding of any view but their own. I thought afterwards that she may also have felt nervous about seeing me after so long and had mustered her friends to bolster her confidence. If I had been alone with her for a week it would have been different. We did have some talks about the old days when glimmers of the Decca of the past came through. The bright spot was Dinky. She was—is—beautiful and practical, taking charge of Decca and looking after the boys far better than she herself had been looked after by Decca. It was no wonder that she chose nursing as her profession when she left home. Her patients were the lucky ones.

When Decca came to England in 1955, her first visit since the war, she must have been stunned by the changes she found. In California she had talked of her relations and English friends as if they were just as she had left them in 1939. In spite of the loss of her beloved Esmond it was impossible for her to understand what the vast upheaval of six years of war had meant to the people and places she had once known.

My next visit to the Americas was very different. In 1955 I went to Brazil for the Carnival in Rio de Janeiro as a guest of Aly Khan. I had first met him at a party in London and often saw him on the racecourse. We had become friends and he was the easiest of company. His wife, Rita Hayworth, was one of the four most beautiful women I have ever seen (the others were Elizabeth von Hofmannsthal, Madame Martinez de Hoz, wife of a South American diplomat, and my sister Diana). Her features were perfect, her mass of truly auburn hair sprang straight from her forehead and cascaded down to her shoulders, and she moved like the dancer she was.

When I arrived at the airport in Rio after the long flight via Dakar, I was held up at immigration; the trouble was the rigmarole on my passport: 'Her Grace Deborah Vivian Cavendish Duchess of Devonshire'. 'Yes, that's me,' I said. The official looked again. 'Where are all the others?' he asked. He took a bit of convincing that I was the one and only, but eventually allowed me to enter. While Aly travelled the country looking at thoroughbred stud farms, I stayed with polo-playing friends of his and went racing with them. In their drawing room where in England there would have been a fireplace with chairs and a sofa, there was a pool instead. But there was no writing table, no writing paper and no way of buying stamps. My hosts could not understand why I wanted these things— necessities for me that seemed positively eccentric to them. Muv began to panic when she heard nothing from me. I explained to her later that they would say things like, 'We'll go to São Paolo tomorrow and buy some', but tomorrow came and we never went.

When Carnival in Rio began we did go and it was everything it is cracked up to be: a stream of beating drums, music that stayed in the head long after it was over, wildly extravagant costumes, nearly naked dancing girls with fruit, flowers and feathers piled on their heads and the male equivalent dressed (or not dressed) in anything they fancied. This uninhibited crowd paraded the streets all night. It was good-natured and happy, with a few hours of semi-quiet after dawn while the revellers gathered strength for a repeat performance. The heat was as extreme as the enjoyment.

We were having dinner at a restaurant one evening when in stumbled a South American polo team dressed as English governesses. Wobbling on court shoes with heels they could not manage, these athletic and gloriously good-looking young men wore demure navy-blue crêpe de Chine dresses with elbow-length sleeves and white cuffs, flat straw hats plonked on their heads, a string of decorous beads, black lace gloves stretched over their huge hands and square, white handbags dangling from their hairy arms. They had all grown up with English governesses so knew exactly how to dress. The tallness and masculinity of these young men made their get-up supremely comical, the best fancy dress ever.

On my last day we flew to a remote stud farm where we rode on cowboy ponies over mountains and ravines where you would not dream of taking an English horse. There were bridges made of two planks, and paths so steep I had to cling to the horse's mane so as not to slide off. We rode for four hours, the last in the tropical dark that falls so suddenly, with fireflies, jungle noises and the delicious smells of flowering trees all around us. We galloped home behind our guide. I asked him afterwards why there had been such a hurry. 'Because of the vampires,' he said.

I also stayed at Aly's house in Neuilly, a mile or so from the centre of Paris. We went to marvellous nightclubs and restaurants, including Maxim's, and turned night into day, sometimes with friends of his, sometimes on our own. Aly took for granted the glamour of this round of pleasure and I was fascinated to see the Continental version of what I already knew in London. But he also had duties, which he took seriously, and there was a group of Ismailis sitting patiently in the hall of his house at all hours waiting for an audience.

You never knew who you were going to meet at Château de l'Horizon, Aly's house on the sea near Cannes, where fellow guests ranged from beautiful women friends to international racing people, with a sprinkling of showbiz thrown in. Ray Stark, the film producer, was there one year with his wife, Fran, a daughter of Fanny Brice, the original 'Funny Girl'. Ray and I were fellow sufferers in not being able to speak a word of French. He was trying hard to learn and was delighted with his progress. 'I know that *glace* is not "glass" and that *chocolat* is "chocolate". Today I discovered that *eau* isn't "oh!" it's water. But I can't imagine why the shops have notices saying *soldes* when a sale is going on. No point in going in if everything is sold.' He was to leave a book in my room. 'Which is your room? I know, the one with the star on the door.' I was stunned by such flattery and missed the Starks and the daily bulletin on his linguistic progress when they left.

One day Aly arranged for me to dine with his father, the old Aga Khan, and his stately Begum, who lived in the hills behind Cannes. As I drove to the house through what seemed to be acres of bedded-out begonias I wondered what I was going to find. I was lucky: the old Aga (whom Nancy referred to as 'Father Divine') made me feel as if I had known him all my life. As I left, he gave me a book and told me very definitely to read it. A far cry from the Ismaili tract I had expected, it was a novel called *In Love*. At 2 a.m. the telephone by my bed rang. It was the Aga: 'How are you getting on with that book?' he asked.

Another friend from that period was Ann Fleming—whose shining life was so sadly cut short by cancer. Many friendships were made in her sunny house on a corner of Victoria Square in Westminster. Ann could seat only eight in her small dining room (we did not know her in her palmy days when she was married to Lord Rothermere and lived at Warwick House), so there was no room for passengers. I sometimes heard her say, 'I would love to ask so-and-so, but I can't sink his boring wife at my table.' She was a dab hand at getting her chosen ones to talk, prodding them into an argument, or anyway a spirited discussion, on every subject under the sun. Andrew loved the arguments and stayed till the early hours.

Lunch or dinner with Ann never failed to be entertaining: politicians, writers, painters, poets, lawyers, Oxford dons and actors, a *Who's Who* of their professions, were all bundled together with no holds barred. More arrived after dinner and the talk got louder. The politicians were mostly Labour: Hugh Gaitskell (who was in love with our hostess), Richard Crossman, Anthony Crosland and Roy Jenkins were all regulars. I never shared Ann's admiration for Arnold Goodman, Harold Wilson's solicitor and adviser, who adored her and on whom she came to rely.

The historian Robert Kee and Lucian Freud were often at Victoria Square, and Francis Bacon too if you were lucky. He did not speak much but commanded attention just by being himself. His face, sad in repose, lit up when he gave his one-sided, wholly captivating smile. One person I often saw but never got to know was Ann's husband, Ian Fleming. He let himself into the house after dining elsewhere. We heard the front door shut and a second later he would put his head round the dining-room door and scan the table. Not liking what he saw, he shook his head and went upstairs to bed.

13

Lismore

The first sight of Lismore Castle as you come over the Knockmealdown Mountains in County Waterford makes your jaw drop. A place of mystery and romance, the huge grey castle—half giant, half fairy—rises from the rocks above the banks of the River Blackwater. 'Built by King John, lived in by Sir Walter Raleigh and plumbed by Adele Astaire, it looks like a castle out of *Le*

Morte d'Arthur,' wrote Paddy Leigh Fermor, a frequent visitor. Steeped in history, it has been the colourful background to tragedies and rejoicing, from civil wars to fantastic festivities, for over eight hundred years.

Andrew's uncle, Charles Cavendish, was given Lismore Castle with its surrounding estate and superb salmon fishing in 1932 as a wedding present by his father, the Ninth Duke. (It had been the Devonshires' Irish home since 1753.) Charlie died in the castle twelve years later, aged thirty-eight, a hopeless alcoholic—the generally accepted reason for his early death. Charming, good-looking and shy, he was loved by all who knew him. After Cambridge, where too much drink and a succession of bad falls in point-to-point races weakened his health, his parents thought a spell in America would do him good and sent him to New York to work in a financial firm. His time there coincided with Prohibition and his health, far from improving, was made worse by the illegal hooch.

Charlie came back to England and fell in love with Adele Astaire, the dancer and entertainer who, partnered by her brother Fred, had taken London by storm in *Lady Be Good*, *The Band Wagon* and *Funny Face*. Adele retired from the stage at the height of her fame to marry Charlie and, as time went by, having once been the more famous of the two siblings, she referred to herself as Fred's sister. Charlie and Adele made their home at Lismore, travelling a great deal and leading a whizzing social life, but always in the shadow of his addiction.

Adele was a fascinating creature of irrepressible vitality but she was also capricious and used a torrent of bad language. 'Oh Dellie, oh Dellie, oh *Dellie*,' her mother, Ann Astaire, used gently to reprimand her from the other end of the dining-room table, but it did not stop Lady Charles Cavendish's all too vivid descriptions of friends and foes. By the time war broke out Charlie was unfit to join up and remained at Lismore, leading the half-life of an alcoholic, assisted by his wickedly complicit butler who gave him whisky camouflaged in a mug. Ann Astaire, a wonderful woman who is still fondly remembered at Lismore, stayed at the castle and did what she could for the ailing Charlie, while Adele went to London and delighted the GIs at the American Red Cross centre.

The castle and its estate had been an outright gift from the Ninth Duke to Charlie, and would have gone to one of Charlie's children in due course, but that was not to be. Adele and Charlie had a daughter in 1933 and twin sons in 1935, all three of whom were premature and died soon after birth. After Charlie's death, Lismore was left to Adele for her lifetime or until she remarried. In 1947, she married fellow American Kingman Douglass, and Lismore came to Andrew. Andrew nearly put his foot in it with Adele when we were married: she sent us a coffee service for a wedding present and as he had just been commissioned in the Coldstream Guards and had other things on his mind, he forgot to write the necessary thank-you letter. Adele was furious and told him she would get Charlie to leave the place to a cousin. The threat produced the required flowery note and all was well.

I first went to Lismore in the autumn of 1947; it

seemed to me like a dream on that visit and remained so ever after. For nearly fifty years Andrew went for the opening of the salmon fishing season in February and we both spent every April there. In 1947 there was still a station at Lismore and the train from Rosslare stopped a few hundred yards from the castle. You could do the last bit of the journey from London on foot, walking up the short drive—or avenue as it is called in Ireland—between the walls of the upper and lower garden. This brought you to the ancient arch of the gatehouse, so low that I used to fear for the butcher boy's head when he stood up in the pony trap that delivered the meat to the castle. The courtyard walls, which are at odd angles to each other, looked for all the world like an Oxbridge quad. The avenue of tall yews, whose branches met high overhead to form a dark tunnel, was, according to Miss Bolton (my sister-in-laws' governess), where Sir Walter Raleigh had walked and she saw his ghost whenever she went to that bit of the garden.

If by some magic I could be transported blindfold from where I am sitting now to the high-ceilinged hall of the castle, the first intake of breath would tell me I was at Lismore. The vague smell of peat and wood, just the general feel of that loved place, would bring nostalgia for the unchanging sights and sounds of half a century. In spite of its size, the castle was as welcoming as can be. Kathleen Nevin, the castle cook, is the world's best. Every morsel of her food had to travel from the kitchen, along a passage, up a flight of steps and across Pugin's extravagant banqueting hall with its star-covered ceiling and chandeliers copied from those in the

House of Commons (or is it the other way round?), until it arrived, still perfect, in the dining room. The brass stair-rods were polished to brilliance. The water ran blue from the copper pipes, staining the baths the colour of a swimming pool. In one of the bathrooms, photographs of Fred Astaire dancing in his top hat, white tie and tails hung next to photos of King Edward VII arriving at the castle in a grand carriage in 1904. The hall with its huge fireplace led to a small sitting room perched high above the river with dreamlike views over woods and far-distant mountains. In the Irish climate the outlook was never the same two days running and the light could change by the minute.

The views from the adjoining drawing room were even more dramatic. King James II spent a night at Lismore in 1689 and is said to have approached the huge bay window then started back in surprise when he saw the sheer drop below. The other window looked east, downstream over the Fifth Duke of Devonshire's beautiful bridge, the arches of which span both the river and The Inches, the fields on the far side that are often flooded. From the window you had the strange experience of looking down on the backs of swans flying below. On the edge of the river, year after year, a heron stood like a sentinel in a little pebble-bottomed inlet watching his stretch of the water. I hardly ever saw him catch a fish but he must have thought it worth his while waiting there patiently on one leg, and I wondered if it was always the head heron that inherited that spot. Tony and Bindie Lambton came to stay for long visits and Tony, who was a renowned shot, used to aim an apple at the heron from the drawing-room window. He never hit it, but the bird would fly off slowly in the lumbering way of herons, to prove that it was untouched.

As if all this were not enough there was Lismore itself, its shops, Protestant and Catholic cathedrals and its people. There were few cars in the town and on Sundays and Fair Days the donkey carts and pony traps followed in single file across the bridge to double park along Main Street. Until the 1960s, horses, goats and donkeys were hobbled as they grazed the Long Acre, the grass on the roadside verges. Travellers and tinkers were plentiful (though how they existed I cannot tell). For us, coming from austerity England, the fact that meat and other food was not rationed added to the unreal atmosphere. There was heady excitement when we discovered on the counter of the Arcade, the draper's shop, rolls and rolls of the top-quality black cloth worn by priests, and we bought lots of it to take home to make coats and skirts.

Living near by in a house belonging to the castle dairy farm was Mrs Feeney, who cooked all her food in an iron pot that hung on a chain over an everlasting fire. Her daughter, Mary, who became a great friend of mine, told me that the taste was second to none, which I can well imagine as the goodness lay in all the ingredients being combined in one pot. Mary Feeney, who made many of the curtains at Lismore Castle, had been taught dressmaking by Ann Astaire and excelled at it. I wore her creations at both the grandest and humblest occasions and always felt happy in them. Norah Willoughby behind the counter of the newsagent's shop knew her customers well and gave them a tremendous welcome when they came in one by one to buy their paper. The town's ancient doctor came to visit me once when I was pregnant. Dressed in curious old-fashioned hunting clothes of green breeches and shiny black leather gaiters, he glanced at the letter sent by my English doctor, looked at me and said, 'The woman doesn't *always* die from this disease', and then left to join the hunt.

* * *

There was plenty of room at Lismore for friends. They arrived with children and dogs off the Fishguard–Rosslare boat. Our old friends Richard and Virginia Sykes came with their family, including Tatton, the eldest, aged about five. He was a bit namby-pamby and held up his spoon (kept in the usual damp cupboard), and whined to Diddy, 'My spoon's rusty.' 'Rusty?' said Diddy. 'That's iron. It will do you good.' Robert Kee was always a welcome guest. His interest in Ireland, which gave rise to his histories of 'that most distressful country', was inspired by his love for Oonagh Oranmore, one of the three blonde Guinness girls, granddaughters of Lord Iveagh. Robert is strikingly handsome, strikingly clever, articulate like no other, and as good a writer as he is talker. *The Green Flag* is generally accepted as being the best of a long list of his works on Ireland. He slid into television naturally and *Panorama* was lucky to have him as its presenter during that programme's most influential years. As an interviewer he was penetrating without being rude and he never interrupted or bullied his victims.

In 1958 Robert brought his friend Cyril Connolly

to stay. I was intrigued to meet this famous writer and critic, who was admired by his peers and apparently loved by women. Cyril had put about the idea that he wanted to buy a house in Ireland, but I soon realized it was just an excuse to see inside some of the houses in the neighbourhood. This resulted in embarrassing telephone calls and visits to people who had no intention of selling. If the plasterwork and proportions were not up to Cyril's expectations, he got as far as the hall then lost interest, leaving me to look at the other rooms and thank for the invasion and obligatory drink. Cyril was said to be a gardener and to understand plants. The climate at Lismore allows all sorts of wonders to be grown that would perish in Derbyshire. Andrew and I were able to plant mimosa and different kinds of magnolia, including the best *Magnolia sprengeri* 'Diva' I have ever seen. We also planted a *Magnolia delavayi*, whose growth was so rapid that, like the hedge in *The Sleeping Beauty*, it would have obliterated the door to the lower garden had it not been drastically cut back every year. When Cyril came to stay, the lower garden was planted for spring and the *Chaenomeles* along the wall was quite a feature. The pink form of the shrub is called 'Apple Blossom'—muddling, but anyone who knows about plants knows the confusing habit plant breeders have of calling a daffodil 'Buttercup' or a nectarine 'Pineapple'. Cyril duly admired it. 'Oh yes,' said Emma, conversant from an early age with such botanical traps, 'Apple Blossom.' 'No,' said Cyril sententiously, 'it's a *Chaenomeles*.' Emma gave him a pitying look and that was that as far as Cyril was concerned.

Paddy Leigh Fermor came to Lismore for the first time in April 1956. He described his visit in a letter to our mutual friend Daphne (ex Bath, then married to Xan Fielding).

The whole castle and the primeval forest round it were spellbound in a late spring or early summer trance; heavy rhododendron blossom everywhere and, under the Rapunzel tower I inhabited, a still, leafless magnolia tree shedding petals like giant snowflakes over the parallel stripes of an embattled new-mown lawn: silver fish flickered in the river, wood pigeons cooed and herons slowly wheeled through trees so overgrown with lichen they looked like green coral, drooping with ferns and lianas, almost like an equatorial jungle. One would hardly have been surprised to see a pterodactyl or an archaeopteryx sail through the twilight, or the neck of a dinosaur craning through the ferns and lapping up a few bushels out of the Blackwater, which curls away like the Limpopo, all set about with fever-trees . . .

Paddy provided all the entertainment anyone could wish for and has been the quickest and funniest companion for more than half a century. The classical scholar, famed writer and acclaimed war hero spent his time bang down to earth when he was at Lismore. He took up the idiotic songs that Decca and I had invented as children and whirled and twirled round the dining room singing this gibberish loudly. To one who had translated 'Widdecombe Fair' and 'John Peel' into Italian (and sings them at the drop of a hat), such nonsense verses came naturally and he entered into the spirit of things with gusto. Taking a cork from a wine bottle, he shut one eye, studied it close up with the other and said, 'What Irish newspaper am I?' The *Cork Examiner*, of course.

Andrew loved Paddy and they went on walks and climbing expeditions in the Pyrenees, Greece and Peru. When he was at Lismore Paddy and I went on long rides, seeing no one all day, up and around the mountains and through the woods to the Grand Lodges, neo-Gothic extravagances that were built as the entrance to a house that never was. Royal Tan was in the stables. A five-times runner in the Grand National (he came second in 1951, won in 1954 and was third in 1956), he had been given to me by Aly Khan, who bought him from Vincent O'Brien's stable when his owner, Joe Griffin, went bust. By the time the old fellow came to me, he had had enough of travelling and refused to enter a horse box. He also did things his way, stopping in the road for no apparent reason and no one could make him budge. Enticements, threats, a lead from another horse, nothing was any good. This exasperated Paddy but he had to concede defeat. 'The trouble with Royal Tan,' he said ruefully, 'is he doesn't like riding.'

When Mrs Hammersley came to Lismore, she brought a travelling companion to help during the journey. On one of her visits the novelist L. P. Hartley filled the role. I hoped he had enjoyed his stay and was disillusioned when in one of his books I read a description of his bedroom at Lismore, down to the smallest detail—and it was not flattering. The sting in the tale was 'a pair of soapstone bookends with no books between them'.

Another of Mrs Ham's carriers of shawls and bags was the Bloomsbury painter Duncan Grant, who was amused by her gloomy forecasts and used to egg her on to describe all the horrors she believed lay in store. (Some of which have come to pass, such as the degradation of art and the appalling misuse of the English language.) Irresistible to both men and women, and with a charm to floor the crustiest of human beings, Duncan became a good friend of Andrew's and mine. He was middle-aged by the time we knew him but still wickedly attractive, with turned-up eyes that disappeared when he laughed. He brought his paints when he came to stay and was the easiest of guests, working away wherever he happened to be. Modest as he was, Duncan would be amazed by the prices his paintings fetch at auction today and by the pleasure his and Vanessa Bell's decorations give to visitors to Charleston, their once very private Sussex home, now open to you and me.

Mrs Ham provided a wonderful subject for Duncan and his two portraits of her are among my treasured possessions. I wish I owned another portrait he made while staying with us. It is of Margaret Murphy, a little red-haired girl who was one of a big family living at the Grand Lodges. Heaven knows how her widowed mother managed with so many children to feed and no husband as breadwinner, but manage she did and was always cheerful and hospitable when I took visitors to call on her at the not-so-grand Grand Lodge, where there was no running water, or any other of the amenities judged necessary today. The Mrs Murphys of this world are the ones who ought to be given medals.

Harold Macmillan came to stay with his wife, Dorothy, who adored Lismore, having spent early springs there when she was a child. Uncle Harold had a lot of the actor in him and to entertain us one evening he played the punter to Porchy Carnarvon's bookmaker. Without rehearsal and dressed in whatever they could find in the hall, including loud-checked caps and binoculars, they gave us a sketch worthy of any theatre. Uncle Harold liked walking alone. One day we dropped him some miles from the castle and he made his way home, deep in thought, with no one to bother him. He had been trudging along a lonely lane for about an hour when he saw a donkey leaning its head over the roadside wall. Uncle Harold, who was getting weary, stopped and said, 'Ass, how far is it to Lismore?' The donkey took no notice but a man emerged from behind the wall, curious to see the daft fellow who had asked a question of a donkey. Little did he guess he was looking at a former Prime Minister of Great Britain and Northern Ireland.

*   *   *

Our weeks at Lismore were enlivened not only by a stream of visitors from abroad but also by neighbours, including a number of friends and relations who, disenchanted with England and its Socialist government, had decided to emigrate. Pam and Derek were among our first guests and they fell for Ireland. Derek was attracted by its lack of bureaucracy and bossiness, not to mention Attlee's penal taxation, and decided to buy

Tullamaine Castle in County Tipperary, where he set up a racehorse training establishment. He and Pam entertained a great deal—too much for Pam to manage single-handed—and they employed a succession of cooks. None of them came up to Pam's high standards and she used to come over to see me and regale me with her kitchen woes. 'Stublow, ordering with Mrs B is a nightmare,' or 'Isn't game soup the richest and loveliest soup you ever laid hands on? Well, a milky affair came up.' This said in a dramatic voice that grew lower and more urgent until the last sentence might have been recounting a world-shaking disaster. To Pam it was. Between cooks she produced the meals herself. I telephoned one day to ask if she could come to lunch. 'No, of course I can't,' she said crossly, 'I'm much too busy making egg mousse for sixty.' (I had forgotten it was the day of the Tipperary point-to-point that was run over the Tullamaine farm.)

Derek was a human time-bomb ready to explode and was not cut out for an enduring marriage. As time went by and he had no success with the racing venture, he began to grow restless and miss his scientific work—a part of his life that was impossible to share with the Tipperary locals. Robert Kee, knowing of Derek's brilliance, once said to him, 'I'm afraid all I know about maths is that two plus two equals four.' Derek thought for a bit and said, 'I've often wondered.' In the 1945 General Election I asked him if he was going to vote Conservative. He exploded and, hardly able to get out the words, said, 'How can I vote for a man who speaks of the *third alternative*?' A rare grammatical error from Winston cost him Derek's vote.

Derek had always been unpredictable, darting off to left and right, and he now spent more and more time away from home, leaving Pam with the racehorses as well as a large house to look after. It became obvious that their years of marriage were at an end. As always when life seemed to conspire against her, Pam faced the separation with courage. After Derek left, she must have had an impossibly difficult time but carried on as best she could and never complained to her sisters, though Diana and I were aware how unhappy she was.

Tullamaine was sold in 1958 but Pam stayed on as a tenant until 1960. We all knew she was careful, but sometimes her watching of the pennies was so comical it has to be recorded. She told her new landlord that the house needed rewiring. He obeyed and sent round some workmen. Pam then said she must have a cow to provide milk for the workmen's tea. He sent round a cow that gave four gallons a day. The workmen only used a pint, so Pam bought four piglets and fed the milk to them. Even they could not get through it all so she sent the rest to the creamery. She was staying with friends when a cheque for £10 arrived from the creamery. Her host, who happened to be a land agent and versed in such matters, said, 'I suppose you're going to pass it on to the landlord.' 'OH NO!' cried Pam. 'After all, *my* gardener milks the cow. But for me his workmen would have to *buy* their milk.' So she kept the cheque, the cow, the pigs and the workmen.

Sophy's first stay at Lismore came when she was a year old. The older children's cot and all that went with it were long gone, but I knew that Pam would still have the cot that Diana's sons slept in when they lived with her during the war. I wrote to ask if I could borrow it. She answered at once to say yes but suggested I get it painted as it was obviously in a poor state. She had some perfectly good blankets, she said, with a few moth holes, and added, 'If Miss Feeney cut them into the right size leaving out the eaten parts she could put some pretty ribbon to bind them and this would save a lot.' She also offered linen sheets: 'Some large double bed sheets which are rather worn but here again Miss Feeney could find plenty left to make cot sheets.'

In the same letter, she reminded me that the sale of the contents of Tullamaine was about to take place. It is wonderful what a country house sale can produce. The glasses she had bought at Woolworths in Clonmel sold for four times their purchase price, even though the exact same ones were available in Woolworths down the road. She included a lot of eggs in the sale that had been stored in Ali Baba pots of brine since the spring flush of the year before. Diana and I teased her that they were all bad and would go off at intervals like pistol shots. But everything went for tiptop prices and several times I heard her announcing loudly, 'Nothing is to go out of this house till it's paid for.'

After she left Ireland, Pam went to live in Switzerland. She took her dogs with her and decided to stay there until they died, not just because of the quarantine regulations but, as she explained in an interview to a German magazine, because she thought they would prefer to spend their old age on the Continent. She made many friends in Switzerland. Diana said that she was the local star and when she walked down the street in Zurich she was greeted by gnomes of high degree with, 'PAMAILAH. How are you? How *vonderful* to see you!' She was loved and appreciated for her unique qualities, and her friends listened open-mouthed to her oft-told tales of childhood. She shared a house with her friend Giuditta Tommasi, an Italian riding teacher. Today any such relationship is immediately connected to sex, and two men or women who choose to live in the same house are said to be homosexual. In some cases no doubt they are, but in many others they are just friends who share a roof. In either case, it is of secondary interest. I find this guessing about the sex life of friends or relations tiresome in the extreme. It is the people who matter; their private lives should be their own.

In 1951 the Mosleys also came to live in Ireland, at the Bishop's Palace (a grand name for what Diana described as 'a pretty old house') in Clonfert, near Ballinasloe in County Galway. The house needed re-roofing, heating, bathrooms and the rest of the necessities for modern comfort. In the unhurried way of Ireland, these additions took some time and it was three years before it was finished to Diana's high standards. On a cold December night in 1954 an ancient beam in a chimney that had been dried out by the new central heating caught fire and before help could arrive the house and most of its contents were well alight. The desperate whinnying of horses in the nearby stables woke the family and, miraculously, no one died in the conflagration. Diana described how all that was left of her four-poster bed, newly trimmed with pale blue silk, were a few red-hot springs. Portraits of her by John Banting and Helleu, drawings by Augustus John, Tchelitchew and others, were reduced to cinders. Diana, her husband and their two sons, Alexander and Max, were homeless.

Andrew immediately lent them Lismore Castle where they spent Christmas in mourning for Clonfert. When a house called Ileclash, 1½ miles from Fermoy and overlooking the Blackwater, came up for sale, although it was a poor substitute for Clonfert, they bought it. This was good news for me as it was only about twenty miles away. We were both busy, but not too busy to meet halfway in the village of Ballyduff (called Ballyduff Cooper by us, of course). The Ballyduff Cooper summits became a feature of life and we would sit enclosed in the privacy of the car, talking to our hearts' content. Diana used to walk from Ileclash to the shops in Fermoy. A necessary part of a visit to that busy town was to lean on the bridge that overlooked the broad Blackwater and watch the torrent below. Diana leant and watched. She was aware of a man next to her doing the same and they stood there together for some time. ' 'Tis all going to the sea,' he said at last. ' 'Tis,' she replied, after some thought.

Eddy Sackville-West moved to Ireland in 1956 mainly to escape the responsibility of Knole, his family home in Kent, and all that went with that great house. He bought Cooleville in the village of Clogheen, the other side of the Knockmealdown Mountains from Lismore, and made it his own creation. Nancy often stayed with Eddy, combining it with a visit to Lismore. (I think she preferred

Cooleville.) Eddy was unmarried and what my father called a 'literary cove', a lover of music and books. Andrew enjoyed his company and he became a regular dinner guest at Lismore. He arrived one evening when no one had been in to tidy and everything was lying about. His first words, in a trembly voice, were, '*Secateurs* on the *mantelpiece*, *saws* on the *hall table*.'

At the time we had a craze for an after-dinner billiard-table game called Freda. It was not athletic and dangerous like Billiard Fives but it did involve running round the table at vital moments. For this, his only attempt at such sport, Eddy brought a little case with daytime trousers and shirt—to save his dinner jacket from possible damage. A convert to Roman Catholicism, he fitted well into the Irish landscape but his romantic view of the country sometimes caused him to invest his duller neighbours with imaginary qualities. When he laughed, which often happened when he was describing one of them, he drew his knees up to his chin. But even he was brought down to earth by the food they served when it was their turn to entertain him. 'There is no excuse,' he wailed with emphasis on each word, 'for coarsely mashed potatoes.'

Andrew's uncle, David Cecil, came to Lismore several times. He was a great friend of Elizabeth Bowen and asked me one day if she lived near by. I had heard of the novelist but knew nothing of Bowen's Court, the family house in County Cork that she inherited in 1930. I asked David if I should invite her to lunch. 'Yes, do,' he said. Elizabeth came and we all fell for her big-boned charm and hesitant speech that came out with such good stuff. She invited us back to Bowen's Court, the archetypal Irish house: dilapidated, beautifully proportioned and freezing cold, except for the sitting room where you could imagine happily spending days in her company. On the top floor of this big and almost empty house was a long broad gallery—unusual in a house of 1776 as it harped back to an Elizabethan plan. At either end of the gallery, which had floorboards as wide as an old oak would allow, there were tall windows and on the south window, engraved with a diamond, was: 'Baby Bowen 1899', commemorating Elizabeth's birth. The floor of the yard that led to the garden was made of the knuckle bones of sheep— something I have never seen before or since. Like everyone who had known the house, I was appalled when I read that Elizabeth had had to sell it and that a few months later the new owner knocked it down. Poor Elizabeth. When she returned to Ireland it cannot have been with pleasure.

We all loved Betty Farquhar, a fierce hunting lady who lived at Ardsallagh, a small, well-proportioned house that stood on a rise near the town of Fethard. She was a product of the Shires and the world of the Quorn, Belvoir and Cottesmore hounds—those legendary packs that she had hunted with six days a week before the war. I once asked her what it was like. 'Ow, just like going to the office,' was the reply. She could dismay a stranger when introduced to him by turning and asking at the top of her voice, 'Who is this *ghastly* man?' Her house was a surprise, with its pieces of stained glass by Evie Hone and paintings by Irish artists of the 1930s and 40s that would fetch a king's ransom today. Her garden was immaculate, as was her appearance; unlike some ex-pats she never went to seed or lowered her standards.

Twice widowed, Betty had no children and fell in love with Ireland through Sylvia Masters, the friend who shared her life and who had grown up at nearby Woodruffe. A legend of courage and originality, Sivvy was Master and Huntsman of the Tipperary hounds long before any woman dreamed of such a thing. She won 101 point-to-points, riding against men who gave no quarter because of her sex. Sivvy was quiet but stood out in a crowd with her straight, daffodil-yellow hair and large eyes. Children adored her and she encouraged them in everything their parents forbade, slipping fags into their hand as soon as the grown-ups were out of sight. Her brother, the actor and playwright John Perry, was a great friend of Binkie Beaumont, the theatrical impresario who ruled the London stage for thirty years. Thus Sivvy and her brother covered a broad spectrum, from hunting hounds to *The Winslow Boy* and *The Little Hut*.

Clodagh Anson, the most loved of spinsters, was a distant cousin of Andrew (their grandmothers were sisters). She lived alone in a damp house across the river 'belonging to the castle'; an eye-catcher among the trees for our north-facing rooms, it carried evidence of the Troubles in the form of bullet holes here and there. Clodagh was the only person I knew of Anglo-Irish background who was accepted by the inhabitants of Lismore, and beyond, as one of them. Unworldly to the last degree, she was the antithesis of a snob and the best of company; it did not matter who was staying with us, she captivated the lot. Tall, ugly and with charm to beat the band, she had lived through the 'bad times' in Ireland and her throwaway tales of her experiences as a girl could have come straight from Somerville and Ross. When she was eighteen her mother, Lady Clodagh Anson, took her to London and made a half-hearted attempt to bring her out as a debutante. Lady Clodagh devoted herself to down-and-outs and their London house was a refuge for beggars. When returning from a grand ball, her daughter had to pick her way over sleeping tramps in the hall, all described in Lady Clodagh's two volumes of memoirs, *Book* and *Another Book*, which are among my unstealables.

At Lismore, Clodagh kept unusual hours and did not wake till lunchtime. From the castle kitchen I could see the blind of her bedroom window pulled firmly down till 12.45 p.m., even when she was lunching with us at 1 p.m. She loved her garden but it was often dark before she was ready to start work so she weeded and dug by the headlights of her ancient car and when the battery failed she wore a miner's lamp so as to be able to garden late into the night. She was a regular churchgoer to the magnificent Church of Ireland cathedral in Lismore. When the service started at 10.30 a.m. Clodagh was always half an hour late and came in with a clatter of banged doors and dropped books. It was decided to start the service at 11 a.m., to give her a chance. She made the same noisy entrance at 11.30. The service was not delayed further or the congregation would have had no lunch.

In 1987 Hubert de Givenchy and Philippe Venet came to stay. I asked Clodagh to lunch and told our unworldly neighbour a bit about them beforehand, how they were leading couturiers in Paris and therefore the world. Over lunch, I heard Clodagh tell Hubert that she was going to stay with her brother in Rome. 'I believe you are a dressmaker,' she said. 'Should I have the hems of my cotton frocks taken up or let down this summer?' With impeccable manners, Monsieur de Givenchy turned to her and said, 'Madame, I cannot advise you, but I would like to make you something to wear when you go to Italy.' We went to measure her. (Hubert and Philippe wore gumboots because they had heard her house was damp.) Clodagh was top-heavy and walked headfirst, her jutting nose hanging over clicking false teeth, and her big hands those of a gardener. She stooped and had a pronounced dowager's hump, which meant that the measurement between her shoulders was some inches longer than that of her long-forgotten bosom. Hubert and Philippe could not help smiling as they made a note of these measurements, but Clodagh was unaware of it. A few weeks later a couple of strong cardboard boxes, with the magic name of Givenchy attached, arrived at Clodagh's house. She had no idea how lucky she was but her friends were jealous of her windfall trousseau from the Avenue George V.

Wendy (nothing to do with Peter Pan but short for Wendell) Howell was a grand American gone native ('How yer *dawgs*?') whom I prized as a friend because she did not take to just anyone and made an exception for me. She liked whippets and whisky and had too many of both. Lots of husbands (including a Roosevelt) had come and gone and she eventually settled with a lady vet in one of those Irish cottages which were rare then and now only happen on postcards. It had an earth floor and stable doors and, in the sitting room, a vast opening for the fireplace where, if you bent down to look up the chimney, you could see a big patch of sky. At the entrance to the cottage was a sculpture of two whippets, old friends to me as they were an echo of a similar model by Gott at Chatsworth. Wendy held a pilot's licence but luckily never offered to take me for a spin.

Obbie, the Twelfth Duke of St Albans, lived at beautiful Newtown Anna, by Clonmel. He had converted his garden shed into a sitting room, 'the finest room in Europe,' he announced. It still had a lot of the garden shed about it and reminded me of my father's at High Wycombe. Like Farve, Obbie had fought in the Boer War, the First World War and joined the Home Guard in the Second. And, like Farve, he had refused promotion to Corporal saying he did not want the responsibility. Another trait they had in common was unpredictability. Obbie once telephoned my mother-in-law and, with no preliminaries, said, 'Moucher, you're not a has-been, but a has-been has-been,' and put down the receiver. During the Second World War, when food was rationed and it was strictly against the law to ask anyone in a neutral country to send any, Obbie delighted in sending postcards, open for all to read, from neutral Ireland to his niece Betty Salisbury, whose husband Bobbety held, at various times during the war, the posts of Paymaster General, Secretary of State for Dominion Affairs, Colonial Secretary, Lord Privy Seal and Leader of the House of Lords. The postcards read, 'I will send the *ham*, *butter*, *bacon* and *steak* you asked for tomorrow,' and arrived at intervals throughout the war.

Another reason for enjoying Lismore was the company of our land agent, John Silcock. When he was a young man and had just finished his training, he had a farewell chat with the Norfolk landowner on whose estate he had been working. 'I'll give you two pieces of advice,' said the landowner. 'Don't go to Ireland and don't marry your principal.' John did both and it was through Irish connections that he came to run Lismore, spending two days a week in the estate office. He was the best of company and got on well with the people who worked at Lismore, which made life smooth for all concerned. I spent hours with him, touring the farm and woods, listening to his tales of working in Ireland. I used to say to Andrew, 'You know, John is wonderful.' This was repeated so often that he became 'Wonderful John', later shortened to 'Wonderful'.

A surprise is always around the corner in Ireland. There was an elephant skull by a bend in the road to Cappoquin and at Ballynatray human bones were dug up in the little churchyard and scattered to allow a new coffin to be buried there. In our early years at Lismore, the beautiful house of Ballynatray belonged to Horace Holroyd-Smyth. The billiard table served as the dining table, with the remains of breakfast at one end, teacups at the other and lunch in the middle. I am not sure about dinner but I remember thinking what a good idea it was. The silver cups won by Mr Horace's point-to-pointers were shiningly clean and obviously prized far beyond anything else in the house. Mr

Horace and his fiancée loved hunting so much that in the closed season they listened to a gramophone record of a hunting horn: 'Gone Away', 'The Find', 'A Kill', all blown to perfection by an expert; and the response of the hounds was tantalizing to hear in the off-season. The hounds were fed on salmon, the cheapest food available because they were caught in a trap at the bottom of the garden as they swam up the Blackwater.

Social life dies hard in Ireland. During the war when there was no petrol for cars, Mr Horace went out to dinner on his tractor dressed in his dinner jacket. In the 1930s Ballynatray took paying guests and Penelope Betjeman and Joan Eyres Monsell (later to marry Paddy Leigh Fermor) slept there on a riding tour. One of the party discovered an unwelcome object far down in the bed: the mustard plaster worn by someone who had died of pneumonia. I cannot help wondering if this was true or whether John Betj invented it. It would have been typical of that house—and of John. The last time I went to Ballynatray, three pigs and a couple of hounds were asleep in the sun, guarding the front door.

*   *   *

Careysville, sixteen miles upstream from Lismore, had some of the best salmon fishing in Ireland. It had been rented by my father-in-law during the 1930s and when it came up for sale soon after the war, he bought it. Andrew took his fishing friends there for the first two weeks of February. They spent the day on the river and usually stayed at Lismore but sometimes at Careysville House which in my father-in-law's day was so cold that it was normal procedure to pick up the rug off the floor and put it over the thin eiderdown. The soil was good and snowdrops in the garden grew so thick and tall that the hounds drew them for a fox.

A green and white hut, more of a cricket pavilion than a fishing hut, stood on the flat ground by the riverbank and was where we had lunch. The food was carried in baskets down the steep steps by beautiful Irish maidens whose job it was to do just that. The fare was always exactly the same: cold meat, salad, hot baked potatoes, a rich Christmas pudding and cheese (usually the squashed up kind in silver paper). Had there been any deviation from this menu there would have been a revolution among Andrew's guests. I never took to fishing—a terrible waste when I could have had the best—but there was always a queue of aficionados for the limited number of rods, so it was just as well.

Careysville produced its own unforgettable people. John O'Brien, the head ghillie, was Andrew's friend and was one of the reasons Andrew loved the place so much. The two men talked to each other all day long of much more than fishing and any rare moments of silence were without awkwardness. Sport produces a unique friendship and Andrew was deeply affected by O'Brien's death in 1964. He was crossing the river with two other ghillies when their boat overturned in turbulent water and all three non-swimmers were drowned. Andrew never felt the same about Careysville again.

Billy Flynn was another ghillie remembered by all. His charm and funniness and tales of the fishery were Ireland at its most beguiling. With his lifelong experience, he hardly needed scales to tell the weight of a fish and a 29½ pounder was brought up to the magic 30lbs by Billy stuffing plum pudding into its mouth. One day the children and I had been talking about ghosts and I asked Billy if he had ever seen one. He thought for some time and said, 'Sure, I saw a sow where never a sow there was.' I went to visit him in hospital when he was dying of a horribly disfiguring cancer of the face; his grossly enlarged cheek and jaw were awful to see and he could only whisper. He wanted to tell me something. I bent down and could just hear, 'Will there be fishing in heaven?'

Our weeks in Ireland had their sombre side. The years of the Troubles in the north had their repercussions in the south. Alfred and Clementine Beit were attacked by thieves at Russborough, their house in County Wicklow, and locked in separate cellars while the gang made off with the best of Alfred's world-famous pictures. Lord and Lady Donoughmore were kidnapped, bundled into a car, driven for miles in the dark at speed and held hostage for four days. Andrew was not put off by these attacks, but after Bloody Sunday in 1972 the Irish government increased the number of Garda looking after him—up to fourteen at any one time—and a police car travelled in front and behind him wherever he went. Three different routes take you from Lismore to Careysville and on the orders of the Garda he had to decide at the last minute which he would take, and several men stayed with him all day on the riverbank. In 1979, after Lord Mountbatten and three members of his family were murdered, even I was given a policeman. He must have been bored walking to the shops, the farm and endless times round the garden. He pointed to a stone sundial one day and asked me what it was. 'A sundial,' I said. 'Oh, does it still work?' It does, but its hours on duty are not long in Ireland.

The time came when all the old friends had departed from our Irish life and Andrew himself was not well. He was no longer able to walk up and down the steep steps from Careysville House to the river, and his failing eyesight made it difficult to cast over the wide water. The death of John O'Brien, the spirit of Careysville, and the loss of other friends made the place too full of ghosts and he stopped going. The castle was made over to Stoker and we retreated from Ireland, where we had had such happy times.

14

Moving to Chatsworth

Soon after my father-in-law died, Andrew said to me, 'Chatsworth may not go on as a family home, but I don't want to be the one to let it go.' He was thinking not only of the house itself, the garden, stables and everything else that goes with Chatsworth, but of what selling would mean to the people who belonged there. This was a major consideration in the struggle to keep it going.

The 1950s were grim for this country. Rationing did not end until 1954, nine long years after the end of the war, and recovery was painfully slow. In our case it was not recovery but a downward slope we were facing. Many beautiful and useful buildings all over England were being destroyed and supplanted by monsters. No one believed that a house like Chatsworth would ever be wanted again, let alone lived in by the descendants of the family who built it. It was a period of limbo. No major decisions were being taken at Chatsworth but nevertheless a five-hundred-year legacy was beginning to come undone.

Hugo Read, who was the land agent during the time when the estate was in debt to the government, had a position of considerable influence as Andrew was often away and left many of the day-to-day decisions to him. I tried to prevent some of the worst desecrations, but the argument for knocking down old buildings and replacing them with new ones, which needed less maintenance, often won. I was talking to Hugo one day about Pilsley, a village on the estate, where he planned to pull down a row of semi-detached cottages called South View. 'Why?' I asked. 'Well, they're only Victorian,' was the answer. Luckily there was no money and the cottages with their remarkable gardens are still there.

The exuberantly Victorian Barbrook House, built by the Sixth Duke's head gardener Joseph Paxton for himself and his family, was not so lucky. It had been the home of the land agent till 1939 but was left unoccupied at the outbreak of the war. By the late 1940s it was used for storage; potatoes and wheat were shovelled into the dining and drawing rooms and it was riddled with dry rot. With so many outstanding repairs on the estate cottages hanging over us—few had indoor lavatories let alone bathrooms—there was no question of restoring such a white elephant and the house became a victim of the times. It was succeeded by an ugly and useful warehouse, designed by Hugo Read. Only the pretty lodge is left to remind us of the former grandeur of Paxton's days, which had included a nine-acre kitchen garden with innovative hot houses, melon pits and pineapples.

It was not just visible signs of the past that were disappearing, morale was also low as no one could envisage a day when the place would be free of debt. The one bright spot in an otherwise dismal period was that the house and garden at Chatsworth were open to the public and, in spite of petrol rationing, visitors came. Hugo Read was wiser and more far-sighted in his views on the future of Chatsworth itself than of Victorian cottages. He believed that in spite of all the difficulties, the family—Andrew, me and our (then) two children—should move into the house. It was nearly twenty years since Eddy and Moucher had taken their belongings—which they had barely unpacked—back to Churchdale, and on the face of it, Hugo's idea seemed wild, a complete reversal of all our efforts at scrimping and saving to pay off death duties. But Hugo, like Francis Thompson, who had emphasized the necessity of a family presence in his letter to my father-in-law in 1947, believed that Chatsworth and its family were inseparable. Both men warned that without a welcoming host the house would become a museum, as arid and lifeless as so many others.

Andrew's initial reluctance to live there may have stemmed from unhappy memories of his grandfather's last years, and perhaps from his parents' attitude towards the house after Billy's death. For a while we considered moving to Hardwick Hall when Granny Evie had had enough. Its astonishing beauty was a strong pull, but the disadvantages of extreme cold (tits pecked at the lead round the little window panes till they fell out and made cruel draughts) and the lack of bathrooms with nowhere obvious to put them, always brought us back to the homelier Chatsworth. By 1957 Andrew was convinced that moving was the right thing to do. I had been longing to live there and was thrilled. In the past when we had walked through the park, I had often said to him, 'Oh, look at that lovely house. I wonder who lives there.' And he would say, 'Oh, do shut up.' But now he threw himself wholeheartedly into the plans.

*   *   *

Once the major decision to move into Chatsworth was made, life changed gear and there were daily decisions to be taken. Even though it looks so big, the house and all its different rooms were surprisingly easy to get to know. First we debated which rooms to use. When it came to choosing our bedrooms, we always came back to the west-facing rooms that the dukes and duchesses had traditionally inhabited. After that it was a question of which should be the drawing room, dining room and kitchen. We looked carefully at the north-facing rooms on the first floor but the lack of sun was a major drawback and we gravitated naturally to the three, large, cheerful, south-facing rooms on the same floor. Our blue drawing room had been

Andrew's aunts' schoolroom and then the billiard room; the yellow drawing room remained unchanged and what used to be the gold drawing room became our dining room.

Immediately below the new dining room was a light, airy room that had been used by Granny Evie's secretary, and we decided to make it the pantry. It had a painted ceiling of quality, which seemed unwise to leave exposed so we put in a false one. Our chosen space for the kitchen was next to the pantry, but that left us with the problem of how to get the food upstairs. The solution was to put a lift in the old stairwell that sticks out on the east side of the house, but a portrait by Lely of General Monk (founder of the Coldstream Guards), which was fitted into one of the Bachelor (the Sixth) Duke's ornate frames on the walls of the dining room, was in the way of the entrance to the new lift, just where the jib door had to go. There was nothing to do but cut the picture in half, so when the door was opened the old soldier's legs swung round, startling the diners, but when it was shut General Monk appeared complete, legs and all. Our guest bedrooms and nurseries were scattered over two floors. Sophy was two when we moved in. There was no lift in our part of the house, so Diddy humped this toddler along the passages and up the stairs. Arriving in the nursery, poor Diddy sighed, 'Oh dear', and these were Sophy's first words.

We turned the garden path along the west side of the house into a private drive and made our entrance through the west front hall, where it had been before the long north wing was built in the 1820s. This left the grander north front door and hall for people who come to see the public part of the house. Andrew, who insisted that as much of the house as possible should be open, was keen that visitors should arrive at the front door and not be shovelled in through a side entrance, as we had seen in other houses newly opened to paying visitors. The public route was sacrosanct, even though it altered in direction from time to time. For fifty years this scheme served us well and allowed tourists to circulate easily, visit the state rooms and descend the west stairs to the chapel.

Once we had decided which rooms we would use and for what, Andrew left the rest to me. He did not want to hear about domestic details and never questioned my decisions. So now I had a job—big enough to occupy every waking moment. My budget was small and most of it had to be spent on plumbing and wiring. (Later, when I worked on the Cavendish and Devonshire Arms hotels I had become used to this squeeze on what I was allowed to spend, but it made me wary of builders' estimates.) People ask me how I did it. The answer is partly that when you are young you think you can do anything, but also—just look at the help I had. There can never have been a better group than the staff I worked with, for whom nothing was too much trouble. The head of the household was the comptroller—an old-fashioned job description meaning being in charge of the domestic staff and the fabric of the house, stables and garden buildings. W. K. Shimwell was comptroller when we moved in; Dennis Fisher succeeded him; followed by Eric Oliver, who in turn was succeeded by his brother John. Eric and John were the third generation of their family to serve the estate; both had graduated from being head house carpenter to comptroller.

We made six flats for staff, which included a night watchman, a telephone switchboard operator and the head of the sewing room. They kept the house alive with their comings and goings, and their eyes and ears were extra security. Telephones were installed in rooms that had never seen such a thing, replacing the bells that had called the maids and valets who no longer existed. The trickiest and one of the longest operations was putting in central heating and the plumbing for seventeen new bathrooms where there had never before been running water ('Who is my sister going to wash in all those baths?' asked Nancy).

There were unexpected complications with the new bathroom that served the red velvet bedroom on the first floor. I wanted the ceiling lowered. This was beautifully done, as were all such alterations, but the coved wall above the window had been painted white and was visible from across the park. So it was repainted a dirty grey like the Derbyshire sky and does not show at all. The painting was done by a Chesterfield firm; their foreman, Eddie Greenwood, and I worked closely together, choosing colours. He was always smiling, even when he swallowed a mouthful of tintacks that he had rashly parked between his lips while using both hands to hang some lining paper. We all waited anxiously for news of the tintacks and were relieved when a message came the next morning to say that there was no longer any need to worry.

As work progressed, I spent more and more time at Chatsworth. I put a chair on the corner of the busiest passage where furniture movers, painters, decorators and sewing room people were bound to pass, and where we could talk about what and where and why. The dogs got to know this and gave up following me round the house for the hundredth time; they knew the walk would not lead out of doors but that sooner or later I would pass this spot, pick them up and at last we would go out. As well as woollen stockings, jerseys, gloves and a master key, an essential piece of equipment was a carpenter's measure. These precious objects disappeared like summer snow, especially when there were carpenters about who slipped them into their pockets without thinking.

I did not employ a decorator; I was too mean to pay for something I could do myself and cannot imagine living surrounded by someone else's taste; and besides, I loved every minute of it. Best of all was seeing plans I had agonized over take shape. Sometimes almost nothing seemed to be happening and then suddenly, like a conjuring trick, it was all there. I was pleased when Nancy Lancaster, who was one of our first guests and whose decoration of Ditchley had been such an influence when I was growing up, said to Andrew, 'My God, you're lucky. If I had done this house for you, you would have had to sell it to pay me.'

Part of the fun was opening drawers and finding things that had been hastily put away when my parents-in-law left. I once looked in a chest of drawers and discovered a miniature of Georgiana Duchess, a Women's Institute programme of 1932, a bracelet given by Pauline Borghese to the Bachelor Duke to hide a crack in the marble arm of a statue of Venus, and a crystal wireless set. It was like finding Christmas presents wherever we went.

Right: At the races with Andrew, September 1938

Below left: With Unity (*left*) at Mill Cottage, Swinbrook, 1940

Below right: My brother Tom. Munich, 1935

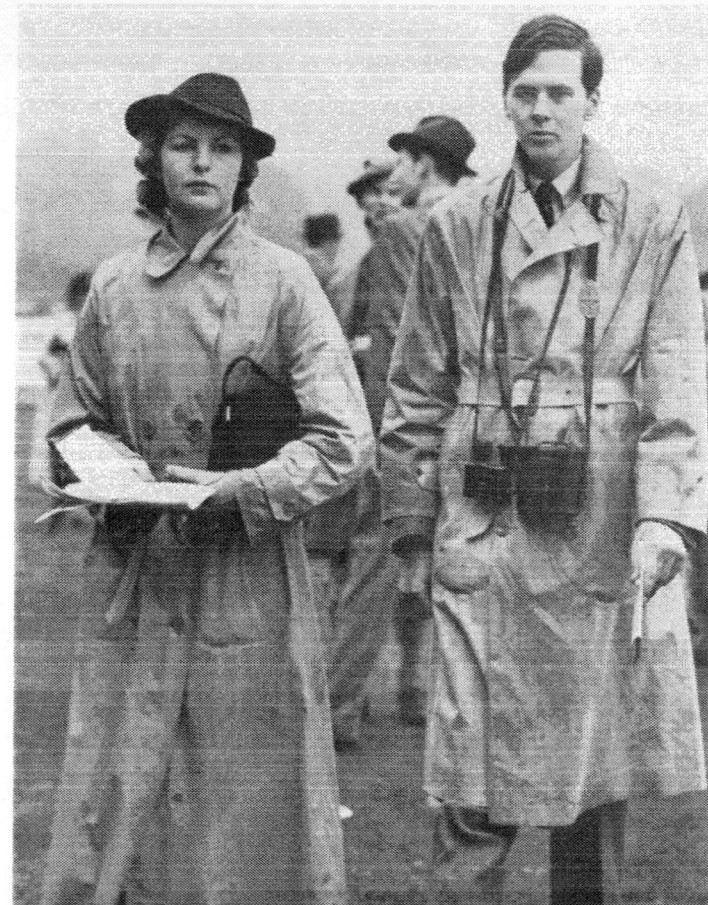

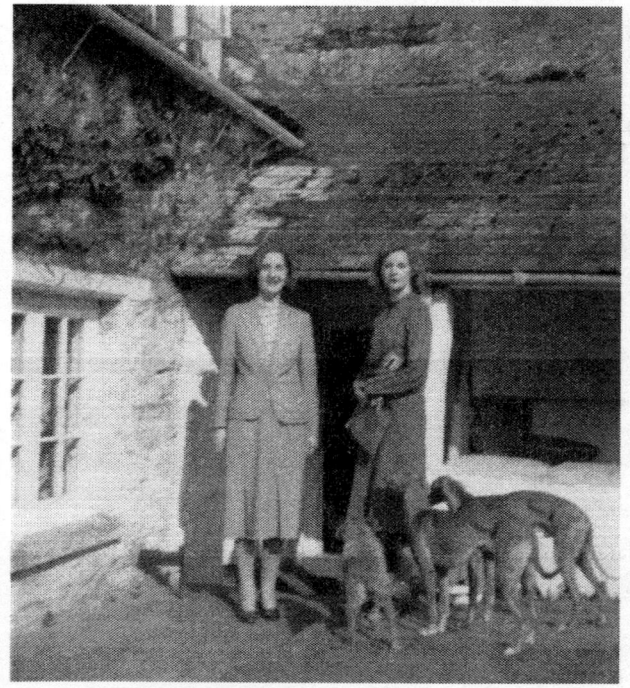

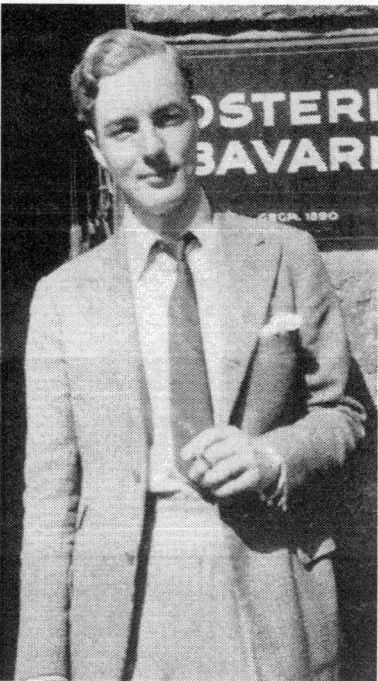

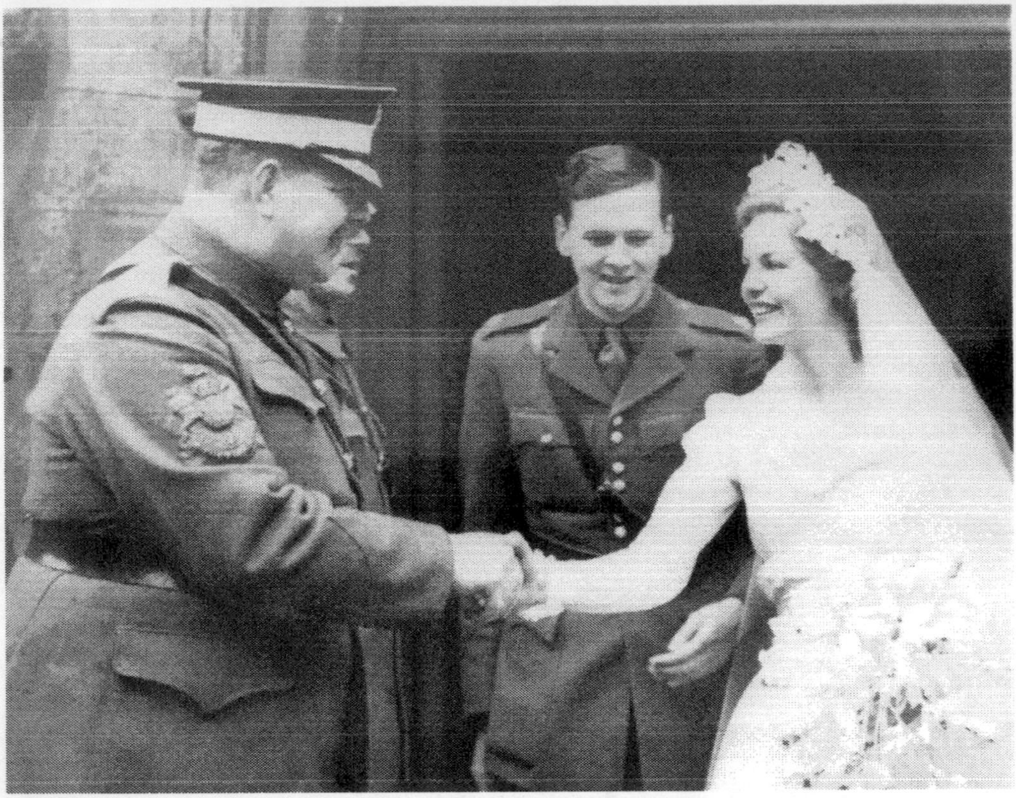

Greeted by Sergeant Major Brittain after our wedding, 19 April 1941

Getting about in a show wagon during petrol rationing. Churchdale Hall, 1943

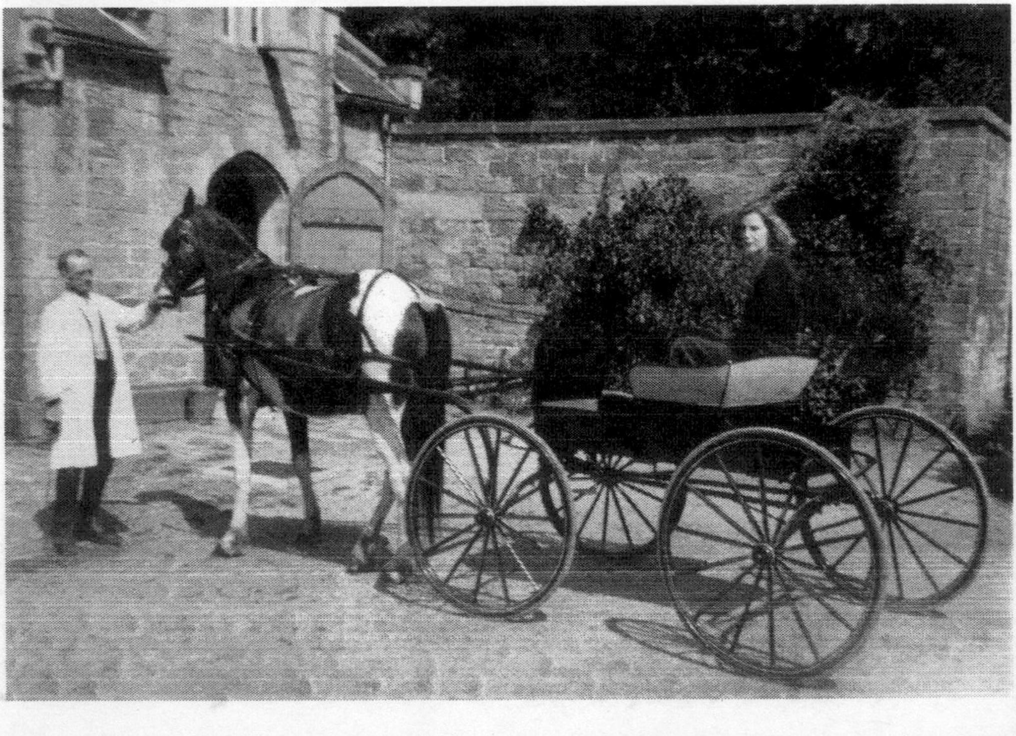

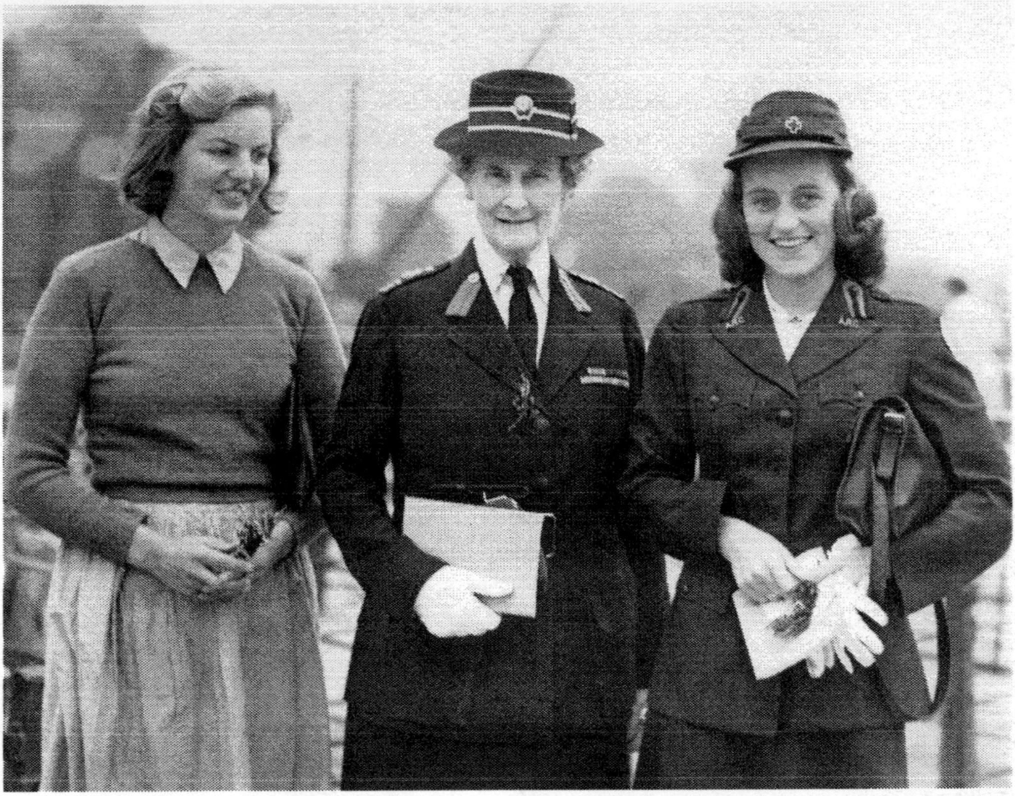

With Andrew's grandmother, Evelyn Devonshire (*centre*), and Kathleen Hartington (Kennedy) (*right*), 1944

Canvassing with Andrew during the 1945 General Election

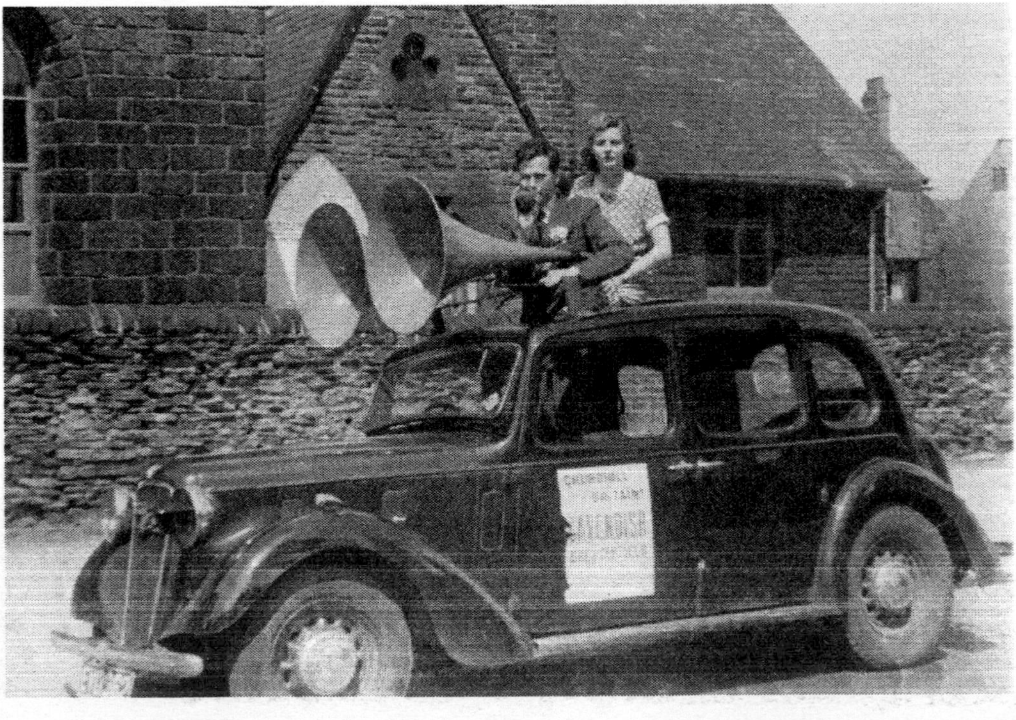

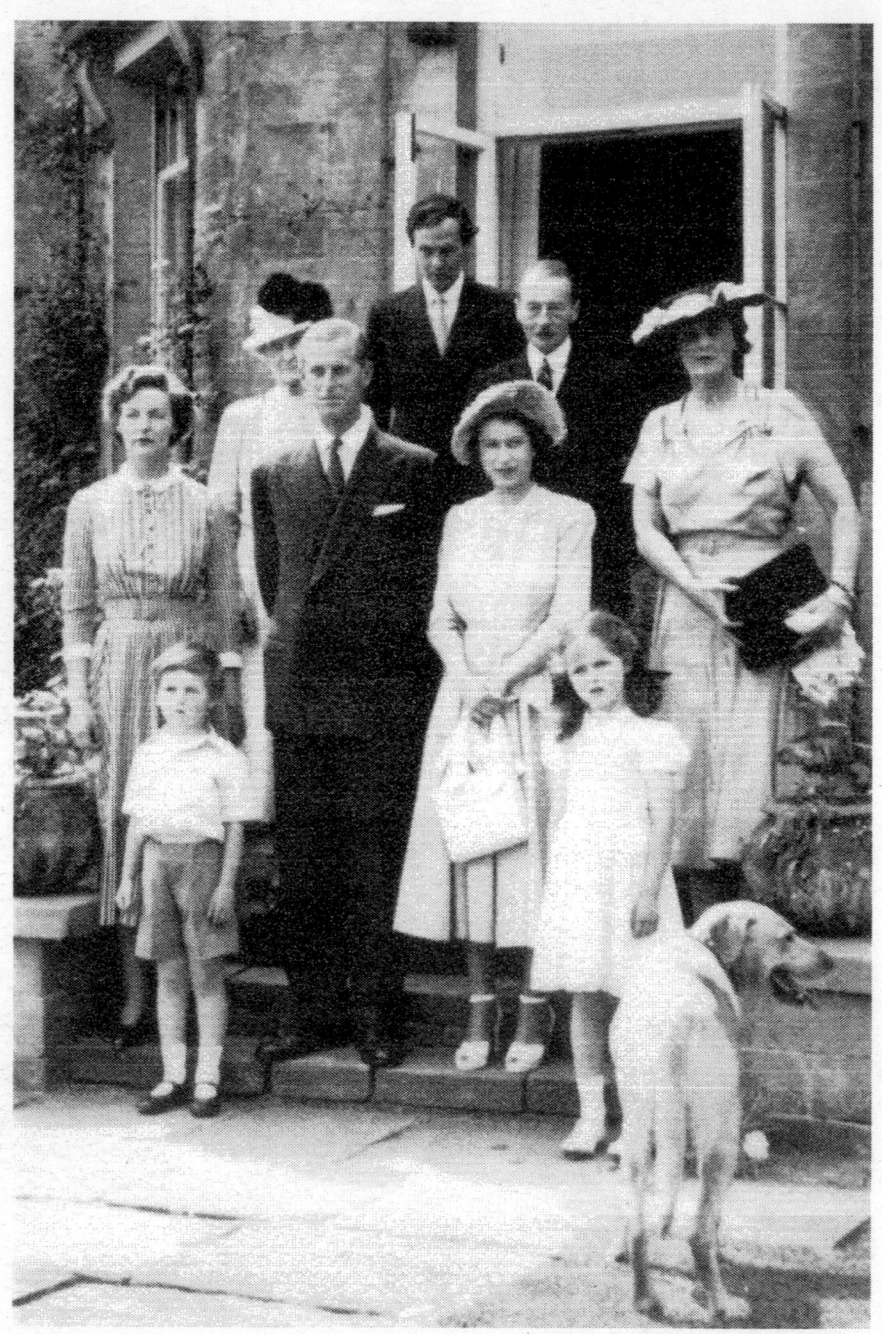

At Edensor House, 1948 (*l. to r.*) DD, Stoker, Evelyn
Devonshire, Prince Philip, Andrew, Princess Elizabeth,
Eddy Devonshire, Emma, Mary Devonshire.
By kind permission of Ron Duggins

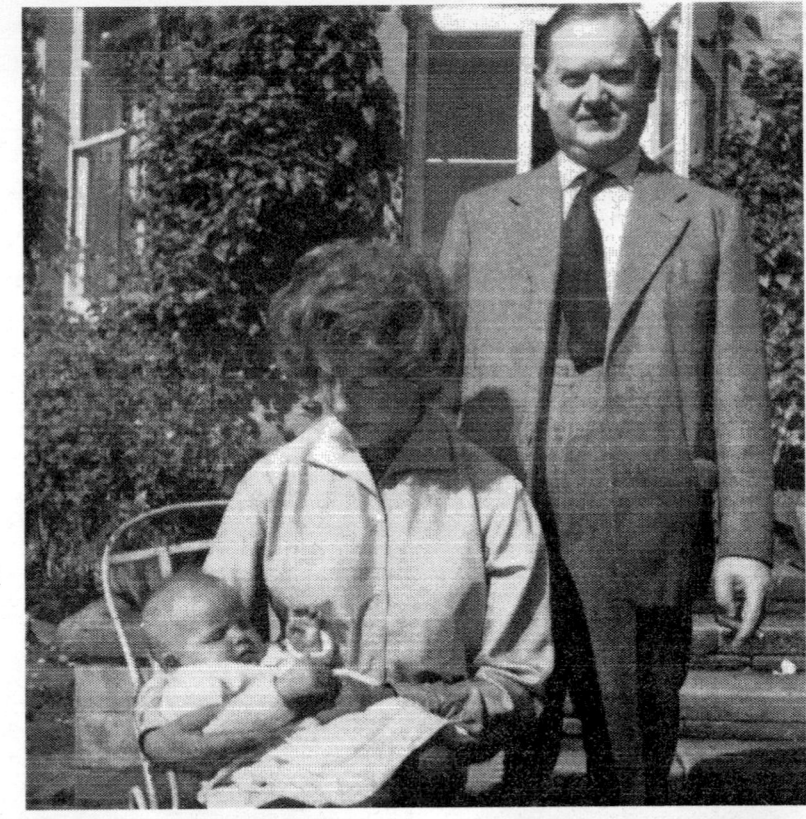

Right: With Sophy and Evelyn Waugh. Edensor House, 1957

Below left: Wearing the hat bought in Paris by Evelyn Waugh

Below right: Kitty Mersey, 1953

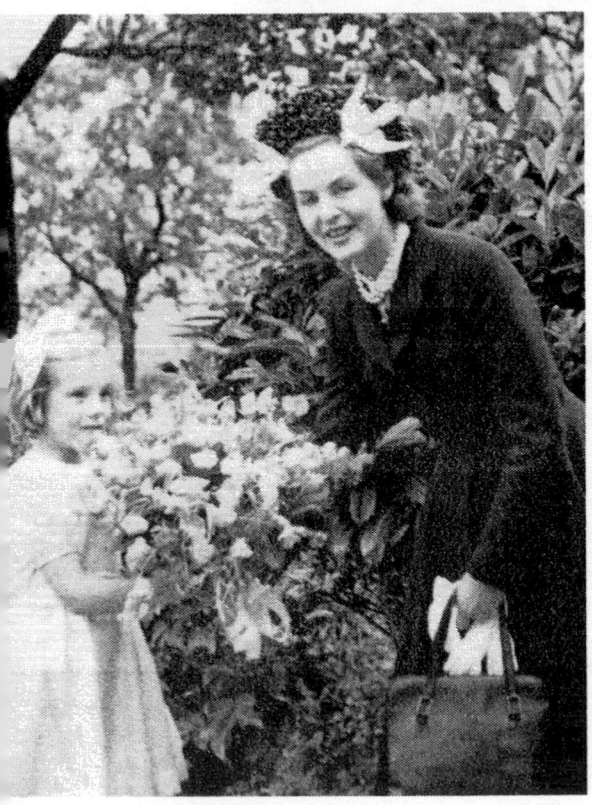

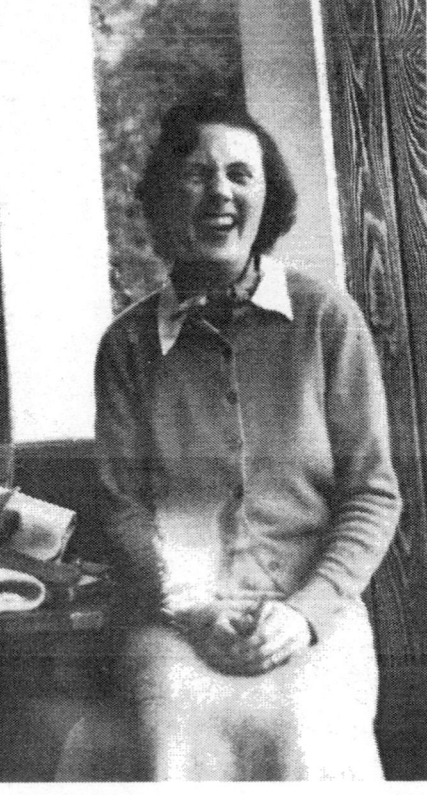

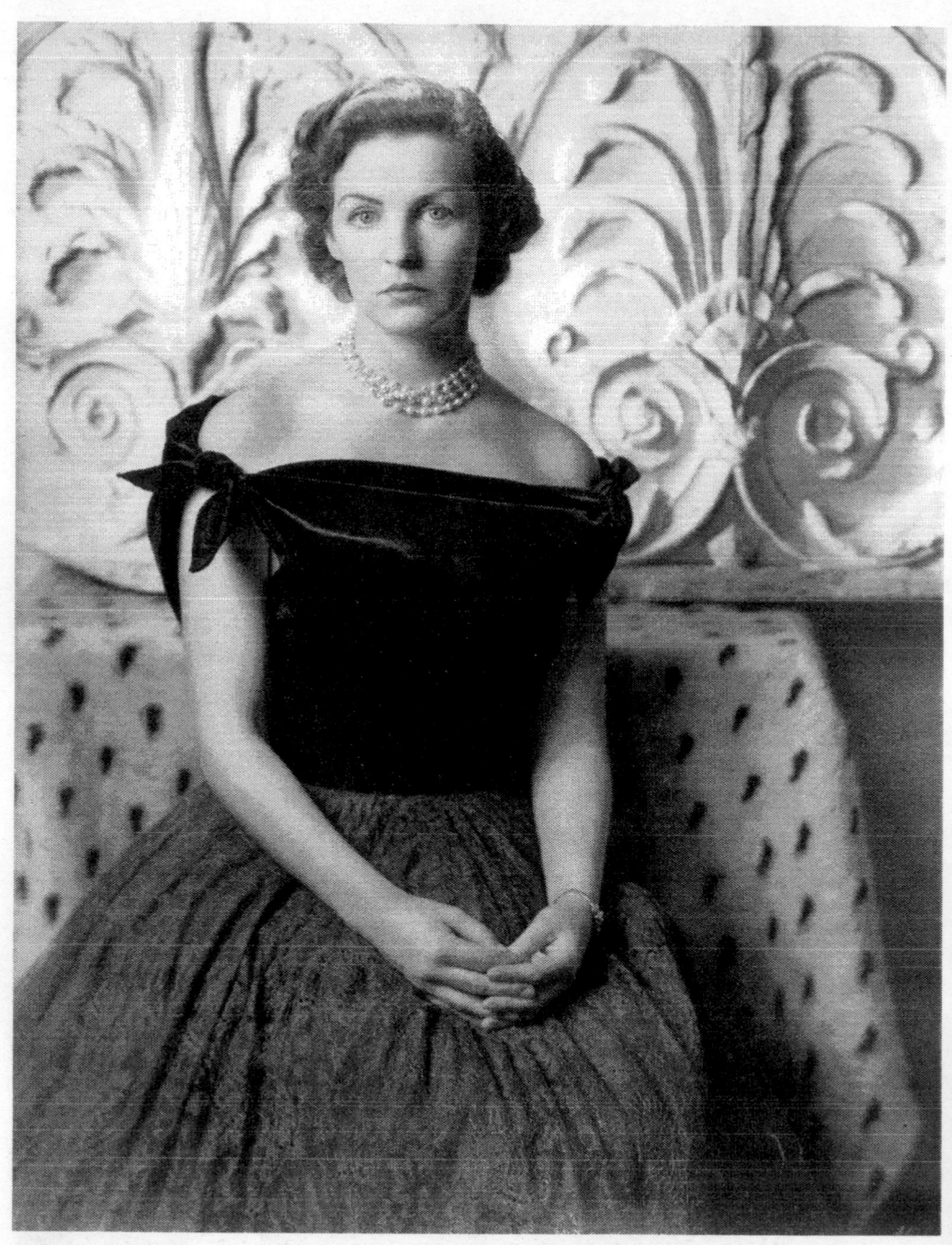

DD, 1950. *Courtesy of the Cecil Beaton Studio Archive at Sotheby's*

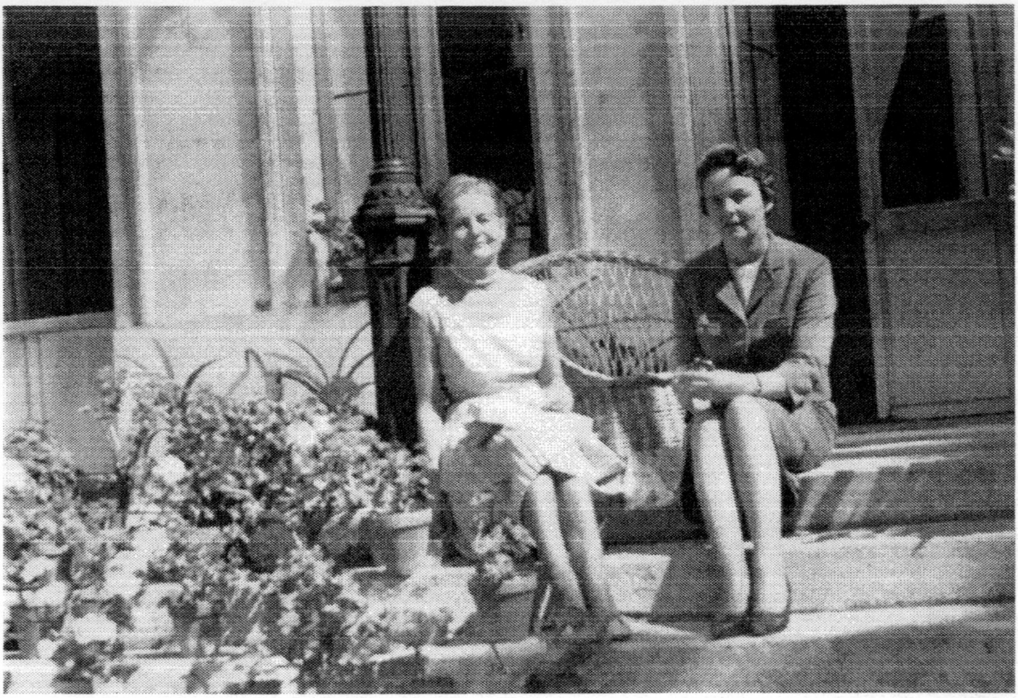

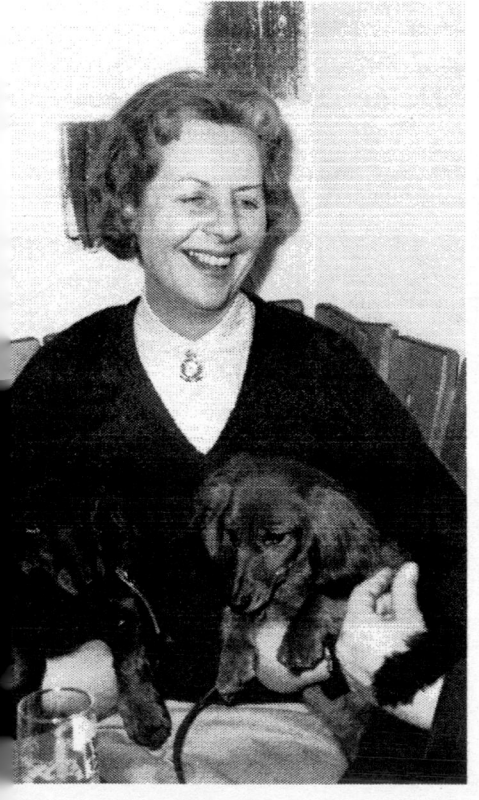

Nancy (*left*) and Decca at Rue Monsieur, Paris

Pamela with her
dachshunds. Zürs, 1964

Diana and Oswald Mosley.
Venice, 1955

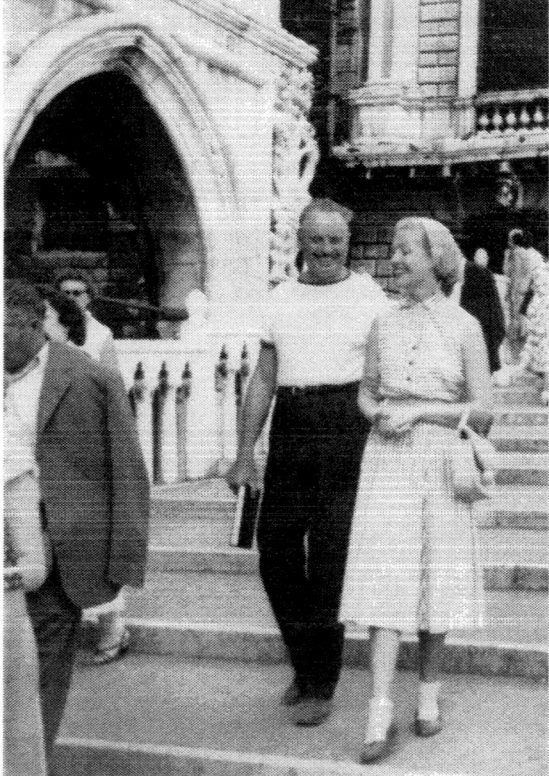

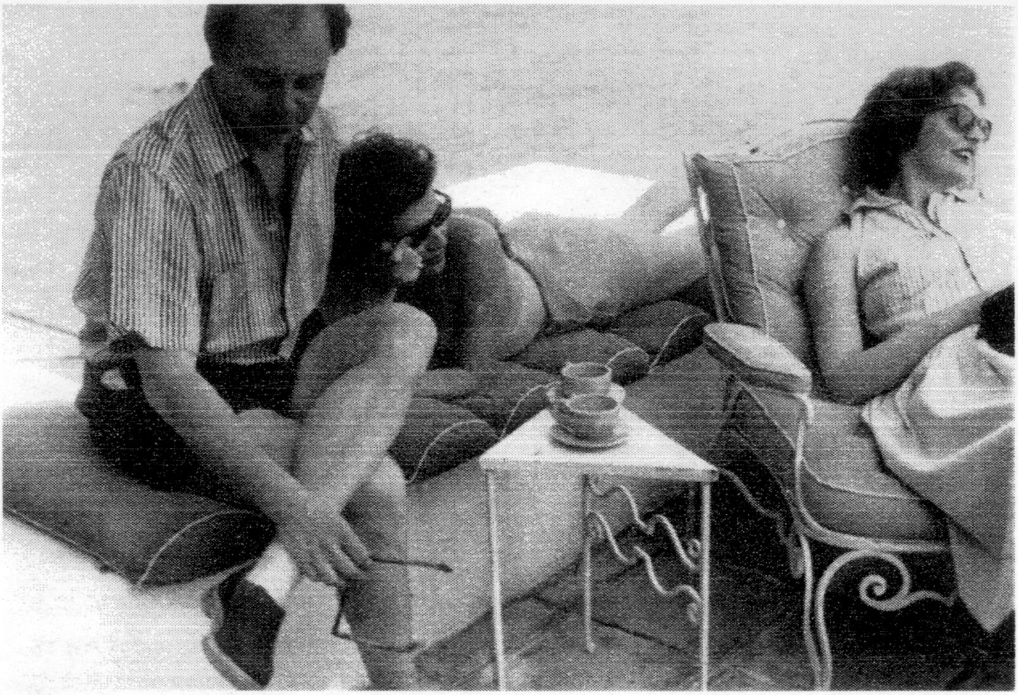

Aly Khan, Teresa de Sousa Campos (*centre*) and DD. Rio de Janeiro, 1955

DD (*left*) and Nancy on the Lido, Venice. *By kind permission of Marina Cicogna*

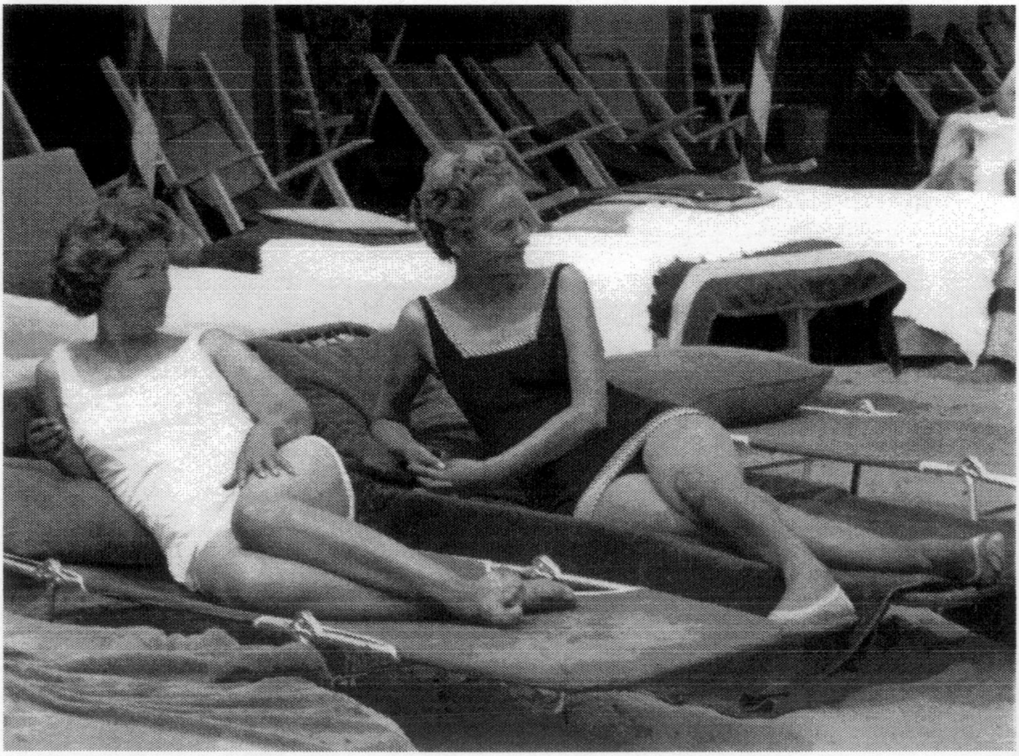

Excitement grew as the rooms began to look cheerful and became fit backgrounds for the furniture, pictures and carpets. Much of these came from other Devonshire houses: Chiswick Villa, Churchdale Hall, Hardwick Hall, Devonshire House and a few beauties saved from Compton Place. It was a motley collection but an extraordinary one from which to be able to choose. W. K. Shimwell, by then the clerk of works and head of the building yard, had an intimate knowledge of the house (where he had served since the age of eleven when he was errand boy and ran to Edensor post office with telegrams). He and Mr Maltby, who had been a house carpenter in London and at Chatsworth since 1910, remembered where various pieces had been previously, which was invaluable. On one occasion Mr Maltby came to me bearing carved wooden draperies which he said Granny Evie had thrown out because they were Victorian, a period she could not abide. Regilded, they were mounted above the blue drawing room windows, for which they had been made.

The actual work, including redecorating the grubbiest and dingiest leftovers from Penrhos School's occupation, took just under two years (and rewiring the rest of the house a further three winters). We eventually moved across the park in November 1959. After all the anticipation, the move seemed quite natural. As soon as I arrived, I felt Chatsworth was home and a perfectly ordinary home at that. I realize now that it was anything but, yet that is how it felt—the obvious place for Andrew and his family to be. Waking the first morning in the bed I was to come home to for the next forty-six years was a joy and I never tired of the incomparable view west across the park. In all those years, I never took the place for granted, but marvelled at it and the fact that we were surrounded by beauty at every turn, both in and out of doors.

*   *   *

Andrew and I used to talk about having portraits painted to join the parade of family likenesses at Chatsworth, but knew that that would have to wait until things looked brighter financially. Then Andrew decided that he wanted to make an exception and asked the Florentine portrait painter Pietro Annigoni, who came to London from time to time and worked in a studio in Edwardes Square, to paint me. In 1954 I spent a month sitting for him, sometimes twice a day. He admired the dark-haired Italian girls by whom he was surrounded and usually painted them or their beautiful northern counterparts. I felt a bit of an imposter and said, 'Sorry about my face, I know it's not what you like.' 'Oh, it's not your fault,' he said, throwing his eyes to heaven (all this through an interpreter as neither of us could speak the other's language). After hours of staring, he decided to paint me in a high white collar and red velvet coat. 'You see,' he said, 'your clothes aren't *à la mode* so it doesn't matter.' The telephone often rang during the sittings. He wanted me to answer it and I was to say he was busy. But the girls soon rang back, hoping to plan a meeting. In spite of not being able to talk, I got fond of Annigoni's presence and his portrait is considered a success.

In the late 1950s I started sitting for Lucian Freud in his Paddington studio. He was a friend and only painted people at his own suggestion. I do not know how many sessions the portrait took, but time had no meaning for him and on it went. Whenever I was in London I used to arrive at the studio at 10 a.m. and sit as still as I could till lunchtime. During the sittings we sometimes talked and sometimes remained silent. Lucian made it obvious that I was not supposed to look at the canvas in the early stages but every now and again, walking round the room during a short break, I caught a glimpse of it. He started painting one eye, and slowly, very slowly, the rest of my face and hair appeared.

At last *Woman in a White Shirt* was ready for Andrew to see. Lucian was out when he called. Andrew hurried up the stairs and made his way between the rickety bedstead and rusty iron bath, almost the only furniture in the studio, to find he was not alone: two men were sitting there. Andrew went to the easel and gazed at 'me', all greenish khaki and with the resigned expression of one who had sat still for hour after hour. After a while one of the men said, 'Who is that woman?' 'It's my wife,' said Andrew. 'Well, thank God it's not mine,' was the bailiff's answer, for that was the profession of the two strangers.

Andrew was an admirer of Lucian's work and was pleased to possess the portrait, which is liked or disliked according to taste. (When Diana Cooper came to stay, she stuck envelopes all over the glass so she could not see it.) For myself, I am glad it was done by an artist who is still a friend and who is acclaimed by critics as 'the greatest living painter' whenever his work is shown. And I believe that as I have got older, so my likeness to the portrait grows.

Lucian was our first guest at Chatsworth; he came to paint a tiny bathroom next to the Sabine bedroom. The idea was to cover the whole of the bathroom walls with cyclamen like the walls in the bedroom next door, which are covered with paintings by Thornhill of Sabine women being tweaked by Roman soldiers. But Lucian is a slow worker and greeted me most mornings with, 'I've had a wonderful night taking out everything I did yesterday.' After five days, the pull of London became too strong and off he went, so the bathroom was never finished.

I had a black Mini which I kept in London and Lucian borrowed it several times. One day he arrived at Chesterfield Street, where we had our London house, swinging the key on his finger. 'This is all that's left of your car,' he said. It had been stolen and that was that. Being driven in London by Lucian was hazardous; Marble Arch was terrifying, Hyde Park Corner even worse. He was Mr Toad, scarf and all, in his old but powerful car. He weaved its long body in and out of the swirling traffic, avoiding buses, bicycles and angry taxi drivers by inches. When I shouted, 'Slower. STOP. PLEASE,' he said, 'It's all right. They've all got brakes.'

Twenty years after painting me, Lucian made a portrait of Andrew. The lengthiness of the sittings shows. Andrew, who was not well at the time, is slumped in a chair and has either nodded off or is staring at the floor—it is impossible to tell which as eyelids take the place of eyes. Lucian also painted

Moucher, Stoker and my sisters-in-law, Elizabeth and Anne. When hung together these portraits span several decades of his work and reflect the changes in his style.

In 1974, Andrew was painted by Theodore Ramos, dressed in the robes of Chancellor of the University of Manchester. It is a good likeness but the clothes are a far cry from his usual frayed silk shirt, pale trousers and tweed coat. Eighteen years later when he was painted by the Glasgow artist Stephen Conroy, in a portrait commissioned by Stoker, he was wearing his everyday clothes, and there stands Andrew to the life.

*   *   *

It was a daily pleasure to live among the pictures at Chatsworth. Gazing at Velasquez' *Lady with a Mantilla* in my sitting room, for example, was a real help when I was trying to do something difficult. There seemed no obvious place to hang Rembrandt's *Portrait of an Old Man*—it has to be studied close to and it is no good muddling it up with other pictures—so Andrew put it on an easel to be examined at leisure. Reynolds' portrait of Georgiana, Duchess of Devonshire and her baby daughter, and Batoni's portraits of the Fifth Duke (looking supercilious) and his younger brother Richard Cavendish (looking drab as befits a second son) suited the blue drawing room. Liotard's pastels of the great actor Garrick and his wife stood out against the deep colour of the red velvet room, and at the same time were protected from too much light as this visitor's room was not often used. It was the same with the furniture:

certain pieces slotted into certain rooms, mixed up without a thought of dates or nationalities. I loved this mongrel arrangement.

Domestic trials were few, but they existed. One was brought about by Nobby, a delightful, selfish and knowing whippet, who wanted to go out in the night; he insisted and there was no escape. So it was on with a thick dressing gown, down thirty-four steps to open the heavy front door and wait in the hall. Sometimes this coincided with the night watchman's thrice-nightly tour of the house. His heavy tread and powerful torch picked me out on my innocent mission. 'It's all right, only me and Nobby,' I would say. We passed the time of day, no—night, and on he went on his round. Nobby whined at the door and thirty-four steps later I got thankfully back into bed. The collie dog was not so demanding, but he made his own trouble. At a coffee morning for a local charity where people had paid a stiff price for a ticket, a Chatsworth man said to me in a low voice, 'There's been an incident. Collie has bitten a lady.' The said lady had refused to be rounded up, which Collie thought was his duty, and she had paid for it with a bitten ankle. She was a good sport and did not sue, but such 'incidents' happened from time to time.

Owning a large house and land brings with it the feeling of being part of a whole, of being in it together with the many people who work there, living cheek by jowl and respecting each other's expertise. At Chatsworth, these people formed an organization unmatched in the country, including cooks, cleaners, archivists, art historians, educationalists, needlewomen, accountants, plumbers, joiners, electricians, lodge porters, security guards, retailers, lecturers, night watchmen, firemen, a computer expert, a photographer and a silver steward. This human kaleidoscope produced the philanderer, the drunk, the saint, the beauty, the troublemaker, the pourer of oil, the flirt, the bore (and Bore Emeritus), the talker and the doer, the observer and the instigator. Some had to be begged to take a holiday; others, like the unnamed artists of the fifteenth century who were known from the subjects of their work as the Master of the Legend of St Ursula or the Master of the Holy Kinship, could be aptly described as the Master of the Unfinished Job. The mixture was fascinating and the people in the different departments made me wonder at their knowledge and interest in the place. Something about Chatsworth makes people want to do their best for it—just as visitors return again and again to discover more.

My role, which was never defined in the way a job would be now, was a woolly Human Resource Last Resort. The knock at my sitting-room door came often enough to make me aware of what I was there for. What people wanted, as we all do, was to talk to someone about their worries, real or imaginary. I only had to listen and out it all came. Sometimes I could 'do something', sometimes I could not, but the fact that the bottled-up trouble was given a hearing was often enough. In the days when the domestic staff lived in, they were at the mercy of their head of department and when things got too much they came to the fount. I did my best, thinking of poor Solomon, but I am sure I often made terrible mistakes. Like my father, I have a weakness in that I have always found it difficult to work with people I do not like. Inevitably in such a large company there were one or two of these, and I am sure I was often unfair when so confronted.

When asked if I found my role difficult, I could always answer no, not really, because I had seen it all my life. From Swinbrook days I was used to farms and to the field sports that go hand in hand with an estate, whether big or small. Farve did not farm himself but I was friendly with the farm tenants and familiar with their stock, crops and calendar. At Chatsworth everything, inside and out, was magnified a hundred times but the underlying feel was the same. It all depended on the people who worked there. There were few demarcation lines between the staff, roles sometimes blurred and melted into the next profession and if one person needed help, the next person lent a hand. It may have been an amorphous organization, run entirely on trust and instinct, but it worked. In all the years Andrew and I lived at Chatsworth, we were let down seriously by only two employees. Our common aim was to leave things better than we had found them. That, I can honestly say, I think we did. And for us, to be surrounded with such beauty and such excellent people was a reward in itself, and the excitement of living at Chatsworth remained with me until I left.

15

Bolton Hall

Bolton hall in Yorkshire was a holiday house, imbued with a holiday atmosphere, where, following family tradition, we spent August for the grouse shooting. There was no formality and only one telephone in a cold cupboard under the stairs. It was a total contrast to Chatsworth. The same six or seven guests came every year for the inside of a week and were replaced by another lot the following week; an annual reunion much looked forward to by all. English sporting events are often marred by bad (another word for appalling) weather, which produces camaraderie like nothing else, and because the same people came to shoot year after year at Bolton, this feeling was magnified. When we were bold enough to invite someone new, he must have felt as though he was starting at a new school or, worse still, joining a new regiment. Englishmen never seem to grow up and, like schoolboys, are wary of a new face. 'Who on earth is that and why have you asked him?' enquires an old boy of the new.

The Bolton Abbey estate had come to the Dukes of Devonshire in 1753, on the death of Lord Burlington, whose only surviving daughter married the future Fourth Duke. Some of the most varied and beautiful landscapes in Yorkshire make up the 30,000 acres of farms, woods and heather moors, well known for the sport they provide. The tall archway topped by a tower in the middle of the

Hall was once the gatehouse to the priory opposite, founded by Augustinian canons in about 1150. The holy men chose a place of spectacular beauty, set in the fertile valley of the River Wharfe. After the Dissolution in 1539, the gatehouse survived when most of the other monastic buildings were knocked down and their stones pillaged. In 1720 the archway was blocked at either end and converted into a house. Extensions were added over the years and in 1843 Paxton enlarged the south wing to make a drawing room with a bedroom and dressing room above for the Duke. Pugin was brought in to decorate the drawing room in fanciful Gothic style. The lofty archway, once the entrance for all traffic to the priory, is now the dining room.

I first went to Bolton in 1946 with my father-in-law and his friends. The only other women in the party were my mother-in-law and Andrew's sisters (no women other than family were ever invited to Bolton—a tradition that Andrew followed). When Andrew was young, he and the other Cavendish grandchildren were boarded out, some in the Bolton Abbey post office, some in the farm across the road and others with tenant farmers. Until rationing came to an end, we stayed in the Devonshire Arms Hotel, half a mile from the Hall. We took it over, filling the bedrooms and queuing for the bath and lavatory. Moucher, Elizabeth, Anne and I rode hill ponies to join the 'guns' at the various heather-thatched lunch huts. This was all very well when the weather was fine, but getting on to a cold, wet saddle in driving rain when you knew there was no chance of being dry till evening was not so good. There was only one motorized vehicle to get the guns up the hill: an ex-army jeep that was usually occupied by the agent, Mr Hay, and his dog—so host and guests walked. A tractor and trailer took the lunch up from the Hall. Now some twenty vehicles trek along the rough tracks—an unheard-of luxury sixty years ago.

Until the early 1950s, when we put it in, there was no electricity at the Hall. The oil lamps often smoked and Pugin's drawing-room ceiling was blackened in places. A row of candlesticks was left out to enable guests to hunt for their bedrooms, up a narrow, winding staircase with ropes for banisters. The house was shabby and lacked the number of baths and lavatories now thought necessary for human habitation. Some of the mattresses were made of hard lumps, some sagged almost to the floor. No one minded. (The grand-looking bed in the King's Room was finally too much and we bought a new mattress.) Two of the bedrooms were pitch dark all day because of the tall yew trees planted a few feet from the house. The others had ancient curtains made of white dimity with long fringes, so there was no hope of keeping out the light.

No one complained. And no one noticed the hole in the drawing-room carpet that got a little bigger each year. Beautiful bits of furniture from Londesborough Hall (where the Earls of Burlington are buried) rubbed shoulders with hard settees covered in hideous cretonne and schoolroom writing tables, their drawers full of silver-framed photographs of King George V and Queen Mary. The King often shot at Bolton in the 1920s and 30s and the house was full to bursting when he came to stay. He brought his own staff, his own post office and a hill pony to carry him to the butts. Queen Mary stayed with her daughter, the Princess Royal, at nearby Harewood House. On 19 August 1921, at 2.00 a.m., a Privy Council was held at the Hall. It was an unusual hour for a meeting, and rare for it to take place in a private house. But the case was an emergency, and the King's formal consent was required before Parliament could be adjourned later that day.

Mrs Canning, our cook in earlier years, came with us to Bolton. A formidable woman of uncertain temper and curious views on life, she had a theory that you could not buy sugar in Yorkshire, so a sack was thrown on to the lorry with all the other comestibles sent from Chatsworth. Mrs White, who had worked under Mrs Canning at her previous job, helped out at Bolton and cooked at Chatsworth when Mrs Canning was on holiday. She was a far better cook than Mrs Canning and unwisely I once said to the latter, 'What a wonderful cook Mrs White is!' 'Huh, well,' said Mrs Canning, 'she could have been, but she only did seven years in the scullery.' There were not enough cooking utensils or linen at the Hall and the lorry from Chatsworth came laden with immense hampers, including 'the Bolton silver' which spent the rest of the year in the safe at Chatsworth. The lorry also brought a set of Derby dessert plates commissioned by the Sixth Duke and decorated with paintings of his houses. For some reason it was thought too risky to use this china at home, but it bumped along the road to Bolton where it formed a traditional part of the dinner table.

The days on the moor were long. The guns often

did not get home till 7 p.m., when they would tuck into tea followed immediately by dinner. The reason for providing tea, however late the hour, was told me by Granny Evie: she thought that if the guns were awash with tea they would drink less whisky later. I cannot say I saw any evidence of this, but we stuck to her rule. When Lord Carnarvon came to shoot, I kept a loaded water pistol by my place at dinner and if the talk got altogether too much, I threatened his velvet jacket with a short sharp shower. The energy of the younger guns inspired the older ones and everyone played desperate games of Billiard Fives late into the night. You would think they would have been too tired, but not a bit of it (though no doubt their shooting suffered the next morning).

There was a large staff at Bolton and the guns often brought their own loaders, usually keepers from their own shoots. This added to the holiday atmosphere and the endless laughter from the low-ceilinged, smoke-filled room where the staff ate (and drank) set the scene for the week. One rare hot August evening after a good supper, a troop of them stripped off and jumped naked into the river. I was terrified that in their high spirits there might be an accident, but mercifully the same number came back as went in.

*   *   *

In Swinbrook days, I had loved going out with Farve and the guns, and had always longed to take part, but knew it was a vain hope. Eddy Devonshire would never have allowed a woman gun at Bolton or Chatsworth, but Andrew had no such prejudice. So at the age of thirty I bought a gun and enlisted the help of Mr Lord, the head keeper at Chatsworth (the famous Mr Maclauchlan had just retired after nearly fifty years' service). Mr Lord and I spent many hours walking the hedgerows, with dogs as beaters to begin with, while I slowly gained enough confidence to take the last butt at Bolton or stand last in the line at a pheasant shoot at Chatsworth. Women guns were rare sixty years ago and initially I was regarded with suspicion all round. Nancy, in her usual way, said that shooting turned me into Farve. 'Better give it up,' she teased, 'it'll ruin your looks.'

It was one of Andrew's many acts of generosity to have kept the shoots going for Stoker and me. He himself had never enjoyed shooting and colour blindness prevented him seeing grouse flying low over the heather. He gave it up soon after his father's death but still enjoyed the organization, having been part of it since childhood. He loved walking and Bolton Abbey gave him the opportunity. Scorning the Land Rovers and ritzy Range Rovers that have replaced legs in the last twenty-five years, he often arrived at a distant line of butts before they did. He sat in their butt with each guest in turn, a folded *Times* in his pocket and Portly, his big, almost white Labrador, by his side. The newspaper was a proper size in those days and when opened its broad white sheets acted as a warning to the grouse, the wildest of birds: STOP, GO AWAY. The presence of their host was inhibiting enough to the guns without the white and off-white deterrents that went with him. (As soon as the drive began Andrew did put the sodden, peaty newspaper back in his pocket.)

The beaters were mostly boys from Skipton Grammar School and they walked for miles through heather and—worse—wet, waist-high bracken. They soon got to know who the guns were and when Uncle Harold was shooting I heard, 'Watch out, lads. There's Uncle Mac up front.' The boys thought that like many old people he might be overconfident and shoot a bit close to the oncoming line of beaters, but there was no need to watch out, he was a good shot. At Bolton Uncle Harold took on the role of the elder statesman, not just of politics but of grouse shooting. Photographs in the local paper of him arriving spawned his 'grouse moor image', which then stuck. He was indulgent to Stoker and his friends, even when, aged sixteen and stumped for something to say to his august neighbour at dinner, Stoker announced, 'Uncle Harold, Old Moore's Almanac says you'll fall in October.' After a suitable pause for thought, the Prime Minister replied, 'Yes, I should think that's about right.'

Our old friend John Wyndham became Uncle Harold's private secretary in 1957. He dreaded the outing to Bolton, especially the rickety ride on the tractor that brought him out to the moor with lunch and any telephone messages that had arrived for his boss that morning. The guns were often late and while they waited John and the farmer who drove the tractor played a game. It was invented by the farmer and involved tossing coins into the heather and retrieving them within a certain time limit. As John was nearly blind and unaccustomed to heather, his opponent always ended with a triumphant, 'I've won.' John was wonderful company and used to make fun of everything to do with the government. At Bolton we watched him throwing top secret Cabinet papers all over the room assigned to Uncle Harold as an office. The typists from Downing Street had never seen such a performance and were half-shocked, half-delighted. Uncle Harold loved John, as did we all. Under the chaos was the sharpest brain in the business.

When Jack Kennedy was President, I often wondered about the messages that went from the Prime Minister at Bolton to the White House. In August 1963, Uncle Harold was staying with us at the same time as David Ormsby Gore, our Ambassador to Washington. Some international crisis was brewing as usual. Uncle Harold summoned David and read him the message he was proposing to send to Jack. It began with a long, flowery account of the day's shooting (something the President had never done) and was larded with such phrases as 'sunlit heather', 'birds plentiful', 'strong north-west wind'. The point of the cable came right at the end of this poetic description. David caught my eye and we started laughing at the idea of the poor puzzled President trying to guess what Uncle Harold was on about. I do not know what found its way to Washington, but I imagine David pruned it somewhat.

Out of the shooting season, Bolton was made thoroughly enjoyable for me by the visits of the architect Philip Jebb, whose company I loved and who worked with me at Chatsworth and at Bolton on the estate buildings. I looked forward to our winter picnics, sitting on crates by an enormous boiler in the beautiful sixteenth-century tithe barn (the only warm place available), surrounded by all the familiar paraphernalia of an estate building-yard. Noël Coward's notion that 'working is so much more fun than fun' was certainly the case with Philip. He was always ready to laugh and we often shared critical views about some of the people we worked with. Philip was in charge of adding the Wharfedale Wing to the Devonshire Arms Hotel, with the help of Harry Moon, a Yorkshire architect, who also became a friend. Working with Philip and Harry was a privilege and it was exciting to see the hotel expand from nine to forty-two bedrooms.

Philip died, aged sixty-eight, in 1995. The loss of his influence and good taste was unlucky for this country; he kept the flag flying during the disastrous 1950s and 60s, when the worst architectural horrors were springing up. Professionally he was second to none and was incapable of designing anything ugly. He ensured that the site and scale of a building fitted the landscape instead of imposing a design that had been dreamt up in an office miles away (which seems to be the easy way out for architects today), and the builders who interpreted his work all agreed his drawings were the most exact they had ever worked from. If only more of his work survived.

16

A Minister's Wife

In 1960 Andrew was made Parliamentary Under Secretary of State for Commonwealth Relations, a job he described as 'not being responsible for making the tea, but for doing the washing up'. In 1962 he was promoted to Minister of State in the Commonwealth Office, a post he held for two years. He enjoyed his four years in government and must have known, by the reactions of all whose paths he crossed, how well he carried out his task. He had a flair for getting on with anyone, no matter who they were or where they came from— the more unlikely the individual the better. His work was not confined to office hours and there was many a diplomatic cocktail party given by the High Commissioner of this or that independent country, and often a dinner as well. Andrew's stamina was tested and he came out with flying colours. The only fly in the ointment was his boss, Duncan Sandys, whom he found abrasive and not easy to work with. More than once, Andrew saw him make senior civil servants cry with his sarcastic, tyrannical ways. He was also very slow in drafting speeches and memos, and Andrew missed train after train for Chesterfield on Friday nights as Duncan agonized over 'and' and 'the'. It is a pity that Andrew only ever had Sandys as his boss; had he had the chance to work for someone else, a friendlier atmosphere would have lightened his load.

I went with Andrew on several official trips to Africa and the Caribbean. Some of it was familiar territory because we had already been to Kenya, Uganda and Rhodesia in 1947, when my father-in-law wanted to invest in land and had asked Andrew to look into the possibilities. In 1947 the flight to Nairobi in a Douglas Dakota took five days, with overnight stops in Brussels, Tripoli, Cairo and Khartoum. From Egypt onwards it was only possible to fly in the mornings, as later in the day the heat had built up too dangerously for the low altitude at which those reliable old planes flew. Over the next three weeks we stayed with nineteen kind hosts, none of whom we had met before—a sure cure for shyness and an experience that I have been grateful for ever since. We enjoyed the free and easy way of life, the beauty of the country and gardens, the richness of the land, and the unfamiliar birds and animals. But I was shocked by the way some of the white women treated their African servants, by their rudeness and the way they talked about their shortcomings in front of them. Independence was a long way off, but resentment was building.

One of our stops was with Lord Francis Scott, a dear fellow and long-time Kenyan farmer. His daughter Pam was the very opposite of the rude women and had started a school and hospital for workers on the family estate. The scandal and mystery of Lord Erroll's unsolved murder, which had taken place among the philandering, hard-drinking Happy Valley set six years previously, was still fresh in everyone's minds. I realized that Lord Francis must have known Erroll, Sir Delves Broughton (the suspected murderer) and the other characters involved. I asked him if he had been in it. 'In it?' he said. 'Of course I was in it up to the neck.' But he was too discreet to enlarge on what he thought about that extraordinary episode.

From Kenya we went to Zanzibar, the island of cloves and giant turtles that moon about on the seashore looking as old and gnarled as Elizabethan oaks. There was no glass in the windows at the Residency and the warm sea breeze came in, as did birds of all kinds. The hospitable Sultana herself made scones for us. Later we went to Uganda in a tiny plane and were met on a grassy airstrip by a young couple from Government House. 'We're only acting,' they told us. 'So are we,' I said, 'we don't usually go on like this.' (Not being versed in diplomatic language I did not know that 'acting' meant playing the role of a superior.) Andrew and I loved the glorious greenness of Uganda and when we returned fifteen years later for Independence we were delighted to see it all again.

My chief recollection of Southern Rhodesia, where we stayed with the Governor General, Sir John Kennedy, and his wife, Bungs, is of Andrew's fury at being made to go to a children's party. The old-fashioned colonial code of conduct still applied to a ridiculous degree: at a reception one night, a woman guest, who had driven miles through the bush, was turned away because she had forgotten her white gloves. On the way home we had a long wait at Benghazi airport while we changed planes. In those days the little airport was not exactly luxurious and we tried to get out of the dust and into the VIP lounge, where we had spotted two deckchairs. We were soon turned out quite roughly and cut down to size by being made to sit on the sand floor till the trusty Dakota was ready to take us to our next stop.

*   *   *

Andrew's time in the Commonwealth Office coincided with the independence of eleven British colonies. In 1961 we went to Nigeria to attend the celebration of that country's first anniversary of Independence. Dr Nnamdi Azikiwe (known as Zik) was Governor General and Commander-in-Chief of the Federation, but Britain retained a High Commissioner in the shape of Antony Head. We stayed with him and his wife, Dorothea, and it was a breath of fresh air to find these old Wiltshire friends (their home was near Salisbury) in Lagos.

The High Commissioner's residence was bang on a lagoon and had been built at vast expense by the architect Lionel Brett. He had had an unequalled opportunity to create a beautiful building—modern architecture is well suited to the tropics—but the result resembled an oversized chicken house. Downstairs was one huge open-plan room for dining and sitting, which looked dangerously like an airport lounge. A staircase sprang from there to what can only be described as nesting boxes, bedrooms with sloping wooden ceilings which gave the feeling they might be lifted at any moment to see if you had laid an egg. They had no balcony—surely the first necessity in a hot climate—and you could only open the windows by climbing on to the high window sills and dragging them down with all your might, like you do in Continental trains.

There was no escape from official duties.

Andrew did his stuff marvellously at the schools, hospitals, universities, maternity homes, slum clearances, housing estates, sports grounds and government offices that we went round till we almost dropped. Antony Head's ADC was Pips Royston, a new face to us and excellent company. Pips banged on the door of our room soon after lunch one day when we were trying to snatch some sleep. 'Hats and gloves at six,' he announced. This was in order to meet Oba Adele II and other local rulers. These exotic gentlemen were not in their first youth and they danced for us half-bare, their extra flesh wobbling in time to the steps. They reminded me of heavy horses displaying at an agricultural show and I immediately liked the look of them.

My crowning moment in Lagos was to have been at a football match when Zik, then at the height of his popularity, invited me to accompany him in his official car for several circuits of the football pitch and present the cup to the winning team. Alas, my moment of glory never came as the match was a draw, but I had an unexpected instant in the spotlight. A huge crowd received Zik with acclaim as we drove round the pitch but by the second circuit they had started to laugh loudly. When we got back to where Antony and Dot were sitting, I asked one of the officials why they were laughing. 'Oh,' he said, 'they thought you were Zik's new wife.' From Lagos, we went to Kano in Northern Nigeria, where the landscape was quite different and the climate hot and dry. We saw extraordinarily beautiful houses built of mud and an Emir sitting under a tree in full white robes, quietly pronouncing judgements.

In August 1962 Princess Margaret represented the Queen at the celebrations to mark the Independence of Jamaica. The British delegation was led by our old friend Hugh Fraser, Secretary of State for Air, who was accompanied by his wife, Antonia. We travelled with the royal party in a Britannia Bristol, a flying drawing-room, for twenty-two hours. When we arrived it was all very formal with the usual programme of official events, which meant hats, gloves and best evening dresses for Antonia and me. Our friend Drue Heinz, generous patron of the arts and the literary world, had kindly offered to lend us hats. By early August the events of the Season when Drue would have needed hers were over, and we took our pick. Trying them on in London turned out to be more fun than wearing them in Jamaica, where it rained enormous drops of warm water that created a sticky, frizzy mess of hair and straw. The American delegation to the celebrations was headed by Vice-President Lyndon Johnson, who was disappointed that Princess Margaret was the centre of everyone's attention and did his best to steal her thunder. At the celebratory ball Andrew offered £10 to the first of our delegation to dance with the Vice-President. I am sorry to say that Antonia won hands down and that I never even managed to be introduced.

The Jamaican Prime Minister, Sir Alexander Bustamante, was the living double of Obbie St Albans and whenever I saw one of them, I always thought it was the other. Like Obbie, Bustamante had a teasing nature, which in his case took the form of leading a bloody revolution against colonial rule. In their inimitable way, the British government imprisoned him and then installed him as leader of his country. Bustamante was a great figure in his native land and I found him no less impressive when he came to England for a Commonwealth prime ministers' meeting. I saw him again at a dinner at Buckingham Palace, mischievous as ever.

In October 1962, Uganda was next on the list and we flew there for an unforgettable week of festivities. It was like a fancy-dress party with people wearing national costumes not just from Africa but from all over the world. Jomo Kenyatta, who was staying in our hotel, minced about whisking his fly whisk, and was followed by two tall, sinister-looking bodyguards. He pinched the room that had been given to Lord Carrington, who was leading the British delegation. We gave a dinner party one night when the Princess Royal (theirs not ours), an old lady with a crew cut, came in her slip; we kept thinking she must put on her dress soon, but the slip was the dress.

The Kabaka (Major General Sir Edward Frederick William David Walugembe Mutebi Luwangula Mutesa II KBE), King of Buganda, was a most attractive man, with that indefinable quality that drew all eyes towards him. He lived on top of a hill in a palace made of bamboo. Two of the big parties were held there and on both occasions the Ugandan electricity (never very reliable) failed, the lights went out and the Kabaka minded—a diplomatic party in the dark is hard to manage. The Kabaka's son and heir, Prince Ronnie, was seven years old at the time and we were delighted to find that his tutor was Mark Amory, an Oxford friend of our daughter Emma. Never knowing who you were going to meet next was what made these outings such fun, and Mark was a big help in explaining the locals and their way of life.

In December 1963 we were in Kenya to see the British flag being lowered. It was another case of poacher turned gamekeeper: Kenyatta was made leader of the country after being imprisoned for seven years by the British. The Duke of Edinburgh represented the Queen at the celebrations and there was the usual confusion along narrow mud roads; we were following Prince Philip's car and it looked for a moment as though we would be late for the flag ceremony. At the ball afterwards Andrew danced with Kenyatta's wives, two black and one white. As we left, the new President presented him with a fly whisk, a traditional honour to an official visitor, which Andrew always kept on his desk. The name Devonshire was well remembered by the new Kenyan government because in 1923, Andrew's grandfather Victor Duke, in his capacity as Secretary of State for the Colonies, had issued a White Paper declaring that, 'Primarily Kenya is an African territory . . . the interests of the African natives must be paramount.'

All the independence ceremonies followed roughly the same pattern: celebratory lunches, dinners, garden parties, cocktail parties, a grand ball, and then the lowering of the British flag and the hoisting of the 'new' country's own. Inevitably, there was an element of tragicomedy about these events, and emotions were mixed; the initial surge of elation and optimism that followed the lowering of the flag was often the signal for an outburst of violence and corruption. It reminded me forcibly of the triumphant British coal miners who, after the 1945 General Election, basked for a moment in the feeling 'we are the masters now', only to find themselves back underground with nothing changed. On our way home to England from one of these ceremonies, we were waiting at Kano airport with some newly ex-District Officers when one of their wives, horrified by her omission, suddenly gasped, 'Oh! I forgot to take down the portrait of the Queen.' I thought it a sad and telling remark; it was indeed the end. What was the future for these excellent people, who had worked so hard to build something that was so soon to be undone?

Let no one get the impression that these trips abroad were anything but work all the way. Andrew had to stick to a government brief in his speeches, which he did not find easy because he preferred speaking off the cuff. There was endless talking to strangers and having to change clothes several times a day, according to what was on the programme. 'You try a few protracted dinners between the Canadian Minister of Labour and the Jamaican Minister of Education,' I wrote to a friend. But in spite of these drawbacks there was always, without exception, some amusing incident; we met outstandingly interesting individuals who eased the way, added to which was the excitement of seeing new countries. Although it was always a relief to get home, I would not have missed it for the world.

Andrew's job involved not only travelling but also looking after the new Commonwealth heads of state when they came to England. In 1964 it was the turn of Sir Ahmadu Bello, the Sardauna of

Sokoto, for an official visit. As often happened, the Commonwealth Office was at a loss as to what to do with him over the weekend. Answer: send him to Chatsworth. We invited Bobbety and Betty Salisbury and other friends to meet the Sardauna, and expected him and his entourage for lunch at 1.00 p.m. We waited and waited and waited. At 3.30 p.m. the cars finally appeared. Out piled not six people, as we had been told to expect, but thirteen. The only extra food I knew we had in the house was ham. Goodness knows what Mrs Canning found for our Muslim guests, but it could not have been the 'accursed' pig.

The Sardauna was friendly and his robes smelled deliciously of herbs. The 3.30 p.m. lunch passed off well, we thought, and the party went round the house afterwards. They stopped by the portrait of Henry VIII and the guide told them about his six wives. This was met with indulgent laughter—the Sardauna had quite a crowd himself. To our surprise, after a late tea the party began to say goodbye—we had been expecting them to stay the night. We later discovered that they preferred the floor to the comfortable four-posters that had been made up for them and, thinking we might be insulted, had decided to leave rather than risk offending us.

Another visitor was the Shah of Persia. He was inspecting factories round about and it was thought by his hosts that a visit to Chatsworth might end the day satisfactorily. This quiet, handsome, serious man arrived for tea in a helicopter. My mother-in-law, who was staying, said to me, 'He'll be tired, you must offer him a bed so he can have a rest.' The Shah was in the prime of life and would, I think, have been astonished if I had done as she advised, so I quietly forgot about it and we got on with tea. I had always admired the Shah's beautiful wives. Farah Diba, a vision in Dior and a worthy queen of the Peacock Throne, was voted one of the world's best-dressed women several times. I was disappointed that she was not with him on this visit.

The President of India, Dr Radhakrishnan, came to stay at Chatsworth in 1963. He was a silent academic whose religion did not allow him to eat meat, fish, chicken, eggs, milk or cheese. That left little but peas, pulses and fruit. It was not easy to devise two dinners and a lunch for him, but we managed somehow. Andrew and I took Dr Radhakrishnan round the house, pointing out objects that might interest him. He never uttered a word—neither a comment, nor a question—until we reached the Orangery at the end of the tour, at which point he turned to Andrew and asked, 'Has the Queen been here?'

After the 1964 General Election when Harold Wilson's Labour government came to power, Andrew was offered the job of Shadow Minister of Transport in the House of Lords. As he could not drive a car, he thought this was not a good idea and retired from active politics in the Conservative cause. He continued to attend the House of Lords but never again held a senior job.

17

The Kennedys

When Joseph P. Kennedy arrived in England on 1 March 1938 to take up the post of United States Ambassador to the Court of St James's, it was not Joe who grabbed the headlines but his wife, Rose, mother of nine, whose youthful appearance and figure were the subject of much attention from the press and the envy of her English contemporaries. Mrs Kennedy, her eldest daughter Rosemary, and second daughter, Kick, were presented at Court on 11 May, heralding the start of their London season, which was also mine. Rosemary was mentally retarded and not able to join in the round of dances and other entertainments, but she did manage the curtsey at Buckingham Palace.

The Kennedys were masters of entertainment and the dinner-dance they gave on 2 June was one of the very best. Joe Jr and Jack Kennedy were not there as they did not arrive in England until the Fourth of July, just in time for a dinner given at the embassy on that important date in the American calendar. The two brothers were thrown in at the deep end but they soon mastered the routine, making friends as easily as Kick had. Twenty-three-year-old Joe Jr was as attractive and full of vitality as the rest of the family and made an immediate impact. He was his father's chosen one to go into politics and make a name for himself. I was always aware of his presence but hardly knew him as he preferred the company of more sophisticated women to eighteen-year-old debutantes. Jack was two years younger and a shadow of his brother. He suffered from poor health and it showed.

Towards the end of July 1938, Andrew and I went to the races with Kick, Jack, Jean and Margaret Ogilvy, Hugh Fraser and David Ormsby Gore. There was no particular significance to this outing except that it was the start of the friendship between Jack and David, which was to play such an important part when, twenty-three years later, Jack became President and David was appointed Ambassador to the US.

David was a first cousin of Andrew and a lifelong friend. When he was up at Oxford, all he liked was jazz, racing and his future wife, the beautiful Sylvia (Sissie) Lloyd Thomas. Learning and lectures were not on his list and he spent his university days lying on the sofa in his St Aldate's lodgings, tapping a foot in time to Nat Gonella on a wind-up gramophone. He did no work and to his father's dismay managed a dismal Third. It was run-of-the-mill to all of us, who were used to our friends just scraping through or failing altogether when the crunch came with exams. David, who with Andrew and the Astor boys was the best company going, was quick to prick any balloon of pomposity, a trait that never deserted him, even in the important Foreign Office roles he played so well in later life. Like his elder brother, Gerard, and Sissie before him, he was killed in a car accident and I mourn them to this day. Years later Jack reminded me of that outing to the races—I had quite forgotten about it. Perhaps he remembered it better than so many other enjoyable days that summer because it was when he first met David.

From their arrival in England, Ambassador Kennedy kept his sons busy with the serious side of life and made sure they learned something of British politics and politicians, industry and the City. As well as sampling the delights of the Côte d'Azur, they also did a whistle-stop tour of European capital cities, gaining a greater knowledge of Europe than most American politicians, storing away these experiences for future use. Jack's time in England at an impressionable age must have influenced the 'special relationship' that he fostered during his years in office. He told me that when he was in hospital as a teenager he read widely and that after reading John Buchan's biography of the seventeenth-century Scottish general, his hero became the great Montrose.

Joe Kennedy Sr was pessimistic about England and France's chances of defeating Hitler and was viscerally opposed to America entering the war. His isolationism cost him his English friends. Joe Jr adopted his father's attitude while Jack remained more detached, but both brothers enlisted before Pearl Harbor. In spite of back pain and generally ailing, Jack somehow passed fit into the US Navy. In March 1943 he was in the Pacific when the boat he was in was rammed and cut in half by an enemy destroyer. After clinging to the wreckage for many hours, the survivors, commanded by Jack, reached a small island. It was not until five days later that they were rescued, and for his heroism Jack was awarded the Navy and Marine Corps Medal.

Joe Jr was an officer in the US Navy Air Corps.

He volunteered for a perilous mission to attack a flying-bomb launch site near Calais and was killed on 12 August 1944 when his plane blew up before reaching its target. He was posthumously awarded the Navy Cross, the highest decoration. His death added to the list of catastrophes that took so many of our friends and family during July and August that year. On receiving the news, Kick, who had been married to Billy for just three months, left for America to attend his memorial service. Wartime journeys across the Atlantic were difficult to arrange, but as the daughter of the US Ambassador she managed it. Three weeks later, Billy was killed and Kick immediately returned to England.

In his letter of condolence to Moucher, Jack wrote that the news of Billy's death was:

about the saddest I have ever had. I have always been so fond of Kick that I couldn't help but feel some of her great sorrow. Her great happiness when she came home which even shone through her sadness over Joe's death was so manifest and so infectious that it did much to ease the grief of our mother and father. It was so obvious what he meant to Kick and what a really wonderful fellow he must have been that we all became devoted to him, and now know what a really great loss his is. When I read Captain Waterhouse's letter about the cool and gallant way Billy died, I couldn't help but think of what John Buchan had written about Raymond Asquith 'Our roll of honour is long, but it holds no nobler figure. He will stand to those of us who are left as an incarnation of the spirit of the land he loved . . . He loved his youth, and his youth has become eternal. Debonair and brilliant and brave, he is now part of that immortal England which knows not age or weariness or defeat.' I think that those words could be so well applied to Billy. I feel extremely proud that he was my sister's husband.

After Billy's death Kick, who was devoted to Eddy and Moucher and to her sisters-in-law, Anne and Elizabeth, wanted to be among the friends in England that she had known since she was eighteen. She bought a house in London, No. 2 Smith Square, Westminster, and for the next four years divided her time between England and America. Her old suitors returned: William Douglas Home was still enamoured of her, Anthony Eden was a friend, as were Richard Wood and Hugh Fraser (who had also been particularly fond of her sister Eunice), but as soon as Kick met Peter, Eighth Earl Fitzwilliam, he became the only contender. But there was a serious obstacle: Peter was married.

Kick had already made a major concession when marrying Billy and agreeing that any sons of theirs would be brought up as Protestants. She knew that her parents would never condone marriage to a divorcee and, indeed, Kick's mother warned her that she would be banished from the family if she went ahead. Hoping to talk her father round, Kick made a plan to meet Ambassador Kennedy in Paris on her way back from a few days with Peter on the Côte d'Azur. The pair set off for Cannes in a chartered plane on 13 May 1948. They hit a violent thunderstorm over the Rhône Valley and after being buffeted in the air for thirty minutes, the plane crashed into a mountainside, killing all on board.

Kick's body was brought to England and she was buried in the Cavendish plot at St Peter's Church in Edensor. I had never been to a funeral before and the solemn words affected me profoundly. She and I were both twenty-eight, not the time of life when you think about death, yet that most vital of human beings had been taken from us. Bert Link, the head gardener, lined her grave with pale mauve wisteria—the sweet-smelling, short-lived flowers so fitting for a life cut short so tragically. Ambassador Kennedy was the only member of her family able to get to the funeral. He wore a bright-blue crumpled suit, which was all he had with him, and this surprising colour accentuated the anguished misery of his face, an image engraved for ever on my mind.

*   *   *

We kept in touch with the Kennedys. When they came to England they always telephoned and we sometimes met in London, but we did not see much of them until 1961 when, to our surprise, Andrew and I were invited to Jack's presidential inauguration. Andrew was intrigued by the invitation and realized what an honour it was to be asked. I did not want to go. There were engagements I was looking forward to at home, including the last shoot of the season. But it was so good of them to think of us that we accepted.

We stayed with the British Ambassador, Sir

Harold Caccia, and his wife, Nancy, and those three days we spent in Washington were among the most extraordinary of our lives. The warmth of the welcome from the Kennedy family, now happy and glorious, was something Andrew and I never forgot. We were given the best seats at all the events, far above anything we expected, and the bitter cold and unrelenting snow made it all the more dramatic. I realized these were events of historic importance and jotted down some notes at the time, which cover the sublime and the ridiculous about equally. These appeared in my book *Home to Roost*, and are reprinted here as an appendix.

Back at Chatsworth, before the week was out, Andrew got a handwritten letter from Jack thanking us both for being present at 'the changing of the guard'. 'I was grateful for the kind letter from the Prime Minister,' he continued, 'I wish you success in your service with him and I hope very much that you and Debo can both come here soon again. Best, Jack.' When you think of the number of letters he had to write thanking his political supporters, to include us seemed incredible. Two weeks later Jack wrote to me suggesting that I accompany the Prime Minister (Uncle Harold) when he went to Washington in the spring to 'cement Anglo-American relations'. I was immensely flattered, but had things planned that I could not change and proposed a date later in the year, which seemed to suit him.

It was at their first meeting in March 1961 that Uncle Harold and Jack decided on David Ormsby Gore for the post of British Ambassador to Washington. David's sister, Katherine, was married to the Macmillans' only son, Maurice, and Uncle Harold had known David for years. David was duly appointed on 26 October 1961. The relationship between ambassador and president was a much closer one than usual and Jack and David met often informally. David was the link between Jack and Uncle Harold, who also struck up a close friendship, and Jack was soon referring to the Prime Minister as Uncle Harold like the rest of us. The friendship surprised some of their aides, but it seemed obvious that the much older, more experienced man, with his classical education and great intellect (who nevertheless always saw the joke), would make a good ally for the young President.

I went to Washington in December 1961 and stayed with David and Sissie in the embassy. The evening after my arrival I dined at the White House for the first time. There were Jack, two men friends of his and me. We sat in the gallery for drinks and when dinner was announced, being the only woman and a foreigner, I went without thinking to the open door. On the threshold Jack threw out his arm and said, 'No, not you. I go first, I'm Head of State.' 'Good heavens,' I said, 'so you are,' and we sat down to dinner.

The Washington round was hectic: lunches and dinners here and there, including enjoyable ones at our embassy. I dined one night with Joe and Susan Mary Alsop before a gala reception at the National Gallery of Art. Joe, a distinguished political journalist, was friends with all at the White House. Twenty people had sat down to dinner when the door opened and in walked the President, unexpected. Joe Alsop got a chair, sat him down and we went on as if nothing had happened. To please its director, Johnny Walker, who was a friend of mine, Jack agreed to make a quick visit to the National Gallery; he had never been there before. I went with him in his car and it was raining when we arrived. As Jack got out to shake hands with the welcoming party, he turned to me and whispered, 'They think I like art. I hate it.' One of our delegates to the United Nations was Lady Tweedsmuir. She found an unexpected opportunity to buttonhole the President on some (to her) pressing matter. 'Not now,' he replied, 'it's your turn tomorrow.' He had got rid of her, but in such a good-natured way that she could not take offence.

From Washington I flew to New York on the same day as Jack ('I go presidential, you go commercial,' he said, putting me in my place). He gathered up various friends and relations in New York to see that I was not left alone for long and they did his bidding, however inconvenient it must have been for them.

Jack added enormously to any entertainment. He was such good company, so funny and straightforward—a mixture of schoolboy and statesman, and you never knew which was coming next. He was the only politician I have ever known who could laugh at himself and did. He never spoke of the posts he had held—as in my experience English politicians always do, starting conversations with, 'When I was Home Secretary . . .' or 'When I was Parliamentary Under Secretary for Health . . .' so that your attention immediately wanders. Jack could say 'I don't know' (which our politicians never do) and in answer to questions he was direct, instead of beating round the bush. The atmosphere was refreshing after London officialdom. When the Shah of Persia was on a state visit to Washington, the press asked those present at Jack's welcoming speech what they thought of the visiting sovereign. One man, who was not a politician but a friend of Jack's, thought for a bit and said, 'Well, he's my kind of Shah.' It was this sort of remark that made Jack's White House so enjoyable and surprising. All the Kennedys had a trait of irreverence and fun. Some years ago when Eunice was in London, she fancied a ride in Rotten Row. Not caring that she had no riding clothes, she hired a horse and off she went in a full-length mink coat and sandals with two-inch heels over her nylon tights—an apparition—without a nod to convention.

In October 1962 Andrew and I went to America for the opening of an exhibition of Old Master drawings from Chatsworth at the Washington National Gallery. Again, we stayed at the embassy. Johnny Walker saw to it that we were fêted in the hospitable way of American museums. Francis Thompson, keeper of the collection at Chatsworth, was not well enough to travel so Tom Wragg, his deputy, oversaw the hanging of the drawings. The Cuban missile crisis was at its height and the world on the brink of nuclear war, but this did not deter the art lovers of Washington and its neighbourhood from flocking to the Gallery. Jackie Kennedy was not able to attend the official opening reception but came during the first day of the exhibition.

We dined at the White House on 21 October, the night before Jack's address to the nation when he told Americans about the situation in Cuba and called on Russia to remove the missiles or face retaliation. He was his usual self, showing no outward signs of the strain he must have felt. In the room where we met for drinks before dinner, photographs of the now infamous missiles (rhymed with 'thistles') were lying on a table and were being picked up and put down by the dinner guests as though they were holiday snaps. I suppose some of us did not realize how near to a world disaster we were; certainly the atmosphere in the White House was unchanged from the previous year—a tribute to steady nerves.

At one point Jack suggested, 'Why don't you call your sister in California?' He asked his switchboard to put me through and wandered off to do something more important. Decca and I talked for a bit but, brought up as we were not to use the telephone for long chats, Decca suddenly became aware of the cost of this long-distance call and said, 'Hen, are you on your own phone?' I had to admit I was not and we went on chatting. Over dinner Jack and I talked about his family's years in London before the war and about old friends. I described how Vice-President Johnson had tried to upstage Princess Margaret at the independence ceremonies in Jamaica and told Jack that Hugh Fraser had been at the head of our delegation. 'Not *our* Hugh Fraser?' he said. 'Yes, of course it was our Hugh Fraser,' I replied. He roared with laughter at the idea, just as Hugh would have laughed at Jack's elevated position.

On another evening in Crisis Week, Jack and I were sitting talking and laughing about the old days, about his sisters Kick and Eunice, and the girls he had met twenty-four years before. He asked about the home life of various politicians, Bobbety Salisbury, for instance. We moved on to war heroes and he wanted to know about Paddy Leigh Fermor and his capture of the German General on Crete in 1944. Suddenly he said, 'Tell me about Perceval.' 'Perceval?' I said. 'I don't know anything about him except that he was the only British Prime Minister to be assassinated.' Jack stayed quiet for a while and then we went back to chit-chat. I knew what he was thinking, and our conversation came back to me when I heard the news on 22 November 1963.

Towards the end of our stay, knowing that he would be interested, Jack found time to show Andrew the White House garden. The only event cancelled during the whole week was a dance that was to have been held at the White House on 22 October, the night of Jack's address to the nation. Uncle Harold and the President were in constant touch by telephone about the situation. It was evident that Jack was seeking advice from the old boy and the fact that they were by now such friends made a difference. As the crisis deepened so the night-time calls became more frequent. In the past, references to SEATO and NATO had often been followed by, 'How's DEBO?' then back to the serious stuff. This time there were no jokes.

At the end of that week of knife-edge diplomacy, Andrew went home on the Sunday night. On the Monday morning the President asked me to go for a last swim at the White House pool, where he swam every day to help his back. Again we talked of old times and especially of Kick. Afterwards I lunched with Eunice, Jean and Ethel before leaving for New York, where there was a festive atmosphere and everyone was breathing a sigh of relief.

When I got home, Jack sometimes telephoned with a question about Uncle Harold or another member of the government or just for a chat, usually in the early hours of the morning. It was a convenient time for him but I was dead asleep when the telephone rang at 3 a.m. 'Do you know it's the Fourth of July?' he began one of these calls. 'Is it?' I said, barely conscious. 'Have you got all your loved ones with you?' he asked. 'No,' I said. 'Why?' and so on. On another occasion he sounded exasperated. 'I was put through to a tavern called the Devonshire Arms. It was closed.' He was always full of Uncle Harold and ready for any stories I could tell about him.

On an official visit to Europe in June 1963, Jack was to have talks with Uncle Harold at Birch Grove in Sussex, and came to visit Kick's grave on his way. Kick was generally agreed to have been his favourite sister and the two had been very close. Edensor was full of Secret Service men during the days before the President's arrival and one of them asked me what sort of people lived in the village. At that moment, Francis Thompson emerged from his house on two sticks, looking as old as the hills. 'That's the sort of person,' I was able to say. The visit was kept secret and our local police on duty had no idea why they had been summoned to this backwater.

Air Force One took Jack to Waddington RAF base in Lincolnshire and a helicopter brought him on to Chatsworth, landing as near as possible to the churchyard. Andrew and I were there to meet him. He came down the steps, obviously suffering from the back pain that plagued him but was never mentioned. A temporary wooden bridge had been built over the ha-ha that divides the park from the churchyard; we went across it together and then left him on his own by Kick's grave.

When Jack joined us at the car, he said he would come to Chatsworth, which he had never seen. This was against the wishes of the Secret Service who said they could not ensure his security because it was open to the public. On the short drive to the house, Jack described the helicopter that had brought him. 'It's even got a bathroom,' he said proudly. 'A bathroom? What on earth for?' I said. 'You couldn't possibly need a bath on that short trip.' What he meant was that it had a lavatory. When we arrived at the house, we joined the public who were making their way up the stairs. They looked at Jack, looked back at each other and looked at him again in a classic double-take, astonished to see the President of the United States sharing their staircase.

Jim and Alvilde Lees-Milne were staying with us, as was Yehudi Menuhin (the latter surprised me by practising scales for four hours at a time, which I could hear coming from his bedroom. I thought he knew all that and would not have to bother). There was time for a quick cup of tea then back to the helicopter and its bathroom. Jack was late for his appointment with the Prime Minister and a headline in the newspapers read, 'MAC MADE TO WAIT'. The next day I was talking to an Edensor resident. 'Wasn't it exciting to see the President?' I said. 'I didn't think so,' came the reply, 'that helicopter blew my hens away and I haven't seen them since.'

Andrew and I were in London on 22 November 1963. I heard the news of Jack's assassination on the wireless and, like the rest of the world, could not believe it. Andrew had to make an after-dinner speech that night; he kept the engagement but wrote in his memoirs, 'Whatever I was saying was of no consequence since all our minds were elsewhere.' We went to the funeral, which was arranged in three days and was, not surprisingly, rather chaotic. We were offered a lift to Washington in the plane chartered for Prince Philip, who was representing the Queen. Also on board were the Prime Minister, Alec Douglas-Home, and the Leader of the Opposition, Harold Wilson. Just as at the Inauguration, Andrew and I were included as part of the Kennedy family. We were closer to the tragic events, therefore, than almost anyone else present—certainly closer than heads of state who had come from all over the world to attend. We were both aware, once again, of our privileged position among the late President's friends. I made notes immediately after the funeral and these, too, appear in an appendix to this book.

*   *   *

Over the years, various members of the Kennedy family came to visit Kick's grave. Bobby stayed with us at Edensor in 1948, shortly after her death. It was summer and he wore shorts and ankle socks; I had never seen the combination and thought Bobby Socks must have been named after him. I loved Bobby, his directness, his blue eyes fastening on the person he was talking to, his quick questions, fired as though from a gun, about old times in England or anything else that came into his head. Like Jack, he was a mixture of childlike lack of sophistication and tough political acumen and, like Jack, he was a schoolboy until you hit the steel.

When visiting Ireland in 1966, I saw the dire state of the finances of the Queen's Institute of District Nurses of Eire. It occurred to me that Bobby might consider a donation to a charity that gave such important service to the people of Ireland. I boldly wrote to him and got a series of comical letters back. 'Dear Debo,' he replied, 'I am at last working on your project . . . I am sorry I have delayed but I love you and I hope it is ~~still~~ mutual. Bobby.' There was a note in the margin pointing to the crossed-out 'still', which said, 'I thought this might be a rather unfair assumption.' He then more or less instructed the regional director of the United States Post Office, Sean Keating, who was about to retire, to hand over the proceeds of the retirement luncheon being given in his honour.

Sean Keating kindly agreed but wrote to Bobby that he had spent many sleepless nights since receiving a copy of my letter, and that if his patriotic ancestors knew that he was having anything to do with a project called the QUEEN'S Institute of District Nursing, they would turn into the 'whirling dervishes of their respective cemeteries'. He ended, 'With the devout prayer that God and my sainted ancestors will forgive me.'

I got another letter from Bobby. 'Good news!' it began:

Sean Keating who is going to raise all the money for your ~~damn~~ nurses is going to Ireland. He would like to go fishing at our family estate which is presently in your name. Could he? Would you let him? He will raise even more money.

You would love him although I don't know if you will even be in Ireland at the time of his visit. Obviously that would not be necessary. He just wants to fish + he says all the fish in Ireland are kept by the British + especially by the Devonshires.

Lots of Love,
Bobby

The correspondence went to and fro between Bobby, his secretary, Miss Novello, Sean Keating and me. The retirement luncheon raised over $10,000 and Bobby duly sent me a cheque, with a covering letter: 'Why the hell do you write Miss Novello & Sean Keating and not me? I like to receive letters from you. Love Bobby.'

When Bobby was assassinated in 1968, I could not go to the funeral but Andrew felt he should represent the family. Moucher thought it important for the Kennedys to know he was there, so on the train that carried the coffin to Washington after the Mass in New York, Andrew made his way down the carriages to take his place among other mourners waiting to have a few words with Rose Kennedy. He found her composure extraordinary. 'We talked of Bobby and Jack and of other members of the family,' he wrote in his memoirs.

She did not mention the actual assassination, but rather talked around it. When I felt my time was up I made my farewells and found Mrs Martin Luther King waiting to make her courtesy call. I have often thought about that afternoon, and I believe her amazing resilience in the face of the family tragedies was entirely a matter of her religious faith. No matter how shocking the events of this world that had overtaken her family, they were secondary to the expectations of the next.

Rose stayed at Chatsworth in July 1969. Andrew found her interesting to talk to and the time passed quickly, but not without a minor incident. At lunch she waved away the dish I had planned, saying, 'I'll have roast chicken.' There was nothing to be said but, 'I'm awfully sorry, Mrs Kennedy, but there isn't any.' For some reason, people often thought Chatsworth was like a hotel and could produce anything on demand. She wanted to go for a walk, but not in the way most of us would, to see something in the park or garden: for her it was a question of counting the steps the doctor had ordered and hardly looking up at what Chatsworth had to offer. Andrew took her to see Hardwick Hall and from there to catch a train from Chesterfield. They found themselves with half an hour to spare, so he walked her round the town which he knew well from his days as a parliamentary candidate. Rose's political antennae were sharpened and she became animated as he pointed out the various public buildings: town hall, school, hospital and the rest.

Teddy Kennedy came to Chatsworth more than once. The last time coincided with a visit from the Prince of Wales. They each planted a lime at the end of the avenue that borders the drive to the Golden Gates and marks the three hundredth anniversary of the creation of the Devonshire dukedom. Looking back, it is a strange quirk of fate that we should have had such a long connection with the Kennedys, who had such powerful political influence yet were visited and revisited by tragedy.

18

Public Life

The organizers of charities, both local and farther afield, often asked Andrew and me to open their money-raising events. As there were so many of these, we soon learned that it would be better to divide them between us. Where possible, I interested myself in charities close to home and was well aware that in the beginning I was invited because of whom I had married and not because of any merit of my own. People were used to female members of the Cavendish family being involved and I was simply following the tradition. Andrew had his own list, which stretched to Eastbourne and London. He was brilliant at public speaking: no matter what the subject or who the audience, he held them in the palm of his hand. Instead of finding a stuck-up fellow full of his own importance, they found themselves laughing at his self-deprecating words; the barriers came down and they sat back and enjoyed it.

One of the first charities I took on was the Children's Society and I soon found myself president of five different committees: Bakewell, Buxton, Chesterfield, Burton-on-Trent and Ashbourne, and a week was set aside for their AGMs. Then every church in the district seemed to be in trouble: the roof was leaking, the heating was broken, so was the organ (things do not change), or the Red Cross needed support. Events to raise money were ever in search of someone to open them and, as a result, Saturdays in summer and those leading up to Christmas were quickly booked up. The events were arranged months in advance, so you were pinned down if something thrilling turned up on the same day.

The local Women's Institute was a top priority. I inherited a love of the WI from Muv. She founded the Asthall and Swinbrook branch and gave talks on her three favourite subjects: Queen Victoria, Nelson and Bread. I was president of the Chatsworth WI for twenty-one years—a rule now stipulates that no one can be president for more than three, a much better plan. For those who do not know about the WI, it is to the country what the Townswomen's Guilds are to towns. Ten years ago it hit the headlines when delegates from rural England gathered in the Royal Albert Hall in London for their Annual Meeting and slow handclapped the speaker, who was none other than Prime Minister Tony Blair. He had broken one of the WI's basic rules, which is No Politics. He was not accustomed to such treatment, especially from women, but was up against it that day and his discomfiture showed.

The WI is a great teacher. Once a year, every officer has to stand and sum up the year's activities, which is a marvellous lesson for anyone frightened of talking in front of a crowd, however small and familiar. It certainly helped me. Granny Evie, who was founder and president of the Derbyshire branch of the Red Cross, used to get in a terrible state of nerves before opening a fête or bazaar in one of the neighbouring villages. This was in spite of the fact that the Red Cross devotees were delighted to see her; it was not like electioneering where you could be heckled and hustled about or be the target of a bad egg. For two days beforehand Granny Evie was fidgety and unhappy, and sometimes took to her bed. Once the ordeal was over, she was a different person. There was no way of helping her overcome her nervousness and she never grew out of it. It seemed to me extraordinary that the daughter of a Viceroy of India, brought up to public life, married to a man who had been Governor General of Canada, mother of seven, the chatelaine of four enormous houses in England and a castle in Ireland, who was Mistress of the Robes to Queen Mary for forty-three years, should nevertheless have been terrified of the platform and a friendly audience.

I did not realize that I would be just as nervous myself, and I did not have Granny Evie's experience of public life to fall back on. I knew I had to do it but, like her, I dreaded even the smallest event when I had to talk to an audience. The worst moment came after the flattering introduction, so well meant but which made me squirm and go pink with embarrassment. There would be a silence and then the fatal sentence, 'Now I will ask Lady Hartington to say a few words.' All eyes on me, just what Nanny said would never happen ('It's all right, darling, no one's going to look at *you*'). My mouth went dry and my legs felt like giving way.

Clutching my bit of paper, I began: 'Mr Mayor, Madam Mayoress, Chairman of the County Council', or whatever organization was represented, 'Thank you so much for inviting me . . .' then heard myself trotting out, 'Best of good causes', 'obvious hard work of the organizers', 'please spend' and other tired expressions, before sitting down with relief to listen to a fulsome speech of thanks by someone else on the platform. My voice sounded all the more ridiculous in front of an audience of Derbyshire folk, who have their own, more harmonious way of talking. I was made acutely aware of this when speaking too loudly one day to a friend in the garden at Chatsworth. I was stopped by a stranger. 'I've read about a 30s voice,' he said, 'but I've never heard it before. Please go on talking.' So I did and we were doubled up with laughter at 'lorst' and 'gorn' and other old-fashioned pronunciations.

One day I was thrown in the deep end. I was staying in Sussex with Kitty Mersey, who was secretary of her local WI. On the day of their meeting, the speaker failed. '*Please*,' said Kitty, 'you must talk to them. Tell them about Chatsworth.' No prep, no notes (something I had never before been without) and off I launched. I cannot say I enjoyed it and cannot believe the audience did either—in deepest Sussex they had never heard of Chatsworth—but it passed off all right and I realized for the first time that I could make people laugh. (It is easy when the audience laughs with you but it is out of your hands if they laugh at you.) When we got home, Kitty showed me the programme and the topic on which the real speaker was to have spoken: 'Ramblings of an Old Woman'. Exactly. The experience encouraged me and I dared to follow it up with after-dinner speeches to various agricultural organizations. The first, at the Oxford Farming Conference, was especially frightening as the guests were scientists, lecturers and heads of this and that.

I have given many talks since but always had to have the words in front of me and the nightmare of leaving my speech behind still haunts me. The nearest I ever got to disaster was to forget my specs; bad enough for me and maddening for the audience. Other hazards lurk. One evening I was to give a talk for charity to an audience that had paid what seemed to me vast sums to hear my twaddle. No sooner had I started than I realized the projector was not working. My talk about Chatsworth was useless without slides and while everyone excuses the odd upside-down picture, when the whole apparatus seized up I felt I was drowning. I sat and stared at the impatient rich people in the rows in front of me kicking the floor and feeling for their car keys, while one or two amateurs pushed and pulled at plugs—all to no avail. A few pictures eventually came through but it was no pleasure to anyone; the thread had been broken and could not be repaired. It was a miserable experience.

American audiences are indulgent. They are

interested in Chatsworth, both the house and the garden, and one year I boldly accepted an invitation to talk at the Metropolitan Museum of Art in New York. This was thanks to Jayne Wrightsman who knows more about the contents of museums worldwide than most professors and who, with her late husband, is one of the Met's munificent benefactors. The event was merciful in that I was not introduced; I just walked on to the stage alone, like Elvis, and started.

It was on this occasion that I realized an odd thing: the larger the audience, the less frightening it is. The lecture hall at the Met held some seven hundred people and to my astonishment it was sold out. A huge black space stuffed with faces is so anonymous that you can imagine there is no one there, but a drawing room with, say, twenty-five friends of the host, who have been told they must come whether they want to or not, is terrifying. This happened to me in San Francisco and, in spite of the audience's kindly good manners, I sensed at once that they were neither interested nor amused. But I had to battle on. I have found talking in public easier as I have got older, perhaps because I no longer care what I look like or whether my stockings are straight. But, oh, the apprenticeship is hard! I love the questions, some so deadly serious on a light-hearted subject; but they keep the audience awake. Recently I gave a talk about my childhood and someone asked me, 'Your sisters are buried at Swinbrook, are you going to join them there?' She did not add the word 'soon' but that is what she meant.

It seems that people now prefer showbiz to open their events. It has taken a long time but even the dimmest actor in the dimmest soap now draws a crowd. I saw the first signs of this many years ago when the chairman of a bazaar in north-east Derbyshire said in his introductory speech, 'We asked Mrs Dale of *Mrs Dale's Diary*, but there was to be a charge. We asked Dr Finlay of *Dr Finlay's Casebook* and he wanted a fee. So we had to ask the Duke of Devonshire.' One organizer said to me about showbiz, 'It's great when they come, but "charge and chuck" is the risk you take.' Apparently showbiz has no compunction in chucking (with the shining exceptions of Alan Bennett and Tom Stoppard who do what they promise). Luckily the formality of the old days is fast fading and events now open themselves: simpler for all concerned.

*   *   *

In 1972 the Royal Smithfield Club held its annual conference in Buxton and Andrew was invited to be the guest speaker. He already had an engagement that day and, knowing of my interest in food and farming, handed me their letter and suggested I go in his place. It was the beginning of my happy association with that triumvirate of farmers, butchers and makers of agricultural machinery. I visited their Show and was hooked, and for many years Earls Court was my destination for four days in late November and early December. On my first visit I saw a tractor with a price tag of £15,000, which made my jaw drop. Today my jaw would fall off should I see the price tag on one of its vast successors.

The Carcase Hall was a carnivore's dream, with

expert butchers on hand to point out the excellence of the prizewinners. To the uninitiated the names of some of the classes were puzzling: 'Carcase Cattle Alive' (to which they could have added 'But Not for Long') and 'Combined Live/Dead Butchers' Sheep'. The pig section showed the cream of the porcine world. One pen had two lively prime baconers with a side of bacon displayed overhead and a notice that read, 'Litter Mate on the Hook'. (It was just as well those pigs could not read.) As for sheep, a girl was spotted coming out of the nearby tube station wearing a shaggy sheepskin coat with a red splodge on the lower back—a sure sign that the original owner of the skin had received the close attentions of a ram in his raddle harness. The townee wearer was oblivious of the reason for the merriment of the group of farmers following her.

I was president of the Royal Smithfield Show from 1972 to 1974 and president of the Royal Smithfield Club in 1975. The Queen Mother honoured the Show with her presence and it was my good fortune to look after her during the more private moments of her day-long visits. The Show was just up her street and she was as at home with the butchers and stockmen as they were with her. I followed in her wake as she toured the stands, and I watched the amazing effect her charm had on all those to whom she talked or happened to meet on her path.

Afterwards, we were shepherded by the exhibition manager—Gerry Kunz, son of Charlie Kunz, the famous dance pianist of my youth—to a room called G9 (no relation of G8 or G20 and I never discovered where rooms G1–8 were). G9 had what are described as 'facilities' where we were meant to 'tidy'. It also had a cupboard with every alcoholic drink under the sun and we were able to settle down and chat, oblivious of Gerry and the other officials waiting outside to take us to lunch. During one of these chats, the Queen Mother told me of her pre-war visits to Chatsworth when Granny Evie was in charge, and how on her last visit, on the eve of the Abdication, she and the Duke of York had been acutely aware of the profound change about to take place in their lives. The association with this troubled time went so deep that, in spite of many invitations, she never came to stay at Chatsworth with us.

G9's drinks cupboard was on the floor, so it was hands and knees for me to find the necessary Dubonnet and gin. I soon learned the drill, kneeling again to pour a second helping—in the wrong proportions no doubt, but with no complaint from the consumer. I loved those moments and the memories. At lunch the Queen Mother asked the assembled company, 'What has happened to mutton? We always get lamb, but never mutton.' As a result, one of the farmers kept on some wether lambs for a second year, and twelve months later we fell on the mutton, caper sauce and all. The Queen Mother was president of the Royal Smithfield Show in 1983 and again in 1987–2001. Tradition has it that one who has held this office remains a vice-president for life and wears a large porcelain brooch to proclaim this. The Queen Mother, who had never been 'vice' of anything, was a little surprised at the wording on the brooch she was expected to wear. She looked at me quizzically, head on one side, and said, 'Shall

I put it on?'

*   *   *

My eight-year association with Tarmac, the international building conglomerate, came about by chance. Eric Pountain, chief executive of John McLean & Sons, a building firm based in Wolverhampton, had a friend who bred Haflingers, the small horses that I too bred. Eric gave a cup to be presented at the Haflinger Breed Show and delivered it to the Chatsworth home farm one day when I happened to be there. We had a chat and off he went to a more important engagement. Soon after this, he invited me to join the board of McLean. Perhaps he asked me because I was a woman (it was starting to be the thing to do to have a female on the board) or perhaps because my name was vaguely known in the Midlands. I did not know what to expect and went to the first meeting full of trepidation (Eric's people must have been equally surprised at my arrival). I kept quiet but soon learned the business language of the house builder: land bank, gearing, leverage, etc. McLean was doing well at the time and the company was looking forward with confidence to a great future.

In 1974 McLean was taken over by Tarmac; a shrewd acquisition as McLean was pounding ahead. Various things had gone wrong at the top of Tarmac and a new chief executive was required. Eric was the outstanding man and obvious choice. Again, a woman was required on the board and, as I had been a few years with McLean, I got promotion and became a non-executive director of

Tarmac plc in 1984. This led to journeys to South Africa and America with Eric and Nicholas Henderson, a fellow non-executive director. Nicko was a lucky appointment for many reasons, perhaps the chief one being that he could speak French, an accomplishment not shared by most of the top brass of the construction industry. The fact that he had been our Ambassador in the United States also helped and we were welcomed wherever we went.

Tarmac expanded into ten US States and our jaunts to America, including crossing the Atlantic on Concorde, were part of our education. One expedition stands out in my memory. Nicko and I were in Virginia and were sent in a helicopter to look at the quarries along the James River. We wanted to dip down to see the famous eighteenth-century plantation houses on this stretch of water; they have been so often written about and photographed and we were curious to see them in reality. The pilot, however, stuck to his instructions to show us the quarries and we managed only tantalizing glimpses of the houses. All the while the helicopter door kept flying open, which did not seem to matter and no one took any notice.

Nicko was chairman of the Channel Tunnel Group in 1985–6 and was instrumental in the run-up to, and making of, the tunnel. The work was done by a consortium of British construction companies, including Tarmac, in conjunction with their French counterparts—with whom Nicko was able to talk with the familiar ease of one who has lived in France. We went with the other directors on an exciting expedition under the sea when our side was about to meet the French tunnellers. The machines were like something out of a giant's toy box and I still have—given to me as a memento of the day—one of the claws that played its part in opening up this underground highway to the Continent.

In the late 1980s Tarmac gave a dinner in a private room at the Connaught Hotel where Andrew and I found ourselves in the company of princes of industry. Also present was Denis Thatcher and I sat next to him. When the Chairman tapped his glass and asked all present for their views on the political situation, two memorable things took place: Andrew predicted the future danger of escalating Muslim extremism, showing, once again, how he grasped the world situation before many others did. When it came to Denis Thatcher's turn to speak, I turned towards my neighbour to find that he had slid down in his chair and that his chin was almost on the table. Eric had the tact to pass quickly to another guest.

*   *   *

One day in 1988 I got a letter from the three directors of the auction house Bonhams, Nick Bonham, Christopher Elwes and Paul Whitfield, inviting me to go and see them. The Bonham salerooms in Montpelier Street were well known to me from Rutland Gate days when we passed them every time we walked through the Hole in the Wall to Brompton Road (often ending up at 'Wicked Old Harrod'). I had haunted their salerooms in the early 1980s looking for portraits of bulls to hang in the Devonshire Arms Hotel at Bolton Abbey and in the wild hope of finding a likeness of 'The

Craven Heifer', a vast creature for whom the doors of her shed at Bolton had had to be widened.

Intrigued by Bonhams' invitation, I went to see them. After polite exchanges, I settled into my chair and they suggested I join the board. 'That is very nice of you,' I said, 'but do you realize I am very old?' 'Oh yes,' they said. 'We know you're very old, but we are very young and it will do quite well.' So I joined and looked forward with pleasure to the prospect of learning about another new world, based on an old family business in which the Bonham family was still represented. I stayed with the company till 1995 when, having done nothing for them, I thought I should make way for someone more spry.

In the same year that I joined Bonhams, I received a letter from Dr Steve Dowbiggin, principal of Capel Manor College in Enfield, inviting me to be patron. I was already too much occupied, but the idea of a College within the boundary of the M25, which taught all aspects of gardening, was too attractive to dismiss out of hand. Besides which Dr Dowbiggin's writing paper was decorated with a drawing of a fritillary growing up one side. So I accepted. It has been fascinating to watch the College develop over the years from 400 students based in an eighteenth-century manor house, to its present position in the world of horticulture with 2,600 students and five satellites in and around London.

The College owes its success to Steve (a man who talks you into doing just what he wants) and his brilliant heads of department who have been with him for many years. People who live in the city have an irrepressible need to get closer to the earth, to learn about it and dirty their hands in the process. The only Good Thing I did for Capel Manor was to introduce Steve to Andrew Parker Bowles. Andrew's family, which includes E. A. Bowles, the famous gardening writer, has many connections with Enfield. Forty Hall, where Capel Manor is planting London's first commercial vineyard, belonged to Andrew's family for many years. He has done more for the College than I ever did.

We had some memorable days with various distinguished visitors. Mrs Thatcher came when she was Prime Minister. Gardening is not her chief interest but she did the rounds of the show gardens and the classrooms, all in a day's work. What made her visit unforgettable was the Force 9 gale that was blowing. I soon looked like the Wild Woman of the West, hair all over the place, as did the other women in the party. But not a hair on the PM's head moved. I was so interested in this phenomenon I could not pay attention to anything else. When Mrs Thatcher left, as tidy as when she arrived, I gave her half a dozen of my best dark brown Welsummer eggs as a thank-you. She looked rather surprised and I wondered if she threw them out of the car window (before it was against the law to scatter unwanted eggs on the road).

In 1993 the Prince of Wales, who chairs the committee responsible for the Royal Collection, invited me to join it. A more fascinating 'job' cannot be imagined. The range of what Sybil Cholmondeley, chatelaine of Houghton Hall, called 'Things' that the committee look after is unequalled in the world, and the dedicated experts involved in the care of them are specialists in a class of their own. It was my good fortune to be a trustee for six years. One of the first projects the committee addressed was the extension to the Queen's Gallery at Buckingham Palace, and I was present at the meetings which decided what the building should look like and which architect should be appointed. It was no easy task to adapt an old building, already fully occupied, to one that could be used for temporary exhibitions of all kinds, but the difficulties were somehow resolved and the new Queen's Gallery feels as if it has always been there. (This was a criterion we tried to follow at Chatsworth when converting beautiful old buildings to a purpose different from that for which they were built.)

Another subject for discussion at meetings was the countless requests from all over the world for loans of works of art. At other times an object—a plate, a knife and fork, or even a chair from a set— that had escaped from one or other of the royal houses appeared in the saleroom. It was the committee's task to decide on their importance and whether to bid for them to gather them back into the Collection.

A complete inventory of everything not personally owned by the Monarch—and therefore belonging to the Royal Collection—was being undertaken and this apparently endless task was like Lewis Carroll's seven maids with seven mops sweeping sand from the seashore. The Collection does not stand still. Some departments, such as photography, were added to almost daily, as were presents from heads of state to the royal family. By the end of 2008, a total of 639,908 items had been inventoried and this database must have made the work of Sir Hugh Roberts, director of the Collection, and others in charge of the various departments more manageable.

Only on rare occasions did Andrew and I attend public events together. Most of these were in the early 1950s when Andrew was Mayor of Buxton, the spa town in the Peak District of Derbyshire. It was an office his father had held in 1920, the year Andrew was born, and 'Buxton' was added to his Christian names. In the early 1950s the popularity of the spa was declining, but Buxton was an up-and-coming conference town with many hotels from the days when an endless supply of warm water made it a popular destination. (Mary, Queen of Scots benefited from the springs during her captivity at Chatsworth, probably the only time she was warm in the cruel climate of north Derbyshire.)

Food and petrol were still rationed in 1952 and a proper regard for the way public money was spent made the fare served at the mayor's welcoming dinners rather odd. We and our visitors all dressed in our best: white tie for Andrew, full evening dress with long white gloves for me. I grabbed anything that shone to pin on before I left home to drive the seventeen twisty miles to the Pavilion Gardens where many of the dinners were held. The first reception that Andrew gave as mayor was for three hundred commercial travellers. The main course at dinner was sausage rolls, followed by chocolate biscuits for pudding and coffee with the milk already in it—all handed round with appropriate formality. The three hundred commercial travellers, and the three hundred hairdressers we entertained the next night, had to eat this menu only once. We soon grew accustomed to it.

At these public events Andrew said that he often heard men say, 'That was before my little do.' He soon learned that this enigmatic statement referred either to a minor heart attack or to some charitable event that the fellow had organized (usually the former). It was this sort of remark that lightened what were sometimes dim occasions. On the whole we enjoyed our more than fifty years of public life. It was the people we met who made the job so intriguing and it gave us an insight into lives and organizations that we would otherwise never have known. Even when faced with a seemingly dull evening, there were always one or two people who made it enjoyable and reminded me of my luck at being present.

19

Orphan

After the war, when Farve went to live at Redesdale Cottage with Margaret Wright (now married to a Mr Dance), we had little contact with him. If we rang him, Margaret answered and we knew she would be standing over him while he talked, so we seldom telephoned. Failing eyesight had made it difficult for him to write. My letters to him do not survive but a reminder from the distant past turned up in the back of a drawer not long ago. It was one of Farve's stiff, top-quality blue envelopes, the sort that cuts your thumb when you rip it open. On it is written, 'Thorn removed from the foot of Stubby's dog.' He does not say which dog, but he understood the prime importance of such a thing to me.

Except for Decca, we all occasionally went to see him at Redesdale. On one of my last visits I took Kitty Mersey, who had been longing to meet him. We sat in his room, surrounded by metal filing cabinets ('mechanically sound, Stubby') and other purely functional furniture, the opposite of what Muv would have chosen. Unopened letters and magazines lay in piles around us. He was old and obviously ill, his one lung still battling with a continuous onslaught of gaspers. The classic features were still there but diminished, and 'my good dentures' were too big for the rest of his face. He was the ghost of what he had once been and had little interest left in life. Kitty said, 'You're not at all what I expected—a fierce person who might not have let me in.' 'Lady Mersey,' he replied sadly, 'I've no savagery left in me.'

Muv, Diana and I went to see him for his eightieth birthday and stayed at the Redesdale Arms (the inn with a sign 'Last Pub in England' on one side and 'First Pub in England' on the other). Diana wrote in her memoirs: 'I shall never forget the expression on Farve's face when Muv appeared at his bedside, and his smile of pure delight.' It was a comfort to me that my parents' last sight of each other seemed to turn back the years to how I remembered them as a child. Farve died four days later, on 17 March 1958. He was cremated and his ashes buried in Swinbrook churchyard. I could hardly believe my eyes when a little box was produced with all that was left of him; his beauty,

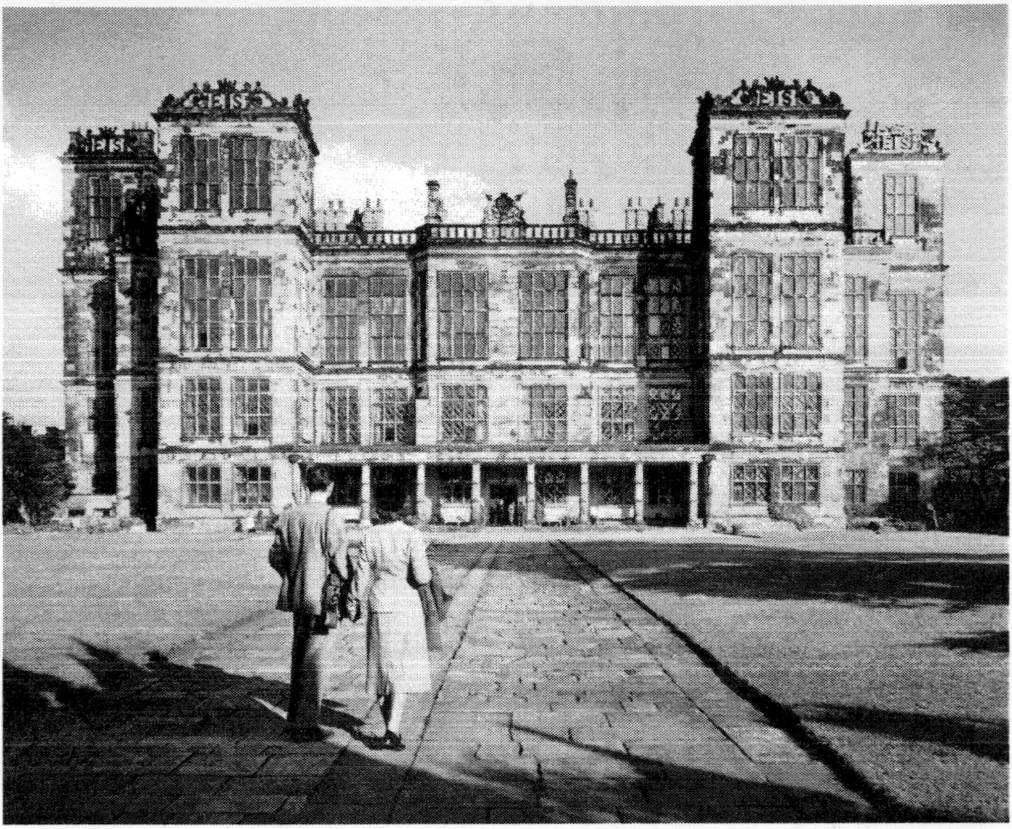

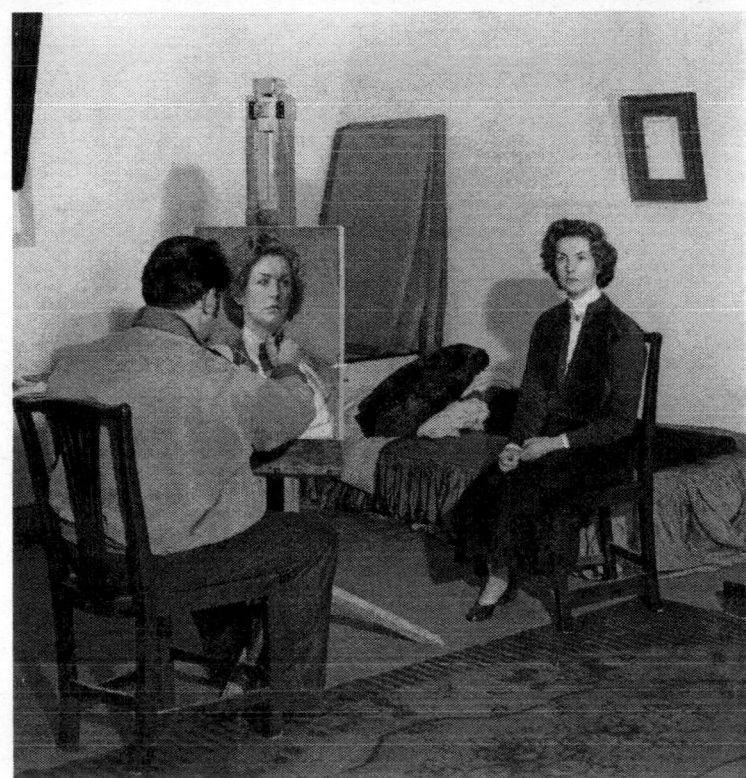

Above:
Hardwick Hall

Right: Sitting
for Pietro
Annigoni, 1954

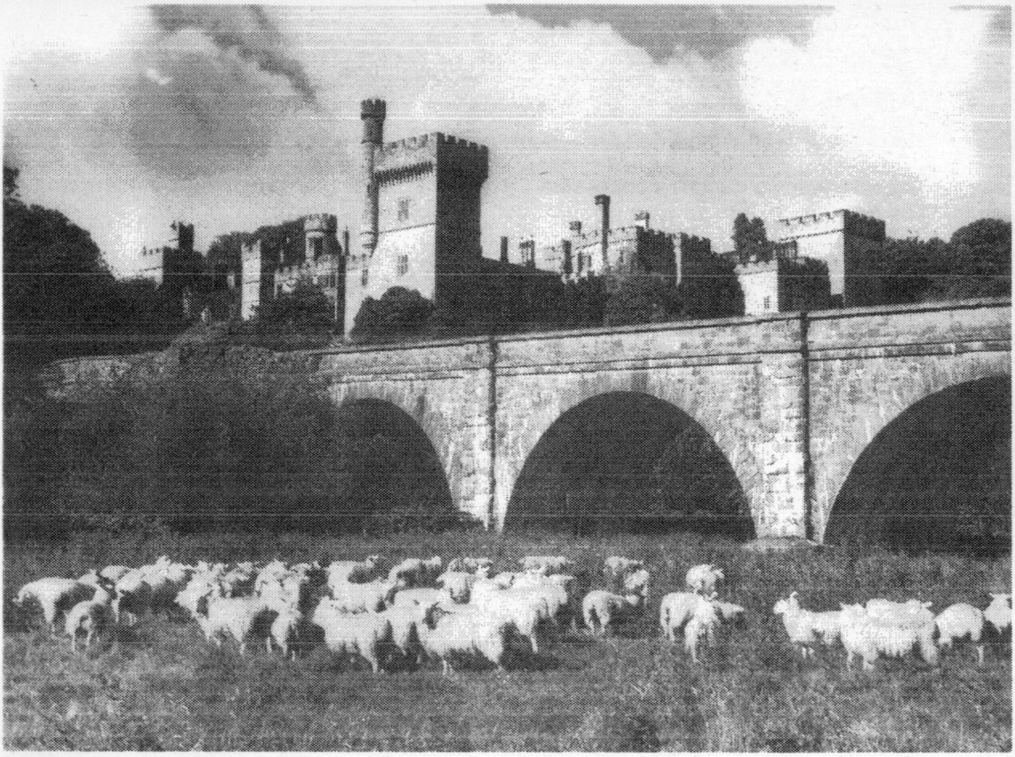

Lismore Castle

With Royal Tan, winner of the 1954 Grand National

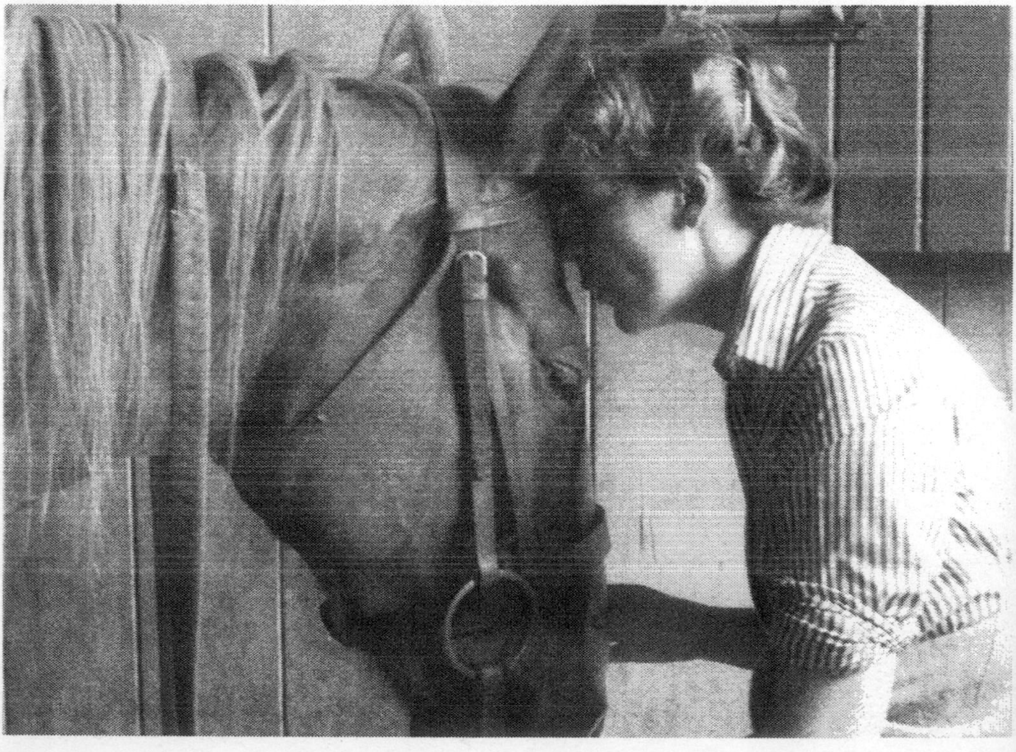

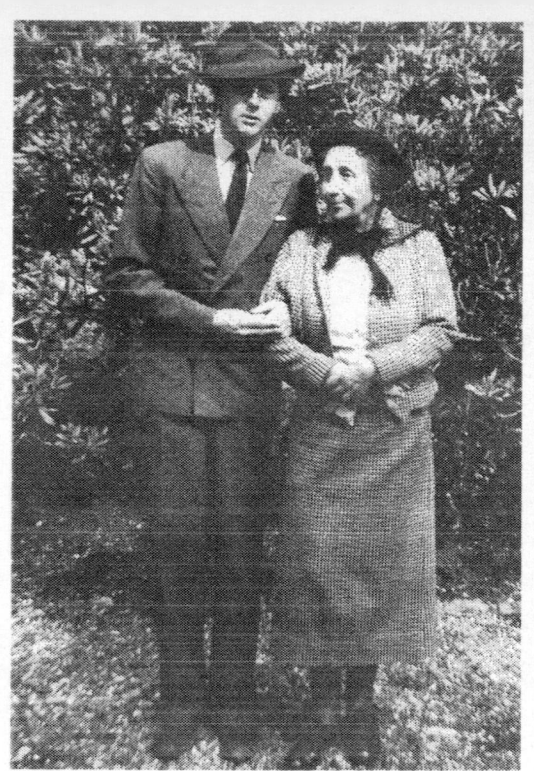

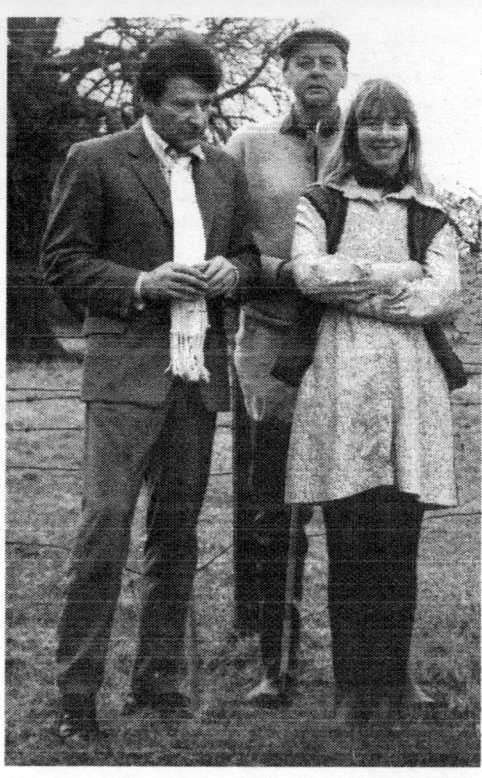

Andrew and Violet
Hammersley. Lismore, *c*.1950

Lucian Freud, Andrew, Penny
Cuthbertson. Careysville,
1972

Robert Kee and Patrick Leigh Fermor. Lismore, 1960

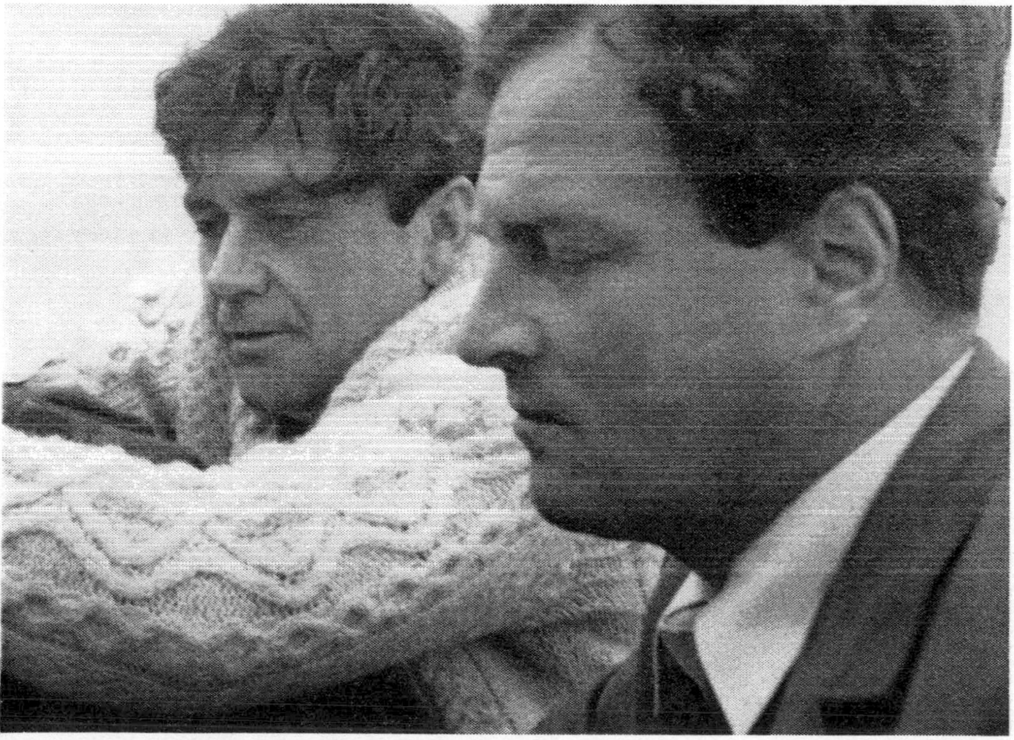

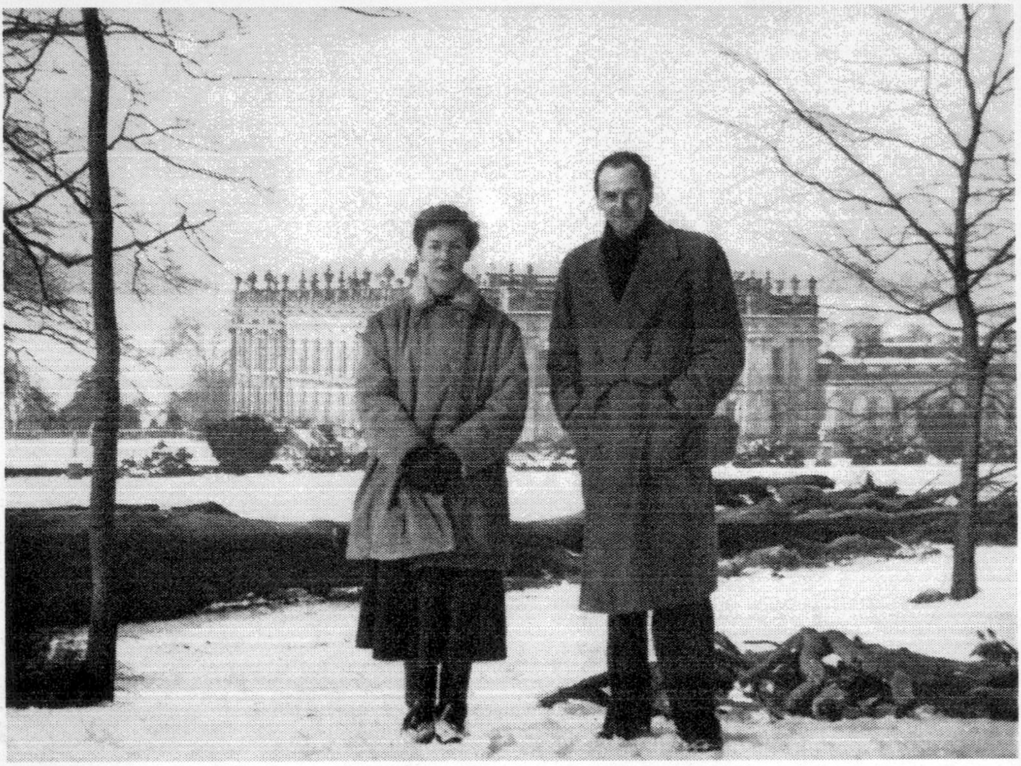

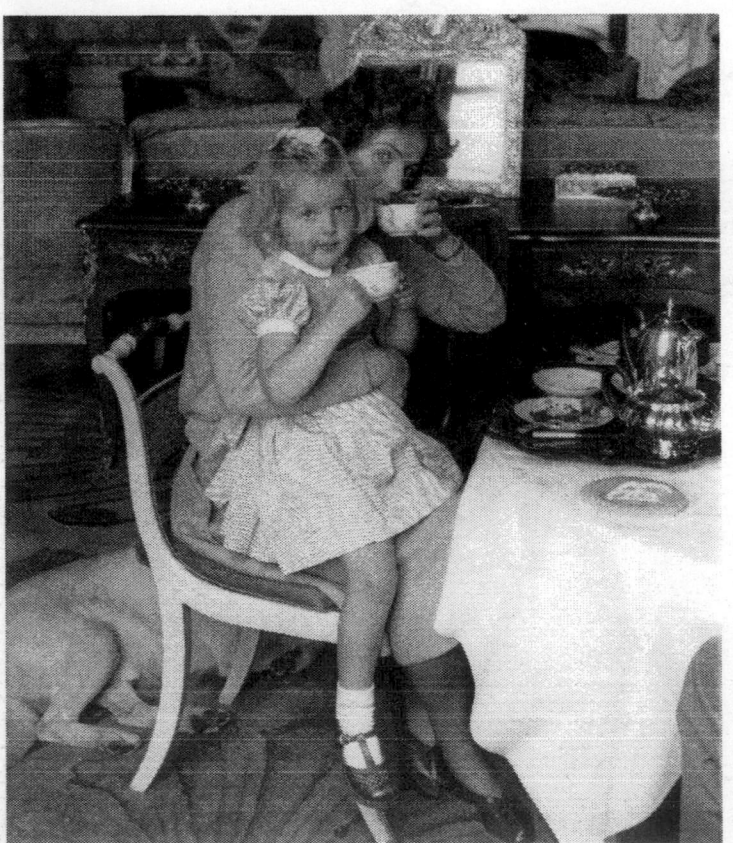

Above: With Andrew in the garden at Chatsworth

Left: With Sophy in the yellow drawing room. Chatsworth, 1960

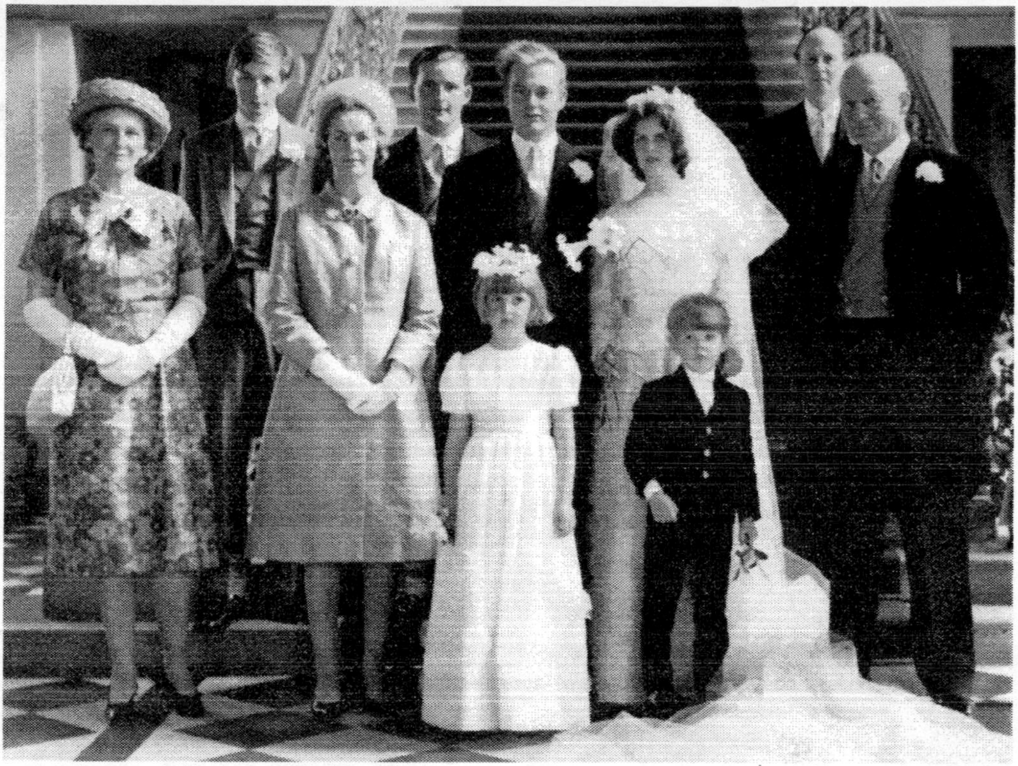

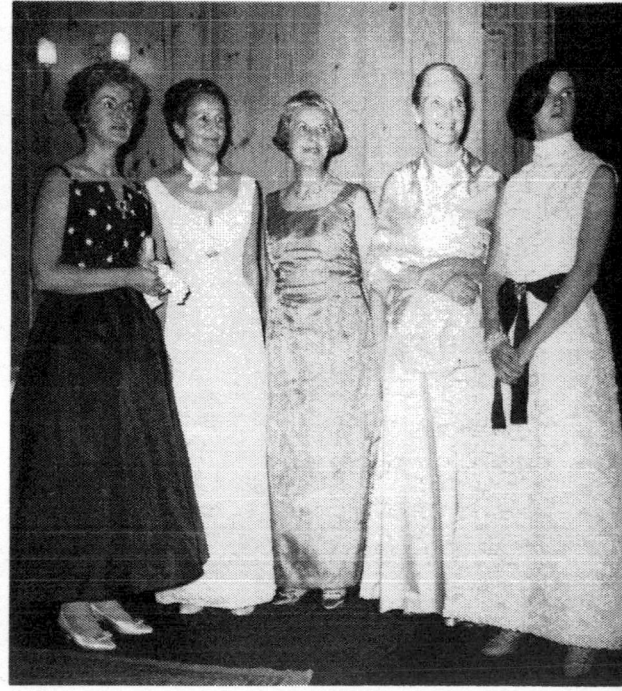

Emma's wedding to Toby Tennant. Chatsworth, 1963 (*l. to r.*) Mary Devonshire, Stoker, DD, David Skailes, Sophy, Toby, Emma, Matthew Yorke, Andrew, Christopher Glenconner

With Cecil Beaton, 1969

At Stoker's wedding, 1967 (*l. to r.*) DD, Nancy, Pamela, Diana, Emma

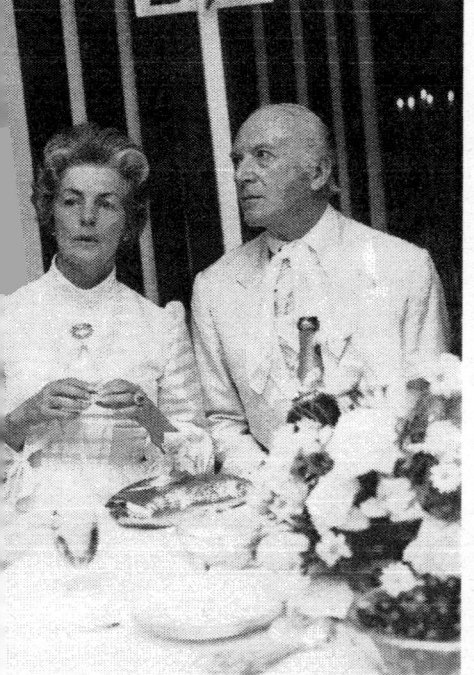

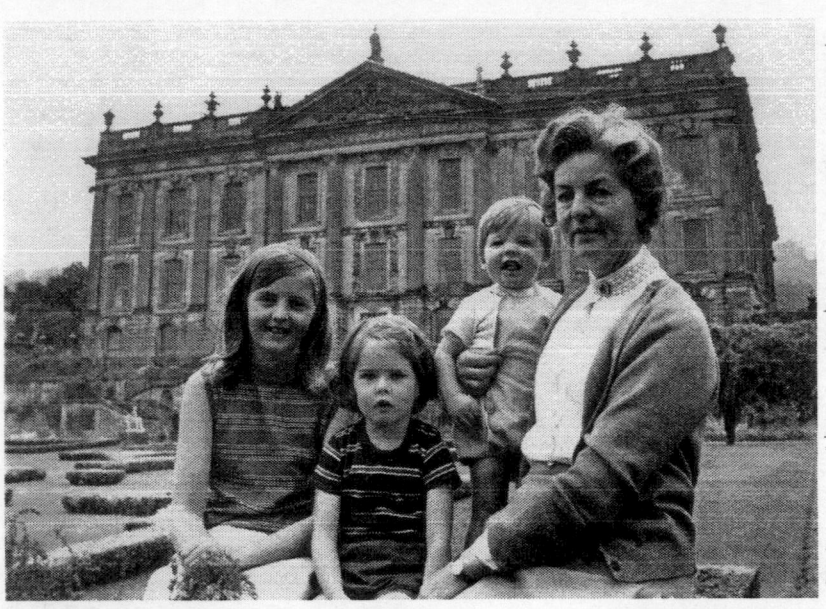

Left: In the west garden with Sophy (*left*) and grandchildren Isabel and Eddie Tennant, 1968. *By kind permission of Ron Duggins*

Below: My bedroom at Chatsworth. *By kind permission of Simon Upton*

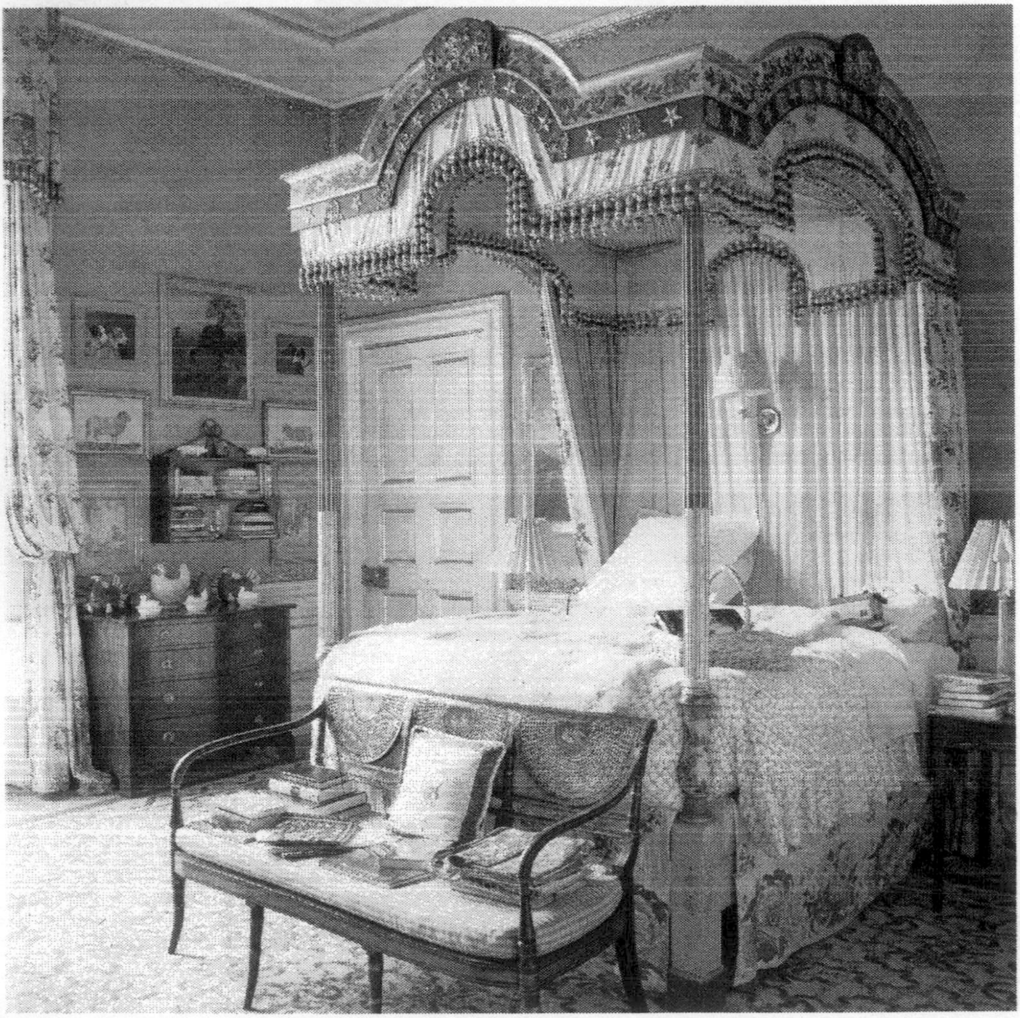

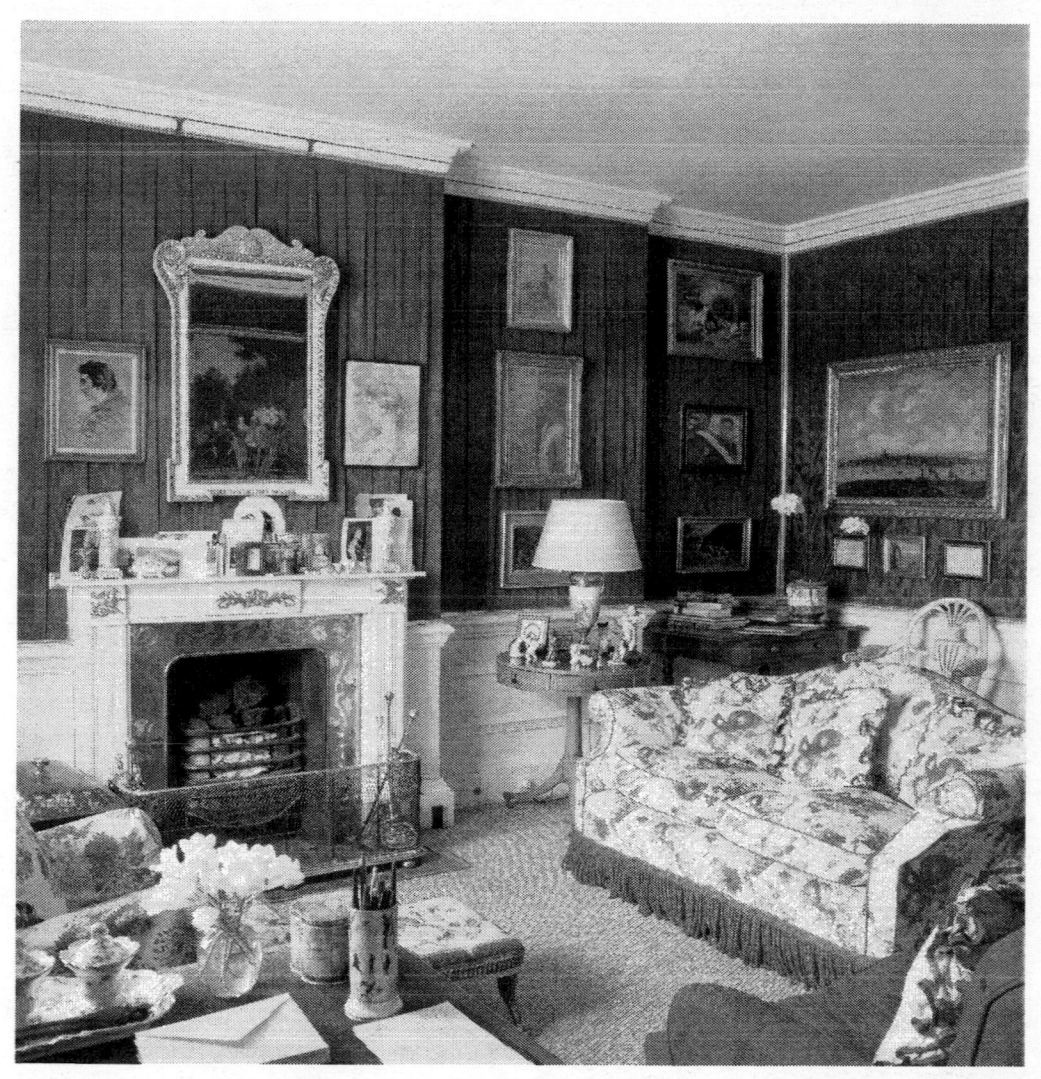

My sitting room at Chatsworth. *By kind permission of Simon Upton*

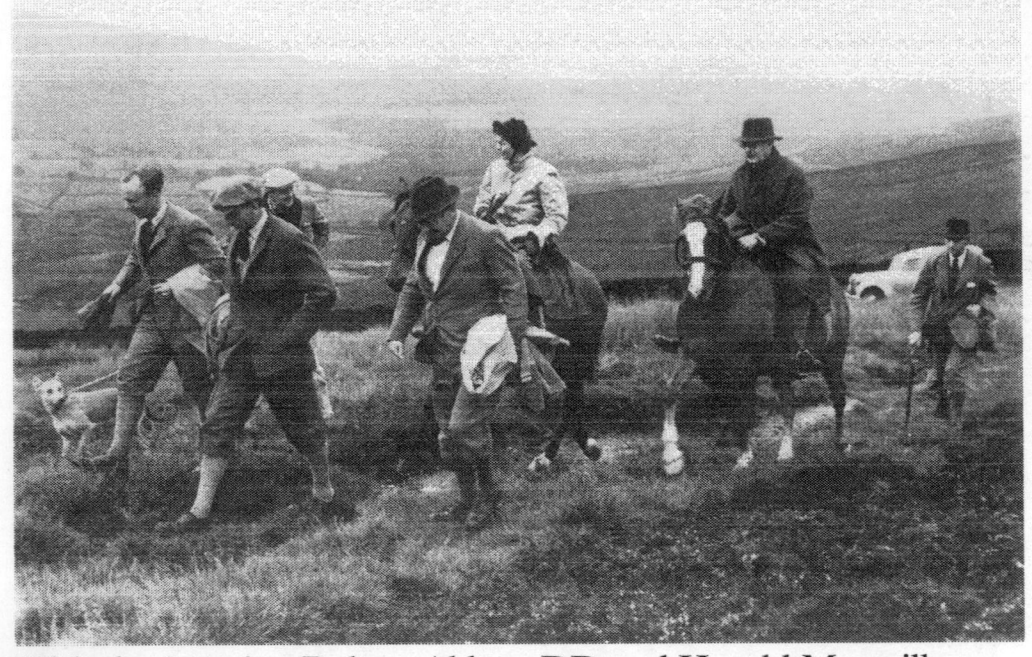

With the 'guns' at Bolton Abbey. DD and Harold Macmillan mounted, early 1960s

Shooting at Chatsworth, 1960. *By kind permission of Snowdon*

With Stoker at the Game Fair. Chatsworth, 1966

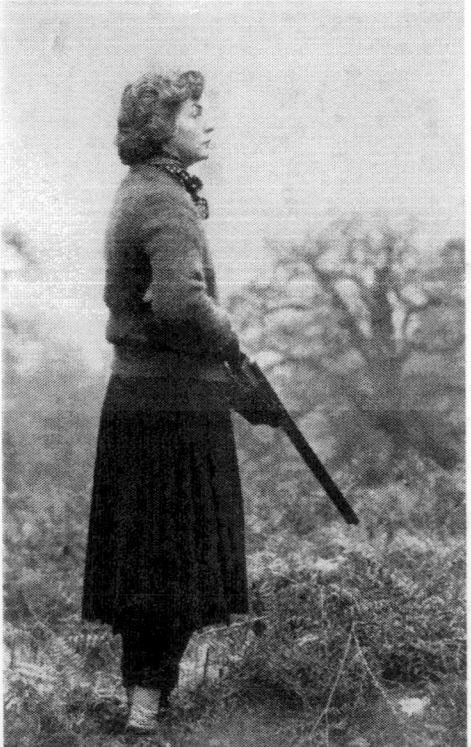

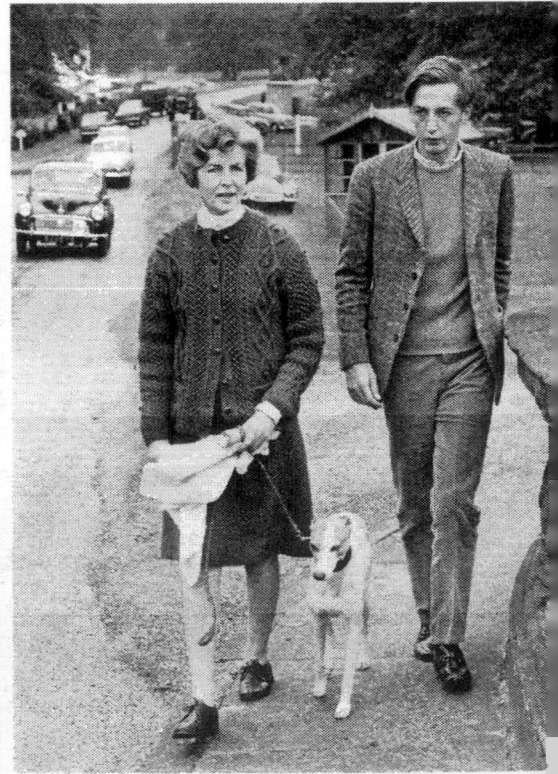

funniness, charm and fury all gone for good, and with it my childhood.

In contrast to Farve's, Muv's last years were spent surrounded by loving family and friends. She lived mostly in London and spent the summer months on Inch Kenneth, where the rigours of island life never seemed too much for her. The complications of transport were exemplified by the cows. Getting them to the bull to produce a calf (and hence some milk) is worth recording. There was a bull at Gribun, on Mull, and at the first sign of a cow being in season, a rope was put round her head and she was led to the jetty at high tide. The dinghy awaited her, oars at the ready, not as a passenger but to tow her. She was pushed into the deep water with an almighty shove and across the channel to Mull they went, the cow swimming behind with no difficulty. The sea had to be calm, of course, which added another factor to this tricky procedure. With luck, all went well at the first service but should she 'turn' at her next heat, the process had to be repeated or there would be no calf—and no milk.

Things got easier when Muv took goats to Inch Kenneth, pedigree British Saanens—quiet white creatures which produce a quantity of milk and are a delight to look after. A long-awaited kid was born. I telephoned Muv to ask whether it was a billy or a nanny. 'Well, darling,' she said, 'I'm afraid it's neither one thing nor another,' her way of saying that it was a hermaphrodite. The goats suited Muv and the island, being smaller, friendlier and easier to deal with than cows.

In old age Muv developed Parkinson's disease. She was stoical and saw the ridiculous side of her uncontrolled movements. When playing Scrabble, which she loved, her shaking hand made the placing of letters uncertain so with her right hand she used to seize her left, which was grasping the air and maddening her, and say, 'Stop it,' half laughing.

Although she was not a classical musician as Tom had been, the piano had always been important to her but now she could no longer control her fingers on the keyboard. Before the disease struck, she used to sing and play popular songs, and was amused by the liberties taken with some of the rhymes: 'I'm bidin' my time/That's the kinda guy I'm'. She loved jazzed-up versions of the classics such as Mendelssohn's 'Spring Song Swung' and Handel's 'Water Music' (renamed 'Mind the Handel's Hot'). *The Daily Express Community Song Book* provided old songs from the Boer War, and classics from the First World War such as 'Keep the Home Fires Burning'. The Irish revolutionary song, 'The Wearing of the Green', was a favourite, as were the inimitable 1930s songs 'Mean to Me', 'Miss Otis Regrets', and 'Goodnight Sweetheart'—so well remembered from Café de Paris days. After the war Muv sometimes used to sing Irving Berlin's sad song, 'Say It Isn't So', and I often wondered if she was thinking of herself when that one came along.

Muv and I were talking one day about old age with Tony Lambton. Knowing that she would not mind, Tony asked her how old she was. 'Nineteen,' she said. 'No, sorry, seventy-three.' I loved the idea of her being forever nineteen inside her ageing body. (She always said that the body is just an old sack—it does not matter what happens to it after death, and she could never understand why people made such a fuss about where and how they were buried.) 'So what's it like being old?' Tony pressed her. Muv thought for a minute and said, 'You aren't followed in the street any more and it's no fun trying on a hat.' Being followed in the street in her day was considered normal, though what outcome the poor followers hoped for I do not know. Perhaps they just appreciated beauty and wanted to see more of it.

*   *   *

The first months of 1963 were some of the coldest for years and frosts kept the ground iron-hard long after there should have been signs of spring. The park at Chatsworth was white with snow and the rabbits were dying of starvation. (Diddy said their corpses were like empty knitting bags.) The weather was bad, if not worse, in Scotland, but Muv travelled as usual to Inch Kenneth in early May. A few weeks beforehand, Nancy had accompanied her to the wedding of our cousin Angus Ogilvy to Princess Alexandra and said how wonderful Muv had looked, 'Got up in black velvet, lace and diamonds . . . the most elegant person there by far.' Coming from Nancy this was extraordinary praise.

Muv was delighted to be back on the island but soon after arriving she collapsed and her daughters were sent for. Nancy, Pam, Diana and I got there as soon as we could but the journey to the Inner Hebrides was never straightforward and the various waits and loss of connections were even more frustrating than usual because of the urgency and the uncertainty of what we would find. Decca was in California. As always in a crisis, my good Old Hen wanted to come, but the journey from San Francisco would have taken at least two days and as the doctor thought Muv might die at any moment, it was likely she would arrive too late.

The cold was bitter, even for the hardy Black Face sheep. There was not a blade of grass for them to eat and dead ewes and their newborn lambs lay beside the road from Salen to Gribun—a pitiful sight. We found Muv in bed and weak. She could talk, but eating and drinking were painfully slow because the muscles in her throat had all but given up. She was pleased to see us and knew why we had come: 'Of course I know why you're here,' she said, 'I'm dying.'

The next two weeks were all alike; she slept most of the time but had some hours of wakefulness, sometimes in extreme discomfort when she was beset by what she called her 'horrors' and was unable to lie still. It was awful to watch and it brought home to me how it is often as difficult to die as it is to be born. There was little we could do to help but it was a comfort to her that we were there. We got a routine going. Pam did the cooking while Nancy, Diana and I sat with Muv. We took it in turns to be with her in the night when she wanted a hand to hold. Every now and again she made us laugh and kept saying how she would be loving it all if she were well. 'Somewhere you'll find my ridiculous will,' she said, 'do change it if you want.' We said we would like to but feared we would go to prison if we did. 'Oh, so you will,' she said and relapsed into sleep. The two young and cheerful nurses from the mainland made the whole difference; not only was their presence a comfort, they could explain to us what was happening.

For the fortnight, while Muv's life drew to an end, we had the intense pleasure of being all four sisters together for the first time since I was a child. It was an unexpected bonus of those sad days and it was never to happen again. Of course we laughed and went back to the old jokes and teases. Nancy complained that her clothes were dirty. 'I'm going to make Woman teach me to wash,' she said, 'and I'll stand and look on while she does.' It worked like a charm. We all knew what the other was thinking and (like my old Collie dog) knew what the other was going to say before she said it. I wondered how anyone could die without at least four daughters at their bedside.

It was only a month from the summer solstice and daylight came early. After one of my turns for sitting with Muv, I went upstairs to bed to hear the crash of the dawn chorus and wondered what on earth the birds were thinking of in this freezing weather. The song of the larks was dominant and when I hear a lark now it takes me straight back to the stairs at Inch Kenneth.

We kept a coal fire going in Muv's bedroom night and day, and finally the coal ran out. It was delivered every two years and it was months before the next load was due. (It used to arrive on a coal boat and was tipped on to the beach at high tide, shovelled into wheelbarrows as quickly as possible and pushed to the coal shed before it could be claimed by the sea.) We took it in turns to scour the beaches at low tide for driftwood. Our eyes soon grew accustomed to picking out the battered white wood from the rocks and stones, and we carried it home in triumph. Sometimes the white object turned out to be the bone of some unfortunate cow that had toppled over the cliff in search of something to eat, and we were disappointed as it was no good on the fire. Soon our food began to run out. At last Diana was able to cross to Mull and drive to Tobermory with a long list of groceries. She returned victoriously some hours later carrying a ham on her head.

No one knew how long our vigil would last. The outside world was so far away it did not exist; only frequent telegrams to and from Decca brought us down to earth. I felt for her being so far away. Over the years her attitude to Muv had changed, as her reactions in those final days of telegrams and letters showed. After Muv's death, she wrote to Nancy that having loathed Muv when she was growing up, she then became 'immensely fond of her, really rather adored her'. She also loved Inch Kenneth, which had been hers since 1959. (After Farve's death, she had bought out Pam's, Diana's and my shares in it, and Nancy had made her a gift of hers.) Decca's love for the island pleased Muv greatly and it was a bond between them.

Three times during those days we thought Muv had gone, but each time she rallied. On one occasion her voice strengthened and she appeared to have a vision: she spoke of bright lights and many people she had known, and said, 'Perhaps, who knows, Tom and Unity?' She slipped into unconsciousness and died on 25 May, aged eighty-three. It was a relief that her 'horrors' were over and that the end was peaceful, but hard to believe in the finality of her death. We held a service over her coffin and took her over the water to Mull, with a piper playing and the flag of the *Puffin* at half mast. The funeral was held at Swinbrook. The winter had relented in the south and the beauty of the churchyard, with its rush of cow parsley and buttercups and the song of thrushes and blackbirds, took me straight back to the mayfly hatching on the Windrush and the sound of Farve's reel in pursuit of a rising trout.

In a lucid moment a week before she died, Muv said to us, 'Now, children, you'll cry at my funeral and then you'll start laughing.' We did. Our sorrow came in waves but so did the laughter. There has to be relief after sorrow, no one can manage without it. Even the saddest, most painful moments do not last, however difficult it is to believe it at the time.

20

Midway

The years of middle age passed in a misty dream. Luxury was a day with nothing written in the diary and such days were rare. All householders know the problems, big and small, but magnify them by the size of Chatsworth and its environs, and you have the picture. The major problems went straight to Andrew, the day-to-day to me. As soon as the house and garden staff had started work, some at 8 a.m. and some at 9 a.m., the telephone began to ring: something had arisen in a faraway place that required an immediate decision or at least on-the-spot consideration. I was needed by the head housemaid on the private side of the house, the housekeeper on the public side, by the sewing room, the head gardener, head house-carpenter, cook, butler's pantry, signwriter, farm manager, head keeper, farmyard, house shops, farm shop or restaurant. When Roger Wardle became land agent I was able to refer to him on all estate matters and on the rare occasions when there was a fiery disagreement between two Chatsworth men, both certain they were right, he was able to settle the dispute to the satisfaction of both parties. I saw him in action on several occasions and came away impressed by his tact.

I loved all this activity, largely because of the pleasure of working with some of the most remarkable people I have ever met. One Chatsworth special was Mr Clegg, who seemed to spend all his days scrubbing the stone passage leading from the back door to the kitchen and elsewhere. The water he scrubbed and mopped with got browner and browner but it did not seem to matter. One Christmas, Mr Clegg volunteered to do lodge duty, which involved opening and shutting the gates to the private drive. I went to visit him in the narrow room of the lodge, where whoever was on duty sat keeping an eye out for the intruders who never came. Mr Clegg was not watching but was deep in a book. I asked him what he was reading. He turned to the title page: *Advanced Algebra*—a lesson to me that you cannot put people into categories.

Maud Barnes, who came from several generations of Cavendish family employees—her father had been the clerk of works at Hardwick—was another of the Chatsworth 'characters'. She did not marry, being one of the thousands of dutiful women who stay at home to look after an ailing parent, but when she was eventually free to do as she pleased, she came to Chatsworth. Her ill-defined job was to clean and tidy my rooms and wash and iron. The mezzanine above my little sitting room was where she carried out these tasks. She had a frightful fox terrier called Spot or Scott (I never discovered which) that ruled her life and made lots of washing—or sending to the cleaners, more likely—of the loose covers where he had, *pour encourager les autres*, lifted his leg.

Maud was neither clean nor tidy, but she was intelligent, well read, excellent company and willing to join in any fun on offer. In the early 1960s the Chatsworth WI put on an entertainment at an open meeting (where non-members are welcome). I went as the Oldest Miss World in the World, decked out in the Devonshire Parure—seven prickly and monumental pieces of jewellery, including a tiara, necklace and stomacher—which, until you look closely, might have been pulled out of the dressing-up box. Diddy, the children's nanny, whose shape reminded me of the kind of bread you can no longer buy: a round dollop sitting atop a larger round dollop, and who always gave the best of her unselfish nature, went as the Sugar Plum Fairy in a white tulle tutu and tights. Waving a wand wrapped in tinsel, this beloved creature, then in late middle age, pirouetted, jumped, flumped and pointed her toe at the audience. Maud went as Ringo Starr under a black Beatle wig that suited her classical features; to see and hear her drumming was sublime. I do believe that she, Diddy and I were the stars that night.

During the holidays my mother-in-law stayed at Moor View (home to the Suicide Squad in our Edensor days) and I loved having her close by. She had a cross cook who shouted at her and everyone else, and talked loudly to herself in the little kitchen. There was a hole in the wall between the kitchen and dining room through which she used to push the food with a furious shove. Moucher's guests always included her brother, David Cecil, and sister, Mima Harlech. The three of them loved each other's company better than anyone's and made the most of their days together, talking, talking as only Cecils can. They did not understand stacking so when they had finished eating and the dirty plates were ready to go back through the hole in the wall, they passed them round and round the table. No one thought to stop and make a pile of them—they were too interested in what they were saying. This display of their unpractical ways was one of the comic entertainments of the year for me.

*   *   *

However enjoyable my job at Chatsworth, it was often like walking on eggshells, not only because I never knew exactly where my remit ended, but because Andrew was a victim of alcoholism and his reactions had become increasingly unpredictable. Had he not written so openly about it in his memoirs, I would not have mentioned my side of the story, but it may be of interest to others to read a first-hand account of what it was like.

Andrew was addicted to alcohol for much of his adult life, a weakness that ran through the

Cavendish family and had also descended to some of his first cousins. Drinking had contributed to his father's premature death at the age of fifty-five and to his uncle Charlie Cavendish's at thirty-eight. Perhaps in Andrew's case things were exacerbated by underlying guilt at having what his brother should have had, and by the pressures and enormous responsibilities that came with this inheritance. After Billy's death, although he enjoyed many things in life, he was driven by a sense of guilt and duty in equal parts.

Living with someone with an addiction of any sort, be it gambling, drugs, alcohol or even compulsive spending—anything done to excess—is wearing. If you have never had the experience it is hard, almost impossible, to understand what it is like. The character of the sufferer changes, in Andrew's case from Dr Jekyll to Mr Hyde and back again with little warning, and to pretend that life is normal is to deny reality. To me *in vino veritas* was the very opposite of what happened: *in vino* brought out the nasty side; it was without the vino that Andrew was himself.

Although he was never physically violent when drunk, some of his actions—now unbelievable and best forgotten—were directed at those closest to him, which I believe is usual, and the effect on his relationship with our three children was dire. When we had people to stay I often found it difficult to concentrate on those next to me at dinner as I always had half an eye on Andrew and his neighbours at the other end of the table, knowing that a flare-up could come at any moment and that they might suddenly be the recipients of his anger. On several occasions he simply left the table and we went on as if nothing had happened.

Sixty years ago none of this would have been discussed; it would have been swept under the carpet by the addict's family in the pretence that it was not happening. I saw my mother-in-law do this and observed her unhappiness. In an attempt to keep Eddy away from his club, where drinking too much was usual among some of the members, she tried to distract him by inviting people she thought would interest him. She did not succeed. For an alcoholic, as with other addicts, the time of euphoria gets shorter and the hangover longer; depression lifts momentarily only to return worse than ever. Today, at last, addicts are treated as ill and are openly spoken of as such. It is understood that sufferers need help in order to free themselves from the bonds of whatever addiction allows them to escape, however fleetingly, from life and its troubles.

Andrew was surrounded by five loyal employees. Not knowing that it was the worst thing they could do, they made a cocoon around him of which I, unwittingly, was part. So successful were we at hiding Andrew's problem that even a senior member of the estate staff who joined in 1981 was unaware of his trouble. Concealing it was a double-edged sword: had it been exposed, Andrew might have sought help earlier, but at the time none of us who thought we were protecting him knew any better. I have now learnt that there is only one course of action, a method developed in America that has been successful all over the world. It comes at a price—the patient has to reach rock bottom, to go so low as to cry for help, and this is painful to watch—but it is a price well worth paying, as the success of Alcoholics Anonymous testifies.

I took advice from counsellors who told me that it was essential to remove Andrew's props and bring his problem out into the open. So I asked the heads of department at Chatsworth to come and see me; we stood in the passage by my room and I was afraid of breaking down as I told them that Andrew was ill and that the nature of his illness was alcoholism. I could see, as these old and trusted friends walked slowly away, that they understood the necessarily harsh nature of the treatment. Henry Coleman, our butler who had been with us since 1963, must have understood it better than most, having been so close to Andrew and me during those difficult times.

Time dims the unpleasant or sad events in life and dates run into each other in a muddled way. What I do know is that Andrew twice made the mighty effort to give up drinking. The first, in the 1970s, lasted for two years and then he started again. In the early 1980s, he went to some counsellors who had treated his cousins with success and this encouraged him to agree to try their method. The cure should have lasted six weeks but after two he rang his sister Anne, who lived near the clinic, and told her he could stand it no longer and would she please fetch him. 'If I had stayed the full six weeks,' he wrote in his memoirs, 'it would have destroyed me.'

Having no wish to see my family and friends I went to a hotel in Eastbourne. My hair—what there was of it—seemed to be even more shocked than I was. It stopped growing for three months. My spell in Eastbourne coincided with Wimbledon fortnight and I have never been able to watch the tournament on television since.

He came back to Chatsworth, doubtful of the success of what he had endured, and started drinking again. Matters reached a head in September 1983. We had guests staying for four days' racing at Doncaster and Andrew's behaviour was out of control and frightening to watch. After two days I telephoned the counsellor in despair and asked her what to do. Without hesitation she told me to tell the guests to leave. (Three close friends immediately understood the desperate situation; the others said they were Andrew's guests and were staying.) She instructed me to cover my bedroom and sitting room with dust sheets and leave the house. The idea was to give Andrew a shock, to make him think that I had left for good—and for all I knew I had.

Stoker and Sophy were indispensable to me during those knife-edge times. Emma and her husband Toby were stalwart supports and asked me to stay for an unlimited time, but in the event Stoker and Amanda took me to Bolton Hall. After a few days, the telephone rang with an agonized request from Andrew, 'Please will you come back?' I said I would if he would give up drinking once and for all. 'The miracle occurred,' he wrote. 'I realized that apart from all the suffering I had caused, I was not my own master. I decided this slavery must stop once and for all.' He went into a nursing home for four days to ensure that no alcohol remained in his blood and started to take

Antabuse, the pill you cannot mix with alcohol without feeling extremely ill.

For all of us at Chatsworth it was indeed a miracle. Andrew slowly got better physically, which must have helped him resist the longed-for drink. Those of us who have been spared such craving cannot understand how hard it must be to give up a lifelong habit. But Andrew did it and for two decades, until the day he died, he never had another drink. My optimistic nature had faith in his resolve and I was proved right. A laden drinks tray was always in his study, to the astonishment of friends who knew his medical history, but he never went near it. The nightmare was over. People he had been unable to face came back as though nothing had happened and he began to take an interest in things he had avoided for years.

The turnaround was all the more remarkable as he was beginning to go blind. Eventually he could not see to read, a terrible deprivation, and radio and television could not take the place of books. As his eyes got worse, he could no longer recognize faces, so the endless engagements in Derbyshire and elsewhere, which he had started to honour again, must have been difficult, and people thought he was cutting them when he failed to speak to them. Yet in spite of the effort it cost him, he continued to play his part to the full until shortly before he died.

*   *   *

Despite the worry of Andrew, which was always in the background, I enjoyed entertaining at Chatsworth; not the official sort where hosts ask people off a list and guests accept because it is part of their job, but having friends to stay. Not long after we moved into the house Cecil Beaton came for a night or two. I was proud of a new border outside the Orangery which was planted with clashing bright-red plants and a few orange flowers—a startling antidote to the pastel colours then favoured by garden designers. I took Cecil to see it. 'It's *arful*,' he bleated. 'It's a *retina irritant*.' Cecil lived at Reddish House in Broadchalke, one of those Wiltshire houses that are so pretty and easy to live in that you feel nowhere could be as good. It was stuffed full of anything that had caught his eye, and because it had caught his eye it became fashionable. Baubles, china objects, ornaments, shawls, bronzes were scattered over every surface, including in the conservatory where watering the plants must have been a tricky job. I stayed at Reddish when Sophy was at nearby Hanford School, and when I fetched her back for lunch my heart was in my mouth as the ten-year-old swung her heavy winter coat, narrowly missing the piles of precious objects.

Cecil was a wonderful host, taking *petits soins* everywhere for the comfort of the guest. Perhaps it was a bit too theatrical, but theatre was part of his trade. During the war Rex Whistler, Lady Juliet Duff, Cecil and several other talented and sophisticated people who lived near the Pembrokes at Wilton House, got up a pantomime. *Heil Cinderella* was made unforgettable by Cecil as an Ugly Sister. Wearing an unadorned black velvet dress—no brooch, no necklace, nothing but a thin, long-sleeved slinky creation described by dressmakers as a 'sheath'—he swayed about, tall and maiden-auntish, singing, 'Don't look now, there's Hitler close behind you.' It was one of the best things I have seen on stage.

In 1976, Lady Bird Johnson, widow of President Johnson, brought her daughter Lynda Bird to Chatsworth. We laid on a tour of neighbouring houses, gardens, villages and public buildings in an attempt to show our part of England at its best. Andrew and I were delighted to have the chance to get to know our guests: a more easy-going, charming pair you could not hope to find. Before they left, Lady Bird told me that she was going to Greece that summer and was reading up on its ancient history. 'I'm trying to figure out ... who ... slew ... who,' she said, very slowly, in her lovely Southern accent. As their car was about to drive away, I said to Lynda Bird, 'Do stop at Sudbury on your way south, it is so well worth it.' 'We can't,' she said. 'Mother is just about Housed Out.'

In 1979 an exhibition, 'Treasures from Chatsworth', travelled to several American museums. I was asked to the opening at the Kimbell Art Museum in Fort Worth and Lady Bird invited me to visit the Johnson Ranch in Austin— all new worlds to me and exciting. The foreword to the exhibition catalogue was written by Professor Sir Anthony Blunt, keeper of the Queen's pictures. He had been to stay at Chatsworth to see the works of art and I had looked forward to his visit. Nancy and Diana had been to one of his lectures in Paris and had fallen for him, and I knew he was revered by his pupils.

In the event I was disappointed and found my guest difficult to talk to. Andrew was away, and dinner on the two nights Sir Anthony stayed seemed to drag on. Perhaps he had expected me to invite people to meet him; he was certainly bored. I was thankful when the time came for him to leave and take his cold eyes and unpleasant personality with him. What followed was unexpected. Waking in my hotel bedroom in Fort Worth on the morning of the opening at the Kimbell, I turned on the television and there, filling the screen, was Sir Anthony's thin, gloomy face and the scandal of his exposure as a traitor. The telephone started ringing. In view of this extraordinary development, should we withdraw the catalogue from sale? After much discussion, it was decided not to. The catalogue sold out and more attention was paid to it and its disgraced author than to the finest exhibits Chatsworth could provide.

Lady Bird Johnson gave a great deal of her time to me and took me to the Harry Ransom Center in Austin, where I saw letters by Evelyn Waugh in his neat little handwriting, and many works by my hero, Edward Lear. Anyone who can write a poem like 'The Akond of Swat' or paint such landscapes as *The City of Syracuse* at Madresfield Court, is worthy of reverence. After poring over these treasures I happened to look up and see, on top of a display cupboard, three cardboard boxes marked 'Jessica Mitford' in large letters. I asked if I could look at them. The librarian told me apologetically that the contents were unsorted, but he brought one down and in it were random notes in my Old Hen's writing—dinner engagements, shopping lists and the like. When later I asked Decca how they had got there, she told me that the Center had paid a huge sum for what she was about to throw away. Wonders will never cease, but I was delighted to find a bit of home in that distant land.

Back at the Ranch after dark, Lady Bird took me to the garden to show me her jacuzzi, the first I had ever seen. We got in and splashed about, lit by searchlights and surrounded by security guards. Neighbours came for dinner and arrived in their own planes. Late at night we stood and waved goodbye as the neat little jets took off into the starry Texan sky, as if it were nothing out of the ordinary. The next morning, Lady Bird asked me if I would like to go with the cowboys to round up some cattle. Of course I would. I was not disappointed by the handsome men, dressed as I had often seen them in films with Stetson hats, check shirts, leather chaps, cowboy boots and spurs, but I was surprised when they pointed to a helicopter instead of a horse, and up and off we went with a cowboy at the controls. The Hereford cattle were driven along by this noisy machine, which dipped and wove as it herded the beasts into the open gates of the corral. I enjoyed this new experience, but wondered why the cowboy pilot had bothered to put on his spurs.

* * *

When Uncle Harold was very old he came to stay for weeks on end. By then he was becoming infirm and walking was not easy. I met him one afternoon in a passage looking rather anxious and forlorn. 'The trouble with this house,' he said, 'is you have to throw double sixes to get out.' He slept in the red velvet bedroom, which opens on to a busy first-floor passage, and sometimes liked to go to bed early with tea and bread and butter for supper.

One evening he heard us talking outside his bedroom and could not bear to miss the chat. A figure in pyjamas and dressing gown emerged, demanded champagne and spent a cheery evening with people generations younger than himself. He knew his lines and spouted them to his audience. Sophy often longed to be anywhere else as she had heard it all before, reminding me of Jeremy Tree at glorious Ditchley during the war. Winston Churchill used to stay there at full moon, when Chequers and Chartwell were easy targets for enemy bombers, and held forth at the dinner table. Most of the guests were spellbound, but not Jeremy, who longed to go to bed and whose wide yawns while the oracle spoke did not go unnoticed.

After lunch with us Uncle Harold retired to a chair in his bedroom, holding a cigar over a wicker wastepaper basket—can you imagine anything more dangerous? He was nearly blind and had taken to Talking Books, especially Trollope, which he must have known by heart. One day he told me in a very serious voice that something odd had happened to Trollope and he could not make it out. I looked at the packet and saw it was *Lucky Jim* by Kingsley Amis. When Andrew was in London, I was often alone with Uncle Harold. No good at politics, I was nevertheless fascinated to hear about the people he had known and worked with for years. Such were his good manners that he never hinted that he would have preferred a more intelligent dinner companion and treated me as if I were a fellow ageing ex-PM. He was easy to laugh at, but also easy to laugh with. When Mrs Thatcher became Prime Minister, she asked him to go and see her. 'That was a good idea,' I said. 'Did you talk?' 'No—she did.'

It was to have private talks with Uncle Harold that the Prince of Wales came to stay in June 1984. What Uncle Harold told him I do not know, but they made good friends and the Prince felt his time was well spent. He reminded me recently that he had asked for a reading list to fill the gaps in his knowledge, and that Andrew and Uncle Harold had scoured the bookshelves to produce one. He says it is invaluable to him still. Thereafter, the Prince stayed at Chatsworth whenever he had an official engagement near by and he was often able to stay on and fit in a day's hunting with the Meynell. In December he used to bring sack loads of Christmas cards to sign—a chore which meant putting an extra table in his room for the seemingly endless piles. The Prince liked the freedom of being able to walk in the woods and over the moor, exploring unknown country. If he did meet one or two walkers and they recognized him, they respected his privacy, greeted him and walked on. One winter weekend I drove him to see the beautiful, late eighteenth-century mill at Cressbrook. A 'Road Closed' sign stopped us just before we reached our destination. The Prince got out of the car and knocked at the door of a nearby cottage. After a while, a man answered and the Prince asked him if we could drive on. The man scratched his head, stared at the visitor and said, very slowly, 'Haven't I seen you somewhere before?'

There was usually a big party of friends when the Prince came to stay and we enjoyed it to the full, but there was no opportunity to get to know him well in a crowd of people who all wanted to talk to him. In March 1988, however, the Prince was in a party of skiers holidaying in Klosters when an avalanche overtook them. He narrowly escaped death but two of his close friends were buried, one of whom died. It was a shattering experience. When the mourning survivors got home, it occurred to me that the Prince, whose diary is crowded with hardly an hour to spare, now had a few days ahead of him with nothing planned. I talked to Andrew and we decided that I should ring up the Prince's private secretary and say how pleased we should be if the Prince would come to Chatsworth to do just what he liked—walk, talk, be with us or stay alone—and to our delight he accepted. It was during those days of slow recovery from shock and the death of his friend that I got to know him. Our friendship has lasted through good times and bad for both of us, and I value it more than I can say.

From the early 1990s my New York friend Jayne Wrightsman, the designer Oscar de la Renta and his wife, Annette, stayed with us every summer. As they always came at the same time of year, there was a limit to the variety of flowers that the Chatsworth head gardeners, Jim Link and later Ian Webster, could produce for the dining-room table. Good and spectacular though the rambler roses were, we soon got through Bobby James, Himalayan blush-pink and the like, so I tried chickens. A Buff Cochin cock was washed for the occasion and sat on some hay in one of the rectangular glass containers made many years ago for the batteries of the turbine house. He was a steady old fellow and made no objection to his new surroundings. A couple of hens of uncertain ancestry occupied another glass container and, as luck would have it, there had been a hatch of Welsummer and White Leghorn chicks that morning so just before dinner I put them in little china baskets lined with hay to keep them warm. The Paul Storr silver wine-coolers were filled with brown and white eggs, and our driver, Alan Shimwell, who was helping with the chicken side of things, slipped an egg into the so-called nest which held the two hens. Our efforts had the desired effect on our American guests, but the old Cochin cock remained unmoved by their loud reactions to his and his consorts' presence; and the chicks presumably thought it was all quite normal as they had only been alive for twelve hours.

The following year I had to think of something better. Piglets. The glass containers were pressed into service again and half a dozen piglets, replete from a long drink of milk from the sow, lay sound asleep on their straw beds in the middle of the dining-room table. The decoration did not last long. 'This really is too much,' said Andrew after the first course. 'Henry, take those pigs off the table.' So Margaret Norris, manager of the Chatsworth Farmyard, who had arranged the *mise-en-scène*, came back, packed up her beloved piglets and took them home to their mother. The following year there was no more livestock; I had done my best, but that was it. I resorted to Old Master drawings on miniature easels in front of each place, which I thought might appeal to our guests as both Jayne and Annette are the recognized backbone of the Metropolitan Museum, which goes in for that sort of thing. I do not believe the Raphaels, Rembrandts and Co.

were splashed by gravy or ice cream, and after dinner they returned to their cold, unwelcoming, air-conditioned, thrice-locked shelves. I would rather be one of Margaret's piglets any day.

Entertaining is full of pitfalls. The Spanish Ambassador to London, Santiago de Tamarón, and his wife, Isabella, came to Chatsworth one summer weekend. Santiago is an admirer of Paddy Leigh Fermor—who he said was his reason for wanting to come to England—so we had a bond. He had given a memorable party for Paddy at the embassy where all Paddy's fans and would-be imitators recited, sang at the top of their voices and jostled for attention. Paddy himself was in Greece so we asked some other friends to meet the Tamaróns. I was about to introduce them to Isabella when my mind went blank. Her name had gone out of my head and, in a panic, I said, 'May I introduce you to . . . Mrs Thing?' Instead of leaving in a bait Isabella was amused. We have remained friends and she now signs herself 'Thing'.

I met the sculptress Elisabeth Frink when I was staying with Edward and Camilla Cazalet, old friends who live in Sussex. Army-bred, blue-eyed, beautiful and quick to laugh, Lis was not at all what I expected and had that larger-than-life personality that has to be felt rather than described. Some of it survives in her work and the pieces I love best are her animals—horses and dogs of such exceptional quality and character. The pick of the horses, I thought and still think, is *War Horse 1991*, which I fell for when I first saw it in plaster in her Dorset studio. I have always preferred heavy horses to thoroughbreds, Shires and Shetlands to racehorses, and here was the epitome of all I admire: tail plaited, ears back, head and eye giving warning that he is about to strike and bite. I wanted so much to see him at Chatsworth and knew where I would put him. After the usual hurdle of persuading the Trustees to buy him, *War Horse* arrived, as did his maker, keen to approve his situation and to supervise his installation. He had travelled in a horse box (what else) and was transferred to the bucket of a JCB that trundled through the garden, driven by Brian Gilbert, the precision expert. Brian could move a china war horse without damaging it and this bronze fellow presented no difficulty. Lis approved of the spot at the south end of the canal, facing out over the Old Park where his ancestors must have grazed. I was thrilled by the whole performance and by the fact that Chatsworth now possessed a monumental example of Lis's art. I too own a couple of her works, thanks to the sales of a book or two: dogs that are to the life.

Lis and I shared a love of poultry and she wrote to me one day telling me that her favourite cock, Reggie, had been unwell and that she had taken him to the vet. It conjured up such a picture: a distinguished Dame of the British Empire, Companion of Honour and Royal Academician, sitting, cock on lap, in the queue in the vet's waiting room. It was to no avail: Reggie died. Lis herself was already mortally ill when she came to see *War Horse* installed and, to my lasting regret, soon followed Reggie into the next world.

In all the years I lived in Derbyshire, Andrew and I went out to dinner in private houses only four times; in each case it was to a dinner given by the

High Sheriff for the High Court judges when on Circuit in the county, one of the duties of the holder of that ancient office. Other dinners—civic, charitable, annual celebrations for clubs and associations, from Rotary and WI to golf—came thick and fast, but they were not held in private houses. We had what could be described as a 'full social life', both in London and with friends in the country, and when at home there was already too much to do without going out to dinner. Once in every fifteen years was enough.

One of these dinners stands out. It was at Calke Abbey, near Ticknall, in 1961 when Charles Harpur Crewe was High Sheriff of Derbyshire. Charles was a recluse who lived an intensely private life in an intensely private house, in his own little kingdom hidden in a vast park in the south of Derbyshire. The dinner for the judges must have been a huge effort for him. Owing to an engagement in London, Andrew could not come, so I went alone. Full of curiosity as to what I should find, I put on my best evening dress and settled into the car to be driven to Ticknall on a damp November night with the prospect of fog.

After some forty miles, we reached the entrance to the park. There were no more white lines or cat's eyes; the secret road was the same colour as the dead grass, and the oaks, stricken with age, seemed to threaten my invading car. The fog swirled round us as we crawled along the seemingly endless drive, skirting uncomfortably close to ponds and avoiding ghostly fallow deer on the narrow twists and turns. I thought we were lost when, round a corner, a dim light appeared. The curtains were drawn back on the ground and first floors of Calke Abbey and the rooms were lit only by candles, something I had never seen in a house of that size before; not even oil lamps reinforced the flickering flames. The judges must have thought they had arrived in a fairy story. I certainly did.

I was led through the cold and stony hall, its walls decorated not with the usual antlers but with heads of Longhorn cattle, whose tapering horns nearly met over their muzzles and must have touched the ground when they had bent to graze, almost preventing their tongues from reaching the grass. How these cattle managed to eat I do not know. Our hosts consisted of Charles, his younger brother Henry and their sister Airmyne. The dining-room table was set with more candles—the only light in that high-ceilinged room, which I imagine had not been used for years. The first course was melon, followed by cold beef, then melon for pudding.

After dinner Airmyne led the women guests back to the drawing room, leaving the men to their port. 'Would you like to see Nanny?' she whispered. I was flattered to be singled out for this honour and we set off up a magnificent flight of shallow, mahogany stairs, along a passage and through a bedroom door. I could just make out a tiny, ancient creature, curled up fast asleep in bed. Airmyne roused her. One eye opened and she just managed, 'Good evening.' We left her in peace and as we trekked back to the drawing room, Airmyne said, 'She was the Kaiser's Nanny' (presumably nanny to the Kaiser's son, Little Willie).

Airmyne had been kicked in the head by a re-mount at the Melton Mowbray cavalry depot at the beginning of the Second World War and Henry told me that she had a silver plate in her skull. The wretched accident had affected her personality and she was never quite the same again. She lived for the animals who were her friends: her horses, dogs and poultry, including a goose. 'Would you like to see the stables?' she said. Of course I would, with Airmyne for guide, but the judges were in court the next day and the fog was thickening. We returned to the drawing room, had a last talk with the other guests and set off home after the strangest evening I can remember.

Charles Harpur Crewe died suddenly in 1981. He was found in his beloved park, apparently setting mole traps. His brother Henry succeeded him and, in 1985, after complicated negotiations to raise the necessary capital endowment, he ceded Calke Abbey to the Treasury in settlement of death duties and it was handed to the National Trust. The house is now open and the Trust has tried its best to preserve the spirit of the late owners. The clutter that filled the house from hall to attic, including a remarkable collection of natural history objects accumulated over centuries, is still there, and the four-poster state bed—a wedding present to the Fifth Baronet and Lady Caroline Manners from Princess Anne, daughter of George II—has been unpacked. (It had been in its packing cases since it arrived from London in 1734.)

Henry remained in a tiny part of the Abbey, which gave it a whiff of the past in the same way that Granny Evie did at Hardwick. Both ex-owners were treated as Exhibit A and visitors were thrilled to find them *in situ*. Henry gradually cast off his shyness and took to social life with enthusiasm. We met at all sorts of Derbyshire functions and his unexpected point of view on any subject was refreshing after what was often banal social chat. It was a joy to find him in Washington in 1985 when he accompanied the now-famous bed to the 'Treasure Houses of Great Britain' exhibition. I was with him when the art correspondents from serious American periodicals questioned him as to why the bed had never been unpacked. 'Oh, I don't know,' he said, 'I suppose they had something else to do.' A friend who was also present reminded me how worried the curator looked when I said, 'Do get into bed, Henry, just to show everyone that it is real.' The Harpur Crewe siblings were the only true eccentrics I have ever met. They have all gone now and with them the mystery; in spite of the Trust's best efforts, Calke Abbey is a lovely house containing an exhibition of curiosities but no Harpur Crewe among them.

21

Living Above the Shop

It is a popular misconception that it was thanks to me that Chatsworth was 'saved'. It is not so. When my father-in-law died and the near-lethal blow of death duties had to be faced, it was Andrew who was determined to keep Chatsworth independent. He turned down overtures from the V&A and Manchester University, who wanted to buy the house and its contents, and he chaired all the meetings that were held to decide how best to pay the bill. He wanted it to stay as it had always been without adding a zoo or safari park. He was proved right and people come to walk, run, talk, shout, play games, bring their dogs and their children, picnic anywhere, and do what they like (the only private area is the Old Park to the south of the house, where the deer have their fawns and calves undisturbed). I believe this freedom is one of the reasons that visitors love the place and I get letters from many people who tell me how peaceful and comforting they find Chatsworth. Even when there is a big crowd, you only have to walk a little way to be on your own, in tranquillity. The house itself has always drawn people, many of whom find it hard to believe that it could be anyone's home; a few come to see the works of art; all come in search of beauty, indoors and out, and most seem to find it.

I think that Andrew would have liked the public to see round the house for nothing, but he knew it was an impossible dream given the expense of its upkeep. In 1980, in order that Chatsworth could continue to be kept open to visitors, Andrew, Stoker and the family's legal advisers created a charitable foundation, the Chatsworth House Trust, whose object is 'the long-term preservation of Chatsworth for the benefit of the public'. An endowment fund was created from the sale of works of art from the private side of the house and from other family resources. The income from this trust fund goes towards the upkeep of the house, garden and park, which are the responsibility of the Council of Management of Chatsworth House Trust. (The first official position I had at Chatsworth was when I was invited to become a member of this council in 1981, thirty-one years after the death of my father-in-law.)

Andrew had an instinct for what was right for the estates, and was always concerned for the people who worked at Chatsworth, as well as for its visitors. It was his idea, for example, to provide the much-used heated indoor swimming pool, tennis court and gymnasium for the staff. He insisted on a free car park at the south (Beeley) end of the park; he made access agreements with the local authorities for paths across the grouse moors, at Bolton Abbey as well as Chatsworth; and out of his own pocket, he provided electric buggies for the disabled to be able to drive on the paths through Chatsworth's 105-acre garden, and also up to the Strid at Bolton Abbey. He was always looking for ways to ensure the survival of Chatsworth. When it was realized that we had many regular visitors—not just numbers in a survey but people who had become well known to our staff—Andrew suggested the 'Friends of Chatsworth' scheme and it has been a success. In 2001, when the house had to delay opening for three weeks because of the threat of foot and mouth disease, it was his idea to try to make up some of the deficit by keeping the house open till 23 December with the public route decorated for Christmas. I thought this would fail but I did as he asked and, thanks to the enthusiasm of the staff, it was—and is—a great draw, with people coming from all over the country to see it.

My own involvement started with Dorothy Dean, our housekeeper from 1968 to 1981, who was the first person to realize that people wanted to take something home from Chatsworth, a souvenir to remind them of their visit. We talked about it and she set out guidebooks, postcards, playing cards, matches and bonbons on a trestle table in the Orangery, a lofty glass-roofed room in the north wing of the house, and, after working all morning with the cleaners, she changed her clothes from housekeeper to shopkeeper and stood behind the table. Sales rose steadily and in 1978 she reported that the takings from the Orangery and a small kiosk in the garden selling plants and ice cream had enabled her to bank £75,000 that season. The Orangery Shop was on its way. Philip Jebb designed stalls in the shape of bookcases, which stood in a circle in the middle of the room around the enormous marble copy of the Medici vase. It all looked very pretty, but the space was almost immediately too small and the stalls were moved against the walls to make more room.

I loved the shop and often served behind the counter. I was so interested in what people wanted and why—shades of Muv's ambition to be the woman behind the till in a French restaurant. We printed better guidebooks, improved our range of postcards, laid in stocks of the ubiquitous tea towels, and out they all flew. We ordered various items with pictures of the house and its contents, an expensive outlay that took some persuading of the Management, of which I was not yet a part. The tinware, our most successful line, generated cash like nothing else. Why? Because the trays, bowls and tea-caddies were pretty, eye-catching, useful *and* were decorated with views of the house, painted by the artist Patricia Machin. The only drawback was the number we had to order at a time—the minimum quantity for trays, for example, was 20,000—but each one we sold was a silent advertisement for Chatsworth, and worth far more to us than just their cash value. The trays became quite famous and sold through the General Trading Company and other London outlets; today they turn up in antique shops at many times their original price.

We introduced a line of knitted garments made from the wool of the Jacob Sheep that grazed in the park. People were intrigued by these four-horned creatures (even the ewes sport this decoration) and snapped up the brown-and-cream coloured jerseys, hats, scarves and gloves until demand exceeded supply. One of the knitters became so obsessed with her work, knitting all day and most of the night, that she lost track of the patterns. Garments of the strangest proportions appeared, either too long or too short or with sleeves a mile long and little else. She was a 'case' and I knew that if we stopped taking her work, it might tip her over the edge, so we gave up the hand-knitted garments and turned to other wares.

We commissioned porcelain manufacturers to make a few items of exceptional quality, also decorated with pictures of the house, and expensive reproductions of seventeenth-century delftware tulip vases at Chatsworth. While these were still for sale they provided high-quality decoration for the shop and even though they were the most expensive items, they did eventually go (you have to sell many postcards to generate the same turnover). At the other end of the scale, for ten pence children could buy colouring-in sheets showing scenes of Chatsworth and the Duchess of Devonshire's Ball of 1897. In a quiet way the

Orangery Shop became well known and in 1983 we engaged a professional manageress. For some years I went to the Birmingham and Harrogate gift fairs, but I soon discovered that our trusted buyers, sisters Sue and Jane Brindley, liked the same things as I did, so I gave up, knowing their eyes would work better than mine.

*   *   *

In the 1960s and early 70s, I received many letters from teachers asking for information to give to their pupils about our farms and woods. The teachers themselves were often ignorant about farming practices, knowing little about the use of common arable crops, for example, let alone about the animals they saw out of the bus window. I was aware of the growing division between town and country and wanted to do something about it. We thought long and hard and decided to convert the disused building-yard near the house into a farmyard, so that children could see cattle, sheep and free-range hens close up—just the opposite of a safari park.

When the educational Farmyard became reality and not just a dream, it grabbed my attention as a new baby would have done and I spent hours there, trying to get it all right. I feel pleased that today about 200,000 people, mostly children, come to enjoy and, I hope, to learn from it every year. It was not designed to be a collection of pets but to show the unsentimental facts about the life cycle of commercial farm stock. Life-size diagrams of butchers' cuts are pinned up in the pigsties and cattle yard, in case there is any doubt as to the animals' fate.

The Farmyard opened in 1973 with pigs, goats and a Shire horse, as well as the unavoidable lavatories and tea shop. Before tractors, Shires were the only source of power on the land (except for steam engines that did the threshing before combine harvesters took over) and Andrew's grandfather's stud was famous. There is great excitement when our Shire mare is about to foal; she has obliged several times with a daytime birth and this is watched with fascination by all. The daily highlight, however, is the milking demonstration. The cows are milked, one at a time and sideways on—the better to show the operation—in front of an incredulous young audience. Watching the children watching the milking is better than any theatre; they remain riveted to the spot until a teacher or parent insists on moving them on. I asked one little boy from a school in the middle of Sheffield what he thought of this performance. 'It's the most disgustin' thing I've ever seen,' he said, vowing never to touch milk again.

We began to hold Open Days in the park for children and teachers. The men from Elm Tree Farm, an arable farm seventeen miles from Chatsworth, brought bundles of half-grown wheat, barley, oilseed rape and potatoes. Few teachers and even fewer children could guess from the leaves which crop was which. The keepers from Chatsworth brought their dogs, guns and a batch of pheasant chicks with their surrogate mothers: broody hens. There were displays of clay-pigeon shooting; some of the teachers tried their hand at it (against the law now, no doubt) and I imagine some of the children would have liked to have a go too—at the teachers. Shepherds and their sheepdogs showed off their skills; it was before *One Man and his Dog* had become so popular on television, but our audience loved it. Foresters were there to explain that trees are a crop and, like other crops, have to be planted, weeded, thinned and eventually harvested—in other words cut down. 'What? *You cut down trees?'* said a furious teacher, who had been brought up to think it a crime. The children were interested in the giant saws and watched David Robinson, a born teacher himself, climbing a tree in the harness used by tree surgeons. Afterwards, teachers and children all piled into their buses and back to their built-up surroundings, but we hoped that a little of what they had seen had rubbed off. I felt that if they understood that the very grass they walked on was a crop, then we had gone a little way towards explaining the use of the land.

If the aim of the Farmyard was educational, the aim of the Farm Shop was purely commercial. Agriculture was in the dumps and I feared for the future of the in-hand farm at Chatsworth and for the men who worked on it. Both were an integral part of the whole. The idea of a farm shop came to me during the Royal Smithfield Club's conference in Buxton in 1972; I was listening to the farmers and butchers and it occurred to me that selling our farm produce direct to the public might help change the farm accounts from red to black. This was long before the public at large had started taking an interest in local food, but instinct told me that the same people who came to Chatsworth to walk in the fresh air and enjoy the glorious landscape would also be attracted by the idea of buying beef and lamb straight from our farm. No doubt too in the back of my mind were memories of Muv's poultry farm of long ago, of her passion for fresh, wholesome fare, and Uncle Geoffrey's campaign for 'unmurdered food—nothing added and nothing taken away'. The Smithfield farmers and butchers, acknowledged experts in the livestock and meat for which these islands are renowned, not only became lasting friends but were also generous with their advice. 'You'll sell all the fillet steak and be left with the forequarters,' they cautioned, and warned of other pitfalls of the trade that they had learned the hard way.

I presented my idea to the Trustees of the Chatsworth Settlement, who did not take me seriously. It was depressing to be met with a no. After years of death duties and debts, the estate office staff seemed to be suffering from inertia; 'anything for a quiet life' was their motto and new ideas were looked on with suspicion. 'We are an agricultural estate,' the land agent explained to me, 'with village property, minerals and woods, and that is what we understand. We have no experience in retailing food.' I was aware of all this but did not give up. I knew that nostalgia for the past was a big attraction for the visitors who came to the house and that the same 'feel' would entice people to a farm shop. Tears at home and arguments elsewhere eventually won the day and we set about getting planning permission.

Andrew wanted the winter months when the house was closed to be quiet, so the only suitable building was the Stud Farm at nearby Pilsley, which was built in 1910 for Victor Duke's Shire horse stallions. Planning permission seemed to take for ever but finally, in 1976, we were granted permission to market produce from the Chatsworth farm and from our tenant farmers. We were allowed to sell freezer packs of meat only, the smallest quantity of beef being one-eighth of a beast, and half of a pig or lamb. We made sausages in a second-hand machine, sold game, including venison, in season, and the arable farm supplied potatoes and flour.

I wanted the shop to be the opposite of a shiny, American-style supermarket with wire shelving and to look like a rough and ready farm outbuilding, with shelves of thick wooden planks and as little metal as possible. Refrigerators do not make tempting showcases, but we had to have some (more is the pity) and I wanted the service to be human and friendly. All went well for a time, then demand dropped, the shop began to lose money and the Trustees said it would have to close unless it turned to profit within a few months. It was saved by Jean-Pierre Béraud, the whirlwind French chef who came to cook at Chatsworth in 1978 and who took over the Farm Shop in 1984.

Jean-Pierre was a born entrepreneur as well as a marvellous chef, but putting him in charge was something of a risk as he could speak little English, did not know the difference between a pound and a kilo and once told me that he had sacked a waitress because he could see from the way she walked that she was no good. He used to storm into my room without warning and sound off loud criticisms of the estate office and anyone who stood in his path. But Chatsworth, and I, never had a better friend. He rescued the dying Farm Shop by installing a kitchen and selling cooked (value-added) food and soon made his presence felt further afield. Cooking demonstrations have become popular and we recently had a visit from Claire Macdonald from the Isle of Skye. She has a glowing reputation as a cook and is a first-rate demonstrator. To the surprise of our audience, she was generous with the double cream and there were mutterings about health risks and cost. 'Well,' she said, 'they sell skimmed milk in my supermarket but I couldn't look a cow in the face if I bought that.' Excellent woman.

If I say the Chatsworth Farm Shop was the first of its kind, I shall get a hundred letters saying, 'No, we were', but it was certainly ahead of the game and is still a leading player. In 2004, the year of Andrew's death, it employed 48 full-time and 52 part-time staff, the turnover was just short of £5 million and it had won many awards. The Farm Shop, like the Orangery, slowly changed from a cottage industry to a serious business, thereby losing much of its charm for me. I prefer the WI way of people making jam, marmalade, bread and cakes in their own kitchens, supplying eggs from their own hens, and knitting garments from a herd of Jacob Sheep. I despair at the current regimentation, the wild rules over hygiene and the insidious and, to my mind, dishonest practice of 'Own Label', which gives the false impression that goods are made on the premises when in fact they come from a factory that supplies the same product to many other shops. There seems to be no way of going back to giving real food, made by real people, to the public on a large scale; it is thought to be too dangerous.

Until 1975, the catering at Chatsworth was a cold water tap by the lodge, now relabelled 'Water for Dogs'. I tentatively suggested to Dennis Fisher, the comptroller, that we should try to offer something more like tea to our visitors. He answered that it would be unpopular with the owners of the tea shops in nearby villages, who relied on the custom of our visitors. And, anyhow, where would we put it? I retreated, but demand was persistent and I eventually made an amateurish attempt to please visitors by persuading some of the local ladies to serve tea, coffee and cake in the stables, where the customers were squashed together in the old horse stalls, perched on iron-hard benches. It pleased nobody and we had to do better. Jean-Pierre came to the rescue again; we invested in some second-hand equipment and he and his staff set up their kitchen underneath the hayracks. Jean-Pierre never allowed anything to be fried, so we were spared the High Street smells, and I am happy to say his edict still holds.

The ever-higher expectations of our visitors began to make us look for a way to expand the restaurant and in 1986 Philip Jebb produced plans for a new building incorporating the old game larder, which was built in 1910 to hang pheasants and was a short distance from the entrance to the house. Two designs were submitted to the planners, but neither suited them, so Jean-Pierre, Bob Getty (the clerk of works), Derrick Penrose (the land agent) and I went to plead our case to the Royal Fine Art Commission, chaired by our old friend Norman St John-Stevas. It was an odd experience. We were not asked to sit down, so we stood like children awaiting a beating from the headmaster. And we got it: permission was refused. 'Have another look at the stable block,' they said. Andrew and I were angry with all concerned, and I still have the formal typed letter from Lord St John refusing us permission. (At the bottom, out of sight of the typist, he has added 'With love from Norman' and three kisses.)

The stable block at Chatsworth was designed in about 1760 by the architect James Paine for the Fourth Duke of Devonshire. Philip, Jean-Pierre, Bob and I explored every nook and cranny of this magnificent building, from the blacksmith's shop and brew house to the horse stalls, loose boxes and harness room. The Victorian carriage house, added by the Sixth Duke in the 1830s, was a possibility but did not look inviting: it was being used as a garage and housed all sorts of cars and clutter, including the Yellow Peril, Victor Duke's 1914 Humber. There was a glass-roofed area where cars were washed, and the pools of oil on the floor in the main building reminded me of Rutland Gate Mews. It took a great deal of imagination to picture what it could become, but my colleagues had that ability in spades and when we were satisfied that we had solved all practical difficulties regarding the kitchens, cold rooms, prep rooms, washing up, heating, lighting, lavatories, delivery space and rubbish disposal, we put in for planning permission again. This time it was granted.

The arches of the covered ride, originally an exercise track for the horses in bad weather, were glazed in so people could sit and eat in comfort. Heavy chains were hung between the pillars to stop too many noses being broken on the new glass.

Bobby Jones, far and away the most skilled in his profession, tiled the walls of the ladies' lavatories with camellias and the gents' with horses. It won a Loo of the Year award and Jean-Pierre and I went to London to receive it from a minister, which we found very pleasing. I had to admit the planners were right: the stables would never again be neglected, their new role was too important for the comfort of our visitors. The conversion of the Carriage House Restaurant was finished to our entire satisfaction in 1991, a year ahead of schedule and within budget. Swallowing what was left of our pride, we asked Lord St John to open it.

*　　　*　　　*

The Peacock Inn in Baslow—so called because it had once belonged to the Duke of Rutland whose family emblem is a peacock—came in-hand in 1972. It was run down and needed a complete overhaul. The Chatsworth Trustees decided to invest in its long-term future and Philip Jebb was invited to redesign the hotel so that the bedrooms should all face south over the home farm. I worked closely with him and, when the time came, it was my responsibility to oversee the decoration and furnishing, which I did with pleasure, using furniture in store at Chatsworth. Perhaps I was given the job because I had done up Chatsworth itself when we went to live there and was thought capable, and perhaps also because I did not cost the Trustees a penny. Had I not done it, they would have had to employ a professional decorator, which would have been a shock to their system. (When we added ten new bedrooms to the inn, in 1986, there was more budget trouble, and I had to go for the cheapest materials scoured from wholesale shops north of Oxford Street.) Eric Marsh took the lease when it opened in 1975 as the Cavendish Hotel and he still runs it thirty-five years later. Under his aegis the hotel has thrived, largely patronized by people who come to see Chatsworth.

The enlargement of the Devonshire Arms at Bolton Abbey in 1982 was a bigger project and produced an unexpected bonus for me, Chatsworth and, I hope, for John and Christine Thompson. Christine was one of three people who answered my advertisement for someone to make the soft furnishings. The applicants brought samples of their work to the interviews and hers were the best. She carried out the job to everyone's satisfaction, on time and on budget, and a few months after the hotel was finished, I got a letter from Christine saying that if we needed four willing hands at Chatsworth—John Thompson was a French polisher and could turn his hand to anything—they would be interested. 'I'm thirty-five years old and I'll work for you for twenty-five years, then I'll retire,' said Christine. A woman of her word, that is what happened—except that she and John completed twenty-six years.

In 1980 Andrew got a letter from Tom Harvey, an old friend who lived in Norfolk, whose wife, Mary Coke, a daughter of Lord Leicester, had been brought up at Holkham Hall. Tom said that the Country Fair at Holkham was extremely successful and suggested that we should hold one along the same lines at Chatsworth. Andrew passed me Tom's letter, saying, 'This is more up your street than mine.' Tom introduced me to Andrew Cuthbert, who was in charge of the team of volunteers who ran the Fair, and my Andrew agreed to give it a try. When our first Country Fair opened the next year there was something for everyone. You could buy gumboots, gloves, garlic and guns, fishing tackle, ferrets, fudge and frocks from the best shops from all over the country. In successive years there were massed pipe and military bands from the Household Cavalry, the Gurkhas, and the Royal Horse Artillery with their horse-drawn gun carriages, as well as terrier and ferret racing, clay-pigeon shooting, archery and sheepdog trials.

The Fair was a success from the start and has become an increasingly popular annual event. Its appeal is twofold: it attracts people from the industrial conurbations surrounding Chatsworth, as well as country people who enjoy fishing, shooting and hunting; and it is a rendezvous for those whose livelihoods depend on country sports. Andrew Cuthbert, who retired in 2002, was indefatigable. I used to look out of my window at daybreak and see him, hours before anyone else turned up, marking out the positions of the various tents and tracks. Thanks to him and his team of Red Socks (worn for instant identification) the Country Fair not only makes a major financial contribution to the upkeep of Chatsworth but also creates an immeasurable dollop of goodwill between Chatsworth and its public.

In 1956 we had followed Badminton and Burghley in staging annual horse trials in the park. Horse trials had become so popular and their calendar so crowded that a date was difficult to find, but early October was eventually chosen. The competitors and spectators loved the course, with its steep hills and turf that had never been ploughed, and all went well till 1988 when, at the end of the first day, a mighty storm devastated the tents and the ground was flooded. Dragging out the heavy vehicles ruined the look of the park and, as it was so late in the year, it took many months for the ground to recover. Regretfully the trials were cancelled, but in 1999 Stoker's wife, Amanda, who is devoted to the sport, reinstated them, the same year she won the three-day event at Badminton with Jaybee, ridden by Ian Stark. With Amanda's experience and support to ensure its success, this event now takes place at Chatsworth in May and once again horse-trial followers come to enjoy this demanding test of horse and rider.

In the early 1980s my friend the designer David Mlinaric told me that several of his clients had been looking without success for classic garden furniture of the kind found in old established gardens. There were several highly skilled joiners at Chatsworth, as well as the enthusiastic Bob Getty, so we thought we would try our hand at making some. Many of the models sought after by the new generation of garden owners were to be found in J. P. White's early twentieth-century *Catalogue of Garden Furniture*. We chose a selection of sturdy, unassuming benches, which would look good in gardens from Northumberland to Cornwall, and took a stand at the annual RHS Chelsea Flower Show.

I loved selling and for each of the twenty-one years that we went to Chelsea, I was on our stall Tuesday, Wednesday, Thursday and Friday, and got to know the showground, exhibitors and organizers well. Garden designers favoured our products and we exported them to the United States, France, Switzerland and Ireland. Our carpenters' workmanship was second to none and we soon had designs of our own, some copied from seats at Chatsworth and one from the popular wheelbarrow seat at Mount Congreve, reproduced with the permission of Ambrose Congreve, whose County Waterford garden has a grove of pink magnolias as tall as forest trees.

The largest seat of all was the 'Chiswick', a faithful copy of what must surely have been a William Kent design for Chiswick Villa. Copies by new manufacturers, light-heartedly named the 'Lutyens', are flimsy ghosts of the real thing. The Kent design was a much sturdier, long-lasting version of extreme beauty with rounded arms and slatted back. Our best sellers were classic plant tubs with fibreglass linings to hold large shrubs. We also did well meeting the revived fashion for wooden lavatory seats, whose middles we made into cheeseboards. We supplemented these products with items from the Orangery Shop. The Chatsworth tin trays flew off the stand—handing them over was like feeding the birds. The shop staff from Chatsworth came to help, as did Bob Getty and Wendy Coleman from the building-yard office. Alan Shimwell was invaluable, carrying boxes of trays from the car park till the string nearly cut off his fingers.

One year our stand was opposite a sandwich bar and a trail of old women, seeing somewhere to sit at last, plonked themselves down on our expensive benches, making it impossible for customers to look, measure and ponder. I had not the heart to move them on, but I was pleased that the sandwich bar had gone the following year. Nicko Henderson came to help on the stall, giving the Chatsworth staff a chance to go round the show. He put on the blue apron, tied at the neck and waist, which we all wore. Several people who had served under him in one or other of his embassies glanced at the tall figure in the apron, could not believe their eyes, walked on, came back to make sure and, still astonished, stayed for a chat. He was a brilliant salesman, but when we checked the pockets of his apron at the end of the day, his inexperience as a shop assistant was exposed and we found hundreds of pounds of forgotten tray money in notes and coins that he had thrown with his apron into the laundry pile as he left.

It is pleasing to look back at our successes, but there were failures as well. Chatsworth Food, a company selling jams, chutneys, biscuits and cakes, which were supposed to make Chatsworth's fortune, was a dismal flop. The management was useless and it quickly went out of business. One good thing came out of it for me, however: Helen Marchant. I did not have a secretary till 1986, when the secretary for Chatsworth Food worked part-time for me. By then the piles of paper on the floor of my little sitting room were toppling. When the business failed and she left, I moved my piles of paper to the ground-floor flower room, where it was easier for people to find me, and began to pester Helen, who was Andrew's secretary, for help with some typing. I was deeply appreciative of Helen's help—and still am.

The most expensive failure was the Chatsworth

Farm Shop in Elizabeth Street, in London's Belgravia. It started with a bang. I took a cockerel on a lead to welcome the Prince of Wales, who had kindly agreed to open the shop, but in spite of this and a daily crowd of customers, the cost of twice-weekly vans taking the meat and other specialities 160 miles from Pilsley to London and back, as well as the difficulty of finding reliable staff, were too great. The shop lost money and sadly had to close.

Few people realize how a house like Chatsworth, the land and the people who live on it are interdependent. Families, some of whom had been with the Cavendishes for generations, were traditionally able to find jobs as disparate as butchers, housemaids, gamekeepers, seamstresses, accountants or librarians—all with the same employer. In the nineteenth century Joseph Paxton, who came to Chatsworth at the age of twenty-three as head gardener, developed skills under the generous patronage of the Sixth Duke that later allowed him to become an MP, director of the railways and the designer of the Crystal Palace. In the twentieth century, Tom Wragg, the Edensor school master's son, became keeper of the collection; Sean Feeney, the smiling butcher whose health prevented him standing for long hours, got a job as a river bailiff. Everyone knew that an effort would be made to accommodate people's needs—something that was seldom possible for other big employers. This created a 'family' atmosphere, which I have never met elsewhere. To me it was spoiling, because starting with new people is something I find difficult. Luckily this seldom happened at Chatsworth; most of the old people remained till they retired and were usually replaced—sparing the bother of advertising—by the next-in-line from their department.

22

Distractions

Life at Chatsworth seemed to leave hardly a moment unoccupied, but thanks chiefly to the wonderful staff, my role there was flexible, and hobbies could be fitted in as well as friends. There was often no defining line between work and other interests, and sometimes one of the organizations connected to a hobby would ask me to become involved in an official way. When this happened there was a danger that what had once been fun would become work and, however enjoyable, would pin me down and I would have to sit at a table listening to everyone mumbling their thoughts. The Bakewell Show was an example. My sisters-in-law and I looked forward keenly to the Thursday after August Bank Holiday. We entered our ponies without a thought of winning and loved every moment of the parade of cattle, sheep, goats, Shire horses, hunters and successful children's ponies. When I was asked to join the committee, it became work; I still enjoyed the Show but it was different.

I have nevertheless been lucky in my life to be able to pursue several interests purely for pleasure. In middle life, grouse shooting ruled the month of August, and pheasant shooting much of November, December and January. I loved all that went with a shoot: the reunion of friends, seeing a new bit of country or finding the same patch of dying leaves beneath my feet, well remembered from the year before. Drive fifty miles in this country and you find different crops, different stone and different voices. Even the BBC has not succeeded in levelling out the latter and listening to the beaters you know if you are in Derbyshire or Devon, Somerset or Sussex, Aberdeen or Anglesey. I liked the battle with the weather, the layers of clothes and the discovery of Derri boots, after which I never had cold feet again. I loved the company of the loader—as long as he made no comment on my shooting. Alan Shimwell, who has done nearly sixty years' service at Chatsworth, both on the farm and in the garden, as well as thirty-three years of chauffeuring, never said a word as chance after chance flew over our heads with nothing to show for it. He was the perfect companion on the long car drives and so popular with our hosts that my theory was that one day they would say to me, 'Don't you bother to come next year, let's just have Alan.'

A shoot is bait for persuading people to travel a long way for a winter weekend. When I had had enough practice for friends to realize I was not intent on murdering their other guests, they invited me to shoot. An annual treat was Keir, Bill Stirling's Perthshire home, where we sometimes had five days' shooting on the trot, a sporting highlight that became known as The Festival. The same team of guns gathered every year, with Bill's sons, Archie and Johnny, representing the younger generation. The same old jokes were repeated—we would have resented any new ones. General Sir

George Collingwood, Royal Artillery, was part of The Festival scene, as was Lord Sefton, the legendary Lancastrian owner of Croxteth in Liverpool and Abbeystead in the Forest of Bowland. Collingwood was not a good shot and after a drive in which he had failed to distinguish himself, Lord Sefton said with mock scorn, 'Call yourself a gunner?' One icy morning our convoy was driving along a main road with a nasty drop on the left. Archie's Land Rover skidded and landed upside down in the field below. His father saw it happen and drove on. 'The stupid boy will be late for the first drive,' is all he muttered. Of such were the Stirlings made. Bill's brother David has gone down in history for founding the Special Air Service, and when Bill led the 2nd Special Air Service Regiment, the SAS was known as 'Stirling and Stirling'.

After two or three days, Bill, who was the most restless man I have ever known, would disappear to Greece, Abu Dhabi or wherever his business interests took him, and we carried on without him. The head keeper at Keir was Jimmy Miller. He was as square as a wrestler (which he was in his spare time) and I would not have liked to meet him on a dark night if I were up to no good, but as a guest of Bill's I could do no wrong. When Archie was about ten and at a loose end in the holidays, he said to Jimmy, 'Shall we go to the cinema this afternoon?' 'Nature is the best cinema, Mr Archie,' came the reply.

Through Ann Fleming, I got to know Sybil Cholmondeley. The second time we met she said, 'I believe you are fond of shooting, would you like to come to Houghton in December?' I would. Sybil was already old, but brimful of energy, opinions and brilliance. She was born Sassoon and she and her brother Philip were of Middle Eastern origin, which gave them a touch of the exotic. A product of pre-First-World-War Paris and London, Sybil had acted as her father's hostess from the age of seventeen and her upbringing had given her the impeccable manners of her generation and kind. I have seen her sitting bolt upright, in apparently rapt attention, being talked at by a thumping bore. She was an example to us all.

After marriage in 1913 to the Marquess of Cholmondeley, Sybil took on Houghton Hall, the magnificent eighteenth-century Norfolk house built for Sir Robert Walpole. Rock Cholmondeley, who was beautiful looking—and aware of it—was a sportsman, soldier, landowner and hereditary Lord Great Chamberlain. He was not fond of social life and as Sybil was of a generation of women who arranged their lives around their husbands, they did not invite many people to stay. Sybil took to country life, learned about the farms, woods and the people who looked after them, and soon joined Rock in the excellent shooting the estate provided. It was unusual for a woman to shoot in the 1930s but Sybil quickly became proficient, as she did in everything that interested her.

I had never seen Houghton before and, like everyone else, was knocked sideways by its unique beauty and by the Cholmondeleys themselves. The approach to the house is past rows of white estate cottages, through a display of white iron gates by a white lodge and into the park; more white comes as ghostly fallow deer pass to and fro under the great oaks. William Kent's opulent rooms were the ideal background for Sybil. On an easel in the sitting room, which was hung with yellow silk, was Holbein's *Lady with a Squirrel*. In the room next door, Oudry's *White Duck* overlooked the French furniture that Sybil described in a throwaway line as 'My brother Philip's things, the best of their kind'. The portraits of her mother and herself by Sargent and one of her by William Orpen ('Old Orps' she called him) positively glowed. Whatever she said was made important by her precise enunciation and clipped tones, lips closing on the last word and often followed by a laugh. When talking one day of diminishing congregations in country churches, she said, 'The trouble is that they don't understand what "verily verily" means.' You soon got to know who 'our neighbours' were— the royal family at Sandringham. The Queen Mother told me that one evening after dining with the said neighbours, Sybil looked for her sable coat in the hall. 'Where's my weasel?' she said to a bemused footman.

I was the only guest on that first visit—the other guns were local Norfolk farming friends—and I felt honoured to be there. We set off in a white Land Rover to see country unknown to me but which was to become familiar over the years. An east wind straight from Russia can make waiting in a field of frozen plough uncomfortable, but at Houghton there were no long waits because the pheasants were wild and got up as soon as the beaters entered the woods—unlike reared birds that are apt to flush. Sybil was impervious to wind or rain and wore a miserable little pair of short gumboots. 'Naval issue,' she announced proudly (she had helped to found the WRNS during the

First World War and rose to be a much respected Commander during the Second). She knew the army of beaters by name and fully appreciated their efforts, which involved tramping through wet kale up to their waists, to provide the sport she loved. Like all well-mannered hosts she was often the 'walking gun', dealing with the birds that fly back over the beaters. She shot with a pair of 16-bore 'over and unders' and missed few. I was impressed and remained so every time I saw her in action.

Sybil came to Chatsworth to shoot, complete with loader, guns and heavy luggage. She went up to change for dinner but could not find her jewel box. There was a frantic search. Where could it be? It transpired that the box was so big and heavy that the pantry staff had mistaken it for her cartridge case and taken it to the gunroom. Andrew asked her what she would like for breakfast, always plentiful before a cold winter's day in the open air: 'I like lifting the lids,' was the answer.

I was visiting a friend in King Edward VII hospital one day and as I was leaving an ambulance drew up. I stepped aside for the stretcher to go in and realized its burden was Sybil. She had broken an ankle tripping up in her hurry to answer the telephone. 'Stay and talk,' she said, so I followed the stretcher into her room. A nurse with a clipboard came to take her details. 'Hello,' she said breezily. Not used to being addressed in the modern manner with such familiarity, Sybil gave a withering look and said, 'What is all this HELLO?' and dismissed the nurse with, 'I will ring when my friend has gone.'

* * *

Andrew's family had been connected to the Sport of Kings for centuries and racing was one of his great loves. I had been passionately interested when I was growing up but the reality of owning a racehorse was different from my dreams as a sixteen-year-old and I never saw the point of it. Had the stud been at Chatsworth, it would have been a different story and we would have known the horses since they were foals. As it was, they were bought, trained and sent to stud by A. N. Other. It was remote control and therefore not attractive to me, though of course I understood the thrill for Andrew whenever he had a winner, and I still keep a keen interest in the progeny of Bachelor Duke and Compton Place, two of his horses that were good enough to stand as stallions.

Race meetings were part of the social round which we both enjoyed. In 1948, and again in 1950 and 1953, we were invited to stay at Windsor Castle for the Royal Meeting at Ascot. During those bleak post-war years, these visits were the most cheering days I can remember. It is uplifting to see something arranged and carried out to perfection, down to the most minute detail. The invitation was for five nights (Monday to Saturday) and four days' racing. The weather is always a gamble and had to be taken into consideration, but somehow four daytime outfits for the races and five best evening dresses were gathered up.

Andrew and I were allocated a bedroom, dressing room and even a sitting room looking out over the Long Walk—the straight double avenue of trees that leads to the famous copper horse. The day's plans and the times when we had to be ready were typed out and left on our writing table each morning—all very helpful in an unfamiliar world. The welcome and 'putting at ease' by the ladies-in-waiting and equerries made everything immediately enjoyable. One year I had not been well and was allowed breakfast in bed. The tray was as big as a table and apparently made of cast iron—a knee-breaker—but the exquisite set of china and the delicious things on it reminded me that it was old-fashioned and therefore desirable. A band played under our window every morning and also in the room next to the drawing room where we sat (or rather stood) in the early evenings.

The drawing rooms were brilliantly decorated with lashings of gold leaf and the furniture, which was upholstered in bright green in one room and bright red in the next, was polished to such a degree that it nearly outshone the guests and their diamonds. The King and Queen and the Princesses Elizabeth and Margaret were the last to enter so there was plenty of time to gaze at the scarlet, six-foot-high standard fuchsias growing in Sèvres tubs. There were about twenty-four guests at dinner and the King and Queen sat opposite each other in the middle of the long table. If an owner or trainer had a winner whilst a guest at the castle, it was traditional for him or her to say a few words after dinner. Jeremy Tree, who was successful from the start of his career as a trainer, turned out a winner and was so worried about having to speak that he was unable to eat a morsel, most unusually for him—as his figure showed. The superb china plates followed by gold ones were whisked away from him as clean as they arrived. But his speech passed off well and I expect he had double helpings for breakfast the next morning.

On our second visit to Windsor, I found sitting next to the King at dinner a rather difficult and frightening experience. No doubt because of frustration at his increasing frailty, his mood was uncertain and at one point he banged his fist on the table so hard that the glasses trembled, and so did I, thinking I had said or done something wrong. The Queen, opposite, gave me reassuring glances. No doubt the King's anger was a symptom of the illness about which we knew nothing then. It must have been an ordeal for him to sit through all those dinners and if we had been told how unwell he was, we would have understood the outburst.

To be driven in a carriage as part of the procession down the racecourse at Ascot was a fascinating experience. As well as the obvious fun of it—the jockey's-eye view of the course and the intoxicating smell of horses and harness—it had an unexpected side. We were taken by car through the park from Windsor Castle to join the carriages. Trotting down the narrow lanes to reach the racecourse, our route was lined with onlookers who, I imagine, had no idea that whatever they said could be heard by the occupants of the carriages: 'Doesn't she look awful in that hat?' 'Who's *he*?' as well as admiring words for the Queen. When it was our turn to drive between the lines of critics, there was an audible 'Ohhh', a groan of disappointment when they realized that all the royals had passed and they were left with a few unknowns, not even a movie star.

Some forty years later when Stoker became Her Majesty's Representative at Ascot, I stayed with him and Amanda in the 'tied house' that goes with the job. The house is just behind the racecourse stands and one can see the legions of workers arriving in the early morning. Stoker took me round the private boxes used by the most prosperous owners. These were decorated in a way new to me, with walls covered in a loose backing on which hung rows of waterproof pockets. Once the florists had finished filling these, the walls were solid with lilies, roses and other midsummer blooms—the last word in sweet-smelling luxury— and they looked like extravagant chintz. It was as entertaining to see these preparations as to watch the racing itself—the best horses in the world competing for the glory of winning (as well as for prize money).

On Epsom Derby Day, racing affects the English public across the board—as the old saying goes, 'All men are equal on the turf and under it.' Four-in-hand coaches and gypsies with their coloured horses join open double-decker buses in the jostling crowds. When the Derby was run on a Wednesday, things seemed to come to a full stop in government and elsewhere, and anyone who could headed for Epsom. Andrew's cousin Betty Salisbury (married to Bobbety, who joined his House of Lords colleagues at Epsom) was not a regular racegoer. In 1968, when the American-owned horse Sir Ivor won, a friend asked her if she had seen Sir Ivor. 'Sir Ivor who?' she said. There was a long walk from the members' enclosure to the paddock, all of it in full view of what is called 'the general public'. I often thought that when the

Queen and the royal family walked down to the paddock they were as close to their sporting subjects as they would ever be, drawn together by a shared enthusiasm (today the paddock is immediately behind the stands). One year when Uncle Harold, the popular Minister of Housing at the time, and Aunt Dorothy were walking to the paddock, the crowd seemed extraordinarily vociferous in their welcome, clapping and cheering him all the way. He took off his top hat and smiled at these devoted supporters. What he did not know was that immediately behind him were the newly wed Aly Khan and Rita Hayworth.

In 1965 Andrew achieved his ambition of owning a top-class horse. Park Top had cost five hundred guineas as a yearling when she was bought by Andrew's friend and trainer, Bernard van Cutsem, for another of his owners. The owner thought the filly too cheap and decided he did not want her, so Bernard offered her to Andrew—a proof, if proof were needed, of the part played by luck in racing. Andrew had to be patient; Park Top did not run as a two-year-old, but Bernard saw a future for her and she went on to be a successful three-, four- and five-year-old, winning the Coronation Cup at Epsom, the Hardwicke Stakes, the Ribblesdale Stakes and the King George VI and Queen Elizabeth Stakes at Ascot, among other important races, as well as coming second in the Prix de l'Arc de Triomphe.

Andrew's book, *Park Top: A Romance of the Turf*, which was published in 1976, revealed as much about him as it did about the mare. The ease and speed with which he wrote it were amazing: he went to a hotel in the north of Scotland for a weekend and came back with the manuscript as good as finished. In 2003, when he began work on his memoirs—drawn from notes he had made over a period of twenty years—it was a different story. He was unwell and found it difficult to concentrate for more than an hour or so at a time. Had it not been for Helen Marchant, who persuaded him to produce a little more each day, and his publisher, Michael Russell, *Accidents of Fortune* would have fizzled out unfinished. As it was, his two helpers were in constant touch and wove his words into a highly readable, honest account of his life. It is too self-deprecating but people can read between the lines, especially when it comes to his account of war service in Italy.

*   *   *

In the 1960s, Shetland ponies became of paramount interest to me. Muv had bought two mares and a stallion to run on Inch Kenneth and their first foal, Easter Bonnet, was born a few days before Muv died. She bequeathed the ponies to Sophy and they came to Chatsworth, but Sophy was more interested in riding ponies than in showing them and so I took them on. Their numbers grew as foals were born and purchases made; at one point I had fifty-five Shetlands, both standard-height blacks and coloured miniatures.

The ponies were looked after by Tommy Jones, a Welshman who came to Chatsworth for a few weeks in the late 1930s to walk a Shire stallion and stayed for the rest of his days. After the advent of tractors, he had had the dismal task of taking the magnificent Shire stallions, pride and joy of

Andrew's grandfather, to be shot and hauled away for dog meat. From Shires to Shetlands was a downgrade in Tommy's eyes, but our success in the show ring made up for it, and he and his wife, Emily, became part of the Shetland scene. I bought a big horsebox with a sleeping compartment, which became known as The Queen Mary by fellow exhibitors. Tommy and Emily stayed in it and gave tea and drinks all round. We showed the ponies all over the country and in 1973, our best year, three of my Shetlands took the championships: 'Chatsworth Darkie' at the Royal Welsh, 'Chatsworth Drogo' at the Royal, and 'Wells Erica' at the Royal Highland.

In 1969 Tommy drove The Queen Mary to Austria and came back with Maximillian, a Haflinger stallion, and two mares—some of the first of the breed to be imported into this country. To announce their arrival to the British horse-loving public I took a stand at the Royal Show where they created a tremendous amount of interest. My sister Pam and I hired a caravan, parked it behind the horses' stalls and spent the week there. Pam made lunch for crowds of friends, we sat on straw bales and were totally happy. Across the grass was the caravan of the renowned show jumper Harvey Smith and his early morning ablutions became of increasing interest as the days went by. The Haflingers soon grew in popularity and numbers, their quiet temperament and sturdy shape making them suitable for heavy riders and disabled adults. I like the heavier type of Haflinger, capable of hauling thinnings in woods too steep for tractors. These were set to work at Chatsworth but I soon realized that the handlers needed training as well as the horses. A young man on our forestry staff, who had never led a horse or pony, put his foot in the way and was trodden on. After this the head forester thought it wiser to withdraw the horses from service.

A regular in the sheep lines at the Royal Show was Araminta Aldington, founder of the Jacob Sheep Society. Araminta lives, breathes, dreams, sleeps, shears, feeds, doses and eats her sheep. Her clothes are made from their fleece and it is sometimes hard to tell the shepherdess from her flock. There she would be in her caravan, talking to visitors who had never heard of Jacobs. A flock have run in the park at Chatsworth since they were first documented in 1762 and when Araminta asked me to join the Society, I happily accepted. The breed had always been of interest to a few owners but until Araminta took charge of the Society they were just park ornaments. With her at the helm, I knew it would do well but I had no idea just how successful it would become and how the quality of sheep would improve; Jacobs have long since been erased from the Rare Breeds list. In 1971 I was invited to be the Society's first president. Our inaugural meeting was held in a room in the old Farmers' Union building in Knightsbridge. A group of 'fanciers' were shuffling around, uncertain quite where to sit and what to do, when the door opened, a man put his head in and said, 'Are you Watercress?'

Poultry has been important to me since childhood. I thought there should be something alive in the garden at Chatsworth and hens were the answer. Stately Buff Cochins waddled around the greenhouses and when threatened by visiting dogs and toddlers crept under the branches of the yew trees that trailed to the ground. The legs of Buff Cochins are feathered down to the feet and they do not like getting wet, so the flower beds were spared their scratching. They were free to go wherever they liked and must have been the most photographed poultry in the British Isles. Meanwhile more and more pens went up to house various rare breeds of chicken.

I realized that the game larder, rejected as the site for a restaurant, would be a handy place to keep a flock of commercial hens. The feeding of the game larder hens was a daily entertainment for the visitors. Sometimes some of their children helped me to collect the eggs and it was a required expedition for my own grandchildren, who called it 'The Granny Show'. The new flock had 1,000 acres of park at their disposal but soon congregated around the visitors' cars, having discovered that the occupants were apt to bring picnics. They became increasingly tame with the car-borne humans, snatching sandwiches and hopping into the cars in the hopes of finding the source of the picnics. All was well until twenty of my dear ones got into a school bus, to the delight of the children. They were not noticed by the staff until they had reached the other side of the bridge, when a teacher shooed them out, expecting them to find their own way home. A fox came in daylight and murdered for fun, as these serial destroyers do. The corpses were photographed, mostly headless with feathers all over the place. I hung the photos in the Farmyard to show the children the nature of this random killer.

The eggs went to the Chatsworth Farm Shop and

sold out as soon as they arrived. A television camera came. 'What do you feed them on?' the interviewer asked. 'Pellets, wheat, maize and kitchen scraps,' I said. The next day a fellow turned up, the double of Hodges, the ARP Warden in *Dad's Army*: 'Is it true you give your hens kitchen scraps?' he asked me. 'Yes,' I replied. 'Well, it's against the law and you must stop at once,' he said. 'Don't you think that the food we eat is good enough for them?' I ventured. He went off, muttering, 'Next time . . .' which I suppose meant prison.

I still have a varied flock: Welsummers and enigmatic Burford Browns for their dark brown eggs; pretty, shy, idiotic Light Sussex; even stupider White Leghorns who dash around on long yellow legs; and neat, clever, sociable little Warrens. My Warrens do not know their luck— they had been destined for an intensive poultry farm. The pecking order rules among the flock: there is a general, some colonels, captains galore, and private soldiers who get out of the way of their superiors at feeding time. The carry-on of this all-female cast is as good as a play and, like a play, is repeated, word for word, gesture for gesture, every day—with the odd matinee thrown in. (Alan Bennett and Tom Stoppard please note: you are welcome to come any day for copy.)

Border Collies are said to be the cleverest dogs in the world and mine was certainly the cleverest dog I ever had. His mother belonged to a Chatsworth shepherd and he was born in a shed at Dunsa, the farm buildings nearest to Edensor. The puppies in the litter were all spoken for except one and the shepherd agreed to let me have him. I

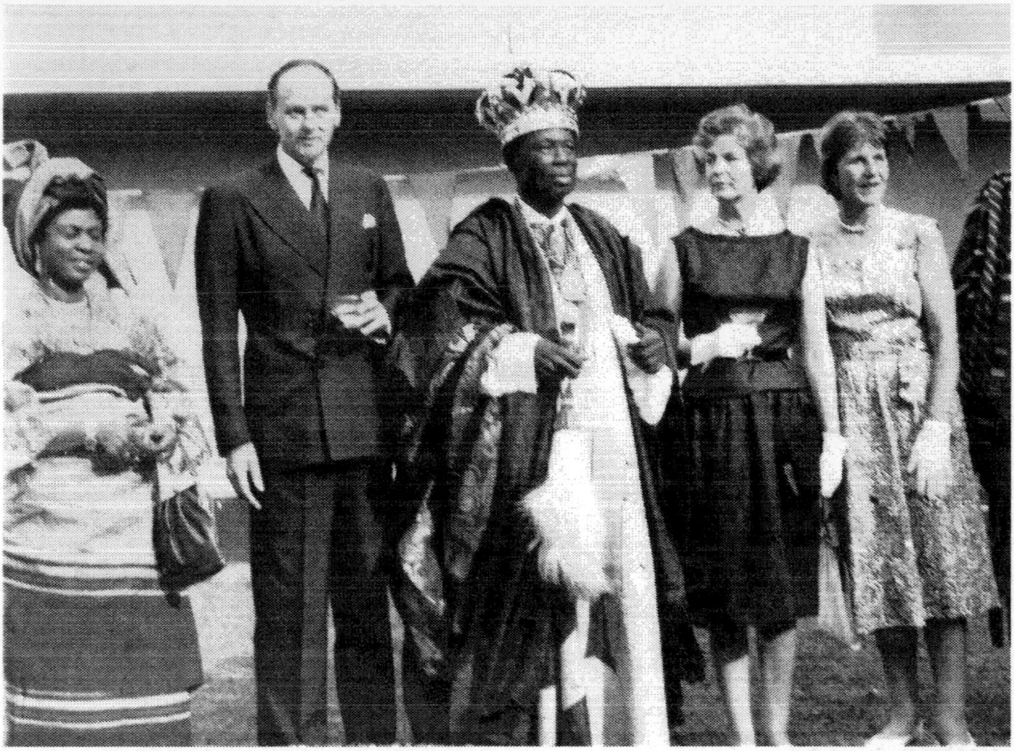

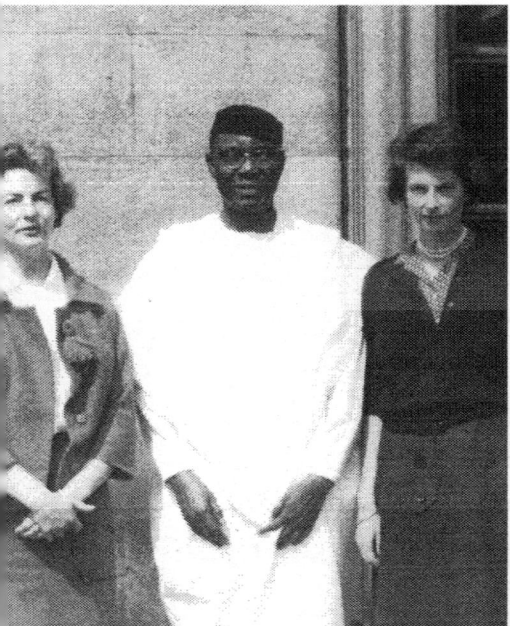

Lagos, 1962 (*l. to r.*) the Olori of Lagos, Andrew, the Oba of Lagos, DD, Dorothea Head

With Dr Nnamdi Azikiwe (Zik) and my sister-in-law Elizabeth Cavendish. Chatsworth, 1961

Visit of the Shah of Persia to Chatsworth

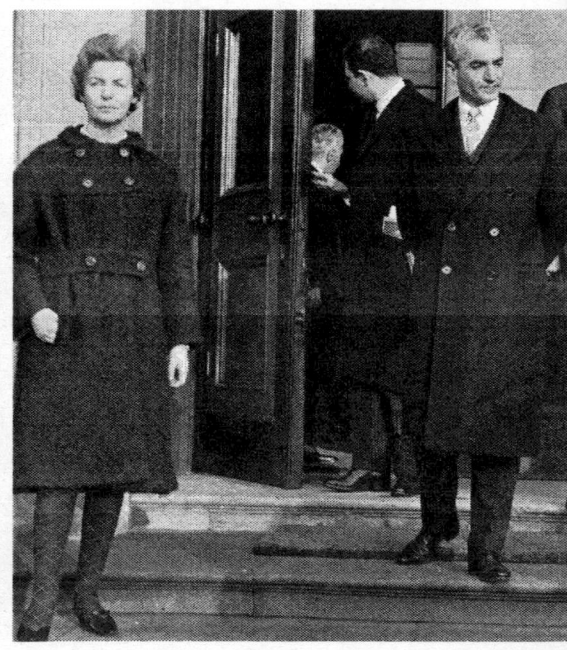

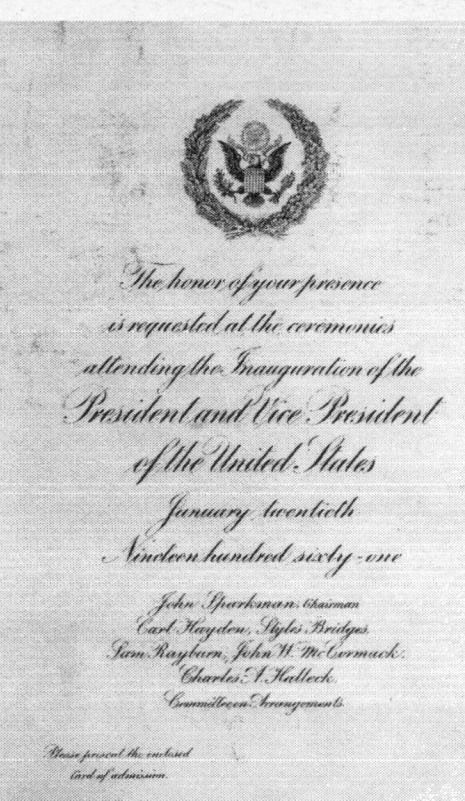

Left: Invitation to the Inauguration of President John F. Kennedy

The honor of your presence is requested at the ceremonies attending the Inauguration of the *President and Vice President of the United States* January twentieth Nineteen hundred sixty-one

John Sparkman, Chairman
Carl Hayden, Styles Bridges,
Sam Rayburn, John W. McCormack,
Charles A. Halleck,
Committee on Arrangements

Please present the enclosed
Card of admission.

Below: Greeting Robert Kennedy on his visit to Chatsworth in 1964 (Eddy Sackville-West is immediately behind me). *By kind permission of Ron Duggins*

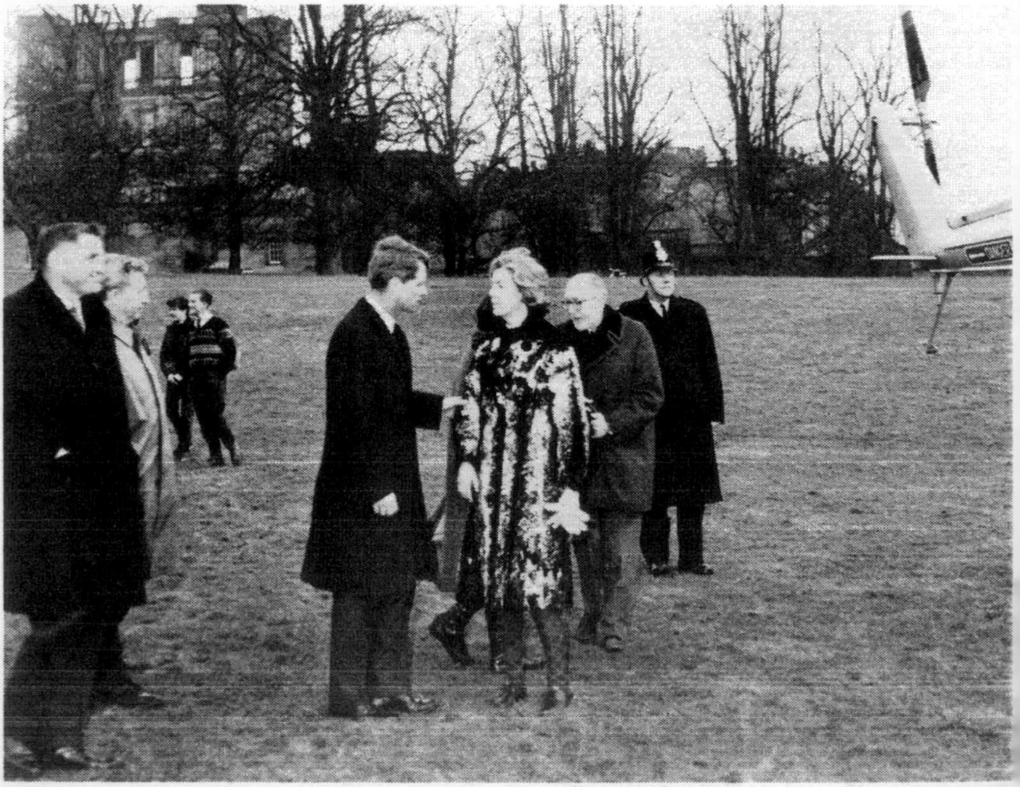

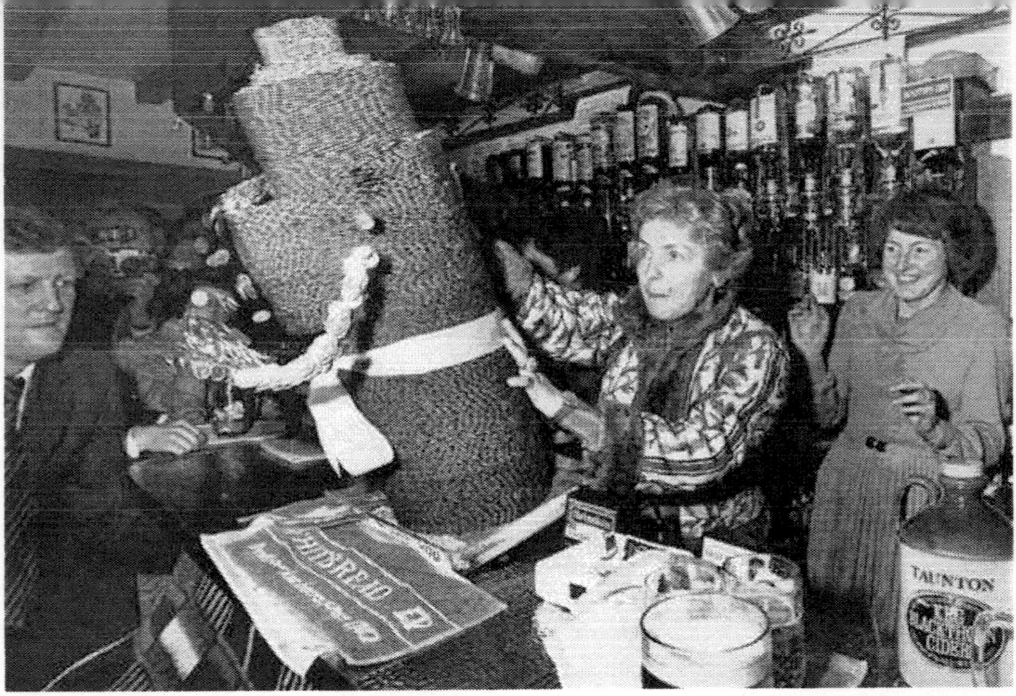

Pushing over a pile of pennies at a charity event in Whitwell, Derbyshire

Serving behind the counter at the Orangery Shop at Chatsworth

With Sophy at the Countryside March, 1997

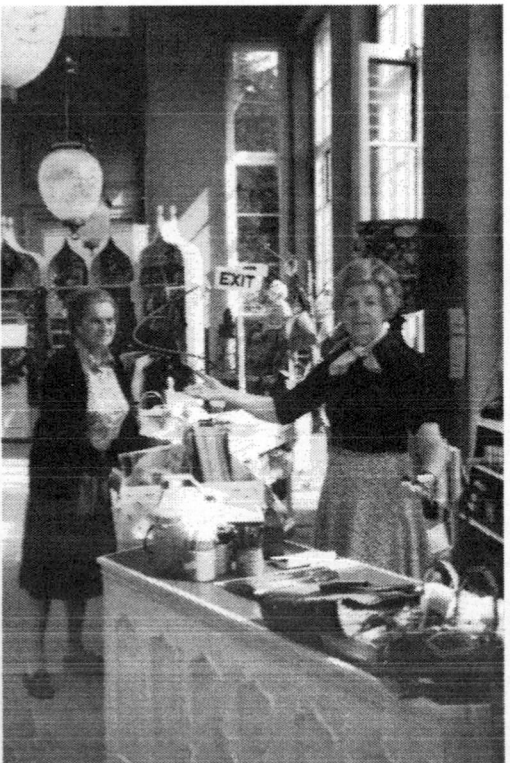

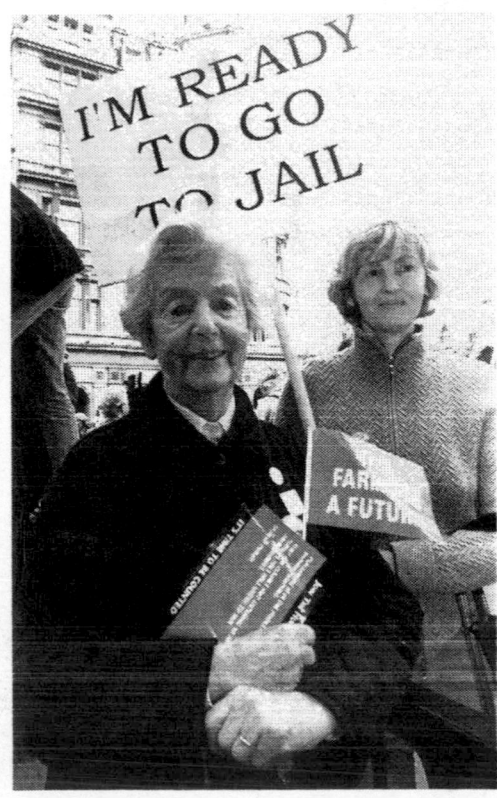

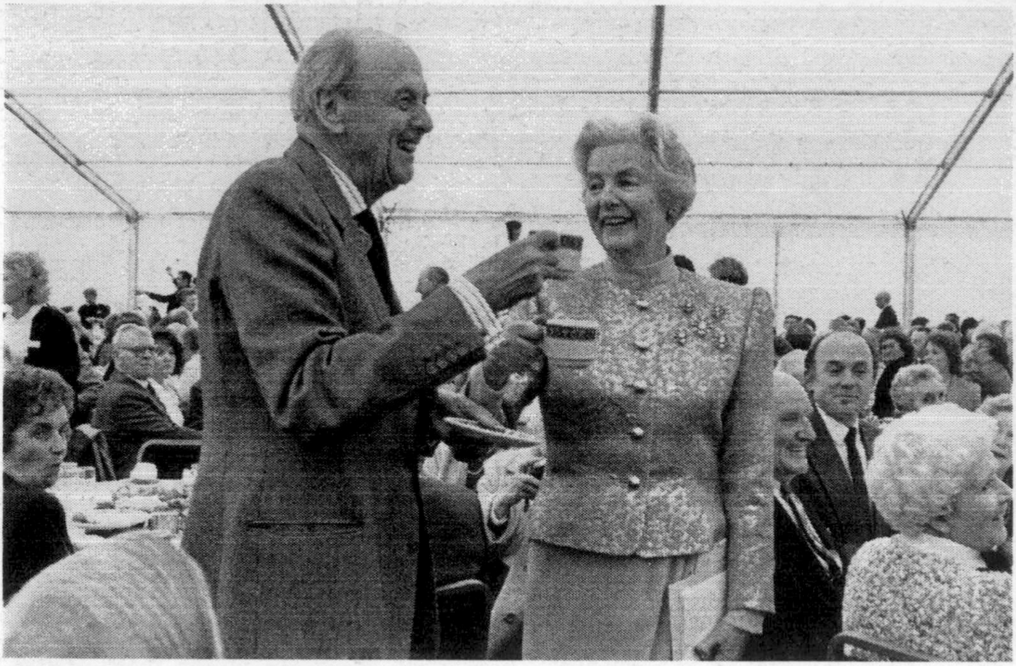

Celebrating our Golden Wedding at Chatsworth with over 1,000 couples from Derbyshire who also married in 1941. *By kind permission of Ron Duggins*

Tercentenary of the dukedom. Chatsworth, 1994

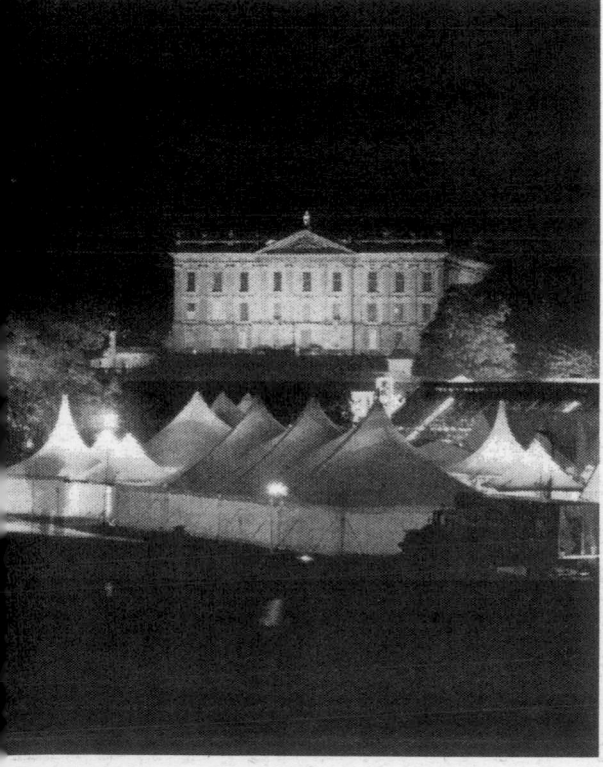

With the Prince of Wales, 2000

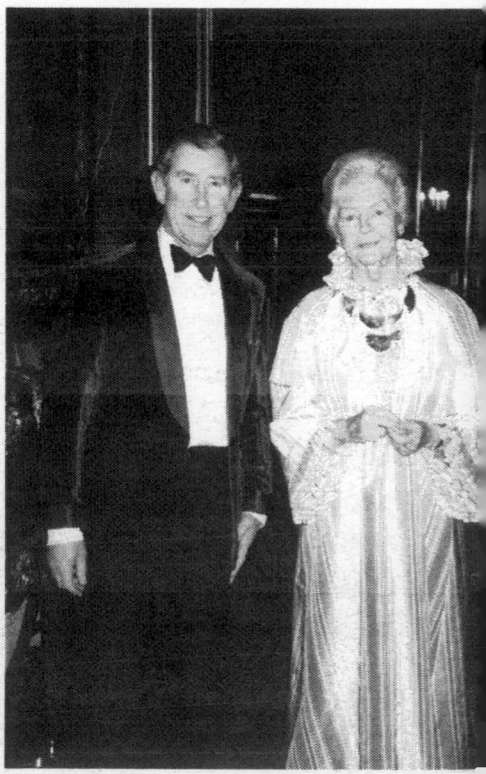

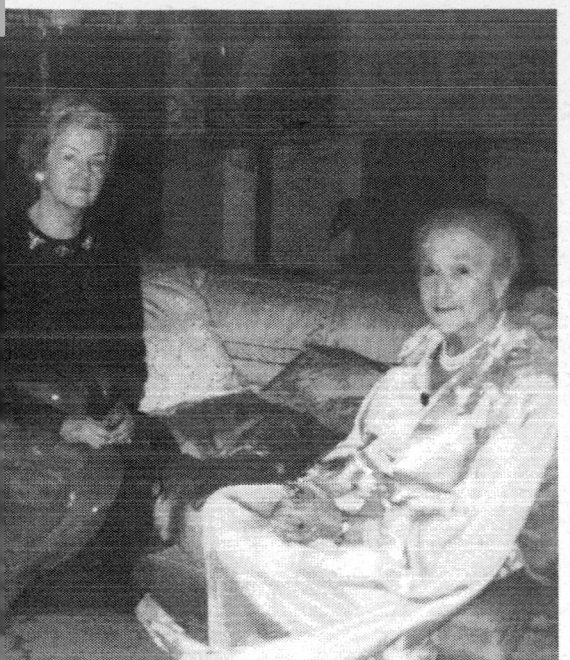

With Sybil Cholmondeley at Houghton

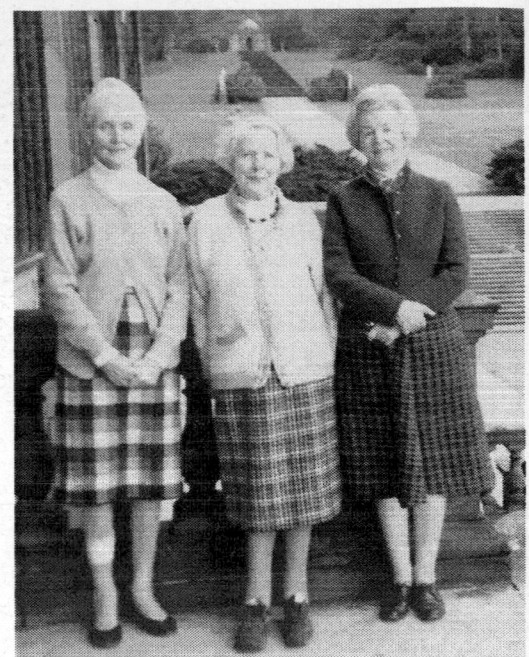

Diana, Pamela and DD at Chatsworth

With Jean-Pierre Béraud, chef and entrepreneur, wearing his fortieth birthday party wig, 10 August 1996. He was killed in a car crash two months later

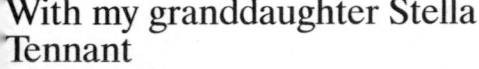

With my granddaughter Stella Tennant

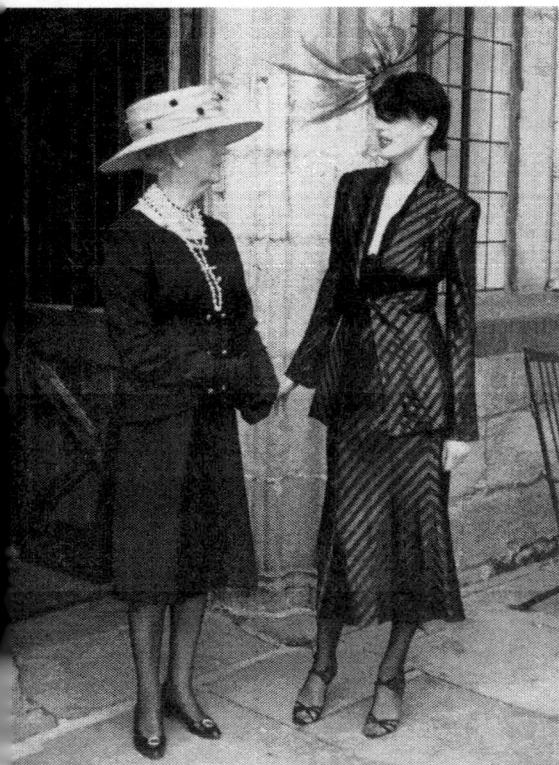

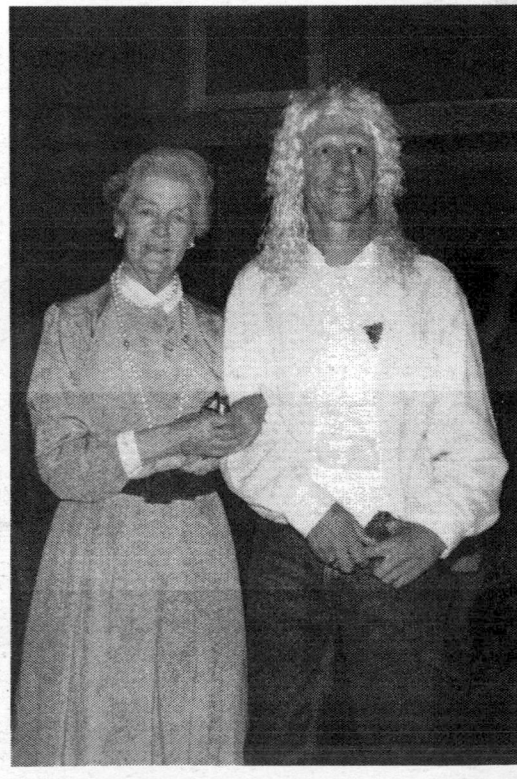

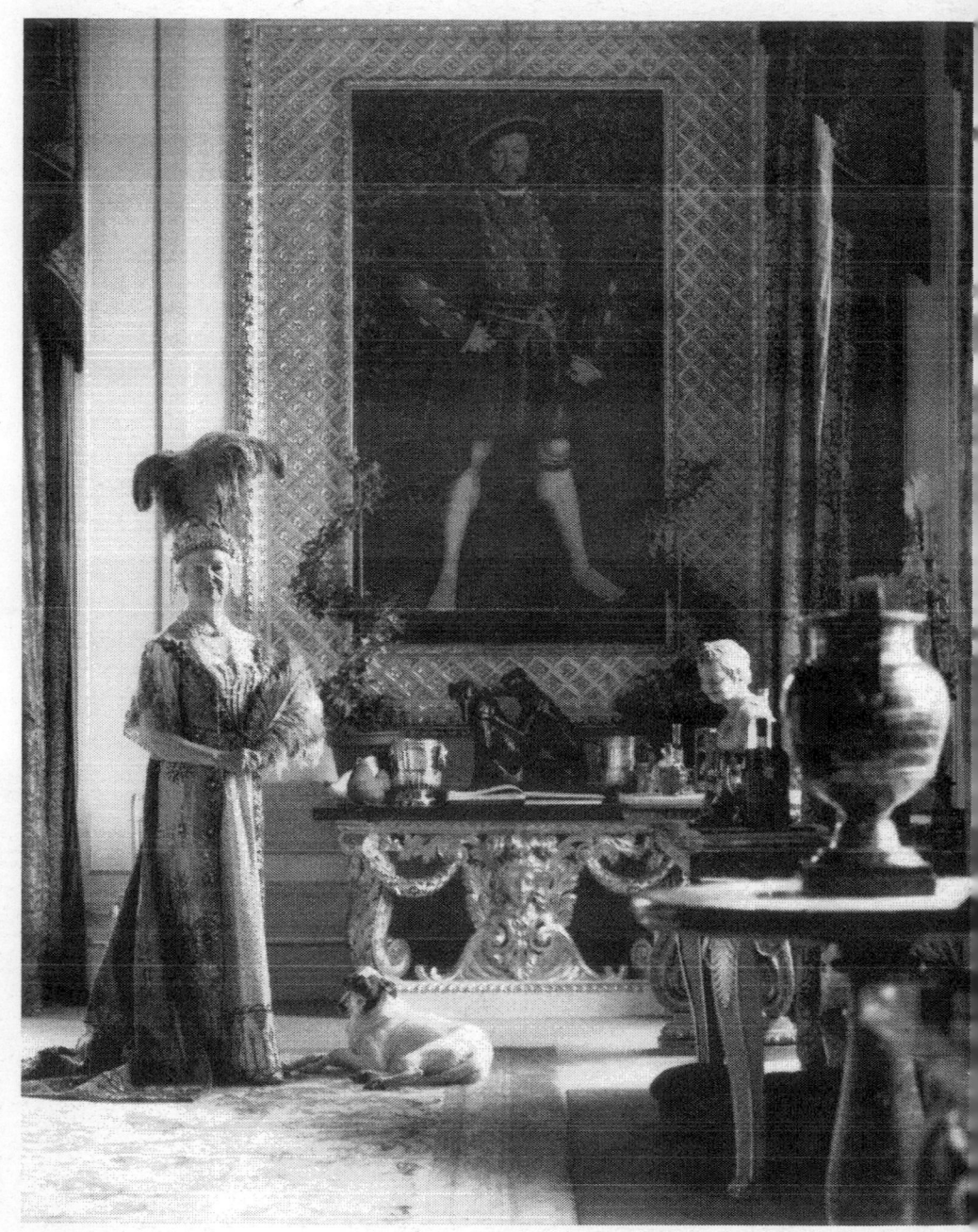

At Andrew's and my eightieth birthday party in the dress made by Worth for Duchess Louise for the Devonshire House Ball in 1897. Chatsworth, 2000. *By kind permission of Simon Upton*

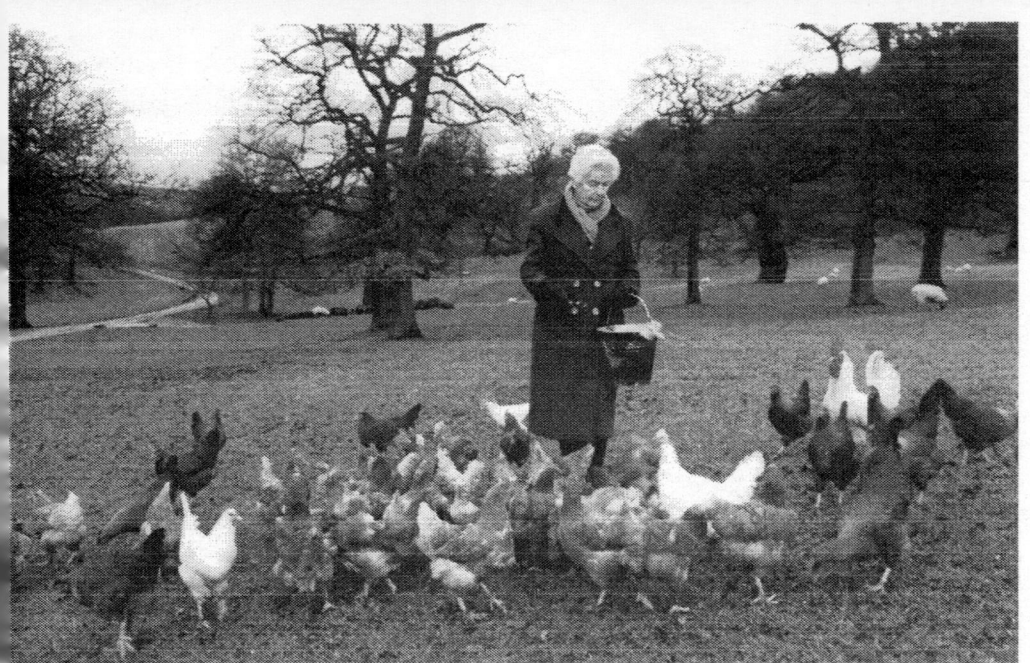

Feeding the hens. *By kind permission of Bridget Flemming*

With my great-grandchildren in 2009 (*l. to r.*) Barney Dunne, Rosa Tennant, Jake Carter, Lily Hill, Victor Hill, Marcel Lasnet, Cecily Lasnet, Alfie Carter, Harry Tennant, Ned Carter, Georgia Tennant, Jasmine Lasnet, Iris Lasnet, Willa Carter, Cosmo Dunne, Isla Tennant, Maud Cavendish.
By kind permission of Charlotte Bromley-Davenport

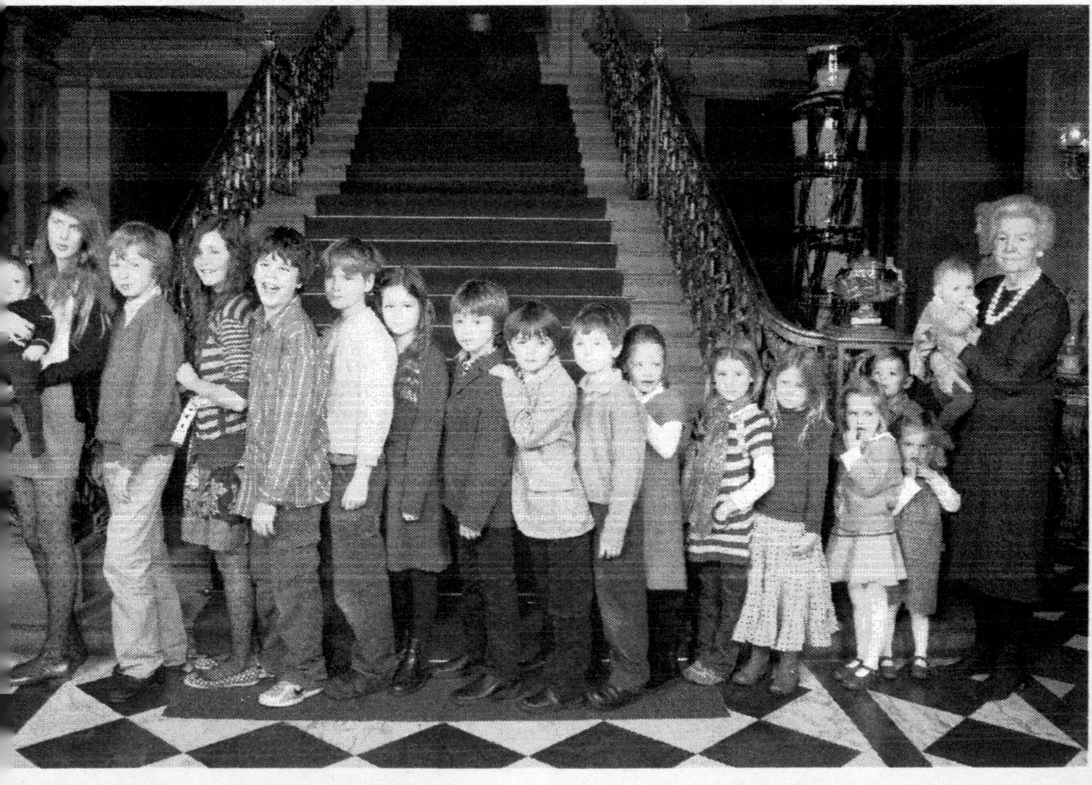

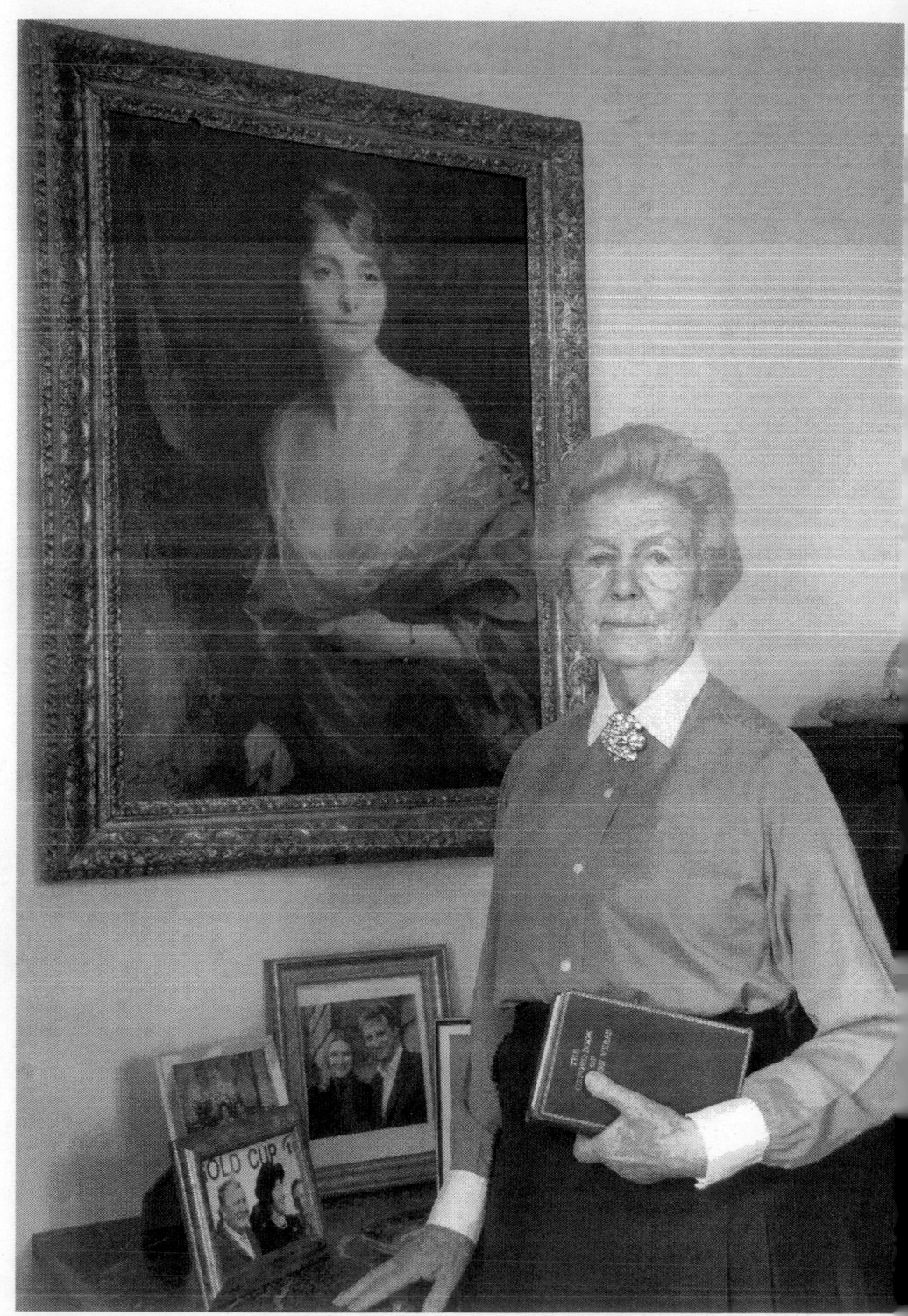

Aged ninety at the Old Vicarage, 2010, under the portrait of Muv painted by Philip de Laszlo in 1916—four years before I was born. *By kind permission of Bridget Flemming*

soon understood that Collies are different from other breeds. They yearn to work but not all come up to the necessary standard to be of use to shepherds. I realized that I needed lessons before I could co-operate with Collie (his name as well as his breed). My tutor was Chris Furness, trainer of many winners at sheepdog trials. Chris came to give me one-to-one tutorials (or one-to-two in this case) but it was soon evident that I was more in need of teaching than my dog.

The first lesson showed the strength of instinct in a Collie, whose ancestors have been bred to work sheep for generations. We were in a paddock with thirty ewes. Collie was getting excited and was eyeing the sheep in a threatening way so I had him on a lead. 'Let him go,' said Chris. Heart in mouth, I did as I was told and off to my right went Collie. He knew to get behind the sheep and obeyed my shout of 'Lie Down' (which we had already practised in the sheep-free garden at Chatsworth). The ewes trotted past us and Collie stayed prone, watching their every move. His behaviour during that first lesson gave me confidence and we went on practising the orders, 'Come Bye' (for go to the right) and 'Away' (for go to the left). I never mastered the whistle with two fingers stuck in the mouth, so I cheated and bought a little metal one. I lived in terror of swallowing it but never dared say so. The rapport between handler and dog is uncanny and after a while Collie often anticipated the command I was about to give. The tone of voice is enough to tell the dog when he has overstepped the mark; I was not immediately forgiven when I ticked off the headstrong but touchy workman and Collie sulked.

When the International Sheepdog Trials were held in the park at Chatsworth, I took Collie to watch. The poor dog sat intently, paws on the chair in front, so longing to join in that I had to wind his lead round and round my hand to hold him. He hated the clapping (sheepdogs' ears are super-sensitive and can hear commands and whistles over long distances) and he did not appreciate the stands full of onlookers, friends and relations of the competitors, to whom the outcome meant so much. Collie and I never became proficient enough to enter a trial, but we had fun at home. I was sitting in my car in a stationary queue one day, waiting to cross the bridge in front of Chatsworth. Visitors are polite to the cattle and sheep that get in their way on the drive and I realized that there were some sheep standing in front of us. They could not go forwards because of the fence and cattle grid, and would not turn back because there were pedestrians on the bridge. I got out of the car and Collie was off in a flash, doing his job of bringing them back. The visitors were entertained by this unexpected cabaret turn that enabled them to reach the house. After Collie, I always wanted a sheepdog by my side, but Andrew thought the rounding up of children in the garden was not a good idea as the nipped ankle of a child (going in what Collie thought was the wrong direction) was a bit too much for the mothers of our young visitors. So I have never had another of these canine geniuses.

*   *   *

In 1995, to my joy and amazement, I was invited to

be president of the Royal Agricultural Society of England. Had I been told in my caravan years that this honour would come my way, I would never have believed it. The distinguished members of the Council, who could teach good manners to all and sundry, allowed me hours in the Poultry Tent, the Sheep Pens, the Rare Breeds Survival Trust stand, the Shetland Pony lines and other treats. I had one small triumph as president: persuading those illustrious gentlemen to ride on the miniature railway around the showground. I have some photos of them, in bowler hats, of course, knees up to their chins, pretending to enjoy this new experience. The last Royal Show has now taken place and it is sad that it is all over. I have no doubt, however, that good will arise from the ashes and that the Stoneleigh site will be put to use for excellence in everything to do with the land, albeit in a different form.

I lost my nerve out hunting when I was nineteen. A new horse turned out to be one of the clumsy few more likely to fall at an obstacle than clear it. Two days on this crasher was enough and to my lasting sorrow I have never been out hunting on a horse since. I am, however, still passionate about field sports. The march organized by the Countryside Alliance to demonstrate against the banning of fox-hunting and other field sports was the highlight of 1997. Chatsworth provided a bus to take gamekeepers, river bailiffs, foresters, gardeners, office staff, cleaners and other field-sports supporters who wished to join in this unique outing. Some had only ventured to London once or twice in their lives; one had never set foot so far south before or seen a motorway service station.

Our land agent, Roger Wardle, who went with the Chatsworth group, told me that when they got on the tube at Wembley, the train was empty. It started to fill as they drew closer to Central London and a passenger, staring at this noisy, hairy, tweedy crowd, turned to Roger and said, 'Who are all these people? Gay Rights?' The Chatsworth party enjoyed the march and the company of men and women of like mind, but were thankful not to live in such a squashed-up place.

Sadly, Sophy and I, who had set off from Chesterfield Street, never found them. Perhaps this was not surprising as some three-quarters of a million people from rural England, Wales, Scotland and Northern Ireland had flocked to London to show the strength of their feelings. Talk about a cross-section: farriers and fishermen, dukes and drainers, all marching for the freedom to enjoy the sports of their forefathers. There were velvet-capped huntsmen and whippers-in from all over the country, from the Quorn to the Blencathra (John Peel's Lake District pack), from the Devon and Somerset Stag Hounds to the Banwen (the South Wales miners' pack)—picking up the Duke of Beaufort's on the way. All accents mixed—a merry crowd on a serious mission. Sophy and I crossed Park Lane into Hyde Park where there was a stand for the speakers. We were in time to hear Baroness Mallalieu, the Labour life peeress who adores hunting, give her impassioned speech: 'Hunting is our music. It is our poetry. It is our art. It is our pleasure. It is where many of our best friendships are made. It is our community. It is our whole way of life.' She understands.

Sophy carried a banner saying, 'I'M READY TO

GO TO JAIL'. Another slogan spotted was, 'EAT BRITISH LAMB, 50,000 FOXES CAN'T BE WRONG'. We left Hyde Park for Piccadilly where we paused to collect a badge from David Hockney that said, 'END BOSSINESS SOON'. Sound advice indeed. With Piccadilly Circus and the Haymarket behind us, we turned right into Trafalgar Square and down Whitehall where for centuries groups of demonstrators from every conceivable minority have marched for justice or recognition. In spite of the passionate feelings of the marchers that day, there was no trouble with the police. When we reached Downing Street (which was well fortified against us) I pointed out the sign to the Welshmen who had become our companions. They stopped as if shot and started shouting insults at the Prime Minister to awaken the dead—but not Mr Blair, he had gone to ground.

Parliament Square, where the tall, handsome keepers from Keir suddenly appeared, was so full of people we could hardly move. Having, we hoped, made our point, Sophy and I walked home through St James's Park, past the Horseguards, up the Duke of York's Steps and into Pall Mall. The famous gentlemen's clubs had opened their doors, even to women, and were handing out sandwiches to anyone who asked for them. Then we had a stroke of luck. One of the Hambro family was walking with us up St James's Street and said, 'Where are you going to have lunch?' and we joined him at Wilton's, a haven after the excitement and the long walk.

One incident from the march remains in my mind. Emma (my grandson Eddie Tennant's wife) was born and brought up in Northumberland where she went out hunting from an early age. She was detailed by the organizers to stand at the top of the moving stairs of the tube station to meet the demonstrators from Northumbria. The first person to emerge was astonished to see 'Our Emma'. 'Oh,' he said, 'I thought London was a big place and the first person I see is you.' No doubt there were many such stories, but one that particularly pleased the organizers was that this vast crowd left no litter.

*   *   *

Writing was an interest that came unexpectedly into my life. I wonder what my sister Nancy would have made of the efforts of the 'nine-year-old' (the mental age beyond which she said I never developed) whose fist, according to her, was incapable of holding a pen. There would no doubt have been a torrent of scorn, but I think she would have liked some of the jokes sprinkled in my books. I am often asked where my sisters' and my urge to write comes from. I cannot answer, unless it is from our grandfathers. Grandfather Redesdale wrote half a dozen books, including *Tales of Old Japan*, an anthology of short stories that is still in print a century or more after it was first published. Grandfather Bowles was not only the founder of *The Lady* and *Vanity Fair*, he was also a prolific author on many subjects.

I began writing at Uncle Harold's bidding. He was looking at the *Handbook of Chatsworth and Hardwick*, written in 1844 by the Bachelor Duke, and said, 'You ought to write down what has happened to the house and garden since.' So I did. I enjoyed the work, in spite of the fact that Andrew did not like the idea. He would have done it brilliantly himself and perhaps thought that Uncle Harold should have asked him and not me. As it was, he retreated from the scene, which made things tricky for me. My mentor and editor was Richard Garnett, whose patience and all-seeing eye meant everything to me. *The House: A Portrait of Chatsworth* was published in 1982 as a bumper guide to Chatsworth. I described how we lived in the house, which looks so grand and is so friendly, and included extracts from the *Handbook*, with a lot of family history and old jokes thrown in. Sales were extraordinary and for one heady week it topped the *Evening Standard* best-seller list.

I felt a bit more confident after this and realized that there was a captive market for books about Chatsworth and the family in 'my' shops. *The Estate: A View from Chatsworth* came about because I was conscious that people thought Chatsworth—the house, park and garden—was the full extent of the Cavendish family's land ownership in Derbyshire. I wanted to give a larger view and wrote about the farms, woods and other properties that constitute the background to Chatsworth. I loved doing *Chatsworth: The House* (the sequel to *The House*: *A Portrait of Chatsworth*). It is a large book, profusely illustrated with Simon Upton's remarkable photographs, and because Chatsworth is so big and varied I found plenty of new ground to cover. The record of the interior of the house as it looked in the last decade of the twentieth century is already an historic document as the changes that are now being made to it are far-reaching. For the same reason, I am pleased that I wrote *The Garden at Chatsworth*, a record of Andrew's and my years in charge.

Pens and pads of ruled paper were in my basket during my last twenty years at Chatsworth. Often lost for days on end, the basket would eventually be discovered by a seat in the garden or camouflaged in a seldom-visited attic room filled with jettisoned furniture. These hazards made progress slow. Deadlines frightened me because something unexpected might turn up and the lined pages of the notebook remain blank.

Writing the weekly Diary and other articles for the *Spectator* was good fun, and for six months I did a regular piece for the *Telegraph*, mainly about life in the country. I was flattered to be asked. Another magazine commissioned an article of 1,000 words—about what I forget—and I duly handed it in on time. The editor telephoned and, after beating about the bush a bit, said, 'Could you add a few more words please?' I said I could, but that I had produced the required number. 'Yes, I know,' he said, with embarrassment, 'but they are all so short we have got a lot of space left.'

I enjoyed doing these occasional articles; it did not seem to matter what was noted down and some pieces found a more permanent home in *Counting My Chickens* and *Home to Roost*. Readers often wrote to me, pulling me up for mistakes or saying that something I had written reminded them of their own experience. Do not believe it when people say that letter writing is finished (although having an address so easy to remember perhaps encouraged it in my case). Writing becomes a habit. Although my eyes are failing, I still go about with a pen in my hand. I wish I could type and use the internet, but that is beyond me now.

*   *   *

I became an Elvis fan by chance. In 1977 I was looking for a television programme on a different subject when I pressed the wrong button and there was the phenomenon. I was riveted by what I saw and heard. I knew about him, of course, but thought he was just another American pop star. Now I understood why he was the most famous man in the world. It was too late to see and hear him in the flesh but some years later I went to a clever resurrection of him in an arena in Manchester, where members of his band, including some of his girl backing singers, the Sweet Inspirations, and the pianist who played such wonderful introductions to the songs, were performing. The girls in their black dresses, covered in sparkles of every description, had grown into ample reincarnations of their earlier selves. In the middle of the stage was a vast screen and there was Elvis singing his best-loved songs, his incredible voice ringing out into the huge arena. The audience went wild, among them many Elvis impersonators, beautifully turned out in the sequinned jumpsuits we all knew so well.

Thanks to the generosity of a friend who lent us a plane to go to Memphis for the day from New York, I was able to visit Graceland. Jayne Wrightsman, Blanche Blackwell and Ashton Hawkins of the Metropolitan Museum were three of the party. It was a cold, bright day in January and the Graceland summer crowds were absent.

Excitement mounted as we went through the gates decorated with musical notes and into the house. We were accompanied by the audio-guide spoken by Priscilla, Elvis's wife, who gave an excellent picture of what it was like when they lived there together. The 1950s furniture and decoration must be some of the few examples left of those years of spindly tables and chairs, and shag carpets so deep you lost your shoes in them.

In some rooms, carpets covered the ceiling as well as the floor. White pianos and giant ancient television sets filled one room while next door in the Jungle Room the arms of the chairs were carved crocodile heads. Elvis saw this bizarre furniture out of the corner of his eye as he was driving past a shop window and was so intrigued that he went back and bought it. His gold discs lined a passage, evidence of his world-wide fame, and the people from the Met put on their specs and studied them closely as if they were seventeenth-century vermeil. His grave in the garden was obliterated by flowers and other tributes that arrived daily at the shrine from his fans. There can be nowhere like Graceland—students of the decorative arts should see it as part of their education, lovingly conserved as it is, whether they are Elvis fans or not.

Back in New York I had an engagement to talk at a lunch arranged for ten influential journalists who wrote about tourism. The idea was for me to tell them about Chatsworth and for them to entice their readers to Derbyshire. I told my journalist neighbours at lunch about the Graceland trip and how moved I had been by it. They looked at me in amazement. Then it was my turn to be amazed:

none of them had been there, and they seemed almost embarrassed to think that I had—in their eyes—sunk so low. Graceland is the second most-visited house in the United States after the White House, and I was left pondering on what they and their readers had missed.

23

Festivities and Celebrations

Andrew's generous nature made him want people to enjoy themselves and he pushed out the boat whenever there was an excuse for a party. These extravagances, some unique in concept as well as execution, were entirely his idea, fired by his wish to give a good time to others.

The first big party we gave at Chatsworth was in 1965 for Stoker's coming-of-age and to celebrate the restoration of the house. A special train brought guests from London to Matlock; some stayed in local hotels, others put up with neighbours, and the house itself was full to bursting. We had wanted to use the state dining room to dance in but the floor would have collapsed, so we used the great dining room instead. Supper was in the sculpture gallery and guests could wander round the house, upstairs to the state rooms and in and out of the private drawing rooms. Many of the young men there that night have remained good friends with Stoker and come back to Chatsworth as hoary seventy-year-olds. Three memories stand out from that night forty-five years ago. Stoker and Amanda Heywood-Lonsdale dancing together; I thought then, perhaps . . . and indeed they were married two years later. I remember Uncle Harold taking Oswald Mosley, his old political adversary, by the arm and the two of them walking through the state rooms for all to see. They came of a generation that could lash each other with words in the House of Commons and dine together the following night as if it were perfectly ordinary, which it was. My third memory is of several uninvited guests being discovered fast asleep in two attic rooms the next afternoon.

Stoker and Amanda were married at St Martin-in-the-Fields on 28 June 1967 and were among the first married couples to have a party on the evening of their wedding instead of disappearing after the reception, or 'going away' as my generation called it. Hubert de Givenchy made Amanda's dress and she wore the Cavendish tiara, which lived in the vaults of a London bank. She went to try it on, accompanied by her mother and Hubert—ever the perfectionist. The three of them squeezed into an underground room where they could scarcely turn round and Hubert was much amused when the only available mirror was a small pocket one from Amanda's bag. In spite of this, the results of his efforts were lovely and the bride looked radiant.

At the dinner party after the wedding, my sister Pam sat next to Lord Mountbatten, a friend of Amanda's family. The last Viceroy of India and Commander-in-Chief of Allied Forces in South East Asia had been briefed about his dinner partner. He turned to her and said, 'I believe you are called Woman by your family?' 'Yes, I am,' she answered, looking at him with her bright blue eyes. 'And may I ask who you are?' Mountbatten was floored by this question and turned to his other dinner partner. When I heard of this comical exchange I said, 'Oh Woman, you MUST have known that face.' 'Well,' she said, 'if he had got all his medals on I might have recognized him.' One of the wonderful things about Pam was how unimpressed she remained by names, money, titles, reputation or any of the world's extras attached to some people.

Over the years, the usual family events—births, marriages and deaths—were duly celebrated. Andrew was one of twenty-one grandchildren on his father's side and in 1988 he invited all his surviving Cavendish cousins and their progeny to lunch at Chatsworth to mark fifty years since they had last been together under the same roof. We had never met many of the children before so had fun matching parents to their offspring. The latter were unruly in the extreme and the next day the housekeeper said to me in a solemn voice, 'Would you like to see the damage your guests did yesterday?' They had had free run of the house, including the state rooms, and some of the damage was indeed interesting.

On 6 July 1990 the coming-of-age of Stoker's son, William, was the incentive for another celebration. It was—I can say it myself because I had little to do with it—perhaps the best party we ever gave. The house remained open to the public throughout the preparations as Andrew was always delighted for visitors to see anything that was going on, private or public. The garden was floodlit for several days before and after the party, and visitors were able to enjoy the floral extravaganzas, including a giant copy of the family crest—a knotted serpent—made with green and yellow flowers.

The south side of the house was unrecognizable: a tent was stretched over the steps that lead down from the first-floor drawing room and went out to the Sea Horse pond, making room for 250 diners. The sides were painted with Derbyshire landscapes and banks of flowers lined the perimeter. The inner courtyard was tented over and became a dance floor with a live band; a tented disco went up on the south lawn and another tent held a flight simulator and bucking bronco machine. I saw Andrew Parker Bowles, Silver Stick-in-Waiting, being neatly bucked off and I decided not to hang around for any more accidents. The Prince of Wales lent us his Arab tent for sitting out, which we covered with a weatherproof outer tent as its exotic contents would have been damaged had it rained. The Prince and Princess of Wales were to have come but he had broken his arm in a polo accident a few days before and they had to cancel.

As well as the beauty of the house, there was something wonderful to look at wherever you turned. Shortly before midnight we were summoned by figures on stilts dressed in costumes inspired by Inigo Jones designs for a royal masque. Their height lent them authority and we trooped after them, through the tent on the south lawn—where tables were now laid for breakfast—to the canal. A firework display began at midnight, synchronized with Beethoven's Fifth. It was the first time I had seen and heard fireworks set to music and the effect astonished the company. As the display came to an end, up rose Jimmy Goldsmith's helicopter into the night sky with another kind of firework on board. I was delighted with a gatecrasher in the elegant shape of Jerry Hall (brought by Christopher Sykes), so easily recognizable that she turned all heads.

On 19 April the following year we celebrated our golden wedding anniversary. Andrew decided to ask everyone in the county whose golden wedding fell in 1991 and we advertised in the *Derbyshire Times* to compile the guest list. A nun from the convent in Matlock wrote to say she had been a bride of Christ for fifty years and could she come. Of course Andrew said yes. (There was a great deal of speculation as to whether she would bring her bridegroom, but in the event she came with her brother.) Every couple was invited to bring a keeper, just in case, and our children and grandchildren came too. We thought we might get a few hundred people, but 3,700 sat down to tea in the biggest tent yet. The local newspaper produced a special celebration issue and Andrew commissioned a souvenir plate from Crown Derby to give to each couple.

The tercentenary of the dukedom fell in 1994 and Andrew went to town. A stage was built on the banks of the River Derwent, west of the house, and tiered seating for 3,000 was erected on the opposite bank. Richard Evans, a professional actor and son of our former doctor, wrote a pageant that spanned the years from Bess of Hardwick to the present day. The Pilsley school children and dozens of local amateur actors were roped in, while professional actors, some of whom also took leading roles, directed the pageant. 'Queen Victoria' drove through the Great Conservatory in a horse and carriage, just as she had done in real life in 1843, and Donald Sinden's voice rose out of the water as 'The Spirit of the Derwent'. The centuries came to life as other ingenious inventions unfolded. On the first night we invited employees, tenants and pensioners from Chatsworth, Bolton Abbey, Lismore, Eastbourne and London. The second night was held in aid of the Children's Society. The events took place in May and it was none too warm, so each guest was given a silver space blanket that folded to the size of a pocket handkerchief—a life-saver on such occasions.

Suddenly Andrew and I were eighty. It was also the year of the millennium: two reasons for a party. Up went another huge tent and a revolving stage on which John Hyatt, the husband of Tristram Holland who edited four of my books, performed a wonderful rendition of Elvis. The invitation said 'fancy dress', and there were plenty of other Elvises, men in gold lamé suits whom I never thought to see in anything so uninhibited and shiny. I wore the gown designed by Worth of Paris for Louise, Duchess of Devonshire to wear at the Devonshire House Ball in 1897. It is made of green and gold shot-silk gauze, with a velvet train embroidered with jewels, metalwork and gold and silver thread, and weighs a ton. The original headdress had disappeared so I wore the largest of the three family tiaras, adorned with ostrich feathers for added impact.

A party the following night was held for what is

loosely described as 'the great and the good' of Derbyshire. Some were neither great nor good but they all seemed to enjoy themselves, even though they were decidedly sticky compared to the rumbustious company of the previous night—black tie keeping inhibitions well in check. Tony Benn, MP for Chesterfield, and Dennis Skinner, MP for Bolsover, neatly avoided being tainted by coming to a party at Chatsworth and did not answer the invitation. It all looked very pretty and music was provided by young local talent. Another incredible firework display was accompanied by a screen of water over the canal on to which photographs of our lives were projected.

Our diamond wedding was in 2001. The list of our golden wedding guests was unearthed, which produced the survivors of sixty years of marriage. The party should have taken place in April, to coincide with our anniversary, but had to be postponed until September because of foot and mouth disease; it was dangerously close and we feared for the park deer and farm animals. The theme of the party this time was 1941. We laid out a week's wartime food rations on a trestle table and our astonished younger guests could hardly believe what they saw. 'Two ounces of bacon for one week?' 'Two ounces of butter? Impossible!' But that is how it was. Utility clothing was not easy to find as it had been worn to death and thankfully thrown away when clothes rationing came to an end, so the staff dressed up in RAF, Royal Navy and Army uniforms of the period. Few knew how to fasten a Sam Browne or on to which uniform it should go; Sergeant Major Brittain who greeted us outside the church after our wedding would have had apoplexy, and I think Andrew, with his military training, was close to putting the offenders on a charge.

The New Squadronaires Orchestra, inspired by the original RAF Dance Band, played songs made famous by Vera Lynn: 'We'll Meet Again', 'There'll be Blue Birds over the White Cliffs of Dover' and 'I'll be Seeing You'. Our ancient guests joined in the singing with gusto and 1941 seemed like yesterday. Andrew commissioned a porcelain loving cup for each celebrating couple and when they eventually tottered off home, a forest of sticks and an array of wheelchairs, with Chatsworth staff at the ready in case of falls, an old gentleman said to me, 'Goodbye and thank you. See you in ten years.' It would have been a small, but extra-special tea party. Sadly it was not to be.

*   *   *

As well as giving parties, we went to some marvellous balls and celebrations given by other people. The first—and perhaps the best ever—grand ball after the war was given in September 1951 by Charles de Beistegui, heir to a Mexican silver fortune, to celebrate the restoration of his magnificent Palazzo Labia in Venice. The extravaganza gave rise to green-eyed jealousy over invitations and was the talk of London, Paris and New York for months. Andrew and I were lucky enough to be invited. He went in eighteenth-century costume and I wore a simple, white muslin dress with a pale blue satin jacket, copied from a portrait of Georgiana, Duchess of Devonshire, by John Downman.

The ball was an unforgettable theatrical performance with entrées of men and women in exquisite costumes. M. de Beistegui, in a vast wig of cascading golden curls and a lavishly embroidered brocade coat, stood on stilts so as to be easily recognized. Daisy Fellowes, regularly voted the best-dressed woman in France and America, portrayed the Queen of Africa from the Tiepolo frescoes in Würzburg. She wore a dress trimmed with leopard print, the first time we had seen such a thing (still fashionable today, sixty years on), and was attended by four young men painted the colour of mahogany. So many women threatened to be Cleopatra that the host decided to settle it himself and named Diana Cooper for the role.

One memorable entrée was Jacques Fath, the Paris couturier, who came as Louis XIV in a headdress of white ostrich feathers as tall as himself, and a shimmering white satin jacket and skirt—like a doublet and hose—embroidered with gold. Cecil Beaton, dressed as a French curé and dancing with Barbara Hutton, was worth watching. Wine, food and entertainment were provided on the public square outside the palazzo for the citizens of Venice. At least one Frenchman of noble birth, who thought he should have been asked to the ball, enjoyed himself among the crowd who were climbing greasy poles for chickens and hams, and he was visited every now and again by the glamorous figures from the palazzo. As this extraordinary night turned into dawn, we splashed our way down the Grand Canal back to our hotel, having had the time of our lives.

In 1953 Moucher was made Mistress of the

Robes to the new young Queen. One of her duties was to arrange the rota for the ladies-in-waiting and I can see her, head clasped in hands, saying, 'I must get through'—the expression for telephoning —'about the Waitings.' Hers is an important job, even in everyday life at Court; at a coronation the role is vital. I was not planning to go to the ceremony as I was pregnant with my fifth baby, due around the end of June. When the baby was born too soon and did not survive, I was not in the mood for celebration and stayed quietly at home trying to recover. As weeks went by someone suggested it might be cheering for me to go after all, especially since Stoker was to be page to Moucher and carry her coronet during the procession. To allow Stoker to take such a prominent role was a big concession on the part of the Earl Marshal, who was in charge: the minimum age for pages was twelve and Stoker was only just nine, but he was considered 'reliable'. Moucher and Andrew encouraged me to go and I am so glad that they did.

Then came the problem of what to wear, as obviously Moucher was to have the robes that had been carefully put away by Granny Evie in 1937 after King George VI's coronation. Chatsworth, as always, came to the rescue. There were a number of tin boxes containing old uniforms and other relics. In the vain hope of finding something for me, we started going through them and, lo and behold, from beneath a ton of tissue paper in the box that had held Moucher's, appeared a second crimson peeress's robe. The velvet is of exceptional quality, so soft your fingers hardly know they are touching it, and of such pure, brilliant crimson as to make you blink.

Miraculously the robe fitted; we had found what we were searching for. But there was a hitch: unlike other peeresses' robes it was cut off the shoulder. Moucher or Andrew asked the Queen's permission for me to wear this irregular style and it was granted. Stoker wore the uniform last worn in 1911 at the coronation of George V, and it was not a bad fit.

In for a penny in for a pound: Andrew and I despatched the Chatsworth state coach to London so we could arrive at the Abbey in style. The coach was tested for roadworthiness, a pair of stout grey horses and a coachman were hired from the Red House Stables in Darley Dale and two burly Chatsworth farm men crammed into Devonshire livery to ride as attendants at the rear. The coach was taken by train to London and the horses stabled at Watney's Brewery. Although it looks large, the coach has surprisingly little room for passengers. On that cold, wet June morning Andrew and I could just squeeze Stoker on the seat between us as we trundled down Park Lane to Piccadilly. We waited for Gerry Wellington's coach to reach us from Apsley House then processed at a stately pace to St James's Street, where the crowd was treated to the sight of the handsome Henry Bath (on his own as he was between marriages) in a well-sprung yellow coach, a faster version than ours, drawn by a pair of Hackneys, smart as paint and stepping out. The people waiting in the empty, rainy streets, many of whom had been stationed there all night, were pleased to have something to look at.

Our route took us to Victoria Street and then we were lost. Neither the coachman nor our farm men knew London and our only communication with them was by a string attached to a button on the coachman's coat. Energetic jerking told the coachman something was wrong but not what. Poor Andrew was sweating with anxiety that we would be late and Stoker would not find Moucher. He lowered his window, a tricky business as it was made of thin real glass and the leather strap that held it was so highly polished it could have slipped from his hand. He put his head out, craning round so the coachman could hear his instructions, 'Turn right, turn left'—a scene that delighted the crowd—till at last we arrived at the entrance to the Abbey.

All was then plain sailing and the organization faultless. Stoker was whisked away to find his Granny, while I joined the female side of the congregation and Andrew the peers. I have never seen a photograph of the massed peeresses and it is a pity if there is none because, young and old, they made an extraordinarily beautiful sight. They had worked hard to look their best: the country ones had been to the bank to get out the family diamonds and the town ladies had spent early hours at the hairdresser with splendid results. Everyone was dressed alike (except for me with my bare shoulders) and the effect was like the chorus in a sumptuous film production.

All eyes were on the monarch, who was dedicating herself to the service of her people. When the Archbishop of Canterbury placed the crown on her head the peeresses put on their coronets and the sea of arms in white gloves rising in unison was unforgettable. The Abbey was lit for television cameras and the dimmest corners were visible for the first time. It was a spectacular and moving combination of splendour and solemnity, a bringing together of Church and State. (I wondered what the Californian communists, my companions of the previous year, would have made of it all.) Moucher carried out her part to perfection. I had never seen her stand so straight before and it enhanced her beauty. Stoker was indeed reliable, except for one enormous yawn which happened to be caught by a photographer. I have no recollection of what happened to us afterwards, how we got home or how we spent the rest of the day, but I was keenly aware of my good fortune at being in the Abbey with history being made in front of my eyes.

Twenty-eight years later Andrew and I were invited to the Prince of Wales's wedding to Lady Diana Spencer. Celebrations began two nights beforehand with an evening party for hundreds of people at Buckingham Palace. Emma, Andrew and I dined at Chesterfield Street, where we were joined by Father Harry Williams, who had been Dean of Chapel at Trinity College, Cambridge, when Prince Charles was an undergraduate. Harry was worried about his clothes: an old grey cotton overall worn over a short black cassock that stopped well above his ankles and gave him the droll appearance of an overgrown French schoolboy.

There are two entrances at Buckingham Palace when big parties are held and the invitation clearly stated our time of arrival, but the whole of London seemed to be making for the palace at the same time and there was a long queue to get in. We were fortunate in having an 'entrée' pass, given to diplomats, government officials and a few others, so we were able to go through a side door by the Queen's Gallery where we found a milling throng and an apparently stationary queue waiting to get up the stairs. We spotted the Archbishop of Canterbury, Alec Douglas-Home and Quintin Hailsham, the Lord Chancellor, who was wearing old-fashioned court dress with lace ruffles and knee breeches and looked like a mischievous boy with his hair scraped down. We were all staring sadly at the queue when some knowing person said, 'Let's take the lift.' So this strangely assorted company, including portly Father Williams, took the lift and when the door opened we found ourselves spat out just where the Queen and Prince Philip were receiving their guests.

The spectacle was better than any film. The women had all made an effort to look their smartest—rare today—and were wearing new, or anyway clean, dresses, and had got out anything that shone to put in their hair. The men, some in unfamiliar foreign uniforms, looked splendid, and there was the usual sprinkling of Africans in multi-coloured robes. The palace brings in outside staff for these occasions and some of the footmen's uniforms did not exactly fit. I often saw old friends among the retired butlers and looked out for Henry Bennett, who had been a footman at Chatsworth before going to be page to the Queen. (The Queen called him 'Bennett' and I called him 'Henry', which made me feel in the swim.) I did not see him that evening—he was probably in the rarefied atmosphere of the supper room where the Queen and the royal family were entertaining their foreign guests.

At 1.30 a.m. Andrew announced, 'We'll go home now.' His sight was beginning to fail and parties had become a strain. Once he had decided he wanted to go home, home it was with no waiting about. But that night it was not so easy. The crowd was still huge and I could not remember which stairs to make for to reach our waiting car. I was almost desperate when I spied Lord Maclean, the Lord Chamberlain, whom I had known when he was Chief Scout. I collared him and said, 'You're a Boy Scout, how about your good turn for the day? Show us the way out.' He looked surprised but, good Scout that he was, took us downstairs and shoved us into the passage that eventually led to the side door.

The next day I was sorry we had not stayed longer. Emma did, and at the very end of the party some high-ranking soldier cut down the balloons from the ceiling with his sword. There was a stampede of dowagers, fighting like mad for the blue and white souvenirs to take home for their grandchildren. Emma managed to get three, one for each of her children.

The following night we joined a vast expectant crowd for the firework display in Hyde Park. Part of the magic of those days and nights was the warm, still weather—the first fine days of a miserable summer—and going out at night was like going out in a southern country. It seemed to take for ever to get dark but when at last the fireworks began they were spectacular. Getting away, however, in a surging mass of half a million people was difficult. The crowd was not pushing deliberately but could not help doing so as they were being pushed from behind and several people were crushed against a barrier on Park Lane.

As we were being swept along in this human tide, I nearly fell over a small old woman. I asked her if she was all right and whether she had anyone with her. She was naturally very frightened and said she was alone. Andrew and I got her between us and waited behind a tree while the crowds surged by. She told us she lived in Brixton and I asked her how she was going to get home. 'I'm not going home,' she said, 'I'm going to spend the night on the pavement in the Strand to see the Prince go by tomorrow.' The last I saw of her was walking purposefully towards Piccadilly, determined not to miss any of the fun. She was typical of many of the people in the crowd that day: a Londoner and an ardent royalist, and nothing was going to prevent her from showing her colours on such an occasion.

Another memorable celebration of that decade was Sybil Cholmondeley's ninetieth birthday, which was held in great style at Houghton in 1984. 'You simply can't imagine the beauty of it all,' I wrote to Paddy Leigh Fermor:

That staggering Stone Hall set up for such an entertainment made me think I should never see anything so beautiful again, gold plate dug from the cellar by D Rocksavage, orchids on every shelf because the present-givers mostly plumped for flowers & somehow Sybil IS orchids, daffs wouldn't do, Sèvres china and the room itself, decor-ated & yet hardly because of it all being one colour viz. stone. Oh heavens it was wonderful. All their old servants came out of cotton wool to do the job & do it they did most wonderfully.

Cake [Queen Mother] wore something shimmering as per, Pss Alexandra a terrific tartan thing in silk with huge sleeves, Dss of Kent came dressed as a clergyman—black silk with white collar & cuffs—we all made a monster effort, jewels galore &, a rare thing, there was exactly the right number of people. Surrounded by the Oudry *White Duck*, many a Gainsborough, Sybil's mater by Sargent, the Holbein of a squirrel & *'my brother Philip's Things'* positively gaudy among the indigenous Kent kit, French clocks surrounded by sort of diamonds, eastern this & that all one size too small but adding a lot, the royal people, seven minutes of block busting non-stop fireworks seen through the fat glazing bars & the old glass which is full of swirls & distortions, fires & flowers everywhere. Oh do try & picture the scene. SHE wore a pink cut-velvet & satin dress made for her mother in 1901. The Duke of Grafton said some good words after dinner, & she, swearing after that she had no inkling anyone was going to do that, answered most brilliantly. She quoted from Horace Walpole something about dowagers being as common as flounders. The fact that the Queen & all the rest of her push were there made the dreamlike feeling more so. Those rooms were made for all that & so was Sybil. I kept thinking how lucky I was to be there.

Five years later, on Boxing Day, Sybil was found propped up in bed, specs on nose, book in hands, dead. Oh how I loved her.

In 1996, the Queen honoured Andrew with the Order of the Garter, which dates to the fourteenth century and is in the personal gift of the monarch. It is the highest accolade of all and I have never known Andrew so thrilled or so moved. We were at Lismore when the letter from Buckingham Palace arrived, and he waved it above his head in joy. I thought back to the thousand and one things he had done for every kind of organization in Derbyshire, to the years of public service he had given elsewhere and to the countless evenings he had spent at functions when he might have been in his book-lined sitting room, and I thought how well deserved this honour was.

The ceremony in the Queen's ballroom at Windsor Castle is witnessed only by those being admitted to the Order, its existing members and their spouses. Andrew and Timothy Colman, the two newly appointed knights, were presented one by one. I described what followed to my sister Diana:

They get dangerously close to the Queen who does something with a 'collar' & something else with a sort of dressing gown cord. She is highly practical, quick & neat & of course the 'presenters' are not and fumble with the cord etc etc till she grabs it herself to get on with the job. The language is thrilling, ancient & frightening, nothing but battling with things & people. All v. moving, partly because it has happened since Edward 3rd & partly because of the slowness of each movement, like a slow-motion film.

Then a long wait for disrobing. All of us round the walls while the Queen says how-d'you-do to everyone, followed by Prince Philip, Friend [Prince of Wales], Cake [Queen Mother] & Pss Anne. Another long wait & drinks & cigs for Denis [Thatcher] then lunch in the Waterloo Chamber. I drew husband & son, & Andrew 2 queens. I had exactly the same Nature Notes talk to Prince P that we had done 2 months ago when I last sat next to him. I wonder if he noted it, not I suppose or he'd have thought of something else. Friend sweet as always.

Then, after fairly ages, the wives & Denis went out into the brilliant sun to walk down to St George's Chapel between the crowds of people who had tickets to be on the walking route.

I greatly looked forward to the annual Garter ceremony and to lunch afterwards, with the long table, the flowers down the middle, the speed with which the delicious food came—no hanging about for a slow eater—and the lottery of whom I would sit next to. I used to pray that it would not be Ted Heath but, with luck, Field Marshal Lord Bramall, with his long and distinguished army career; a man in a million. But whoever my neighbour was, it all passed too quickly. The procession from the castle to St George's Chapel was like a scene from some ancient drama, the knights in their velvet robes and black hats with white feathers, and the heralds dressed as playing cards. The Order is limited to twenty-four non-royal knights. As the gift is for life, many of them are old and there are always a couple of wheelchairs. Andrew's driver told him that the other drivers ran a sweepstake, betting on which of these venerable ladies and gentlemen would be the next to create a vacancy. Lord Longford used to arrive in a London taxi, which looked funny squeezed between the Bentleys. He climbed in and out with difficulty and the danger of some important bit of his clothes coming off was ever-present.

As with so many English ceremonies, the men in their finery made even the smartest women look dim. We hen pheasants walked down the hill to the Galilee Porch and had a moment to glimpse the invited crowd on either side of the road—I seldom managed to pick out the Chatsworth contingent but knew they were there—before trooping into the Chapel and settling ourselves in the stalls of the Quire. Above us hung the Garter banners and you needed a doctorate in heraldry to know which coat of arms was whose. Back up the hill to Windsor Castle for tea and proper iced coffee, then off home to real life until the following year.

I go to far fewer parties today, but the one given in 2009 by Sister Teresa Keswick, someone I have loved since she first came to Chatsworth as a friend of Stoker's in the early 1960s, was a corker. Held at the Carmelite Monastery in Quidenham, Norfolk, it was to celebrate Teresa's twenty-five years in the Carmelite Order. As a girl, Teresa was immensely popular, throwing herself wholeheartedly into whatever was happening, and making it 'go'—the opposite of many of her contemporaries, most of whom were silent and hidden under a curtain of hair, their jerseys pulled up to their ears. They were no help to me, poor old hostess, and I had to carry the whole thing—except when Teresa came. Now, for a quarter of a century, she had led a monastic life of prayer, toil and fasting.

Sister Teresa has three brothers and countless cousins, many of whom stayed the night before the party at Hatfield House, as did I. The joy of that night with Robert and Hannah Salisbury was made all the more remarkable for me as I could remember the old days at Hatfield when Roman Catholics were frowned upon. The people who mounted the steps of the bus that took us to Teresa's celebratory Mass could not possibly have gathered together under that roof when I first knew the place in 1943.

The chapel was full when we arrived. Teresa was the only nun visible and the service was taken by priests. I do not remember much of what was said, my mind was full of thoughts of Teresa as a young woman. Even now, forty years later, I still feel her absence whenever there is a gathering of her contemporaries. After Mass, we left the chapel and stood outside on the gravel. The guests fell silent while Teresa's eldest brother, Henry, began to speak. Teresa stood next to him holding a large bell.

Henry's words were full of teases and memories of old days and suddenly the two of them were back in the nursery. Teresa was listening, laughing and crying in turn, and when she sensed that Henry was about to say something out of bounds, she rang the bell loudly to muffle his indiscretions. It was a sublime performance on both their parts. After these formalities, Teresa whirled around making sure her guests were fed and given champagne. When it was all over, she retreated into her silent life of prayer.

24

The Others

After Muv died, Nancy wrote to Gaston Palewski, 'I have a feeling nothing really *nice* will ever happen again in my life, things will just go from bad to worse, leading to old age and death.' Those words were a rare exception to her usual effervescent cheerfulness. She never had the happiness that most women seek; luck plays such a big part in meeting the right person at the right time and that luck eluded her. She made her own way through her own efforts and was rewarded with the enormous success of her books, but she never had the wholehearted love and support of a husband, lover or children.

Even her sisters were ignorant of her innermost thoughts, and her disappointments remained private. She never complained and gave an everlasting impression of light-heartedness and jokes. After *Don't Tell Alfred* she said she had run out of plots for novels and turned, with equal success, to history. *Voltaire in Love* demanded serious research and she worried about her eyes and the long hours of reading tiny print; *Madame de Pompadour* and *The Sun King*, both best-sellers, were acclaimed by historians and the reading public alike. Of her last book, *Frederick the Great*, she said to me, 'It's not only the best book I have written, it is the best book I have read,' which was greeted by 'Oh, shut up,' from me, as she knew it would.

Nancy's annual visits to Venice were as regular as clockwork. While writing her history books, she stayed in a small hotel on Torcello and spent the day in her room working. Day-trippers invaded the island but as soon as they had gone, Nancy went out to look for a discarded Continental *Daily Mail*. In latter years she stayed with Anna Maria Cicogna in her house on the Grand Canal and went every day to the Lido where she lay baking in the sun, venturing from time to time into the tepid sea. Could that annual overdose of sun have led to the cancer that eventually killed her?

Nancy had a wide circle of friends including Field Marshal Montgomery. It was an unlikely friendship on the face of it, but you did not need much imagination to see that he had a great deal of Farve in him. Added to these familiar traits was a comic side that came to the fore during his television interviews when one could not help laughing at his certainty that he was always right. (It is high time the BBC gave us a repeat of his unique performance.) Nancy used to lunch with the Field Marshal at Fontainebleau when he was Deputy Supreme Commander of NATO forces in Europe, and she recounted these visits in some of her funniest letters to Evelyn Waugh:

He is terribly like my Dad—watch in hand when I arrived (the first, luckily) only drinks water, has to have the 9 o'clock news and be in bed by 10, washes his own shirts, rice pudding his favourite food. All my books by his bed and when he gets to a daring passage he washes it down with Deuteronomy.

The world saw Nancy as a town person: she was always elegant and, even when alone and working, never looked sloppy. But underneath all this she loved the country, the seasons and the people who worked the land. In January 1967 she left Paris for her adored Versailles where she bought a house with a garden, something she longed for. Two years later she was diagnosed with cancer. The news coincided with the announcement of Gaston's marriage to his long-standing love, Violette de Talleyrand Périgord. None of us knew what this meant to Nancy. She made a joke, of course, of what must have been a shattering blow—her way of dealing with bad news. Gaston had always told her that his political career would be ruined if he married a divorced woman, thereby ruling Nancy out. And then he did just that.

Nancy's last illness has been described by her biographers and, most poignantly, by Nancy herself in her letters. Suffice it to say that for four and a half years, from March 1969, when a malignant lump was removed from her liver (she said, 'Of course, it's my white-bearded twin brother'), to when she died at the end of June 1973, she was rarely out of pain. She had several spells in hospitals in Paris and London, including ten weeks at the Nuffield in Bryanston Square where fashionable doctors brought her flowers but did nothing to improve her condition. She saw twenty-nine doctors in all, ranging from famed surgeons to quacks. After seeing a new one she would say, 'The doctor tells me I'll be much better in three weeks,' but she never was. During days free of pain she would say 'I'm cured', but the raging torment soon returned.

When her housekeeper Marie retired another prop went and Nancy missed her homely countenance. As the pain got worse we tried to visit her in turn. Diana never failed her and drove the fifteen miles from Orsay at all hours of the day and night. Decca made the long and expensive journey from California several times. I went to stay with her as often as I could, or I stayed at Orsay with Diana and we would spend the day with Nancy. But Pam was the sister Nancy most wanted when she was ill—just her presence was a comfort. All childhood teases were forgiven and forgotten as Pam recounted tales of her dogs, her household affairs and Derek's eccentricities during their married life.

It was not all gloom. The garden, an imitation of a hay meadow of her youth, gave Nancy pleasure. Such plots were all the fashion in England until their owners realized that Mother Nature needs a lot of help to keep the garden looking 'natural', and that, without it, the meadow readily turns into a beige tussocky desert in July. Nancy wrote hilarious descriptions of the mating tortoises in the garden and her dismay at the flowering of a plastic-pink cherry tree, which she longed to cut down but never dared as Marie and her neighbours admired it so.

When Decca came over from America to see Nancy, she and Diana met for the first time since 1936. I shall never forget the look of wonderment on Decca's face. After Unity, Diana had been Decca's most adored sister as a child and there she was, her beauty unchanged. They embraced and the past seemed to evaporate. They even exchanged a letter. But Decca told me that it was impossible to recreate her love of Diana; it had been too important to her in childhood and it was better not to try. They never saw each other again.

I visited Nancy a few days before she died. It was very hot and she was lying on her bed, covered by a sheet that did not conceal her pitifully thin body. The years of pain had crushed even her spirit and at last she was ready to go. I sat in silence near her and after a while she stirred and opened her eyes. 'Is there anything, *anything* I can do?' I asked her. 'No, nothing,' she said. 'I just wish I could have one more day's hunting.' She died on 30 June and was buried next to Unity in Swinbrook churchyard.

Pam came back to live in England in 1972. Woodfield—the house in Gloucestershire that she had bought when Tullamaine, her Irish house, was sold—was let and while she waited for it to become available she came to stay at Chatsworth. She moved into a flat on the third floor with grand views across the park and soon made the rooms feel like home. Friends used to make their way up to the flat (christened 1A, Chatsworth Buildings by Nancy) to sit by the fire with her. She was the inspiration behind the making of the kitchen garden at Chatsworth. She had often talked about the possibilities of a neglected plot above the stables, known as the Paddocks, and a few years later it was transformed into the kitchen garden of my dreams. I got into trouble with the estate office because I forgot to tell the budgeting people about it, and it was not cheap. Never mind, there is a kitchen garden at Chatsworth now.

I loved staying with Pam at Caudle Green and often think it was her happiest home. Woodfield House stands close to the village green, and to the south it has a stupendous view over a deep valley with a stream, both sides lined with the old trees of the Miserden Woods. It had eight acres of land, pigsties, stables and a cowshed. It was the ideal house for anyone who loves the Cotswolds. Pam's presence there felt exactly right: the house, garden, paddocks and owner all suited each other.

When you walked through the back door of Woodfield (I never saw anyone use the front door) you were met with a delicious smell of herbs—Pam's trademark, to be found wherever she lived, and the stone passage behind the kitchen held it as a welcome. The single bedroom where I slept had a bedside table with *Lark Rise to Candleford* on it and this, admittedly excellent, reading matter remained there for the next twenty years. In the kitchen–dining room was a blue Rayburn stove where Pam produced the best soups, roasts and stews imaginable. (When Nancy heard of the Rayburn she pretended to think it was a room hung with portraits by the famed Scotch artist.) I often asked Pam, 'How *do* you make this soup?' 'Oh, out of my head,' was always the answer. She was a careful shopper and discussed his trade with her butcher. 'Mrs Jackson *selects*,' Diana's driver, Jerry Lehane, used to say.

The kitchen garden was Pam's heaven and the vegetables cherished far above orchids. Her guests sat down to eat to tales of where the seeds were from, how they had been planted and the rest of their life history. Gerald and Gladys Stewart were her next-door neighbours and became her dear friends. She was lucky to have the services of Gerald in the garden and I wish she had lived to see his autobiography, *Pipe Lids and Hedgehogs*, with its evocative descriptions of life in the Cotswolds seventy-five years ago.

In the nicest possible way, all Pam's geese were swans. 'Look, Stublow, my tree peony,' she once said to me, 'isn't it wonderful?' as if I were being introduced to the plant for the first time. She was not boasting, just celebrating excellence. In 1977 Caudle Green marked the Queen's Jubilee in its own way. Pam took charge of the celebrations and wrote to Diana that the village residents were thrilled with her plan and that most had accepted the invitation when they heard that it was to be in her cowshed. Even the few dissidents bold enough to refuse had 'caved in' eventually. The cowshed, where she kept her chickens, was described by Pam as the room with 'the great west window'—in fact a rusted iron contraption with ill-fitting panes. Pam forged ahead and ordered (spelling was not her strong point): 'Sausages from the Moncks and rolls from the Nudist Colony.' There was also to be 'a real Cheddar cheese in its own skin, a barrel of jolly beer' and some Appenzeller eggs pickled in vinegar. 'Oh Debo,' Diana wrote, '*why* weren't we there.'

Life for Pam at Caudle Green went steadily on, ruled by the seasons and her black Labrador, Beetle, who was an improvement on the yapping dachshunds and a popular guest wherever she went. On a spring weekend in April 1994 Pam drove to London to stay with her friend Margaret Budd. They did the shops, had dinner with another friend, Elizabeth Winn, and more shopping the next day. That evening while they were having drinks with a neighbour, Pam fell down some steep stairs and broke both bones in her right leg below the knee. I wrote to Decca:

Ambulance men perfect & very quick ('we've got an English *lady* here' they said—rare bird, true enough), hospital at once—wonderful in every way, new, off Fulham Road. Spent a dopy night & next A.M. was operated on to put plate in the usual way. All went well & on waking she asked what won the Grand National. I spoke to her (asked for the nurse & got her) THAT EVENING, still a bit sleepy but quite OK. That was Sat. Sun & Mon never better, seen by E. Winn who said she looked v. pretty in bed & was in fine form & very funny. Tues A.M., Andrew & I went to London from Cork, punctual, drove to Margaret's where we found her outside her door saying quick, they've just telephoned to say come at once. So we dashed. Found curtains round the bed, I said I'm her sister I must see her & the Sister said talk to the Dr. He took us to a little room which I suppose ought to have been a sign of the seriousness, he said all the technical things which had happened in her poor body & I said so what's her future & he said she died 10 minutes ago. Hen. Please picture. After a bit we went to see her, so odd, just a bod with no one there.

The loss of Pam meant more to me than I ever thought it could. She seemed so permanent, so rock-steady. One who was impressed by her outward calm was the author Brian Masters, who wrote to me after her death, 'Your sister Pamela did not mind being laughed at. There was a rare kind of serenity, almost floating above life rather than fighting through it.' But, as with Nancy, there were rumblings of anxiety in Pam that she never allowed the outside world to see. She would sometimes say to one of us, 'I worry terribly about . . . ' but not if we were in company. Margaret Budd, who had been a friend since her husband, George, and Derek were in RAF 604 Squadron together, told me that she stayed with Pam at Tullamaine soon after Derek had left. Margaret told Pam how she admired her keeping cool at such a difficult time. 'If only you knew,' Pam said, 'I may seem calm but everything is churning underneath.'

*　　　*　　　*

After Muv's death, Decca's visits to England became longer and more frequent, and each time she seemed increasingly reluctant to leave. Her London friends, including the television presenter Jon Snow and human rights lawyer Helena Kennedy, saw a good deal of her when she was over. She and Bob stayed at Chatsworth but I got the feeling they were delighted when the time came to leave, taking with them a store of anecdotes so easily gathered from the Chatsworth way of life and relayed with much derisory laughter to their London friends. Decca could be spiky and took offence easily, not on her own account but when her politics were challenged. Andrew was as hospitable as he knew how, but the truth was that none of the brothers-in-law liked each other (except for Andrew and Sir O who both got on well with Derek), and it was a question of family duty when they did meet.

Decca's courage was never in doubt. She and Bob worked tirelessly for civil rights campaigns, often in the face of danger. In the spring of 1963 she published *The American Way of Death*, an exposé of the powerful funeral industry. It flew immediately to the top of the best-seller list and remained there until President Kennedy was assassinated, when it disappeared. It was a wonderful book, funny and shocking, a remorseless attack on the undertakers who took advantage of the recently bereaved, played on their emotions and persuaded them to fork out for the most expensive coffins and elaborate burials. Embalming was encouraged, even when the body was being buried without delay, and the poor corpse, dressed in his or her best clothes, was made to look ready to spring from the coffin.

Decca's descriptions of the technicalities involved were disgusting and she enjoyed keeping me informed:

Dearest Henny,

Glad you liked Practical Burial Footwear. Yes there are some other fascinators: such as New Bra-Form, Post Mortem Form Restoration, Accomplish So Much for So Little. They cost $11 for a package of 50, Hen you must say that's cheap, shall I send you a few? There's also The Final Touch That Means So Much, it's mood-setting casket hardware. Hen do you prefer a gentle Tissue-

Tint in yr. arterial? It helps regain the Natural Undertones. It's made specially for those who prefer a fast Firming Action of medium-to-rigid degree.

Hen I bet you don't even know what is the best time to start embalming, so I'll tell you: Before life is quite extinct, according to the best text-book we've found on it. They have at you with a thing called a Trocar, it's a long pointed needle with a pump attached, it goes in thru the stomach and all liquids etc. are pumped out. Thence to the Arterial. I do wish the book was finished, it seemed to be going along well for a bit but now it's all being totally reorganized.

Decca's first volume of memoirs, *Hons and Rebels*, was, and still is, a huge success. At times imagination takes over from the truth—which is more amusing, of course, but unfair on the uncles, aunts and other figures of our youth who never did us any harm but stumped up at Christmas without fail. But that was Decca. These two books set her on the road to fame: universities asked her to be visiting professor, or some such title, her pupils adored her and invitations proliferated. She and I were talking one day about her second book of memoirs. 'What's the title?' I asked. 'The Final Conflict,' she replied. 'A Fine Old Conflict?' I said, having only half-listened to the answer, and that is what she called it.

Decca was the only sister who drank spirits and smoked, and in her seventies these two habits caught up with her. In 1994 she fell and broke an ankle. She realized the trouble that her drinking was causing her family and stopped that very day. She did it without any help, just steely determination. Two years later she was diagnosed with lung cancer and even she could not prevent the disease from spreading. Her daughter, Dinky, a trained nurse, was with her and the doctors gave her six to nine months to live. I was about to set off for America to see her when Dinky rang to say it was too late. She died on 23 July 1996, aged seventy-nine.

Decca had made arrangements for the simplest and cheapest possible funeral: a cremation, no ceremony and her ashes scattered at sea. Her friends in San Francisco arranged a joke funeral with six black, plumed horses drawing an antique hearse, which she had once laughingly said she had wanted, and her friends in London arranged a send-off in a theatre where they recited eulogies. I could not face it so stayed at home with my own thoughts about my remarkable dear old Hen.

Diana's memoirs, *A Life of Contrasts*, were published in 1977 and she was interviewed on television by Russell Harty. The camera stayed on him for a few seconds longer than usual at the end of the interview and he wiped his brow and said 'Phew', so unusually impressed was he by his subject's reactions to his questions. The trouble for him was Diana's honesty: she told him exactly what she thought and why, in intelligible English, without guile, hesitation or exaggeration. Her beauty and serenity coupled with honesty was a bit too much for Harty. The media, even then, were unaccustomed to such truthfulness. This was Diana's strength, but it was also what made her unpopular in many circles.

Diana loved the Temple and was completely happy there, able to go to Paris whenever she wanted in the knowledge that she had that beautiful place to return to. Her garden was the source of much satisfaction and never failed to produce flowers for the house. There was no greenhouse, so she grew annuals but was never quite sure what would come up. One year she forgot to order ahead and filled the flower beds with zinnia plants, much to the amusement of Les Amateurs de Jardin, who were regular visitors. In one corner of the garden was a long, narrow swimming pool designed for exercise and, like everything of Diana's, it fitted its place perfectly. The walls of the pool were painted a dark colour— so much nicer to look at than the usual bright blue—and a shed provided shade in the summer.

Sir O was a persuasive talker and as a politician had been not just a speaker but an orator of the first order. On the platform his words poured out of him with passion and he took his audience with him willy-nilly. I only once saw him addressing a meeting but the memory of his delivery and his electric personality when aroused for a cause stayed with me. He liked to hold forth at meals. Sometimes our chat got too silly for him. When Diana and I were describing something we had seen and could not quite remember, we would spin it out, to hold the other's attention, with a lot of 'If you see what I mean . . . kind of . . . well, sort of . . . you know', and Sir O took this up himself— very much in inverted commas. Diana's way of talking was unique. One day when she was driving with Sir O along the Riviera he had to turn the car round, which involved backing it dangerously close to the cliff. 'Vaguely whoa,' she said quietly, as he got nearer and nearer to the edge.

Sir O was always kind to me and I was fond of him, but I realized that as he got older he was a full-time job for Diana. He demanded all her attention and anything that took her away from him was not well looked on. This made life difficult and a climax was reached when Nancy was ill and needed Diana's constant support. Diana told me that there were times when she drove over to Versailles early in the morning and rushed back to the Temple to be there when Sir O woke up. She had suffered from intermittent migraines since the 1950s and these got progressively worse, making it impossible for her to plan ahead with certainty. They became so serious at one point that she had to lie in a darkened room sometimes for a day or more at a time. The doctor prescribed Cafergot, a strong drug that alleviated the pain but did not make it disappear altogether.

Sir O died suddenly at the age of eighty-four on 3 December 1980. Diana was devastated and felt that life without him was not worthwhile, a state of mind she never really shook off. She slowly came back to what seemed normality but she was, in fact, inconsolable and, every year, the first week of December brought what she described as her 'dark days'. In 1981 she had what was thought to be a stroke which left her semi-paralysed. The doctors in France said that nothing could be done and simply suggested suitable nursing. Diana's son Max asked Professor Sidney Watkins, head of the Formula One on-track medical team, if he would see her. Max hired an ambulance plane to take Diana to England and on arrival at the London

Hospital the Prof diagnosed a brain tumour. It was removed and mercifully proved to be benign.

I went to see Diana in intensive care; she was conscious and shivering and begging for a blanket. It was awful not being able to get her one, but the orders were to keep her temperature low. She came to Chatsworth to convalesce and I put her in the centre dressing room with a bed near the window so she could see the view across the river to the end of the park, which she found comforting. No one appreciated beauty more than Diana and I believe her time at Chatsworth helped her to recover. It was wonderful for me to have her pinned there so I could go in and out for a chat. She had been my confidante since the end of the war (our correspondence would fill a library of its own), and at difficult times I do not know what I would have done without her.

Diana never burdened people with her sorrows or disappointments. In her late eighties the upkeep of the Temple became too much and she decided to sell the house she had loved for fifty years and move to Paris. She left without a murmur, never turning to look back, but what a terrible wrench it was. Her daughter-in-law Charlotte was her prop and stay and found her a flat. She also found Elo, the Filipino housekeeper of whom Diana became very fond, and in return Elo gave Diana her complete devotion. The flat became the centre for Diana's friends and family; it was easier to get to than the Temple and the welcome was just the same.

Diana seemed ageless, as beautiful as ever and generally in good health. Her flat was near the offices of *Vogue* magazine and she was oblivious of the fact that the girls inside pressed their faces to the windows to watch this elegant, upright great-great-granny walk by. As she grew older she had become cruelly deaf, an affliction that was doubly hard on her as there was nothing in the world she liked better than chat; she also missed music, which had always meant a great deal to her. She was plagued by hymn tunes, dredged up from her youth, which went round and round her head. We laughed about it, of course, but they went on troubling her.

The heatwave that hit France in August 2003 was too much for Diana, now aged ninety-three. I made a dash to see her in the suffocating heat; we pulled the blinds, shut the windows and opened the inner doors in the wild hope that the air would move and bring some relief. The air may have moved but it was hot air to hot air. I have never experienced anything similar—it was like Africa. On 11 August, when a loved granddaughter was in the room with her, Diana slipped away. Never was there such a loss to me, perhaps the closest of her relations, and to everyone who was lucky enough to know her. For months afterwards I picked up a pen to write to her only to throw it down again when I remembered there was no point.

Muv, Farve, Nancy, Pam, Unity and Diana are all buried in the churchyard at Swinbrook, lately joined by Diana's grandson, Alexander Mosley, after his tragic death in 2009. The graves seem to be a magnet for people who have enjoyed Nancy's and Diana's books and every time I go there I find flowers on one or other of them; sometimes a single stalk, sometimes a bunch with a note attached. The other day I saw people gazing at the gravestones and being addressed by a lecturer. I hurried away but could not help wondering what she was saying.

25

The Old Vicarage

Andrew's decline in health was long. For some years he had been nearly blind and was finding getting about increasingly difficult, but I never once heard him complain about his lot. Towards the end he did not want to go out of doors or even leave his room. He stayed in bed, eating nothing, sometimes for days on end. When he did get up to walk to the dining room, and later when he was pushed there in a wheelchair, he sat at the table shaking his head at everything that was offered him. All he wanted was to go back to bed, where he literally turned his face to the wall. No radio, no television—just silence. The only people he wished to see, other than me, were Helen Marchant and Henry Coleman. Nothing sparked his interest; politics, racing, it was all over. He had lost the will to live.

Seeing him so deeply depressed and unhappy about the various indignities of his physical condition, no one could have wished him to go on living. During the last two days, Henry seldom left him and stood at the end of his bed, watching in case he wanted some little thing. When Andrew slipped into unconsciousness and quietly left this world it was almost a relief. He died late on the evening of 3 May 2004, aged eighty-four. The finality of death hits only long after the event, but everyone at Chatsworth realized immediately that the old order had gone.

Andrew's funeral took place seven days later at St Peter's Church, Edensor. Because there were to be three memorial services I thought that it would be a quiet country funeral attended by the family, a few friends and the people who lived round about. In his wisdom, John Oliver, the comptroller, knew otherwise. Thousands came. It was the first beautiful day of spring and the park was at its best, the pale green of the trees half-transparent against the richer green of the grass. John Oliver led the procession from Chatsworth to the church and walked the whole mile without once raising his head. The route was lined on either side by members of staff, pensioners, friends and strangers, who stood, heads bowed, in silence. The newspaper chose to publish photographs of the waitresses from the Carriage House Restaurant, in their black dresses, white aprons and caps, and described them as our 'parlourmaids'—another reason for not believing everything you read in the papers. Guardsmen from the Coldstream Guards, Andrew's old regiment, soldiers from the Royal British Legion, with which he had had long connections, and from the Worcestershire and Sherwood Foresters, with their ram mascot, lined the churchyard path.

I went in Andrew's car, driven by his long-time driver Joe Oliver (of that indispensable family), accompanied by my sisters-in-law, Elizabeth and Anne. Stoker and Amanda walked behind the hearse, leading the enormous crowd of mourners.

Paddy Leigh Fermor, aged nearly ninety, walked with the family—to which he almost belongs. We were too many to be seated in the church and there were tents for the overflow, but the beauty of the day meant they were not necessary. At the exact moment the coffin was lowered into the grave a group of Derbyshire Microlights, of which Andrew was patron, passed overhead making wispy, whining noises. For me, the whole event was like something being enacted, not real. However much you realize that death is inevitable, when it happens to someone you have known so well for so long, it does not seem possible.

John Oliver and Helen Marchant arranged the wake, which was held in our last big tent to go up on the south lawn. When they saw the procession walking back to the house for tea, the regular Chatsworth visitors, who come to the park in search of freedom and beauty, joined in. Ramblers with backpacks, women with babies, men in shorts and little else mingled with bishops and members of the House of Lords. No one was turned away and it became a party after Andrew's own heart. Again I had a dreamlike sensation as I watched the people arrive, wondering what it was all for, then suddenly remembering.

I was astonished by the number of condolence letters I received—over three thousand. When answering the kind things people said, I learned more of Andrew's many acts of generosity over the years. The three memorial services held later that summer at Bolton Priory in Yorkshire, the Guards Chapel in London and St Carthage's Cathedral, Lismore, each reflected different aspects and events in his life and brought back many memories for those of us who were there.

A year after Andrew's death, I went with my daughter Emma to visit friends in the south of England. I probably overdid it and shortly after getting home I suffered a 'transient ischaemic attack', lost consciousness and was hurried off to the Hallamshire Hospital in Sheffield in an ambulance with the siren ringing and lights flashing (or so they told me afterwards). I woke up a few hours later to find my bed surrounded by doctors from all corners of the earth and wondered why these busy fellows were staring at me as I felt perfectly all right. They ordered a brain scan, then went about their business. The nice black porter who pushed me in a wheelchair along the endless passages called me 'Darling' and that encouraged me. The scanner made a noise like a rattling London tube train, only much louder. I was shown the photos immediately afterwards: one looked like an inaccurate map of Europe, another was an exact replica of a hotel carpet. I would have preferred a landscape by Atkinson Grimshaw but the camera could not lie. The friendly porter wheeled me back to my room with its view of all Sheffield, and I soon went home (fetched by my grandson Eddie Tennant), humbled by the kindness and skill of all concerned at the Hallamshire.

I stayed on at Chatsworth for eighteen months after Andrew died, but the passages began to seem long and the stairs steep. It was time to move, to make way for the next generation. Stoker and Amanda had made their home at Beamsley Hall, near Bolton Abbey, but in the knowledge that they would come to Chatsworth in due course. They have settled with enthusiasm into the house—the heart of the Chatsworth 'business', which is what country estates now are.

* * *

In December 2005 I moved to the Old Vicarage in Edensor, the village where Andrew and I had lived sixty years earlier. The house has no architectural merit, but its atmosphere makes it a happy place— the influence, I believe, of the devout men who occupied it for two hundred years. Parts of it had been built on and knocked down in a haphazard sort of manner, and it was in poor condition. After the builders had done their work of rewiring, plumbing and heating, of moving walls, stripping paint and putting in new windows and floors, it was ready for decorating. David Mlinaric, a friend in need if ever there was one, was an indispensable help with the placing of electric points, light switches, baths and so on; these are easy to take for granted but you rue the day if you get them wrong, and he gets them right.

David made another important contribution: I wanted to reinstate the fireplace in my bedroom that had been blocked up in the 1950s on the orders of the Chatsworth land agent, so David went to the building-yard with Malcolm Hulland, the clerk of works, to have a look at the old grates and other bits and pieces stored there. With his infallible eye, he spotted some small white tiles like the ones on my bedroom floor. He brought them back and, to our satisfaction, they were the ones that had been removed fifty years earlier.

I chose the colours and arranged the furniture—

as I had done many times before in houses big and small. My essential tools were an Old-Vicarage-sized tape measure (rather than the builders' ones I had used and lost by the dozen at Chatsworth) and a picture in my mind's eye of what I wanted. A bonus from my short stay at the Hallamshire was the plastic bracelet they put on every patient's wrist. It was a thrilling cerulean blue and I held on to it for the colour of a guest bathroom at the Old Vic. This bathroom, which is bristling with FACILITIES (including a bed covered in towelling—muddling for guests), seems to be a success, thanks to my unexpected spell of unconsciousness.

Amanda and Stoker were generosity itself and allowed me to take whatever pieces of furniture I liked from Chatsworth. I have never regretted my choice, and being able to bring these old friends with me made the move easier. I am especially happy to have the pair of Wellingtons (not boots) that used to be in my sitting room at Chatsworth. These tall, narrow, red leather-fronted drawers, replicas of those that the Iron Duke took with him on his campaigns, are a godsend for storing papers and add the necessary *coup de rouge* to my new drawing room. (Paddy Leigh Fermor says this means a glass of red wine, but to me it is the essential bit of colour that gives something extra to a room.)

The house has several guest bedrooms, which seem to be elastic, and it is a joy to be able to have my children, grandchildren and great-grandchildren to stay. From the first night that I slept in my bedroom, where I now write, I felt as if I had been here for years. A new window to the east lets me see the unwilling winter dawn through the trees in my neighbour's garden and it is a daily treat. The other window looks south. Before I moved in, a bank came right up to the front door of the house and, spoilt as I was by the views at Chatsworth, I found it too close for my liking. A bulldozer scooped out a semicircle, giving more light and a feeling of space.

Much of the garden was a building site for the first winter (the ground takes a season to settle) but the flower beds had to be planted with lightning speed in spring, a method described by Jim Link, the retired head gardener at Chatsworth, as 'cheque-book gardening'. Jim, Alan Shimwell and Ian Webster (the present head gardener) are walking, talking, living garden encyclopaedias. I call these three founts of knowledge 'the apprentices', to the amusement of Adam Harkness (a generation or two younger), who now looks after the garden at the Old Vic. My favourite part is the kitchen garden. How I wish my sister Pam were here to see my sorrel and herbs. She would be full of criticism, of course: 'Stublow, you're doing that *all wrong*.' Nancy would think my chosen marigolds perfectly frightful, adding, perhaps, 'For a nine-year-old the garden looks quite nice.' Decca would not look but would head straight indoors to the fire, clasping her dress—too thin for the Derbyshire summer—tightly around her. As for Diana, if only she were still here to spend weeks with me.

In extreme old age you suddenly find you are unable to run uphill, two buckets full of hen food are heavier than they were and the cheerful scream of hearing aids, proving that they are working, is a welcome sound. Other things go wrong. Paddy Leigh Fermor, aged ninety-four, came to stay, got into the bath, looked down at the tap end and to his dismay saw that both feet had turned black. 'Oh God,' he thought, 'Teeth, ears and eyes are wonky and now my feet.' He need not have worried. He had got into the bath with his socks on.

Twenty years after the Bible's allotted span of three score years and ten, faces also change and nature warns you that more than a little powder is necessary. A photographer was coming to take snaps for publicity for a book. I thought some make-up might mask the stalactites and other horrors that appear from nowhere on old faces, so I called on the services of Victoria Noakes, a trained beautician and the daughter of my old friend John Webber, hairdresser. John has driven over the moor from Chesterfield every week for forty-five years to do my hair ('Go on, get up and shake,' he says when he has cut it) and has never once cancelled because of bad weather. Helen Marchant telephoned him: 'How much sand and cement does she want?' he asked. I do not know what Helen answered, but Victoria arrived armed with 'Industrial Strength Concealer'. All this was good for the character, and my head, swollen by fan letters about *Home to Roost*, shrank to normal size. Victoria made me look positively decent, the 'Industrial Strength' did a great job—many untoward bits were concealed—and I faced the photographer with confidence.

I love being back in the village of Edensor. 'Sleepy' it is not: it is as animated as the cross-section of people who live in it. Some are very old like me, some are still hard at work, and there is a troop of children who keep it all alive. My sister-in-law Elizabeth lives at the top of the village; we telephone each other daily and, like in *Mapp and Lucia*, often meet for lunch. I open the Old Vic for people to visit on 'Edensor Day', which is held as close as possible to 29 June, St Peter's patronal festival. We hold a village fête in the garden with stalls, teas and races for the children, and the look round my house is popular. Every nook and cranny is on show: the bathrooms, my shoe cupboard, the kitchen with scones fresh from the oven, the downstairs lavatory lined with silver paper and portraits of Elvis, the incubator in the old laundry where chicks are hatched—the lot. One or two customers are disappointed: 'I came to see the chandeliers and all I found was Habitat.' What is wrong with Habitat? Anyway, the disappointing lantern was from Conran and is just what I wanted.

Now that I am ninety, I suppose things ought to slow down but it does not seem to happen. There is life in the Old Vic yet and, far from feeling 'a lilac relic of bygone days' (which is how I was described recently by a journalist I have never met), there is rarely a blessed day with nothing written in the diary. I do not feel cut off from the past, the present or the future, and there are innumerable occasions that take me to London or elsewhere for a night or two. Old friends and their children come to stay, as do all my descendants. On Boxing Day 2009 a photograph was taken of me with my then seventeen great-grandchildren. They lined up beside me like so many carriages attached to an engine, in similar formation to Victor Duke and sixteen of his twenty-one grandchildren in a photograph taken in 1931. The differences are interesting: the straight partings, buttoned gaiters and shine on the shoes of the obedient, pre-war children are in contrast to the stockinged feet and tousled hair of my lot. Both Victor Duke and I are holding a baby, but the Duke has a cigarette in his mouth with the ash about to drop on his youngest grandchild.

Great age is a question of luck not skill and yet you are congratulated or rewarded as if you had done something clever. During the last month of being eighty-nine I had the sort of treats that anyone of any age would dream of. I received a lifetime achievement award from the Derbyshire tourist board, which delighted me. Stoker and Amanda gave a dinner-dance for 910 guests: pensioners and estate employees with their spouses, from Chatsworth, Bolton Abbey and Lismore. This coincided with the Chatsworth long-service awards when my old associates Alan Shimwell and Henry Coleman and I were given enviable presents (our combined years at Chatsworth added up to nearly 170). The stable yard was tented over for the event, and the Carriage House Restaurant, Jean-Pierre's Bar and every table in the old covered ride were full of people enjoying themselves. Andrew would have loved it.

A birthday treat of a different kind was an invitation from the Prince of Wales and the Duchess of Cornwall to see *La Fille Mal Gardée* at Covent Garden. I was allowed to bring four guests and took two grandchildren, a great-nephew and his girlfriend. We sat in the Royal Box with our host and hostess, drinking in the atmosphere of the place that I had first visited with Adrian Stokes, and Nanny Blor as chaperone, in 1936. I hope it was the start of a love of the ballet for my grandchildren. The next day was a book launch at Claridges with the best mix of people I have ever seen at such an event. It was given by *Tatler* and Dior for Penguin's relaunch of Nancy's novel *Wigs on the Green*, first (and last) published in 1935. Such parties did not take place when Nancy was writing and she would have been surprised at the outpouring of admiration for her work. As her literary executor, it gives me pleasure to see how she still makes people laugh in this strange new world we live in.

These galas coincided with the unveiling of the changes, both structural and decorative, made by Stoker and Amanda over the last two or three years to the house and garden at Chatsworth. Although I no longer have a role there, I am still interested in all that happens. The reviews in the press and on television were without a dissenting voice: there was nothing but praise, summed up by the *Sun* as 'See Chatsworth before you die'.

This brought home to me the astonishing change of heart that has taken place over the last sixty years towards places like Chatsworth. The attitude in the old days was: 'Pull it down, it's dirty, damp and of no interest. Tax the owners (19/6 in the pound—97.5 per cent) till the pips squeak and till neither house nor garden survive.' Neglect and decay of large houses was the order of the day and nature made sure that lack of maintenance resulted in snow and rain finding their way through weak places in roofs and broken windows. Dry rot and deathwatch beetle invaded the interiors, while self-sown sycamores and rampant brambles made sure the garden walls fell to bits. Chatsworth, Hardwick Hall, Compton Place, Bolton Hall and Lismore Castle were what is now described as 'at risk', along with hundreds of other houses, gardens and estate villages all over the country. It was not until 1974 (twenty-four years after Andrew inherited his father's possessions along with the eighty per cent death duties they carried) that an exhibition at the V&A, 'The Destruction of the Country House', drew attention to the numbers of such places that are lost and gone for ever. It may have been the turning point in public opinion.

Slowly, slowly, hostility towards owners who had been struggling to maintain their old homes turned, first to grudging admiration of their efforts and then to adulation if they had managed to keep their roofs on. I have watched with incredulity this turn of events, from the days when coal was dug from opencast mines within a few yards of the front of Wentworth Woodhouse in Yorkshire (the largest private house in England), when no English women would do domestic work at a place like Chatsworth and when it was rumoured that Derbyshire County Council intended to run the A6 road along the river in front of the house, to the present, when pride and delight is taken in what is now called our 'heritage'—the word itself reflecting the sense of proprietorship felt by many people.

These developments are near the heart to me and mean a great deal to the people who live round about. The fact that so much survives at Chatsworth is in large measure due to Andrew, and I believe that his liberal attitude towards our visitors may have played a part in turning the general view upside down. I have also enjoyed watching some of my own ideas come to fruition: the Farm Shop (which opened against all professional advice), the house shops and catering (the latter employs the largest number of people in any one department) and the Farmyard (which plays its part in linking country and town). The reputation of these ventures spread and many owners of other houses open to visitors came to Chatsworth 'to see how to do it', and then went home to put something similar into practice—the highest form of flattery.

In spite of Andrew's assertion that I did not know the difference between turnover and profit, the businesses have prospered in a most satisfactory way, and make a significant contribution to the Chatsworth House Trust and the Chatsworth Settlement Trustees. When I left Chatsworth in 2005 they had a combined turnover of £7.6 million and employed 269 people—51 per cent of the estate payroll. It goes without saying that without the support of the staff none of this would have been possible.

My new house and garden are a continual delight and I find twenty roses just as interesting as two hundred, and so on down the line. I am sure that, with the affection and encouragement of my children, my grandchildren and my great-grandchildren, together with that of my most valued friends, there is lots more to come.

For now, I look back on a wonderful life watching other people work.

Appendices

Appendix I describes a joyous celebration, Appendix II is stark tragedy. After half a century these events are part of history. Andrew and I were lucky to see them close to, in a way that only the Kennedy family did.

The immediacy of the notes I made is the reason for adding them here, because of our privileged places at both events. This is why I have repeated them after they were published in Home to Roost *(John Murray, 2009).*

I

President Kennedy's Inauguration, 1961

The jumble of impressions of the last three days is so thick with oddness and general amazement it's very difficult to put them in any sort of order. The utter sweetness of our Ambassador, Andrew hopping about being humble and saying that his job as parliamentary under-secretary makes him a very junior minister, the deliciousness of the brekker, the warmth of the embassy, the dread coolth of outdoors, the friendliness of the Kennedys and the extraordinary informality of the most solemn moments. My word, it is an odd country.

Thursday 19 January
The first day was mercifully quiet after the journey, which was very long (we came down at

Shannon for some strange reason, also the plane from New York was late so we arrived at the embassy at what was 4.30 a.m. for us, having left London at 2 p.m. the day before—fourteen and a half hours).

They raked in some embassy people for lunch, so that was easy. Then it started to snow and it snowed and snowed, and although Snow Plans A, B, C *and* D were put into operation, the capital city of the USA pretty well seized up, as they are not prepared for such an eventuality. Cars were abandoned in the middle of streets; engines chuck it very easily it seems and snow gets packed under the mudguards so that the wheels won't go round.

We were given tickets for the gala performance which was to raise money for the Democrats, who are $4 million in debt after the election (seats $1,000). So we buggered off to the place called the Armory, which is about twice the size of Olympia and the same idea. The embassy gave us a car while we were there, a very old-fashioned English thing called an Austin Princess. It took two and a half hours to get to the blooming Armory. It should have taken twenty minutes but the traffic was solid and so many cars broke down in the queue to get there. Our heater broke and I had only a fur cape, my word it was bitter. Andrew panicked all the way as the tickets said we had to be there at 8.30 and the President Elect was due at 9.00. At about 10.00 he said we'd better give it up and go home but luckily we couldn't as we were hemmed in on all sides by dread cars. The cold was extreme, about twenty degrees of frost, snowing hard and a bitter wind.

We finally loomed and by a miracle arrived at a

very good time, viz. about ten minutes before the Kennedys. We needn't have worried as people were coming and going all the time, which we weren't to know. I thought it would be like a royal do in England but it was far from it.

We had marvellous seats, next to the Kennedys' box and between two very grand senators and their wives, who looked slightly down their noses at two complete strangers having such good places, till various Kennedys came and were fearfully nice, especially Bobby (who turns out to be attorney general with a staff of 35,000) who hugged us. Old Joe Kennedy, that well-known hater of England and the English, was very welcoming, and to crown all Jack came and said hello, to the astonishment of our senatorial neighbours.

The performance included all my favourites: Frank Sinatra, Jimmy Durante, Nat King Cole, Ethel Merman, Tony Curtis, Ella Fitzgerald, to mention a few, also Laurence Olivier and the chief American opera singer called Helen Traubel, who sang in a huge voice some ridiculous verses about the Kennedys' baby. It was WONDERFUL, especially at the finale when they had all done their turns and they ended up doing skits on popular songs with topical words. So unrehearsed were they that they had to read their lines and somehow it *was* so funny, just like Women's Institute theatricals at home, but when one looked again, there were all those famous faces. I adored all that.

We got home at 3 a.m. The heat in the house was fantastic. I opened all windows and slept with one blanket but it was still BOILING.

Friday 20 January

Next day was the actual inauguration. Left the embassy about 10 a.m. in order to be in our places at 11. Long queues of cars as we neared the Capitol. Anyone of note—ambassadors, senators, governors of States—had their name or country on the side of the car. We were next to some ratty-looking souls from Bulgaria in one traffic block, it made one think.

Eventually arrived at the Capitol. Horrid getting out as it was so cold with a cruel wind. The ambassadress had given me some long nylon stockings and knickers combined, also some rubber boots to put over my shoes. It was fearfully cold *with* these things—without them, heaven knows, I think I would have frozen to death. They gave Andrew a flask of whiskey but he still shivered throughout and put his scarf round his head (like the Queen). We were told to wear top hats and smart things—both absolutely unnecessary as people were dressed for the Arctic. Some women had come in ridiculous flowered hats, which they soon covered up with scarves, rugs and anything to hand.

It was difficult to find our seats, no one knew where anything was, not even the few policemen who were about. When we eventually found our places they were very good for seeing—we were on street level, immediately in front of the Capitol where the ceremony was to take place, on a large balcony, high up but all plainly visible. Our seats were wooden strips, no backs, no floor and snow everywhere. No numbers or reserved places, one just sat where one liked on forms like at a school treat. Next to us were two Pakistanis with cameras.

Just in front of me was old Mrs Roosevelt who had arrived an hour before we did and must have been terribly cold. The organization seemed so vague I was afraid it would all be very late and we would be pillars of ice but in fact it started only a quarter of an hour after the appointed time.

The balcony of the Capitol was full of senators and congressmen sitting either side of the roofed pavilion from where Jack was to speak. The Capitol is faced with gleaming white marble and looked fine against the blue sky and snow, though the dome is painted just off-white, which slightly spoils the brilliant effect. Various members of the Kennedy family arrived. The girls—Eunice, Pat and Jean—were without hats, which seemed surprising for such a formal event. One could pick out the Eisenhowers, Trumans—Margaret and hubby—old Joe and Mrs Kennedy, but they were about the only people I knew by sight. Nixon and Mrs soon joined them.

Tension was mounting for Jack's arrival but it was badly arranged from a dramatic point of view—so different from things in England. No proper path was made for him through the crowd—people started shouting and suddenly there he was. Jackie looked very smart indeed in plain clothes of pale beige; the only woman who looked dressed at all.

There was a long pause after his arrival. People were cold and were stamping their feet. The star was there but nothing was happening. Eventually, the master of ceremonies announced some tune by the band and a famous gospel singer, Mahalia Jackson, whom I'd never heard of, sang 'The Star-Spangled Banner'. Then the swearing-in and four prayers—Roman Catholic cardinal, Jewish rabbi, Greek Orthodox priest and a Protestant—all much too long and not at all moving or impressive. Nobody paid the slightest attention and even the senators took photographs throughout, moving about to get in better positions. Some people in our row didn't stand up for the prayers. My Pakistani neighbour, at the third one, gave me a wink and said, 'Let's sit this one out', which I was going to do anyway as the rug fell in the snow every time we stood up.

Jack's speech was wonderful, the *words* were so good, almost biblical. Everyone was thankful to get up and move when it was over as we could only think of getting out of the cold and wind. We were told there was a bus reserved for the Kennedy family which we were to get on, but it seemed impossible to find. No one knew anything and there was no official-looking person to ask. After pushing and shoving and, in desperation, even stopping to ask a police car, we found it at last and the relief of getting into an overheated bus was wonderful.

In the bus we found Eunice and her husband (whose Christian name is Sargent, if you please, *fearfully* nice though). We were driven to a hotel for lunch with the family and close friends. Lots of grandchildren milling about, lots of delicious buffet food. Jack and Jackie, and Bobby and Ethel had lunch in the Capitol with the Cabinet, so weren't there. Back into the bus (which had a label on it 'Kennedy Family' like 'Chatsworth Tours') and through the guarded gates into the garden of the White House, whereupon all the people in the bus gave a loud cheer, led by Eunice, and shouted

'Here we are'.

As I got into the hall of the White House, a Marine stepped forward, gave me his arm and armed me all the way through the house to the President's stand, from where we watched the parade. Andrew and I had seats several rows back. (All the seats were marked with people's names. The Marine asked me mine, I said, 'Devonshire', so he said, 'Mrs Devon*shyer*, you are heeere.') Next to us were Mr and Mrs Charles Wrightsman, who never turned up because they thought it too cold. The box had a roof and was enclosed at the sides with perspex but it was still extremely draughty and bitterly cold, even though there were army rugs on each seat.

The stands were gimcrack and the decorations practically nil, just a few small flags. Queer for such a rich country. The diplomats were next to us, sitting on raised forms, completely in the open. The Eastern ones looked so cold I felt terribly sorry for them as there was no escape and they couldn't leave till the parade was over.

The parade itself was an extraordinary mixture of Army, Navy and Air Force with girls' bands, majorettes in fantastic uniforms with long legs in pink tights, crinolined ladies on silver-paper floats, horses from the horsy states all looking a bit moth-eaten, army tanks, dread missiles (rhymes with 'epistles') on carriers, bands everywhere. One man marching by in an air-force contingent broke ranks, whipped out a camera, took a photograph of the President and joined in again. Imagine a Coldstream guardsman doing the same at the Trooping of the Colour.

The television cameras and a host of other

photographers were immediately opposite the President's stand. The cameras were on him the whole afternoon. The informality was so queer— the President drinking coffee and eating a biscuit as the parade marched by. But he stood there for over three hours.

After about an hour and a half a message came, Would I go and sit beside him. It was the oddest feeling I've ever had, finding myself a sort of consort, standing by this man, talking to him during lapses in the parade. The telly people were stumped by the advent of a strange English lady; they knew the politicians and the film stars but not ordinary foreigners. We told Sir Harold Caccia when we got back and he said no English woman had ever done that before, so I *did* feel pleased.

Jack Kennedy has got an aura all right and he was obviously enjoying it all so much. After about three-quarters of an hour he said would we like to go with his father to the White House for tea, which I took to mean I'd been there long enough. The White House is very good inside, big rooms covered in silk, one dark red, one dark green, a huge creamish-coloured ballroom and a rather awful round room covered in a horrid blue Adam-design silk, which everyone seemed to like best. The diner is green, I'm sorry to say, painted solid gloomy green, pillars and all. Pictures of presidents all over the shop, all ghoulish.

We didn't see the President again as he was still at the parade when we left after tea. Got back to the embassy about 6.15 to be told dinner at 7.15, so I rushed to dress for the ball. Luckily I didn't take a tiara, which various people said I ought to have done, as no one wore one and I would have looked like a daft opera singer dressed up for Wagner. Mercifully only the Caccias for dinner. Afterwards we were taken by them to a party given by some cinema people. Lots of ambassadors and grandees there, a sort of after-dinner cocktail party. They don't mind the press like we do, and no wonder as they write in a very different way from ours, perfectly friendly and no sting in it.

Then back to the Armory for the Inaugural Ball. This time no traffic jam and we arrived without difficulty. All the seating at floor level had been removed and a vast dancing floor put in its place. Shown to the President's box again, where we sat until someone said there was drink and a telly in a room at the back. So we made off there and saw Mrs David Bruce, a friend of Nancy [Mitford]'s, rather beautiful and probably coming to London with her husband as ambassador. Without any warning, the President suddenly walked into the room and was taken off to a television interview next door. Meanwhile we watched his inaugural speech again on the telly.

Back to the Presidential box to watch the dancing, which didn't happen because everyone stood looking up at the box, waiting for Jack to appear. When he did he got terrific applause. He didn't go down to the dance floor but talked to various people along his row. Wherever he goes he is like a queen bee, surrounded by photographers, detectives, nexts of kin and worshippers. By this time, we were sitting in the topmost tier just below the roof. As Jack came back along the first row, fenced in as usual by humans, he saw us, broke away and climbed over seven rows of seats to say goodbye, to the utter astonishment of the people sitting either side of us. A photographer who had got, as he thought, a very bad place and who had been grumbling, was now able to take the closest close-up of all.

I told Jack about Unity [Mitford]'s letter of twenty-one years ago saying how he was going to have a terrific future. I also asked him if he knew Harold Macmillan and he said he was going to see him soon. We said how we were loving everything that had been arranged for us, to which he replied that we'd stuck it well. He and Jackie then left. We waited till some of the crush had dispersed and thought we'd leave too. Andrew went out into the bitter night to look for the chauffeur—no sign of him. Eventually he was found, the car had broken and there we were with no hope of getting home. After an hour and a half the chauffeur suggested we take Labour leader Mr Gaitskell's car and send it back for him. By a miracle we saw Gaitskell among the 10,000 people there and thankfully squashed into his car, me sitting on a drunken lady who answered 'balls' to everything I said.

Saturday 21 January
We went to the Senate the next day, taken by a new senator's wife who had lunched at the embassy. Hideous place; they each have a desk and chair, like in school. Andrew went into the Chamber (they have a reciprocal agreement with members of certain foreign governments) and two senators immediately launched into speeches of welcome. I was sweating in case he would make one back but he only bowed. Good old Andrew.

The upshot of the whole outing is two new bodies to worship—Sir Harold Caccia and Jack Kennedy. I've written him a letter beginning 'My dear Jack'. I do hope I won't have my head cut off for impertinence. One of the comical things was that Andrew had some secrets from Harold Macmillan to tell the ambassador and nothing was said until we all went to bed on the last night, when I heard them talking in the passage outside my room for hours. I can see that's the way things are done in high life, very odd.

II

President Kennedy's Funeral, 1963

Sunday 24 November
Left Chatsworth with Andrew at 12.40 to drive to London airport. Found Mr Wilson in the VIP lounge. Talked to Marie-Louise de Zulueta, who had come to see her husband off. The PM and his wife arrived soon afterwards. Prince Philip arrived exactly on time. We got into the plane at 4.50 and took off at 5.10. There were headwinds of 140 mph that slowed us up and the flight took nine hours.

It was a huge Boeing 707. There were 150 empty seats behind us—something I have never seen before. Prince Philip called us up to his seats in front and asked Mr Wilson to join him for dinner. I sat next to Wilson with the Prince opposite, and Andrew sat with the Douglas-Homes on the other side of the aisle.

My lot started talking about aeroplanes (a safe subject, I suppose) in such an incredible, almost technical, way that it was quite impossible to listen to them and I found my mind wandering. Wilson had such dirty fingernails it put me off dinner. I wished I was with Andrew and the Homes but kept thinking how extremely odd the company and that I ought to be interested, but it was impossible to be so. Wilson has a level, grating voice and podgy face with a too small nose. After dinner tried to sleep a bit.

When below was all lights on the east coast of America, the sad reason for the journey hit me again and I dreaded arriving. We were met by a 'mobile lounge', a vast bus-like thing with room for many more people than we were. Our Ambassador, David Ormsby Gore, and his wife, Sissie, looking red-eyed and worn out, the Secretary of State, Dean Rusk, whose face was puffed up, and some others welcomed us on the tarmac and joined us on the bus.

At the terminal were the Commonwealth ambassadors, including nice George Laking from New Zealand with whom I'd had tea on my last visit. Television cameras and lights, then a procession of about six cars with police sirens at front and rear. Twenty-two miles into Washington and no stopping at red lights. It was a strange feeling arriving at the embassy. We had a drink and short talk in the drawing room before, thankfully, going to bed.

David said that Bobby Kennedy was taking the brunt; not only was he bitterly sad himself and having to deal with arrangements that were chaotic because of everything being at such short notice, but also he was the one person who could comfort Jackie. He said that General de Gaulle was the only Head of State who had demanded to see Jackie, so she said she would see them all. Jack's belongings have already been removed from his office and bedroom and the White House has taken on a deserted look.

Sissie said that Mass at the White House for friends and the Catholics who worked there was the most tragic thing she ever saw—everyone crumpled with grief.

Monday 25 November
Prince Philip, the Prime Minister and David left for St Matthew's Cathedral before we did, as they were to walk in the procession from the White House. Andrew and I, Sissie, and Prince Philip's ADC left at about 11 a.m. Brilliant sunshine, frosty day with bright blue sky. We arrived at the Cathedral without a hitch. It is not very big and has only about 2,000 seats. We were all seated separately as the pews reserved for friends were already full. I was on an aisle, having arrived late, and the people already in the pew moved up for me. Prince Philip seemed very far towards the back of the church. Apparently he had no seat and the Douglas-Homes had moved to make room for him.

When I could bring myself to look round, I saw Jayne Wrightsman and behind her Fifi Fell, as beautiful as ever. There was no music for a long time. I never saw so many sad faces and when Jack's great friends came in—Bill Walton, Chuck Spalding, Evelyn Lincoln, Charles Bartlett, Arthur Schlesinger, MacGeorge Bundy—it was too much. Then the family arrived with Jack's two little children. Rose Kennedy looking small and hunched and Bobby too. Eunice, Jean and Pat with no veils but wearing black-lace mantillas, their faces set and staring and so so sad.

The coffin was carried by eight soldiers. It was impossible to believe that the vital, fascinating and clever person was shut up in that box. Quite impossible.

The service, luckily, was incomprehensible and the cardinal faced the altar most of the time. No agonizing hymns, so it seemed far away and impersonal. There was Communion in the middle and quite a lot of people besides the family went up to the altar. On our way into the church, the Scotch pipers had played very fidgety music, as had the military band. We heard afterwards that it was because they do not do a slow march here, so it does not sound nearly as solemn as in England.

On the way out of the church, the overseas visitors stopped several times and for a full minute General de Gaulle stood next to me. He has the strangest appearance I ever saw—very tall, yet collapsed somehow and a long ugly nose. Haile Selassie looked fine—small and beautiful. The rest looked as they do in their photographs.

Our car arrived wonderfully quickly and we followed the procession to the cemetery. When it began to go at a slow pace, the secret service men—who were guarding Prince Philip, Alec Douglas-Home, De Gaulle and the Canadian Prime Minister, Lester Pearson—all got out and walked three-a-side of each car. There were crowds all the way for the three miles to the cemetery, which is on the side of a hill and beautiful. We arrived just as the last part of the service had begun. Aeroplanes flew overhead, including the President's plane that we'd seen at

Lincolnshire airport in June when Jack came to Chatsworth. Prince Philip was jostled to the back again, behind a lot of soldiers, so he was not among the foreign visitors when they came away from the grave. The Russians were completely enclosed by secret service people. I saw Colonel Glenn and that ghastly Queen of Greece with her dangling earrings, and many famous faces mixed up with police and hangers-on, who were all ambling about in the bright sun waiting for cars. Jackie looked tragic, with tears glistening on her veil, and Rose so very pathetic. The Kennedys are so good when things are going well but they are not equipped for tragedy.

We drove back to the embassy through thinning crowds. There was a great sense of sorrow and emptiness everywhere. We drank a lot of tea. I was very tired, as were all—we had left at 11.00 and got back about 4.00. Andrew went up to change and pack. Prince Philip went to Lyndon Johnson's reception at the White House. We watched it on television and, as usual, De Gaulle hogged the limelight. He arrived late so there was much speculation as to where he was and, when he did arrive, all was focused on him. The TV commentator was not too nice about Prince Philip or Sir Alec. Andrew and the Prince left for New York in an air-force jet and then on to London on a scheduled flight, Mr Wilson in tow.

The Canadians came for dinner—Ambassador Charles Ritchie with his talkative wife, Lester Pearson and his wife and their foreign secretary, Paul Martin, who had to go to the lav in the middle of dinner. David and Sissie looked slightly better, I thought. The very fact of having to have people in the house is probably a good thing; having to go on with ordinary life, though the outlook here is very bleak for them. They came and talked for ages in my room. Very, very sad, but we talked about other things. I wonder so much what David will do. No doubt he will have to stick out another year as ambassador here, which must be an awful prospect. It will be very difficult working with the new administration—no intimacy, no shared memories and no jokes.

Tuesday 26 November

The Prime Minister went to see Lyndon Johnson and came back saying he was friendly, tried to make a good impression and said that he would carry out Jack's foreign policy, etc. David said the White House was completely changed. Jackie had wanted to move by today but has put it off till Friday.

I went over to Eunice and found her perfectly extraordinary, laughing almost as if the thing had never happened, yet talking about everything in the past tense. We walked round her house about twelve times. How awful to live in a place where you can't go for a proper walk. Horses and dogs everywhere and one little boy aged about three. Bill Walton came for lunch, so nice, and both were wonderfully cheerful and talking about a memorial for Jack and what it should be. They suggested a long street from the White House to the Capitol, paved in different colours and with graded heights so people could see processions etc.

It seems Jackie has been extraordinary, planning everything with Bobby to do with the funeral. She was even laughing about going to see Johnson as the widder woman with lowered eyes and asking him to carry on various things Jack had been interested in. She is going to live in Georgetown it seems.

I left with Bill, having telephoned Bobby who said I could go and see him. His house is near the road and had a few sloppy policemen outside it. A man opened the door in his shirtsleeves. Jack's special assistant, Kenny O'Donnell, was there. Bobby and Ethel have built on a big drawing room, a lovely room, where there was a cot for the new baby. Ethel came in looking about seventeen—it's impossible to believe she has eight children. She's so terribly nice and good. I love her. Then Bobby arrived in a dressing gown which did not reach his knees and all hairy like an animal from top to bottom, but a v. lovable face and stout legs. I did not stay long. The house was in turmoil, telephones going everywhere.

Back to the embassy. Much chatting with Elizabeth Home, who is cast in the same mould as Dorothy Macmillan—a large reassuring body and great niceness pervading all. Johnny Walker, director of the Washington National Gallery, and his Scottish wife came for drinks. Then the Russian Ambassador, Anastas Mikoyan, suddenly turned up with interpreters. An odd roomful.

For dinner came Joe and Susan Mary Alsop, Ted Sorensen—Jack's special counsellor—and his girlfriend and Bill Walton. Sorensen scarcely spoke all evening. Sissie says he is one of the worst affected of all. I sat next to the Prime Minister. He says his brother, William Douglas-Home, has written a play about a peer who gives up his title to become PM. What a surprise. Had a talk with Joe Alsop after dinner about Mollie Salisbury and Pamela Egremont and their different roles in life. Everyone left quite early and we went to bed because of the early start. Somehow the atmosphere has lifted a bit but I would not stay here for *anything* and long to get out of it.

Wednesday 27 November
Called at 6.45. Quick breakfast downstairs with everyone. Sissie and David came to the airport in an overheated mobile lounge and suddenly the atmosphere was like that at our arrival. Did not say much. Felt David so overwhelmed again with pent-up emotion. He kissed me goodbye— something he has never done before. I feel a strong bond with him. He loved Jack so much and saw the funniness better than anyone.

I do not know what I remember most about these strange two days, which is all it was though it seemed like three months. Perhaps it was three-year-old John Kennedy leaving the church, touching the flag on the coffin and being led away by some huge man, followed by a sobbing nanny; or General de Gaulle standing just by me as he waited for the heads of state to leave the church; or Prince Philip's stern blue look as he stood in the same place while tears poured down my face; or Dean Rusk all crumpled when he came to meet our PM; or Chuck Spalding and Bill Walton as they arrived at church; or Fifi Fell's beautiful face in a trance at the end; or David and Sissie, blotchy and thin—I came away feeling so terribly sorry for them that words were impossible. The light has gone out for so many people and for David and Sissie it has been a hammer blow.

Besides the secretaries, there were only the Douglas-Homes, Liberal leader Jo Grimond and me in the PM's vast chartered plane on the way home. Went across the aisle to talk to Mr Grimond, who is charming and woolly and hopeless but sees the point, very quick. The four of us had lunch together. It was dark outside because of the time change. Any strain there may have been soon wore off. We had a friendly talk as politicians do with people of opposing convictions, yet there sat the man, Grimond, who is probably going to do-in any chance Home has of getting back at the next election. Sir Alec's sweet string vest showed through his shirt. He has a strange, saintly streak, so quiet and calm and good. When Elizabeth Home and Jo Grimond were talking, the PM said he had wanted to make David OG foreign secretary but Rab Butler had said he wouldn't serve unless he was given the job. Home evidently has a tremendous regard for David. His patience is extraordinary.

About half an hour before we were due into London, a message came to say there was fog and that we would have to land at Prestwick or Manchester. I said do let's go to Manchester and all come to Chatsworth for the night. They politely said they must get back to London whatever happened. In the end we made for Manchester. I repeated my invitation and sent messages for cars to meet us.

We arrived at Chatsworth at about 11 p.m., after what seemed an endless journey. House floodlit. Dennis, Bryson and Henry standing at the door. It all looked warm and welcoming. The only sad thing was no flowers in the rooms. Jo Grimond, Harold Evans—the PM's public relations adviser—Timothy Bligh and Philip de Zulueta all turned up. Sir Alec said if he crept into bed and lay very still we would not have to change the sheets for Princess Margaret who was coming the next day.

I so wished they could have stayed the weekend but they were called at 6.30 and to catch the 7.24 train. They arrived and left in the dark.

Acknowledgements

My grateful thanks are due to my children Sto, Emma and Sophy; and to Mark Amory, Sally Ball, Stuart Band, Claire Barlow, Patrick Beresford, Mrs P. Blackett, Henry Coleman Sr, William Cumber, Julie Davison, Peter Day, Gerard Dempsey, Caroline Dick, Ian Else, Richard Evans, Bridget Flemming, the Venerable David Garnett, Breda Geoghegan, Fortune Grafton, Linda Gustard, Ben Heyes, Tristram Holland, Derek Latham, the late Peter Maitland, Mary Marsden, Edward Marshall, Patricia E. Martin, Denis Nevin, Phonsie O'Brien, Dr Margaret O'Sullivan, Jane Ormsby Gore, Jaime Parladé, Andrew Peppitt, the Reverend Richard Pyke, Hugh and Janie Roberts, Christine Robinson, Douglas and Sue Seel, Claudia Severn, Iola Symonds, Mark Terry, Roger Wardle and Marie-Lou de Zulueta.

As for Charlotte Mosley and Helen Marchant, I am not sure if they are aware that without them there would be no book. Thank you to both.

I would also like to thank the following for granting me permission to quote from copyright material: the John F. Kennedy Library Foundation for John F. Kennedy's letter; Maxwell Taylor Kennedy for Robert F. Kennedy's letters; Constancia Romilly Weber for Jessica Mitford's letter; and Brian Masters for his letter about Pamela Jackson.

Unless otherwise credited, the illustrations are privately owned. Most are securely fixed into family albums and are the property of the Mitford

Archive; it has not always been possible to identify the photographers, for which I offer my apologies. I am extremely grateful to the following for giving permission to use their work: Charlotte Bromley-Davenport, the Cecil Beaton Studio Archive at Sotheby's, Marina Cicogna, Ron Duggins, Bridget Flemming, Tony Snowdon and Simon Upton.